FIFTH CANADIAN **EDITION**

An Invitation to Health

DIANNE HALES
LARA LAUZON
University of Victoria

NELSON

NELSON

An Invitation to Health, Fifth Canadian Edition

by Dianne Hales and Lara Lauzon

VP, Product and Partnership Solutions:
Anne Williams

Publisher, Digital and Print Content:
Jackie Wood

Marketing Manager:
Terry Fedorkiw

Content Development Manager:
Jacquelyn Busby

Photo and Permissions Researcher:
Carrie MacGregor

Production Project Manager:
Jaime Smith

Production Service:
MPS Limited

Copy Editor:
Maria Jelinek

Proofreader:
MPS Limited

Indexer:
May Hasso

Design Director:
Ken Phipps

Higher Education Design PM:
Pamela Johnston

Interior Design:
Trinh Truong

Cover Design:
Ken Cardinouche

Cover Image:
shapecharge/Getty

Compositor:
MPS Limited

Printed and bound in Canada
3 4 5 6 22 21 20 19

For more information contact Nelson Education Ltd., 1120 Birchmount Road, Toronto, Ontario, M1K 5G4. Or you can visit our Internet site at nelson.com

Library and Archives Canada Cataloguing in Publication

Hales, Dianne R., 1950-, author
An invitation to health / Dianne Hales, Lara Lauzon, University of Victoria.—Fifth Canadian edition.

Includes bibliographical references and index.
ISBN 978-0-17-665719-2 (softcover)

1. Health—Textbooks. 2. Self-care, Health—Textbooks. 3. Textbooks. I. Lauzon, Lara, 1955-, author II. Title.

RA776.H216 2017 613
C2016-907616-4

ISBN-13: 978-0-17-665719-2
ISBN-10: 0-17-665719-3

To my husband, Bob, and my daughter, Julia, who make every day an invitation to joy, and in loving memory of my parents, Henry and Lucille Plucinnik.
Dianne Hales

To my students who inspire me every day and my son, Lindon, who inspires me to "live well."
Lara Lauzon

Brief Contents

Contents

CHAPTER 5 Personal Nutrition 105

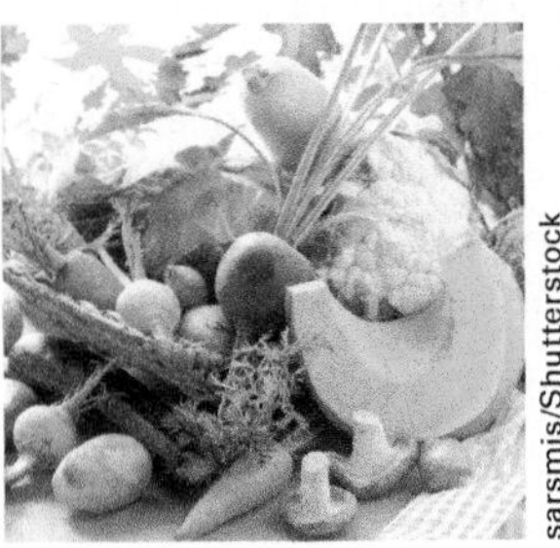
sarsmis/Shutterstock

CHAPTER 6 Managing Your Weight 135

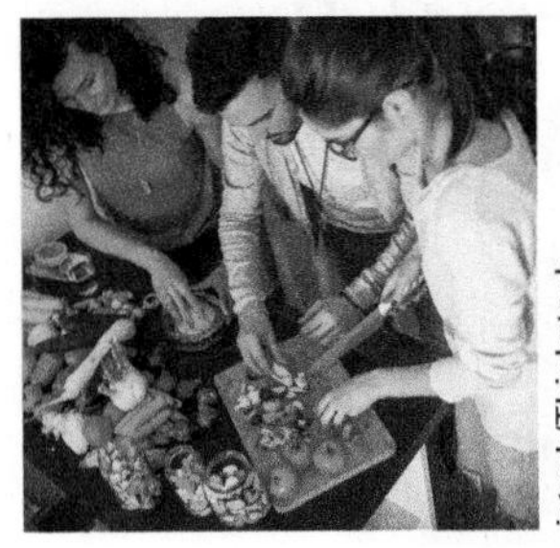
istock/Thinkstock

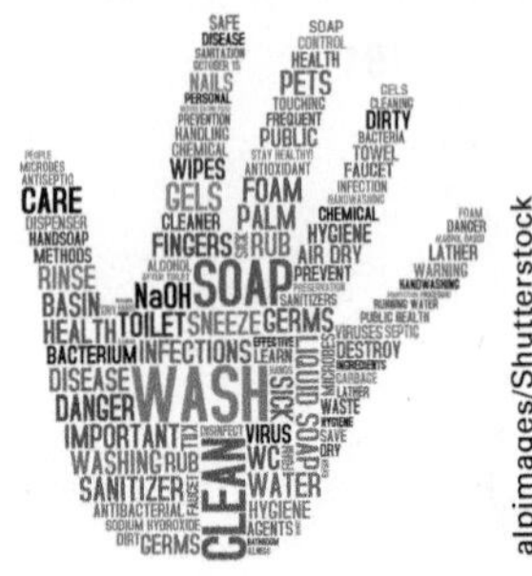
alpimages/Shutterstock

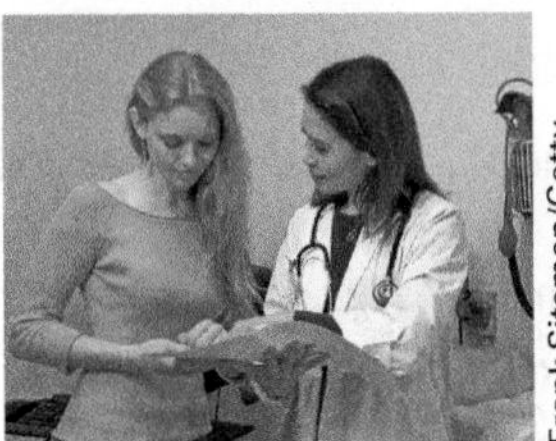
Frank Siteman/Getty

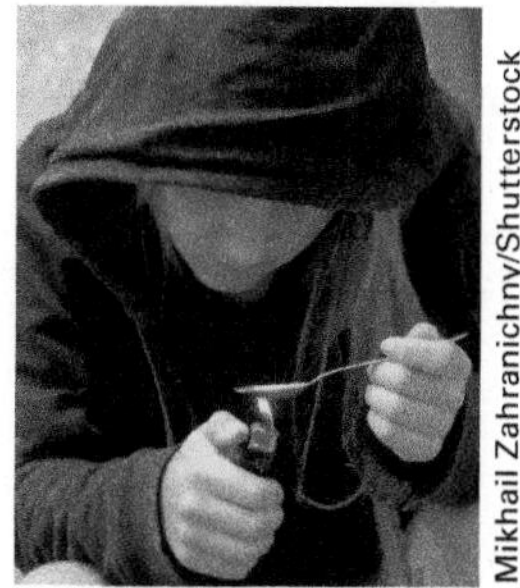
Mikhail Zahranichny/Shutterstock

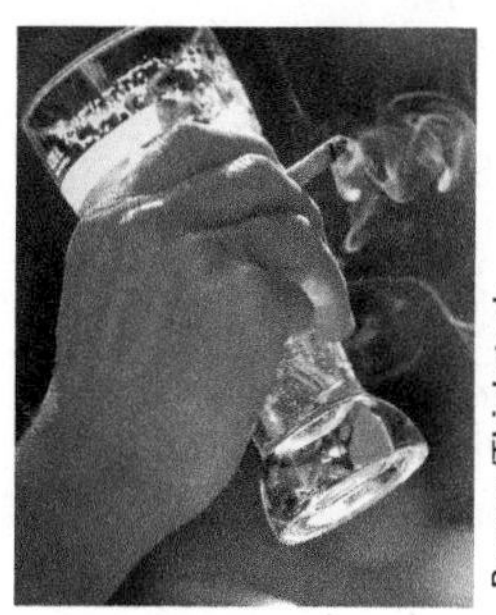
Bunyos/Thinkstock

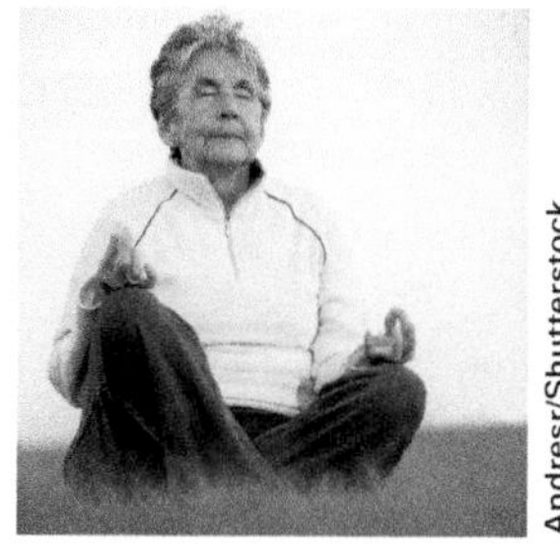
Andresr/Shutterstock

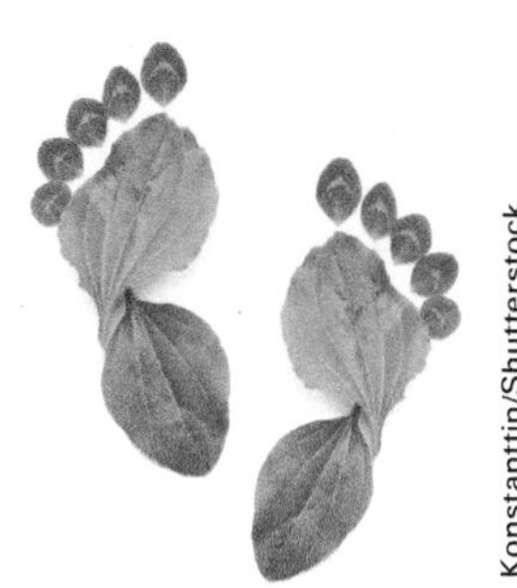
Konstanttin/Shutterstock

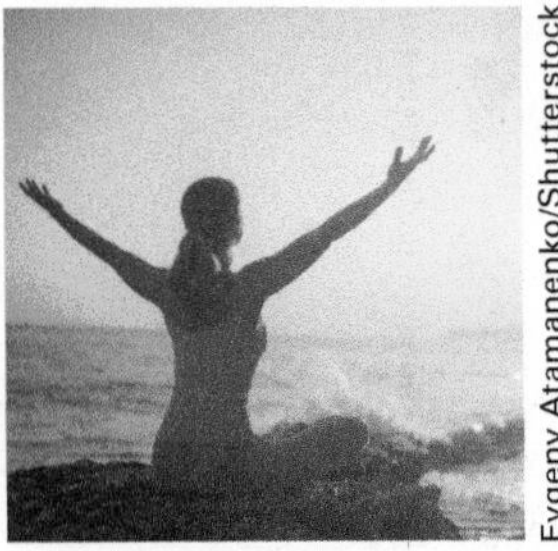

Evgeny Atamanenko/Shutterstock

Key Features

Strategies for Change

Strategies for Prevention

X and Y Files

Self-Surveys

Self-Responsibility—Social Responsibility

Human Potential

Preface

TO THE STUDENT

Health + Wellness = Potential. This textbook is an invitation to learn about health and wellness concepts that can enhance and help you reach your potential. It is an invitation to embrace a healthy and well way of living. The knowledge you acquire in this textbook will assist you in making better choices, or maintaining the healthy choices you already have adopted—ones that can have a direct impact on how you feel and function, now and for decades to come.

As you read through this textbook, ask yourself the following questions:

- How healthy or well are you?
- Are you emotionally intelligent? Are you able to cope with emotional upsets and crises?
- Do you participate in regular physical activity?
- Do you understand how nutrition plays a role in healthy living?
- Are your relationships with others solid and supportive? Are you conscientious about birth control and safe-sex practices?
- What do you know about your risk for infectious diseases, heart problems, cancer, or other serious illnesses?
- Do you use medications wisely and say no to illegal drugs? Do you use alcohol responsibly? Do you smoke?
- How much do you know about the Canadian healthcare system and complementary and alternative medicine?
- What steps have you taken to ensure your personal safety at home, on campus, and on the streets?
- What can you do to live a long and healthy life?
- What are you doing today to assist with global wellness?
- Are you spiritually connected? Are you living a meaningful and purposeful life?

Self-care, self-responsibility, and social responsibility are also important concepts when it comes to personal and professional health and wellness. Over time, your priorities and needs will inevitably change, but the important connections between your body, mind, and spirit will remain the same. The values that guide you through today can keep you mentally, emotionally, physically, and spiritually well throughout your lifetime.

An Invitation to Health, Fifth Canadian Edition, provides you with information, advice, recommendations, and research so that you can start or continue to take charge of your own health. However, knowledge alone can't assure you a lifetime of well-being. The skills you acquire, the habits you form, the choices you make, and the way you live day by day will all shape your future. We hope you will embrace health and wellness so that you have the opportunity to live a fulfilling life and realize your potential.

This is our invitation to you.

—Dianne Hales
—Lara Lauzon

TO THE INSTRUCTOR

As health and wellness educators, we have the opportunity to encourage our students to become aware of the importance of taking personal responsibility for their health and acquiring the knowledge and skills they need to support their well-being, prevent serious health problems, and reach their potential.

An Invitation to Health, Fifth Canadian Edition, offers many features and elements designed to inspire and involve students in making healthy lifestyle choices. Every chapter incorporates some research on Canadian college and university students. Numerous tables and graphs provide recent data on the health, habits, and concerns of Canadians. We have included the most recent health and wellness research available. We describe health and wellness as a process of discovering, using, and protecting all possible resources within the individual, family, community, and environment. We encourage students to use *An Invitation to Health*, Fifth Canadian Edition, as an owner's manual for their bodies, minds, and spirits. By using this book and taking your course, students can acquire the power to make good decisions, to assume responsibility, and to create and follow a healthy lifestyle. This textbook is our invitation to them to live what they learn and make the most of their health and their lives.

OVERVIEW OF THE FIFTH CANADIAN EDITION

The fifth Canadian edition of *An Invitation to Health* presents a wealth of new research, references, and features. The basic themes are health and wellness education, personal responsibility, commitment to prevention, practical applications of knowledge, and a focus on behavioural change and social responsibility. All chapters have been updated to keep the textbook as current as possible and to honour requests by students and reviewers.

WHAT'S INSIDE

An Invitation to Health, Fifth Canadian Edition, includes everything your students need in a streamlined text. Dianne Hales and Lara Lauzon are known for the way they speak *with* students—not at them. Students' comments about this textbook are very positive.

The many new figures throughout the textbook provide current Canadian-focused information and data on physical activity behaviour, nutrition, and statistics on overweight Canadians; cancer rates and diabetes; drug and alcohol use; health expenditure and serious injury rates; greenhouse gas emissions and global temperature statistics; and attendance at religious or spiritual services.

Tables have been updated or replaced in many chapters. For example, students can access information about national, provincial, and territorial health and wellness initiatives; national and provincial nutrition initiatives; current legislation for driver distraction and distracted driving laws in Canada; and environmental initiatives on Canadian campuses.

One of the things we are most proud of is the use of current research to support the information we present. Over 780 references were either updated or are brand new. The majority come from primary sources, including professional books; medical, health, physical activity, and mental health journals; health educational periodicals; scientific meetings; federal and provincial agencies and consensus panels; publications from research laboratories and universities; and personal interviews with specialists in a number of fields. Whenever possible, Canadian references are used. We think it is important to share with our students information that is grounded in leading-edge research.

We continue our commitment to include First Nations and Aboriginal health and wellness information in the textbook. In Chapter 1, we present a new First Nations Perspective on Health and Wellness model developed by the First Nations Health Authority. We think it is a wonderful way to celebrate indigenous knowledge. We have also added an environmental dimension of wellness in Chapter 1 to bring attention to the importance of global wellness. In Chapter 2, there is new information from the American Psychiatric Association and the *Diagnostic and Statistical Manual of Mental Disorders* (DSM-5). We have added the new Brazilian Food Guidelines and an updated section on genetically modified organisms (GMOs) to Chapter 5. In Chapter 6, there is an updated section on global obesity, a revised skinfold measurement section, and an updated fad diet section. Chapter 7 includes a new section on muscle dysmorphia, and in Chapter 8, we have added information on the male birth control pill. In Chapter 9, there is a new section on the Zika virus. It was also important to include a new section on physician-assisted dying in Chapter 15. Chapter 16 has updates about the Paris agreement, as well as new sections on the ecological determinants of health and on microplastics and microbeads.

Human potential stories are such an important part of our textbook. These moving stories are about individuals who have faced great challenges or who have made a difference to the lives of others. They show the connection between healthy lifestyle choices, the ability to leave legacies, and social responsibility. These stories inspire students and faculty members to ponder about their own potential while celebrating the potential of others. In the fifth Canadian edition of *An Invitation to Health*, you will meet a group of amazing students from the University of Manitoba who designed a campus health and wellness course with assistance from one of their professors; their story is in Chapter 1. Two new stories are also presented in Chapters 7 and 10. An update to the human potential story in Chapter 8 is poignant and meaningful.

Some new self-surveys are included in this edition; the one in Chapter 1 is titled *Planning Your Journey to Wellness: A Road Map*, which was developed by the First Nations Health Authority. We are excited to share this survey with students and believe it can be a catalyst for goal setting and planning for personal well-being. A new, thought-provoking spirituality self-survey is in Chapter 17.

New key terms were added to many chapters and include **exergaming, HITT, genetically engineered organisms (GE), muscle dysmorphia, drunkorexia,** and **microplastics.**

We have included a new Check-in feature in each chapter to encourage students to incorporate what they have learnt into their lives. We have continued to include a special Self-Responsibility/Social Responsibility text box and a Chapter Summary at the end of each chapter. These elements give students the opportunity to reflect on how they might embrace lifestyle changes and test their understanding of the key concepts in the chapter. Other features include the chapter FAQs, Strategies for Change, Strategies for Prevention, and the X and Y Files. In addition, the Web Links sections present reliable Internet addresses where students can turn for additional information.

A TEXT FOR THE CANADIAN STUDENT!

SELF-RESPONSIBILITY—SOCIAL RESPONSIBILITY

SELF-RESPONSIBILITY

It seems ludicrous to prepare a student for a lifetime career in their area of interest and not prepare them for the responsibilities of maintaining their life.[85]

Dr. Bill Hettler

Education can be an important step toward making healthy lifestyle changes. As you read through this textbook and debate health and wellness concepts with your classmates, friends, families, and professors, think abo... ...ou might take responsibility for lifestyle changes that will enhance your health, well-being, and personal potential. Begin by asking yourself what Stage of Change you are in.

SOCIAL RESPONSIBILITY

It's our responsibility to pass on what we inherited, not to squander it, but to build on it.

Christine Gregoire

Taking care of ourselves allows us to be better able to take care of others. What can you do to make your campus healthy and well?

Self-Responsibility/Social Responsibility Boxes. To enhance behaviour change, this element has been designed to help Canadian students reflect on the Stages of Change model throughout every chapter.

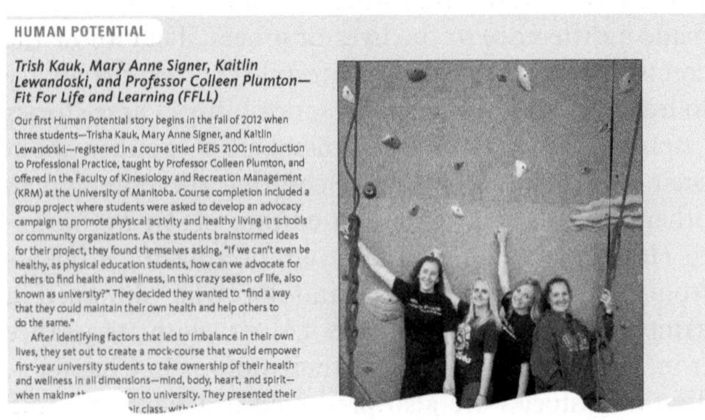
HUMAN POTENTIAL

Trish Kauk, Mary Anne Signer, Kaitlin Lewandoski, and Professor Colleen Plumton—Fit For Life and Learning (FFLL)

Our first Human Potential story begins in the fall of 2012 when three students—Trisha Kauk, Mary Anne Signer, and Kaitlin Lewandoski—registered in a course titled PERS 2100: Introduction to Professional Practice, taught by Professor Colleen Plumton, and offered in the Faculty of Kinesiology and Recreation Management (KRM) at the University of Manitoba. Course completion included a group project where students were asked to develop an advocacy campaign to promote physical activity and healthy living in schools or community organizations. As the students brainstormed ideas for their project, they found themselves asking, "If we can't even be healthy, as physical education students, how can we advocate for others to find health and wellness, in this crazy season of life, also known as university?" They decided they wanted to "find a way that they could maintain their own health and help others to do the same."

After identifying factors that led to imbalance in their own lives, they set out to create a mock-course that would empower first-year university students to take ownership of their health and wellness in all dimensions—mind, body, heart, and spirit—when making ... ...on to university. They presented their ...ir class, ...

Human Potential Stories. These special box features, found in every chapter, relate stories about Canadians who have faced challenges and made a difference in the lives of others. These stories help to illustrate the link between health and wellness and human potential.

Canadian-Related Research. The most up-to-date health research and research on Canadian students and students from other countries appears in every chapter.

Other Outstanding Features and In-Text Tools! With outstanding, interesting features and in-text tools designed to help students take charge of their own well-being, *An Invitation to Health*, Fifth Canadian Edition, truly stands above the rest! The authors are unmatched in their ability to inspire and convey how attainable learning and living a healthy lifestyle can be.

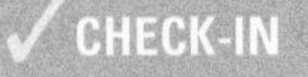

Do you want to change a health behaviour? If so, what stage of change are you in?

The **Check-In Feature:** We have added a new Check-in feature for our fifth Canadian edition. Throughout every chapter the students will find questions to consider. This feature will encourage critical thinking about chapter information.

X AND Y FILES

Men, Women, and Stress

Women, who make up over half of today's college and university students in Canada, experience greater psychological distress than men. Authors of a study of college students on stress, sex differences, and coping strategies found that female students reported higher levels of overall stress, family responsibilities, social relationships, and daily troubles. They also reported a greater level of stress with regard to finances. In comparison to male students, female students showed a higher use of self-help to cope with their stress levels.[25] Results from another study found that female college students experience greater stress than ...le college students with regard to the quality of their

The X and Y Files. Topics related to sex and gender differences in health are highlighted in this special feature, including "Men, Women, and Stress" and "Men and Women as Healthcare Consumers."

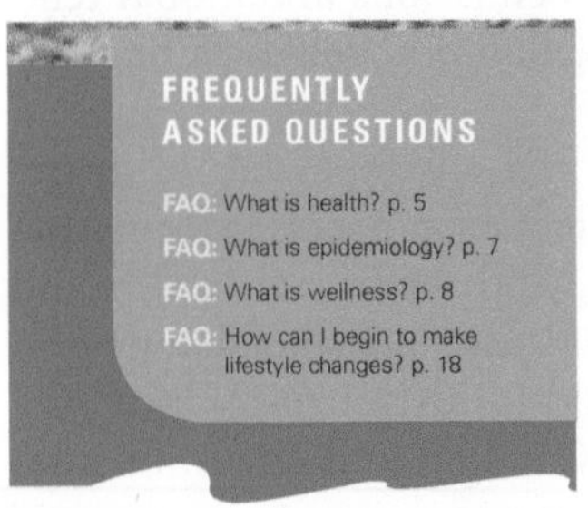
FREQUENTLY ASKED QUESTIONS

FAQ: What is health? p. 5

FAQ: What is epidemiology? p. 7

FAQ: What is wellness? p. 8

FAQ: How can I begin to make lifestyle changes? p. 18

FAQs. Frequently Asked Questions appear at the beginning of each chapter and engage students with answers to the most commonly asked questions. Page references are included after each question signalling where the answer can be found.

STRATEGIES FOR CHANGE

More Options for Change

- **Modelling—**Observing other people and emulating their behaviours, successes, or positive lifestyle choices. Look around your community and find people you admire, and who represent your beliefs and values. Watch them carefully. Try to model their behaviour and success. Ask them if they would be willing to mentor you.
- **Positive visualization—**Creating a mental picture of a goal or a behaviour change and visualizing yourself making that change. Watch yourself achieve that goal through your own eyes. Make the image a full-length movie and replay it over and over. Research has shown that positive visualization can help you manifest your goal.

Strategies for Change and Prevention. Appearing throughout the book, the Strategies for Change boxes provide practical checklist-style behavioural change strategies for achieving better health. The Strategies for

Prevention boxes provide effective, practical checklists for preventing health problems and reducing health risks.

SELF-SURVEY

Ultimately you have more control over your health than anyone else. Use this course as an opportunity to commit to at least one healthful behaviour and improve on it. Earlier in this chapter, you explored a First Nations Perspective on Health and Wellness (see Figure 1-1.) The First Nations Health Authority has also created the self-assessment below, which is an excellent resource for everyone. Answer the questions to gain insight that will help you navigate your personal journey to wellness.

Planning Your Journey to Wellness—A Road Map

Commitment

What is your present level of commitment to addressing any changes needed that relate to your lifestyle? Rate from 0 to 10, 10 being fully committed:

0 1 2 3 4 5 6 7 8 9 10

Strength

What behaviours or lifestyle habits do you currently engage in regularly that you believe support your health?

____

____

What behaviours or lifestyle habits do you currently engage in regularly that you believe are self-destructive?

____

Support

Who do you know that will sincerely and consistently support you with the beneficial lifestyle changes that you will be making?

____

____

Manage

What is your present level of stress (psychological, physical, workplace)?

Rate from 0 to 10, 10 being totally stressed out.

0 1 2 3 4 5 6 7 8 9 10

What do you love to do?

____

Wellness Self-Assessment

How often have you been physically active this week (30-minute intervals of moderate [walking] to intense activity)?

0 1 2 3 4 5 6 7

How many 8 oz (1 cup) glasses of water did you drink yesterday?

0 1–3 4–7 8–10

How many servings of fruits/vegetables did you have yesterday (1 serving = 1 half cup)?

Self-Surveys. Self-Surveys at the end of each chapter link directly to chapter content. They provide an opportunity for students to assess their knowledge and understanding of course concepts, thereby encouraging personal reflection and increasing student engagement in course material.

Chapter Summary

1. How can health promotion be defined?
   a. mutual aid, self-care, and healthy environments
   b. a way of thinking about the social and economic forces that shape health
   c. the process of enabling people to increase control over and to improve their health
   d. the absence of disease and infirmity
2. What is the definition of wellness?
   a. purposeful, enjoyable living, characterized by personal responsibility and enhancement of physical, mental, and spiritual health
   b. a state of complete physical, mental, and social well-being

   b. provincial government commitment for healthy policies and programs
   c. federal government commitment for national health programs and services
   d. encouragement from friends to ignore inherent risks linked to unhealthy lifestyle choices

7. Which of the following factors do NOT shape positive behaviours?
   a. reinforcing factors, which involve external recognition for achieving a goal
   b. lifestyle choices that include misuse and abuse of substances
   c. predisposing factors, which include knowledge,

Chapter Summary To test their knowledge, students are invited to review important chapter material through a format of multiple-choice questions.

WEB LINKS

Canadian Institute for Health Information
www.cihi.ca
Access information about national health indicators and standards, health spending, current health research, and the Canadian Population Health Initiative (CPHI).

Canadian Institutes for Health Research
www.cihr-irsc.gc.ca/
Learn about Canada's lead federal funding agency and funding opportunities for health research in four areas: biomedical, clinical, health systems and services, and population and public health.

Health Canada
www.hc-sc.gc.ca
A federal government website where health information can be found. Check out *The Daily*, a special page that keeps Canadians on top of current health issues.

First Nations and Inuit Health, Health Canada
www.hc-sc.gc.ca/fniah-spnia/index-eng.php
Discover public health and health-promotion services for First Nations and Inuit people in Canada.

First Nations Health Authority
www.fnha.ca/what-we-do/health-and-wellness-planning
The first and only provincial First Nations Healthy Authority in Canada. Check these Web pages for tips, guides, and resources for health and wellness planning.

University of Toronto–Scarborough, Health and Wellness Centre
www.utsc.utoronto.ca/hwc/wellness-campus
This website provides an example of health and wellness programs and initiatives being offered at the University of Toronto–Scarborough. Support for students includes a Wellness Peer Program and a Mental Health Network.

Web Links Updated interactive websites include Canadian sources and encourage students to use these resources for additional information and learning.

CRITICAL THINKING

1. What is the definition of health according to the text? Does your personal definition differ from this? Does it differ from your definition of wellness? If so, in what ways? How would you have defined the terms "health" and "wellness" before reading this chapter?
2. Talk to classmates from different racial or ethnic backgrounds than yours about their culture's health attitudes. Ask them what is considered healthy behaviour in their culture. For example, is having a good appetite a sign of health?
3. Where are you on the wellness–illness continuum? What variables might affect your place on the scale? What do you consider your optimum state of health to be?
4. Think about a behavioural change you have made in your life in the past two years. How did your "change process" link to the six stages of the trans-theoretical model of change? In what ways would you like to change your present lifestyle? Where are you now on the Stages of Change continuum?

Critical Thinking Questions. At the end of each chapter, students are asked to consider some applications of the chapter's coverage or weigh in on a health-related controversy.

INSTRUCTOR RESOURCES

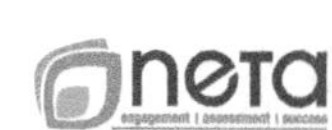

The Nelson Education Teaching Advantage (NETA) program delivers research-based instructor resources that promote student engagement and higher-order thinking to enable the success of Canadian students and educators. Visit Nelson Education's **Inspired Instruction** website at nelson.com/inspired/ to find out more about NETA.

The following instructor resources have been created for *An Invitation to Health*, Fifth Canadian Edition. Access these ultimate tools for customizing lectures and presentations at nelson.com/instructor.

NETA Test Bank This resource was written by Brenda Bruner, Nipissing University. It includes over 550 multiple-choice questions written according to NETA guidelines for effective construction and development of higher-order questions. Also included are 280 completion questions, 170 matching questions, and 138 essay questions.

cognero® Full-Circle Assessment™ The NETA Test Bank is available in a new, cloud-based platform. **Nelson Testing Powered by Cognero®** is a secure online testing system that allows instructors to author, edit, and manage test bank content from anywhere Internet access is available. No special installations or downloads are needed, and the desktop-inspired interface, with its drop-down menus and familiar, intuitive tools, allows instructors to create and manage tests with ease. Multiple test versions can be created in an instant, and content can be imported or exported into other systems. Tests can be delivered from a learning management system, the classroom, or wherever an instructor chooses. Nelson

Testing Powered by Cognero for *An Invitation to Health* can be accessed through nelson.com/instructor.

NETA PowerPoint Microsoft® PowerPoint® lecture slides for every chapter have been created by Brenda Bruner, Nipissing University. There is an average of 40 slides per chapter, many featuring key figures, tables, and photographs from *An Invitation to Health.* NETA principles of clear design and engaging content have been incorporated throughout, making it simple for instructors to customize the deck for their courses.

Image Library This resource consists of digital copies of figures, short tables, and photographs used in the book. Instructors may use these jpegs to customize the NETA PowerPoint or create their own PowerPoint presentations. An Image Library Key describes the images and lists the codes under which the jpegs are saved. Codes normally reflect the chapter number (e.g., C01 for Chapter 1), the figure or photo number (e.g., F15 for Figure 15), and the page in the textbook; C01-F15-pg26 corresponds to Figure 1-15 on page 26.

NETA Instructor Guide This resource was written by Karen McLaren. It is organized according to the textbook chapters and addresses key educational concerns, such as typical stumbling blocks student face and how to address them. Other features include discussion questions, suggestions for guest speakers and panel presentations, in-class activities, and other resources for further study.

MindTap Offering personalized paths of dynamic assignments and applications, **MindTap** is a digital learning solution that turns cookie-cutter into cutting-edge, apathy into engagement, and memorizers into higher-level thinkers. MindTap (adapted by Roberta Panchuk of the University of Saskatchewan) enables students to analyze and apply chapter concepts within relevant assignments, and allows instructors to measure skills and promote better outcomes with ease. A fully online learning solution, MindTap combines all student learning tools—readings, multimedia, activities, and assessments—into a single Learning Path that guides the student through the curriculum. Instructors personalize the experience by customizing the presentation of these learning tools to their students, even seamlessly introducing their own content into the Learning Path.

STUDENT RESOURCES

MINDTAP Stay organized and efficient with **MindTap**—a single destination with all the course material and study aids you need to succeed. Built-in apps leverage social media and the latest learning technology. For example:

- ReadSpeaker will read the text to you.
- Flashcards are pre-populated to provide you with a jump-start for review—or you can create your own.
- You can highlight text and make notes in your MindTap Reader. Your notes will flow into Evernote, the electronic notebook app that you can access anywhere when it's time to study for the exam.
- Self-quizzing allows you to assess your understanding.

Visit nelson.com/student to start using MindTap. Enter the Online Access Code from the card included with your text. If a code card is *not* provided, you can purchase instant access at NELSONbrain.com.

Acknowledgments

It is exciting, as the Canadian author, to be celebrating our fifth Canadian edition of *An Invitation to Health.* It hardly seems possible that my work on the first Canadian edition of the textbook began in 2004. It has been quite a journey and I am so proud of all the advances and improvements in every edition. Thanks must first go to Dianne Hales, the author of *An Invitation to Health*, Brief Third Edition, which was published in the United States in 2004 and used as a template for our first Canadian edition of the textbook. Thanks must also go to Jackie Wood, Publisher, Higher Education, who continues to champion this textbook. I value her wise counsel and trust in my abilities. Thank you also to Lenore Taylor-Atkins, Publisher, Higher Education, who facilitated the review process for the fifth Canadian edition. Her connection with the reviewers resulted in many thoughtful suggestions, which I was able to integrate into this edition. I also want to acknowledge Jacquelyn Busby, our content development manager. She provided encouragement and support throughout the writing and revision process. Her enthusiasm and assistance allowed for the inclusion of new material that we hope students will enjoy and learn from.

I worked very closely with Christina Maria Jelinek, who was our copy editor for the third, fourth, and now fifth Canadian editions. I knew I would enjoy working with her when I received a note letting me know she was passionate about her work. She was and it made all the difference. We work so well together. Her attention to detail has made every manuscript so much better.

Thanks must also go to Trinh Truong for the cover design; Christine Gilbert and Jaime Smith, our production project managers; Carrie McGregor, our freelance permissions coordinator and photo researcher; and Daniela Glass, our project manager, rights acquisition and policy. Our senior project manager for this edition was Naman Mahisauria from MPS Ltd. and we were fortunate to have him on board for the final production process. I work with an amazing group of dedicated people who understand the concepts of health, wellness, and potential. I know that a textbook cannot be produced and published without committed team members who help an author through the key phases of production.

Finally, I would like to thank the reviewers for this edition as well as the previous Canadian edition. Their comments were honest, valuable, thorough, and helpful. They challenged me to do my very best work. Their willingness to share their ideas and resources has made *An Invitation to Health* a first-class textbook. They are

Andrea Bedard, University of Winnipeg
Diana Bedoya, Simon Fraser University
Katrina Blacklock, Norquest College
Brenda Bruner, Nipissing University
Sylvia Emmorey, Durham College
Garreth Jones, University of British Columbia–Okanagan
Meredith Lowe, Georgian College
Linda McDevitt, Algonquin College
Robin Milhausen, University of Guelph
Jeremy Noble, University of New Brunswick
Linda Nykolyn, Norquest College
Roberta Panchuk, University of Saskatchewan
James Wendland, Capilano University
Tammy Whitaker-Campbell, Brock University

Lara Lauzon

About the Authors

LARA LAUZON

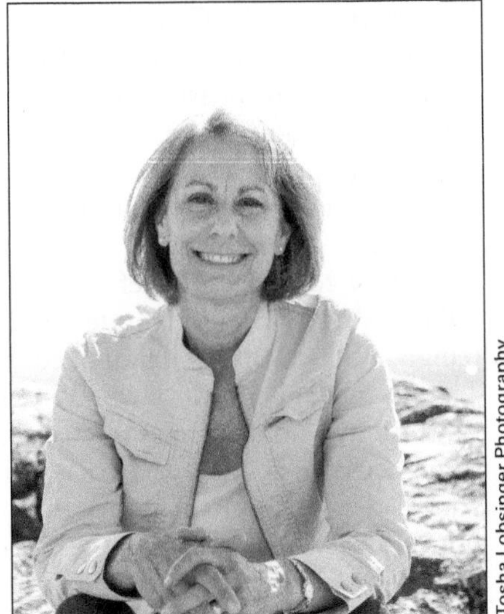
Tosha Lobsinger Photography

Lara Lauzon is an Associate Professor at the University of Victoria in British Columbia. Her teaching focus in the School of Exercise Science, Physical and Health Education is student health, wellness, and personal potential. Her research specialty is in teacher wellness. She is also a consultant specializing in workplace wellness and leadership. She has worked for not-for-profit, municipal, provincial, and private health and fitness agencies. She co-produced and hosted an internationally syndicated health and fitness show called *Body Moves* for seven years. She has won many awards, including a Faculty of Education Teaching Excellence Award (University of Victoria), a Graduate Student Award for Teaching Excellence, the Victoria "Y" Women of Distinction Award for the fitness and health category, the B.C. Promotion Plus Leadership Award for promotion of girls and women in fitness and sport, a B.C. Paraplegic Association Award for the production of two fitness videos for persons with disabilities, and a Community Wellness Award for outstanding contribution to the field of community wellness. She accepted an honorary membership to the Golden Key International Honour Society at the University of Victoria. She has written hundreds of fitness and health columns for newspapers and health magazines and has published a number of fitness and health journal articles. She is a co-author of *Leadership for Recreation, Leisure and Parks Services*, Fourth Edition, and also has a chapter titled "A Work In Progress" included in a collaborative work called *Wise Women Speak: Changes Along the Path*. She is a popular keynote speaker and continues to present health and wellness workshops in Canada and the United States.

DIANNE HALES

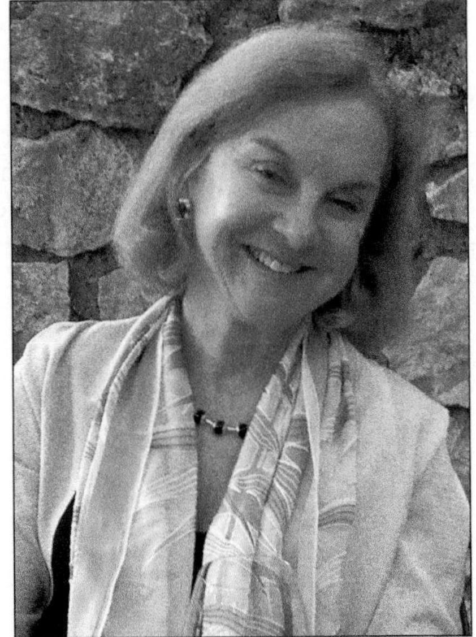
Julia Hales

Dianne Hales, a contributing editor for *Parade*, has written more than 2000 articles for national publications. Her trade books include *Just Like a Woman: How Gender Science Is Redefining What Makes Us Female* and the award-winning compendium of mental health information, *Caring for the Mind: The Comprehensive Guide to Mental Health*. Dianne Hales is one of the few journalists to be honoured with national awards for excellence in magazine writing by both the American Psychiatric Association and the American Psychological Association. She also has won the EMMA (Exceptional Media Merit Award) for health reporting from the National Women's Political Caucus and Radcliffe College, and numerous writing awards from various organizations, including the Arthritis Foundation, California Psychiatric Society, CHAAD (Children and Adults with Attention-Deficit Disorders), Council for the Advancement of Scientific Education, National Easter Seal Society, and the New York City Public Library.

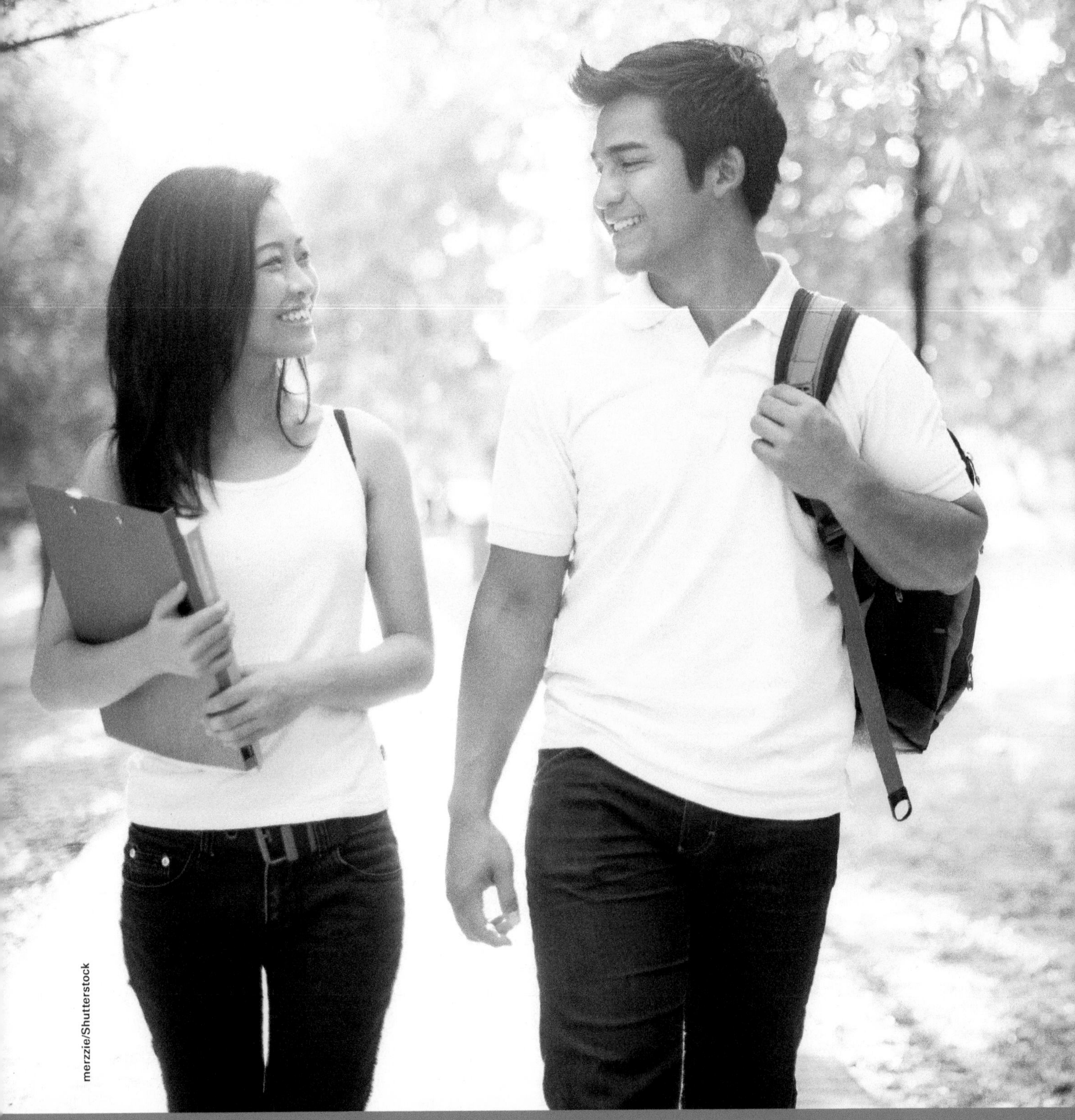
merzie/Shutterstock

AFTER READING THIS CHAPTER, YOU WILL BE ABLE TO:

- **define** health and wellness
- **describe** and **discuss** health-promotion and wellness models
- **identify** the seven dimensions of wellness and **describe** how they relate to total wellness
- **list** and **describe** the social determinants of health
- **recognize** the factors that shape the development of positive health behaviours
- **describe** how beliefs and attitudes influence behaviour
- **apply** a behaviour-change theory to a personal health and wellness action plan

An Invitation to Health and Wellness

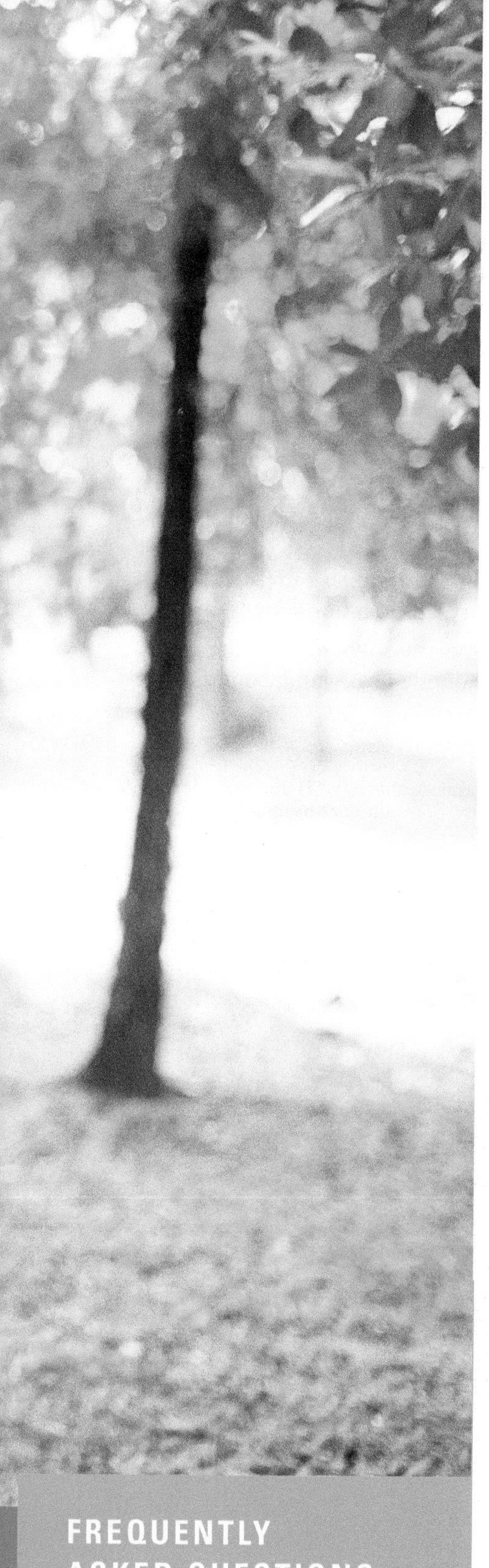

FREQUENTLY ASKED QUESTIONS

"How are you?" You may hear that question many times each day. "Fine," you answer, without thinking. But how often do you ask yourself how you really are? How do you feel about yourself and your life? Are the lifestyle choices you are making supporting your personal well-being and career goals?

Being healthy and well includes a connection between body, mind, and spirit. Health and wellness are also dependent on the community, society, and environment in which you live. This edition of *An Invitation to Health* is an invitation to embrace a "well" way of living and an opportunity to reflect upon the link between healthy lifestyle choices and your own personal potential.

As you read through this book, you will discover the importance of emotional and physical well-being. You will be encouraged to think about the benefits of physical activity and healthy food choices. Drug, alcohol, and tobacco use is discussed as well as such topics as sexuality, reproductive choices, and lowering your risk of major diseases. You will also find out about environmental issues that affect global wellness and the spiritual dimension of holistic living.

Establishing the basis for good health now can support a healthy way of living in your future. We begin with an introduction to health and wellness.

HEALTH AND WELLNESS

There has been much discussion among health and wellness advocates as to whether health equals wellness or wellness equals health. For many, being well is essentially the same as being healthy. For others, there is a distinction between the two terms. Many health and wellness programs are based on similar health risk–reduction strategies. In this section, you will be introduced to definitions of *health* and *wellness*. You will also discover some health promotion and wellness models. You are encouraged to adopt or adapt whatever terms and models you find meaningful.

Travelling back to ancient Greece, we meet our earliest and most enduring icon of medicine and health and wellness—that of the Greek god of health and father of medicine, Asklepios, also known by his Roman name, Aesculapius. Two of Asklepios's children also became celebrated healers. His daughter Panacea believed that the best way to help people was to treat illness. Her sister Hygeia believed that it was important to teach people how to live so that they did not become ill.[1] Their legacy is our understanding of the words **panacea**, which means "a remedy for all ills or difficulties,"*[2] and **hygiene**, meaning healthy: "a science of the establishment and maintenance of health; conditions or practices conducive to health."*[3]

First Nations and Aboriginal Health and Wellness

In Canada, we do not have to return to ancient Greek mythology to be educated or inspired about health and wellness. Instead, we can look to the worldview of First Nations and Aboriginal Peoples to gain an understanding of health and well-being, in which the emphasis on the interconnectedness between the physical and spiritual world, between individuals and their environment, and between the mind, body, and spirit guides the concept of **holism**.[4]

Kulchyski, McCaskill, and Newhouse say that "at the heart of most elders' stories and teachings is the idea that it is important for an individual to attempt to live Bimaadiziwin, 'the way of good life' or 'everyday good living' in accordance with the teachings of the Creator."[5] They suggest that "it is through an understanding of the reciprocal relationship between ourselves and Mother Earth and living in a balanced way that we are provided with the sustenance, both physical and spiritual, necessary for life."[6]

First Nations Medicine Wheels assist in the teaching of Bimaadiziwin. Although there are many different but related versions, they share traditional theology, philosophy, psychology, and the teachings of the Creator. The First Nations Health Authority (FNHA)—guided by First Nations in BC, traditional teachings, and approaches from healers and Elders and other health partners—has created a visual image of a First Nations Perspective on Health and Wellness (see Figure 1-1). A description of the visual depiction helps us to understand the meaning and vision of wellness.[7]

There are five inner circles:*

- The Centre Circle—reminds us wellness begins with taking responsibility for our own health and wellness.
- The Second Circle—encourages us to balance mental, emotional, spiritual, and physical aspects of wellness.
- The Third Circle—links the values of respect, wisdom, responsibility, and relationships.
- The Fourth Circle—portrays where we come from and who we are surrounded by—land, community, family, and nations.

*Source: First Nations Health Authority, "Traditional Healing," http://www.fnha.ca/what-we-do/traditional-healing.

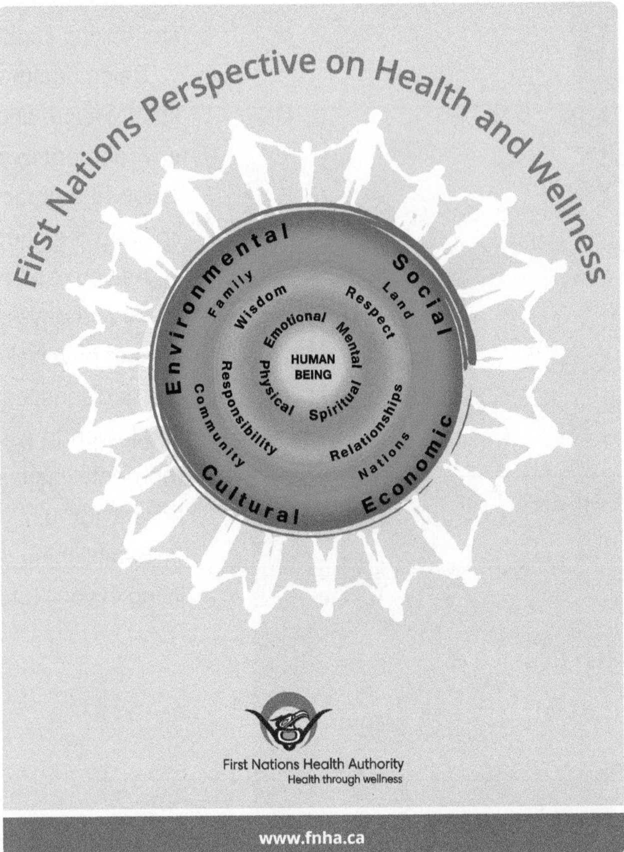

Figure 1-1 **First Nations Perspective on Health and Wellness**

Source: First Nations Health Authority. (2016). A First Nations Perspective on Health and Wellness. Wellness and the First Nations Health Authority. www.fnha.ca/wellness/wellness-and-the-first-nations-health-authority/first-nations-perspective-on-wellness.

*By permission. From Merriam-Webster's Collegiate ® Dictionary, 11th Edition © 2016 by Merriam-Webster, Inc. (www.Merriam-Webster.com).

- The Fifth Circle—represents the important influences of the social, cultural, economic, and environmental determinants of health and well-being.
- The Outer Circle—illustrates children, families, elders, and people in all communities standing together, with respect for one another, building relationships.

A more in-depth description of the First Nations Perspective of Wellness can be found on the First Nations Health Authority website at www.fnha.ca.

HEALTH AND HEALTH PROMOTION

What Is Health? Another view of health has its beginnings in the World Health Organization (WHO), an agency that has shaped our understanding of health as many Canadians know it today. The World Health Organization emphasized the importance of the preventive side of health, and a declaration was adopted that stated that "the enjoyment of the highest attainable standard of health is one of the fundamental rights of every human being."[8] The WHO's definition of **health** as "a state of complete physical, mental, and social well-being and not merely the absence of disease or infirmity" was adopted on April 7, 1948.[9] This was the beginning of a new era in health care.

In 1974, an important document titled *A New Perspective on the Health of Canadians* presented epidemiological evidence for the focus of lifestyle and environmental factors on health. Often referred to as the Lalonde Report,[10] this breakthrough work presented a conceptual framework called the Health Field Concept, which included four main elements: human biology, environment, lifestyle, and health-care organizations. The report was influential in persuading medical leaders to rethink current medical practices based on treatment-focused medicine and acknowledge that vast sums of money were also being used to treat diseases that could have been prevented.

The definition of health continued to broaden as we moved from measuring our nation's health status only by **morbidity** (disease) and **mortality** (death) rates to viewing health as a part of everyday living. In 1986, the first International Conference on Health Promotion, organized by the WHO and hosted in Ottawa, Ontario, by The Hon. Jacob (Jake) Epp, the federal minister of health and welfare at that time, was held as a response to growing expectations for a new public health movement around the world. An international agreement known as the *Ottawa Charter for Health Promotion*[11] was signed at this conference. The agreement helped build healthy public policy through health promotion:

> ***Health promotion** is the process of enabling people to increase control over and to improve their health. To reach a state of complete physical, mental, and social well-being, an individual or group must be able to identify and realize aspirations, to satisfy needs, and to change or cope with the environment. Health is, therefore, seen as a resource for everyday life, not the objective of living. Health is a positive concept emphasizing social and personal resources, as well as physical capacities. Therefore, health promotion is not just the responsibility of the health sector, but goes beyond healthy lifestyles to well-being.**

A follow-up report titled *Achieving Health for All: A Framework for Health Promotion*[12] identified three national health challenges: reducing inequities, increasing the prevention effort, and enhancing people's capacity to cope. The three mechanisms to health promotion were identified as **self-care**, the decisions and actions individuals take in the interest of their own health; **mutual aid**, the actions people take to help each other cope; and **healthy environments**, the creation of conditions and surroundings conducive to health. Implementation strategies included fostering public participation, strengthening community health services, and coordinating healthy public policy. This health promotion framework is still used today as a foundation for planning, implementing, and evaluating health promotion programs and education.

Many more health models have been developed over the past few decades. The Health Belief Model, originated by Hochbaum, Kegels, and Rosenstock in the 1950s, was developed to help explain and predict health behaviour. This model considers social, ecological, and environmental factors that can influence our behaviour.[13] A more detailed description of this model is found on page 17 of this chapter. The Precede-Proceed model for health program planning and evaluation was developed and adapted by Green and Kreuter over a 40 year period of work and education in community health promotion.[14] The purpose of the model is to provide a guide to improving our health through a socio-ecological approach. The authors of this model encourage us to think about our own individual health behaviours and choices within the environment we live in. They also encourage health experts and planners to support a population health approach and improve conditions at a community level that will support individual behaviour change. (See Figure 1-2 for a Canadian English adaptation of the model).

---

*Source: World Health Organization, "The Ottawa Charter for Health Promotion," found at http://www.who.int/healthpromotion/conferences/previous/ottawa/en/.

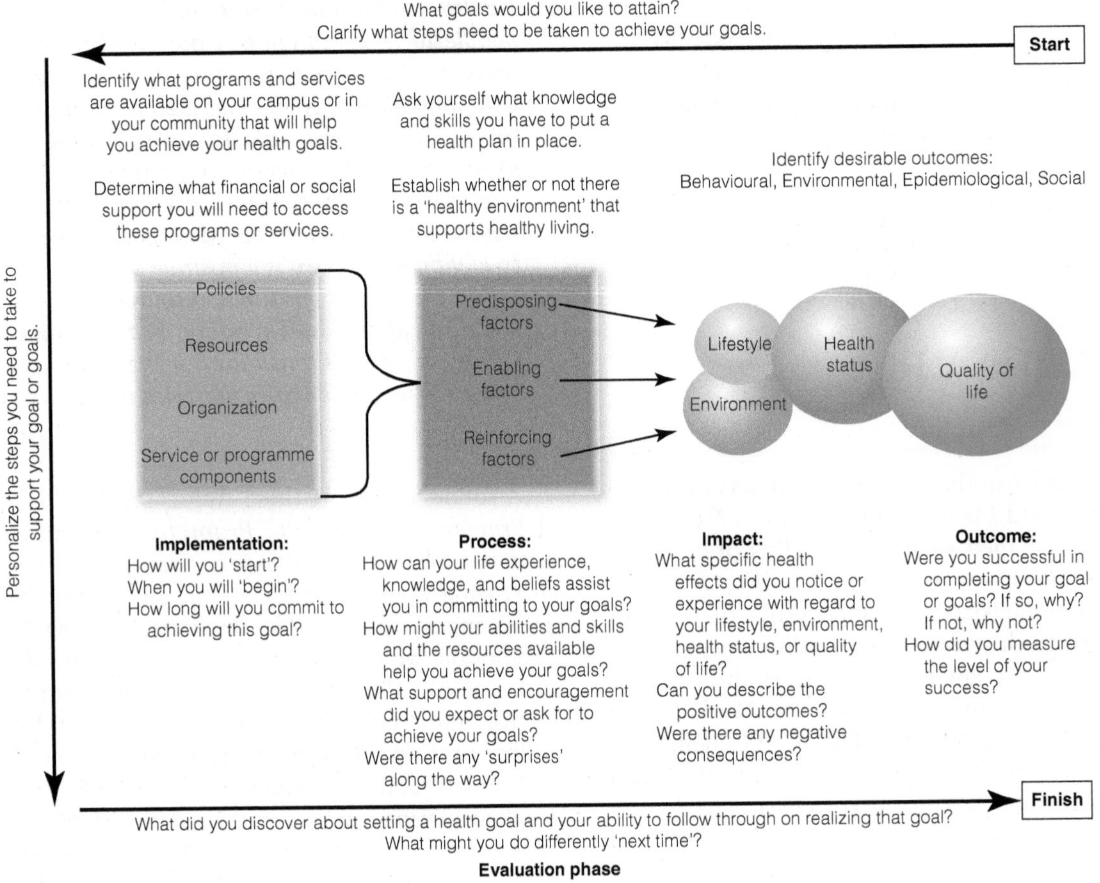

Figure 1-2 **Precede-Proceed Model for Health-Promotion Planning and Evaluation**

Source: Adapted from L.W. Green. (2009, May). A Resource for instructors, students, health practitioners, and researchers using: The Precede-Proceed model of health program planning & evaluation. A Canadian Adaptation of the Model. Available at http://lgreen.net/precede.htm; and Lawrence W. Green and Marshall Kreuter, *Health Program Planning: An Educational and Ecological Approach*, 4th edition. (New York: McGraw-Hill, 2005).

The Quality of Life Model, developed in Canada at the Quality of Life Research Unit at the University of Toronto, is another helpful tool for individuals or communities wanting to enhance their health and well-being. This model has three life domains—Being, Belonging, and Becoming—with each domain having three subdomains (see Table 1-1). Quality of life is measured as the degree to which a person enjoys the important possibilities of his or her life.[15] The model emphasizes an individual's physical, psychological, and spiritual functioning; the connections with his or her environment; and the opportunities for maintaining and enhancing skills.

Health professionals, researchers, and recreation and school educators working in numerous national, federal, and provincial agencies support the health and well-being of Canadians, too. A short description of some of these agencies and the programs and services they provide are shared here.

The Canadian Institute for Health Information (CIHI) is an independent, not-for-profit organization that provides information about national health indicators and standards, health spending, and current health research. One example of a special project of CIHI is the Canadian Population Health Initiative (CPHI).[16] **Population health** is a way of thinking about the social and economic forces that shape the health of Canadians. It builds upon public health and health promotion but goes beyond our more traditional understanding of the causes of health and illness.

The Public Health Agency of Canada works closely with provinces and territories to keep Canadians healthy and reduce healthcare costs. Headed by the chief public health officer, who reports to the minister of health, this national agency focuses on efforts to prevent chronic diseases and responds to health emergencies and infectious disease outbreaks. Its mission is to renew the public health system in Canada and support a sustainable healthcare system.[17]

The Canadian Institutes of Health Research (CIHR)[18] is a federal agency that funds health research in Canada. New health knowledge gained from the research is then made available to health, recreation, and school professionals and practitioners so that

TABLE 1-1

Quality of Life Model

Being	Who One Is
Physical Being	• physical health • personal hygiene • nutrition • exercise • grooming and clothing • general physical appearance
Psychological Being	• psychological health and adjustment • cognitions • feelings • self-esteem, self-concept, and self-control
Spiritual Being	• personal values • personal standards of conduct • spiritual beliefs
Belonging	**Connections with One's Environment**
Physical Belonging	• home • workplace/school • neighbourhood • community
Social Belonging	• intimate others • family • friends • co-workers • neighbourhood and community
Community Belonging	• adequate income • health and social services • employment • educational programs • recreational programs • community events and activities
Becoming	**Achieving Personal Goals, Hopes, and Aspirations**
Practical Becoming	• domestic activities • paid work • school or volunteer activities • seeing to health or social needs
Leisure Becoming	• activities that promote relaxation and stress reduction
Growth Becoming	• activities that promote the maintenance or improvement of knowledge and skills • adapting to change

Source: Quality of Life Model. Developed at the Centre for Health Promotion. Permission to use the model granted by The Quality of Life Research Unit. Department of Occupational Therapy, 500 University Avenue, Rm. 914, Toronto, Ontario, M5G 1V7. Found at www.utoronto.ca/qol/concepts.htm.

health services, programs, and products can help to strengthen our healthcare system.

The First Nations, Inuit & Aboriginal Health branch of Health Canada[19] supports the delivery of public health and health-promotion services to First Nations, Inuit, and Aboriginal peoples on reserves and in Inuit communities in all parts of Canada. Information about nutrition; outdoor adventure leadership; diabetes; fetal alcohol syndrome; injury prevention; and alcohol, drugs, and tobacco is also available through this agency.

ParticipACTION, a national not-for-profit organization created in 1971, closed in 2001, and revitalized in 2007, is the voice of physical activity and sport in Canada. ParticipACTION's mission is to inspire and support Canadians to "move more." Using a combination of public messaging, social marketing strategies, and partnerships between health, medical, recreation, and sport bodies, ParticipACTION's vision is to ensure an active Canadian society.[20]

If you are planning to work with children in a school or recreation setting, you will find the work that Physical and Health Education Canada (PHE Canada)[21] is doing to be helpful and inspiring. This organization, first named the Canadian Physical Education Association (CPEA), was founded in 1933 by Dr. Arthur Lamb of McGill University. Advocating for and educating about quality physical and health education programs such as Quality Daily Physical Education (QDPE) and Comprehensive School Health (CSH) in both school and community environments has become its mission.

Many provincial and territorial governments in Canada have also developed health reports, initiatives, and programs. Table 1-2 lists some of them.

✓ CHECK-IN

How would you define health?

What Is Epidemiology? **Epidemiology** is the "study of how often diseases occur in different groups of people and why."[22] Epidemiology can be used to evaluate health strategies and prevent certain illnesses. It is also used to guide doctors and healthcare providers in the management of patients who are dealing with specific diseases. If you were to engage in epidemiological research, you might find yourself studying in any of the following areas: infectious disease, neuroepidemiology, chronic disease, or epidemiology of aging.

Epidemiological research uses a variety of methodological approaches including environmental, clinical, genetic, molecular, social, life course, pharamacoepidemiology, and surveillance epidemiology. Researchers can examine the distribution of disease in a specific population, known as descriptive epidemiology, or investigate a hypothesized causal factor by conducting a study that relates to the exposure of interest to the

TABLE 1-2

National, Provincial, and Territorial Health and Wellness Reports, Initiatives, and Programs

Province	Initiative	Website
British Columbia	Stay Active, Eat Healthy BC Recreation and Parks Association (BCRPA)	http://stayactiveeathealthy.ca/
Alberta	The Alberta Centre for Active Living	www.centre4activeliving.ca
Saskatchewan	Saskatchewan in Motion	www.saskatchewaninmotion.ca
Manitoba	Manitoba Healthy Living	www.gov.mb.ca/healthyliving/index.html
Ontario	The Ontario Federation of School Athletic Associations Healthy Active Living	http://www.ofsaa.on.ca/resources/healthy-active-living
Quebec	Government of Quebec Going the Healthy Route at School	www.education.gouv.qc.ca/en/teachers/going-the-healthy-route-at-school/
New Brunswick	Government of New Brunswick—Social Development	www2.gnb.ca/content/gnb/en/departments/social_development/wellness.html
Prince Edward Island	Department of Health and Wellness Healthy Living	www.gov.pe.ca/health/wellness
Nova Scotia	Nova Scotia Health and Wellness—Active Living Branch	http://novascotia.cioc.ca/record/DHW0002
Newfoundland	Department of Health and Community Services—Health Promotion and Wellness	www.health.gov.nl.ca/health/wellnesshealthyliving/index.html
Yukon	Yukon Health and Social Services Pathways to Wellness	www.yukonwellness.ca/
Northwest Territories	Northwest Territories Health and Social Services—Community Wellness	www.hss.gov.nt.ca/social-services/community-wellness
Nunavut	Nunavut Department of Health—Healthy Living	www.livehealthy.gov.nu.ca/en
Canada	Health Canada: Healthy Living	www.hc-sc.gc.ca/hl-vs/index-eng.php

disease, known as analytical epidemiology. There are many exciting careers in epidemiology. You can find out more about workshops, national conferences, and volunteer opportunities for students at the Canadian Society for Epidemiology and Biostatistics website at http://csebca.ipage.com/wordpress/.

WELLNESS AND THE WELLNESS MOVEMENT

What Is Wellness? **Wellness** can be defined as purposeful, enjoyable living or, more specifically, a deliberate lifestyle choice characterized by personal responsibility and optimal enhancement of physical, mental, and spiritual health. More than freedom from disease, it means taking steps to prevent illness and involves a capacity to live life to the fullest. A healthy and well individual has a greater capacity for personal potential. To understand how the concepts of wellness and health fit together, we will review the history of the wellness movement.

Dr. Halbert Dunn, considered a pioneer of the wellness movement, was a physician and Chief of the United States National Office of Vital Statistics from 1935 to 1950. He believed health care should be more than the treatment of disease. His definition of wellness was based on that of the World Health Organization; however, he believed that health was *a passive state of homeostasis or balance*, whereas wellness was *a dynamic process of continually moving toward one's potential for optimal functioning*. Wellness, for Dunn, was dependent on three criteria: (1) direction and progress toward a higher potential of functioning; (2) the total individual, which includes physical, mental, emotional, social, and spiritual components; and (3) functioning and adapting for daily living and in times of crisis.[23]

In 1974, while Canadians were moving toward a new perspective on health care, Dr. John Travis, inspired by Halbert Dunn, founded the first Wellness Resource Center in the United States in 1975. A medical doctor by training, Travis decided to shift his focus from disease care to self-responsibility and prevention. His wellness model, the Illness/Wellness Continuum, is seen in Figure 1-3. Travis suggests that many of us are at the neutral point where we are not ill but have much more potential to be well. His definition of wellness includes the belief that wellness is a choice, a decision you make to move toward optimal health, and a lifestyle you design to achieve your highest potential for well-being.[24] He continues to write about wellness, with a new focus on global wellness, and children and wellness. His website can be accessed at www.thewellspring.com.

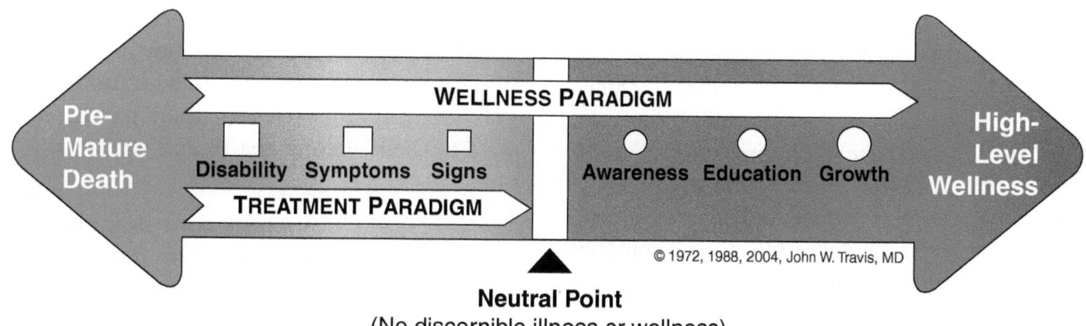

Figure 1-3 **Illness/Wellness Continuum**

Source: *Wellness Workbook*, 3rd edition, by John Travis, MD, and Regina Sara Ryan, Celestial Arts, Berkeley, CA. © 1981, 1988, 2004 by John W. Travis. www.wellnessworkbook.com.

Another influential wellness expert, Dr. Bill Hettler, the co-founder of the National Wellness Institute, began his work in the wellness field at the University of Wisconsin–Stevens Point in the 1970s. Hettler believed that health care could be improved with health-promotion activities and educational opportunities that encouraged self-care. He created a Lifestyle Assessment Questionnaire (LAQ) that has been redesigned as TestWell, a self-scoring wellness assessment, which is available for personal or organizational use.[25] A short version is now available online at www.nationalwellness.org. Click on Resources—Testwell—Sample Testwell Assessments. There are college and adult versions of this inventory.

Hettler also developed the Six Dimensions of Wellness model (see Figure 1-4). This model has been used in many corporate health and wellness programs around the world. A brief overview of the six dimensions is presented here.

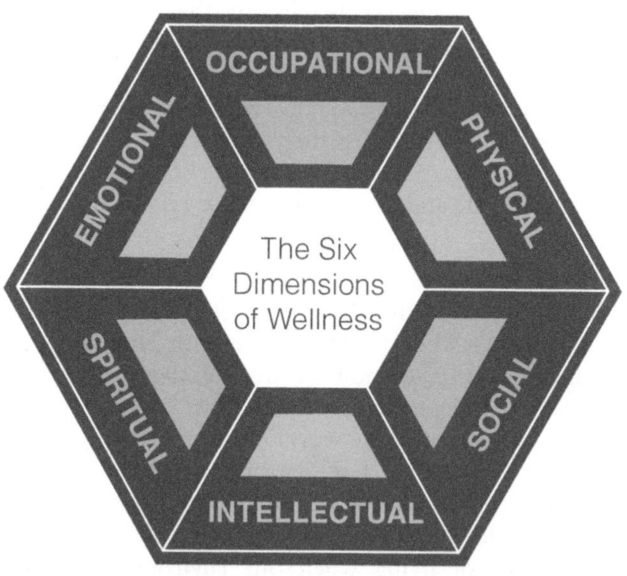

Figure 1-4 **Six Dimensions of Wellness**

Source: B. Hettler, National Wellness Institute (1993). Testwell, Pg. i. Copyright 1979 by Hettler, © 1993 by National Wellness Institute, Inc., WCB Brown & Benchmark Publishers. Also available at www.nationalwellness.org/ index.php?id_tier=2&id_c=25. Permission granted by National Wellness Institute.

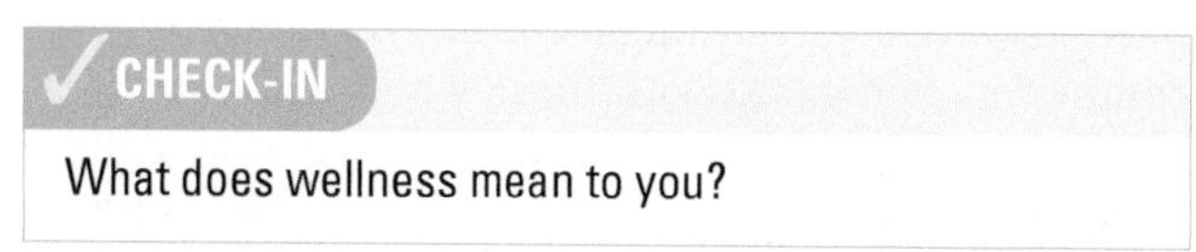

CHECK-IN

What does wellness mean to you?

Social Dimension This dimension encourages a collectivist view of the world—that of contributing to society, helping others, and valuing the concept of interdependence between ourselves and our environment. By embracing the social dimension of wellness, we begin to take an active part in improving our world by actively seeking ways to enhance personal relationships, celebrate friendships, and build healthy communities.[26] Examples on a college or university campus would include peer helping; special event planning; establishing smoke-free policies for academic buildings, residences, and dining areas; promoting a safe campus; and enforcing alcohol laws and policies.

Health educators are placing a greater emphasis on the social dimension of wellness. Research has shown that social support influences health and well-being. Individuals who have a sense of connection to others are more likely to have a secure attachment style and benefit from supportive relationships.[27]

Occupational Dimension Finding enrichment through our work or vocation can enhance our well-being. A "well" occupation is consistent with personal values, interests, and beliefs. It is also the attitude we hold about our work. In a well work environment, you contribute your skills and talents to your community and enjoy work that is meaningful and rewarding. Occupational wellness follows the tenet that it is healthy to balance work and other life commitments.[28]

As you begin to plan for your career or to reflect upon the career choices you have made, an understanding of the importance of occupational wellness can direct you in your choice of profession, ensure job satisfaction, help you to define your career ambitions, and assist you in evaluating your personal performance on the job.

Spiritual Dimension Identifying our basic purpose in life; learning how to experience love, joy, peace, and fulfillment; and helping ourselves and others achieve our potential are all aspects of the spiritual dimension. Spirituality has been described in many ways. Definitions include transcendence, connectedness, a power, a force, or energy.[29] Reyman, Fialkowski, and Stewart-Sicking suggest that "creating a core spiritual dimension among students may help the students be healthy in all dimensions."[30] Nelms et al. also found significant relationships between self-reported levels of spirituality and the health of college students.[31]

Additionally, spirituality can mean a connection to a formal religion or faith. Research shows that people who regularly attend religious services are twice as likely to have a very strong feeling of belonging to their community compared with those who do not attend at all.[32] Current research has also shown that cancer patients who attend religious services or who believe in a spiritual source report better physical health.[33] And in an extensive review of literature, Nichols and Hunt suggest that spirituality can help people with chronic illness.[34]

Physical Dimension Physical wellness is met through participation in regular physical activity. Aerobic conditioning includes walking, running, cycling, and swimming—activities that help to keep our hearts healthy. Exercises such as strength training and calisthenics help to improve muscle strength and endurance. Stretching exercises keep us flexible.

Being physically active helps us maintain a healthy body weight or body mass index. To be physically well, we also need to make healthy food choices and avoid harmful behaviours such as tobacco use, drug misuse, and excessive alcohol consumption. It is important to get medical attention when needed and take care to use medical interventions such as prescription drugs properly. As physical wellness is pursued, a heightened awareness of the connection between body, mind, and spirit is experienced. In a study by Melton, Hansen, and Gross,[35] college students who took part in physical activity programs felt that their participation contributed to their lifelong health and wellness.

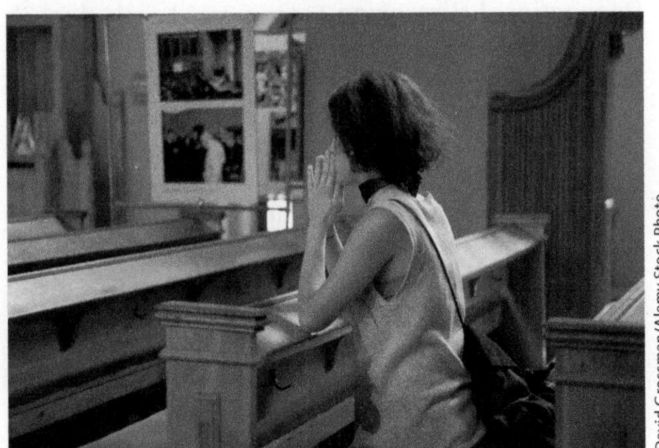

David Grossman/Alamy Stock Photo

In every culture, religious and spiritual rituals play an important role in the lives and health of individuals.

Intellectual Dimension Your brain is the only organ capable of self-awareness. Every day you use your mind to gather, process, and act on information; to think through your values; and to make decisions, set goals, and figure out how to handle a problem or challenge. Intellectual wellness refers to your ability to think and learn from life experience, your openness to new ideas, and your capacity to question and evaluate information. Throughout your life, you'll use your critical thinking skills, including your ability to evaluate health information, to safeguard your well-being.

A well person cherishes intellectual growth and stimulation. When we embrace this dimension of wellness, we stretch and challenge our minds with intellectual and creative pursuits and become more productive.[36]

Emotional Dimension Emotional wellness includes the degree to which one feels positive and enthusiastic about oneself and life.[37] It also involves awareness and acceptance of a wide range of feelings in oneself and others. When you are emotionally well, you have the capacity to express and manage your own feelings. You make choices and decisions based upon the connection of feelings, thoughts, philosophies, and behaviours. You become aware of limitations and personal and professional stressors but are able to effectively work around those limitations and cope with the stressors.[38]

Emotional wellness also means that we have the capability to work independently but recognize the importance of being able to ask for help or support when needed. An emotionally well individual knows that there are times when there is a benefit to working interdependently with others and celebrating the commitment, trust, and respect that those relationships are based on.

Environmental Dimension—The Seventh Dimension of Wellness We are adding a Seventh Dimension of Wellness in this edition of our textbook (see Figure 1-5). Climate change and global warming have made people around the world aware that many of the natural resources we have become dependent on are limited. Air, land, and water quality are being compromised due to human action. It is difficult to adopt a "well" way of living when our environment is not healthy and well. Environmental wellness includes being respectful of and attempting to live in harmony with nature. It means ensuring the stability and longevity of our natural resources. It demands leadership

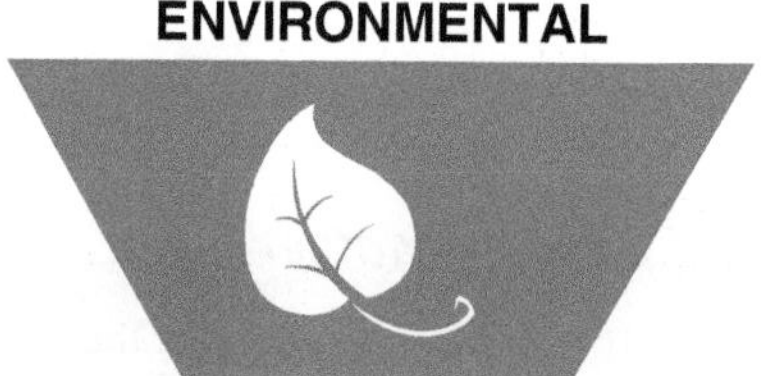

Figure 1-5 **Environmental Dimension—The Seventh Dimension of Wellness**

Adapted from: University of Guelph. (2016). Seven dimensions of health. Student Services. Seven Dimensions of Wellness: https://www.uoguelph.ca/studenthealthservices/wellness-centre/seven-dimensions-wellness; University of Regina, Recreation Services—Dimensions on Wellness: http://www.uregina.ca/recservices/wellness/dimensions.html.

and a long-term coordinated effort from all of us. Students, faculty, staff, and administration at numerous colleges and universities across Canada are recognizing that we all have a personal and societal responsibility for making an effort to create sustainable campuses. Some examples of campus environmental initiatives include the development of sustainability offices or units, bus passes, recycling programs, bike racks, the protection of green spaces, water bottle refill stations, composting, vegetarian food options, and energy conservation.[39]

Are you doing your part for the environmental dimension of wellness? We all have the ability to make a positive impact with regard to our environment. Reflecting on our personal choices is the first step. Putting an action plan into place is the second step.

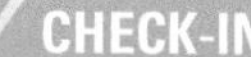

How do you rate yourself on each of these dimensions of wellness?

HEALTH CHALLENGES

Demographic Growth The study of demography focuses on many areas. Research in this field includes studies on the size, growth, and age of a population. It also includes studies on geographical distribution of human populations, and births, deaths, marriages, and how and where people migrate. Trends in demographic growth affect the demand for healthcare services.

According to Statistics Canada, the estimated population in 2014/2015 increased by 0.9 percent from 2013/2014, to 35.9 million Canadians. This is the lowest growth rate noted since 1998/1999.[40] However, it continued to be the strongest growth rate among the G7 countries (the group of seven major advanced economies). Figure 1-6 illustrates the population growth rate by province and territory for 2013/2014 and 2014/2015. The main source of the increase in population was international migration. Eighty-five percent of immigrants settled in Ontario, Quebec, Alberta, and British Columbia.[41] People also moved from one province to another. This is known as interprovincial migration.

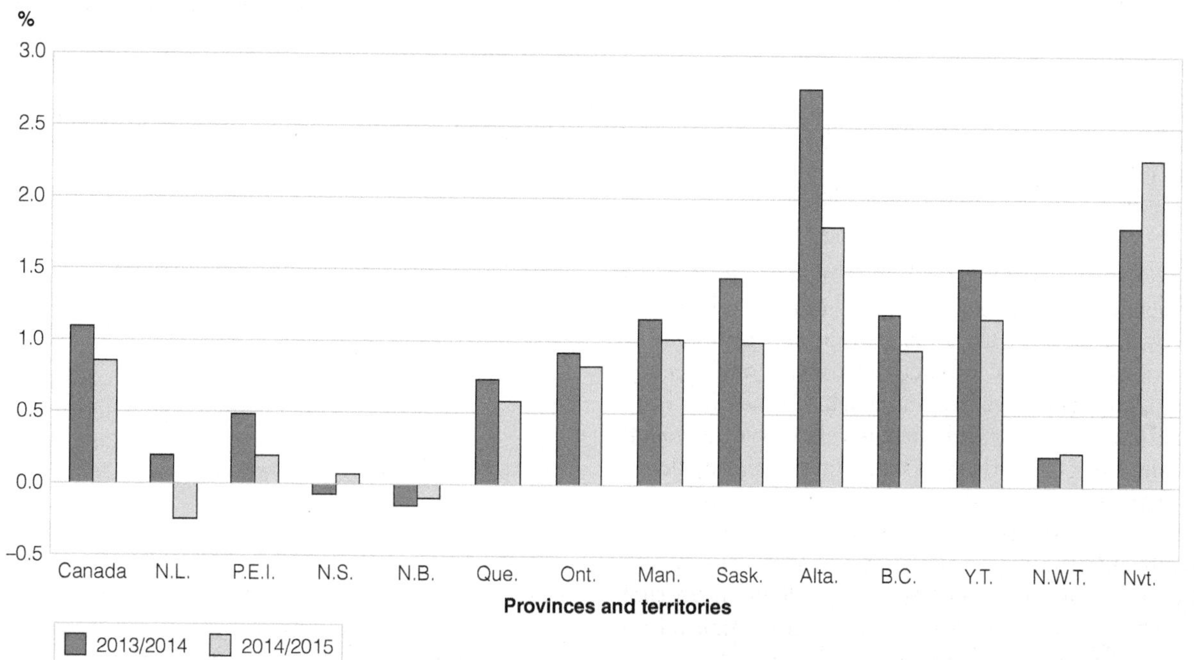

Figure 1-6 **Population Growth Rate, 2013/2014 and 2014/2015, Canada, Provinces and Territories**

Source: Ministry of Industry. (2015, September). *Annual demographic estimates: Canada, provinces and territories*. Statistics Canada. Demography Division. (p. 18) Available at http://www.statcan.gc.ca/pub/91-215-x/91-215-x2015000-eng.pdf.

When the population increases, healthcare costs are often inevitable.

- Rising costs have been associated with the two leading causes of death for Canadians—cancer and heart disease. Direct costs such as drug therapy, physician assistance, and hospital costs are also increasing as Canadians deal with lower respiratory diseases and a massive increase in the onset of type 2 diabetes.
- Hypertension, or high blood pressure, is a major contributor to poor health and affects one in five Canadians. Costs for supporting health care in this regard are growing.
- Research indicates that where we live can have an impact on our lives too. The years of potential life lost (YPLL) are greater if you live in the northern regions of Canada. Research shows that unintentional and self-inflicted injuries are also higher in these regions.
- Mental health issues are also a concern. Just over 5 percent of Canadians report having experienced symptoms consistent with a major depressive episode over the past year. Demand for mental health services increases overall healthcare costs.

In 1900, the average woman could expect to live to be 50.9 years of age, compared with 47.9 years for a man. Infectious diseases, such as smallpox and tuberculosis, claimed tens of thousands of lives, particularly among the young and the poor. A high percentage of women died during childbirth or shortly afterward.

The good news is that we are now living longer. Between 1995 and 1997 the combined average life expectancy for males and females was 78.4 years.[42] According to the WHO, the combined life expectancy for males and females born in 2013 was 82 years of age. For males born in Canada in 2013 the average life expectancy was 80 years of age. For females it was 84 years of age.[43] Living longer has many societal benefits; however, healthcare costs rise greatly as Canadians age. The availability of healthcare services can also be a challenge.

Social Determinants While health and wellness is dependent on self-care, other factors must also be taken into consideration. Health is determined by complex interactions between our environment, our genetic makeup, and where we live and work. Canada has been a world leader in research that is related to the **social determinants of health (SDOH)**, but there is evidence that there is a growing inequality in social and economic status between groups of Canadians. According to Raphael,[44] the larger the gap, the lower the health status of the overall population. He is convinced that we still have much to do to secure and to maintain a healthy Canadian population.

Different agencies define and describe health determinants in various ways. The World Health Organization (WHO) focuses on inequities such as

X AND Y FILES

Do Sex and Gender Matter?

Sex does matter. That was the conclusion of the Institute of Medicine Committee on Understanding the Biology of Sex and Gender Differences in the first significant review of the status of sex and gender differences in biomedical research.

Sex, the committee stated, is "a classification, generally as male or female, according to the reproductive organs and functions that derive from the chromosomal complement." *Gender* refers to "a person's self-representation as male or female, or how that person is responded to by social institutions on the basis of the individual's gender presentation." Rooted in biology, gender is shaped by environment and experience.

The experience of being male, female, or transgender in a particular culture and society can and does have an effect on physical and psychological well-being. This realization is both new and revolutionary. For centuries, scientists based biological theories solely on a male model and viewed women as shorter, smaller, and rounder versions of men. We now know this simply isn't so (see Figure 1-7). Sex begins in the womb, but sex and gender differences affect behaviour, perception, and health throughout life.

Gender differences persist in sickness as well as in health. Before age 50, men are more prone to lethal diseases, including heart attacks, cancer, and liver failure. Women show greater vulnerability to chronic but non-life-threatening problems such as arthritis and autoimmune disorders. Women are twice as likely to suffer depression; men have a fivefold greater rate of alcoholism. Women outlive men by approximately five years, yet they are more prone to age-related problems, such as osteoporosis and Alzheimer's disease. Health behaviours—patterns of drinking, smoking, or using seat belts—also are different in men and women.

More women than men have a regular physician. Men have fewer dental as well as medical checkups. They're less likely to seek psychiatric services, to have their cholesterol levels and blood pressure checked regularly, and to undergo some form of screening for colon cancer. More women than men are overweight, and fewer women are physically active. Although college and university men are among those at highest risk of testicular cancer, three out of four do not know how to perform a self-examination. Male undergraduates are much less likely to examine their testicles than female students are to examine their breasts. College- and university-age men also are significantly more likely to engage in risky and physically dangerous behaviours and to suffer more injuries, including fatal ones, as a result.

Recognition of these gender differences is transforming medical research and practice. A new science called *gender-specific medicine* is replacing one-size-fits-all health care with new definitions of what is normal for men, women, and transgender, more complex concepts of disease, more precise diagnostic tests, and more effective treatments.

Sources: Committee on Understanding the Biology of Sex and Gender Differences. (2001). *Exploring the biological contributions to human health: Does sex matter?* Washington, DC: Institute of Medicine, National Academy of Sciences; D. Hales. (2001). *Just like a woman*. New York: Bantam; D. Hales. (2002, September). Biology shows women and men are different. *Mayo Clinic Women's Healthsource 6*(9), 1; Public Health Agency of Canada. (2012, October 26). The Chief Public Health Officer's Report on the State of Public Health in Canada. (2012). *Influencing Health—The Importance of Sex and Gender*. www.phac-aspc.gc.ca/cphorsphc-respcacsp/2012/index-eng.php.

He

- averages 12 breaths a minute
- has lower core body temperature
- has a slower heart rate
- has more oxygen-rich hemoglobin in his blood
- is more sensitive to sound
- produces twice as much saliva
- has a 10 percent larger brain
- is 10 times more likely to have attention deficit disorder
- has an attention span of 5 minutes, as a teen
- is more likely to be physically active
- is more prone to lethal diseases, including heart attacks, cancer, and liver failure
- is five times more likely to become an alcoholic
- has a life expectancy of 80 years

She

- averages 9 breaths a minute
- has higher core body temperature
- has a faster heart rate
- has higher levels of protective immunoglobulin in her blood
- is more sensitive to light
- takes twice as long to process food
- has more neurons in certain brain regions
- is twice as likely to have an eating disorder
- has an attention span of 20 minutes, as a teen
- is more likely to be overweight
- is more vulnerable to chronic diseases, like arthritis and autoimmune disorders, and age-related conditions like osteoporosis
- is twice as likely to develop depression
- has a life expectancy of 84 years

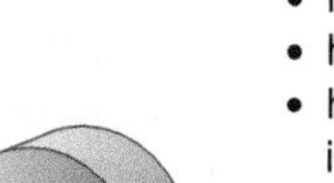

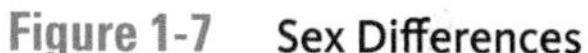

Figure 1-7 Sex Differences

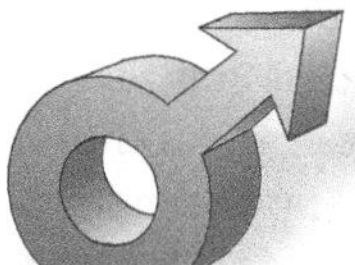

Men and women are different in many ways.

Sources: Committee on Understanding the Biology of Sex and Gender Differences. (2001). *Exploring the biological contributions to human health: Does sex matter?* Washington, DC: Institute of Medicine, National Academy of Sciences; D. Hales (2001). *Just like a woman.* New York: Bantam; D. Hales (2002, September). Biology shows women and men are different. *Mayo Clinic Women's Healthsource*, 6(9), 1; World Health Organization (WHO). (2016). Statistics. Countries. Canada.

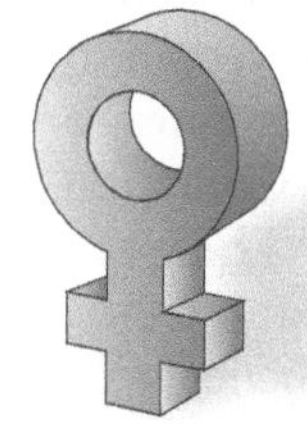

unemployment, unsafe workplaces, lack of access to health systems, and women and gender equity.[45] The Public Health Agency of Canada lists 14 social determinants of health,[46] which include income and social status, education and literacy, and healthy child development. A more in-depth look at the 14 social determinants based on the work of Mikkonen and Raphael[47] in their *Social Determinants of Health, The Canadian Facts* report will be presented in this section.

Income and Income Distribution The poverty gap has widened over the past decade in Canada. A report from Statistics Canada determined that in 2012, families who were in the top income bracket held 47 percent of the overall total of household wealth. Canadian families who were in the bottom income bracket held only 4 percent of the total household wealth.[48] Low income predisposes people to greater social deprivation resulting in the inability to afford basic food, clothing, and housing. It also limits participation in recreational, educational, and cultural activities. Raphael found that children brought up in socio-economically disadvantaged households often suffer from a range of diseases as an adult. They also die earlier than children raised in more economically well-off households.[49]

Education When people have a higher level of education, they tend to have better health and better access to job training and opportunity for gainful employment. In a study comparing education, sex, and race in 93 counties in the United States, researchers discovered that in more than 70 percent of the counties, education was a predictor of poor or fair health and poor mental health days.[50] In Canada, Aboriginal students have lower rates of high-school graduation, and their attendance at postsecondary schools is well below the national average. Korpal and Wong encourage "culturally appropriate and community-based educational interventions . . . that redefine education as empowering for the health of First Nations people."[51]

Unemployment and Job Security Many changes in the workforce have occurred because of **globalization**—the increased transnational movement of capital, goods, people, and political systems and a rapid turnover of ideas and images through new communication technologies. This has resulted at times with layoffs and an increase in temporary, part-time, casual, contract, and self-employment work situations. Half of working Canadians experience some sort of income and job insecurity. In January 2016, unemployment rates rose to 7.2 percent—the highest it had been since December of 2013.[52] Unemployment can also increase the likelihood of making unhealthy lifestyle choices such as smoking and misuse of alcohol.[53]

Employment and Working Conditions Working hours, physical conditions at the workplace, time pressures, and unrealistic work demands can cause high levels of "work stress."[54] Stress at work can lead to health issues such as mental and emotional conditions, high blood pressure, and cardiovascular disease. High-stress working conditions can also lead to workplace injuries. When other social determinants are considered, lack of education and lack of job security can lead to lack of job opportunities, thus leading to low income, and then the circle continues.

Early Childhood Development Children who have limited opportunities for learning at an early age are often at risk later in life due to cognitive and emotional immaturity. This can lead to lower educational attainment. Research shows that children living in disadvantaged households are sometimes at greater risk for health problems associated with improper nutrition, high stress levels, and social deprivation. Access to daycare also contributes to health and well-being. Only 17 percent of Canadian families have access to regulated daycare.[55] There are numerous studies suggesting that while high-quality, early childhood education has many positive benefits for society, total spending on daycare spaces has dropped.

Food Insecurity Food is a basic human need and one of the most important social determinants of health. Reports suggest that 8.3 percent of Canadian households encountered food insecurity between 2011 and 2012. People in Nunavut suffered the highest rate of food insecurity—36.7 percent—which is over four times the Canadian average. Single-parent families also struggle with 22.6 percent reporting food insecurity.[56] Malnutrition has long-lasting effects on children and can result in heart disease, diabetes, food allergies, and high blood pressure during childhood or later life. Research also shows that there are psychological impacts on families dealing with food insecurity that are linked to behavioural, emotional, and academic problems.

Housing There continues to be a housing crisis in Canada. When many Canadians spend more than 30 percent of their total income on rent or housing costs, money is not available for food, health care, or recreation.[57] Reports indicate that 3.3 million Canadian households can be considered unaffordable, overcrowded, or below acceptable standards. In 2014, approximately 235 000 people experienced homelessness. About 1 out of 5 households spend over 50 percent of their low income on rent.[58] Again, we can see the connection between the social determinants of health. Low-paying jobs and lack of job security result in individuals who cannot afford housing. Individuals who are under-housed or homeless are at greater risk for numerous health issues.

Social Exclusion Social exclusion can be defined as the lack of opportunity to participate fully in society. Social exclusion is often based on gender, age, ability, sexual orientation, race, ethnicity, and religious beliefs. Public health experts suggest that socially excluded Canadians are often denied participation in civil affairs, access to certain goods and services, the opportunity to participate and contribute to social and cultural activities, and access to well-paying jobs or economic resources.[59] Discrimination against specific groups of people in Canada is systemic and gives rise to powerlessness and hopelessness. Social problems and health inequities continue as one disadvantage causes further disadvantages.[60]

Social Safety Net A social safety net includes programs, services, and benefits that help individuals and families during various life transitions or unexpected events. In Canada, employment insurance programs provide some support, but changes to the eligibility requirements of these programs shows that only 40 percent of Canadians are now eligible to receive benefits even if they have been paying into the program.[61] In November 2015, Statistics Canada announced the largest increase (up 9.2 percent) in the total number of people accessing Employment Insurance since February 2010. Approximately two-thirds of the overall increase was found in Alberta.[62]

Health Services Although the *Canada Health Act* requires provincial governments to support citizens through a public healthcare insurance program, there are serious issues of access to care across Canada. Rural versus city access is of concern. Research also shows that low-income earners are more likely to have to wait for medical care or appointments with a physician as compared to high-income earners, and less likely to see a specialist when needed. Low-income earners or unemployed individuals are also less likely to fill prescriptions or access other required treatments due to cost.[63]

Aboriginal Status Canada's First Peoples face many challenges when it comes to health. The average income of Aboriginal men and women is much lower than the average income of non-Aboriginal men and women. Food and housing insecurity are important concerns. Chronic diseases and infection rates are much higher in the Aboriginal population than the rest of the Canadian population. As already mentioned above, education levels differ for Aboriginal students compared with other Canadian students. The concern is that the much lower graduation rates for Aboriginal peoples compared to non-Aboriginal peoples occur whether or not they are living on or off the reserve.[64]

Gender Gender refers to a person's self-representation as male or female. The experience of being male or female in a particular culture and society can and does have an effect on physical and psychology well-being. When it comes to gender, Canadian females are at greater risk with regard to the social determinants of health than are males. They are less likely to have full-time employment, are less likely to be eligible for employment insurance, and often have lower-paying jobs, and the majority of women take on more responsibilities with regard to child care. Their earning power is often compromised because of child-care issues or lack of job opportunities, and wages are not always equal even when women find well-paying jobs.

However, males are also at risk for other reasons. Their suicide rate is four times higher than that of females. They are also more likely to be victims of assault or be involved in crime than females. Social and economic resources do impact both males and females and are intertwined in the health of both genders.[65]

Race We are a multicultural society. Citizens and landed immigrants in Canada have come from all parts of the globe. However, race, one of the social determinants of health, impacts individuals and families in many ways. Canadians of colour experience higher unemployment, economic returns for immigrants are not forthcoming for many, and the health status of recent immigrants and refugees appears to deteriorate over time once they have settled in Canada. An increase in mental health issues of immigrants has also been noted by public health experts.[66]

Disability Canada does not have a good track record when it comes to supporting Canadians with disabilities. Compared to other members of the Organisation for Economic Co-operation and Development (OECD), Canada provides the second lowest compensations and benefits to citizens who are disabled. In fact, Canada has some of the strongest restrictions with regard to successful application for disability benefits. While there is an attempt on federal and provincial levels to integrate persons with disabilities into the workforce, there are many employers who are just not willing to make modifications to the workplace to accommodate people who have special needs.[67] We have much work to do to address this social determinant of health.

Taking Action All is not doom and gloom in Canada, however. Six key strategies to enhance the social determinants of health have been adopted by a number of health agencies and provincial governments. They are

1. adopting a framework for social inclusion;
2. promoting full employment, job security, and healthy working conditions;
3. protecting universal access to our high-quality health system;
4. protecting Canada's high-quality public education system;
5. ensuring the right of all Canadians to adequate housing and food; and
6. reducing income disparities by ensuring minimum wages and levels of social assistance.

The health and well-being of Canadians depends on a commitment from individuals to adopt healthy lifestyles in partnership with municipal, provincial, and federal governments to support healthy lifestyle choices for everyone.[68]

✓ CHECK-IN

How have the social determinants impacted your health and wellness?

THE HEALTH OF COLLEGE AND UNIVERSITY STUDENTS

Universities Canada reported that undergraduate enrolment for both full- and part-time students exceeded over 1.7 million in 2015. Full-time students in 2014–2015 numbered 979 000. There were 312 000 part-time students.[69] We also welcomed about 89 000 full-time international undergraduate students on campuses across Canada (approximately 11 percent of full-time undergraduates) and 44 000 full-time international students in graduate programs (almost 28 percent of all graduate students).[70]

Investing in a university or college education to prepare for a career has many benefits. However, a career cannot be sustained if individuals are not healthy. With regard to lifestyle choices, college and university students sometimes engage in behaviours that put them at risk for serious health problems. Davis et al. found that college-age men are more likely than women to engage in risk-taking behaviours—to use drugs and alcohol; to engage in risky sexual behaviours, such as having multiple partners and having sex while under the influence of alcohol; and to drive dangerously. Men also are more likely to be hospitalized for injuries and to commit suicide. Three-quarters of the deaths in the 15–24 age range are men.[71]

College or university living can be hazardous to your health, too. Dormitories have proven to be breeding grounds for serious infectious diseases such as meningitis. Second-hand smoke can present a long-term threat to smokers' roommates. Binge drinking imperils not only the drinkers but also those in their immediate environment, including anyone on the road if an intoxicated student gets behind the wheel of a car.[72]

Undergraduates also face risks to their psychological health. In a Canadian survey, college students reported more distress than the general Canadian population or their peers not enrolled in college.[73] Nearly a third of more than 7500 undergraduates surveyed had significantly elevated psychological distress—women more than men, younger students more than upper-level students.

First year seems to take the greatest toll on college and university students. In an American study, a survey of 3680 students interviewed at the beginning and end of their first year found significant drops in physical and emotional well-being. As entering freshmen, 51 percent rated their physical health as "above average." At the end of the year, only 41 percent did. The percentage of students reporting above-average emotional health dropped from 52 percent to 45 percent.[74]

However, despite potential health risks, the great majority of students survive and thrive at college and university and also increases their chances of a long and healthful life. Many risk factors for disease—including high blood pressure, elevated cholesterol, and cigarette smoking—decline steadily as education increases, regardless of how much money people make. Education may be good for the body as well as the mind by influencing lifestyle behaviours, problem-solving abilities, and values. Individuals who earn college and university degrees gain positive attitudes about the benefits of healthy living, learn how to gain access to preventive health services, join peer groups that promote healthy behaviour, and develop higher self-esteem and greater control over their lives.

✓ CHECK-IN

How do you think your current health behaviours may affect your future?

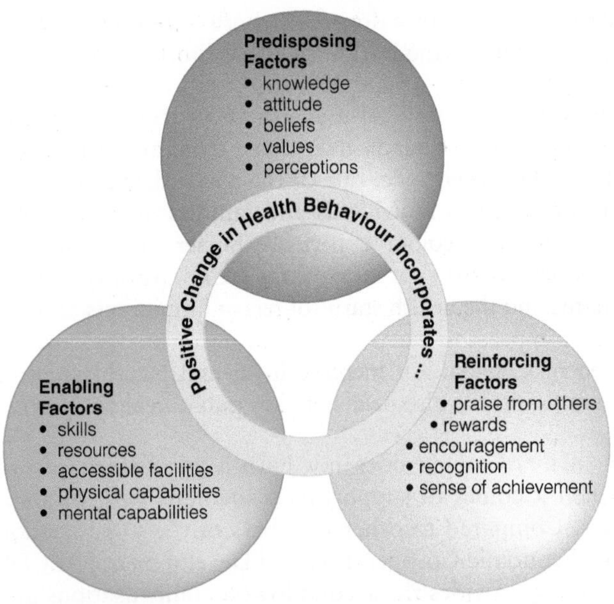

Figure 1-8 Factors That Shape Positive Behaviour

MAKING HEALTHY CHANGES

Your choices and behaviours during your university or college years can influence how healthy you will be in the future. When it comes to lifestyle choices, you are the one who is in charge. Ask yourself what aspects of your life could use some attention and improvement. Use this textbook and course as an opportunity to embrace healthy living. Take time to learn about how you can make healthy decisions every day. The following sections discuss some of the processes you might go through to make a successful change for the better.

Understanding Health Behaviour Behaviours that affect your health include exercising regularly, eating a balanced nutritious diet, seeking care for symptoms, and taking the necessary steps to overcome illness and restore well-being. If you want to improve health behaviour, it is important to realize that change isn't easy. Between 40 and 80 percent of those who try to kick bad health habits lapse back into their unhealthy ways within six weeks. To make lasting beneficial changes, it helps to understand the three factors that shape behaviour: predisposing, enabling, and reinforcing (see Figure 1-8).

Predisposing Factors The use of the term "predisposing factors" with regard to health behaviours is best known from Green and Kreuter's Precede-Proceed Model for Health Program Planning and Evaluation[75] (see Figure 1-2, p. 6). **Predisposing factors** encourage a behaviour change or inhibit us from changing. They include knowledge, attitudes, beliefs, values, self-efficacy, behavioural intentions, and existing skills. Other predisposing factors that play a role in a lifestyle change process include our age, sex, socio-economic levels, ethnicity, family background, healthcare access, and level of education. Take a moment to think about the predisposing factors in your life. What is your current understanding of living a healthy lifestyle? What family values have shaped your perception of health and wellness? And, while predisposing factors can lead to behaviour change, remember that without enabling and reinforcing factors, the change might be short-lived.

Enabling Factors Within the Precede-Proceed Model, enabling factors make it possible or easier for people or populations to change their behaviours. Positive **enabling factors** include individual physical capabilities and mental capacities, resources, living conditions, societal support, and accessible facilities, programs, and services. They also include developing skills, which are in addition to any predisposing existing skills that an individual already possesses. Examples are learning how to access medical advice and procedures, learning more about healthy nutrition practices, and developing exercise routines that assist in desired behaviour change. Watch out for negative enablers such as people who encourage you to choose unhealthy lifestyle options, or health programs and services that have not been proven to be beneficial.

Before you initiate a change, assess the means available to reach your goal. No matter how motivated you are, you'll become frustrated if you keep encountering obstacles. Breaking a task or goal down into step-by-step strategies is important in behavioural change.

Reinforcing Factors **Reinforcing factors** may include praise from family and friends, rewards from teachers or parents, or encouragement and recognition for meeting a goal. They can also include healthy community policies such as smoke-free facilities, the availability of an on-site workplace health and wellness program, or even the option of registering in a health and wellness course at a college or university.

While these reinforcing factors are very important, lasting change depends not only on external rewards but also on an internal commitment and sense of achievement. To make a difference, reinforcement must come from within too. A decision to change a health behaviour needs to stem from a permanent, personal goal, not from a desire to please or to impress someone else. If you lose weight for a special occasion, you're almost sure to regain the weight afterward. But if you shed extra weight because you want to feel better about yourself or get into shape, you're far more likely to keep off the weight. As you begin to make lifestyle changes, think about ways you can reinforce the adoption of a new way of living. Determine how you will reward yourself for successes, and consider ways in which you might accept small failures or relapses that will most likely occur.

Decision Making Every day you make decisions that have immediate and long-term effects on your health. You decide what to eat, whether to drink or smoke, when to exercise, and how to cope with a sudden crisis. Beyond these daily matters, you decide when to see a doctor, what kind of doctor, and with what sense of urgency. You decide what to tell your doctor and whether to follow the advice given, whether to keep up your immunizations, whether to have a prescription filled and comply with the medication instructions, and whether to seek further help or a second opinion. The entire process of maintaining or restoring health depends on your decisions; it cannot start or continue without them.

The small or large decisions of everyday life can be broken down into manageable steps:

- **Set priorities.** What matters most to you? What would you like to accomplish in the next week, month, or year? Look at the decision you're about to make in the context of your values and goals.
- **Inform yourself.** The more you understand, the better you'll be able to make healthy decisions. Gathering information may involve formal research or informal conversations with teachers, counsellors, family members, or friends.
- **Consider all your options.** List as many options you can think of, along with the advantages and disadvantages of each.
- **Tune in to your intuitive feelings.** While it's not infallible, your sixth sense can provide valuable feedback. If something just doesn't feel right, listen to this inside voice. Are there any fears you haven't dealt with? Do you have doubts about taking a certain path?
- **Consider a worst-case scenario.** When you've come close to a final decision, imagine what will happen if everything goes wrong—the workload becomes overwhelming, your partner betrays your trust, your expectations turn out to be unrealistic. If you can live with the worst consequences of a decision, you're probably making the right choice.

The Health Belief Model Decision making also depends on your attitudes and beliefs. A well-known model to explain and predict health behaviours, originally developed in the 1950s and updated in the 1980s, is the **health belief model (HBM)** (see Figure 1-9).[76] This model focuses on **attitudes,*** "a feeling or way of

*By permission. From Merriam-Webster's Collegiate ® Dictionary, 11th Edition © 2016 by Merriam-Webster, Inc. (www.Merriam-Webster.com).

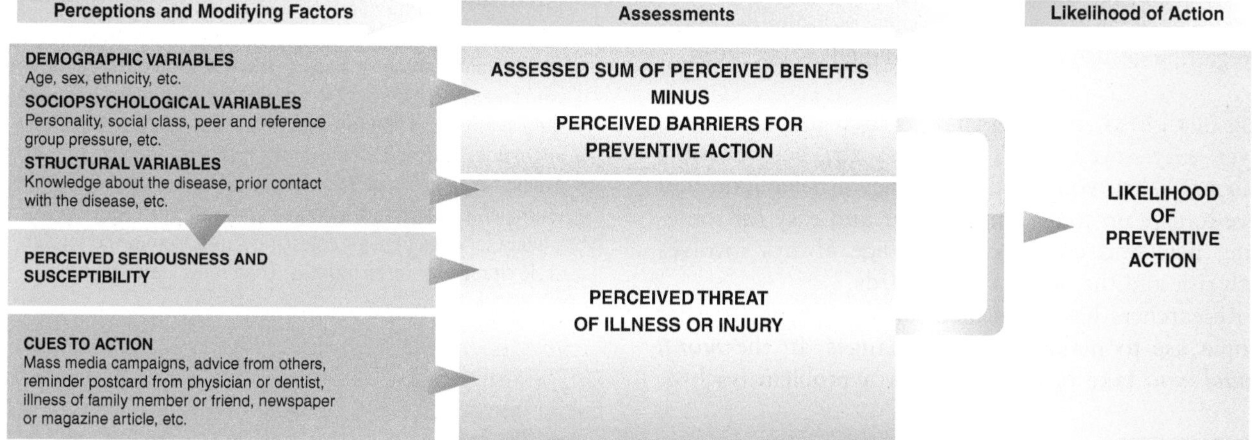

Figure 1-9 Health Belief Model

Source: Adapted from *Health Psychology: Biopsychosocial Interactions*, Edward P. Sarafino. © 1990 John Wiley & Sons. Reproduced with permission of John Wiley & Sons.

thinking that affects a person's behavior,"[77] and **beliefs,*** "a state or habit of mind in which trust or confidence is placed in some person or thing."[78] Your attitudes and beliefs are predisposing influences on your capacity to change. According to this model, people will take a health-related action based on the following factors:

- **Perceived susceptibility.** People will change their health behaviours only if they believe they are at risk; for example, they begin to notice they are coughing a lot after every cigarette they smoke.
- **Perceived severity.** The probability that an individual will change depends on how serious he or she believes the consequence of not changing is; for example, they begin to find it difficult to climb up a set of stairs or play a game of pick-up soccer with friends.
- **Perceived benefits.** People change when they truly believe there is "something in it for them"; for example, a friend quit smoking, is feeling better, has more money for healthy lifestyle choices, and is choosing to be with other non-smoking friends.
- **Cues to action.** People will change when they notice or experience something that helps them move from thinking about changing to actually making the change; for example, (1) a relative is diagnosed with lung cancer and he or she was a long-time smoker; or (2) the information on cigarette packages that now includes health warnings "hits home."
- **Self-efficacy** (added to the model in 1988 and found to be one of the most important factors). A person's belief that he or she has the ability to make and follow through on a lifestyle change process increases the likelihood of a change in behaviour; for example, a person knows he or she is able to explore strategies to quit smoking, is not afraid to ask for help from friends and medical experts, and values himself or herself enough to actually quit smoking.

Over the years the health belief model has been used to help people change unhealthy behaviours, such as smoking, overeating, and inactivity, or to encourage them to take positive health actions, such as using condoms and getting needed vaccinations and medical checkups.

How Can I Begin to Make Lifestyle Changes? Change is never easy—even if it's done for the best possible reasons. When you decide to change a behaviour, you have to give up something familiar and easy for something new and challenging. Change always involves both risk and the prospect of rewards.

Researchers have identified various approaches that people use to make beneficial changes. In the *moral model*, you take responsibility for a problem (such as smoking) and its solution; success depends on adequate motivation, while failure is seen as a sign of character weakness. In the *enlightenment model*, you submit to strict discipline to correct a problem; this is the approach used in Alcoholics Anonymous. The *behavioural model* involves rewarding yourself when you make positive changes. The *medical model* sees the behaviour as caused by forces beyond your control (a genetic predisposition to being overweight, for example) and employs an expert to provide advice or treatment. For many people, the most effective approach is the *compensatory model*, which doesn't assign blame but puts responsibility on individuals to acquire whatever skills or power they need to overcome their problems.

Before they reach the stage where they can and do take action to change, most people go through a common process. First, they reach a level of accumulated unhappiness that makes them ready for change. Then they have a moment of truth that makes them want to change.

*By permission. From Merriam-Webster's Collegiate ® Dictionary, 11th Edition © 2016 by Merriam-Webster, Inc. (www.Merriam-Webster.com).

STRATEGIES FOR PREVENTION

Setting Realistic Goals

Here's a framework for setting goals and objectives, the crucial preliminary step for prevention. The framework is based on the SMART model[79]—your goals and objectives need to be Specific, Measurable, Achievable, Realistic, and Trackable or Time-Based.

- **Specific**—Determine your goal or objective. Define it in words and on paper. An overarching goal may be to "eat healthier." Establish a specific goal: increase vegetable and fruit intake on a daily basis.
- **Measurable**—Determine how you will measure your success. If your goal is to increase your vegetable and fruit consumption, make a commitment to eat the recommended 8 to 10 servings per day set out by *Canada's Food Guide*.
- **Achievable**—Think in terms of evolution, not revolution. If you want to change the way you eat, start by changing your vegetable and fruit consumption two days a week. Work toward eating the recommended servings every day.
- **Realistic**—Identify your resources. Do you have the knowledge, skills, finances, time—whatever it takes? Find out from others who know. Be sure you're ready for the next step. List solutions for any obstacles you foresee. Where can you purchase fresh vegetables and fruits? How much is this going to cost?
- **Trackable (and Time-Based)**—Keep track of your changes. Try journalling. Start a nutrition journal and record your daily or weekly servings of vegetables and fruits. Commit to this lifestyle change for three months. Then reevaluate your goal.

✓ CHECK-IN

What SMART Goals can you make to enhance your health and wellness?

Social and cultural **norms**—behaviours that are expected, accepted, or supported by a group—can make change much harder if they're constantly working against a person's best intentions. You may resolve to eat less, for instance, yet your mother may keep offering you homemade brownies because your family's norm is to show love by making and offering delicious treats. Or you might decide to drink less, yet your friends' norm may be to equate drinking with having a good time.

If you're aware of the norms that influence your behaviour, you can devise strategies either to change them or adapt to them. Another option is to develop relationships with people who share your goals and whose norms can reinforce your behaviour.

Stages of Change There are many theories and models that have been developed to assist people who want to make lifestyle changes. One of the well-recognized models is the trans-theoretical model of change, developed by Prochaska, Norcross, and DiClemente in the 1980s.[80] These researchers discovered that individuals tend to progress through a sequence of stages as they make a change. Certain activities and experiences, called *change processes*, help individuals progress through these stages (see Figure 1-10). As you read each chapter of this textbook, refer to this model of change to determine if you are ready to make a lifestyle change and where you are in terms of your readiness to make that change.

STRATEGIES FOR CHANGE

More Options for Change

- **Modelling—**Observing other people and emulating their behaviours, successes, or positive lifestyle choices. Look around your community and find people you admire, and who represent your beliefs and values. Watch them carefully. Try to model their behaviour and success. Ask them if they would be willing to mentor you.
- **Positive visualization—**Creating a mental picture of a goal or a behaviour change and visualizing yourself making that change. Watch yourself achieve that goal through your own eyes. Make the image a full-length movie and replay it over and over. Research has shown that positive visualization can help you manifest your goal.
- **Shaping—**Building desired behaviour in small steps and rewarding positive behaviour changes over time. Set yourself up for success. Start slowly. Change one thing at a time. Gradually make further changes, but keep the pace of change realistic and achievable. Be willing to adapt if change is not working.

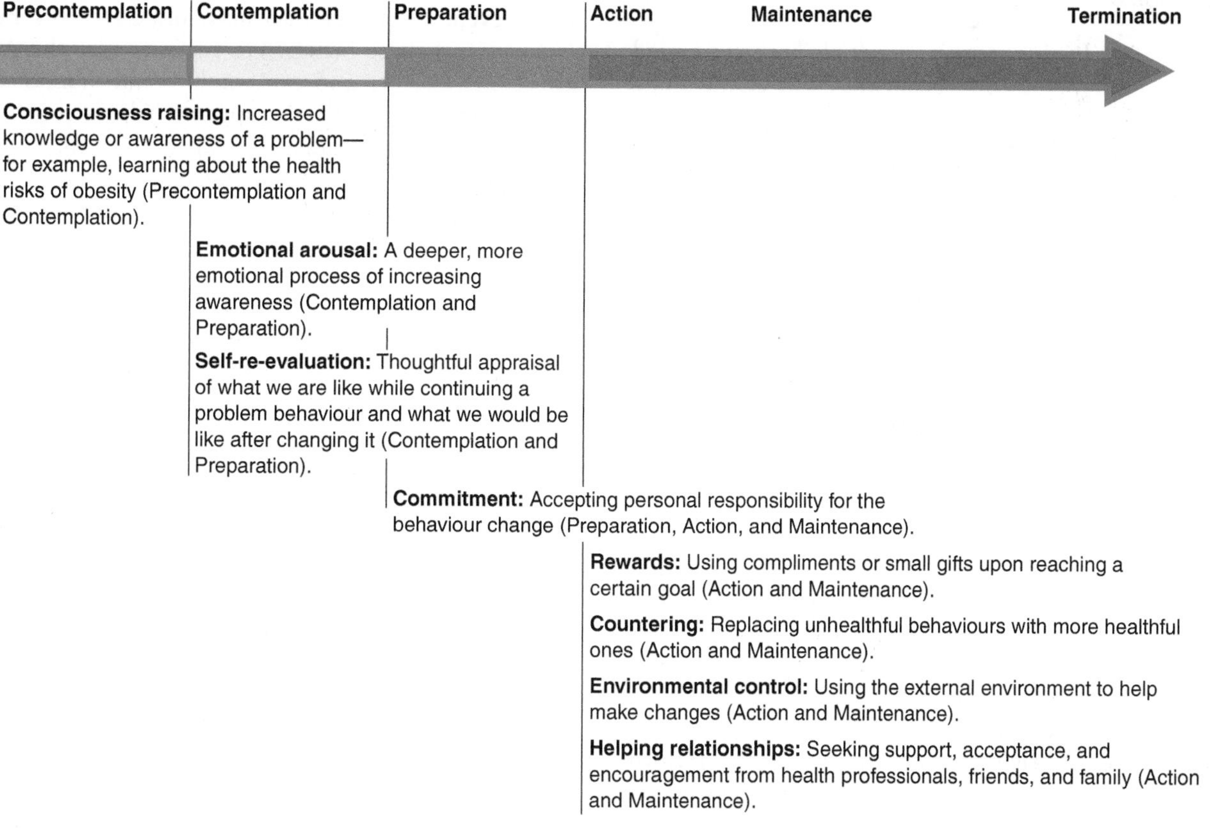

Figure 1-10 The Stages of Change and Some Change Processes

Source: Reprinted from Petrocelli, J.V. (2002). Table 1: Processes and stages of change: Process of change and their descriptions. *Journal of Counseling and Development*, Vol 80, Issue 1, Pg. 24. The American Counseling Association. Reprinted with permission. No further reproduction authorized with out written permission from the American Counseling Association.

Precontemplation Individuals at this stage are often not even aware that they have a problem, whereas others around them might. They have no intention of making a change.

Contemplation Individuals in this stage are aware they have a behavioural problem and begin to consider making a change. Feedback from family members or friends, or increased personal knowledge about the benefits of changing can move someone from precontemplation to contemplation. However, they may be torn between the positives of the new behaviour and the amount of energy, time, and other resources required to change. Some people settle in this stage for years, but Prochaska et al. discovered that a shift to the next stage of preparation usually occurs within the next six months.

Preparation People in this stage intend to change a problem behaviour within the next month. Some focus on a master plan. They might look into fitness classes or gym memberships. They might start by making small changes, such as walking to classes rather than driving their car.

Action People at this stage are modifying their behaviour according to their plan. This stage requires a commitment of time and energy. Changes made during this stage are visible to others. For instance, they might be jogging or working out at the gym three times a week.

Maintenance In this stage, individuals have continued to work at changing their behaviour. The change may take from six months to a lifetime. New exercisers are likely to stop during the first three to six months. Some lapses may be temporary.

Termination While it may take two to five years, a behaviour can become so deeply ingrained that it becomes a new habit and a person can't imagine abandoning it.

✓ CHECK-IN

Do you want to change a health behaviour? If so, what stage of change are you in?

Successful Change Some people find it helpful to sign a contract—a written agreement in which they make a commitment to change—with their partner, parent, or health educator. Spelling out what they intend to do, and why, underscores the seriousness of what they're trying to accomplish.

As described briefly in the section on the Health Belief Model (see page 17), change also depends on self-efficacy, the belief that you can and will succeed. In his research on self-efficacy, psychologist Albert Bandura[81] found that the individuals most likely to reach a goal are those who believe they can. The more strongly they feel that they can and will change their behaviour, the more energy and persistence they put into making the change. Other researchers have linked positive health change with optimism.

Another crucial factor is **locus of control.** If you believe that your actions will make a difference in your health, your locus of control is internal. If you believe that external forces or factors play a greater role, your locus of control is external. Individuals with an external locus of control for health are less likely to seek preventive health care and are less optimistic about early treatment.

Reinforcements, either positive (rewards) or negative (punishments), can also play a role. If you decide to set up a regular exercise program, you might reward yourself with a new tracksuit if you stick to it for three months or you might punish yourself for skipping a day by doing an extra ten minutes of exercises the following day. Small, regular rewards are more effective in keeping you motivated than waiting for one big reward after a long period of time. Take note of immediate rewards too. Do you feel better? Are you more rested? Are you more physically able?

Your **self-talk**—the messages you send yourself—also can play a role. Mental health professionals have recognized the conscious use of positive self-talk as a powerful force for changing the way individuals think, feel, and behave. Ellis's **rational-emotive therapy (RET)**[82] includes an ABC approach. A stands for activating events, B stands for beliefs, and C stands for consequences of these beliefs. He suggests that the ABCs affect one another and can combine into irrational or neurotic thoughts. RET therapy can help us cope when life events do not unfold as we expect them to.

Meichenbaum, a Canadian researcher, has carried out numerous studies on **self-instructional methods** where he discovered that individuals who practise instructional self-talk appear to cope better with stressful situations. Further research determined that therapists can also significantly influence or modify what clients share in a therapy session based on this method.[83]

One other method of self-talk is to practise blocking negative thoughts. "We have a choice about how we think," explains psychologist Martin Seligman, Ph.D., author of *Learned Optimism*. By learning to challenge automatic negative thoughts that enter our brains and asserting our own statements of self-worth, we can transform ourselves into optimists who see what's right rather than pessimists forever focusing on what's wrong. "Optimism is a learned set of skills," Seligman contends. "Once learned, these skills persist because they feel so good to use. And reality is usually on our side."[84]

✓ CHECK-IN

How "internal" or "external" do you rate your locus of control?

HUMAN POTENTIAL

Trisha Kauk, Mary Anne Signer, Kaitlin Lewandoski and Professor Colleen Plumton—Fit For Life and Learning (FFLL)

Our first Human Potential story begins in the fall of 2012 when three students—Trisha Kauk, Mary Anne Signer, and Kaitlin Lewandoski—registered in a course titled PERS 2100: Introduction to Professional Practice, taught by Professor Colleen Plumton, and offered in the Faculty of Kinesiology and Recreation Management (KRM) at the University of Manitoba. Course completion included a group project where students were asked to develop an advocacy campaign to promote physical activity and healthy living in schools or community organizations. As the students brainstormed ideas for their project, they found themselves asking, "If we can't even be healthy, as physical education students, how can we advocate for others to find health and wellness, in this crazy season of life, also known as university?" They decided they wanted to "find a way that they could maintain their own health and help others to do the same."

After identifying factors that led to imbalance in their own lives, they set out to create a mock-course that would empower first-year university students to take ownership of their health and wellness in all dimensions—mind, body, heart, and spirit—when making the transition to university. They presented their advocacy campaign to their class, with the Dean of KRM, Dr. Jane Watkinson, in attendance. She was fully supportive of the idea of a "healthy campus." Trisha, Mary Anne, and Kaitlin recount that they were "intimidated and terrified, but also felt empowered." This was their first major university presentation as undergraduate students. Despite nerves and excitement their presentation was a big success. As it turned out that was not the end of their story.

Though they had successfully completed the course, they decided they wanted to be "real agents of change." In 2014, in consultation with their professor, Colleen, and other faculty members, the students submitted a proposal to the University of Manitoba in connection with the *Teaching and Learning Enhancement Fund;* they were successful in receiving a grant of 11 000 dollars to create a pilot course for Fall 2015 to coincide with the opening of the new Active Living Centre. The students stated that "while the entire [grant application] process was tiring and at times discouraging—we had no idea how many hoops we'd have to jump through and often asked each other, 'Is this actually ever going to happen?'—it was so unbelievably rewarding!" The experience taught them to never give up and keep persevering to achieve their dreams.

They established a development team that consisted of themselves and faculty members. A curricular team provided advice with regard to the incorporation of Indigenous perspectives within the course and identified learning outcomes related to the moving, feeling, thinking, and being "body." A curriculum consultant helped develop experiential learning outcomes and activities that would introduce students to the supports and resources available on campus. A content expert helped to prepare the online and face-to-face seminars that provided the theoretical foundation for the course. The students knew that the course

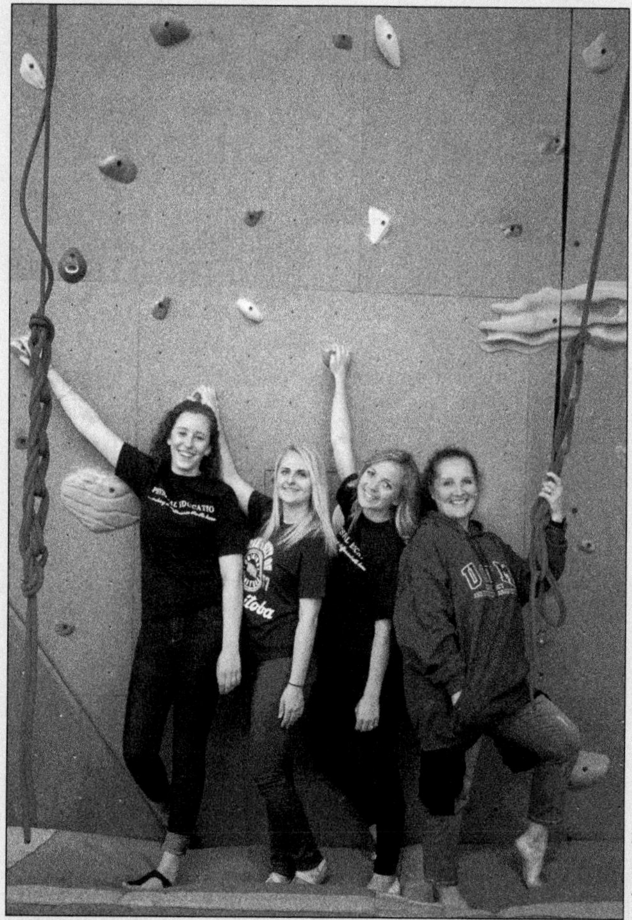

Taylor Gould

Trisha Kauk, Mary Anne Signer, Kaitlin Lewandoski, and Professor Colleen Plumton—University of Manitoba celebrating the Fit for Life and Learning Course (FFLL) they developed for first-year University of Manitoba students.

needed to incorporate a blended learning format to increase student engagement. The result was content that included medicine wheel teachings, which were introduced in the teepee at Migizii Agamik, the Aboriginal House on the campus; general health and wellness information; stress management techniques; personal nutrition; life skills (financial literacy); mental health (U of M Mental Health Strategy); and alcohol and tobacco use. The curriculum also provided an opportunity for students to participate in a variety of physical activities, on a weekly basis, at the Active Living Centre. Options included progressive relaxation, group fitness sampler, yoga, power circuit, rock climbing, skating, and traditional games.

A pilot course was launched in the fall of 2015. The course was offered to a group of wonderful students who were the perfect combination of individuals whose reason for taking the course was to "get healthy" and "increase their daily physical activity levels." The last class was a celebration with a feast and an opportunity for students to reflect on what the course meant to them and how they would move forward with their healthy living plan. The benefits of

(Continued)

offering the Fit for Life and Learning course were the life changes that each of the students made as a result of taking the course. They discovered the many resources and supports on campus that could assist with their healthy living journey.

Reflections from Trisha, Mary Anne, and Kaitlin show that developing and piloting the course meant a lot to them too. "Imagine a course designed by university students! We never truly thought when we launched our idea that it would become a reality. The most amazing part was the deep friendships that we developed. It began with our need for a connection with people who share the same passions and dreams . . . that is, changing the world through movement and wellness in all dimensions. Our amazing professor, Colleen, often reminded us of a quote by Henry Ford: 'Whether you think you can or whether you think you can't—you're right!' We now know we can and did make this happen and will continue to be advocates for healthy living throughout our lives!"

Trisha is completing her After-Degree Bachelor of Education program at the U of M (physical education and biology), Mary Anne accepted a teaching position in rural Manitoba, and Kaitlin is completing a Master of Occupational Therapy at U of M. Professor Colleen Plumton continues to do what she is best at—inspire, motivate, care, and trust in her students through teaching at the U of M.

Health and Wellness Education In the past, health and wellness education focused either on individual or organizational change. Today, many educators are using a framework in which individual behaviour change occurs within the context of the environment of a person's life. Its primary themes—prevention of health problems and protection from health threats—can establish the basis for good health now and in the future.

The Power of Prevention No medical treatment, however successful or sophisticated, can compare with the power of prevention. Preventive efforts have already proved helpful in increasing physical activity, quitting smoking, reducing dietary fat, preventing sexually transmitted diseases and unwanted pregnancy, reducing intolerance and violence, and avoiding alcohol and drug abuse.

Prevention can take many forms. Primary or before-the-fact prevention efforts might seek to reduce stressors and increase support to prevent problems in healthy people. Consumer education provides guidance about how to change our lifestyles to prevent problems and enhance well-being. Other preventive programs identify people at risk and empower them with information and support so they can avoid potential problems. Prevention efforts may target an entire community and try to educate all of its members about the dangers of alcohol abuse or environmental hazards, or they may zero in on a particular group (for instance, seminars on safer sex practices offered to teens) or an individual (one-on-one counselling about substance abuse).

In the past, physicians did not routinely incorporate prevention into their professional practices. But times have changed. Medical schools are providing more training in preventive care. A growing number of studies have demonstrated that prevention saves not only money but also productivity, health, and lives. Many deaths caused by cardiovascular disease, strokes, and cancer could be avoided or delayed by preventive measures. Eliminating smoking and changes in diet could prevent even more.

The Potential of Protection There is a great deal of overlap between prevention and **protection**. Some people might think of immunizations as a way of preventing illness; others see them as a form of protection against dangerous diseases. In many ways, protection picks up where prevention leaves off. You can prevent sexually transmitted infections (STIs) or unwanted pregnancy by abstaining from sex. But if you decide to engage in potentially risky sexual activities, you can protect yourself with condoms and spermicides. Similarly, you can prevent many automobile accidents by not driving when road conditions are hazardous. But if you do have to drive, you can protect yourself by wearing a seat belt and using defensive-driving techniques.

The very concept of protection implies some degree of risk—immediate and direct (for instance, the risk of intentional injury from an assailant or unintentional harm from a fire) or long term and indirect (such as the risk of heart disease and cancer as a result of smoking). To know how best to protect yourself, you have to be able to realistically assess risks.

✓ CHECK-IN

What steps are you taking to protect your health and wellness?

Assessing Risks We all face a host of risks, from the danger of being the victim of violence to the hazards of self-destructive behaviours like drinking and using illegal drugs. At any age, the greatest health threats stem from high-risk behaviours—smoking, excessive drinking, not getting enough exercise, eating too many high-fat foods, and not getting regular medical checkups, to name just a few. That is why changing unhealthy habits is the best way to reduce risks and prevent health problems.

Environmental health risks also need to be assessed. Every year brings calls of alarm about a new hazard to health: electromagnetic radiation, fluoride in drinking water, hair dyes, silicone implants, radon, and lead, for example. Here are some key factors to consider:

- **Are there possible benefits?** Advantages—such as the high salary paid for working with toxic chemicals or radioactive materials—may make some risks seem worth taking.
- **Is the risk voluntary?** All of us tend to accept risks that we freely choose to take, such as playing a sport that could lead to injuries, as opposed to risks imposed on us, such as threats of terrorism.
- **Is the risk fair?** The risk of skin cancer affects us all. We may worry about it and take action to protect ourselves and our planet, but we don't resent it the way we resent living with the risk of violence because the only housing we can afford is in a high-crime area.
- **Are there alternatives?** As consumers, we may become upset about cancer-causing pesticides or food additives when we learn about safer chemicals or methods of preservation.
- **Are lives saved or lost?** Our thinking about risks often depends on how they're presented. For instance, if we're told that a new drug may kill one out of every 100 people, we react differently than if we're told that it may save the lives of 99 percent of those who use it.

THE FUTURE OF HEALTH AND WELLNESS

Medical science is moving ahead at an astonishing speed. Every week seems to bring a new discovery or breakthrough. But with all the advances in medical science, it is still important to make healthy lifestyle choices that support all the dimensions of health and wellness. You have that choice.

SELF-SURVEY

Planning Your Journey to Wellness—A Road Map

Ultimately you have more control over your health than anyone else. Use this course as an opportunity to commit to at least one healthful behaviour and improve on it. Earlier in this chapter, you explored a First Nations Perspective on Health and Wellness (see Figure 1-1.) The First Nations Health Authority has also created the self-assessment below, which is an excellent resource for everyone. Answer the questions to gain insight that will help you navigate your personal journey to wellness.

Commitment

What is your present level of commitment to addressing any changes needed that relate to your lifestyle? Rate from 0 to 10, 10 being fully committed:

0 1 2 3 4 5 6 7 8 9 10

Strength

What behaviours or lifestyle habits do you currently engage in regularly that you believe support your health?

____

____

What behaviours or lifestyle habits do you currently engage in regularly that you believe are self-destructive?

____

____

Support

Who do you know that will sincerely and consistently support you with the beneficial lifestyle changes that you will be making?

____

____

Manage

What is your present level of stress (psychological, physical, workplace)?

Rate from 0 to 10, 10 being totally stressed out.

0 1 2 3 4 5 6 7 8 9 10

What do you love to do?

____

Wellness Self-Assessment

How often have you been physically active this week (30-minute intervals of moderate [walking] to intense activity)?

0 1 2 3 4 5 6 7

How many 237 ml (8 oz – 1 cup) glasses of water did you drink yesterday?

0 1–3 4–7 8–10

How many servings of fruits/vegetables did you have yesterday 125 ml. (½ cup)?

0 1–3 4–7 8–10

How many servings of traditional foods have you had this past week? (Consider foods from your own cultural background.)

0   1–3   4–7   8–10

Do you need to quit smoking?

☐ Yes   ☐ No

Wellness is a balance of many factors. Using the circle below, shade your level of satisfaction in each area of your life. Use the considerations below to determine your satisfaction in your physical, spiritual, emotional, and mental health and wellness. For example, if you are 60% satisfied in your career, shade the first six levels of the career slice. Do the same for each area, starting from the centre point radiating outward.

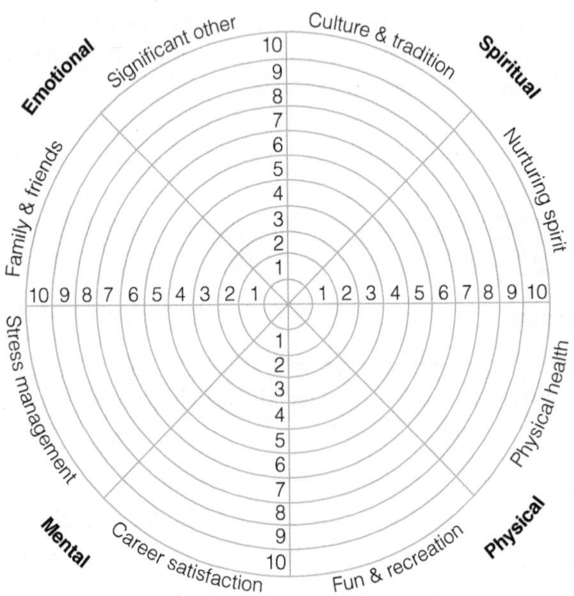

Use the guiding questions below to fill in your wellness wheel. While examples are provided, this is your journey; feel free to interpret each quadrant as you see fit.

A Perfect Balance?

HOW BALANCED IS YOUR WELLNESS WHEEL? What does your wheel reveal about how you spend your time? Do you find that you are focused only on your strengths? What aspects do you need to focus on to achieve balance?

Goal Setting

What goals would you like to achieve this year in terms of your personal health and wellness? A great way to set goals is to begin by writing them down. It's also a good idea to share your goals with trusted family and friends who will support you on your wellness journey. Listed below are a few questions that may assist you in thinking about some goals you may consider working towards this year.

Ask Yourself...

What do you want more of in your life?

____

If you had ____________ how would that make you feel?

What physical activity, healthy eating, mental wellness, and spiritual wellness activities will help you get more of what you want?

____

My Goals:

1.
2.
3.

Set Smarter Goals that are

SPECIFIC I will walk every day.

MEASURABLE I will walk 10,000 steps a day.

ACHIEVABLE/ATTAINABLE I will walk in the rain, snow or hail.

REALISTIC I will walk to and from work each day.

TRACKABLE/TIMEFRAME I will walk to and from work for the next month and will re-evaluate this goal after the month.

Physical	Spiritual	Emotional	Mental
PHYSICAL HEALTH Do you have any health conditions that currently are affecting you? If you have no health concerns you would shade in 100% of the slice.	CULTURE/TRADITION Are you satisfied with the amount of participation you engage in your culture or your traditions?	SIGNIFICANT OTHER Are you satisfied with the intimate relationship you are in?	CAREER How satisfied are you in your job/career? Are you achieving an ideal work/life balance?
FUN/RECREATION Are you satisfied with the amount of time you have for your hobbies and sports?	NURTURING YOUR SPIRIT Are you taking care of your spirit? (ceremonies, religion, meditating, creative expressions, etc).	FAMILY & FRIENDS Are you satisfied with the relationships you have in your life?	STRESS MANAGEMENT Are you managing your stress? (yoga, deep breathing, physical activity, being on the land, etc.)

EVERYBODY CARES I will share my goals and desired changes with trusted family and friends.

RESOURCES I will make a list of the things I need to add or take away from my routine in order to help me achieve my goals.

Healthy Habits

Whenever you set a goal to remove an unhealthy habit, you need to add a healthy habit (e.g., if you are going to stop drinking pop, replace the habit with drinking herbal teas such as peppermint tea).

FNHA Wellness Assessment

Nurturing Spirit

These are the aspects of your life that give you a sense of purpose, make you feel connected, and make you smile.

How balanced do you feel in the mental, emotional, spiritual, and physical aspects of your life?

- ☐ Very balanced .... Low health risk
- ☐ Sometimes .... Reduced health risk
- ☐ Not balanced at all .... Elevated health risk

Do you feel connected to family and/or friends?

- ☐ Very much .... Low health risk
- ☐ Sometimes .... Reduced health risk
- ☐ No .... Elevated health risk

Do you ever feel sad or unhappy?

- ☐ Rarely .... Low health risk
- ☐ Sometimes .... Reduced health risk
- ☐ Often .... Elevated health risk

Being Active

These are the aspects of your life that get your body moving for fun, fitness, or holistic health.

I do 150 minutes of moderate to vigorous aerobic physical activity every week.

- ☐ Yes, most of the time .... Low health risk
- ☐ Some of the time ....Reduced health risk
- ☐ Not often .... Elevated health risk

I do muscle and bone strengthening activities at least 2 days per week.

- ☐ Yes, most of the time .... Low health risk
- ☐ Some of the time .... Reduced health risk
- ☐ Not often .... Elevated health risk

I limit my recreational screen time to no more than 2 hours per day.

- ☐ Yes, most of the time .... Low health risk
- ☐ Some of the time .... Reduced health risk
- ☐ Not often .... Elevated health risk

I limit my sedentary (motorized) transportation and sitting for long periods of time.

- ☐ Yes, most of the time .... Low health risk
- ☐ Some of the time .... Reduced health risk
- ☐ Not often .... Elevated health risk

Maintaining A Healthy Body Weight

Has your weight changed unintentionally in the past 6 months?

- ☐ Yes, I have gained more than 2.2 kg (5 pounds) .... Elevated health risk
- ☐ No, my weight has stayed within a few kilograms (pounds) .... Reduced health risk
- ☐ Yes, I have lost more than 2.2 kg (5 pounds) .... Elevated health risk
- ☐ I don't know .... Risk unknown

Have you tried to change your weight?

____

____

Do you ever feel that your weight is affecting your overall wellness?

____

____

Eating Healthy

These are the aspects of your life that impact the food available to nourish your body and soul.

How many vegetable and fruit servings do you eat in a day? (A serving is about 125 mL (½ cup) or one small vegetable or fruit, the size of a tennis ball.)

- ☐ 7 or more servings per day .... Low health risk
- ☐ 4–6 servings per day .... Reduced health risk
- ☐ 3 or less servings per day .... Elevated health risk

I often worry that food will run out before month end.

- ☐ No.. Reduced health risk
- ☐ Yes .... Elevated health risk

How often do you eat traditional foods? (Consider foods from your own cultural background.)

- ☐ Almost daily .... Low health risk
- ☐ 2–3 times per week .... Reduced health risk
- ☐ Not often .... Elevated health risk

What are some aspects of your eating pattern that are benefiting your wellness?

____

____

What are some aspects of your eating pattern that you would like to change?

____

____

Optimizing Health

These are other aspects of your life that can impact your holistic health and wellness.

Blood Pressure (mmHg)

- ☐ Less than 130/85 .... At target
- ☐ 130/86–139/89 .... Slightly elevated
- ☐ 140/90–159/99 .... Elevated
- ☐ 160/100 or higher .... Too high—see Dr.

Blood Glucose (mmol/L): Fasting

- ☐ Less than 6.1 .... At target
- ☐ 6.1–6.9 .... Elevated—see Dr.
- ☐ Greater than 7.0 .... Too high—see Dr.

Blood Glucose: Random

- ☐ Less than 7.8 .... At target
- ☐ 7.8–11.0 .... Elevated—see Dr.
- ☐ Greater than 11.0 .... Too high—see Dr.

Hemoglobin A1c (%)

If you have not previously been diagnosed with diabetes:

- ☐ Less than 6.0 .... At target
- ☐ 6.0–6.4 .... Elevated—see Dr.
- ☐ Greater than 6.5 .... Too high—see Dr.

If you have previously been diagnosed with diabetes:

- ☐ Less than 7.0* .... At target
- ☐ Greater than 6.5 .... Elevated—see Dr.

* 7.1–8.5 for some people—discuss your target with your doctor

Total Cholesterol/HDL-C Ratio

- ☐ Less than 4.0 .... At target
- ☐ 4.0–4.9 .... Slightly elevated
- ☐ 5.0–5.9 .... Elevated
- ☐ Greater than 6.0 .... Too high—see Dr.

Medical Health

Do you have a family doctor?

____

____

If yes, do you have regular visits with your family doctor for routine medical care?

____

____

If no, when was the last time you saw a doctor?

____

____

____

Dental Health

Do you have access to dental care in your community or in a nearby centre?

____

____

Do you receive regular dental care?

____

____

Respecting Tobacco

When tobacco is used in a traditional way, it benefits the spirit and strengthens the ties to one's culture. Tobacco used in a non-traditional manner, like smoking cigarettes or chewing tobacco/snuff, can increase your risk of premature death and illness such as lung diseases, heart disease, certain types of cancer, and pregnancy risks. These questions refer to tobacco that is used in a non-traditional manner.

- ☐ I have never smoked .... Low health risk
- ☐ I quit smoking more than 2 years ago .... Reduced health risk
- ☐ I quit smoking less than 2 years ago .... Elevated health risk
- ☐ I don't smoke, but I am exposed to second-hand smoke .... Elevated health risk
- ☐ I smoke a pipe, cigar, and/or chew tobacco .... High health risk
- ☐ I smoke 10 cigarettes or less per day .... High health risk
- ☐ I smoke 11–19 cigarettes per day .... High health risk
- ☐ I smoke more than 20 cigarettes per day .... Very high health risk

If you use tobacco in a non-traditional manner and are a current smoker, or use pipes, cigars, or chewing tobacco, answer the following questions:

Have you attempted to quit previously? If yes, how many quit attempts have you made?

____

____

Are you interested in quitting?

____

____

What resources or supports do you believe would help enable you to quit?

____

____

Chapter Summary

1. How can health promotion be defined?
   a. mutual aid, self-care, and healthy environments
   b. a way of thinking about the social and economic forces that shape health
   c. the process of enabling people to increase control over and to improve their health
   d. the absence of disease and infirmity
2. What is the definition of wellness?
   a. purposeful, enjoyable living, characterized by personal responsibility and enhancement of physical, mental, and spiritual health
   b. a state of complete physical, mental, and social well-being
   c. attitudes and beliefs that contribute to a healthy state of mind
   d. the absence of physical or mental illness
3. What is epidemiology?
   a. the study of the six dimensions of wellness and how they can be used to lower rates of mortality
   b. a combination of life choices, chances, and circumstances
   c. the study of health and wellness
   d. the study of how often diseases occur in different groups of people and why they occur
4. Which statement about sex and gender differences is true?
   a. A man's core body temperature runs higher than a woman's.
   b. A man's heart beats at a higher rate than a woman's.
   c. Men are more likely to be physically active.
   d. More men than women are overweight.
5. Which of the following are social determinants of health?
   a. income and income distribution, unemployment and job security, housing and education
   b. medical treatment, new health products, and drug therapy
   c. depression, sleep problems, and family concerns
   d. environmental stressors, short- and long-term stressors, and social stressors
6. Which of the following is NOT required for support for people who want to adopt healthy lifestyle choices?
   a. municipal government commitment for healthy communities
   b. provincial government commitment for healthy policies and programs
   c. federal government commitment for national health programs and services
   d. encouragement from friends to ignore inherent risks linked to unhealthy lifestyle choices
7. Which of the following factors do NOT shape positive behaviours?
   a. reinforcing factors, which involve external recognition for achieving a goal
   b. lifestyle choices that include misuse and abuse of substances
   c. predisposing factors, which include knowledge, attitudes, and beliefs
   d. enabling factors, which are related to an individual's skills and capabilities to make behaviour changes
8. If you want to change unhealthy behaviour, which strategy is least likely to promote success?
   a. believing that you can make the change
   b. rewarding yourself regularly
   c. during self-talks, reminding yourself about all your faults
   d. accepting that you are in control of your health
9. According to the Stages of Change in the trans-theoretical model of change, which statement is NOT correct?
   a. In the maintenance stage, individuals have avoided relapse for six months.
   b. In the contemplation stage, individuals are considering changing a problem behaviour in the next six months.
   c. In the action stage, individuals are actually modifying their behaviour according to their plan.
   d. In the preparation stage, individuals intend to change a problem behaviour in the next six months.
10. Which statement is NOT correct?
    a. Prevention involves specific actions taken after participating in risky behaviour.
    b. You can prevent health problems by educating yourself about them and then avoiding the risky behaviours that can lead to these problems.
    c. An example of a preventive measure is to avoid driving in icy, snowy conditions, and an example of a protective measure is to put chains on your tires.
    d. In assessing risks, ask the following two questions: Is the risk voluntary? Are there alternatives?

Answers to these questions can be found on page 29.

SELF-RESPONSIBILITY—SOCIAL RESPONSIBILITY

SELF-RESPONSIBILITY

It seems ludicrous to prepare a student for a lifetime career in their area of interest and not prepare them for the responsibilities of maintaining their life.[85]

Dr. Bill Hettler

Education can be an important step toward making healthy lifestyle changes. As you read through this textbook and debate health and wellness concepts with your classmates, friends, families, and professors, think about ways you might take responsibility for lifestyle changes that will enhance your health, well-being, and personal potential. Begin by asking yourself what Stage of Change you are in.

SOCIAL RESPONSIBILITY

It's our responsibility to pass on what we inherited, not to squander it, but to build on it.

Christine Gregoire

Taking care of ourselves allows us to be better able to take care of others. What can you do to make your campus healthy and well?

CRITICAL THINKING

1. What is the definition of health according to the text? Does your personal definition differ from this? Does it differ from your definition of wellness? If so, in what ways? How would you have defined the terms "health" and "wellness" before reading this chapter?
2. Talk to classmates from different racial or ethnic backgrounds than yours about their culture's health attitudes. Ask them what is considered healthy behaviour in their culture. For example, is having a good appetite a sign of health?
3. Where are you on the wellness–illness continuum? What variables might affect your place on the scale? What do you consider your optimum state of health to be?
4. Think about a behavioural change you have made in your life in the past two years. How did your "change process" link to the six stages of the trans-theoretical model of change? In what ways would you like to change your present lifestyle? Where are you now on the Stages of Change continuum?

WEB LINKS

Canadian Institute for Health Information
www.cihi.ca
Access information about national health indicators and standards, health spending, current health research, and the Canadian Population Health Initiative (CPHI).

Canadian Institutes for Health Research
www.cihr-irsc.gc.ca/
Learn about Canada's lead federal funding agency and funding opportunities for health research in four areas: biomedical, clinical, health systems and services, and population and public health.

Health Canada
www.hc-sc.gc.ca
A federal government website where health information can be found. Check out *The Daily*, a special page that keeps Canadians on top of current health issues.

Public Health Agency of Canada
www.publichealth.gc.ca
Find credible and practical e-health information gathered from federal, provincial, and municipal agencies; university libraries; and community groups.

First Nations and Inuit Health, Health Canada
www.hc-sc.gc.ca/fniah-spnia/index-eng.php
Discover public health and health-promotion services for First Nations and Inuit people in Canada.

First Nations Health Authority
www.fnha.ca/what-we-do/health-and-wellness-planning
The first and only provincial First Nations Healthy Authority in Canada. Check these Web pages for tips, guides, and resources for health and wellness planning.

University of Toronto–Scarborough, Health and Wellness Centre
www.utsc.utoronto.ca/hwc/wellness-campus
This website provides an example of health and wellness programs and initiatives being offered at the University of Toronto–Scarborough. Support for students includes a Wellness Peer Program and a Mental Health Network. Check out health and wellness programs and services at your college or university.

Please note that links are subject to change. If you find a broken link, use a search engine such as www.google.ca and search for the website by typing in keywords.

Key Terms

The terms listed here are used within the chapter on the page indicated. Definitions of terms are in the Glossary at the end of the book.

action 20
attitude 17
belief 18
contemplation 20
enabling factors 16
epidemiology 7
globalization 13
health 5
health belief model (HBM) 17
health promotion 5
healthy environments 5
holism 4
hygiene 4
locus of control 20
maintenance 20
modelling 19
morbidity 5
mortality 5
mutual aid 5
norms 19
panacea 4
population health 6
positive visualization 19
precontemplation 20
predisposing factors 16
preparation 20
prevention 22
protection 22
rational-emotive therapy (RET) 20
reinforcements 20
reinforcing factors 17
self-care 5
self-instructional methods 20
self-talk 20
shaping 19
social determinants of health (SDOH) 12
termination 20
wellness 8

Answers to Chapter Summary Questions

1. c; 2. a; 3. d; 4. c; 5. a; 6. d; 7. b; 8. c; 9. d; 10. a

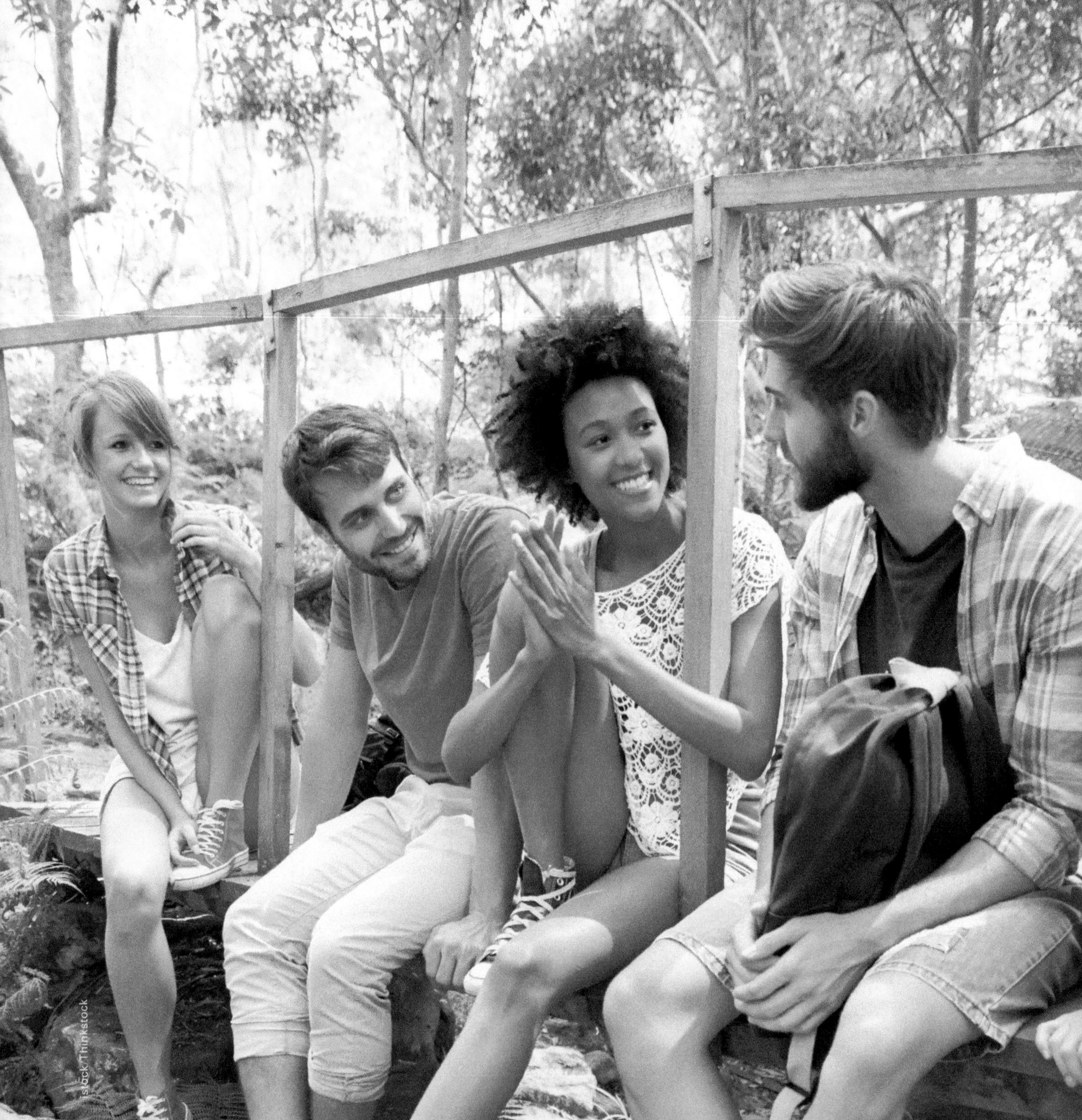

AFTER READING THIS CHAPTER, YOU WILL BE ABLE TO:

- **identify** the four dimensions of psychosocial health—emotional, mental, social, and spiritual
- **discuss** the concepts of emotional and spiritual intelligence
- **describe** the relationship of needs, values, self-esteem, and a sense of control to psychosocial health
- **determine** ways in which you can live a fulfilling life
- **explain** the differences between mental health and mental illness, and **list** some effects of mental illness on psychological and physical health
- **describe** the major mental illnesses—anxiety disorders, depressive disorders, attention disorders, and schizophrenia—and the characteristic symptoms of each type
- **discuss** some of the factors that may lead to suicide as well as strategies for prevention
- **describe** the treatment options available for those with psychological problems

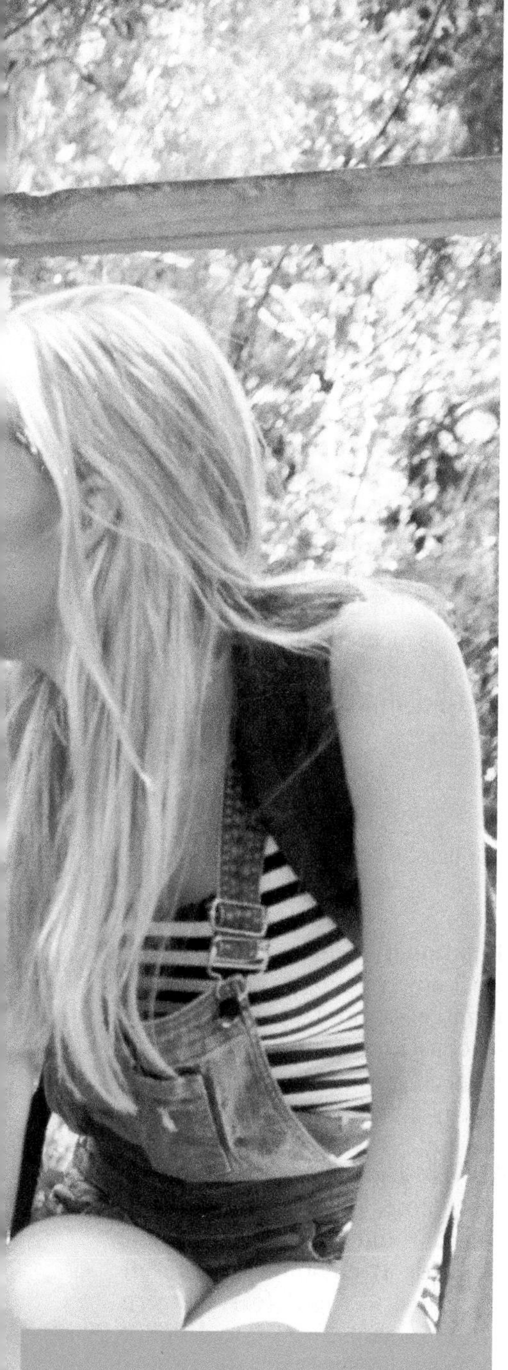

2

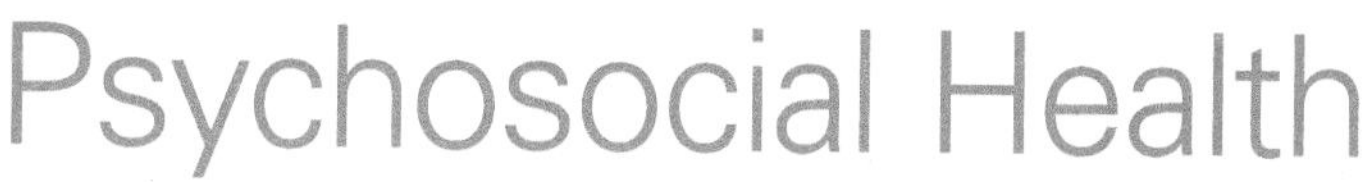

Psychosocial Health

Enjoying a high level of psychosocial health can make the difference between facing life's challenges with optimism and confidence or feeling overwhelmed by expectations and responsibilities. There have been numerous studies that suggest this is true for many college and university students.[1,2] Living away from home for the first time, taking on greater responsibilities with regard to both academic and personal lives, and dealing with emerging adulthood can be both exciting and challenging. Returning to college or university as an older adult student can be difficult and daunting. Attempting to balance work, family commitments, parenting, elder care, and education can stretch one's ability to stay psychosocially well.

Young adulthood is also a time when many serious mental health issues such as anxiety disorders, bipolar disorders, major depression, personality disorders, and schizophrenia often develop. The sad fact is that many people do not realize they can feel better. Only one of every five men and women who could use treatment ever seeks help. Yet 80–90 percent of those treated for psychological problems recover, most within a few months.[3]

By learning about psychosocial health and psychological disorders, you may be able to enhance your overall well-being while recognizing early warning signals so you can deal with potential difficulties or seek professional help for more serious problems.

FREQUENTLY ASKED QUESTIONS

WHAT IS PSYCHOSOCIAL HEALTH?

"A sound mind in a sound body is a short but full description of a happy state in this world," the philosopher John Locke wrote in 1693. More than 300 years later, his statement still rings true. However, modern theorists suggest that while healthy minds and bodies are essential for total wellness, our **psychosocial health** is actually a complex interaction of processes or factors that are both psychological and social in nature and encompass our emotional, mental, social, and spiritual states.[4] While they can and will be described separately in this chapter, all of the dimensions are inextricably linked.

There are many ways to engage in lifestyle choices that support your psychosocial health. The three tools listed below have been suggested by experts from *Live Your Life Well*.[5]

- *Connect with others*. Being concerned about other people, building meaningful relationships, and being comfortable giving and receiving care and attention are benchmarks of psychosocial health. Brown-Fraser et al., in a study on the development of a community organic vegetable garden, found that university student volunteers not only learned about fruit and vegetable production and consumption, but also that interactions between the students and community members were "positive, productive and engaging."[6]
- *Stay positive*. People who experience a range of human emotions such as joy and fear, love and jealousy, and happiness and anger—yet cope with these feelings in a healthy way—are psychosocially well people who take life's opportunities, challenges, and disappointments in stride. Researchers who studied first-year university students in Queensland, Australia, found that when students reported high levels of optimism they experienced less stress than those who reported lower levels of optimism. They also found that when students believed they had the ability to achieve at university they were better able to adjust and accept the demands of academic life.[7]
- *Deal better with hard times*. The transition from adolescence to adulthood is a major step for many people. Everyone faces challenges at various times in life. Being able to practise self-care, accept responsibility for one's actions, manage time and money appropriately, and plan for the future by making and following through on short- and long-term goals are all aspects of adult life. Current research shows that students with "grit"—a blend of perseverance and passion—realize greater success at university. Students that demonstrate a gritty character also seem to be better at finding direction in their lives.[8]

Of course it is important to remember that psychosocial health will ebb and flow. At times, you will feel comfortable with yourself, enjoy connecting with others, and accept the responsibilities of "growing up." At other times you might not. If you sense an imbalance, take a step back; evaluate where you are at and where you would like to go. Then make a commitment to rebalance.

Mental Health **Mental health** is the "thinking" part of psychosocial health. It describes our ability to perceive reality as it is, to respond to its challenges, and to develop rational strategies for living.[9] Good mental health helps us carry out adult responsibilities, adapt to change, and cope with adversity.[10]

A mentally healthy person doesn't try to avoid conflicts and distress, but copes with life's transitions, traumas, and losses in a way that allows for emotional stability and growth. Staying mentally healthy can prevent the start or relapse of a mental illness or help us deal with mental health issues that are sometimes associated with a physical illness.

✓ CHECK-IN

How do you support your mental health?

Emotional Health **Emotional health** refers to the ability to express and acknowledge one's feelings and moods and exhibit adaptability and compassion for others.[11] Emotions are a conscious mental reaction usually directed toward a specific object or person. They are often accompanied by physiological and behavioural changes in our bodies. Richard Lazarus, an influential psychologist, was a pioneer in the study of emotion and stress. He promoted the importance of the connection between emotion and thought. He identified four types of emotions: 1) emotions that result from loss, harm, or threats (e.g., fear, anger); 2) emotions resulting from benefits (e.g., joy, delight); 3) borderline emotions (e.g., hope, compassion); and 4) complex emotions (e.g., love, grief).[12]

Characteristics of an emotionally healthy person include the following:

- an understanding that the self is not the centre of the universe
- the ability to respond in a suitable way to situations or events that are either distressing or amazing
- a sense of control over the mind and body that leads to health-enhancing choices and decisions
- a high level of optimism
- a passion for work and play[13]

✓ CHECK-IN

How do you support your emotional health?

Emotional Intelligence Emotionally healthy people also tend to have higher levels of **emotional intelligence**—the ability to recognize and manage our own emotions and recognize, understand, and influence the emotions of others.[14] Robert Blank, a registered psychologist, educator, and facilitator who has many years of experience working with students dealing with depression, anxiety, attention deficit disorder (ADD), attention deficit/hyperactivity disorder (ADHD), and general stress issues, suggests that it is important to balance our intellect with our emotions. In an academic environment, cognitive development is highly valued and can be one of our greatest strengths. However, being aware and mindful of the present, or "staying in the now," allows us to come back to the moment, to check in with ourselves and discover what we need to do to support our health and well-being. Blank speaks with passion about education being a process of transformation and a development of our emotional selves.[15] High levels of emotional intelligence may make an even greater difference in a person's personal and professional success.

Psychologist Daniel Goleman identified five components of emotional intelligence (sometimes called *emotional quotient* or EQ): self-awareness; altruism; personal motivation; empathy; and the ability to love and be loved by friends, partners, and family members. People who possess high emotional intelligence are people who truly succeed in work as well as play, and build flourishing careers and lasting, meaningful relationships.[16]

Emotional intelligence isn't fixed at birth. The emotional competencies that benefit students are focusing on clear, manageable goals, and identifying and understanding emotions.[17]

Social Health **Social health** refers to the ability to interact effectively with other people and with the social environment.[18] Social health enhances our capability to function as a contributing member of society while supporting and helping others to do the same. A key foundation for social health in a society is making sure that there is equal access to assistance, goods, services, and programs that help individuals add to the quality of their lives and their communities. Characteristics of social health include

- an optimistic sense of trust in others;
- supportive, constructive, and positive interactions with friends, family, and others;
- the ability to form relationships;
- celebrating our diverse society by accepting differences; and
- being open to new experiences with others.

Two important elements of social health are having social support and social bonds.

Social support refers to the care and security that family, friends, colleagues, and professionals provide us. Cooke et al.,[19] in a study examining the definition of social support, suggests that there are five important types: *emotional* (reassurance), *esteem* (value and respect), *network* (sense of belonging in a group), *appraisal* (positive feedback), and *altruistic* support (perception that doing something for others is worthwhile). Social support can also include *tangible* support such as providing life's basic needs, for example, finances, goods, and housing. Studies have shown that social support is a critical component in maintaining health and well-being. Jackson et al.[20] found that social support on a campus setting increased health self-efficacy and facilitated the adoption and maintenance of health-promoting lifestyles among college students. Brown et al.[21] also discovered that providing social support can be even more beneficial to oneself than others with regard to supporting longevity.

Social bonds can be defined as the degree to which people are integrated into and attached to their families, communities, and society.[22] Hirschi is credited with the development of the Social Bond theory in 1969.[23] He introduced four social bonds that he believed helped to reduce the risk of the adoption of unhealthy lifestyle choices. They are *attachment*, *involvement*, *investment*, and *belief*. Social bonds are significant as socializing agents. They encourage us to follow social norms, act in a respectful way, and make healthy lifestyle choices. Hirschi would go on to shift the focus of his social bond theory to that of social control.[24]

✓ CHECK-IN

Can you describe your social support and social bond network?

Spiritual Health **Spiritual health** involves our ability to identify our basic purpose in life and to experience the fulfillment of achieving our full potential.[25] A spiritually healthy person does not have to follow a specific religious doctrine, but may. In Canada, First Nations spirituality is becoming respected and embraced as a living faith tradition and a way of healing. Holst[26] suggests that the primary reason for this may be that many of us find something lacking in our inherited church communities or in our daily lives. Betty Bastien,[27] a Siksikaitsitapi, Sikapinaki (Black Eyes Woman) from the Blackfoot peoples in southern Alberta, says that Ihtsipaitapiiyo'pa—the sacred power, spirit, or Source of Life whose manifestation is the sun—helps her identify the meaning and purpose of her life. Chief Larry Oakes of the Nekaneet First Nation in Saskatchewan focuses on traditional ceremonies, medicines, and healing practices to help people get back in touch with their **culture**—a sense of who we are, where we come from, and what we believe in.[28] The elders also talk about the spiritual connection to animals and the environment.[29]

Spiritual health includes

- a belief in what some call a higher power, in someone or something that transcends the boundaries of self;
- a strong sense of values, morals, and ethics;
- recognizing individuality and self-worth;
- a deep understanding of the interconnectedness of humans with each other and with nature; and
- sharing the virtues of hope, faith, and forgiveness.[30]

Spiritual Intelligence Mental health and medical professionals, counsellors, and spiritual healers have long recognized the power of **spiritual intelligence**. Some would define this term as the capacity to "enhance individual's [our] capabilities and qualities such as compassion, creativity, and wisdom by improving the self awareness and feelings of connection with divine energy."[31] However you define the term, spiritual intelligence does centre on the discovery of an inner wisdom.

There is research that suggests all of us are born with the potential to develop spiritual intelligence.[32] Yet many of us are not even aware of this ability or do little to nurture it. Part of the reason may be that we confuse spiritual intelligence with religion, dogma, or old-fashioned morality. We don't have to believe in God or go to church to be spiritually intelligent. Spiritual intelligence allows us to use the wisdom we have when we are in a state of inner peace. Changing the way you think—by listening less to what's in your head and more to what is in your heart—is one way to develop spiritual intelligence.

A much more in-depth discussion of spiritual health and well-being is presented in Chapter 17, The Spirit of Health and Wellness.

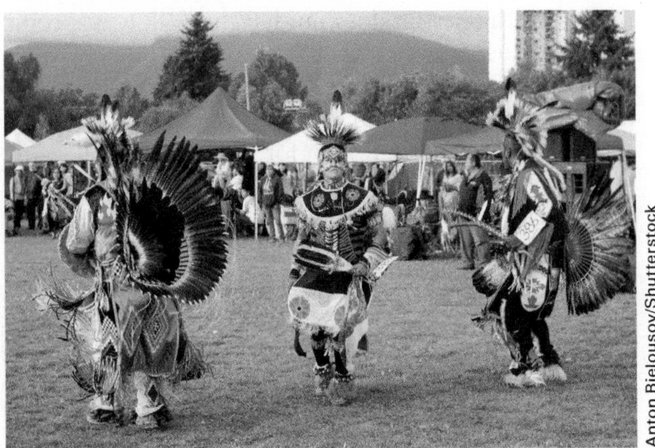

Anton Bielousov/Shutterstock

First Nations powwows celebrate spirituality.

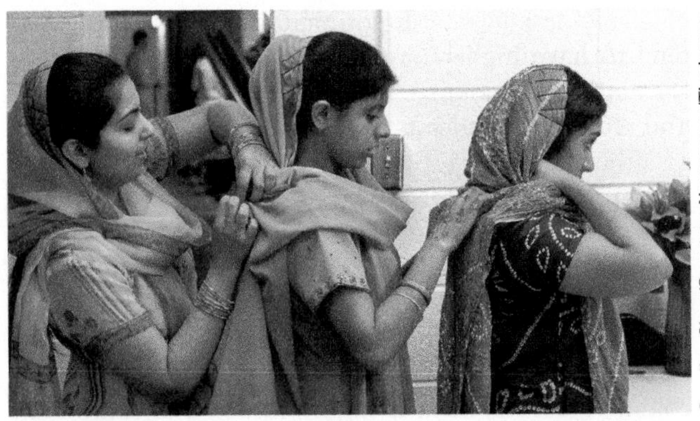

Caroline Chen/Syracuse Newspaper/The Image Works

Campus clubs and organizations provide an opportunity for individuals from different ethnic backgrounds to celebrate their culture and educate others about it.

✓ CHECK-IN

What does spiritual health mean to you?

HOW CAN I LEAD A FULFILLING LIFE?

What's life all about? Most of us ask this question sooner or later. Whether dreams come true or fade away, whether we achieve our goals or not, we find ourselves confronting profound questions about our purpose in life. This next section will present information about how to identify your needs as you take the next steps toward enhancing your psychosocial health as it relates to leading a fulfilling life.

Identify Your Needs We all have psychological and physiological needs. They range from basic common survival needs important for all human beings to social, intellectual, and cultural needs for specific individuals or populations. They differ from "wants," which often include our desires or wishes. Identifying your needs is an important step you can make toward living a fulfilling life. Two psychological models that address the concept of need as it links to personality and psychosocial health are introduced here.

Maslow's Hierarchy of Needs One of the most influential psychologists of modern times, Abraham Maslow believed that human needs are the motivating factors in personality development. His model, Maslow's Hierarchy of Needs[33] (see Figure 2-1), is based on his research of exemplary people. He emphasized positive human behaviour. He was interested in people's possibility for fulfillment of their potential. The human needs are arranged with the most basic human needs at the bottom of the pyramid and the secondary and higher needs placed in ascending order on the hierarchy. Maslow put forward the idea that to become

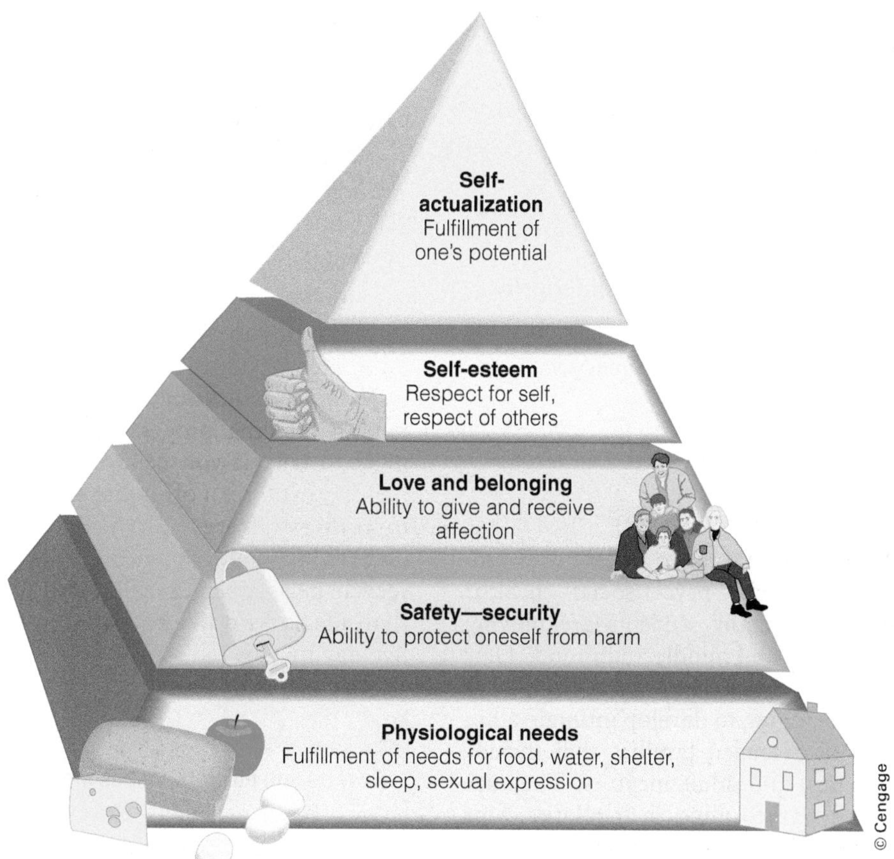

Figure 2-1 Maslow's Hierarchy of Needs

To attain the highest level of psychological health—self-actualization—you must first satisfy physiological, safety and security, love and belonging, and self-esteem needs.

self-actualized, we must first satisfy basic *physiological needs*. These include food, water, air, shelter, sleep, and sexual expression. If these requirements are not met the body cannot function.

Next come the *safety and security needs*. These needs include the ability to protect ourselves from the elements and harm, a focus on personal security and stability, and a freedom from fear. With our safety and security needs met, we then begin to fulfill our *love and belonging needs*. Examples include a connection to family members, building friendships, affection for others, and romantic and intimate relationships. If these needs are not met, loneliness and social anxiety can result. *Self-esteem needs*, which include respect for ourselves and respect for others, fulfill human desires to be valued by others. When these needs are not met the consequence can be a sense of helplessness. *Self-actualization* is the highest level. According to Maslow, few individuals reach this state, in which one derives the greatest possible satisfaction from life. **Self-actualization**,[34] also defined as living to realize one's full potential and function at the highest possible level, is meant to celebrate the uniqueness in individuals and most certainly varies from person to person.

In 1969, Maslow amended his model and added another level to the hierarchy—that of self-transcendence,[35] although this level is not represented on the classical model that is used in textbooks today. This additional level could help us connect psychosocial health and spirituality, but little research has been conducted on the self-transcendence level of his model.

While there are criticisms of Maslow's Hierarchy of Needs model, it has been a useful tool for many people who are trying to determine what factors are holding them back from realizing their potential.

✓ CHECK-IN

Where are you on Maslow's Hierarchy of Needs model?

Erikson's Theory of Psychosocial Development Another well-known theory is Erik Erikson's Theory of Psychosocial Development.[36] Erikson explored three aspects of identity—ego identity (self), personal identity (our peculiarities), and social/cultural identity (the roles we play). His theory describes the impact of social experience on individuals throughout their lifetimes. He determined that we move through varying stages of development as we age, and our experiences during those stages can set us up with a sense of mastery or a sense of inadequacy. Each stage builds on the success of the previous stage. The stages are

- infancy (0 to 1 year)—basic trust vs. mistrust,
- early childhood (1 to 3 years)—autonomy vs. shame,
- play age (3 to 6 years)—initiative vs. guilt,
- school-age (6 to 12 years)—industry vs. inferiority,
- adolescence (12 to 19 years)—identity vs. confusion,
- early adulthood (20 to 25 years)—intimacy vs. isolation,
- adulthood (26 to 64 years)—generativity vs. stagnation, and
- old age (65 to death)—integrity vs. despair.

How does Erikson's theory link to college and university students and their psychosocial health? According to this theory, many students are moving from adolescence to young and middle adulthood. They are in the process of discovering who they are and what they value. They are beginning to develop intimate adult relationships and build extended families that include new friends, workmates, and adult mentors. They are also in the process of transforming their relationships with parents and family members. Adams et al.[37] invited a sample of 351 university students between the ages of 18 and 21 years to complete measures of psychosocial maturity based on Erikson's model. Their findings suggest that family cohesion and a sense of connectedness with family members during this stage of development appear to encourage initiative, effectiveness, competence, and a personal sense of trust in other students.

Older students in the middle and late adulthood stages are reevaluating their lives, dealing with major shifts, struggles, and opportunities. Fostering social support and social bonds seems to be essential for success at these stages too as students continue to gain a clearer sense of self.

Clarify Your Values Your **values**—based on your beliefs—are the criteria by which you evaluate things, people, events, and yourself; they represent what's most important to you.[38] In our complex world, values can provide guidelines for making decisions that are right for you. If understood and applied, they help give life meaning and structure.

Social psychologist Milton Rokeach[39] distinguished between two types of values. *Instrumental values* represent ways of thinking and acting that we hold important, such as being loving or loyal. *Terminal values* represent goals, achievements, or ideal states that we strive toward, such as happiness. Instrumental and terminal values form the basis for our attitudes and our behaviour.

There can be a large discrepancy between what people say they value and what their actions indicate about their values. That's why it's important to clarify your own values, making sure you understand what you believe so you can live in accordance with your beliefs. To do so, follow these steps:

1. Carefully consider the consequences of each choice.
2. Choose freely from among all the options.
3. Publicly affirm your values by sharing them with others.
4. Act out your values.

Values clarification is not a once-in-a-lifetime task, but an ongoing process of sorting out what matters most to you. If you believe in protecting the environment, do you turn off lights and walk rather than drive to conserve energy? Do you vote for political candidates who support environmental protection? Do you recycle newspapers, bottles, and cans? Values are more than ideals we'd like to attain; they reflect the way we live day by day.

✓ CHECK-IN

How do you put your values into action?

Strengthen Your Self-Esteem Each of us wants and needs to feel significant as a human being with unique talents, abilities, and roles in life. A sense of **self-esteem**,[40] or belief and pride in ourselves, gives us the confidence to achieve at school or work and to reach out to others to form friendships and close relationships. Self-esteem is the little voice that whispers, "You're worth it. You can do it. You're okay."

Self-esteem is not based on external factors such as wealth or beauty but on what you believe about yourself. It's not something you're born with; the seeds of self-esteem are planted in childhood and develop over time. It's also not something anyone else can give you, although those around you can either help boost or diminish your self-esteem.

Low self-esteem is more common in people who have been abused as children and in those with psychiatric disorders, including depression, anxiety, alcoholism, and drug dependence. Feeling neglected as a child can also lead to poor self-esteem. Adults with poor self-esteem may unconsciously enter into relationships that reinforce their negative self-perceptions and may prefer and even seek out people who think poorly of them.

One of the most useful techniques for bolstering self-esteem and achieving your goals is developing the habit of positive thinking, talking, and behaving. Psychology, a field that at times concentrated on what was wrong in our lives and minds, has shifted its focus to the study of what goes right. Whereas much research used to focus on **learned helplessness**,[41] blaming others for our failures after we have experienced repeated disappointments and letdowns and transferring our responsibility for adopting healthy lifestyle choices over to society, *positive psychology*[42] emphasizes building on personal strengths rather than treating weaknesses. Negative observations, such as constant criticism or reminders of the most minor of faults, can undermine self-image, while positive affirmations—compliments, kudos, encouragements—have proven effective in enhancing self-esteem and psychological well-being. Individuals who fight off negative thoughts fare better psychologically than those who collapse when a setback occurs or who rely on others to make them feel better.

People who learn to be **optimistic,**[43] who have an inclination to anticipate the best possible outcome, and who are **resilient,**[44] who have the ability to develop and master skills to recover or get through stressful situations, are less likely to suffer from mental disorders and more likely to lead happy, productive lives. If you are optimistic, you are someone who tends to look at life with a "glass half full" attitude. You expect the best. If you are resilient you tend to trust in your ability to figure things out and to ask for help when dealing with difficult situations or complex challenges. Eisenbarth[45] examined the effects of appraised stress and optimism in predicting symptoms of depression and anxiety in 172 male and 181 female college students. His data found solid support for the stress-buffeting effect of optimism in these students.

Lench,[46] in a study of 336 college students, found that simply thinking positively did not always lead to health benefits. However, when students were optimistic they were better able to focus on positive goals and understand what they had to gain when involved in certain experiences instead of focusing on potentially negative consequences.

Self-esteem has proven to be one of the best predictors of college and university adjustment. Students with high self-esteem report better personal, emotional, social, and academic adjustment.[47] However, true self-esteem requires an honest sense of your own worth. In a study of students, psychology professors followed self-enhancers who began their first year with an inflated sense of their own academic ability. These students expected to get much higher grades than might be expected based on their high school grades and test scores. They felt confident and happy for a while; however, they did no better academically and were no more likely to graduate than their realistic peers. In fact, their self-esteem and interest in school declined with each passing year.[48]

✓ CHECK-IN

How optimistic and resilient are you?

Manage Your Moods **Feelings**[49]—bodily or emotional responses that help us realize we are experiencing some type of emotion—can come and go within minutes. A **mood**[50] is a more sustained emotional state that colours our view of the world for hours or days. According to some surveys, bad moods descend upon us an average of three out of every ten days. A few people, about 2 percent, are happy just about every day. About 3 percent report bad moods four out of every five days.[51] Some personality types are prone to longer bad moods, which can lead to health problems.

There are also gender differences in mood management: Men typically try to distract themselves (a partially successful strategy) or use alcohol or drugs (an ineffective tactic); women are more likely to talk to someone (which can help) or to ruminate on why they feel bad (which doesn't help).[52] Learning effective mood-boosting, mood-regulating strategies can help both men and women pull themselves up and out of an emotional slump.

Make a Change The most effective way to banish sadness or a bad mood is by changing what caused it in the first place—if you can figure out what made you upset and why. "Most bad moods are caused by loss or failure in work or intimate relationships," says Larsen. "The questions to ask are: What can I do to fix the failure? What can I do to remedy the loss? Is there anything under my control that I can change? If there is, take action and solve it."[53] Rewrite the report. Ask to take a makeup exam. Apologize to the friend whose feelings you hurt. Tell your parents you feel bad about the argument you had.

If there's nothing you can do, accept what happened and focus on doing things differently next time. Or think about what happened in a different way and put a positive spin on it. This technique, known as *cognitive reappraisal* or *reframing*, helps you look at a setback in a new light: What lessons did it teach you? What would you have done differently? Could there be a silver lining or hidden benefit?

If you can't identify or resolve the problem responsible for your emotional funk, the next-best solution is to concentrate on altering your negative feelings. Try setting a quick, achievable goal that can boost your spirits with a small success. Clean out a closet; sort through the piles of paper on your desk; email or text message a friend.

Be Happy Being happy is an important part of psychosocial health, and "happiness" researchers, backed by thousands of scientific studies, cite mounting evidence that **happiness**—a feeling directly connected to our engagement with family, work, or a passionate pursuit—is not only buildable but also measurable. In cutting-edge research, psychologist Sonja Lyubomirsky, author of *The How of Happiness: A Scientific Approach to Getting the Life You Want*,[54] and her colleagues have fine-tuned proven strategies into practical prescriptions to enhance happiness. "Different methods are a better 'fit' for different people," she explains. "Keeping a daily gratitude journal seems hokey to some people, but writing a letter of gratitude may be very meaningful."[55] Timing and "doses" also matter. Performing five acts of kindness on a single day yields a greater halo effect than a single daily altruistic gesture. She also suggests that to sustain happiness you must make the effort on a daily basis.

Learn to Laugh Humour is one of the healthiest ways of coping with life's ups and downs. Laughter stimulates the heart, alters brainwave patterns and breathing rhythms, reduces perceptions of pain, decreases stress-related hormones, and strengthens the immune system. In psychotherapy, humour helps channel negative emotions toward a positive effect. Even in cases of critical or fatal illnesses, humour can relieve pain and help people live with greater joy until they die.[56]

Joking and laughing are ways of expressing honest emotions, of overcoming dread and doubt, and of connecting with others. They can also defuse rage. Try keeping a file of favourite funny cartoons or jokes. Check out funny quotes of the day. Go to a funny movie. Hang out with people who love to laugh.

✓ CHECK-IN

How often do you laugh?

Move a Little More Often In studies of mood regulation, another good option for managing your moods is to get moving. Exercise consistently ranks very high as an effective strategy for banishing bad feelings. Research has shown that aerobic workouts, such as walking or jogging, significantly improve moods. Results of a study of college students who participated in walking, water aerobics, and yoga indicated that all activities provided psychological benefits, with yoga being the most effective in producing a state of calmness or relaxation.[57]

In another study on first-year Canadian undergraduates, students who were physically active during the transition year from high school to university reported higher levels of vigour and lower levels of tension and fatigue compared to inactive students. The findings of this study[58] and others suggest that students have much to gain in terms of psychological and physiological health by staying active.

Even non-aerobic exercise, such as weightlifting, can boost spirits; improve sleep and appetite; reduce anxiety, irritability, and anger; and produce feelings of mastery and accomplishment. More information about the benefits of physical activity for health is included in Chapter 4.

Sleep! Do you find yourself staying up late cramming for final exams? Do you have difficulty getting up for an early morning class? Do you wonder why you are so tired? The answer might be that you are not getting enough sleep. In the course of a year, 25 percent of the Canadian population suffers from a variety of sleep disorders.[59] The cumulative long-term effects of sleep loss and sleep disorders include an increased risk of hypertension, diabetes, obesity, depression, heart attack, and stroke.

College and university students are notorious for staying up late to study and socialize during the week and sleeping in on the weekends. On average students go to bed one to two hours later and sleep 1–1.6 hours less than students of a generation ago.[60] Numerous studies have been done on the variation of sleep patterns of students. Galambos and Dalton,[61] in a study of Canadian students in their first semester of university, determined that use of alcohol was followed by a loss of sleep time and sleep quality; lower amounts of sleep on a previous night were followed by decreased time on school work; and poorer quality of sleep was followed by increased stress. Another study on sleep and academic performance showed that later wake-up times were associated with lower average grades.[62] Driving while sleep deprived is also a common occurrence reported by adolescents and college-aged students.[63]

Sleep is essential for functioning at your best. The following are some of the key ways in which your nighttime sleep affects your daytime well-being and psychosocial health.

- **Learning and memory**—When you sleep, your brain helps consolidate new information so you are more likely to retain it in your memory.
- **Metabolism and weight**—The less you sleep, the more weight you may gain. Chronic sleep deprivation may cause weight gain by altering metabolism and by stimulating excess stress hormones. Loss of sleep also reduces levels of the hormones that regulate appetite, which may encourage more eating.
- **Safety**—People who don't get adequate nighttime sleep are more likely to fall asleep during the daytime. This can cause falls, medical errors, traffic mishaps, and road accidents.
- **Mood/quality of life**—Too little sleep, whether just for a night or two or for longer periods, can cause psychological symptoms, such as irritability, impatience, inability to concentrate, and moodiness. Poor sleep also affects your motivation and ability to work effectively. Growing evidence suggests that disturbed sleep is associated with increased risk of psychiatric disorders.
- **Cardiovascular health**—Serious sleep disorders such as insomnia and sleep apnea have been linked to hypertension, increased stress hormone levels, irregular heartbeats, and increased inflammation, which may play a role in heart attacks.

- **Immunity/cancer prevention**—Sleep deprivation alters immune function, including the activity of the body's killer cells. Keeping up with sleep may also help fight cancer.

No formula can say how long a good night's sleep should be. Normal sleep times range from five to ten hours; the average is seven and a half. Listen to your body's signals and adjust your sleep schedule to suit them.

✓ CHECK-IN

How much sleep do you usually get?

Feel in Control Although no one has absolute control over destiny, we can do a great deal to control how we think, feel, and behave. By realistically assessing our life situations, we can live in a way that allows us to make the most of our circumstances. By doing so, we gain a sense of mastery. In many surveys, people who feel in control of their lives report greater psychological well-being than those who do not.

Albert Bandura's social cognitive theory of human functioning[64] suggests that **self-efficacy**[65]—our belief that we can influence or produce an effect over events that affect our lives—is a foundation of human motivation, well-being, and personal accomplishments. He suggests that unless we believe we can produce desired results by our actions, we will have little incentive to act or to persevere in the face of difficulties. Efficacy beliefs play a key role in shaping our lives. Our level of self-efficacy influences the types of activities and environments we choose to be in.

Develop Autonomy One goal that many people strive for is **autonomy**,[66] defined as governing ourselves or being independent. While family and society influence our ability to grow toward independence, autonomous individuals are true to themselves. As they weigh the pros and cons of any decision, whether it's using or refusing drugs or choosing a major area of study or a career, they may seek the opinions of others, but they do not allow their decisions to be dictated solely by external influences. Their **locus of control**[67]—that is, where they view control as originating—is *internal* (from within themselves) rather than *external* (from others).

Assert Yourself Being **assertive**,[68] characterized as confident statements and behaviour, means recognizing your feelings and making your needs and desires clear to others. Unlike aggression, a far less healthy means of expression, assertiveness usually works. You can change a situation you don't like by communicating your feelings and thoughts in non-provocative words, by focusing on specifics, and by making sure you're talking with the person who is directly responsible.

Becoming assertive isn't always easy. Many people have learned to cope by being passive and not communicating their feelings or opinions. Sooner or later they become so irritated, frustrated, or overwhelmed that they explode in an outburst—which they think of as being assertive. Assertiveness doesn't mean screaming or telling someone off. You can communicate your wishes calmly and clearly. Assertiveness is a behaviour that respects your rights and the rights of other people, even when you disagree.

Connect with Others While developing autonomy and asserting ourselves can help us feel we have more control in life, connecting with others is another important element in psychosocial health. As we have already discussed, people who feel connected to others tend to be healthier physically and psychologically. College and university students are no exception: those who have a supportive, readily available network of relationships are less psychologically distressed and more satisfied with life.

Covey[69] says that when we develop autonomy or independence, we can then enter into a whole new dimension—that of interdependence. Building rich, enduring relationships with other people allows us to ask for or give help when needed. As we begin to trust in ourselves and others, we begin to think of working or being together as a win–win situation—a mutual benefit.

Become Socially Responsible Becoming socially responsible is a wonderful way to connect with others. Whereas **altruism**[70] is an unselfish regard for people, **social responsibility**[71] is a principle or ethical theory that suggests governments, corporations, organizations, and individuals have a responsibility to contribute to the welfare of society. Research does show that Canadians are good at giving. In a report based on the *2013 General Social Survey on Giving,*

STRATEGIES FOR CHANGE

Steps to Sleeping Better

- Keep regular hours for going to bed and getting up in the morning. Stay as close as possible to this schedule on weekends as well as weekdays.
- Develop a sleep ritual—stretch, meditate, practise yoga, pray, or read a book to ease the transition from wakefulness to sleep.
- Don't drink coffee or caffeinated liquids late in the day. The effects of caffeine can linger for up to eight hours. Don't smoke. Nicotine is an even more powerful stimulant—and sleep saboteur—than caffeine.
- Don't rely on alcohol to get you to sleep. Alcohol disrupts normal sleep stages, so you won't sleep as deeply or as restfully as you normally would.
- Recent studies suggest that having a 30-minute power nap can lower stress and refresh you with no disruption in nighttime sleep. Just be sure it is a power nap!

Volunteering and Participating, 82 percent of Canadians over the age of 15 made a financial donation to a charitable or other nonprofit organization in 2013. While the number of people donating since 2010 decreased by 2 percent, the amount of donations increased by 14 percent, bringing the total amount of donations to 12.8 billion dollars.[72] Approximately 12.7 million Canadians (44 percent of the population) aged 15 years or older volunteered their time for a community group, nonprofit, or charitable organization during 2013, providing almost 1.96 billion hours, which is equal to about 1 million full-time jobs.[73]

Whether you are altruistic on a personal level or participate in a corporate community project, research reveals that people who help other people consistently report increased levels of self-esteem, lowering of physical and mental stress, and a surge of well-being, called *helper's high*, a unique sense of calmness, warmth, and enhanced self-worth. Hans Selye, the father of stress research, described cooperation with others for the self's sake as *altruistic egotism*, whereby we satisfy our own needs while helping others satisfy theirs. College students who provided community service reported changes in attitude (a greater degree of thankfulness for personal opportunities) and behaviour (a greater commitment to do more volunteer work).[74]

Service learning has been shown to help students reflect on the health disparities evident in their own communities and assist them in making healthy lifestyle choices so that they are better prepared to help others.[75] The focus on "others" sometimes helped them move from a focus on self-referral to that of doing something purposeful and meaningful for others. Researchers have also discovered that when students perceive their community service experience as being of high quality, they feel a sense of civic responsibility and are more likely to continue volunteering.[76] Business school students are asking for curriculum that helps them understand the financial benefits of social responsibility. They are beginning to understand that working for companies whose business plans align with their own personal values of caring for others will lessen their stress as they move into career-oriented jobs.[77]

The options for volunteerism and giving to others are limitless: serve a meal at a homeless shelter, collect donations for a charity auction, or teach reading in a literacy program, for example. Volunteer opportunities are often available on college and university campuses. Women's centres, intercultural clubs, peer mentoring, and study groups are just a few options.

Many businesses across Canada and around the world have adopted a social responsibility mandate as part of their strategic planning process. The Government of Canada, through the Innovation, Science, and Economic Development department, promotes Corporate Social Responsibility (CSR) because it makes companies more innovative, productive, and competitive. CSR often overlaps with corporate citizenship or sustainability initiatives.[78] Hurst reports that approximately "33 percent of volunteers employed by Canadian companies said their employer had a program or policy to encourage volunteering."[79] Formal support for volunteering included an opportunity to change or reduce work hours, providing transportation for volunteer activities, and sponsoring specific volunteer events. The benefits of employer-supported volunteering included a higher likelihood of success in their job, gaining relevant work-related skills, and recognition for their volunteer work.

As you ponder your own career path, take time to think about ways you might become socially responsible—a concept that is win-win for businesses and individuals.

✓ CHECK-IN

What social responsibility initiatives are being encouraged on your campus?

Overcome Loneliness According to a *Canadian Social Trends* report, time spent alone has been continually increasing for the last 20 years.[80] For some individuals, being alone and being lonely are two different things. Not all people who spend time alone are lonely. However, loneliness can cause emotional distress when it is a chronic rather than an episodic condition.[81] Findings in another survey showed that people who spent a lot of time by themselves were less likely to be very happy with their lives than those who spent little time alone. Forty-eight percent of those who spent less than two hours alone on an average day were very happy, compared with 37 percent of Canadians who spent eight or more hours by themselves.[82]

To combat loneliness, people may join groups or teams. College and university recreation and athletic departments offer many opportunities for students to connect with each other. However, some students surround themselves with superficial acquaintances and begin participating in unhealthy lifestyle behaviours, while others avoid the effort of trying to connect with other people in person, limiting most of their personal interactions to social networking on the Internet. Some studies are showing that the use of the Internet may actually make people feel lonelier. Dittman,[83] in a study on undergraduate students, found that loneliness is more prevalent in the students who use the Internet more than 40 hours per week and in those who prefer the Internet over face-to-face interaction or talking on the phone.

Odaci and Kalkan[84] also found that problematic Internet use (five hours or more a day) showed a significant association with loneliness and levels of dating anxiety. More recent research suggests that students who constantly feel lonely show greater problematic

Internet use than students who never or only sometimes experience feelings of loneliness.[85]

Kim et al.,[86] in a study on Hong Kong university students, established that students reporting heavy use of the Internet (four or more hours per day) had multiple psychosocial and physical health risks that included skipping meals, sleeping late, having hypersomnia, and being overweight. In yet another study, Odaci[87] found that as problematic Internet use rises, a student's belief in their ability to succeed academically declines. All of these issues can also contribute to feelings of loneliness as students begin to withdraw from social settings.

The access to information and the ability to stay connected are just two of the remarkable benefits of the Internet, but it is important to be mindful of the psychosocial and physiological costs, especially if you are a college or university student preparing for your future career.

Gender can affect the experience of loneliness. Some studies have found that men are lonelier than women. Others find no gender differences in loneliness, but researchers note men, particularly those who score high on measures of masculinity, are more hesitant than women to admit that they're lonely.[88]

The true keys to overcoming loneliness are developing skills to fulfill your potential and learning to reach out to others. Joining a study group, volunteering on campus, coaching children's sports teams, or finding part-time work can connect you with others and lessen the feeling of loneliness you may be experiencing.

Face Social Anxieties Some people are born with a predisposition to shyness. Others become shy because they don't learn proper social responses or because they experience rejection or shame. There are people who are fearfully shy; they experience **social isolation**, in which they withdraw and avoid contact with others and experience a high degree of anxiety and fear in social situations. As well, there are people who are self-consciously shy; they enjoy the company of others but become highly self-aware and anxious in social settings.

Social anxieties often become a problem in late adolescence.[89] Nelson found that relatively shy young men and women were more anxious and depressed, engaged in fewer social events, and experienced reduced relationship quality with their parents, friends, and romantic partners than non-shy peers.[90] About 7 percent of the population could be diagnosed with **social phobia**, a severe form of social anxiety in which individuals typically fear and avoid various social situations.[91] Adolescents and young adults with severe social anxiety are at increased risk of major depression.[92] The key difference between these problems and normal shyness and self-consciousness is the degree of distress and impairment that individuals experience.

If you are shy, you can overcome much of your social apprehensiveness on your own, the same way you might set out to make other lifestyle changes. You can improve your social skills by pushing yourself to talk with a stranger in one of your classes or to a person attending a meeting or gathering. Gradually you'll acquire a sense of social timing and a verbal ease that will take the worry out of close encounters with others. Those with more disabling social anxiety may do best with professional guidance, which has proven highly effective. Over time, most people are able to emerge from the walls that shyness has built around them and take pleasure in interacting with others.

UNDERSTANDING MENTAL HEALTH

Mentally healthy individuals value themselves, perceive reality as it is, accept their limitations and possibilities, carry out their responsibilities, establish and maintain close relationships, pursue work that suits their talent and training, and feel a sense of fulfillment that makes the efforts of daily living worthwhile (see Figure 2-2). Yet, there are people who suffer from mental health disorders who struggle to maintain their mental health.

The World Health Organization reports that mental disorders affect more than 450 million people around the world with 350 million people suffering from depression, 26 million from schizophrenia, 125 million affected by alcohol use disorders, and 24 million from Alzheimer's and other dementias.[93,94] There are calls for increased efforts to recognize, treat, and prevent mental disorders.[95]

What Is a Mental Illness? While people may speak of nervous breakdowns or insanity, these are not

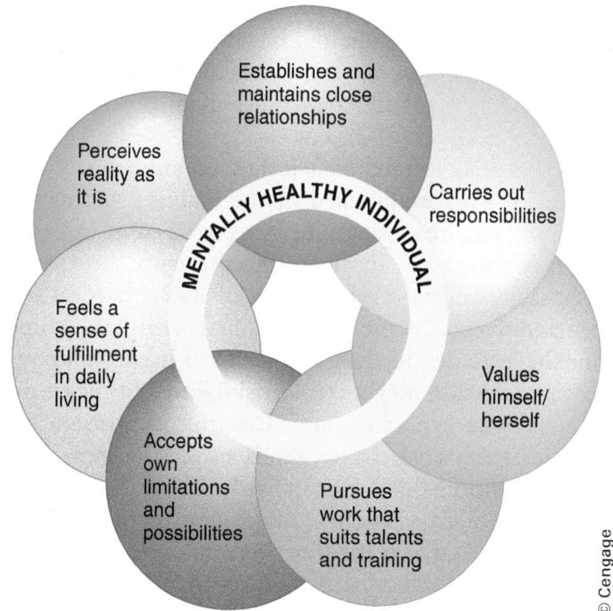

Figure 2-2 Mentally Healthy Individual
Mental well-being is a combination of many factors.

scientific terms for mental illness. The contributors to the *Report on Mental Illnesses in Canada* define **mental illness** as changes in thinking, mood, or behaviour (or a combination of these) associated with significant distress, dysfunction, and impaired functioning over an extended period of time.[96] The symptoms of mental illness vary from mild to severe, depending on the type of mental illness, the individual, the family, and the socio-economic environment. Mental illness includes mood disorders, schizophrenia, anxiety disorders, personality disorders, and eating disorders.

Nearly one in five Canadian adults is affected by mental health issues on an annual basis. This represents about 6.8 million Canadians or approximately 19.8 percent of our total population. Mental illness impacts everyone—individuals, families, communities, and our overall health-care system.[97] Diagnosis of mental health issues often occurs at a young age. It is estimated that almost 28 percent of young people aged 20–29 years of age will experience a mental illness during a given year. As Canadians reach the age of 40 years, one in two people will have been affected by a mental illness.[98]

A study on the economic impact of major mental health problems and illnesses on our Canadian economy suggests that total costs were approximately 50 billion dollars in 2011. About 42.3 billion were spent on providing care, support, and treatment. More than 6 billion dollars were lost due to absenteeism and staff turnover.[99]

Does Mental Health Affect Physical Health? Mental illness affects the mind and the body. **Anxiety**, described as a feeling of apprehension and dread, can lead to intensified asthmatic reactions, skin conditions, and digestive disorders. Stress can play a role in hypertension, heart attacks, sudden cardiac death, and immune disorders. Individuals with mental illness can develop physical symptoms such as weight loss and blood biochemical imbalances associated with eating disorders.

Depression, defined as a feeling of unhappiness and despair, often accompanied by the inability to function normally, has increasingly been recognized as a serious risk factor for physical illness. According to a review of large-scale studies on depression of more than 36 000 men and women, depressed individuals were 1.5–4 times more likely to develop heart problems.[100] In still-unknown ways, depression may increase risk factors for heart disease, such as hypertension.[101] Together, depression and heart disease worsen a patient's prognosis more than either condition alone. One in five heart-attack survivors suffers major depression.[102] They are two to five times more likely to die in the first 6–12 months following a heart attack.[103] Since depression can and often does recur, physicians now view it as a chronic illness with lifelong implications for mental and physical health.[104] Treating mental health problems leads not only to improved health but also to lower health-care costs as it reduces hospitalizations, cuts medical expenses, and reduces work disability.

Diversity and Mental Health Mental illness affects people in all occupations, educational and income levels, and cultures. However, there are some gender and age differences that can be noted. Rates among women are higher than among men in all age groups.[105] (see also X & Y Files: "Sex, Gender, and Mental Illness Issues").

Young adults are also at risk. Research suggests that over one million young Canadians between the ages of 9 and 19 were living with a mental illness in 2011. Studies have also determined that these youth have a high risk of having the same mental illness or developing a new mental illness when they become adults.[106]

Cultural assimilation plays a role in mental health, too. Loneliness, isolation, alien religious rituals, suppression of native language, ridicule, harsh punishment, and sexual abuse experienced at residential schools across Canada have been emotionally devastating to many children of First Nations, Inuit, and Métis descent. Many studies show that the high levels of psychological problems in our Aboriginal communities are a direct result of the abuse suffered.[107]

There are growing reports that people experiencing **homelessness**, which includes absolute homelessness, being at risk for homelessness, or hidden homelessness,[108] are more likely to experience mental health issues. Not having a home is a harsh reality for many Canadians. All groups in our society are affected—youth, men and women, single- or two-parent families, older adults, immigrants, and Aboriginal peoples. There are a growing number of college and university students who also struggle to find affordable and safe housing and depend on campus food banks.[109] The result is increased stress levels and difficulty coping with academic demands. This can lead to an increased risk for mental illness and possible addictions.

Stigma There are widespread misconceptions about mental illness. Individuals suffering from a mental illness are sometimes thought to be weak, lazy, and indecisive and are subject to **stigma**—a severe social disapproval. They are also discriminated against, subjected to violence and abuse, not provided with civil and political rights, and not allowed to participate fully in society. Beliefs about mental illness include the following:[110]

- All individuals with mental health issues are dangerous.
- Mental illness is caused by supernatural forces.
- People with mental health conditions should be housed in facilities far away from local communities.

- Their right to vote should be restricted.
- Their access to employment should be limited.

We all have an important role to play with regard to dealing with mental health issues. You might start by becoming responsible for adopting healthy lifestyle choices so that you lower your risk for mental illness. You can be an advocate for de-stigmatizing mental illness. You might attempt to support others close to you who are dealing with mental health issues. You can begin working with local, national, and international governments and agencies to develop plans and strategies that will provide better services and education for mental health. Presently, Canada does not have a national strategy for suicide prevention, whereas many other countries do.

Anxiety Disorders **Anxiety disorders** may involve inordinate fears of certain objects or situations (phobias); episodes of sudden, inexplicable terror (panic attacks); chronic distress (generalized anxiety disorder); or persistent, disturbing thoughts and behaviours (obsessive-compulsive disorder). About 3 million Canadians (11.6 percent of the population) in 2013 reported that they suffered from anxiety and mood disorders that caused mild to severe impairment.[111]

Generalized anxiety disorder (GAD), an excessive or unrealistic apprehension that causes physical symptoms, can last for six months or longer. It often starts when people are in their twenties.[112] Unlike fear, which helps us recognize and avoid real danger, GAD is an exaggerated, irrational, or unwarranted response to harmless objects or situations. The most common symptoms are faster heart rate, sweating, increased blood pressure, muscle aches, intestinal pains, irritability, sleep problems, and difficulty concentrating.

Chronically anxious individuals worry constantly, about almost everything: their health, families, finances, marriages, and potential dangers. Treatment for GAD may consist of a combination of psychotherapy, behavioural therapy, and anti-anxiety drugs.

Many individuals do not seek treatment for their anxiety. Sometimes the symptoms themselves may interfere with seeking help. Yet, most people who do get treatment, even for severe and disabling problems, improve dramatically.

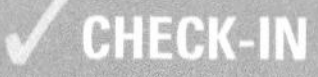

Have you suffered from anxiety disorders?

Phobias **Phobias**—the most prevalent type of anxiety disorder—are out-of-the-ordinary, irrational, intense, excessive, unreasonable, and persistent fears of certain objects or situations. The most common phobias involve animals, particularly dogs, snakes, insects, and mice; the sight of blood; closed spaces (*claustrophobia*); heights (*acrophobia*); air travel; and being in places or situations from which they perceive it difficult or embarrassing to escape (*agoraphobia*). The result of a phobia is the inability to function as usual at school or work or in social relationships.

Although various medications have been tried, none is effective by itself in relieving phobias. The best approach is **behaviour therapy**, which consists of gradual, systematic exposure to the feared object (a process called *systematic desensitization*). Numerous studies have proven that exposure to the actual source of the fear, rather than simply imagining it, is highly effective. *Medical hypnosis*, the use of induction of an altered state of consciousness, also can help.

Panic Attacks, Panic Disorder, and Post-Traumatic Stress Disorder Individuals who have had **panic attacks** describe them as the most frightening experiences of their lives. Without reason or warning, their hearts race wildly. They may become light-headed or dizzy. Because they can't catch their breath, they may start breathing rapidly and hyperventilate. Worst of all is the terrible sense that something horrible is about to happen: that they will die, lose their minds, or have a heart attack. Most attacks reach peak intensity within ten minutes. Afterward, individuals live in dread of another one.

X AND Y FILES

Sex, Gender, and Mental Illness Issues

Research has shown that there are sex and gender differences in the incidence of mental illness in Canada:

- More than twice as many women as men suffer from anxiety and mood disorders.
- Anxiety and mood disorders for women tend to peak while they are in their 20s and for men in their 30s.
- Women are twice as likely to experience depression than men and are one and a half times more likely to be hospitalized with depression.
- Men and women have similar rates of bipolar disorder.
- Men and women are affected equally by schizophrenia, but men often develop the illness earlier than women.
- There are gender biases in the treatment of psychological disorders. Doctors are more likely to diagnose depression in women than men, and if you are a female, you are more likely to be prescribed mood-altering psychotropic drugs than men.
- There is a significantly higher number of women suffering from post-traumatic stress disorder than men.

Sources: Mood Disorders Society of Canada (2009, November; 3rd ed.). *Quick facts: Mental illness and addiction in Canada.* http://www.mooddisorderscanada.ca/page/quick-facts; Mental Health Commission of Canada (2010). *Why investing in mental health will contribute to Canada's economic prosperity and to the sustainability of our health care system.* http://www.mentalhealthcommission.ca/English/document/5210/making-case-investing-mental-health-canada-backgrounder-key-facts

Panic disorder develops when panic attacks recur or apprehension about them becomes so intense that individuals cannot function normally About two million Canadians suffer from panic disorder.[113] Parents, siblings, and children of individuals with panic disorders also are more likely to develop them than are others.[114]

The two primary treatments for panic disorder are (1) *cognitive-behavioural therapy*, which teaches specific strategies for coping with symptoms like rapid breathing; and (2) *medication*. Treatment helps as many as 90 percent of those with panic disorder improve significantly or recover completely, usually within six to eight weeks. Individuals who receive cognitive-behavioural therapy as well as medication are less likely to suffer relapses than those taking medication alone and often can learn to control their symptoms without drugs.[115]

In **post-traumatic stress disorder (PTSD)** individuals re-experience terror and helplessness they have experienced in the past again and again in their dreams or intrusive thoughts. In the past, PTSD was viewed as a psychological response to out-of-the-ordinary stressors, such as captivity or combat. However, other experiences can also forever change the way in which people view themselves and their world. Thousands of individuals experience or witness traumatic events, such as fires or floods. According to research, almost half of car accident victims may develop PTSD. Those who were seriously injured are especially vulnerable.[116] Children, in particular, are likely to develop PTSD symptoms if they have witnessed a loved one or friend being assaulted or have been sexually abused.

Those with pre-existing psychological problems may be the most vulnerable. In the brain, stress hormones linked to powerful emotio[illegible] memories of events. The s[illegible] psychological help, the b[illegible] Behavioural, cognitive, an[illegible] help individuals suffering from PTSD; however, new research suggests that trauma produces changes in the brain that impede a person's ability to think and talk about the events. Traditional therapies can sometimes be debilitating for PTSD sufferers. Belleruth Naparstek, a renowned psychotherapist, suggests that guided imagery uses what is most accessible in the traumatized brain to help with the healing. Often individuals who have PTSD will respond to nonverbal engagement, such as images, symbols, metaphors, drawing, writing, conscious breathing, and movement.[117]

Obsessive-Compulsive Disorder Another type of anxiety disorder is known as **obsessive-compulsive disorder (OCD)**. Some individuals suffer only from an *obsession*, a recurring idea, thought, or image that they realize, at least initially, is senseless. The most common obsessions are repetitive thoughts of violence, contamination, and doubt. Most people with OCD also suffer from a *compulsion*, repetitive behaviour performed according to certain rules or in a stereotyped fashion. The most common compulsions involve handwashing, cleaning, hoarding useless items, counting, or checking (for example, making sure dozens of times that a door is locked).[118] New OCDs added to the American Psychiatric Association *Diagnostic and Statistical Manual of Mental Disorders* (DSM-5)[119] are excoriation (skin-picking) disorder, trichotillomania (hair-pulling disorder), and substance/medication-induced obsessive-compulsive and related disorder.

Individuals with OCD realize that their thoughts or behaviours are bizarre, but they cannot resist or control them. Eventually, the obsessions or compulsions consume a great deal of time and significantly interfere with normal routine, job functioning, social activities, and relationships with others.

OCD is believed to have biological roots. It may be a result of gene abnormalities, head injury, or even an autoimmune reaction after childhood infection with the strep bacteria. Treatment may consist of cognitive therapy to correct irrational assumptions and behavioural techniques such as progressively limiting the amount of time someone obsessed with cleanliness can spend washing and scrubbing, and medication. About 70–80 percent of those with OCD improve with treatment.

Attention Disorders **Attention deficit/hyperactivity disorder (ADHD)** is a psychiatric diagnosis used by the *American Psychiatric Association* to describe individuals who are hyperactive, impulsive, and may or may not have inattentive behaviours. The term **attention deficit disorder (ADD)** is still often used interchangeably with ADHD.[120]

There are three different types of ADHD:

- **ADHD, Predominantly Inattentive Type**—where individuals are inattentive, but not hyperactive or impulsive. They often have difficulty finishing tasks and following directions, and appear to be forgetful and disorganized. They are sometimes slow to respond and have difficulty processing information.
- **ADHD, Predominantly Hyperactive-Impulsive Type**—where individuals are overactive, impulsive, fidgety, and restless. Characteristics include talking excessively, being constantly on the go, and acting before thinking.
- **ADHD, Combined Type**—where individuals are inattentive and also display hyperactive and impulsive symptoms.

The causes of ADHD are complex and include genetic and biological factors. Research has shown that individuals with ADHD often have smaller overall brain volumes than others, particularly in the right frontal region, an area of the brain associated with the processes of paying attention and focusing concentration.[121]

HUMAN POTENTIAL

Christopher Bratseth—The Power of Kindness

Christopher Bratseth, a past graduate student of mine, has faced many challenges along his way but has found meaning in his work and personal life. I hope you enjoy his story.

Sometimes from our darkest moments come our clearest insights about how to live well. During my undergraduate degree, I suffered through periods of depression brought on by test-taking and social anxiety. Although I took part in sports and loved the academic challenge of school, I did not have the resources to cope with the emotional challenges. I still remember one night in my third year when I was overcome by grief and mental anguish. In this moment, I felt like I could empathize fully with the silent suffering of so many people with mental illness. I promised myself then that if I found a way to overcome this pain, I would work to relieve the suffering of others. This intention would shape my life in more powerful ways than I could ever imagine.

I was fortunate to work with a registered psychologist. I spent time in counselling to reduce my fear of public speaking, open up to my family about my depression, and learn how to reduce my anxiety through meditation, physical activity, and cognitive behavioural therapy. Taking these healing steps allowed me to enjoy my last years at university and finish my degree.

After university, I wanted to work in media and find a way to serve others. I began working with three of my closest friends—Erik Hanson, Val Litwin, and Brad Stokes—to create a web-television show called Extreme Kindness. The concept was simple: we would film spontaneous acts of kindness and upload them to our website in the hopes that people would be inspired to be the change they wished to see in the world. Unfortunately, our forward momentum was slowed by a series of challenging events.

The year 2001 was life-altering for our group. Erik, Val, and myself came together to support our friend Brad and his mother, Judy, after she was diagnosed with ovarian cancer. We were there beside Brad and his sister Devon when their mother passed away. During our time with her, Judy taught us about the need to live in the moment and follow our passions for helping others.

One month later, our world was shaken again in the wake of the horror of September 11. It was in our collective moments of reflection that we found our focus. We began to see how kindness connects all people regardless of their social, economic, and religious backgrounds. Kindness was also immediately empowering and accessible to anyone who was suffering. We believed kindness could be an antidote to the disconnection and fear with which people were plagued. Our simple but passion-filled gesture was to build a Kindness Crew—a group committed to connecting the world through kindness.

In the fall of 2002, after a year of planning, we embarked on the road trip of a lifetime. We set out across Canada on the *Extreme Kindness Tour* with a mission to inspire a million acts of kindness. We travelled by motorhome from Victoria, British Columbia, to St. John's, Newfoundland, connecting with others through compassion. In each community we visited, we staged Kindness Marathons—working from dawn until dusk with schools, nonprofits, and businesses on community projects and acts of service.

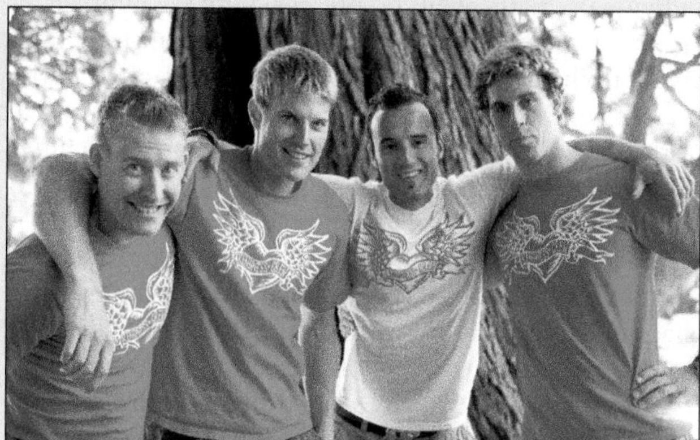

Courtesy of Christopher Bratseth

Brad Stokes, Chris Bratseth, Val Litwin, and Erik Hanson of the Kindness Crew.

From staffing soup kitchens in Calgary and roofing homes in Winnipeg to serving the homeless in Toronto, our acts ranged from the mundane to the magnificent. Our highlights included mobilizing the town of Salmon Arm, British Columbia, to commit over 19 000 random acts of kindness in one day; having the city of Gander, Newfoundland, proclaim November 23 Kindness Day; CNN broadcasting our story across the world; and Catherine Ryan Hyde (the author of the book *Pay it Forward*) flying out to Halifax to join us on our tour. In the end, there was no way to directly measure the impact of the tour; however, as a group we made it our life mission to inspire, educate, and mobilize others toward service.

The tour spawned work with schools, nonprofits, First Nations communities, and Fortune 500 companies. One firm, SAS Canada, was inspired to allow all employees four days off per year to volunteer with their charity of choice. We have also written two books to engage others to be kind: *Cool to Be Kind—Random Acts and How to Commit Them* and *A Call to Arms: Embrace a Kindness Revolution*.

Ironically, I have begun to make a living as an educator. I work as a high-school teacher and share my passion for kindness with youth through a student club called The Compassion Project. In one project the students shot a documentary exploring intergenerational perspectives on compassion. Elders from our community and students shared their thoughts on how compassion can help individuals, connect communities, and improve the school environment.

With the overarching focus of helping others I have found the inner strength to heal and overcome my anxieties. Kindness has become a central virtue in my life, and I am grounded by the words of Theodore Isaac Rubin who eloquently said, "Kindness is more important than wisdom and the recognition of this is the beginning of wisdom." Kindness is also a starting point for living a healthy life. Life still ebbs and flows, but now the main current of my life is filled with a richness that leaves me with a feeling of peace and purpose.

You can check out the Kindness Crew's website at www.extremekindness.com.

Between 40 and 70 percent of youngsters with ADHD do not outgrow this condition. About 4 percent of college and university students have ADHD.[122] Individuals with ADHD present with a number of symptoms that include hyperactivity, impulsivity, and distractibility. Hyperactivity in adults is often more subtle—an internal fidgety feeling rather than a physical restlessness. As people get older, academic difficulties can become much more of a problem. Students with ADHD may find it hard to concentrate, read, make decisions, complete complex projects, and meet deadlines.

Relationships with peers can also become more challenging. Young people with ADHD may become frustrated easily, have a short fuse, and be argumentative, negative, and defiant. Sleep problems are common, and depression and anxiety disorders are higher. However, many students who have ADHD are very resilient and find ways to successfully complete their academic studies. Many Canadian colleges and universities have centres for students with disabilities and provide extra or specialized support for exam writing. Health, counselling, and student services sometimes offer programs and services to support students who need a little extra help. There are also studies that suggest family support can increase academic success for college students with ADHD.[123]

Depressive Disorders Depression, the world's most common mental ailment, affects the brain, the mind, and the body in complex ways. It is the leading cause of years of life lived with disability (YLD).[124] Stress-related events may trigger half of all depressive episodes; great trauma in childhood can increase vulnerability to depression later in life.[125] Approximately 8 percent of Canadian adults will experience major depression at some time in their lives, and the onset of depression usually occurs during adolescence.[126] A nationwide 2012 National College Health Assessment found that about 29.5 percent of college students reported feeling "so depressed that it was difficult to function" at some time in the past year.[127]

Comparing everyday blues to a **depressive disorder**, defined as a psychological disorder involving persuasive and sustained depression, is like comparing a cold to pneumonia. Major depression can destroy a person's joy for living. Food, friends, sex, or any form of pleasure no longer appeals. It is impossible to concentrate on work and responsibilities. Depressed individuals may fight back tears throughout the day and toss and turn through long, empty nights. Thoughts of death or suicide may push into their minds.

But there is good news: depression is a treatable disease. Psychotherapy is effective for mild depression. In more serious cases, **antidepressant** medication, prescription drugs used primarily to treat symptoms of depression, can lead to dramatic improvement in 40–80 percent of depressed patients.

Exercise also is a good way to both prevent and treat psychological problems. Several studies have shown that exercise effectively lifts mild to moderate depression; for some patients with major depression, exercise may be more effective than drug treatment.[128] In a study of 150 individuals diagnosed with major depression, one group was assigned to four months of walking, jogging, or cycling; another took antidepressant medication; and a third both exercised and took medication. At the end of four months, all had improved significantly. Six months later, the exercisers were in better shape physically and mentally—and much less likely to have suffered a relapse. At 10 months, the chance of a patient still being depressed was reduced by 50 percent for every 50 minutes of current weekly exercise.[129] Among older adults, low-intensity exercise that included weight training improved overall mood more than aerobic exercise alone.[130]

Major Depression The simplest definition of **major depression** is sadness that does not end. The incidence of major depression has soared over the last two decades, especially among young adults.

The characteristic symptoms of major depression include

- feeling depressed, sad, empty, discouraged, tearful;
- loss of interest or pleasure in once-enjoyable activities;
- eating more or less than usual and either gaining or losing weight;
- having trouble sleeping or sleeping much more than usual;
- feeling slowed down, or feeling restless and unable to sit still;
- lack of energy;
- feeling helpless, hopeless, worthless, inadequate;
- difficulty concentrating, forgetfulness, not able to think clearly or make decisions;
- persistent thoughts of death or suicide;
- withdrawal from others, lack of interest in sex; and
- physical symptoms (headaches, digestive problems, aches, and pains).

Neuroscience, the study of the brain, has revealed that major depression is as physical as diabetes or heart disease. Dozens of brain-imaging studies have revealed abnormalities in the front part of the brain, which is involved in regulating emotions, and the shrinking of certain brain regions during depressive episodes.[131]

Most cases of major depression can be treated successfully, usually with psychotherapy, medication, or both. Psychotherapy alone works in more than half of mild-to-moderate episodes of major depression. Psychotherapy helps individuals pinpoint the life problems that contribute to their depression, identify negative or distorted thinking patterns, explore behaviours that contribute to depression, and regain a sense of control and pleasure in life. Two specific psychotherapies—cognitive-behavioural therapy and interpersonal therapy—have proven as helpful as antidepressant drugs in treating mild cases of depression, although they take longer than medication to achieve results.

Data from the *2014 Survey on Living with Chronic Diseases in Canada* indicates that 70 percent of Canadians who reported having a mood disorder or anxiety were currently taking prescription medication. Seventy-seven percent of those who were not taking prescription medication at the time of the survey reported that they had done so within the last 12 months.[132] These prescription drugs generally take three or four weeks to produce significant benefits and may not have their full impact for up to eight weeks.

Newer antidepressants that boost levels of the neurotransmitter serotonin have proven equally effective as older medications, but their side effects are different. Patients report higher rates of diarrhea, nausea, insomnia, and headaches.[133] Older drugs are more likely to adversely affect the heart and blood pressure and to cause dry mouth, constipation, dizziness, blurred vision, and tremors. Many people are not aware that the new treatment options may be more effective and tolerable.

Eighty percent of people who have one episode of depression are likely to have another. Because of this high risk of recurrence, many psychiatrists now view depression as a chronic disease and advise ongoing treatment with antidepressants. However, little is known about the long-term effects of these medications.[134] There is also concern about the soaring health costs linked to the widespread prescription of **SSRI (selective serotonin reuptake inhibitor)** antidepressants among Canadians. SSRIs are a special class of compounds used as antidepressants in the treatment of depression, anxiety disorders, and some personality disorders. Janet Currie, in a report about the marketization of depression, reports that Canadians spend billions of dollars on prescription drugs.[135] She wonders why non-drug therapies such as exercise, psychotherapy, and nutrition changes are not being marketed as aggressively.

Paul Andrews, an evolutionary biologist working at McMaster University, found that although antidepressants do relieve the symptoms of depression, risks might include increased digestive problems, problems with sexual stimulation, developmental problems in infants, abnormal bleeding, and stroke and death in the elderly. Antidepressants might also trigger more severe depressive episodes when they are discontinued. Andrews does suggest, however, that when people are undergoing certain types of therapy for diseases such as cancer or recovering from a stroke, the use of antidepressants might be helpful.[136]

For individuals who cannot take antidepressant medications because of medical problems, or who do not improve with psychotherapy or drugs, *electroconvulsive therapy* (ECT)—the administration of a controlled electrical current through electrodes attached to the scalp—remains the safest and most effective treatment. About 50 percent of depressed individuals who do not get better with antidepressant medication and psychotherapy improve after ECT. This type of therapy is still considered controversial by some medical professionals.

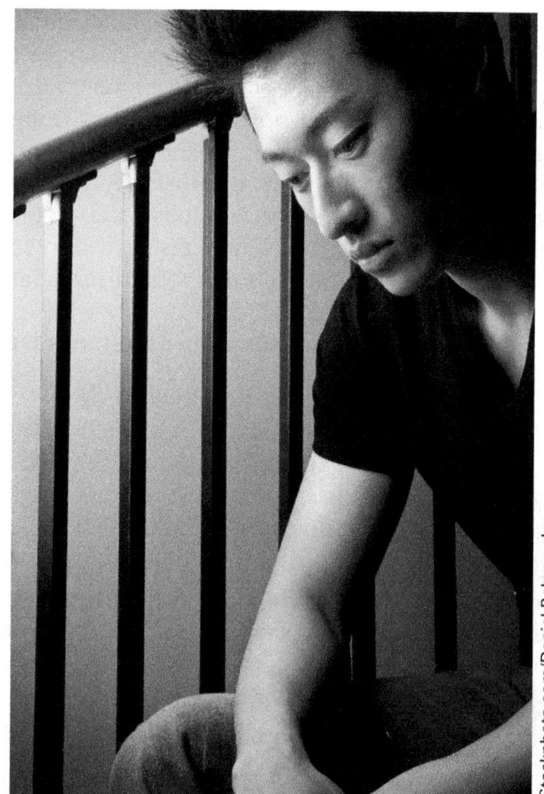
iStockphoto.com/Daniel Bobrowsky

A number of factors can contribute to the development of depression during your college or university years, including stressful events, poor academic performance, loneliness, and relationship problems.

As mentioned above, for some people exercise can be an alternative or an additional support to the use of antidepressants. A study by Dunn et al. found that participation in aerobic exercise for 30 minutes three to five times a week dramatically reduced the symptoms of mild to moderate depression.[137] Due to ongoing research showing that exercise can be a successful individual or support therapy, the American Psychiatric Association has included exercise in their current treatment guidelines.[138]

✓ CHECK-IN

Have you ever experienced symptoms of depression?

Bipolar Disorder (Manic Depression) **Bipolar disorder**, or manic depression, consists of mood swings that may take individuals from *manic* states of feeling euphoric and energetic to *depressive* states of utter despair. In episodes of full mania, they may become so impulsive and out of touch with reality that they endanger their careers, relationships, health, or even survival. One percent of the Canadian population suffers from this serious but treatable disorder, which affects both sexes and all races. For bipolar disorder, it is generally accepted that the ratio between men and women is approximately equal.[139] However, research also shows that women are hospitalized for bipolar disorder at significantly higher rates than men.[140]

The characteristic symptoms of bipolar disorder include

- mood swings (from happy to miserable, optimistic to despairing);
- changes in thinking (thoughts speeding through one's mind, unrealistic self-confidence, difficulty concentrating, delusions, hallucinations);
- changes in behaviour (sudden immersion in plans and projects, talking very rapidly and much more than usual, excessive spending, impaired judgment, impulsive sexual involvement); and
- changes in physical condition (less need for sleep, increased energy, fewer health complaints than usual).

During manic periods, individuals may make grandiose plans or take dangerous risks. But they often plunge from a high to a low depressive episode, during which they may feel sad, hopeless, and helpless and develop other symptoms of major depression. The risk of suicide is very real.

Professional therapy is essential in treating bipolar disorders. Mood-stabilizing medications are the cornerstone of treatment, although psychotherapy plays a critical role in helping individuals understand their illness and rebuild their lives. Most individuals continue taking medication indefinitely after remission of their symptoms because the risk of recurrence is high.

Premenstrual Issues **Premenstrual syndrome (PMS)** and **premenstrual dysphoric disorder (PMDD)** refer to a wide range of physical and emotional symptoms that affect a woman about 5–11 days before she begins her monthly menstrual cycle. Physical symptoms can include bloating of the abdomen, breast tenderness, headache, fatigue, and less tolerance for noise and lights. Emotional symptoms can include feelings of sadness, anxiety, poor self-image, or tension. Behavioural changes can include irritability, hostility, and outbursts of anger toward others. Women suffering from PMDD experience more severe symptoms than those of PMS and they can become debilitated with anxiety issues or major depression.

The exact cause of PMS or PMDD is not known; however, it has been suggested that changes in the brain hormone levels may be one cause, while social, cultural, biological, and psychological factors may also be contributing factors. PMS and PMDD are now included in the American Psychiatric Association's *Diagnostic and Statistical Manual of Mental Disorders*, fifth edition (DSM-5).[141] The addition of this syndrome and disorder has been controversial. Some women appear to function with PMS, but some women cannot function well when struggling with PMDD. Other women develop very severe symptoms of PMS, but are not clinically diagnosed with PMDD. Further information on PMS and PMDD can be found in Chapter 7.

Seasonal Affective Disorder (SAD) **Seasonal affective disorder (SAD)** is a condition that affects 1 to 3 percent of the Canadian population. Compared to clinical depression, where people have severe bouts of feeling down all of the time, low energy, problems with sleep and appetite, and difficulty functioning at home and at work, people with SAD experience these symptoms only during the fall and winter seasons.[142] According to information from the Canadian Mental Health Association,[143] 13–17 percent of people who are diagnosed with SAD have close family members who had SAD too.

Some research suggests that SAD might result from shorter day lengths, where exposure to sunlight is limited. Treatments for SAD include light therapy or phototherapy. Patients with SAD are exposed to bright, artificial, fluorescent light for as little as 30 minutes a day. Use of these special light boxes has resulted in significant improvements in 60–80 percent of SAD patients.[144]

People may experience nausea, headaches, or eye strain when they first begin their treatment. There are no known long-term harmful effects of light therapy, but people with medical conditions such as retinal disease or diabetes should check with their eye doctor before beginning light therapy. People with bipolar disorder should also check with their family physician. Other treatments for SAD include antidepressant medications, counselling, and spending more time outdoors during the winter months.

Schizophrenia

Schizophrenia, one of the most debilitating mental disorders, profoundly impairs an individual's sense of reality. It is characterized by abnormalities in brain structure and chemistry and affects every aspect of psychological functioning, including the ways in which people think, feel, view themselves, and relate to others. According to the American Psychiatric Association *Diagnostic and Statistical Manual of Mental Disorders* (DSM-5),[145] diagnosis of schizophrenia must include at least one of the following three symptoms—disorganized speech, hallucinations, and delusions.

The symptoms of schizophrenia include

- hallucinations—seeing or hearing things that do not exist;
- delusions—false or irrational beliefs;
- inability to think in a logical manner;
- talking in rambling or incoherent ways;
- making odd or purposeless movements or not moving at all;

- repeating others' words or mimicking their gestures;
- showing few, if any, feelings; responding with inappropriate emotions;
- lacking will or motivation to complete a task or accomplish something; and
- functioning at a much lower level than in the past at work, in interpersonal relations, or in self-care.

Schizophrenia affects 1 percent of the Canadian population. Fifty-two percent of hospitalizations for schizophrenia in general hospitals are among adults 25–44 years of age. Current research shows that hospitalization rates for schizophrenia in general hospitals are increasing among young and middle-aged men.[146]

Schizophrenia has a profound effect on an individual's ability to function effectively in all aspects of life. This includes self-care, family relationships, income, school, employment, housing, community, and social life.[147] Researchers have identified early markers of schizophrenia, including impaired social skills, intellectual ability, and capacity for organization.

Schizophrenia might be the result of a failure in brain development that occurs very early in life. The underlying defect is probably present before birth. Schizophrenia has a strong genetic basis and is not the result of upbringing, social conditions, or traumatic experiences.[148] Current research is also showing links between adolescence use of cannabis and a high frequency of cannabis use with an increased risk for schizophrenia.[149]

Minimizing the impact of this serious illness depends mainly on early diagnosis and appropriate treatment and support. A comprehensive treatment program includes antipsychotic medication, education, family support, rehabilitation, cognitive therapy, and integrated addictions programs.

Suicide Suicide (taking one's own life), while not a psychiatric disorder, is often the tragic consequence of emotional and psychological problems. It usually marks the end of a long road of hopelessness, helplessness, and despair. According to the World Health Organization (WHO), approximately 804 000 people died of suicide globally in 2012. This estimation may not be accurate, though, because in many countries suicide deaths are not be reported or counted. In middle- and low-income countries, the ratio of men to women dying of suicide is approximately 1.5–1. This ratio in richer countries is 3–1. For young people aged 15–29, suicide is the second-leading cause of death.[150]

In Canada, 3926 people died from suicide in 2012. Suicide was ranked as the ninth-leading cause of death. Three provinces—Ontario, Prince Edward Island, and the Yukon—had the lowest average suicide rates between 2009 and 2011. Suicides in Nunavut were six times higher than the Canadian average (see Figure 2-3). Research shows that males are three times more likely to die by suicide attempts than females. However, women are 3–4 times more likely to attempt suicide and find themselves hospitalized 1.5 times more often than males. Females are inclined to use less deadly methods when they do attempt suicide.[151]

Concern about Aboriginal youth suicide is also rising. Suicide happens approximately five to six times more among Canadian Aboriginal youth than non-Aboriginal youth. For First Nations youth and adults up to 44 years of age, suicide and other self-inflicted injuries are the leading causes of death.[152]

What Leads to Suicide? Researchers have looked for explanations for suicide yet they have found no conclusive answers. Many influences—mental disorders, personality traits, biologic and genetic vulnerability, medical illness, and psychosocial stressors—can combine in ways that lower an individual's threshold of vulnerability. School pressures, social difficulties, confusion about sexual orientation, family problems, and

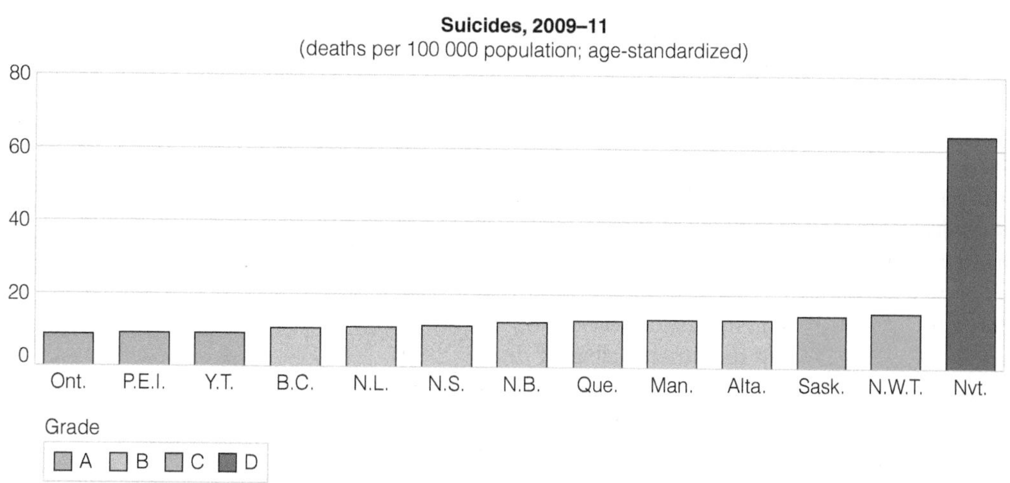

Figure 2-3 **Suicides, Provincial and Territorial Rankings between 2009 and 2011—Deaths per 100 000 Population, Age-standardized**

Source: Statistics Canada, Conference Board of Canada. http://www.conferenceboard.ca/hcp/provincial/health/suicide.aspx.

drug and alcohol use and abuse may also be contributors. The risk of suicide is higher in people who live in cities, are single, have a low income, or are unemployed.[153] No one factor in itself may ever explain fully why a person chooses death.

Some specific factors believed to be linked to suicide are listed here:

- More than 95 percent of those who commit suicide have a mental disorder.
- Many of those who commit suicide drink beforehand and their use of alcohol may lower their inhibitions. Since alcohol itself is a depressant, it can intensify the despondency suicidal individuals are already feeling.
- Drug abuse also can alter thinking and lower inhibitions against suicide.
- Hopelessness and helplessness may be the most common contributing factors in suicide. When hope dies, individuals expect the worst possible outcomes for their problems.
- Investigators have found abnormalities in the brain chemistry of those who complete suicide, especially low levels of a metabolite of the neurotransmitter serotonin. There are indications that individuals with a deficiency of this substance may have as much as a ten times greater risk of committing suicide than those with higher levels.
- Access to guns can add to the risk of suicide.
- Major life crises such as job changes, births, financial reversals, divorce, and recent retirement can increase the risk of suicide.
- Longstanding, intense conflict with family members or other significant people may add to the danger.

Suicide rates among women show three peaks: the late teens (15–19 years), in middle age (45–59 years), and among older seniors (80–84 years). For men, mortality rates rise dramatically in the late teens (15–19 years) and early twenties (20–24 years). They continue to be high until middle age (40–44 years) when they start to decrease.[154]

STRATEGIES FOR PREVENTION

If You Start Thinking about Suicide

- *Talk to a mental health professional.* Counselling is available on all college and university campuses. Make an appointment immediately. Another option—call a suicide hotline.
- *Find someone you trust and can talk with honestly about how you are feeling.* If you suffer from depression or another mental disorder, educate trusted friends or relatives about your condition so they are prepared if called upon to help.
- *Avoid drugs and alcohol.* Most suicides are the result of sudden, uncontrolled impulses, and drugs and alcohol can make it harder to resist these destructive urges.
- *Go to the hospital.* Hospitalization can sometimes be the best way to protect your health and safety.

IF SOMEONE YOU KNOW STARTS THINKING ABOUT SUICIDE

- *Encourage your friend to talk.* Ask concerned questions. Listen attentively. Show that you take the person's feelings seriously and truly care.
- *Don't offer trite reassurances.* List reasons to go on living.
- *Suggest alternative solutions to problems.* Encourage positive action, such as getting away for a while to gain a better perspective on a problem.
- *Don't think that people who talk about killing themselves never carry out their threats.* Most individuals who commit suicide give definite indications of their intent to die.

Where Can I Turn for Help? As a student, your best source for identifying local services may be your college or university's health unit. Medical personnel can tell you about general and mental health counselling available on campus or at school-based support groups, community-based programs, and special emergency services.

You can also access an important document released by the Canadian Mental Health Association in 2004 called *Your Education—Your Future, A Guide to College and University for Students with Psychiatric Disabilities.*[155] This resource focuses on particular aspects of college and university experience and how students who are faced with mood disorders and mental illness can improve their level of self-care while studying at an academic institution. The full report is available online at www.cmha.ca/youreducation. The report includes information about how students can ask for advice on arranging academic accommodations, work out emergency plans, and engage others in advocating on their behalf.

Within the community, you may find help through community mental health centres and local hospitals. You can call the psychiatric or psychological association in your city or province for the names of licensed professionals. Your family doctor may also be able to help.

Types of Therapists Only professionally trained individuals who have met federal or provincial licensing requirements are certified as psychiatrists, psychologists, psychoanalysts, social workers, psychiatric nurses, and marriage and family therapists. Before selecting any of these mental health professionals, be sure to check the person's background and credentials.

- **Psychiatrists** are licensed medical doctors (M.D.) who have training in various forms of psychotherapy and psychopharmacology. They can prescribe medication.

- **Psychologists** have completed a university graduate degree program and required licensing. They cannot prescribe medication.
- **Psychoanalysts** are either psychiatrists or psychologists who have taken special training in psychoanalysis. They assist clients in overcoming past traumas.

Certification or licensing depends on the province.

Other therapists include pastoral counsellors, social workers, stress-management counsellors, and alcohol and drug counsellors.

Options for Treatment The term **psychotherapy** refers to any type of counselling based on the exchange of words, guided imagery, or healing work in the context of the unique relationship that develops between a mental health professional and a person seeking help.

Psychodynamic Psychotherapy **Psychodynamic psychotherapy** takes into account the role of early experiences and unconscious influences in *actively* shaping behaviour. Psychodynamic treatments work toward the goal of providing greater insight into problems and bringing about behavioural change. According to current thinking, psychotherapy can actually rewire the network of neurons within the brain in ways that ease distress and improve functioning in many areas of daily life.

Psychoneuroimmunology is a branch of medicine that acknowledges the interactions between psychological factors, our central nervous system, and our immune function that is regulated by our neuroendocrine system. The techniques used to assist individuals dealing with stress and mental health issues include mind–body interventions such as meditation, guided visual imagery, and therapeutic touch. Professionals that work in this area come from many cross-disciplines such as medical doctors and nurses, naturopaths, osteopaths, Chinese medicine doctors, chiropractors, as well as psychiatrists and psychologists.

Interpersonal Therapy **Interpersonal therapy (IPT)** focuses on relationships in order to help individuals deal with unrecognized feelings and needs and improve their communication skills. IPT concentrates on the current problems of getting along with others.

Cognitive-Behavioural Therapy **Cognitive-behavioural therapy (CBT)** focuses on inappropriate or inaccurate thoughts or beliefs to help individuals break out of a distorted way of thinking. The techniques of CBT include identification of an individual's beliefs and attitudes, recognition of negative thought patterns, and education in alternative ways of thinking. Individuals with major depression or anxiety disorders are most likely to benefit.

Behaviour therapy strives to substitute healthier ways of behaving for maladaptive patterns used in the past. Its premise is that distressing psychological symptoms are learned responses that can be modified or unlearned.

Psychiatric Drug Therapy **Psychiatric drugs** that alter brain chemistry and relieve psychiatric symptoms have brought hope and help to millions of people. Often used in conjunction with psychotherapy and sometimes used as the primary treatment, these medications have revolutionized mental health care.

When taken appropriately, psychiatric agents can alleviate tremendous suffering and reduce the financial and personal costs of mental illness by lessening the need for hospitalization and by restoring an individual's ability to function normally, to work, and to contribute to society. But they do have side effects and must be used with care.

✓ CHECK-IN

Where would you turn if you wanted help with a psychological issue?

Alternative Mind-Mood Medicine Increasingly consumers are trying natural products, such as herbs and enzymes that claim to have psychological effects. Because they are not classified as drugs, many of these products have not undergone the rigorous scientific testing required of psychiatric medications, and some medical professionals are concerned that little is known about their safety or efficacy. Health Canada has put a regulatory framework into place that now oversees regulations for all natural health products. A more in-depth discussion about these regulations can be found in Chapter 13. It is important to remember that "natural" doesn't necessarily mean risk-free. However, there is an increasing number of Canadians that indicate herbs and enzymes have been very helpful in their attempts to deal with mental health issues.

One example of a herb used to help treat depression is St. John's wort (named after St. John the Baptist because the yellow flowers of the Hypericum perforatum plant bloom in June, the month of his execution). It has been used to treat anxiety and depression in Europe for many years. Although more than 24 clinical trials have investigated St. John's wort, many researchers feel that most had significant flaws in design.[156] *Recent research does suggest that St. John's Wort can interfere with certain prescription drugs and important medicines such as antidepressants, blood thinners, birth control pills, heart medicines, and HIV drugs.*[157] *Some side effects include dizziness, abdominal pain and bloating, constipation, nausea, fatigue, and dry mouth.*

SELF-SURVEY

Recognizing Depression

Depression comes in different forms, just like other illnesses such as heart disease. Not everyone with a depressive disorder experiences every symptom. The number and severity of symptoms may vary among individuals and also over time.

Read through the following list, and check all the descriptions that apply to you.

- ☐ I am often restless and irritable.
- ☐ I am having irregular sleep patterns—either too much or not enough.
- ☐ I don't enjoy hobbies, my friends, family, or leisure activities any more.
- ☐ I am having trouble managing my diabetes, hypertension, or other chronic illness.
- ☐ I have nagging aches and pains that do not get better no matter what I do.
- ☐ Specifically, I often experience
  - ☐ digestive problems
  - ☐ headache or backache
  - ☐ vague aches and pains like joint or muscle pains
  - ☐ chest pains
  - ☐ dizziness
- ☐ I have trouble concentrating or making simple decisions.
- ☐ Others have commented on my mood or attitude lately.
- ☐ My weight has changed a considerable amount.
- ☐ I have had several of the symptoms I checked above for more than two weeks.
- ☐ I feel that my functioning in my everyday life (work, family, friends) is suffering because of these problems.
- ☐ I have a family history of depression.
- ☐ I have thought about suicide.

Answers to Self-Survey

Checking several items on this list does not necessarily mean that you have a depressive disorder because many conditions can cause similar symptoms. However, if you have checked a number of items on the list a conversation with your healthcare provider or mental health therapist may be helpful. Even though it can be difficult to talk about certain things, your healthcare provider is knowledgeable, trained, and committed to helping you.

If you can't think of what to say, try these conversation-starters:

"I just don't feel like myself lately."
"My friend (parent/roommate/spouse) thinks I might be depressed."
"I haven't been sleeping well lately."
"Everything seems harder than before."
"Nothing's fun anymore."

If you are diagnosed with depression, remember that it is a common and highly treatable illness with medical causes. Your habits or personality did not cause your depression, and you do not have to face it alone.*

---

*Source: University of Michigan Depression Center, 800-475-MICH, www.med.umich.edu/depression.

Chapter Summary

1. Which statement best describes psychosocial health?
   a. social acceptance, self-acceptance, and interaction with others
   b. physical agility and physical fitness
   c. complex interaction of emotional, mental, social, and spiritual states
   d. firm grasp on reality
2. Which of the following components is encompassed in emotional intelligence?
   a. creativity, sense of humour, scholastic achievement
   b. integrity, honesty, and perseverance
   c. piety and tolerance
   d. the ability and skill to identify, assess, and control your emotions
3. Which of the following activities can be linked to the concept of social responsibility?
   a. participating in a community fundraising event with colleagues through your place of work or in a college or university class
   b. being a regular participant at a party or social gathering
   c. being a regular participant in an Internet chat room
   d. going on a shopping spree
4. Which statement about individuals who have developed a sense of mastery over their lives is true?
   a. They are skilled at controlling the actions of others.
   b. They are usually passive and silent when faced with a situation they don't like.

c. They are aware that their locus of control is internal, not external.
d. They are aware that their locus of control is external, not internal.

5. Which statement best describes a mental disorder?
a. a condition associated with migraine headaches and narcolepsy
b. a condition that is usually caused by severe trauma to the brain
c. a behavioural or psychological disorder that impairs an individual's ability to conduct one or more important activities of daily life
d. a psychological disorder that is easily controlled with medication and a change in diet

6. What is the definition of mental health?
a. four types of emotions: fear, joy, hope, and love
b. a state of emotional and psychological well-being in which an individual is able to use his or her cognitive and emotional capabilities, function in society, and meet the ordinary demands of everyday life*
c. emotional quotient (EQ)
d. the ability to interact with people around us

7. Which statement about anxiety disorders is true?
a. Anxiety disorders are the least prevalent type of mental illness.
b. An individual suffering from a panic attack may mistake her symptoms for a heart attack.
c. The primary symptom of obsessive-compulsive disorder is irrational, intense, and persistent fear of a specific object or situation.
d. Generalized anxiety disorders respond to systematic desensitization behaviour therapy.

8. What are some characteristic symptoms of major depression?
a. difficulty concentrating, lack of energy, and eating more than usual
b. exaggerated sense of euphoria and energy
c. palpitations, sweating, numbness, and tingling sensations
d. talking in rambling ways, inability to think in a logical manner, and delusions

9. In which situation might a person be at higher risk of committing suicide?
a. if he is taking antidepressant medication
b. if he lives in a rural environment and is married
c. if he has been diagnosed with hyperactivity disorder
d. if he has lost his job because of alcoholism

10. Which of the following statements is true?
a. Psychiatric medications do not have any known side effects.
b. Psychiatric medications affect every aspect of a person's physical, mental, and emotional functioning.
c. Psychologists are usually trained in a variety of psychotherapeutic techniques and are licensed to prescribe psychiatric medications.
d. Interpersonal therapy focuses on inappropriate or inaccurate thoughts or beliefs.

Answers to these questions can be found on page 55.

*Source: Copyright © 2016 by houghton Mifflin Harcourt Publishing Company. Adapted and reproduced by permission from *The American Heritage Dictionary of the English Language*, Fifth Edition.

SELF-RESPONSIBILITY—SOCIAL RESPONSIBILITY

SELF-RESPONSIBILITY

When we learn to manage our emotions long enough to stop and shift our attention to the quieter message of the heart, we can gain a wider perspective on any situation, often saving ourselves from hurt, frustration, and pain.

***Doc Childre and Howard Martin,* The HeartMath Solution**

It is not always possible to manage stressful situations with skill, energy, and enthusiasm, but you have to start somewhere. Being responsible for lifestyle choices that enhance your well-being is one step. The other—asking for help when you need it—can assist you in undertaking a challenging goal. Today, ask yourself who might provide support for problems you are facing or future visions you have. This would be an example of moving from preparation to action.

SOCIAL RESPONSIBILITY

When you do nothing, you feel overwhelmed and powerless. But when you get involved, you feel the sense of hope and accomplishment that comes from knowing you are working to make things better.

Unknown

If you have energy and time to help others, find an organization or agency that aligns with your values and do something for someone else. You will be making a difference for others and yourself.

CRITICAL THINKING

1. Would you say that you view life positively or negatively? Would your friends and family agree with your assessment? Ask two of your closest friends for feedback about what they perceive are your typical responses to a problematic situation. Are these indicative of positive attitudes? If not, what could you do to become more psychologically positive?
2. Research has indicated that many homeless men and women are in need of outpatient psychiatric care, often because they suffer from chronic mental illnesses or alcoholism. Presently, in many provinces, health-care dollars are scarce for proper treatment and prevention programs. How do you feel when you pass homeless individuals who seem disoriented or out of touch with reality? Who should take responsibility for their welfare? Should they be forced to undergo treatment at psychiatric institutions?
3. You have been prescribed a psychoactive drug to help alleviate symptoms of a mental disorder. What questions would you ask your family physician or psychiatrist before you begin taking this drug? How could you find out about any reported risks or side effects? How would you know if the medication was working?

WEB LINKS

Canadian Mental Health Association

www.cmha.ca

This site has numerous and current reports on mental illness and mental health as well as links to other sites that provide mental health information.

Canadian Mental Health Association—Your Education Your Future—A Guide to College and University for Students with Psychiatric Disabilities

www.cmha.ca/youreducation

This site provides college and university students with a valuable resource—information gathered from colleges and universities across Canada and from students with psychiatric disabilities. The guide, organized into sections, can help students and families who are interested in finding out more about the rewards and challenges of higher education.

Canadian Psychological Association

www.cpa.ca

From Need a Psychologist? to Psychology Quick Facts and Psychology Works Fact Sheets, you can browse for information about psychology and mental health. There is also information for individuals wanting to discover how to become a psychologist in Canada.

Centre for Addiction and Mental Health (CAMH)

www.camh.net

The Centre for Addiction and Mental Health is Canada's leading addiction and mental health teaching hospital. This site provides you with information about clinical practice, health promotion, education, and research.

Partners for Mental Health: Crisis Centres across Canada

www.partnersformh.ca/resources/find-help/crisis-centres-across-canada/

A national, nonprofit organization dedicated to improving how we all think about, act toward, and treat mental health. Links to numerous agencies and resources are available at this site, including links to crisis centres in your area.

Key Terms

The terms listed here are used within the chapter on the page indicated. Definitions of the terms can be found in the MindTap for An Invitation to Health *at www.nelson.com/student.*

Answers to Chapter Summary Questions

1. c; 2. d; 3. a; 4. c; 5. c; 6. b; 7. b; 8. a; 9. d; 10. b

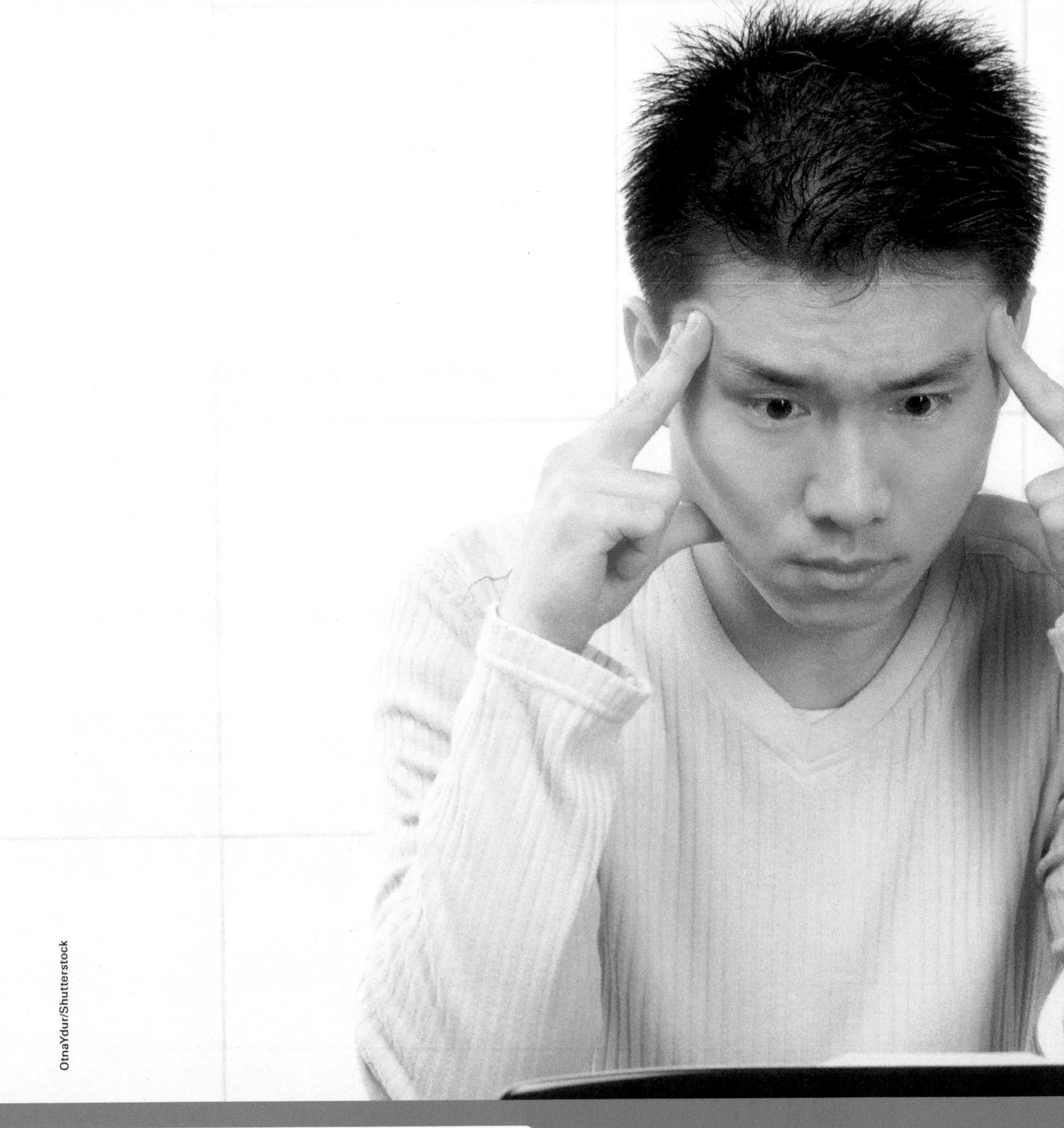

OtnaYdur/Shutterstock

AFTER READING THIS CHAPTER, YOU WILL BE ABLE TO:

- **define** stress and stressors, and **describe** how the body responds to stress according to the general adaptation syndrome (GAS) theory
- **list** the physical changes associated with frequent or severe stress and **discuss** how stress can affect the cardiovascular, immune, and digestive systems
- **explain** how stressful events can affect psychosocial health
- **describe** some personal causes of stress, especially those experienced by students, and **discuss** how their effects can be prevented or minimized
- **discuss** the major societal stressors
- **identify** ways of managing time more efficiently
- **describe** some stress management techniques

3

Personal Stress Management

You know about stress. You live with it every day: the stress of passing exams, preparing for a career, meeting people, facing new experiences. Everyone—regardless of age, gender, race, or income—has to deal with stress, as an individual and as a member of society.

Stress has profound effects, both immediate and long term, on our bodies, our minds, and our spirits. While stress alone doesn't cause disease, it triggers molecular changes throughout the body that make us more susceptible to illness. Its impact on the mind is no less significant. The burden of chronic stress can undermine the ability to cope with day-to-day hassles and can exacerbate psychological problems such as depression and anxiety disorders, which in turn impacts our spirit and prevents us from fully realizing our personal potential.

Yet stress in itself isn't necessarily bad. What matters most is not the stressful situation but an individual's response to it. By learning to anticipate stressful events, to manage day-to-day hassles, and to prevent stress overload, you can find alternatives to running endlessly on a treadmill of alarm, panic, and exhaustion. As you organize your schedule, find ways to release tension, and build up coping skills, you will begin to experience the sense of control and the confidence that make stress a challenge rather than an ordeal.

FREQUENTLY ASKED QUESTIONS

WHAT IS STRESS?

Stress can be defined in a number of ways: "a physical, chemical, or emotional factor that causes bodily or mental tension and may be a factor in disease causation"*[1]; an internal state of arousal; or the physical state of the body to various demands. Dr. Hans Selye, the "Father of Stress Theory" and a pioneer in studying physiological responses to challenge, defined stress as "the non-specific response of the body to any demand made upon it."[2] Dr. Selye, born in Vienna, Austria-Hungary, in 1907, began building his stress research program at McGill University in 1931. He went on to work at the Université de Montréal and was the president and founder of the International Institute of Stress between 1977 and 1982.

When we say that we are "stressed," it usually means that we are reacting to **stressors**—the things that upset or excite us. Stressors can be tangible and include dealing with an angry friend or missing the bus, or intangible and include emotions that arise when we are participating in an athletic competition or challenging ourselves in a new way. Based on many studies over the past 40 years, researchers have distinguished five categories of stressors.

- **Acute time-limited stressors**—Anxiety-provoking situations such as having to give a talk in public.
- **Brief naturalistic stressors**—A more serious challenge such as meeting a deadline for a major student group project.
- **Stressful event sequences**—Difficult consequences of a natural disaster or traumatic occurrence such as a death of a friend or relative. There is a recognition that although stressful at the time, the difficulties will end at some point in the future.
- **Chronic stressors**—Ongoing demands caused by life-changing circumstances, such as a permanent disability caused by an accident or caregiving of a loved one who is dealing with Alzheimers. These stressors do not have any clear end point.
- **Distant stressors**—Traumatic experiences that occurred long ago such as child abuse or work in a war zone. They continue to have emotional and psychological impact.

Not all stressors are negative. Some of life's happiest moments—births, reunions, weddings—are enormously stressful and we weep with the stress of love and joy. Selye coined the term **eustress** for positive stress in our lives (*eu* is a Greek prefix meaning "good"). Eustress challenges us to grow, adapt, and find creative solutions in our lives. He described **distress** as the negative effects of stress that can deplete or even destroy life energy. Ideally, the level of stress in our lives should be just high enough to motivate us to satisfy our needs and not so high that it interferes with our ability to reach our fullest potential. It is important to point out that there are other researchers who suggest that stressors are neither positive nor negative; instead it is our reaction to the stressors that create these labels.

*By permission. From Merriam-Webster's Collegiate® Dictionary, 11th Edition © 2016 by Merriam-Webster, Inc. (www.Merriam-Webster.com).

WHAT CAUSES STRESS?

Of the many biological theories of stress, the best known may be the **general adaptation syndrome (GAS)** (see Figure 3-1), developed by Selye.[3] He discovered that our bodies constantly strive to maintain a stable and consistent physiological state, called **homeostasis.** Stressors, whether in the form of physical illness or a demanding job, disturb this state and trigger a non-specific physiological response. The body attempts to restore homeostasis by means of an **adaptive response.**

Selye's GAS, which describes the body's response to a stressor—whether threatening or exhilarating—consists of three distinct stages:

1. *Alarm.* When a stressor first occurs, the body responds with changes that temporarily lower resistance. Levels of certain hormones may rise; blood pressure and heart rate may increase. The body quickly makes internal adjustments to cope with the stressor and attempts to return to normal activity.

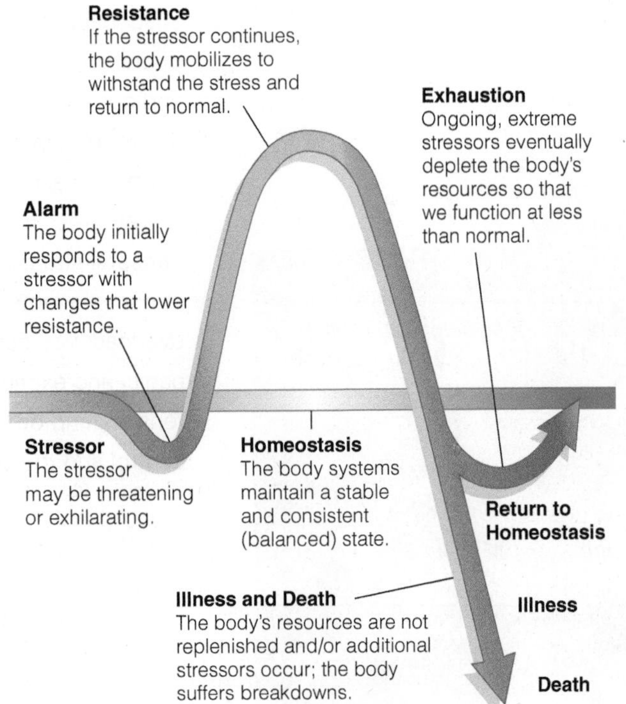

Figure 3-1 General Adaptation Syndrome (GAS)
The three stages of Hans Selye's GAS are alarm, resistance, and exhaustion.

2. *Resistance.* If the stressor continues, the body mobilizes its internal resources to try to sustain homeostasis. For example, if someone you love is seriously hurt in an accident, you initially respond intensely and feel great anxiety. During the subsequent stressful period of recuperation, you struggle to carry on as normally as possible, but this requires considerable effort.
3. *Exhaustion.* If the stress continues long enough, you usually cannot keep up your normal functioning. Even a small amount of additional stress at this point can cause a breakdown.

Among the many non-biological theories is the **cognitive-transactional model of stress and coping,** developed by Richard Lazarus and Susan Folkman,[4] which looks at the relation between stress and health. Psychological stress, according to Lazarus, is a relationship between a person and his or her environment and the power to deal with the demands of that relationship without unreasonable or destructive costs."[5] The model suggests that an event will (1) trigger a *primary appraisal process* where an individual will perceive the event as a threat or a challenge, then; (2) a *secondary appraisal process* will take over and a comprehensive assessment of both the person's ability to manage the threat or the challenge and their coping resources will occur, then; (3) *coping responses* will be initiated and the stress outcomes of the event will depend on the effectiveness of the cognitive appraisal and the person's coping process, then; (4) the stress outcomes will *feed back* into the cognitive appraisal stage if more needs to be done to resolve the situation.

Folkman and Lazarus also discovered that a form of coping such as *planful problem solving* may have a healthy effect on the emotion response whereas *confrontive coping and distancing* may make things worse, at least in some populations and in some contexts.[6] So, an event may be stressful for one person but not for another, or it may seem stressful on one occasion but not on another. For instance, one student may think of speaking in front of the class as extremely stressful, while another relishes the chance to do so.

Stress experts Thomas Holmes, M.D., and Richard Rahe, M.D., devised a scale to evaluate individual levels of stress and potential for coping based on life-change units that estimate each change's impact. People who accumulate more than 300 life-change units in a year are more likely to suffer serious health problems. It is important to remember, though, that scores on the scale represent "potential stress"; the actual impact of the life change depends on your own response (see Self-Survey: "Student Stress Scale," at the end of the chapter).

IS STRESS HAZARDOUS TO PHYSICAL HEALTH?

These days we've grown accustomed to warning labels advising us of the health risks of substances such as alcohol and cigarettes. Medical researchers speculate that another component of 21st century living also warrants another warning label: stress.[7] In recent years, hundreds of studies have shown that stress contributes to approximately 80 percent of all major illnesses: cardiovascular disease, cancer, endocrine and metabolic disease, skin rashes, ulcers, ulcerative colitis, emotional disorders, musculoskeletal disease, infectious ailments, premenstrual syndrome (PMS), uterine fibroid cysts, and breast cysts. It has specifically been linked in a negative way to our immune system, our heart, and our digestive system.

Stress and the Immune System There is a special science called **psychoneuroimmunology (PNI)** that focuses on the relationship between our brain's response to stress and our immune system. Stress triggers complex changes in the body's endocrine, or hormone-secreting, system. It is not the intent in this chapter to provide a detailed biology lesson on the immune system; however, a brief overview will help to show how stress affects us.

When our brain takes note, either consciously or subconsciously, of some sort of stressor, it prepares our body for "fight or flight." This response gets us ready for quick action. The emotional response stimulates the **autonomic nervous system (ANS)**[8] response, which starts in a region of the brain called the cerebral cortex. The ANS is part of the central nervous system and regulates the functions of some of our internal organs such as the heart, stomach, and intestines, and some muscles and glands.

The ANS is comprised of two separate branches. One is the **sympathetic nervous system (SNS)**, which initiates the release of stress hormones that increase our heart rate and respiratory rate—basically speeding everything up. The **hypothalamus**, a section of the brain that acts as our control centre, reacts to stress hormones that have been released by the SNS. In turn, the hypothalamus stimulates the adrenal glands, releasing a hormone called **epinephrine**, which is also known as adrenaline. Epinephrine initiates an increase in blood flow, which causes dilation in the air sacs in the lungs, known as alveoli. This allows for more oxygen to be taken in and a rise in breathing rate. There is also a release of more glucose from the liver that helps to increase muscle contractions.[9]

At the same time, blood begins to be diverted away from the digestive system as a way of saving energy. The hypothalamus also triggers the pituitary gland to release another hormone called **adrenocorticotrophic hormone (ACTH)**. This hormone tells the adrenal glands that they need to release **cortisol**, which is the hormone that helps to release nutrients the body has stored for energy. Other parts of the body release endorphins which help with pain relief.

The other branch of the ANS is the **parasympathetic nervous system (PNS)**,[10] which slows down other systems that were stimulated by the stress response. The main job of the PNS is to restore homeostasis. Though it appears that these two systems are working in opposition to each other, they are actually attempting to help us stay in a state of equilibrium. This is the way our bodies were made to work.

Some researchers who study in the area of psychoneuroimmunology have determined that when our adrenal hormones, of which cortisol is one, stay at high levels for long periods of time, the white blood cells (T cells) in our body lose their ability to keep us healthy. Not all research has found this to be true, but many studies have suggested that when the stress response stays on, with no time to adapt or return to a normal level of functioning, our immune system becomes compromised.

Dr. Gabor Maté, a Canadian physician, has found that even people who have calm, rational "exteriors" but deny their own feelings and needs over a long period of time just to please others tend to have compromised immune systems.[11] In his book, *When the Body Says No: The Cost of Hidden Stress*, he shares stories of his patients who have been on "red alert" for years ignoring or suppressing legitimate feelings. He believes that when we do not address our emotional issues our stress response stays on. The result—our immune system becomes confused and starts attacking itself.

Even minor hassles take a toll. Lazarus has shown that the daily hassles a person experiences can be more harmful to our health than significant life changes. He believes that these daily events are damaging to our health because of how frequently they occur.[12]

Figure 3-2 illustrates how persistent or repeated increases in stress hormones can be hazardous throughout the body. Very prolonged or severe stress can damage the brain's ability to remember and can actually cause brain cells, or neurons, to atrophy and die.

Research has shown that traumatic stress, such as losing a loved one through death or divorce, can impair immunity for as long as a year or longer.

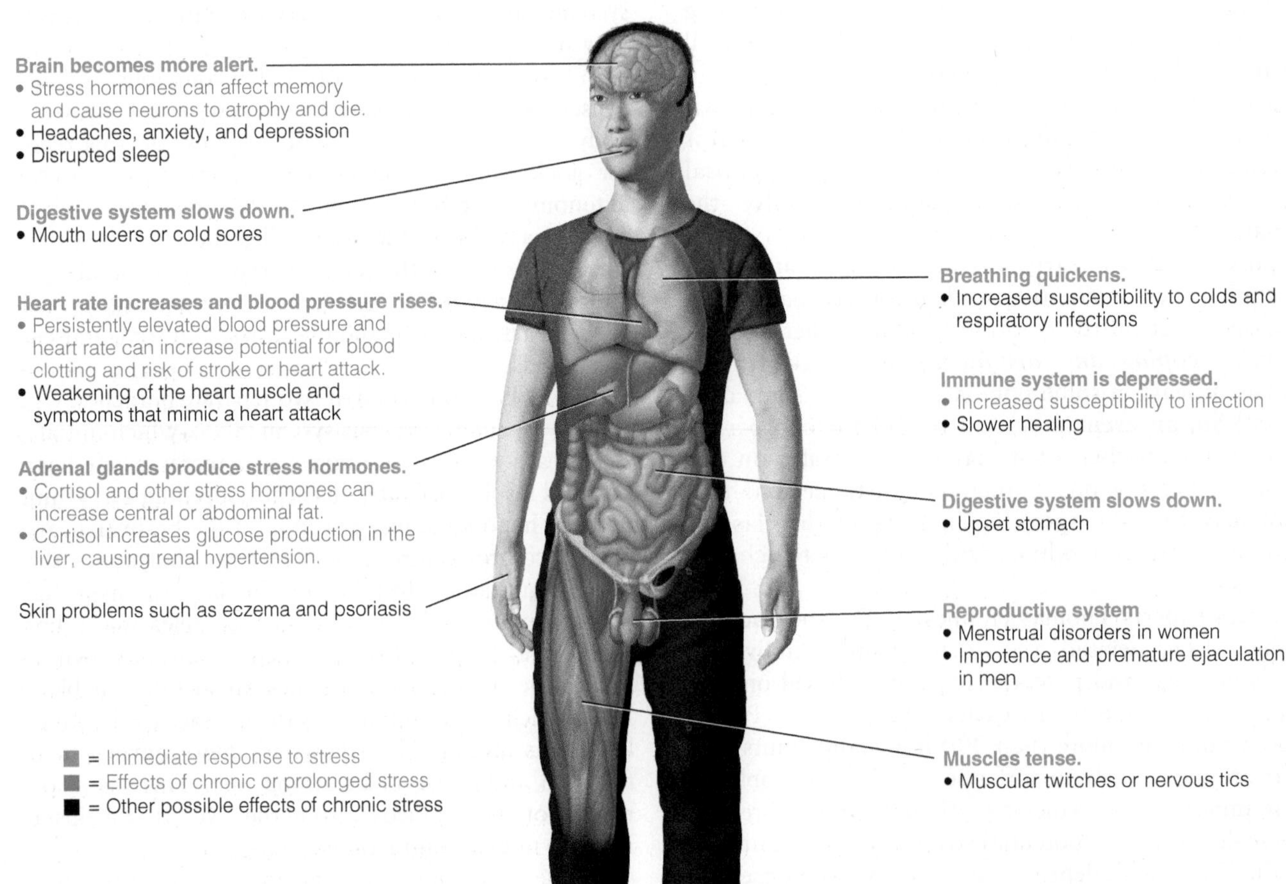

Figure 3-2 Effects of Stress on the Body

Stress and the Heart The links between stress, behaviour, and the heart are complex. One way in which stress increases the risk of heart attack and other cardiovascular problems is the link to negative lifestyle choices. In a study that followed about 6500 men and women for seven years, those with the highest stress levels smoked more and exercised less and had a 50 percent higher rate of heart attacks, strokes, and bypass surgeries.[13] Stress may also be the most significant inherited risk factor in people who develop heart disease at a young age. Family transmission of emotional and psychological stress, specifically anger in young males, greatly increases the likelihood of early heart disease. Young adults whose blood pressure spikes in response to stress may also be at risk of hypertension as they get older.

In the 1970s, cardiologists Meyer Friedman and Ray Rosenman suggested that excess stress could be the most important factor in the development of heart disease. They compared their patients to individuals of the same age with healthy hearts and developed two general categories: Type A and Type B.

Hardworking, aggressive, and competitive, Type As never have time for all they want to accomplish, even though they usually try to do several tasks at once. Type Bs are more relaxed, though not necessarily less ambitious or successful. The degree of danger associated with Type A behaviour remains controversial, as further studies over the past 30 years resulted in both support for and contradiction to Friedman and Rosenman's findings. However, of all the personality traits linked with Type A behaviour, the one that has emerged as the most sinister is chronic hostility or cynicism. People who are always mistrustful, angry, and suspicious are twice as likely to suffer blockages of their coronary arteries. Friedman and fellow researchers[14] also found that altering Type A behaviour, within a controlled experimental design, did reduce cardiac morbidity and mortality in post–myocardial infarction (heart attack) patients.

A major global study, led by Canadian researchers, on the effect of modifiable risk factors associated with myocardial infarction, found that the majority of these attacks may be predicted by nine easily measured risk factors. While the two most important factors were cigarette smoking and abnormal ratio of blood lipids, which together predicted two-thirds of the global risk of heart attacks, other important risk factors in men and women included hypertension, along with psychosocial factors, abdominal obesity, and diabetes.[15]

Stress and the Digestive System Eating on the run, gulping food, or overeating under stress can result in poorly chewed foods, an overworked stomach, and increased abdominal pressure. These habits can lead to stress-related problems. Reaching for sugary snacks to calm your nerves or comfort yourself will send your blood sugar levels on a roller-coaster ride—up one minute and down the next. Coffee, tea, and cola drinks can make your strained nerves jangle even more.

By drinking plenty of water, you replenish lost fluids and prevent dehydration. Fibre-rich foods counteract common stress-related problems, such as cramps and constipation. A regular intake of protein and complex carbohydrates is important, especially in times of stress. Try not to skip meals. If you do, you're more likely to feel fatigued and irritable. You will find more in-depth information about healthy food choices in Chapters 5 and 6.

As mentioned, when you confront a stressor, your body responds by producing stress hormones such as cortisol. This speeds up the conversion of proteins and fats into carbohydrates, the body's basic fuel, so that we have the energy to fight or flee from a threat. This can be a good thing. However, increased amounts of cortisol can also trigger the release of more free fatty acids, or disassembled triglycerides, into the blood. This can then cause excessive central or abdominal fat, deep abdominal obesity, and suppression of the immune system,[16] all which heighten the risk of diseases such as diabetes, high blood pressure, and stroke.[17] Even slender, premenopausal women faced with increased stress and lacking good coping skills are more likely to accumulate excess weight around their waists, thereby increasing their risk of heart disease and other health problems.[18]

IS STRESS HAZARDOUS TO PSYCHOSOCIAL HEALTH?

There has been much debate over the years about the impact of stress on our psychosocial health. Everyone experiences stress. Stress is a normal, everyday experience and within acceptable limits can play a positive role in our lives. Yet there is a difference between everyday stress that has us coping with work demands, family responsibilities, and even playful activities and stress that becomes so great our coping mechanisms begin breaking down.

Social health can be impacted. Your relationship with your family, friends, co-workers, and loved ones affect and are affected by the stress in your life. As described in Chapter 2, social support has proven effective in easing stress, loneliness, and depression in college students. Stress can impact our spiritual health—our search to identify our basic purpose in life and to experience the fulfillment of achieving our maximum potential. But your spirit, when nurtured, can help you both resist and recover from stress.

Even mild stressors can interfere with your intellectual health—the brain's functioning—by impairing sleep, dampening creativity, disrupting concentration and memory, and undermining your ability to make good choices and decisions. Our personal health is also influenced by environmental health and wellness. External forces such as pollution, noise, natural disasters, exposure to toxic chemicals, and threats to your safety can cause or intensify stress in your life.

Stress becomes distress when symptoms such as moodiness, irritability, depression, and anxiety become an everyday occurrence. Some people describe their distress as a feeling of paralysis or numbness. Incapacitating fears can create an imbalance in all the psychosocial dimensions.[19]

Usually intense feelings and behaviours based on fear subside with time. The stressful event fades into the past, and those whose lives it has touched adapt to its lasting impact. But sometimes individuals remain extremely distressed and unable to function as they once did. While the majority of individuals who survive a trauma recover, about 12 percent of the population suffers from **post-traumatic stress disorder (PTSD)** and later develops serious symptoms such as depression, anxiety, and panic attacks.[20]

✓ CHECK-IN

How does stress affect the various dimensions of your health?

TYPES OF STRESSORS

Student Stress Being a student—full time or part time, at any age—can be extremely stressful. You may feel pressure to perform well to qualify for a good job or graduate school. To meet tuition payments, you may have to juggle part-time work and coursework or apply for student loans. You may feel stressed about choosing a major, getting along with a difficult roommate, passing a particularly hard course, or living up to your parents' and instructors' expectations. If you're an older student, you may have children, housework, homework, a job, and eldercare to balance. Your days may seem so busy and your life so full that you worry about coming apart at the seams. One thing is for certain: you're not alone. Stress levels among college and university students have risen, especially among women (see X & Y Files: "Men, Women, and Stress").

Surveys of students at colleges and universities show that stress levels are consistently high and stressors are remarkably similar.[21] Among the most common stressors are the following:

- test pressures
- academic failure
- financial problems
- problems in friendships and dating relationships
- daily hassles
- pressures as a result of competition, deadlines, and the like
- losses, whether caused by the breakup of a relationship or the death of a loved one

In one Canadian study,[22] researchers found that medical students were stressed because of the need to learn a large quantity of new information, time pressure, loss of opportunities for social activities, and going into debt. Another important finding was the discovery that the medical students who previously did very well academically compared to their peers sometimes found themselves to be in the average category when compared to their medical-student peers. Academic excellence at an institution of higher learning can be quite different from that in a hometown school and can also cause stress.

Hamaideh[23] found that the highest stressors experienced by students were self-imposed and were related to specific stressors such as a personal desire to compete and win or a need to be noticed by others. The second most common group of stressors was linked to pressures such as grades, work, and relationships with friends. Hamaideh recommends stress management workshops organized specifically for students to address these stressors and help lower student stress.

Another study showed that perceived stress of college and university students can be linked to a number of physical and mental health problems such as depression and social anxiety. This perceived stress could have a negative impact on academic success.[24]

Many students bring complex psychological problems with them to campus, including learning disabilities and mood disorders such as depression and anxiety. Some have grown up in broken homes and bear the scars of family troubles. Others fall into the same patterns of alcohol abuse that they observed for years in their families or suffer lingering emotional scars from childhood physical or sexual abuse. In some First Nations and Inuit communities, young people have dealt with high rates of suicide and grief over multiple losses and disruptions of lifestyle.[25]

Among college and university students, excessive levels of stress have been linked to increased headaches, sleep disturbances, and colds.[26] Students have said that they react to stress physiologically (by sweating, stuttering, trembling, or developing physical symptoms), emotionally (by becoming anxious, fearful, angry, guilty, or depressed), behaviourally (by crying, eating, smoking, or being irritable or abusive), or cognitively (by thinking about and analyzing stressful situations and strategies that might be useful in dealing with them).

Social support, effective time management, forming close friendships, and meditation programs also reduce

X AND Y FILES

Men, Women, and Stress

Women, who make up over half of today's college and university students in Canada, experience greater psychological distress than men. Authors of a study of college students on stress, sex differences, and coping strategies found that female students reported higher levels of overall stress, family responsibilities, social relationships, and daily troubles. They also reported a greater level of stress with regard to finances. In comparison to male students, female students showed a higher use of self-help to cope with their stress levels.[27] Results from another study found that female college students experience greater stress than male college students with regard to the quality of their friendships, their relationship with their parents, and their love relationships.[28]

Lifestyle choices may help explain why women feel so stressed. One survey revealed that men attending college or university spend significantly more time doing things that are fun and relaxing: exercising, partying, watching TV, and playing video games. Women, on the other hand, tend to study more, do more volunteer work, and handle more household and child-care chores.[29]

At all ages, women and men tend to respond to stress differently. While males react with the classic fight-or-flight response, females under attack try to protect their children and seek help from other females—a strategy dubbed *tend-and-befriend*.[30] When working mothers studied by psychologists had a bad day, they coped by concentrating on their children when they got home. Stressed-out fathers were more likely to withdraw.[31]

The difference in stress responses between men and women may be the result of hormones and evolution. While both men and women release stress hormones, men also secrete testosterone, which tends to increase hostility and aggression. For prehistoric women, who were usually pregnant, nursing, or caring for small children, neither fight nor flight was a wise strategy. Smaller and weaker than males, women may long ago have reached out to other women to form a social support system that helped ensure their safety and that of their children.

stress and compensate for the depressive effects of negative experiences, such as failing a test.[32]

Students between the ages of 18 and 25 must also deal with the emerging adulthood stage. Neuroimaging research has revealed that the brain continues to develop throughout the first quarter-century of life. This affects cognition and problem solving. In dealing with daily stressors the brains of students in this age range rely more on the amygdala, a small almond-shaped region in the medial and temporal lobes that processes emotions and memories. This is one reason any stressor—a poor grade or a friend's criticism—feels as intensely upsetting as a major crisis. As we age, the frontal cortex lobe of the brain matures and plays a greater role and helps put challenges into perspective.

It is important to be aware during this transitional developmental period of life that your brain may not always grasp the long-term consequences of your actions. Drugs and alcohol are especially toxic to the developing brain and can limit the maturity of the frontal cortex lobe.

Campuses are providing more frontline services than they have in the past, including career workshops, study skills sessions, and social and recreation programs to help students manage the stress of making the transition from high school or work to college and university life. Brock University offers a number of individual and community programs that enhance student well-being. One example is the Student Health and Wellness HUB, which offers sessions with a Peer Health Educator and a "Walk Station" where students can book a 30-minute session where they can write their essays while they walk.[33] *The University of British Columbia (UBC) has an extensive Live Well, Learn Well Web page that includes a Student Health 101 magazine, health assessments, a Healthy Minds at UBC Facebook page, and a Twitter@UBC account.*[34] *Check out your college or university student services department to see what is available to support your psychosocial health.*

Relationship Stress In addition to academic work and career preparation, many students begin to establish romantic relationships during their time at college and university. While some of these relationships lead to long-term partnerships, others end because of betrayal, differences in expectations, or varying degrees of readiness for commitment. Some students recognize that relationship issues are quite common as young people move from adolescence to young and middle adulthood. They deal with the preoccupation with their emerging relationships, sleepless nights, feelings of excitement or agitation, joyfulness or sadness, and their inability to focus by talking to family and friends, visiting a counsellor,[35] exercising, or praying,[36] and then take steps to move forward and learn from the experience.

However, there is research that shows other students find themselves dealing with **complicated grief**,[37] an intense and extended period of grief that is also often linked to the loss or death of a family member, friend, or acquaintance. Key characteristics include a sense of disbelief, anger and bitterness, recurrent intrusive thoughts, intense yearning, and preoccupation of thoughts of the person they were involved with. Field et al.,[38] in a study of 192 university students who had experienced a recent breakup of a romantic relationship, reported a number of important findings that link to complicated grief:

- Of students who had experienced a previous relationship breakup prior to the study and those who had not, both groups had difficulty controlling intrusive thoughts and scored high on sleep disturbance scales.
- The female students experienced greater breakup distress.
- The most important predictors for higher scores on the Breakup Distress Scale used in the study were the level of feeling betrayed by the breakup, a shorter time since the breakup had occurred, and a higher rating of the relationship prior to the breakup.

In another study done at Bowling Green State University,[39] students also reported depression, signs of post-traumatic stress disorder, avoiding friends or loved ones, and missing work or skipping classes.

If you are a student who is having difficulty dealing with relationship challenges or breakup stress, know that many other students feel the same way and that there are ways to deal with your grief. Interpersonal psychotherapy, complicated grief therapy, counselling, the support of family and friends, and choosing healthy lifestyle choices can help in significant ways. More information on relationships can be found in Chapter 7.

Financial Stress Financing a college or university education can be difficult. Obtaining adequate funding to cover tuition, books, accommodation, and food is a major concern for many students. A 2015 Canadian Federation for Students report states that between 1990 and 2014, tuition fees in Canada increased over 155 percent on average.[40] Students who access student loans graduate with a national average debt of approximately 28 000 dollars.[41]

According to Statistics Canada, approximately 43 percent of college graduates and 50 percent of university graduates depend on government or non-government student loans to help them complete their undergraduate degrees. The non-government loans include assistance from family and private banks.[42] A study done in the United Kingdom found that in addition to academic studies, many students take on part-time work due to financial necessity. The added responsibilities sometimes result in a lower academic performance.[43]

There are things you can do to manage the financial obligations that a postsecondary education demands.

- Take advantage of financial plans, scholarships, and bursary programs.
- Take advantage of your summer vacations. Look for work internship programs that might support your degree.
- Make a budget. Attempt to stick to it or revise when necessary. Start by writing down all your regular monthly expenses and miscellaneous spending. Be honest! Write down your income. Monitor your spending from the beginning of each term. Create an emergency fund. Money spent on alcohol, cigarettes, drugs, eating out, and social events might be better spent on your education.
- Use credit cards wisely.
- Be resourceful. Use coupons. Share food expenses with friends. Shop wisely.
- Make a plan for repayment of student loans before you graduate.
- Be frugal—this is an important part of financial stress management while you are a student.

In an effort to assist students in managing their finances, a team of researchers at a university implemented a financial intervention strategy. One hundred and seventy undergraduate students[44] tracked all of their spending for an entire term. Income from all sources such as scholarships, jobs, and gifts was also tracked. An online money management and tracking system was used for monitoring spending and summarizing expenses and income. About two-thirds of the participants in the study reported that they changed their spending behaviour or maintained spending patterns that complemented their values. All participants indicated that they had a higher level of awareness of their spending habits as a result of the intervention. At other colleges and universities, peer helpers are assisting students who are attempting to get a handle on their finances. Students are beginning to understand the importance of credit history, balancing budgets, compulsive buying habits, and taking responsibility for their spending patterns. Information from Statistics Canada indicates that in 2013, nearly one-third of university graduates with student loans had paid off their debt within three years after graduation.[45]

Test Stress For many students, mid-terms and final exams are the most stressful times of the year. Results of an Ipsos-Reid survey, conducted on Canadian university

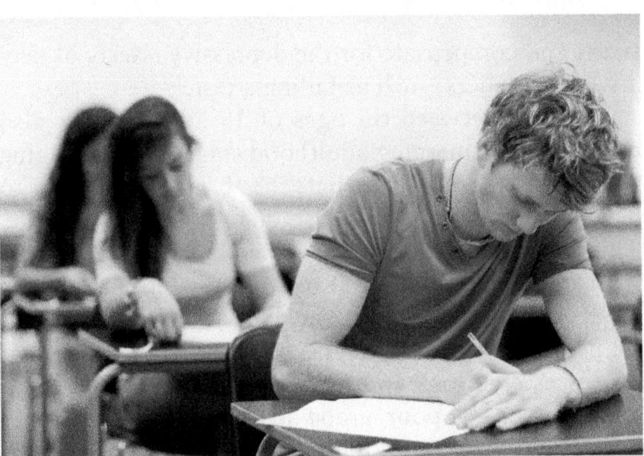

wavebreakmedia ltd/Shutterstock

Tests are acute time-limited stressors that provoke your body's adaptive stress response.

students for Kumon Math and Reading Centres,[46] showed that no students described themselves as free of stress, and 40 percent said they experienced high stress levels when studying for exams. Stress levels were the highest in Saskatchewan and Manitoba at 52 percent, followed by Ontario at 47 percent, and the lowest in Quebec at 27 percent.

Some college and university health services units report that the incidence of colds and flu soar during finals. Some students feel the impact of test stress in other ways—headaches, upset stomachs, skin flare-ups, or insomnia. The university students responding to the Ipsos-Reid survey reported all of these symptoms. Additional examples of exam-related stress ranged from feelings of nervousness and anxiety (29 percent), to difficulty sleeping (27 percent), to fatigue and exhaustion (15 percent). Students also reported having difficulty focusing or concentrating (12 percent), feeling irritable (12 percent), having bad moods (11 percent), and even nausea and vomiting (10 percent).[47] Under exam stress, students can also experience a dip in immune function and a higher rate of infections.

Students most susceptible to exam stress are those who believe they'll do poorly and who see tests as extremely threatening. Negative thoughts often become a self-fulfilling prophecy. As their fear increases, they try harder, pulling all-nighters. Fuelled by caffeine and munching on sugary snacks, they become edgy and find it harder and harder to concentrate. By the time it's test day, they're nervous wrecks, scarcely able to sit still and focus on the exam.

One way to defuse stress is through relaxation programs such as controlled breathing, meditation, mindfulness practice, progressive relaxation, guided imagery (visualization), and yoga. Another way is to learn how to transform stress into resilience. Researchers Steinhardt and Dolbier found that students who participated in a four-week resilience education program had significantly higher resilience scores, more effective coping strategies, higher scores on self-esteem and self-leadership factors, and lower scores on depressive symptoms and perceived stress level in the post-intervention than did the wait-list control group.[48] Another strategy is to begin preparing for mid-terms, finals, and papers early. Sixty-eight percent of students report that they only start studying or preparing for exams at most a week in advance, and another 27 percent admit to staying up all night to prepare.[49]

STRATEGIES FOR PREVENTION

Defusing Test Stress

The following tips might help you beat test stress:

- Get organized and take your time. Establish short- and long-term goals for yourself. Make a study schedule for each course. Set aside a small amount of time every day or every other day to review the course materials.
- Take clear notes. Make your notes work for you. Attend classes. Check for online notes. Complete your assigned readings. Visit with your professor during his or her office hours.
- Maintain a realistic perspective. Consider the bigger picture. How much is your exam worth toward your final mark? Budget your study time well.
- Be positive. Picture yourself taking your final exam. Imagine yourself walking into the exam room feeling confident that you have prepared well.
- Study in 30- to 60-minute intervals. Take 5- to 10-minute breaks regularly. Get up from your desk, breathe deeply, and stretch. Try mini-meditation breaks and deep breathing. You'll feel more refreshed than you would if you drank another cup of coffee.
- Organize a study group with other students. But be sure to study on your own, too.
- Get enough sleep. Your brain will perform better.
- Be satisfied with doing your best. You can't expect to ace every test; all you can and should expect is your best effort.

Other Stressors Centuries ago the poet John Donne observed that no man is an island. Today, on an increasingly crowded and troubled planet, these words seem truer than ever. Problems such as discrimination, environmental disasters, illness and disability, technostress and Internet addiction, and workplace stressors can no longer be viewed only as economic or political issues. Directly or indirectly, they affect the well-being of all of us—now and in the future.

Discrimination Discrimination is a form of a societal stressor. It can take many forms—some as subtle as not being included in a conversation, some as blatant as threats scrawled on a wall, and some as violent as brutal beatings and other hate crimes. Because it can be hard to deal with individually, discrimination is a particularly sinister form of stress. By working together we can challenge the ignorance and hateful assumptions that fuel bigotry, and promote a healthier environment for all.

In the last decade, there have been continued reports of intolerance among young people and a greater tolerance for overt expressions and acts of hatred on college and university campuses. In a recent study by Jewell and Morrison,[50] students at a mid-sized Canadian university were assessed on the frequency and types of negative behaviours directed toward gay men. Results show that discrimination is still apparent. Homonegative behaviour that included telling anti-gay jokes and spreading gossip about gay males functioned as a way to indirectly denigrate gay male students. The researchers also discovered that anti-gay behaviour reinforced traditional male roles and helped to lessen aggressors' feelings of discomfort when in close proximity to gay males.

In another study, researchers found that classroom interventions on college and university campuses must be supported by experiential learning outside the classroom. Brief exposure to gay, bisexual, lesbian, and transgendered issues in the classroom was not sufficient to help some students change homophobic beliefs and attitudes.[51]

Discrimination with regard to culture is also an issue on many campuses. A study done in Canada showed that Aboriginal students who embraced and practised their culture faced frequent experiences of racism from mainstream society. What raised their stress levels even more were the frequency and unpredictability of the racist experiences.[52] As well, some Aboriginal students do not see themselves or their cultures reflected in the curriculum being offered in schools. There are not enough positive role models in the education system.

Many colleges, universities, and workplaces have set up programs and classes to educate people about sexual orientation, cultural differences, women's issues, and physical and mental challenges. It is time to make campuses and communities less alienating and more culturally and emotionally accessible, with programs and polices targeted not only at minorities but the population as a whole.

Environmental Stressors Natural disasters such as blizzards, earthquakes, floods, hurricanes, and volcanoes and man-made disasters such as chemical spills, nuclear reactor meltdowns, oil spills, and wars cause stress for people of all ages all over the world. In the past few years, monumental disasters displaced people and destroyed homes and land masses. Challenges continue as we deal with the aftermath of earthquakes, tsunamis, flooding, and toxic poisoning of rivers, oceans, and land.

Research has shown that environmental stressors can leave deep psychological scars. Walsh describes the outcome of environmental and economic harm caused by environmental disasters such as the BP oil spill disaster in the Gulf of Mexico as a *psychic* toll.[53] Young children's lives were turned upside down, adults lost their source of income, and entire communities were fractured. Lübken and Mauch[54] suggest that natural disasters are remembered for long periods of time and have far-reaching effects. In Canada communities have been impacted by disasters such as the Lac-Mégantic runaway train and derailment in Quebec and environmental concerns emerging from the oil sands production in Alberta. The catastrophic flooding of the Bow, Elbow, Highwood, Red Deer, Sheep, Little Bow, and South Saskatchewan rivers resulted in major flood damage in Calgary, Alberta, and the surrounding area in 2013. In the Polley Lake Mine disaster in 2014, a tailing pond spilled its banks and flooded Polley Lake, Hazeltine Creek, Quesnel Lake, and Cariboo Creek.

Acts of Terrorism Terrorism can also be classified as a stressor. Miller and Heldring, in their integrative review of literature examining the psychological impact of the September 11, 2001, terrorist attack on the World Trade Center in New York, U.S.A., determined that the most commonly occurring psychological symptom reported one year after the attack was post-traumatic stress disorder (PTSD). Other psychological problems that were reported included high levels of anxiety, deep sadness, fear, irritability, anger, sleep disorders, and difficulty concentrating.[55]

De Zulueta[56] suggests that we need to be especially watchful of the mental health consequences of mass violence as it can affect families and entire communities for generations. It appears that cognitive therapy is an effective treatment for PTSD related to terrorism and other civic conflicts.[57]

Illness and Disability Just as the mind can have profound effects on the body, the body can have an enormous impact on our emotions. Whenever we come down with the flu or pull a muscle, we feel under par. When the problem is more serious or persistent—a chronic disease such as diabetes, for instance, or a lifelong hearing impairment—the emotional stress of constantly coping with it is even greater. Most colleges and universities have in place a system for special concessions with regard to academic programs should students become ill. Student ancillary services, the counselling unit, or academic advisors can help.

A common source of stress for college and university students is a learning disability. Some students have one area of difficulty, such as reading or math. Others have problems with attention, writing, communicating, reasoning, coordination, social competence, or emotional maturity—all of which may make it difficult to excel. Asking for help can alleviate much stress that is linked to disabilities. Someone with a learning disability may exhibit the following traits:

- unable to engage in a focused activity such as reading; physically restless
- extremely distractible, forgetful, or absent-minded
- easily frustrated by waiting, delays, or traffic; constantly irritated
- disorganized; unable to manage time efficiently and complete tasks on time
- impulsive, making decisions with little reflection or information
- easily overwhelmed by ordinary hassles
- clumsy, with a poor body image and poor sense of direction

Technostress It may seem as if an expression such as **technostress** would be a relatively new term, but it was defined in a book titled *Technostress: The Human Cost of the Computer Revolution*, written in 1984. The author, Craig Brod,[58] described it as a modern disease of adaptation caused by people's inability to manage with new computer technologies in a healthy way. He suggested that technostress could be either a feeling of anxiety or mental pressure resulting from a struggle to embrace computer technology or stress from overexposure to computer technology.

There is no doubt that we have benefited from technology. One example is the Internet, which has been used in many positive ways as a teaching and learning resource. However, it has also impacted individuals, families, and work environments in negative ways. It is difficult to get away from technology. Cellphones, pagers, laptops, electronic tablets—our personal and professional lives have become intertwined. Some students are never "unplugged."

Symptoms of technostress are brain overload, frustration, feeling overwhelmed, and having a sense of things never being finished. There is always one more email to answer, one more photo to look at on Facebook, or one more voice mail to tend to. For some individuals, technology is becoming an addiction. Problematic Internet use can result in less study time, less socializing with friends in person, and unhealthy lifestyle choices. A study done on university students in Hong Kong revealed that heavy Internet users were twice as likely as others to report poorer eating habits and sleeping behaviours, being overweight, and poorer academic performance.[59]

Video gaming has become pervasive. While a stress release for some, studies have shown that regardless of gender, video game use is linked to greater drug use, heavy drinking behaviours, and a negative impact on the quality of relationships with friends and families.[60] Violent video game use for women has been linked to lower self-worth.[61]

A study on Facebook usage of students at the University of Guelph showed that there was a significant connection between the amount of time spent on Facebook and jealousy-related feelings and behaviours. The students who participated in the study averaged about 40 minutes per day on Facebook and had between 25 and 1000 Facebook friends. Most of the students who were involved in a relationship with someone reported that they had friends on their Facebook page that their partners did not know; 74.6 percent were somewhat likely to add previous romantic or sexual partners as friends. Women were more likely to be jealous than men. As well, the researchers found that people who were considered to be jealous types were more likely to have Facebook jealousy too.[62]

One other aspect of technology that is worrisome is Internet gambling. The availability of 24-hour access has made this type of gaming more addictive and problematic, and is having a negative psychosocial impact. Griffiths and Barnes surveyed university students and found that Internet gamblers were significantly more likely to be problem gamblers than non-Internet gamblers, and that males were significantly more likely to be problem Internet gamblers than females.[63] In yet another study on college students, Internet gambling frequency was significantly associated with poor mental health, increased problems with family members, more missed classes, and problems with anxiety.[64]

How do you know if technology is starting to impact your psychosocial health? If you continually check emails, Facebook accounts, or text messages to the point of it interfering with socializing with others in person, or if you find yourself gaming or gambling instead of focusing on that academic paper that is due, you might be at risk for technostress and addiction. Take care to manage technology or it will manage you.

Workplace Stress More than ever, many people find that they are working up to 55 or 60 hours per week—and enjoying it less. This exhausting cycle of overwork causes stress, which can make us work harder, which leads to more stress. Even the workplace itself can contribute to stress. A noisy, open-office environment can increase levels of stress without workers even realizing it.

According to a report from the Mental Health Commission of Canada (MHCC), 28.4 per cent of Canadians between 15 and 75 years old find that most work days are quite stressful or extremely stressful.[65] Stress in the workplace can be difficult to define because stress impacts individuals in different ways. However, employees' mental, physical, and emotional health are often impacted when they cannot meet work demands. The result can be lower work productivity. In addition to impacting the financial bottom line of an agency, workplace stress also impacts co-workers. Other stressors for Canadian workers included financial concerns, time issues, and family and personal matters such as relationships and parenting.

Yet work in itself is not hazardous to health. Attitudes about your work and habits related to how you work are the true threats. Feeling unappreciated, believing you have no control over your work environment, or resenting requests to upgrade or improve work-related skills can increase your stress levels. A job—stressful or not, enjoyable or not—can be therapeutic. Choose your work wisely. The government of Alberta has created a comprehensive Healthy Workplace website where you can find information on how to begin and sustain a workplace wellness program.[66] There are ideas for everyone, whether you are working part or full time. Companies who want to attract and keep their employees are beginning to understand the importance of a healthy workplace. They see the connection between productivity, loyalty, and employee health. As described in Chapter 1, occupational wellness is an important dimension of overall well-being.

✓ CHECK-IN

What is your greatest source of stress at this moment?

STRESS SURVIVAL

Sometimes we respond to stress or challenge with self-destructive behaviours such as drinking or using drugs. These responses can lead to psychosocial problems, such as anxiety or depression, and physical problems, including psychosomatic illnesses.

Defence mechanisms, such as those described in Table 3-1, are other responses to stress. These psychological devices are mental processes that are sometimes used to help us cope with personal problems. Such responses are not the answer to stress—however, learning to recognize them in yourself will enable you to deal with your stress in a healthier way.

The key to coping with stress is realizing that your *perception* of and *response* to a stressor are crucial. Changing the way you interpret events or situations—a skill called *reframing*—makes all the difference. An event such as a move to a new city is not stressful in itself. A move becomes stressful if you see it as a traumatic upheaval rather than an exciting beginning of a new chapter in your life.

It is important to recognize that balance in life is not a still point—rather, it is a process. In order to manage our unique and individual stressors, we need to be willing to recognize what is disruptive and unbalanced and how we feel physically and emotionally when it happens. Finding ways to regain equilibrium when life presents unexpected challenges can help to lower our stress levels.

How Can I Manage My Stress? There are many strategies and relaxation techniques that can lessen the stress build-up inside your body and help you to regain a sense of calm and control. Deep breathing can relax your body and quiet your mind. Learning to recognize signs that your stress load is getting out of hand can help you de-escalate your stress level and assist you in doing something to calm yourself down. Putting things into proper perspective can help you cope with the situation at hand. Laughter can also counter stress.

Some people find prayer helpful while others relieve their stress and boost their energy level by participating in regular physical activity. More information about the benefits of physical activity can be found in Chapter 4. A healthy diet can ease stress issues that are linked to under-eating, compulsive eating, and emotional eating. Journalling—putting your feelings into words—is another simple, yet effective way to work through stress.

More formal relaxation techniques include progressive relaxation, visualization, meditation, mindfulness, and biofeedback.

Progressive relaxation works by intentionally increasing and then decreasing tension in the muscles. While sitting or lying down in a quiet, comfortable

TABLE 3-1

Common Defence Mechanisms Used to Alleviate Anxiety and Eliminate Conflict

Defence Mechanism	Example
Denial: The refusal to accept a painful reality.	You don't believe that the research about Internet addiction could be true. You are convinced it does not have anything to do with you.
Displacement: The redirection of feelings from their true object to a more acceptable or safer substitute.	Instead of lashing out at a coach or a teacher, you snap at your best friend.
Projection: The attribution of unacceptable feelings or impulses to someone else.	When you want to end a relationship, you project your unhappiness onto your partner.
Rationalization: The substitution of acceptable reasons for the real motivations for your behaviour.	You convince yourself that it is all right to binge drink on the weekends because "everyone in the residence is doing it."
Reaction formation: Adopting attitudes and behaviours that are the opposite of what you feel.	You lavishly compliment an acquaintance whom you really despise.
Repression: Keeping threatening impulses, fantasies, memories, feelings, or wishes from becoming conscious.	You don't "hear" the alarm after a late night, or "forget" to read your course outline so you miss a deadline for a paper.

STRATEGIES FOR PREVENTION

How to Avoid Stress Overload

To avoid stress overload, watch for the following warning signals:

- physical symptoms, including chronic fatigue, headaches, indigestion, diarrhea, and sleep problems
- battling frequent illness or worrying about illness
- self-medicating, including using non-prescription drugs
- having problems concentrating on studies or work; producing poor quality work or not able to complete tasks
- feeling irritable, anxious, or apathetic
- working or studying longer and harder than usual
- exaggerating, to yourself and others, the importance of what you do
- becoming accident-prone
- breaking rules, whether it's a curfew at home or a speed limit on the highway
- going to extremes, such as drinking too much, overspending, or gambling

setting, you tense and release various muscles, beginning with those of the hand, for instance, and then proceeding to the arms, shoulders, neck, face, scalp, chest, stomach, buttocks, and so on, down each leg to the toes. Relaxing the muscles can quiet the mind and restore internal balance.

Visualization, or **guided imagery**, involves creating mental pictures that calm you down and focus your mind. Some people use this technique to promote healing when they are ill. Visualization skills require practice and, in some cases, instruction by qualified health professionals. Another option is guided imagery CDs and MP3 downloads. Check out Health Journeys at http://healthjourneys.com.

Meditation has been practised in many forms over the ages. Brain scans have shown that meditation activates the sections of the brain in charge of the autonomic nervous system, which governs bodily functions such as digestion and blood pressure that we cannot consciously control. Meditation helps a person reach a state of relaxation, but with the goal of achieving inner peace and harmony. There is no one right way to meditate, and many people have discovered how to meditate on their own, without even knowing what it is they are doing. Most forms of meditation have common elements: sitting quietly for 15 to 20 minutes once or twice a day; concentrating on a word, image, or number; and breathing slowly and rhythmically. However, even a few minutes of meditation each day or in times of high stress can be beneficial. Increasing numbers of college and university students are turning to meditation as a way to cope with stress. Research has shown that meditation can reduce college students' experiences of stress, anxiety, depression, and perfectionistic thoughts.[67]

Mindfulness is a modern form of an ancient Asian technique that involves maintaining awareness in the present moment. You tune in to each part of your body, scanning from head to toe, noting the slightest sensation. You allow whatever you experience—an itch, an ache, a feeling of warmth—to enter your awareness. Then you open yourself to focus on all the thoughts, sensations, sounds, and feelings that enter your awareness. Mindfulness keeps you in the here and now, thinking about what is rather than about what if or if only.

Biofeedback is a method of obtaining feedback, or information, about some physiological activity occurring in the body. An electronic monitoring device attached to the body detects a change in an internal function and communicates it back to the person through a tone, light, or meter. By paying attention to this feedback, most people can gain some control over functions previously thought to be beyond conscious control, such as body temperature, heart rate, muscle tension, and brain waves. The goal of biofeedback for stress reduction is a state of tranquility, usually associated with the brain's production of alpha waves, which are slower and more regular than normal waking waves.

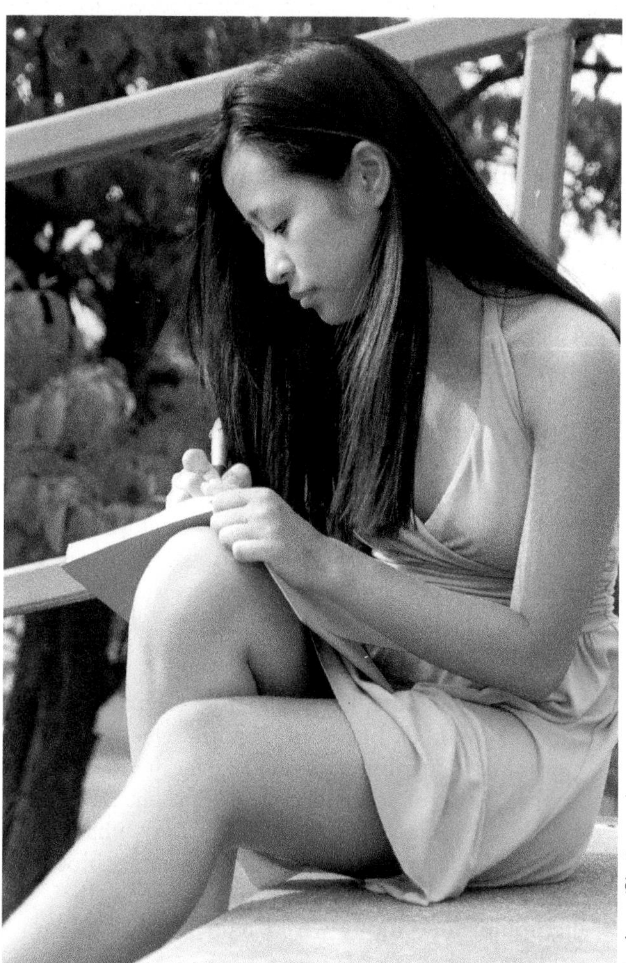

Ken Innes/Shutterstock

Writing in your journal about feelings and difficulties is a simple and very effective way to help control your stress.

STRATEGIES FOR CHANGE

Determining Stressors, Coping Mechanisms, and Activities for Relieving Stress

The following tips from the University of Ottawa might help you beat test stress:

- Take a couple of minutes to write down all the stressors you can think of that are currently present in your life.
- Then write down all of the coping mechanisms or activities you use to relieve the stress caused by the stressors you have listed.
- Now choose two of these coping mechanisms or activities that have worked to decrease your stress in the past.
- Commit to TWO of these coping mechanisms or activities per day for the next week.
- Track your success in using these coping mechanisms or activities—examples might include documenting mindful moments or meditation sessions, using a journal to record positive thoughts, monitoring exercise or physical activity sessions, asking for help, completing a food log for healthy eating, or noting sleep patterns.
- Determine what coping mechanisms or activities helped you manage your stress.
- Continue to use these techniques or try some different activities the next week.

How Can I Organize My Time? We live in what some sociologists call hyper-culture, a society that moves at warp speed. Information constantly bombards us. The rate of change seems to accelerate every year. Our time-saving devices—smartphones, laptop computers, and electronic tablets—have simply extended the boundaries of where and how we work.

As a result, more and more people are suffering from time sickness, a nerve-racking feeling that life has become little more than an endless to-do list. The best antidote is time management—to help us find our way out of the time trap.

Every day you make decisions and the choices about how to use your time that directly affect your stress level. Time management involves skills that anyone can learn, but it takes commitment and practice to be able to put these skills into action. Try some techniques that students have found useful:

- **Schedule your time.** Use a paper or electronic calendar or planner. Beginning the first week of class, mark down deadlines for each assignment, paper, project, and test scheduled that semester. Develop a daily schedule, listing very specifically what you will do the next day, along with the times. Block out times for working out, eating dinner, calling home, and talking with friends, as well as for studying.
- **Develop a game plan.** Allow at least two nights to study for any major exam. Set aside more time for researching and writing papers. Make sure to allow time to type, edit, and print out a paper—and to deal with emergencies such as a computer breakdown. Set daily and weekly goals. When working on a big project, don't neglect your other courses. Whenever possible, try to work ahead in all your classes.
- **Identify time robbers.** For several days keep a log of what you do and how much time you spend doing it. You may discover that disorganization is eating away at your time or that you have a problem getting started. Look for opportunities to save time. An hour spent with a resource librarian familiar with your field of study can save you many hours searching for research or resources on your own.
- **Make the most of classes.** Read the assignments before class rather than waiting until just before you have a test. Go to class. Read your lecture notes at the end of each day or at least at the end of each week. We all have different learning styles, so ask yourself how you learn best: are you an auditory, visual, or kinesthetic learner?
- **Develop an efficient study style.** Some experts recommend studying for 50 minutes, then breaking for 10 minutes. When you're reading, write notes or questions to yourself in the margins to help you retain more information. Even if you're racing to start a paper, take a few extra minutes to prepare a workable outline.
- **Focus on the task at hand.** Rather than worrying about how you did on yesterday's test or how you'll ever finish next week's project, practise mindfulness—focus intently on whatever you're doing at any given moment. If your mind starts to wander, use any distraction—the sound of the phone ringing or a noise from the hall—as a reminder to stay in the moment.
- **Break bigger tasks into smaller ones.** Break down your term paper into a series of steps, such as selecting a topic, identifying sources of research information, taking notes, and developing an outline.
- **Keep your workspace in order.** Even if the rest of your room is a shambles, try to keep your desk clear. Piles of papers are distracting, and you can end up wasting lots of time looking for notes you misplaced or an article you have to read by morning. Try to spend the last 10 minutes of the day cleaning up your desk so you will have a fresh start on the new day. Your workspace also includes your computer. Organize your school, work, and personal files. Back up important files. Take time to delete files or emails you no longer need.

Many colleges and universities offer time-management courses or workshops. York University has an excellent time-management information package available online at http://lss.info.yorku.ca/resources/university-time-management/.[68] You may want to access this site to find out more about the time-management cycle, goal setting, time awareness, and time tracking.

Overcoming Procrastination Putting off until tomorrow what should be done today is a habit that creates a great deal of stress for many students. It also takes a surprising toll. When asked if procrastination ever lowered the quality of academic work (papers or projects), caused them to hand in a paper late or not at all, or resulted in lower exam scores, 42 percent of students admitted that they usually or always were affected in at least one of the three areas. About 33 percent admitted that the quality of their academic work was compromised by procrastination and about 25 percent said it impacted their exam results.[69]

The three most common types of procrastination are putting off unpleasant things, putting off difficult tasks, and putting off tough decisions. Procrastinators are most likely to delay by wishing they didn't have to do what they must or by telling themselves they "just can't get started," which means they never do.

To get out of the procrastination trap, keep track of the tasks you're most likely to put off, and try to figure out why you don't want to tackle them. Think of alternative ways to complete these tasks. If you put off researching for an academic paper, ask yourself if the problem is the research itself or if it is the lack of understanding on how to do an online library search. If you don't know how to search university databases, get help from a librarian. It can be the catalyst to overcoming your procrastination and it will save you time in the long run.

Do what you like least first. Once you have a major task out of the way, you can concentrate on the tasks you enjoy. Build time into your schedule for interruptions, unforeseen problems, and unexpected events. Know that writing academic papers or studying for exams usually takes longer than you think it will.

HUMAN POTENTIAL

Rob Dyke—An Epic Journey: Just Say Yes

Consider competing in Ironman competitions, swimming across the Strait of Georgia from Vancouver to Victoria, B.C., climbing Mount Everest, and attempting to swim around Vancouver Island. Many people would say participating in these events would be very demanding, even nearly impossible. Our human potential story for this chapter is about Rob Dyke, an adventurer. Rob fully embraces what life has to offer and encourages others to put their potential in perspective so that they might fulfill their dreams and visions, too. Here is his story.

I learned about discipline, commitment, and hard work from a long competitive swimming career that took me to the University of Victoria. I also learned that I was swimming for a variety of reasons: for my parents, for my coach, for my school, and for my country, for medals and glory. But I was unaware at that moment that I was meant to do more—something else, something meaningful, something for myself—without losing sight of others' needs.

After my swimming career at UVic was over, I set out to make a difference. After challenging myself with Olympic-distance triathlons and Ironman competitions, I then took on the challenge of swimming across the Strait of Georgia, from Vancouver to Victoria, when a fellow distance swimmer was unable to attempt a first-ever swim to raise funds for sick children. I gave it my best but was pulled out of the water semi-conscious after eight hours of swimming in the Pacific Ocean. I could have been discouraged and given up, but I decided to learn from my mistakes instead. I became the first person to complete the 52-kilometre swim the following year, in 1996. I did so in 10.5 hours—raising funds for the B.C. Children's Hospital. Further adventures included a six-month journey from the Bay of Bengal to a climb up Mount Everest in support of a good friend's dream to summit without oxygen in 2003; attempting a 1400-kilometre swim around Vancouver Island, also in 2003; and another trip up Mount Everest in 2005 as the cook for a British climbing team. Then came another attempt at the almost impossible swim around Vancouver Island in the summer of 2005 for an agency and cause I am passionate about—the Canadian Red Cross. The successful swim continues to raise money for a legacy fund dedicated to reducing the yearly drowning average of 400 across Canada and make remote villages water-safe. The fund has raised more than $150 000 so far.

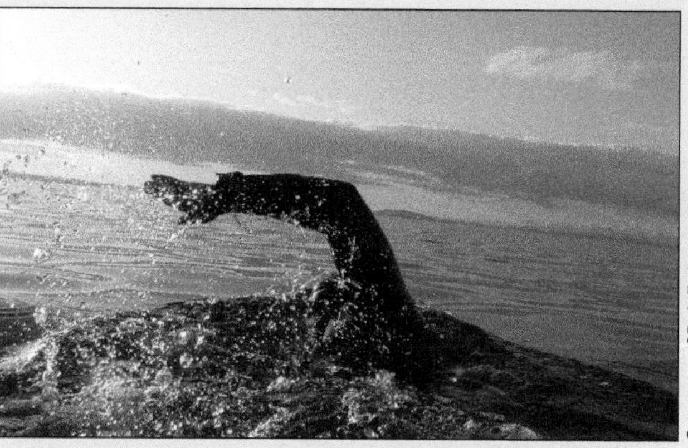

Courtesy of Rob Dyke

Rob Dyke—CEO of The Carbon Solution, motivational speaker, and philanthropist—swimming around Vancouver Island, Canada, raising money for the Canadian Red Cross.

From all of my adventures, I have learned some powerful life lessons. I consider myself an ordinary man who consistently does extraordinary things. I think that there is a hero in us all, but sometimes it gets hidden under layers of unnecessary caution and common sense, buried by stress, fear of failure, and

(Continued)

embarrassment. Preparation for my journeys has been predominantly mental and spiritual. I have spent time in the mountains and with Buddhist monks to find deep inner strength. I have discovered that there is a powerful mind, body, and spiritual connection within all of us, and that when you find something you love to do, you can make doing things you love a habit. Everyone will have their rough days, their stressful times, their doubts and reservations, but when you trust in your abilities you can do amazing things that can sometimes help others.

As one student commented after hearing me speak, "Over the past few months I have been doubting those things that I have always wanted to do, stressing out about my marks, student loans, and my future. Today I have learned that self-doubt can stop you from learning about new things, meeting new people, making a difference in this life. If there is something that you want to do, mental power and positive thoughts are strong enough to help you exceed your limits. I plan to create an experience that is life-changing in my future." And as I have now learned to say, "Just say yes."

Rob continues to deliver Keynote speeches and work in green-economy consulting. He also enjoys assisting start-up companies realize their potential.

SELF-SURVEY

Student Stress Scale

The Student Stress Scale, an adaptation of Holmes and Rahe's Life Events Scale for college-age adults, provides a rough indication of stress levels and possible health consequences.

In the Student Stress Scale, each event, such as beginning or ending school, is given a score that represents the amount of readjustment a person has to make as a result of the change. In some studies, using similar scales, people with serious illnesses have been found to have high scores.

To determine your stress score, add up the number of points corresponding to the events you have experienced in the past 12 months.

	Event	Points
1.	Death of a close family member	100
2.	Death of a close friend	73
3.	Divorce of parents	65
4.	Jail term	63
5.	Major personal injury or illness	63
6.	Marriage	58
7.	Getting fired from a job	50
8.	Failing an important course	47
9.	Change in the health of a family member	45
10.	Pregnancy	45
11.	Sex problems	44
12.	Serious argument with a close friend	40
13.	Change in financial status	39
14.	Change of academic major	39
15.	Trouble with parents	39
16.	New girlfriend or boyfriend	37
17.	Increase in workload at school	37
18.	Outstanding personal achievement	36
19.	First quarter/semester in college	36
20.	Change in living conditions	31
21.	Serious argument with an instructor	30
22.	Getting lower grades than expected	29
23.	Change in sleeping habits	29
24.	Change in social activities	29
25.	Change in eating habits	28
26.	Chronic car trouble	26
27.	Change in number of family get-togethers	26
28.	Too many missed classes	25
29.	Changing colleges or universities	24
30.	Dropping more than one class	23
31.	Minor traffic violations	20
	Total Stress Score	____

Answers to Self-Survey

Here's how to interpret your score: If your score is 300 or higher, you're at high risk for developing a health problem. If your score is between 150 and 300, you have a 50–50 chance of experiencing a serious health change within two years. If your score is below 150, you have a one in three chance of a serious health change. It is important to remember that different people deal with stress in different ways and that stressful situations are a part of everyone's lives at times.

Source: Kathleen Mullen & Gerald Costello, *Health Awareness Through Discovery*. Minneapolis: Burgess Publishing Company, 1981. Reprinted by permission.

Chapter Summary

1. Which of the following best defines stress?
   a. negative emotional state related to fatigue and similar to depression
   b. the physiological and psychological response to any event or situation that either upsets or excites us
   c. the end result of the general adaptation syndrome
   d. motivational strategy for making life changes

2. According to the general adaptation syndrome theory, how does the body typically respond to an acute stressor?
   a. The heart rate slows, blood pressure declines, and eye movement increases.
   b. The body enters a physical state called eustress and then moves into the physical state referred to as distress.
   c. If the stressor is viewed as a positive event, there are no physical changes.
   d. The body demonstrates three stages of change: alarm, resistance, and exhaustion.

3. Over time, increased levels of stress hormones have been shown to increase a person's risk for which of the following conditions?
   a. diabetes, high blood pressure, memory loss, and skin disorders
   b. stress fractures, male pattern baldness, and hypothyroidism
   c. hemophilia, AIDS, and hay fever
   d. influenza, sore joints, and asthma

4. Which symptom might be experienced by a person suffering from post-traumatic stress disorder?
   a. procrastination
   b. constant thirst
   c. drowsiness
   d. terror-filled dreams

5. Which statement about stress levels in college and university students is true?
   a. Stress levels may be high due to stressors such as academic pressures, financial concerns, learning disabilities, and relationship problems.
   b. Stress levels are usually low because students feel empowered, living independently of their parents.
   c. Stress levels are typically highest in fourth-year students because their self-esteem diminishes during the undergraduate years.
   d. Stress levels are lower in minority students because they are used to stressors such as a hostile social climate and actual or perceived discrimination.

6. Which situation is representative of a societal stressor?
   a. Peter is told that his transfer application has been denied because his transcripts were not sent in by the deadline.
   b. Nia and Kwame turn on the television to discover that there has been another suicide bombing in Afghanistan.
   c. Kelli's boyfriend drives her car after he has been drinking and has an accident.
   d. Joshua, who is the leading basketball player on his college varsity team, has just been diagnosed with diabetes.

7. Which scenario best illustrates the defence mechanism of displacement?
   a. You have a beer in the evening after a tough day.
   b. You act as if nothing has happened after you have been laid off from your job.
   c. You start an argument with your sister after being laid off from your job.
   d. You argue with your boss after he lays you off from your job.

8. If you are stuck in a traffic jam, which of the following actions will help reduce your stress level?
   a. deep, slow breathing
   b. honking your horn
   c. berating yourself for not taking a different route
   d. getting angry at the other drivers who are slowing you down

9. Which activity can help people achieve a relaxed, peaceful state of being?
   a. an aerobic exercise class
   b. playing a computer game
   c. meditating for 15 minutes
   d. attending a rap concert

10. Which of these techniques should you try to help you effectively manage your time?
    a. using a calendar or planner
    b. keeping a log of your activities for a week
    c. tackling a large task by breaking it down into a series of smaller tasks
    d. all of the above

Answers to these questions can be found on page 75.

SELF-RESPONSIBILITY—SOCIAL RESPONSIBILITY

SELF-RESPONSIBILITY

If you want to be brave, do not count your fears.

Cree wisdom

During stressful times, it can be difficult to believe in your own possibilities, but possibilities can be healing. If you find your stress levels rising, stop, reflect, seek advice, and quietly find your way. This is the most important time to practise healthy and well ways of living. How can you move yourself from contemplating your stress to preparing a stress-management plan? How can you move from preparation to action?

SOCIAL RESPONSIBILITY

If you find yourself down, the best way to pick yourself up is to do something for somebody else. You can't see your own joy, but you can see someone else's.

Nissa

When you are feeling down, one of the best ways to lighten your own load is to help someone else. How might you lessen someone's stress today? Make them a meal. Help them with a school project. Take them for a walk. Reaching out to others is a proven stress reducer.

CRITICAL THINKING

1. Stress levels among college and university students have reached record highs. What reasons can you think of to account for this? Consider possible social, cultural, and economic factors that may play a role.
2. Identify three stressful situations in your life and determine whether they are examples of eustress or distress. Describe both the positive and negative aspects of each situation.
3. Can you think of any ways in which your behaviour or attitudes might create stress for others? What changes could you make to avoid these?
4. What advice might you give an incoming first-year student about managing stress in college or university? What techniques have been most helpful for you in dealing with stress? Suppose that this student is from a different ethnic group than you. What additional suggestions would you have for him or her?

WEB LINKS

The Canadian Institute of Stress

www.stresscanada.org

The Canadian Institute of Stress (CIS) was founded by Drs. Hans Selye and Richard Earle. The site offers information on personal stress control, distance education and certification, workplace training and consulting, and research and development innovations.

Transitions—Ontario Native Education Counselling Association (CNECA)

http://oneca.com/transitions/

Designed to support First Nations, Métis, and Inuit students as they transition through their education journey and between home and the workplace, this website and its resources provide a wealth of information for anyone.

Health Canada. Healthy Living. Mental Health—Coping with Stress

www.hc-sc.gc.ca/hl-vs/iyh-vsv/life-vie/stress-eng.php

This Health Canada website includes background information on stress, a discussion of symptoms of stress, the health effects of stress, and a section on how to minimize your stress levels. This website also includes links to a variety of other mental health organizations.

York University Learning Skills—Time Management

http://lss.info.yorku.ca/resources/university-time-management/

Learn about the time management cycle, goal setting, taking action, and procrastination. Access online learning resources for reading skills, note taking, test preparation, and stress tips.

Please note that links are subject to change. If you find a broken link, use a search engine such as www.google.ca and search for the website by typing in keywords.

Key Terms

The terms listed here are used within the chapter on the page indicated. Definitions of the terms are in the Glossary at the end of the book.

adaptive response 58
adrenocorticotrophic hormone (ACTH) 60
autonomic nervous system (ANS) 59
biofeedback 69
cognitive-transactional model of stress and coping 59
complicated grief 63
cortisol 60
defence mechanisms 68
distress 58
epinephrine 59
eustress 58
general adaptation syndrome (GAS) 58
guided imagery 69
homeostasis 58
hypothalamus 59
meditation 69
mindfulness 69
parasympathetic nervous system (PNS) 60
post-traumatic stress disorder (PTSD) 62
progressive relaxation 68
psychoneuroimmunology (PNI) 59
stress 58
stressors 58
sympathetic nervous system (SNS) 59
technostress 66
visualization 69

Answers to Chapter Summary Questions

1. b; 2 d; 3. a; 4. d; 5. a; 6. b; 7. c; 8. a; 9. c; 10. d

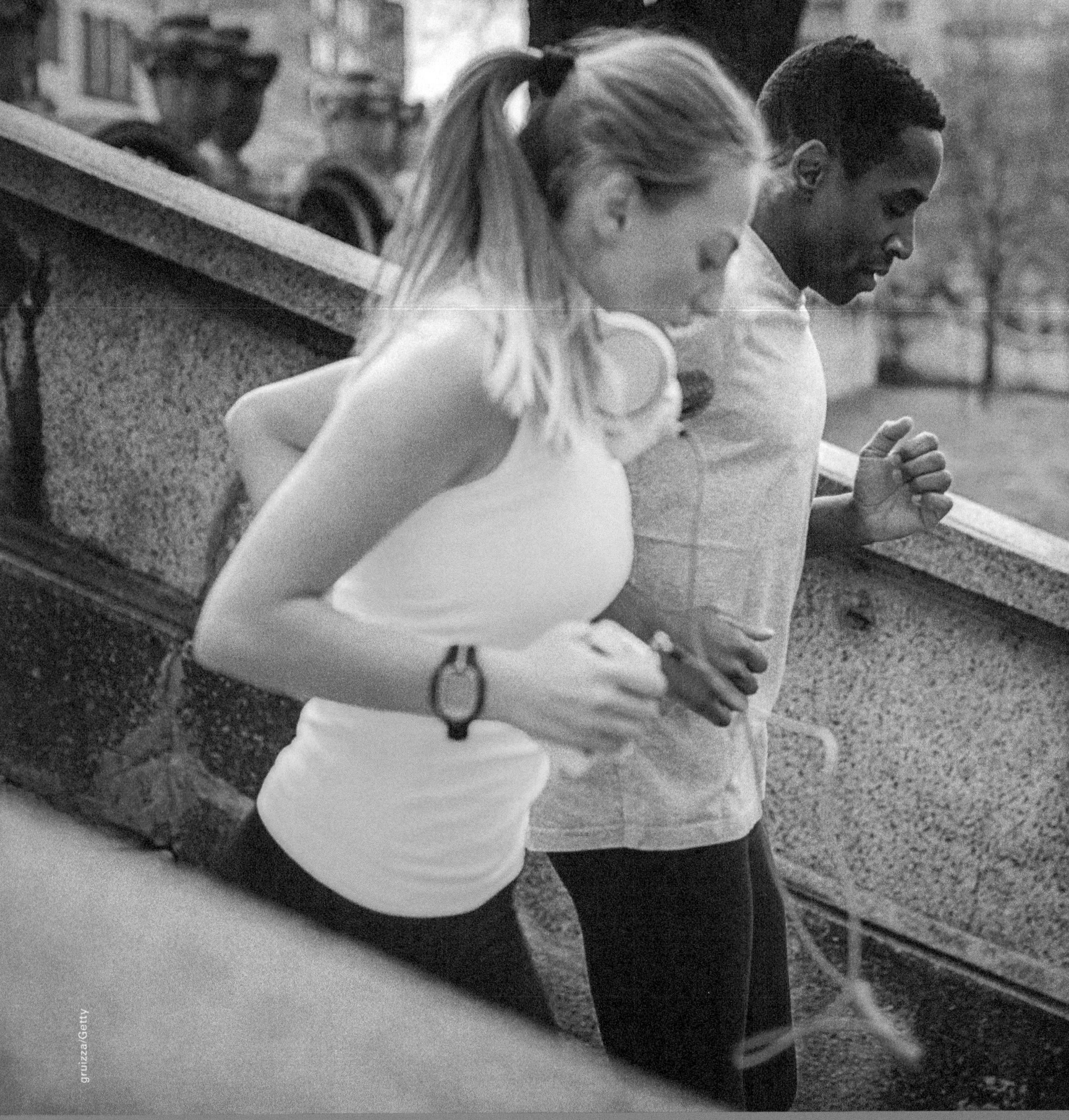
gruizza/Getty

AFTER READING THIS CHAPTER, YOU WILL BE ABLE TO:

- **define** the terms "physical activity," "physical fitness," "exercise," and "sport"
- **list** the five components of health-related fitness
- **describe** the health benefits of regular physical activity
- **list** the different forms of cardiorespiratory, muscular strength, endurance, and flexibility activities
- **design** cardiorespiratory, strength, endurance, and flexibility workouts
- **list** safety strategies for physically active individuals

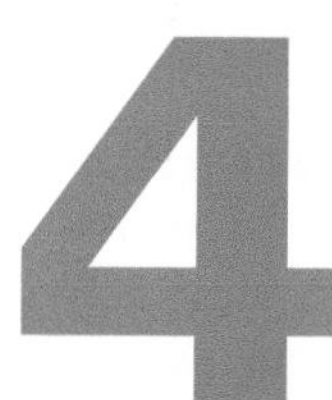

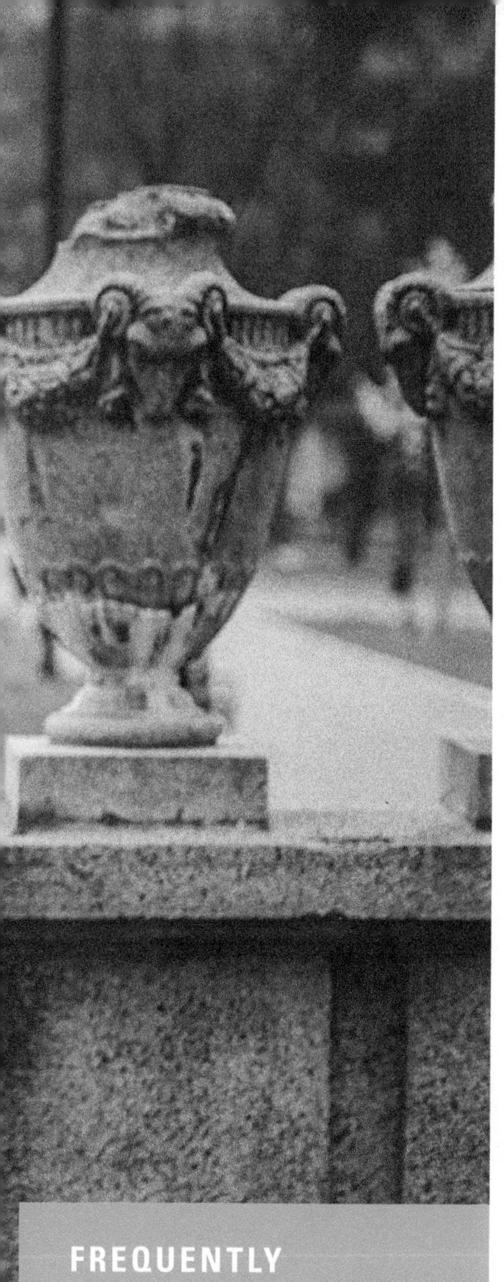

Physical Activity for Fitness, Health, and Athletic Performance

We are designed to move. Our bodies can run, stretch, bend, climb, glide, and stride—day after day and year after year. The human body thrives on physical activity. When we use our bodies, we become stronger and healthier.

As you'll see in this chapter, regular physical activity yields immediate rewards: it boosts energy, improves mood, soothes stress, improves sleep, and makes you feel better. In the long term, physical activity slows many of the changes associated with chronological aging, such as loss of calcium and bone density, and lowers the risk of serious chronic illnesses.

You will also discover that to get these benefits, you do not have to be a fitness fanatic. A study by Tremblay and Chiasson[1] shows that Canadian college students, aged 17–20, whose lifestyles included regular moderate daily physical activity and healthy food choices, improved their level of health.

What else is in this chapter? There is an introduction to *Canada's Physical Activity Guidelines*; an outline of the principles of exercise; and information about aerobic, muscular strength and endurance, and flexibility programs.

FREQUENTLY ASKED QUESTIONS

PHYSICAL ACTIVITY

Physical activity can be defined as any bodily movement produced by the skeletal muscles that increases heart rate and breathing and requires a substantial increase over resting energy expenditure.[2] You can be physically active by participating in health-related exercise such as walking, running, and swimming; leisure pursuits like gardening, bowling, and even household chores; and athletic or sport performance such as basketball, rowing, and hockey.

The benefits of regular physical activity have been known for a long time. Early studies in the 1950s by Morris and Heady[3] demonstrated that people who were physically active at work were less likely to suffer from heart disease and diabetes. Studies by Paffenbarger and his colleagues[4] in the 1970s established that physical activity could protect people from coronary mortality. In a landmark study by Berkman and Breslow,[5] exercising regularly was one of the seven health habits that strongly impacted mortality rates (the others were sleeping seven to eight hours per night, eating breakfast almost every day, rarely eating between meals, drinking alcohol in a moderate way or not at all, not smoking, and maintaining weight near an ideal level). Further studies over the past two decades have concluded that regular physical activity can lower your risk of heart disease, diabetes, high blood pressure, and some types of cancer and can help you maintain a healthy weight.[6,7] The next section of this chapter will describe the associations between physical activity and health, physical activity and fitness, and physical activity and athletic performance.

Physical Activity and Health The Public Health Agency of Canada (PHAC) has a responsibility for improving the health and well-being of Canadians.[8] The goals of this agency are

- funding national healthy living projects;
- improving collaboration between federal, provincial, and territorial governments with regard to healthy living initiatives;
- collecting and sharing knowledge about healthy living so national, provincial, and municipal agencies can make informed program decisions when implementing healthy living strategies; and
- encouraging Canadians to increase their physical activity levels.

These goals have been set because Canada is facing a physical inactivity and obesity crisis that has a major impact on our economy. Janssen,[9] in a study on the health-care costs of physical inactivity in Canadian adults, found that the estimated direct costs in 2009 were 2.4 billion dollars, the indirect costs were 4.3 billion dollars, and the total healthcare costs were 6.8 billion dollars. These values represent 3.8, 3.6, and 3.7 percent of the healthcare costs respectively.

A 2015 report suggests that if just 10 percent of Canadians who do not meet the current recommended physical activity guidelines made a modest improvement in their physical activity levels, there would be a projected reduction of 2.6 billion dollars in healthcare spending on conditions such as diabetes, cancer, heart disease, and hypertension between 2015 and 2040.[10]

Given that physical inactivity has become an epidemic in Canada and the fact that research has shown without a doubt that physical activity helps our bodies function at their best (see Figure 4-1), the Healthy Living Unit partnered with the Canadian Society for Exercise Physiology (CSEP) and provided support for the revisions of the Canadian Physical Activity Guidelines.[11]

For adults aged 18–64 years, the guide recommends an accumulation of at least 150 minutes of moderate- to vigorous-intensity aerobic physical activity (MVPA) per week, in bouts of 10 minutes or more.[12] Canadians are

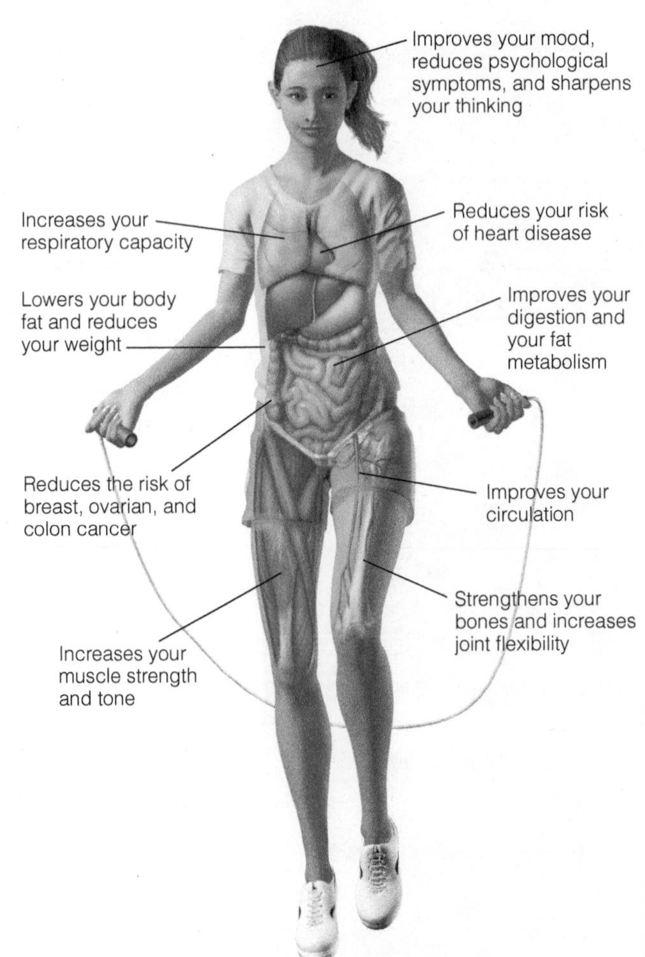

Figure 4-1 The Benefits of Exercise
Regular physical activity enhances your overall health and helps prevent disease.

also encouraged to add muscle- and bone-strengthening activities using major muscle groups, at least two days per week (see Table 4-1). For adults aged 65 years and older (see Figure 15-3 in Chapter 15), the same recommendations are made, but with caution extended to individuals who have poor mobility and a suggestion to perform physical activities to enhance balance and prevent falls.

TABLE 4-1

Canadian Physical Activity Guidelines

FOR ADULTS—18–64 YEARS

Guidelines

To achieve health benefits, adults aged 18–64 years should accumulate at least 150 minutes of moderate- to vigorous-intensity aerobic physical activity per week, in bouts of 10 minutes or more.

It is also beneficial to add muscle and bone strengthening activities using major muscle groups, at least 2 days per week.

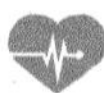

More physical activity provides greater health benefits.

Let's Talk Intensity!

Moderate-intensity physical activities will cause adults to sweat a little and to breathe harder. Activities like:

- Brisk walking
- Bike riding

Vigorous-intensity physical activities will cause adults to sweat and be 'out of breath'. Activities like:

- Jogging
- Cross-country skiing

Being active for at least **150 minutes** per week can help reduce the risk of:

- Premature death
- Heart disease
- Stroke
- High blood pressure
- Certain types of cancer
- Type 2 diabetes
- Osteoporosis
- Overweight and obesity

And can lead to improved:

- Fitness
- Strength
- Mental health (morale and self-esteem)

Pick a time. Pick a place. Make a plan and move more!

☑ Join a weekday community running or walking group.
☑ Go for a brisk walk around the block after dinner.
☑ Take a dance class after work.
☑ Bike or walk to work every day.
☑ Rake the lawn, and then offer to do the same for a neighbour.
☑ Train for and participate in a run or walk for charity!
☑ Take up a favourite sport again or try a new sport.
☑ Be active with the family on the weekend!

Now is the time. Walk, run, or wheel, and embrace life.

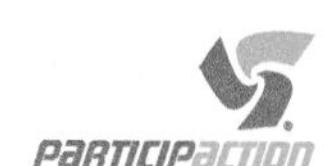

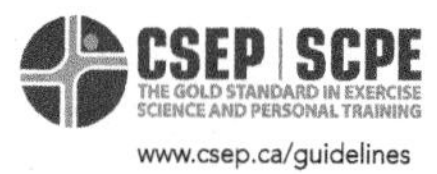

www.csep.ca/guidelines

Source: Canadian Physical Activity Guidelines, © 2011, 2012. Used with permission from the Canadian Society for Exercise Physiology. www.csep.ca/guidelines

✓ CHECK-IN

Do you meet these recommendations for physical activity?

CSEP (Canadian Society for Exercise Physiology) has also developed new Canadian Sedentary Behaviour Guidelines for children 0–4 years and 5–11 years, and youth 12–17 years. These guidelines are meant to help us focus on the 23 hours per day when we might not be engaged in physical activity. For children under 2 years old, screen time such as television and electronic games are not recommended. For children 2–4 years old, screen time should be limited to less than one hour per day or less. For children aged 5–17, recreational screen time should be limited to no more than two hours per day, and extended sitting and time spent indoors should be limited. Research is now being done on the development of sedentary guidelines for adults aged 18–64 years and older adults over 65 years.[13]

Findings from the *2012 and 2013 Canadian Health Measures Survey (CHMS)*[14] show that only about one in five adults and older adults met the recommended 150 minutes of moderate-to-vigorous physical activity sessions in 10-minute periods per week (see Figure 4-2). Thirty-two percent of adults aged 18–39 were more likely to meet the guidelines than adults aged 40–59 (18 percent) or 60–79 (12 percent). Figure 4-3 illustrates the average time adults spent being sedentary and being active in light or moderate-to-vigorous physical activity (MPVA). Adults aged 18–30 were sedentary on average for nine hours and 36 minutes. They were also the most active with an average of 34 minutes of MPVA per day. Adults aged 40–59 were sedentary on average for nine hours and 49 minutes and active for 23 minutes. Older adults aged 60–79 on average were sedentary for 10 hours and eight minutes daily and active for 14 minutes per day.

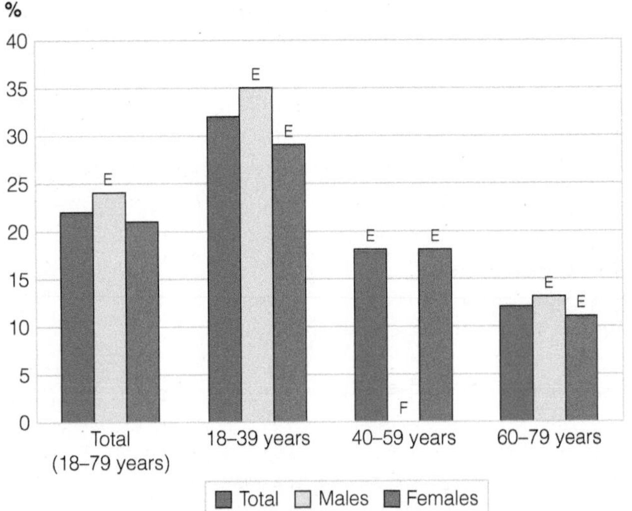

ᴱuse with caution (data with a coefficient of variation from 16.6% to 33.3%)
ᶠtoo unreliable to be published (data with a coefficient of variation (CV) greater than 33.3%; suppressed due to extreme sampling variability)
1. According to the Canadian Society for Exercise Physiology, adults should accumulate at least 150 minutes of moderate-to-vigorous activity in periods of at least 10 minutes per week.

Figure 4-2 Proportion of adults aged 18–79 meeting the Canadian Physical Activity Guidelines by age group and sex, Canada, 2012 and 2013.

Source: Statistics Canada. (2015, November 27). *Directly measured physical activity of adults, 2012 and 2013*. Publications. http://www.statcan.gc.ca/pub/82-625-x/2015001/article/14135-eng.htmarticle/14135-eng.htm

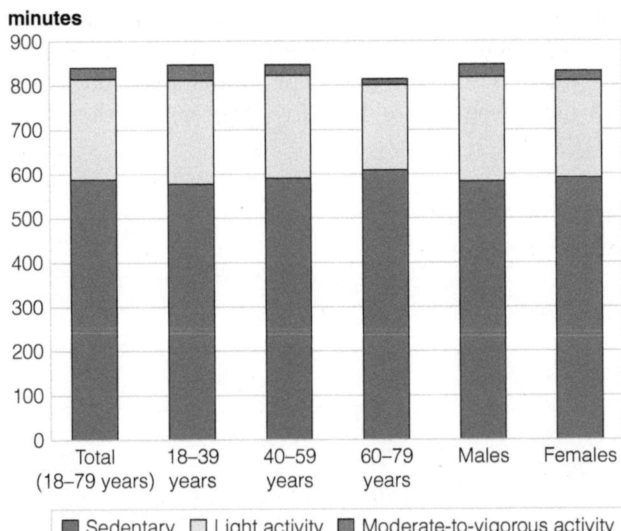

Figure 4-3 Average time spent sedentary, and in light- or moderate-to-vigorous physical activity of adults aged 18 to 79, by age group and sex. Canada, 2012 and 2013.

Source: Statistics Canada. (2015, November 27). *Directly measured physical activity of adults, 2012 and 2013*. Publications. http://www.statcan.gc.ca/pub/82-625-x/2015001/article/14135-eng.htm

Physical Activity and Fitness **Physical fitness** is the ability to respond to routine physical demands with enough reserve energy to cope with a sudden challenge.[15] Consider yourself fit if you meet your daily energy needs, can handle unexpected extra demands, and are protecting yourself against potential health problems, such as heart disease. Fitness is important for both health and athletic or sport performance. **Exercise** is physical activity that you plan, structure, and repeat for the purpose of conditioning your body.[16] Exercise is used to improve health and maintain fitness.

The five health-related components of physical fitness include aerobic or cardiorespiratory endurance, muscular strength, muscular endurance, flexibility, and body composition (the ratio of fat and lean body tissue).

Cardiorespiratory fitness refers to the ability of the heart to pump blood through the body efficiently so a person can sustain prolonged rhythmic activity. Aerobic exercise is any activity, such as brisk walking, jogging, running, swimming, or cycling, in which sufficient or excess oxygen is continually supplied to the body.

To determine a person's level of cardiorespiratory fitness, a VO2 max or maximal oxygen uptake test can be administered. **VO2 max** refers to the maximum amount of oxygen that an individual is able to use during intense or "maximal" exercise. Experts measure VO2 max as millilitres of oxygen used in one minute per kilogram of body weight. The more oxygen you are able to use during high-level exercise, the more energy you can produce. The test can be difficult if a true VO2 max level is to be determined; however, VO2 max can also be estimated by using less strenuous tests. One example is the Bruce Treadmill test.

Genetics, age, gender, and altitude all have an influence on VO2 max. The average VO2 max for a sedentary individual is about 35 ml/kg/min. For the average person, healthy aerobic exercise means working out strenuously without pushing to your VO2 max level or to the point of breathlessness.

Muscular fitness has two components: strength and endurance. **Muscular strength** refers to the force within muscles; it is measured by the absolute maximum weight that a person can lift, push, or press in one effort. Strong muscles help keep the skeleton in proper alignment, improve posture, prevent back and leg aches, help in everyday lifting, and enhance athletic performance. Muscle mass increases along with strength, which makes for a healthier body composition and a higher metabolic rate.

Muscular endurance is the ability to perform repeated muscular effort; it is measured by counting how many times a person can lift, push, or press a given weight. Important for posture, muscular endurance helps in everyday movement as well as in athletics and sports. Both components are equally important.

Flexibility is the range of motion around specific joints. Flexibility depends on many factors: your age, sex, and posture; how muscular you are; and how much body fat you have. As children develop, their flexibility increases until adolescence. Then a gradual loss of joint mobility begins and continues through adulthood. Both muscles and connective tissue, such as tendons and ligaments, shorten and tighten because they are not used through their full range of motion.

Body composition refers to the amount of fat (essential and stored fat) and lean tissue (bone, muscle, organs, water) in the body. A high proportion of body fat has serious health implications, including an increased incidence of heart disease, high blood pressure, diabetes, stroke, gall bladder problems, back and joint problems, and some forms of cancer. More information on body composition is available in Chapter 6.

Physical conditioning (or training) refers to the gradual building up of the body to enhance cardiorespiratory or aerobic fitness, muscular strength, muscular endurance, and flexibility; and a healthy body composition. **Functional fitness**, which is gaining greater emphasis among professional personal trainers, refers to the performance of daily activities. Exercises that mimic job tasks or everyday movements can improve an individual's balance, coordination, strength, and endurance.[17]

Physical Activity and Athletic Performance Many activities demand a special type of athletic performance that includes skill-related fitness such as agility, balance, coordination, and power. Improving skill-related fitness can help people enjoy a higher level of success in lifetime **sport**, which is defined as leisure-time physical activities that are planned, structured, and competitive.

Agility is the ability to change your body position and direction quickly and efficiently and is important in many sports such as basketball, racquetball, and tennis. Agility tests include running forward and backward, then performing crossover steps. **Balance**, the body's ability to maintain proper equilibrium, is necessary in day-to-day life as well as sports such as gymnastics or skiing. A stork stand test, where you stand on one foot and place your other foot on the inside of the supporting knee and hold yourself steady as long as possible without moving, can help you improve your balance.

Coordination, the integration of the nervous and muscular systems, which allows for harmonious body movements, is an important skill in sports that demand throwing, catching, and hitting. **Power**, defined as the ability to produce maximum force in the shortest time, has two components—speed and force. **Speed** is the ability to propel the body or a part of a body rapidly from one point to another. **Force** is an influence that causes movement of a body, often described as pushing or pulling. A combination of these components allows a person to jump, spike, throw, or hit with force. Power is necessary for everyday activities too, such as climbing stairs, lifting objects, and preventing falls.

Plyometrics are specialized, high-intensity training exercises that develop athletic performance skills. Exercises include hops, jumps, bounding movements, and jumping on and off a box. Care must be taken when performing plyometric exercises because they can be risky.

The Health Benefits of Physical Activity If exercise could be packed into a pill, it would be the single most widely prescribed and beneficial medicine in the nation. Many physicians and healthcare providers are now supporting a global movement called Exercise is Medicine™ (EIM) and Exercise is Medicine® Canada (EIMC)[18] where patients' physical activity programs are assessed and reviewed as part of a regular physical examination.

They are also connecting with other healthcare, recreation, and fitness professionals in the community to support active, healthy lifestyles for their patients. In Canada, the goal of this initiative is to increase the number of Canadians of all ages to meet the Physical Activity Guidelines. University and college students registered in medical, exercise science, recreation, and health studies have begun to support this movement too. Serving as ambassadors, students are creating local Exercise is Medicine on Campus clubs; developing physical activity programs and opportunities such as fun runs and educational events; providing basic exercise counselling; and assisting as consultants within Student Health Services units.[19] The Canadian Medical Association (CMA) is positioning the medical profession as a leader in advocating the benefits of regular physical activity. This next section will highlight some of these benefits.

Better Bones Weak and brittle bones are common among people who don't exercise. **Osteoporosis**, a condition in which bones lose their mineral density and become increasingly susceptible to injury, affects a great many older people. According to Osteoporosis Canada, approximately one in three women and one in five men will endure an osteoporotic fracture during their lifetime.[20] Women are more vulnerable because their bones are less dense to begin with. Exercise during adolescence and young adulthood may prevent bone weakening and fractures in old age. Researchers estimate that a minimum of two 45-minute exercise sessions per week may protect the bones of post-menopausal women.[21] Step aerobics and weight-bearing activities can help you maintain bone mass in adulthood.

Better Mental Health and Functioning Exercise is an effective, but underused, treatment for mild to moderate depression and may help in treating other mental disorders.[22] Regular, moderate exercise, such as walking, running, or lifting weights, has proven helpful for depression and anxiety disorders, including panic attacks. Research is showing that exercise and physical activity can be used as a therapy for individuals dealing with both acute and chronic depression.[23] It also eases certain symptoms, such as agitation and hallucinations, in schizophrenic patients.[24] In a study of people with major depression, exercise proved as effective as medication in improving mood and also helped prevent relapse.[25]

Lifelong fitness may protect the brain as we age. Improving cardiorespiratory fitness reduces the harmful effects of aging on brain structures as well as on memory and other functions. In a recent study, men and women with early-stage Alzheimer's disease who were more physically fit had larger brains compared to their less-fit counterparts.[26]

Brighter Mood and Less Stress As described in Chapters 2 and 3, exercise boosts your mood. It also increases energy, improves concentration and alertness, and increases the ability to handle daily stress. During longer exercise sessions, some people have reported an experience called a "runner's high," which may be the result of increased levels of mood-elevating brain chemicals called **endorphins**.[27] Research also shows that even short 20-minute bouts of exercise, regardless of the intensity level of the sessions, lower stress levels.[28]

Enhanced Immunity It appears from numerous studies that there is a link between moderate, regular physical activity and an enhanced immune system. This may be due to the reduction of stress hormones such as cortisol that can dampen resistance to disease.[29] Dr. David Nieman's research showed that moderate exercise repeated on a near-daily basis has a cumulative effect and provides a long-term benefit to our immune system. He also discovered that individuals who walked at 70–75 percent of their V02 max (maximal oxygen uptake) for 40 minutes per day had half as many sick days due to colds or sore throats as those who didn't exercise.[30] While moderate exercise seems to bolster a person's immune system, heavy training may increase the risk of upper respiratory tract infections for endurance athletes.[31]

Healthier Heart and Lungs Sedentary people are about twice as likely to die of a heart attack as people who are physically active. In Canada, cardiovascular disease (CVD) is the second leading cause of premature death.[32] However, researchers have found that people who participate in 150 minutes per week of moderate to intense leisure-time physical activity have a 14 percent lower risk of cardiovascular heart disease compared to people who reported no leisure-time physical activity. When individuals engaged in 300 minutes per week of moderate to intense leisure-time physical activity, their risk of cardiovascular heart disease was 20 percent lower than people who reported no leisure-time physical activity. They also found that even people whose physical activity levels were lower than the recommended levels had significantly lower risk of cardiovascular heart disease than people who had no leisure-time physical activity.[33] Exercise also lowers levels of the indicators of increased heart disease risk, such as high cholesterol and C-reactive protein. As well, heart muscles become strong, blood is pumped more efficiently, heart rate and resting heart rate slow down, and blood pressure may drop slightly too.

In addition to its effects on the heart, exercise makes the lungs more efficient. They take in more oxygen, and their vital capacity (ability to take in and expel air) is increased, providing more energy for you to use.

Longer and More Active Life According to the World Health Organization (WHO), physical inactivity has been identified as the fourth leading risk factor for global mortality, causing an estimated 3.2 million deaths globally.[34] As we have discussed, inactivity increases all causes of mortality, doubles the risk of cardiovascular diseases, diabetes, and obesity, and increases the risk of colon cancer, high blood pressure, osteoporosis, depression, and anxiety.[35] Exercise slows the changes that are associated with advancing age: loss of lean muscle tissue, increased body fat, and decreased work capacity. Capacity for exercise has proven a better predictor of whether elderly people would die in the next few years than other risk factors, such as high blood pressure, high total cholesterol, or smoking.[36]

Exercise also helps older adults retain the strength and mobility needed to live independently. It boosts strength and stamina, lessens time in wheelchairs, and improves outlook and the sense of being in control.[37] Formerly sedentary people, even the elderly, who begin to exercise live longer, on average, than those who remain inactive.[38]

Lowering the Risk of Cancer Research also shows that physical activity can help cancer patients; for instance, it can lower the likelihood of getting some forms of cancer and may lessen the risk of recurrence of a second cancer.[39] Grimmet,[40] in her study on exercise and cancer survivorship, indicates that while all exercise programs should be individualized, with various treatments, symptoms, and contraindications to physical activity taken into consideration, exercise is an effective therapy for reducing a number of secondary cancers. She advocates exercise as part of a treatment protocol because it is a low-cost intervention that has the potential to improve the health and well-being of many individuals dealing with cancer.

Ahn et al.,[41] in a study on exercise therapy and the length of hospital stay of colon cancer patients, found that low- to moderate-intensity post-surgical exercise reduced the length of hospital stay and improved bowel motility after surgery in patients with stages I–III colon cancer. Another study, by Wolin, Colditz, and Lee,[42] provides evidence that people who participate in physical activity can expect to reduce their risk of colon cancer by up to 24 percent.

Physical activity has also been shown to protect against breast cancer in women. Bernstein[43] found that while more research is still needed to determine the optimal type of activity, amount of time, intensity level, and frequency of exercise for women, exercising 30–60 minutes per day at a moderate or vigorous level will lower risk of breast cancer. Activity done during youth appears to be more important than later activity in the prevention of premenopausal breast cancer. The message to all women is to adopt a physically active lifestyle and maintain it for life.

Lowering the Risk of Type 2 Diabetes According to the Canadian Diabetes Association, more than ten million Canadians are living with diabetes or prediabetes.[44] Nine out of ten Canadians with diabetes have type 2 diabetes.[45] Of special concern is diabetes in Aboriginal communities, where Aboriginal peoples are three to four times more likely to acquire type 2 diabetes than non-Aboriginal Canadians.[46]

At this time there is no known way to prevent type 1 diabetes. However, type 2 diabetes can be prevented or at least delayed through lifestyle choices such as participating in regular physical activity, choosing a healthy diet, and weight management. A joint position statement, co-written by the American College of Sports Medicine (ACSM) and the American Diabetes Association (ADA), states that exercise is very important in the prevention and control of insulin resistance, prediabetes, and type 2 diabetes. Recommendations include participating in both aerobic and resistance training. Exercise must be done on a regular basis to realize benefits.[47] More information about diabetes is presented in Chapter 10.

Lowering Weight A 2015 report from the Organisation for Economic Co-operation and Development (OECD) shows that obesity rates among both adults and children in Canada are higher than most other OECD countries. Obesity in all 34 OECD countries tends to be higher among women and in less educated populations.[48] The good news is that in combination healthy eating and physical activity can help people lower their weight. As your body responds to the increased demand from your muscles for nutrients, your metabolic rate rises, the body burns more calories, and body fat decreases. Moreover, this surge persists after exercise, so you continue to use some calories even after you've stopped working out. Called excess post-exercise oxygen consumption (EPOC), this increased metabolism includes oxygen replenishment; lactate removal; and increased ventilation, blood circulation, and body temperature. The body generally takes anywhere from 15 minutes to 48 hours to fully recover to a resting state. The magnitude and duration of EPOC depends on sex and intensity and duration of exercise.[49]

Many college and university students are concerned with weight gain. Cafeteria food, lack of cooking skills, the dependence on fast foods, and a decrease in physical activity for many students all relate to the dreaded "freshman 15." Recreation and athletic services and even some academic courses are now delivering exercise programs designed for weight loss and management for students. In one study, students registered in a bimonthly class where health and wellness information was discussed. They were also required to record their daily walking totals. Participants who completed the program reported increases in general exercise activity, resistance training, and walking behaviour. Findings showed that there were decreases in both body fat and body mass.[50]

X AND Y FILES

Men and Women: Physical Fitness and Physical Activity Levels

While men and women benefit equally from physical activity and exercise, there are gender differences with regard to activity levels.

- Men are more likely than women to fully intend to be active because it is considered to be fun, exciting, or enjoyable.
- More women than men intend to be active to lose weight.
- Agreement may be required from senior members of some households before women can use family financial resources to engage in physical activity.
- Women often have a workload that includes careers as well as caregiving roles for family members, and time available for physical activity is minimal.
- Cultural expectations may limit the participation of women and girls.
- Women's income is often lower than men's and may limit access to physical activity facilities.
- Women are more likely than men to cite lack of time, energy, or skill as barriers to an active lifestyle.
- Women are more likely than men to rate advice on scheduling physical activity into daily life and choosing the most important activities as very important in making it easier for them to be physically active.

According to Statistics Canada, men were more moderately active during their leisure time at 57.6 percent in 2013 than women at 52.8 percent.[51] Males also had a significantly higher level of light activity than females—three hours and 55 minutes for males and three hours and 37 minutes for females on a daily basis.[52]

Physiology needs to be considered, too. On average, men have roughly twice the percentage of muscle mass and half the percentage of body fat. Overall, men are about 30 percent stronger, particularly above the waist. Their lungs take in 10–20 percent more oxygen, so they have a greater VO2 max or maximal oxygen uptake. They also pump more blood with each heartbeat.

Women's body fat is often distributed around the hips and thighs; men carry more body fat around the waist and stomach. The average woman has a smaller heart, a lower percentage of slow-twitch muscle fibres, and a smaller blood volume than a man. Because women have a lower concentration of red blood cells, their bodies are less effective at transporting oxygen to their working muscles during exercise.

Even though training produces the same relative increases for both sexes, a woman's VO2 max or maximum oxygen intake remains about 25–30 percent lower than that of an equally well-conditioned man. In elite athletes, the difference is smaller: 8–12 percent. Because the angle of the upper leg bone (femur) to the pelvis is greater in a woman, her legs are less efficient at running. However, in some endurance events, such as ultra-marathon running and long-distance swimming, female anatomy and physiology may have some aerobic advantages. The longer a race—on land, water, or ice—the better women perform.

In another study, Greaney et al. identified barriers and positive factors for healthy weight management among college students. They found that two of the top four semester goals among the students surveyed included increasing physical activity levels and improving diet, and gaining, losing, or maintaining weight. The other two goals were improving or maintaining their academic standing, and maintaining an active social life. Perceived barriers to achieving their physical activity and weight management goals included lack of discipline, social situations, time constraints, and ready access to unhealthy food. Positive factors included support for regular physical activity on campus, social support for healthy living choices, and healthy food choices in cafeterias.[53]

THE PRINCIPLES OF EXERCISE

The body, superbly designed for multiple uses, adjusts to meet physical demands. If you need to sprint for the bus, your heart rate will speed up and pump more blood. Beyond such an immediate short-term adaption, physical training can produce long-term changes too. Although there are limits on the maximum levels of physical fitness and performance that any individual can achieve, regular exercise can produce improvements in anyone's baseline of fitness. The following principles of exercise are fundamental to any physical activity plan.

Overload Principle The **overload principle** requires a person exercising to provide a greater stress or demand on the body than it's usually accustomed to handling. For any muscle, including the heart, to get stronger, it must work against a greater-than-normal resistance or

STRATEGIES FOR CHANGE

Activating Your Lifestyle

- Add a physical component to passive activities. Stand while talking on the phone. Stretch during television commercials.
- Actively use waiting time. If you have to wait for a delayed appointment, take a quick walk down the hall or up the stairs.
- Create opportunities for getting physical. Go dancing instead of to the movies. Shoot hoops instead of sipping coffee.

HUMAN POTENTIAL

Sam Wade—Pedalers for Prostate and Easter Seals on Wheels

Sam Wade's adventures would fill an entire book. He was born in Richmond, British Columbia, where he grew up playing various sports and most notably was the team captain for his high school rugby team in both Grades 11 and 12.

Heading to university, he had a plan. While working toward a degree in kinesiology, he would also spend time with his girlfriend and play rugby. While the plan seemed to guarantee success, Sam found out that sometimes life happens. Within a couple of months, the relationship ended and an injury left Sam sidelined and unable to play the sport he loved. It was a time of great change in how Sam saw himself and his future. After several months of avoiding social situations, dropping grades, and struggling to get out of bed in the morning he sought out help.

During this time of transition, he became more invested in psychology classes. He also registered in a course focused on personal health, wellness, and potential. After meeting and being influenced by his psychology professors and a number of health and wellness presenters who shared stories of overcoming challenges and contributing to society, Sam began to re-engage in university life. He also participated in a small group community legacy project in the health and wellness class. He discovered that this project changed everything. Through this opportunity he began to realize and experience that the secret to life was about contribution and serving others.

The small community legacy project in one course evolved into monthly community legacy events with a group of friends through a project called *Simple Acts of Charitable Kindness*, or SACKS for short. Sam and his friends donated blood, funded the construction of a well in Africa, planted trees, and collected clothing, food, and books for those in need. "Going to class can only teach you so much," Sam says. "You can't be a passive learner. Education acts a catalyst, and when you combine it with action great things happen."

University life became exciting and meaningful. However, in November 2008, Sam learned his grandfather had been diagnosed with prostate cancer. While he was no longer running due to his rugby injury, Sam knew he could still cycle. He set in motion a plan to bike across Canada, from coast to coast, with a goal to raise money and awareness for prostate cancer research. Sam and the friends he recruited to participate in the ride called themselves *Pedalers for Prostate*. After 75 days and 8000 kilometres of cycling, Sam and his friends raised 13 000 dollars for the Prostate Centre in Victoria, British Columbia.

Sam believes that challenging trips such as the one he went on are an avenue for self-discovery. He says that you learn about what is physically and mentally possible when you have the right reasons, strategies, and supports in place. He credits friends Brian Tong, Tevis Bateman, and Fred Tsai for helping him complete the trip. "It's having someone that shares a dream with you that can give you the momentum and capacity to create lasting change."

The following summer, Sam enrolled in a university co-op program. He was employed as a camp counsellor at the B.C. Easter Seals organization, where children with disabilities have possibly the best week of their year. Tragically, that March he learned that a

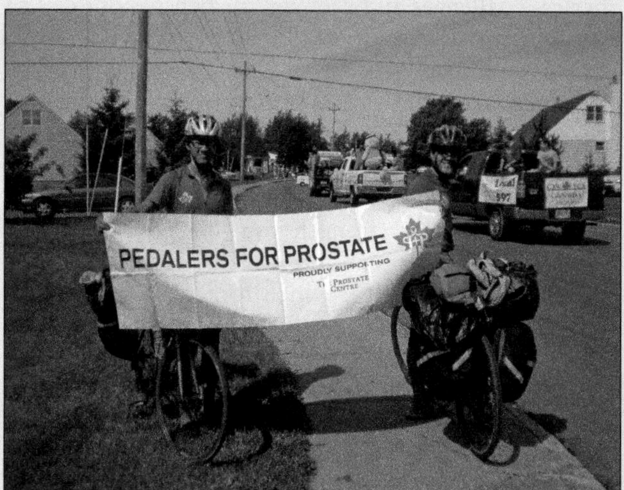

Courtesy of Sam Wade

Sam Wade and friend Brian Tong on their cross-Canada *Pedalers for Prostate* cancer fundraising tour.

friend of his, a boy born with Morquio syndrome who attended the camp, had unexpectedly passed away. So on April 30, 2011, under the banner of *Easter Seals on Wheels*, Sam and Brian began a second bike trip from Vancouver, British Columbia, to Mexico, to honour his friend and raise funds for the organization his friend valued so much. After another 3000-kilometre journey they fundraised 8000 dollars.

One year later, Sam was approached by a friend and previous camper, Luke Galvani. Luke was born with muscular dystrophy and uses a power wheelchair for mobility purposes. He had seen the work Sam had done at the camp and he also wanted to make a difference for the children who attend the Easter Seals Camps. This led to the creation of a second *Easter Seals on Wheels* fundraiser. Together, Sam and Luke decided to compete in three 24-hour Easter Seals relay races in Victoria, Vancouver, and Kelowna in 2012 as a fundraising opportunity. Sam clocked 100 kilometres in two hour-long shifts during the first relay. For the other two relays he ran and also "wheeled" in a manual wheelchair, which tested his physical capacity in a new way. Together Sam and Luke raised 10 000 dollars and were an example for staff, campers, and friends of what is physically possible to achieve, for people of all abilities.

Sam trusts that when you help for the right reasons there is truly unlimited potential in what we can accomplish. He is convinced that there is nothing more powerful than the human spirit. There have been times in his life where he regretted not taking action on something he felt passionate about. He says, "Learning to listen to my heart and taking action manifests life-changing results. A lot of times, when things become difficult we focus too much on the destination, but to me it's really been about the journey, the people you meet, the lives you change. That's what makes it all worth it."

Sam is now a pediatric occupational therapist working in Vancouver, British Columbia. He continues to serve children with disabilities and their families by providing tools and strategies that enable them to participate in all of life's possibilities.

challenge. To continue to improve, you need further increases in the demands—but not too much, too quickly. **Progressive overloading** gradually increases physical challenges and provides the benefits of exercise without the risk of injuries.

Overloading is specific to each body part and to each component of fitness. To improve cardiovascular fitness levels you must overload your cardiovascular system—the heart, lungs, and blood vessels—and walk or run with more intensity or for a longer duration. For muscular strength you must overload specific muscles. You can do this by increasing the tension on the muscles, which forces them to adapt and get larger. This is known as muscle **hypertrophy**. Leg exercises develop only the lower limbs; arm exercises, only the upper limbs. This is why each person needs a comprehensive fitness plan that includes a variety of exercises to develop different parts of the body.

How do you increase **tension** within a muscle—sometimes described as the primary load a muscle experiences when you exercise? You do it by adding resistance applied against the muscle or group of muscles you are trying to strengthen. Using your own body weight as the tension or resistance is one way. Exercise examples include performing push-ups or pull-ups. You can also use barbells, dumbbells, or other weight training equipment.

Whatever exercise you do, there is a level or threshold at which fitness begins to improve; a target zone, where you can achieve maximum benefits; and an upper level, at which potential risks outweigh any further benefits. The acronym **FITT** sums up the four dimensions of progressive overload: *frequency* (how often you exercise), *intensity* (how hard), *time* (how long), and *type* (specific activity).

Frequency To achieve and maintain physical fitness, you need to exercise regularly, but the recommended frequency varies with different types of exercise and with an individual's fitness goals. CSEP suggests that there is clear evidence that supports what they describe as a *dose-response relationship* between increased physical activity and health benefits. However, an extensive review of the exercise literature, conducted to update the Canadian Physical Activity Guidelines, did not show clear evidence that activity needed to be done daily or every other day. So the guidelines, described in the beginning section of this chapter, were revised from recommending activity every day for 60 minutes to recommendations that encourage a weekly amount of aerobic physical activity. As shown in Table 4-1, for 18- to 64-year-olds, CSEP recommends at least 150 minutes of aerobic MVPA per week.

For muscle- and bone-strengthening activities such as weight training, the recommendation is at least two days per week.

Intensity Exercise intensity varies with the type of exercise and with personal goals. To improve cardiovascular fitness, you need to increase your heart rate to a target zone (the level that produces benefits). More information about your target heart rate is included in the Cardiorespiratory section coming up. The Canadian Physical Activity Guidelines recommend moderate- to vigorous-intensity (MVPA) aerobic physical activity.

To develop muscular strength and endurance, you need to increase the amount of weight you lift or the resistance you work against and/or the number of repetitions. More information about resistance training is included in the Muscular Strength and Endurance section.

For enhanced flexibility, you need to stretch muscles beyond their normal length.

Time (Duration) The amount of time, or **duration**, of your workouts is also important, particularly for cardiovascular exercise. As mentioned above, the Canadian Physical Activity Guidelines recommend 150 minutes of moderate to vigorous aerobic physical activity per week. Duration and intensity are interlinked. If you're exercising at high intensity (biking or running at a brisk pace, for instance), you don't need to exercise as long as when you're working at lower intensity (walking or swimming at a moderate pace). For muscular strength and endurance and for flexibility, duration is defined by the number of sets or repetitions rather than total time.

Type (Specificity) The **specificity principle** refers to the body's adaption to a particular type of activity or amount of stress placed upon it. Jogging, for instance, trains the heart and lungs to work more efficiently and strengthens certain leg muscles, but it does not build upper body strength or enhance flexibility. If you want to improve on muscle strength, specific resistance training exercises will have to be performed. If increased flexibility is your goal, stretching exercises or yoga will have to be on your to-do list.

Reversibility Principle The **reversibility principle** is the opposite of the overload principle. Just as the body adapts to greater physical demands, it also adjusts to lower levels. If you stop exercising, you can lose as much as 50 percent of your fitness improvements within two months. If you have to curtail your usual exercise routine because of a busy schedule, you can best maintain your fitness by keeping the intensity constant and reducing frequency or duration. The principle of reversibility is aptly summed up by the phrase, "Use it or lose it."

Recovery Principle It is important to follow the **recovery principle** so that your body can adapt to the loads you put upon it, whether that is aerobic conditioning exercises such as walking, jogging, or running or resistance or weight training exercises such as calisthenics or resistance training. To recover from aerobic conditioning sessions alternate days of training. If you are a beginner walker or runner, start by walking two or three times a week with a day of rest in between walks and runs. Once you are a seasoned walker or runner try alternating walks and runs on a daily basis. Or walk or run shorter distances one day and longer distances another.

For muscle strength allow 48 hours but no more than 96 hours between training sessions. Two or three 30-minute training sessions a week can be sufficient for building muscle strength and endurance. You can train every day, but if you do, design your activity sessions so that alternate muscle groups are being worked on different days.

How Much Exercise Is Enough? The answer to this question is—It depends on your exercise goal: fitness or health. The two are related, but are not the same. Fit people are healthy people with reduced risks of heart disease, hypertension, stroke, and diabetes and a lower mortality rate. Yet it is possible to get nearly all the health benefits of exercise without reaching high levels of fitness. Dr. Steven Blair from the Cooper Aerobic Institute found similar health benefits from a single 30-minute session of moderate exercise as from three 10-minute moderate aerobic sessions throughout the day.[54]

If you're not active at all, any physical exercise will produce some benefits. In the beginning, you are better off starting out *slow and short*, with just a 10-minute walk or bike ride a few days a week, than pushing to do too much and giving up because of injury or discomfort.[55] In a study of 45 healthy office workers, even those who exercised just once a week had lower body weights and lower body fat than those who didn't work out at all.[56] Simply walking one hour a week reduced the risk of heart disease for sedentary middle-aged women, even those who were overweight, smoked, or had high cholesterol.[57]

Should I Check with My Doctor Before I Get Started? If you are unsure about whether or not you should begin a physical activity or exercise program, you might want to complete the Physical Activity Readiness Questionnaire (PAR-Q). This form, developed by the B.C. Ministry of Health in 1978[58] and revised by an Expert Advisory Committee of the Canadian Society for Exercise Physiology in 2002,[59] consists of seven questions that will help you determine if you are ready to begin exercising (see Table 4-2). Also available are the PARmedX, which is used by physicians for individuals who have had positive responses to the PAR-Q, and the PARmedX for Pregnancy, for pregnant women who wish to become more active.[60]

Improving Cardiorespiratory Fitness As defined in the Physical Activity and Fitness section, cardiorespiratory fitness refers to the ability of the heart, lungs, and circulatory system to deliver oxygen to muscles working rhythmically over an extended period of time. Unlike muscular endurance, which is specific to individual muscles, cardiorespiratory endurance involves the entire body. **Aerobic exercise**, which improves cardiorespiratory endurance, is any physical activity that stimulates and strengthens the body's ability to utilize oxygen. Examples include brisk walking, jogging, and running. A person who builds up good aerobic capacity can maintain long periods of physical activity without great fatigue.

In **anaerobic exercise**, the amount of oxygen taken in by the body cannot meet the demands of the activity. This quickly creates an oxygen deficit that must be made up later. Anaerobic activities are high in intensity but short in duration, usually lasting only about ten seconds to two minutes. An example is sprinting 400 metres, which leaves even the best-trained athletes gasping for air.

In non-aerobic exercise, such as bowling, softball, or doubles tennis, there is frequent rest between activities. Because the body can take in all the oxygen it needs, the heart and lungs really don't get as much of a workout.

Am I Working Hard Enough? There are different ways you can determine whether you are exercising hard enough or if you are overdoing it.

Target Heart Rate—Standard Method To use your pulse or heart rate as a guide, feel your pulse in the carotid artery in your neck. Slightly tilt your head back and to one side. Use your middle finger or forefinger, or both, to feel for your pulse. (Do not use your thumb; it has a pulse of its own.) Do not press too hard or you will slow or cut off the blood supply to your brain and heart. You can also use the radial artery along the side of your wrist. Press your forefinger and middle finger down gently on the radial artery until you feel a pulse. Again, do not press too hard. To determine your heart rate, count the number of pulses you feel for 10 seconds and multiply that number by six, or count for 30 seconds and multiply that number by two. The first count is "0".

Your **resting heart rate (RHR)** is usually measured while lying down on your back. Fitness experts suggest that you measure RHR first thing in the morning upon waking. Fitness trainers and coaches also remind us that heart rate response depends on our posture. Peter Dobas, a Community Manager at Obstacle Course Training, suggests that we measure our RHR in the position that is similar to the activity we are about to participate in.[61] A standing RHR, which is often 10–15 beats per minute above a supine RHR, might be a better starting point for individuals who are walking, jogging, or running. A seated RHR might be more appropriate as a baseline measurement for cycling or rowing activities. A supine or lying down RHR might be better for a baseline for swimmers.

For target heart rate, begin taking your pulse during, or immediately after, exercise, when it's much more pronounced than when you're at rest. Three minutes after exercise, take your heart rate again. The closer that reading is to your resting heart rate, the better your condition. If it takes a long time for your pulse to recover and return to its resting level, your body's ability to handle physical stress is poor. As you continue working out, however, your pulse will return to normal much more quickly.

TABLE 4-2

Physical Activity Readiness Questionnaire (PAR-Q)

Physical Activity Readiness Questionnaire PAR-Q (revised 2002)

PAR-Q & YOU

(A Questionnaire for People Aged 15–69)

Regular physical activity is fun and healthy, and increasingly more people are starting to become more active every day. Being more active is very safe for most people. However, some people should check with their doctor before they start becoming much more physically active. If you are planning to become much more physically active than you are now, start by answering the seven questions in the box below. If you are between the ages of 15 and 69, the PAR-Q will tell you if you should check with your doctor before you start. If you are over 69 years of age and you are not used to being very active, check with your doctor.

Common sense is your best guide when you answer these questions. Please read the questions carefully and answer each one honestly: check YES or NO.

YES	NO	
☐	☐	**1. Has your doctor ever said that you have a heart condition <u>and</u> that you should only do physical activity recommended by a doctor?**
☐	☐	**2. Do you feel pain in your chest when you do physical activity?**
☐	☐	**3. In the past month, have you had chest pain when you were not doing physical activity?**
☐	☐	**4. Do you lose your balance because of dizziness or do you ever lose consciousness?**
☐	☐	**5. Do you have a bone or joint problem (e.g., back, knee, or hip) that could be made worse by a change in your physical activity?**
☐	☐	**6. Is your doctor currently prescribing drugs (e.g., water pills) for your blood pressure or heart condition?**
☐	☐	**7. Do you know of <u>any other reason</u> why you should not do physical activity?**

If you answered

YES to one or more questions

Talk with your doctor by phone or in person BEFORE you start becoming much more physically active or BEFORE you have a fitness appraisal. Tell your doctor about the PAR-Q and which questions you answered YES.

- You may be able to do any activity you want—as long as you start slowly and build up gradually. Or, you may need to restrict your activities to those which are safe for you. Talk with your doctor about the kinds of activities you wish to participate in and follow his/her advice.
- Find out which community programs are safe and helpful for you.

NO to all questions

If you answered NO honestly to <u>all</u> PAR-Q questions, you can be reasonably sure that you can

- start becoming much more physically active—begin slowly and build up gradually. This is the safest and easiest way to go.
- take part in a fitness appraisal—this is an excellent way to determine your basic fitness so that you can plan the best way for you to live actively. It is also highly recommended that you have your blood pressure evaluated. If your reading is over 144/94, talk with your doctor before you start becoming much more physically active.

➔ **DELAY BECOMING MUCH MORE ACTIVE:**

- If you are not feeling well because of a temporary illness such as a cold or a fever—wait until you feel better; or
- If you are or may be pregnant—talk to your doctor before you start becoming more active.

PLEASE NOTE: If your health changes so that you then answer YES to any of the above questions, tell your fitness or health professional. Ask whether you should change your physical activity plan.

Informed Use of the PAR-Q: The Canadian Society for Exercise Physiology, Health Canada, and their agents assume no liability for persons who undertake physical activity. If in doubt after completing this questionnaire, consult your doctor prior to physical activity.

Source: Physical Activity Readiness Questionnaire (PAR-Q) © 2002. Used with permission from Canadian Society for Exercise Physiology. www.csep.ca

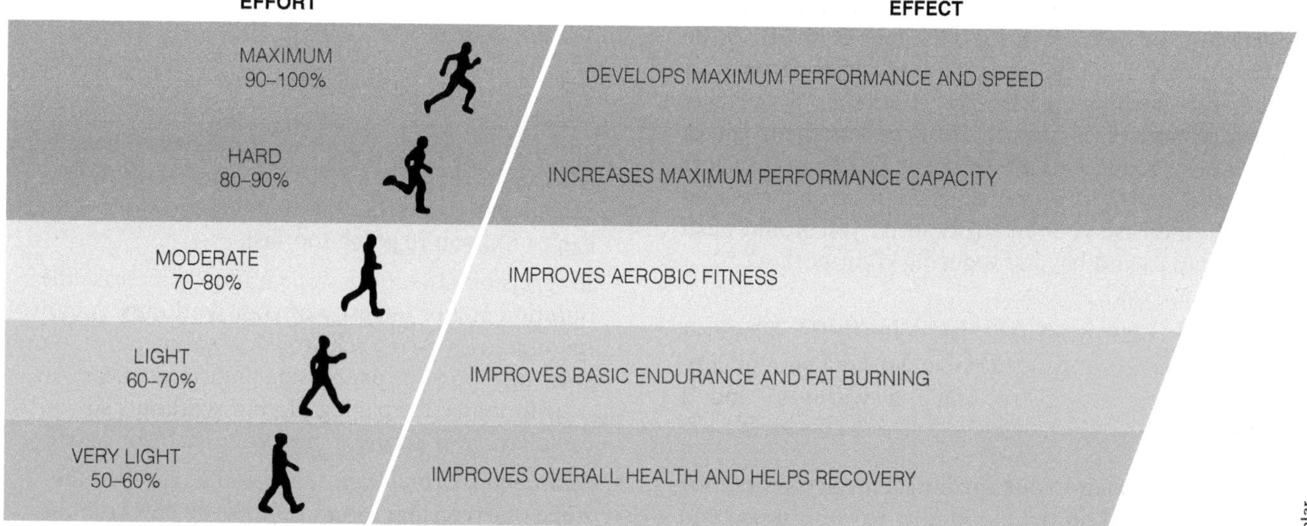

Figure 4-4 **Recommended Target Heart Rate Zones for Various Levels of Activity**

You don't want to push yourself to your maximum heart rate, but fitness experts recommend you exercise at about 55–90 percent of that maximum to get cardiovascular benefits from your training. This range is called your **target heart rate.** If you don't exercise intensely enough to raise your heart rate, your heart and lungs do not benefit as much from the workout. If you push too hard and exercise at or near your absolute maximum heart rate, you can run the risk of placing too great a burden on your heart. Figure 4-4 shows the target heart rates for various zones of exercise intensity. Remember, your heart rate is dependent on many factors such as amount of restful sleep, food and drink choices and amounts, stress levels, and body temperature. Use heart rate monitoring as a guide only.

The following formula can also be used to calculate your maximum and target heart rates (in beats per minute):

1. Estimate your maximum heart rate. Take 220 − your age = (this is your maximum).
2. Determine your lower-limit target heart rate by multiplying your maximum heart rate by 0.55 = ._____
3. Determine your upper-limit target heart rate by multiplying your maximum heart rate by 0.9 = . _____

Your target heart rate range is between your lower and upper limits.

If your goal is losing weight, exercise at 55–70 percent of your maximum heart rate in order to burn fat calories. To improve aerobic endurance and strengthen your heart, work at 70–80 percent of your maximum heart rate. A target heart rate of between 40 and 50 percent of maximum is recommended for individuals who are in poor physical condition. Competitive athletes often train at 80–100 percent of their maximum heart rate.[62]

Target Heart Rate—Karvonen Method Another way to measure heart rate is to use the Karvonen formula. Some fitness experts believe that using the Karvonen method provides a more accurate training heart rate (THR). Whereas the target heart rate calculation method described in the previous section is a common method used, it does not take into consideration the individual differences in resting heart rate. The Karvonen method incorporates heart rate reserve, which is the difference between your maximum heart rate and your resting heart rate.[63]

The Karvonen formula is: THR = ([HRmax − HRrest] × % intensity) + HRrest. HRmax (maximum heart rate) minus HRrest (resting heart rate) equals HRR, or heart rate reserve.

To determine your maximum heart rate (HRmax), use this method:

Women: 226 – your age
Men: 220 – your age.

There are many online Training Heart Rate calculators available. A Canadian option is available at www.ottawarun.com/heartrate.htm[64] where both the Standard method and the Karvonen method are calculated.

Rating of Perceived Exertion (RPE) Another option for monitoring exercise intensity is the **rating of perceived exertion (RPE)**, a self-assessment scale that rates symptoms of exertion, such as breathlessness and fatigue. You can use the RPE scale to describe your sensation of effort when exercising and gauge how hard you are working. The original scale was developed by Gunnar Borg in 1982. His scale had a range of 6–20. The rating of six described "no feeling of exertion" whereas the rating of 20 described a feeling of "very, very hard" exertion. The revised Borg Category-Ratio-10 scale (CR-10) uses a rating scale of 0–10 with 0 being a rating of "nothing at all" and 10 being "extremely strong (almost maximum)." With the modified version of the Borg Scale, you would want to rate your effort between 3 and 7 to be working in an aerobic training zone. To increase your intensity level, you would push yourself up to and beyond 8 during your workout.[65]

How Do I Design an Aerobic Workout? Whatever activity you choose, your aerobic workout should consist of several stages, including a warm-up and a cool-down.

Warm-Up To prepare your cardiorespiratory system for a workout, speed up the blood flow to your lungs, and increase the temperature and elasticity of your muscles and connective tissue to avoid injury, start by moving gently. Walking briskly for about five minutes is a good way to begin. This helps your body make the transition from inactivity to exertion. Follow this general warm-up with some simple strength, balance, and stretching exercises. After reviewing more than 350 scientific studies, the ACSM concluded that preparing for sports or exercise should involve a variety of activities and not be limited to stretching alone.

Aerobic Activity The two key components of this part of your workout are intensity and duration. As described in the previous section, you can use your target heart rate range to make sure you are working at the proper intensity. The current recommendation is to move 150 minutes per week. If you like to participate in daily physical activity, following the Canadian Physical Activity Guidelines over a seven-day period would mean actively exercising about 21 minutes per day. Each activity session should last at least 10 minutes.

Cool-Down There are different views on how individuals should cool down after participating in aerobic activity sessions. After you have pushed your heart rate up to its target level and kept it there for a length of time, it is a good idea to slow the pace of exercise instead of stopping suddenly. Walking for 5–10 minutes at a comfortable pace before you end your workout session can ensure an adequate supply of blood to the heart and prevent blood pooling in your lower extremities. It can also help to lower the level of lactic acid buildup in your muscles; this can alleviate delayed onset muscle soreness, which can occur between 24 and 48 hours after your workout.[66]

Your Long-Term Fitness Plan One of the most common mistakes people make is to push too hard, too fast. Often they end up injured or discouraged and quit entirely. If you are just starting an aerobic program, think of it as a series of phases: beginning, progression, and maintenance:

- *Beginning (4–6 weeks).* Start slow and low (in intensity). If you're walking, monitor your heart rate and aim for 55 percent of your maximum heart rate. Moving at the right pace is also important. If you can sing as you walk, you're going too slowly; if you can't talk, you're going too fast.
- *Progression (16–20 weeks).* Gradually increase the duration and/or intensity of your workouts. Add five minutes every two weeks to your walking time. Gradually pick up your pace, using your target heart rate as your guide. Keep a log of your workouts so you can chart your progress until you reach your goal.
- *Maintenance (lifelong).* Once you've reached the stage of exercising for an hour every day, combine or alternate activities that you enjoy. This can be a form of *cross-training.*

Walking Walking continues to be the most popular physical activity in Canada. In 2013, 72.4 percent of Canadians reported walking during their leisure time in the past three months.[67] The good news is that walking may well be one of the best exercises we can do. Figure 4-5 shows good walking technique.

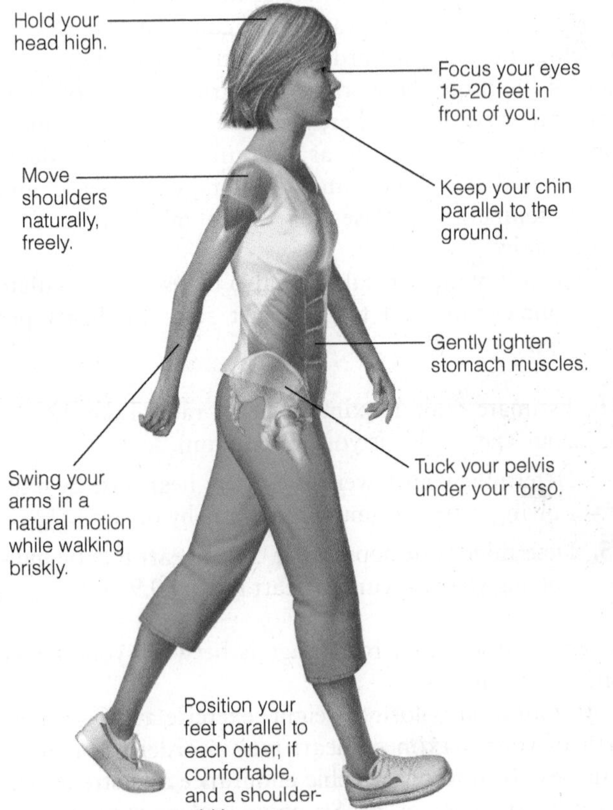

Figure 4-5 Good Walking Technique

Source: Mayo Clinic © Mayo Foundation for Medical Education and Research. All Rights Reserved. www.mayoclinic.com

Research has demonstrated the health benefits of walking for both men and women and for both healthy individuals and those with heart disease. The Women's Health Study found that even walking one hour per week can lower heart-disease risk among relatively sedentary women.[68] Walking also protects men's hearts, whether they're healthy or have had heart problems. In a British study of 772 men, those who regularly engaged in light exercise, including walking, had a risk of death that was 58 percent lower than that of their sedentary counterparts.[69]

The Physical Activity Resource Centre (PARC), managed by the Ontario Physical and Health Education Centre (OPHEA), has a user-friendly toolkit available online called *Walk This Way Users Guide*.[70] You can learn about setting walking goals, how to include walking in your daily life, and how to keep track of your walking program. A *Walk This Way First Nations Kit* is also available. Treadmills are another option. They keep you moving at a certain pace and are a good alternative to outdoor walks. Holding onto the handrails while walking on a treadmill is recommended if you are not familiar with this type of cardio equipment, but it does reduce both heart rate and oxygen consumption, so you burn fewer calories. Experts advise that treadmill training can be used in rehabilitation from strokes or Parkinson's disease.[71]

There is a body of research about *manpo-kei* or 10 000 steps.[72] Some studies suggest that stepping 10 000 times a day can be a beneficial way to increase heart health, lose weight, and feel healthier. Crouteau implemented an eight-week pedometer lifestyle-intervention program with 37 college employees. The results of this study indicated that those employees who used pedometers had a significant increase in average daily step counts as compared to those who did not use pedometers.[73] Tudor-Locke, one of the foremost pedometer researchers, began the First Step Program, a research project funded by the Canadian Diabetic Association. Her findings showed the activity level of older adults in the First Step Program who used pedometers was significantly higher than the activity level of the control group—the participants in the research study who did not use pedometers.[74,75]

The typical adult averages about 5310 steps per day. Children average between 11 000 and 13 000 steps per day. Very active children average about 16 000 steps. How far is 10 000 steps? The average person's stride length is approximately .76 metres long. That means it takes just over 2000 steps to walk 1.6 kilometres or 1 mile. Ten thousand steps are close to eight kilometres or five miles. (See step conversions in Tables 4-3, 4-4, and 4-5). Wearing a pedometer or any of the numerous activity trackers such as Fitbit, Garmin, Misfit, Jawbone, or Microsoft band is an easy way to track your steps each day. Start by wearing your activity tracker every day for one week. Put it on when you get up in the morning and wear it until bedtime. Record your daily steps in a log or diary. Or try one of many new apps available such as Nike+, Strava, My Fitness Pal, or Runtastic.[76] Another option is mapping your route and calculating the distance travelled using online route planners.[77] After one week you can calculate your average daily steps. To increase your step count, add 500 daily steps every week until you reach 10 000 steps per day.

Although a pedometer cannot gauge the intensity of your effort—it counts walking on flat ground the same as hiking up a mountain, and stride length will differ from person to person—the benefits of using a pedometer far outweigh these small limitations.

TABLE 4-3

Step Your Way to Health and Fitness

Step Conversion Chart—Approximate Distance

Steps	Kilometres	Miles
500	0.4	0.25
1000	0.8	0.50
2000	1.6	1.0
3000	2.4	1.5
4000	3.2	2.0
5000	4.0	2.5
6000	4.8	3.0
7000	5.6	3.5
8000	6.4	4.0
9000	7.2	4.5
10 000	8.0	5.0

Jogging and Running The difference between jogging and running is speed. You should be able to carry on a conversation with someone on a long jog or run; if you're too breathless to talk, you're pushing too hard.

If your goal is to enhance aerobic fitness, then long, slow, distance running is best. If you want to improve your speed, try *interval training*, which consists of repeated hard runs over a certain distance, with intervals of relaxed jogging in between. Depending on what

TABLE 4-4

Walking Time and Approximate Step Count Conversion

Minutes	Steps
20 minutes	Equals about 3000 steps
30 minutes	Equals about 3000 to 6000 steps
50 minutes	Equals about 6000 to 8000 steps
60 minutes	Equals about 8000 to 10 000 steps

TABLE 4-5

Adult Step Conversion Chart

Activity Conversion for Adults

ACTIVITY STEPS PER MINUTE	F	M
Aerobic dancing (low impact)	142	127
Aerobics (high impact)	189	181
Aerobics (6–8" step)	236	218
Aerobics (10–12" step)	260	254
Backpacking (on hill with under 4.5 kg or 10 lb load)	189	181
Backpacking (on hill with 4.5–9.07 kg or 10–20 lb load)	212	199
Ballet dancing	118	127
Baseball	142	127
Basketball (leisurely, non-game)	165	127
Basketball (game)	212	145
Basketball (playing in wheelchair)	165	163
Bicycling	212	199
Bicycling (BMX or mountain)	236	218
Bicycling (stationary–general)	189	181
Bicycling (stationary–light)	142	145
Bicycling (stationary–moderate)	189	181
Bicycling (stationary–vigorous)	283	254
Bowling	71	73
Canoeing	94	91
Chopping wood	165	145
Circuit training (general)	212	199
Dancing, ballroom (slow)	71	73
Dancing, ballroom (fast)	118	109
Dancing, country	118	109
Dancing, disco	118	109
Dancing, line	118	109
Dancing, square	118	109
Dancing, swing	118	109
Elliptical jogger (medium)	236	218
Football, tackle	236	218
Football, touch/flag	212	199
Gardening (moderate)	118	109
Gardening (heavy)	142	145
Golf (without cart)	118	109
Golfing (riding in cart)	94	91
Horseshoes	71	73
Ice skating (leisurely)	189	181
In-line skating	200	190
Jogging (general)	189	181
Jogging (in water)	212	199
Judo and karate	260	254
Jumping rope (slow)	212	199
Jumping rope (moderate)	260	254
Jumping rope (fast)	330	290
Kickboxing (moderate)	330	290
Kickboxing (vigorous)	401	363
Kickboxing (very vigorous	472	435
Mowing lawn	142	127
Pilates	94	91
Racquetball (casual)	189	181
Racquetball (competitive)	260	254
Rowing	189	181
Running 12.8 km/hr or 8 miles/hr (7.5 minutes/mile or 4.7 minutes/km)	354	326
Running 16 km/hr or 10 miles/hr (6 minutes/mile or 3.8 minutes/km)	425	399
Scrubbing floors	94	91
Shovelling snow	165	145
Skiing downhill (moderate to steep)	165	145
Skiing cross-country	212	181
Snowshoeing	212	199
Soccer (casual)	189	181
Soccer (competitive)	260	145
Stair climber machine	236	218
Stair climbing (up stairs)	212	199
Stair climbing (down stairs)	71	73
Swimming, backstroke	189	181
Swimming, breaststroke	260	254
Swimming, butterfly	283	272
Swimming, freestyle	189	181
Swimming, sidestroke	212	199
Tennis (doubles)	165	145
Vacuuming	94	73
Volleyball	118	91
Walking	94	91
Washing the car	71	73
Waterskiing	165	145
Waxing the car	118	109
Weight-lifting	71	73
Wrestling	165	145
Yoga	71	54

Source: America on the Move Foundation, Inc., 2008. http://www.toddpost537.org/Documents/POWER/MTS1/HANDOUT-Step_Conversion_Chart.pdf

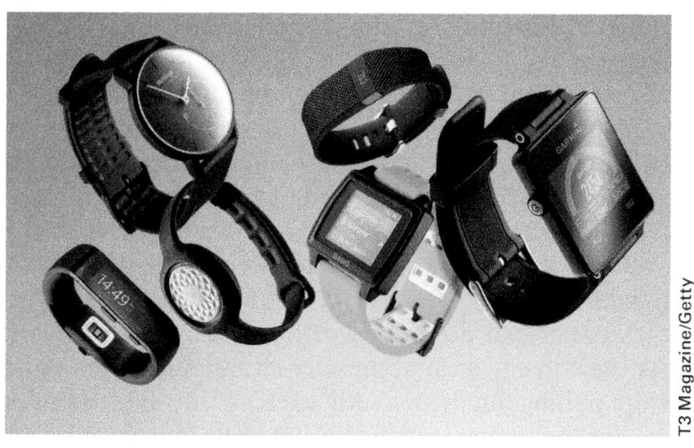
T3 Magazine/Getty

Fitness trackers like these allow you to track your steps, distance, calories burned, and active minutes.

suits you and what your training goals are, you can vary the distance, duration, and number of fast runs, as well as the time and activity between them.

If you have been sedentary, it's best to launch a walking program before attempting to jog or run. Start by walking for 10–20 minutes three times a week at a comfortable pace. Once you can complete a brisk 20-minute walk, alternate fast walking with slow jogging. Continue to alternate in this manner until you can jog for 10 minutes without stopping.

Other Aerobic Activities Many people prefer different forms of aerobic exercise. All of the activities listed below can provide many health benefits. Among the popular options are:

- *Aerobic dance or fitness class.* A typical aerobic class consists of warm-up stretching exercises followed by choreographed movement patterns, often done to music. Some classes include floor exercises such as sit-ups and muscle strength and endurance exercises followed by cool-down exercises.
- *Cardio kick-boxing.* Also referred to as kick-boxing or boxing aerobics, this hybrid of boxing, martial arts, and aerobics offers an intense total-body workout. An hour of kick-boxing burns an average of 500–800 calories, compared to 300–400 calories in a typical step class.
- *Exergaming.* A popular way to "get fit" today is to participate in **Exergaming**, which is defined as the playing of video games that require rigorous physical exercise and are intended as a workout.[78] Participants can race virtual bicycles by pedalling a simulated exercise bike or try out a variety of sports such as tennis, baseball, and boxing programs. The farther along you advance in these games, the more challenging the exercise session becomes. One study on male and female college students found that their participation in interactive computer bike racing games was as effective as traditional exercise in eliciting recommended training heart rates in accordance with the American College of Sports Medicine (ACSM) guidelines.[79] In another study of Taiwanese university medical students, researchers discovered that participation in Kinect Sports video game programs provided a moderate to vigorous level of physical activity.[80]
- *HITT—High Intensity Interval Training.* **HITT** refers to exercise training sessions that consist of up to 10 minutes of intense exercise within a 30-minute training session that includes a warm-up, interval training, recovery periods, and a cool-down.[81] HITT training programs often mix aerobic exercise, calisthenics, and weight lifting. Equipment such as jump ropes, rowing machines, resistance bands, gymnastics rings, plyometric boxes, and kettlebells are used to increase intensity of the workouts.
- *Spinning™.* Spinning is a cardiovascular workout for the whole body that utilizes a special stationary bicycle. Led by an instructor, a group of bikers listens to music and modifies their individual bike's resistance and their own pace according to the rhythm. An average spinning class lasts 45 minutes. Spinning is a popular option for aerobic exercise because people of different ages, skills, and fitness levels can participate in the same class.
- *Step training or bench aerobics.* Stepping combines step or bench climbing with music and choreographed movements. Basic equipment consists of a bench 10–30 centimetres high. The fitter you are, the higher the bench—but the higher the bench, the greater the risk of knee injury.
- *Stair climbing.* Stair-climbing machines are a popular piece of fitness equipment in most fitness centres. Exercisers push a pair of pedals up and down, which is much easier on the feet and legs than many other activities. You can also use the stairs in an office building or dormitory as a way of increasing your

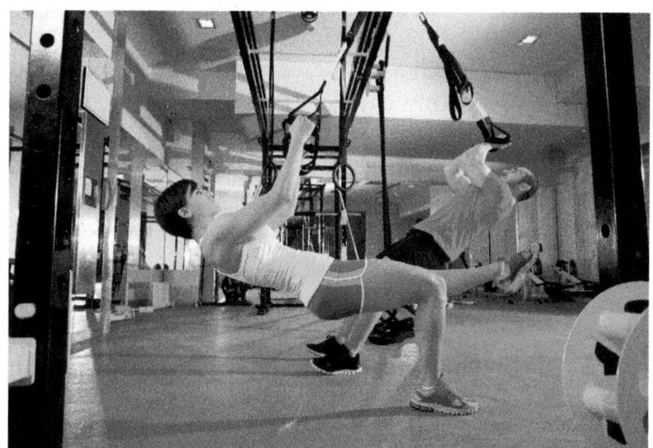
holbox/Shutterstock

HITT (High Intensity Interval Training) consists of bouts of 10 minutes of intense exercise within a 30-minute workout. Workouts include the use of plyometric boxes.

daily physical activity. Climbing just two flights of stairs every day could result in a loss of 2.7 kilograms, or six pounds, per year.[82]

- *Swimming*. For aerobic conditioning, try to keep up a steady pace for 20 minutes that's fast enough to make you feel pleasantly tired, but not completely exhausted. Your heart will beat more slowly in water than on land, so your heart rate while swimming is not an accurate guide to exercise intensity.

MUSCULAR STRENGTH AND ENDURANCE

Muscular fitness workouts are important because they enable muscles to work more efficiently and reliably. Conditioned muscles function more smoothly and contract more vigorously with less effort. With exercise, muscle tissue becomes firmer and can withstand much more strain—the result of toughening the sheath protecting the muscle and developing more connective tissue within it.

The two dimensions of muscular fitness are strength and endurance. As described in the introductory section of this chapter, **muscular strength** is the maximal force that a muscle or group of muscles can generate for one movement.[83] We measure muscular strength by establishing how much weight a person can lift once. Trainers call this your **one repetition maximum**, or **1RM. Muscular endurance** is the capacity to sustain repeated muscle actions.[84] Research on burning fat shows that a good way to reduce your body fat is to add muscle strength and endurance exercises to your workouts. Muscle tissue is your very best calorie-burning tissue, and the more you have, the more calories you burn, even when you are resting. You don't have to become a serious bodybuilder. Using hand-held or free weights two or three times a week is enough.

Prolonged exercise prepares the muscles for sustained work by improving the circulation of blood in the tissue. The number of tiny blood vessels, called capillaries, increases by as much as 50 percent in regularly exercised muscles, and existing capillaries open wider so that the total circulation increases by as much as 400 percent, thus providing the muscles with a much greater supply of nutrients. This increase occurs after about 8–12 weeks in young people, but takes longer in older individuals. Inactivity reverses the process, gradually shutting down the extra capillaries that have developed.

Muscles at Work Muscles that are not used will atrophy, weaken, or break down. If you use them rigorously and regularly, however, they grow stronger. The only way to develop muscles is by demanding more of them than you usually do as described in the section discussing the overload principle on page 84. This is called **overloading.** As you train, you have to gradually increase the number of repetitions or the amount of resistance and work the muscle to temporary fatigue.

You need to exercise differently for strength than for endurance. To *develop strength*, do four to eight repetitions with heavy loads. As you increase the weight your muscles must move, you increase your strength. To *increase endurance*, do eight to twelve repetitions with lighter loads.

Muscles can do only two things: contract or relax. As they do so, skeletal muscles either pull on bones or stop pulling on bones. All exercise involves muscles pulling on bones across a joint. The movement that takes place depends on the structure of the joint and the position of the muscle attachments involved.

In an **isometric** contraction, the muscle applies force while maintaining an equal length. The muscle contracts and tries to shorten but cannot overcome the resistance. An example is pushing against an immovable object, such as a wall, or tightening an abdominal muscle while sitting. There is no movement as the muscle contracts. Push or pull against the immovable object, and hold each muscle contraction for five to eight seconds; repeat 5–10 times daily.

An **isotonic** contraction involves dynamic muscle movement against a constant resistance several times. The actual force exerted by the muscle is not constant because at some point in the movement, the position of the joint will produce a mechanical advantage. Contracting the muscle constitutes the **concentric phase** of an isotonic contraction. Lowering the weight to the starting position of the exercise represents the **eccentric phase** of the lift.

True **isokinetic** contraction is a constant speed contraction. Isokinetic exercises require special machines that provide resistance to overload muscles throughout the entire range of motion. Hydraulic strength training equipment used in some fitness centres such as Curves is sometimes called an isokinetic training program.

How Do I Design a Muscle Workout? A workout with weights should exercise your body's primary muscle groups, including the *deltoids* (shoulders), *pectorals* (chest), *triceps* and *biceps* (back and front of upper arms), *quadriceps* and *hamstrings* (front and back of thighs), *gluteus maximus* (buttocks), *trapezius* and *rhomboids* (upper back), and *abdomen* (see Figure 4-6). Various machines and free-weight routines focus on each muscle group, but the principle is always the same. Muscles contract and relax as you raise and lower a weight, and you repeat the lift-and-lower routine until the muscle group is tired.

A weight-training program is made up of **repetitions** or **reps** (the single performance of an exercise, such as lifting 20 kilograms one time) and **sets** (a set is the number of repetitions of the same movement, such as a set of 20 push-ups).

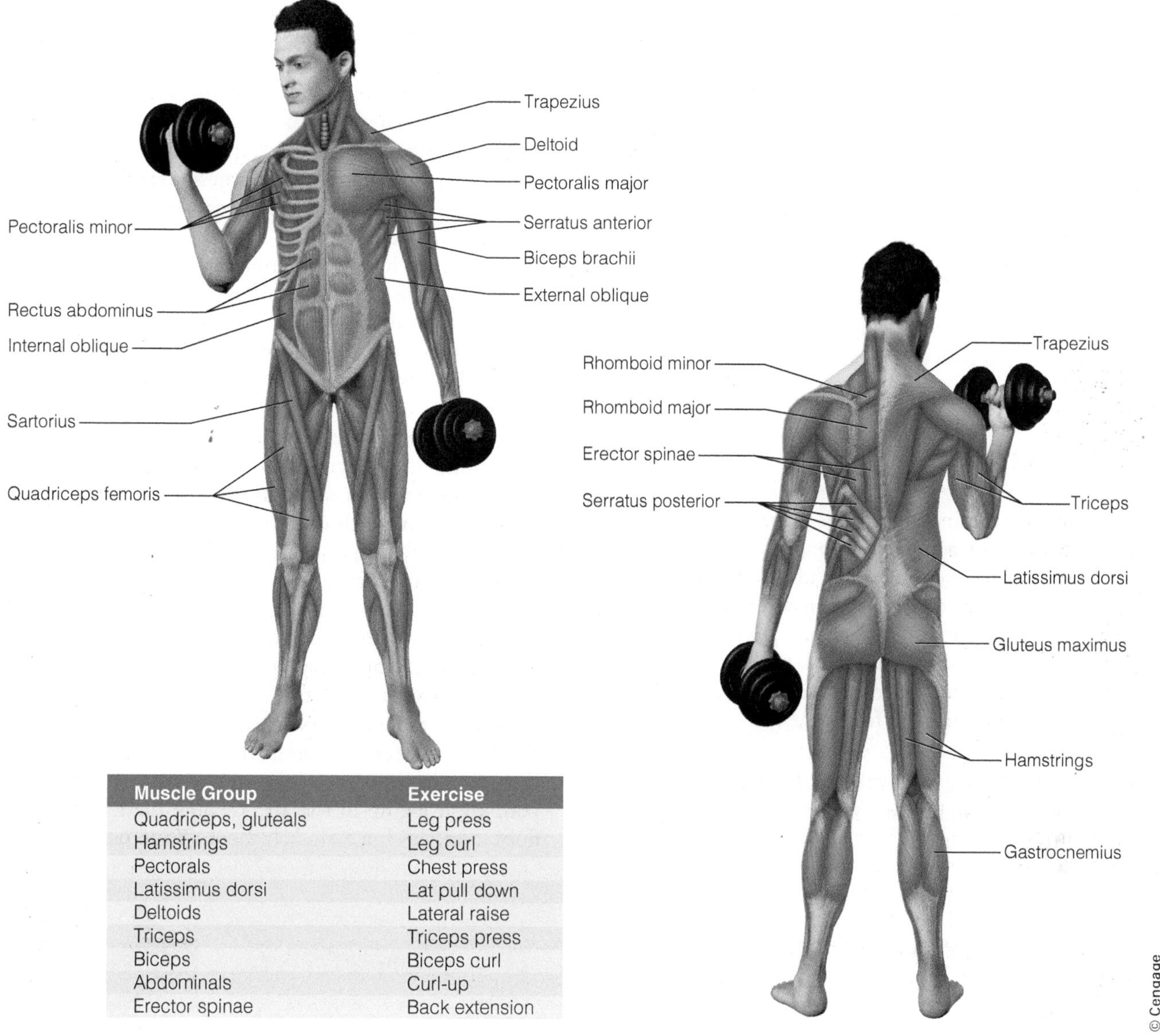

Muscle Group	Exercise
Quadriceps, gluteals	Leg press
Hamstrings	Leg curl
Pectorals	Chest press
Latissimus dorsi	Lat pull down
Deltoids	Lateral raise
Triceps	Triceps press
Biceps	Biceps curl
Abdominals	Curl-up
Erector spinae	Back extension

Figure 4-6 **Primary Muscle Groups**

Different exercises can strengthen and stretch different muscle groups.

Maintaining proper breathing during weight training is crucial. To breathe correctly, inhale when muscles are relaxed, and exhale when you push or lift. Don't hold your breath, because oxygen flow helps prevent muscle fatigue and injury.

No one type of equipment—free weight or machine—has a clear advantage in terms of building fat-free body mass, enhancing strength and endurance, or improving a sport-specific skill. Each type offers benefits but also has drawbacks.

Free weights offer great versatility for strength training. With dumbbells you can perform a variety of exercises to work specific muscle groups, such as the chest and shoulders. Machines, in contrast, are more limited; most allow only one exercise.

However, strength-training machines have advantages, too. They ensure correct movement for a lift, which helps protect against injury and prevent cheating when fatigue sets in. They isolate specific muscles, which is good for rehabilitating an injury or strengthening a specific body part. Because they offer high-tech options such as varying resistance during the lifting motion, they can tax muscles in ways that a traditional barbell cannot.

Core strength conditioning refers to the training of the muscles that support your spine and keep your body stable and balanced. When you have good core stability, the muscles in your pelvis, lower back, hips, and abdomen work in harmony. When your core is weak, you become more susceptible to lower back pain and injury. The major muscles of your core include the transverse abdominis, the deepest of the abdominal muscles; the external and internal obliques on the side and front of the abdomen around your waist; and the rectus abdominis, a long muscle that extends along the front of the abdomen. Strengthening all your core muscles provides stability, improves balance, and protects you from injury. Other types of exercise programs such as yoga, Pilates, and the use of exercise balls, bosu balls, and balance boards provide muscle strength and endurance workouts, too. Beginner to advanced classes are available with certified instructors.

✓ CHECK-IN

What type of strength training exercises do you do as part of your physical activity sessions?

FLEXIBILITY

Flexibility determines the range of motion achievable without injury at a joint or group of joints. Genetics, age, sex, and body composition all influence how flexible you are. Over time, the natural elasticity of muscles, tendons, and joints decreases, which results in stiffness. Girls and women tend to be more flexible than boys and men to a certain extent because of hormonal and anatomical differences.

How Do I Design a Flexibility Workout? There are three ways to stretch: static stretching, PNF stretching, and ballistic stretching.

Static stretching involves a gradual stretch held for a short time (10–60 seconds). A shorter stretch provides little benefit. Since a slow stretch provokes less of a reaction from the **stretch receptors** (sensory receptors found within the belly of a muscle that detect changes in the length of the muscle), the muscles can safely stretch farther than usual. Fitness experts most often recommend static stretching because it is both safe and effective. An example of a static stretch is the knee chest pull for lower back muscles. (See Figure 4-7 (e)). With one leg stretched out (with knee in a soft, unlocked position), gently pull the other leg toward your chest. Hold for 10–60 seconds. Repeat with the other leg. You should feel a pull, but not pain, during the stretch.

In **PNF (proprioceptive neuromuscular facilitation) stretching** your own body, a partner, gravity, or a weight serves as an external force or resistance to help your joints move through their range of motion. PNF stretching techniques can be *passive*—no associated muscular contraction, or *active*—voluntary muscle contraction. You can achieve a more intense stretch and a greater range of motion with PNF stretching. There is a risk of injury, however, because the muscles themselves are not controlling the stretch.

One example of a PNF stretch is the *hold-relax* technique. To stretch your hamstring muscle (the muscle of the upper back of your leg), you lie on the floor and lift your right leg up in the air, keeping the left leg on the floor and the knee slightly bent. Your partner moves

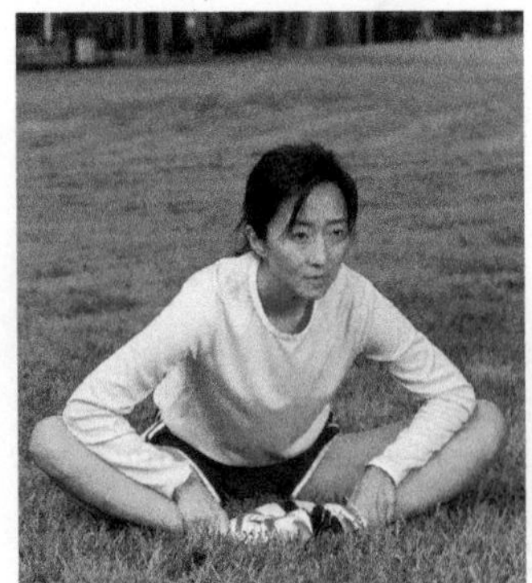

© Matthew Farruggio

(a) Foot pull for the groin and thigh

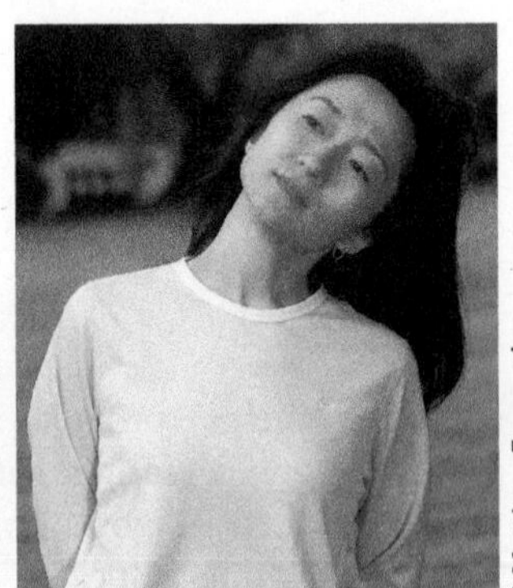

© Matthew Farruggio

(b) Lateral head tilt

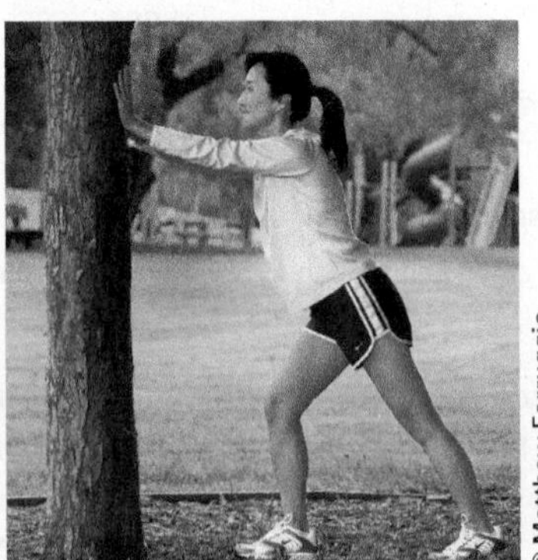

© Matthew Farruggio

(c) Wall stretch for Achilles tendon

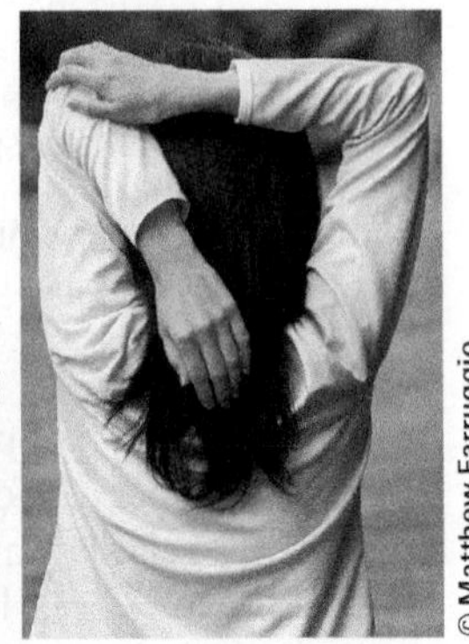

© Matthew Farruggio

(d) Triceps stretch for the upper arm and shoulder

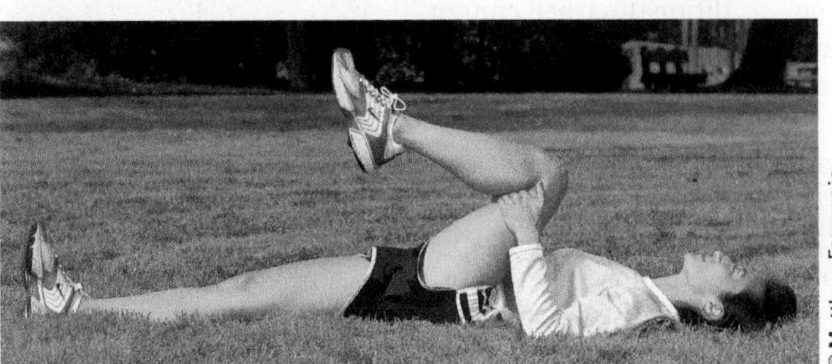

© Matthew Farruggio

(e) Knee chest pull for lower back muscles

Figure 4-7 Some Simple Stretching Exercises

(a) Sit on the ground and bend your legs so that the soles of your feet touch. With your hands on your ankles, sit tall, lean forward, and press on your knees with your elbows. Hold for 10 seconds; repeat. **(b)** Gently tilt your head to each side. Repeat several times. **(c)** Stand one metre (three feet) from a wall or post with your feet slightly apart. Keeping your heels on the ground, lean into the wall. Hold for 10 seconds; repeat. **(d)** Place your right hand behind your neck and grasp above the elbow with your left hand. Gently pull the elbow back. Repeat with the left elbow. **(e)** Lying on your back, clasp one knee and pull it toward your chest. Hold for 10–60 seconds; repeat with the other knee.

the extended right leg toward your body to a point of mild discomfort. You hold this stretch for 10 seconds followed by relaxation. This same PNF stretch is repeated with the left leg. Another PNF stretching technique is the *contract-relax* exercise where, using the hamstring stretch as an example, you lift your right leg off the floor and contract your hamstring muscle against your partner's hand while your partner moves the extended limb toward your body. This is followed by a second stretch where you relax but your partner pushes against the extended leg as in the hold-relax technique.

Ballistic stretching is characterized by rapid bouncing movements, such as a series of up-and-down bobs as you try again and again to touch your toes with your hands. These bounces can stretch the muscle fibres too far, causing the muscle to contract rather than stretch. They can also tear ligaments (strong fibrous cords that connect bone to bone) and weaken or rupture tendons (strong fibrous cords that connect muscles to bones). Because of its potential danger, fitness experts generally recommend against ballistic stretching. However, some sport and fitness trainers encourage the use of ballistic stretching exercises. By simulating a specific movement pattern or motion that athletes would do in their sport, such as high kicking stretches in soccer, they prepare their athletes for the game.

Dynamic stretching involves controlled movements that gradually increase your reach and speed of movement. This type of stretching improves dynamic flexibility and takes you to the limits of your range of motion. It does not force any part of your body beyond its range of motion. It is used in many warm-up activities for programs such as dance or martial arts.

✓ CHECK-IN

What type of stretching exercises do you do to maintain or improve your flexibility level?

The Benefits of Flexibility Flexibility can make everyday tasks, such as bending over to tie a shoe or reaching up to a high shelf, easier and safer. It can also prevent and relieve the ankle, knee, back, and shoulder pain that many people feel as they get older. If you do other forms of exercise, flexibility lowers your risk of injury and may improve your performance.

- *Prevention of injuries.* Flexibility training stretches muscles and increases the elasticity of joints. Strong, flexible muscles resist stress better than weak or inflexible ones.
- *Relief of muscle strain.* Muscles tighten as a result of stress or prolonged sitting. If you study or work in one position for several hours, you will often feel stiffness in your back and neck. Stretching helps relieve muscle tension and enables you to work more effectively.
- *Relaxation.* Flexibility exercises are great stress-busters that reduce mental strain, slow the rate of breathing, and reduce blood pressure.
- *Better athletic performance.* Good flexibility allows for more efficient movement and exertion of more force through a greater range of motion. This is a special benefit for any activity, from gymnastics to golf, where positions beyond the normal range of motion are necessary to perform certain skills.
- *Relief of soreness after exercise.* Many people develop delayed-onset muscle soreness (DOMS) one or two days after they work out. This may be the result of damage to the muscle fibres and supporting connective tissue. Stretching can help to prevent DOMS.
- *Improved posture.* Bad posture can create tight, stressed muscles. If you slump in your chair, the muscles in the front of your chest may tighten, causing those in the upper spine to overstretch and become loose. Stretching the chest muscles can help you sit up straight.

Stretching and Warming Up Stretching is a specific activity intended to elongate the muscles and keep joints limber, not simply a prelude to a game of tennis or a five-kilometre run. The value of stretching varies with different activities. One of the best times to stretch is after an aerobic workout. Your muscles will be warm, more flexible, and less prone to injury. In addition, stretching after aerobic activity can help a fatigued muscle return to its normal resting length and possibly help reduce delayed muscle soreness.

STRATEGIES FOR PREVENTION

How to Avoid Stretching Injuries

- Don't force body parts beyond their normal range of motion. Stretch to the point of tension, back off, and hold for 10 seconds to a minute.
- Do a minimum of two repetitions of each stretch, with equal repetitions on each side.
- Breathe! Don't hold your breath. Continue breathing slowly and rhythmically throughout your stretching routine.
- Don't attempt to stretch a weak or injured muscle.
- Stretch individual muscles before you stretch a group of muscles. For instance, stretch the ankle, knee, and hip before a stretch that works all three.
- Don't make quick, jerky movements while stretching. Since a slow stretch provokes less of a reaction from the stress receptors, the muscles can safely stretch farther than usual.

Warming up means getting the heart beating, breaking a sweat, and readying the body for more vigorous activity. For most sports, light to moderate activity, such as walking at gradually increasing intensity, is a better warm-up than stretching.

MIND–BODY APPROACHES

Pilates, Tai Chi, and yoga programs, increasingly popular on campuses and in community recreation and fitness centres, can help reduce stress, enhance health and wellness, and improve physical fitness.

Pilates Used by dancers for deep-body conditioning and injury rehabilitation, Pilates was developed more than seven decades ago by Joseph Pilates. Pilates exercises improve flexibility and joint mobility and strengthen the core by developing pelvic stability and abdominal control.

There are "mat" or "floor" classes that stress the stabilization and strengthening of the back and abdominal muscles. Fitness centres also offer training on specialized Pilates equipment, primarily a device called the Reformer that consists of a frame and various cables, pulleys, springs, and sliding boards that are attached for a series of progressive range-of-motion exercises. Pilates exercise involves very precise repetitions in several planes of motion.

Tai Chi This ancient Chinese practice, designed to exercise your body, mind, and spirit, gently works muscles, focuses concentration, and improves the flow of qi (often spelled "chi"), the vital life energy that sustains health. Because of its focus on breathing and flowing gestures, Tai Chi is sometimes described as *meditation in motion.*

Yoga One of the most ancient of mind–body practices, yoga comes from the Sanskrit word meaning "union." This popular physical activity program offered at many college and university recreation facilities blends flexibility, strength, endurance, and coordination into the practice. There is also a focus on breathing techniques and mindfulness or spiritual practice that unites all aspects of a person. Yoga has also gained acceptance as part of a comprehensive stress management program. Some studies have demonstrated a number of benefits:

- **Improved flexibility.** Yoga may offer protection from back pain and injuries.
- **Protection of joints.** Yoga postures take joints through their full range of motion, providing a fresh supply of nutrients to joint cartilage.
- **Stronger, denser bones.** Yoga uses weight-bearing postures.
- **Enhanced circulation.** Postures boost the supply of oxygen throughout the body.
- **Lower levels of the stress hormone cortisol.** As discussed in Chapters 2 and 3, cortisol can affect the immune system.
- **Improved balance.** In both recreation and exercise rehabilitation programs, participants have experienced significant improvement in their ability to balance. This could be attributed to the improvement in neuromuscular control that results in strength improvements and allows for increased balance.

Streeter et al., in a study on the effects of yoga versus walking on mood and anxiety, concluded that a 12-week yoga intervention not only improved mood and lowered anxiety, but did so with greater levels of improvement than a walking program.[85] *Another study on college and university students established that yoga was one of the top ten physical activity courses of interest.*[86]

There are many different types of yoga: Ashtanga, Bikram (hot), Hatha, Iyengar, Kundalini, Power, and Vinyasa yoga, to name just some of the more popular ones.

✓ CHECK-IN

Have you ever tried mind–body physical activity approaches?

BODY COMPOSITION

Body composition is another component of fitness. As described at the beginning of this chapter, body composition is the amount of fat versus the amount of lean tissue in our body. The best way to maintain a healthy body composition is to combine regular physical activity and good nutrition. An in-depth description of body composition is included in Chapter 6, Managing Your Weight.

SAFE AND HEALTHY WORKOUTS

Whenever you work out, you don't want to risk becoming sore or injured. Starting slowly when you begin any new fitness activity is the smartest strategy. Keep a simple diary to record the time and duration of each workout. Get accustomed to an activity and then begin to work harder or longer. In this way, you strengthen your musculoskeletal system so you're less likely to be injured, you lower the cardiovascular risk, and you build the exercise habit into your schedule.

How Can I Prevent Injuries? Females and males are equally likely to suffer an exercise-related injury. An estimated one in four women and one in three men discontinue their exercise programs because of injury.[87] **Acute injuries**—sprains, bruises, and pulled muscles—are the result of sudden trauma, such as a fall or collision. **Overuse injuries** are the result of overdoing a repetitive activity, such as running. When one particular joint is overstressed (such as a tennis player's elbow or a swimmer's shoulder), *tendonitis*, an inflammation at the point where the tendon meets the bone, can develop. Another common overuse injury is *plantar fasciitis*, which is an inflammation of the plantar fascia. The fascia, which is a broad band of dense, inelastic tissue that runs from your heel to your toe on the bottom of your foot, has the job of protecting the nerves, muscles, and blood vessels of the foot. When you overuse your foot, the plantar fascia can become tender and painful, usually under the ball of the foot and at the heel. This injury needs immediate attention. Leaving this injury to get better on its own usually results in further injury, and even walking can become too difficult due to the pain. Ice treatments, stretching, and wearing supportive shoes can help.

Other overuse injuries include *shin splints*, *stress fractures*, and *runner's knee*. Shin splints is a term used to describe almost any pain in the front of the lower legs. If you experience pain and inflammation along the inner side of your lower leg, along the tibia bone (shinbone), you might be diagnosed with having shin splints. Stress fractures, which can occur in any bone, are commonly seen in the foot and the tibia bone. They are a more serious injury than shin splints. They are prevalent in runners or athletes who jump on hard surfaces. Runner's knee also describes many different injuries that happen to the knee joint. The most common problem is patella femoral syndrome, where the patella (or kneecap) does not glide over the groove in the thigh bone as it should. A sharp or dull pain is usually felt on the front part of the knee, but may be on the inside or outside, or you may experience a general ache in the knee area. Sometimes there is a grinding or clicking noise. Women tend to deal with this sport injury more often than men because of the angle of their pelvis and femur (thigh bone).

To prevent injuries and other exercise-related problems before they happen, use common sense and take appropriate precautions, including the following:

- Get proper instruction and, if necessary, advanced training from knowledgeable instructors.
- Begin any exercise program slowly and thoughtfully.
- Make sure that stretching and exercises are preventing, not causing, injuries.
- Wear proper footwear.
- Make sure you have good equipment and keep it in good condition. Always check your equipment prior to each use (especially if you're renting it).
- Use reasonable protective measures, including wearing a helmet when cycling, skiing, or skating.
- Take each outing seriously. Avoid the unknown under adverse conditions (e.g., hiking unfamiliar terrain during poor weather or kayaking a new river when water levels are unusually high or low) or when accompanied by a beginner whose skills may not be as strong as yours.
- Never combine alcohol or drugs with any sport.

Overtraining About half of all people who start an exercise program drop out within six months. One common reason is that they **overtrain**, pushing themselves to work too intensely, too frequently. Signs of overdoing it include persistent muscle soreness, frequent injuries, unintended weight loss, nervousness, and an inability to relax. Overtraining for endurance sports such as marathon running can damage the lungs and intensify asthma symptoms. If you're pushing too hard, you may find yourself unable to complete a normal workout or to recover after a normal workout. Rest is just as important as your training program.

Taking Care of Injuries Sooner or later most active people suffer an injury. Although most are minor, they all require some attention. Ignoring a problem or trying to push through the pain can lead to more serious complications.

Price If you develop aches and pains beyond what you might expect from an activity, stop. Never push to the point of fatigue. If you do, you could end up with sprained or torn muscles or ligaments. If you have an exercise injury, follow the PRICE technique:

- Protect the area with an elastic wrap, sling, splint, cane, crutches, or air cast.
- Rest to promote tissue healing. Avoid activities that cause pain, swelling, or discomfort.
- Ice the area immediately, even if you are seeking medical help. Wrap the ice in a cloth. Don't put the ice pack directly on your skin. Repeat every two or three hours for the first 48–72 hours. Cold reduces pain, swelling, and inflammation in injured muscles, joints, and connective tissue. It may slow bleeding if a tear has occurred.
- Compress the area with an elastic bandage until the swelling stops. Loosen the wrap if the pain increases, the area becomes numb, or swelling is occurring below the wrapped area.
- Elevate the area above your heart, especially at night. Gravity helps reduce swelling by draining excess fluid.

After following the PRICE technique, it might be wise to request assistance from a sports medicine professional such as a kinesiologist, physiotherapist, or sports medicine physician. Proper and controlled exercise rehabilitation can help the healing process.

Thinking of Temperature Prevention is the wisest approach to heat and cold problems when you are exercising. Knowing what can go wrong is part of that preventive approach. We are fortunate in Canada to have Dr. Stephen Cheung, our Canada Research Chair in environmental ergonomics, doing some cutting-edge research in the area of temperature control.[88] We already know that having our body temperature stay greatly above normal or below normal for an extended period of time can harm several of our bodies' systems. Examples are changes in the blood flow to our brains, our ability to think properly, and our ability to move. Dr. Cheung is furthering this research and looking at how controlling both regional temperature in parts of our body and our core temperature affects physical and mental responses. This research is helping not only people who exercise in hot and cold weather but also emergency workers who work in extreme conditions.[89] Prevention is the wisest approach to heat problems.

Heeding Heat Always wear as little as possible when exercising in hot weather. Choose loose-fitting, lightweight, white, or light-coloured clothes. Never wear rubberized or plastic pants and jackets to sweat off pounds. These sauna suits don't allow your body heat to dissipate, and they can be dangerous. Drink plenty of fluids while exercising (especially water), and watch for the earliest signs of heat problems, including cramps, stress, exhaustion, and heatstroke.

✓ CHECK-IN

Do you pay attention to proper hydration when working out?

Coping with Cold Protect yourself in cold weather (or cold indoor gyms) by covering as much of your body as possible, but don't overdress. Wear one layer less than you would if you were outside but not exercising. Don't use warm-up clothes of waterproof material because they tend to trap heat and keep perspiration from evaporating. Make sure your clothes are loose enough to allow movement and exercise of the hands, feet, and other body parts, thereby maintaining proper circulation. Because 40 percent or more of your body heat is lost through your head and neck, wear a hat, turtleneck, or scarf. Cover your hands and feet, too; mittens provide more warmth and protection than gloves.

SELF-SURVEY

Are You Ready to Become More Active?

Physical Activity Stages of Change Questionnaire

For each of the following questions, circle Yes or No. Please be sure to read the questions carefully.

Physical activity or exercise includes walking briskly, jogging, bicycling, swimming, or any other activity in which the exertion is at least as intense as these activities.

1. I am currently physically active. NO YES
2. I intend to become more physically active in the next six months. NO YES

For activity to be regular, it must add up to a total of 150 minutes of moderate to vigorous aerobic physical activity per week in bouts of 10 minutes or more. For example, you could take one 30-minute walk or take three 10-minute walks for a daily total of 30 minutes five out of seven days.

3. I currently engage in regular physical activity. NO YES
4. I have been regularly physically active for the past six months. NO YES

Answers to Self-Survey

Scoring Algorithm	Question			
	1	2	3	4
Precontemplation	No	No		
Contemplation	No	Yes		
Preparation	Yes		No	
Action	Yes		Yes	No
Maintenance	Yes		Yes	Yes

Source: Adapted, with permission, from B.H. Marcus and L.H. Forsyth, 2003, *Motivating People to Be Physically Active, 2nd ed.* (Champaign, IL: Human Kinetics), 138.

Chapter Summary

1. Mary Ann takes a step aerobics class three times a week. Which component of physical fitness does her exercise routine emphasize?
   a. muscular strength and endurance
   b. flexibility
   c. cardiorespiratory fitness
   d. body composition

2. Which of the following is one of the benefits of regular physical activity?
   a. decreased bone mass
   b. lowered risk of shin splints
   c. enhanced immune response
   d. altered sleep patterns

3. The Canadian Physical Activity Guidelines for Adults (18–64) recommend what activities?
   a. 30–60 minutes of physical activity per day
   b. 150 minutes of moderate-to-vigorous-intensity aerobic physical activity per week, in bouts of 10 minutes or more, and muscle- and bone-strengthening activities using muscle groups, at least two days per week
   c. 90 minutes of moderate- to vigorous-intensity aerobic physical activity (MVPA) per week, in bouts of 30 minutes or more
   d. 60–90 minutes of physical activity at least three days per week

4. What does the overload principle require?
   a. It requires three to five days of exercise a week.
   b. It requires a person exercising to provide a greater stress or demand on the body than it's usually accustomed to handling.
   c. It requires a person exercising to work at low intensity for longer periods of time to deplete the body's resources.
   d. It requires participating in a specific fitness training program.

5. To improve aerobic fitness at what percentage of your target heart rate is recommended while working out?
   a. 60–65 percent
   b. 70–80 percent
   c. 80–90 percent
   d. 90–100 percent

6. What is the primary benefit of aerobic exercise?
   a. It improves cardiorespiratory endurance.
   b. It helps condition your muscles, enabling them to work efficiently and reliably.
   c. It can enhance weight loss.
   d. It increases the range of motion of your joints.

7. What might an aerobic workout consist of?
   a. 5 minutes of brisk walking, 30 minutes of flexibility exercises, 5 minutes of brisk walking
   b. 15 minutes of resistance exercises followed by 10 minutes of stretching
   c. 10 minutes of sprints, 5 minutes of slow jogging, 5 minutes of stretching, 10 minutes of sprints
   d. 5 minutes of stretching, 5 minutes of brisk walking, 45 minutes of jogging, 5 minutes of slow walking, 5 minutes of stretching

8. Which statement about isometric, isotonic, and isokinetic exercises is true?
   a. Isokinetic exercises usually involve pushing on an object, isometric exercises involve pulling on an object, and isotonic exercises involve lifting an object.
   b. Isometric and isokinetic exercises can be done with free weights, but isotonic exercises require special resistance machines.
   c. Weightlifting is an isotonic exercise, pushing against the wall is an isometric exercise, and isokinetic exercises require special machines that move muscles through their range of motion.
   d. Isotonic exercises are much more effective at contracting muscles than isometric or isokinetic.

9. Which of the following is a benefit of a regular flexibility program?
   a. stronger heart and lungs
   b. relief of muscle strain and soreness
   c. increased strength and endurance
   d. increased bone mass and leaner muscles

10. Which of these is NOT a good suggestion for staying safe when exercising in hot weather?
    a. Wear loose-fitting, lightweight clothes.
    b. Carry a damp towel or cloth to cool yourself down.
    c. Drink plenty of fluids, especially water.
    d. Wear one layer more than you would if you were not exercising.

Answers to these questions can be found on page 103.

SELF-RESPONSIBILITY—SOCIAL RESPONSIBILITY

SELF-RESPONSIBILITY

Clarify, adjust, and take it to completion.

Mark Allen, six-time winner of the Hawaii Ironman

Beginning or maintaining a regular physical activity program takes time, commitment, and energy. You don't have to be an elite athlete like Mark Allen, but you can use his words of advice to get started or to keep going. If you are trying to "get back on track," clarify: ask yourself what is stopping you. Do you prefer group fitness classes or walks or runs on your own? Do you need some instruction from a fitness expert to get you started? Once you figure out what is preventing you from participating in regular physical activity, then adjust. Check out your daily schedule. Find ways to "fit fitness in." Remember, you do not have to spend hours at a fitness facility to realize fitness benefits.

SOCIAL RESPONSIBILITY

Look after yourself. Look after one another.

Right To Play

Once you have begun or rejuvenated your fitness program, take it to completion. Ask yourself what success will look like. Will you plan to compete in an 8-kilometre run, or does attendance at a regular yoga program mean success to you? The wonderful thing about a physical activity program is that you can start one—any time—even if you have stopped in the past. Prochaska's Stages of Change support Mark Allen's model: you contemplate, prepare, take action, and then maintain.

If you have ever thought about doing some volunteer work, consider volunteering for Right To Play. This organization encourages and supports young adults who want to make a difference through physical activity and sport. Check out the many opportunities to link physical activity, sport, health, and children at www.righttoplay.com.

CRITICAL THINKING

1. Allison knows that exercise is good for her health, but she figures she can keep her weight down by dieting, and worry about her heart and health when she gets older. "I look good. I feel okay. Why should I bother exercising?" she asks. What would you reply?
2. Your friend has just been selected to the university varsity soccer team. Practices begin in July. You are aware that a couple of other soccer players have suffered heat-related incidents while practising. What can you do to help your friend protect his health while on the field?

WEB LINKS

American College of Sports Medicine (ACSM)

http://www.acsm.org/

ACSM is the largest sports medicine and exercise science organization in the world. Access this site for up-to-date news releases, publications, and research documents.

Canadian Fitness and Lifestyle Research Institute

www.cflri.ca

This national research agency advises, educates, and informs Canadians about the importance of healthy, active lifestyles.

Canadian Society for Exercise Physiology

www.csep.ca

You can find the Par-Q forms and all of the Canadian Physical Activity Guidelines at this site. Click on the Physical Activity link. There is also important certification information and a comprehensive section on the *Canadian Physical Activity, Fitness & Lifestyle Approach Protocol (CPAFLA)*—an assessment that is administered to one million Canadians each year. Health screening forms are also now downloadable.

Exercise is Medicine, Canada

http://www.exerciseismedicine.org

Exercise is Medicine® Canada (EIMC) is a movement to make Canadians healthier. It is a joint partnership between the American College of Sports Medicine and the American Medical Association. EIMC is based upon the belief that physical activity is an integral part of the prevention and treatment of chronic disease. You can also click on EIMC in Action/EIMC on Campus, a special initiative for college and university students who want to start an "Active U Challenge."

PHE Canada (Physical & Health Education Canada)

www.phecanada.ca

Canada's professional organization for physical educators. Check out this website for a variety of programs, resources, and information on school-based physical and health education initiatives for school-aged children. Up-to-date research is also available.

Please note that links are subject to change. If you find a broken link, use a search engine such as www.google.ca and search for the website by typing in keywords.

Key Terms

The terms listed here are used within the chapter on the page indicated. Definitions of the terms are in the Glossary at the end of this book.

acute injuries 99
aerobic exercise 87
agility 81
anaerobic exercise 87
balance 81
ballistic stretching 97
body composition 81
cardiorespiratory fitness 80
concentric phase 94
coordination 81
core strength 95
duration 86
dynamic stretching 97
eccentric phase 94
endorphins 82
exercise 80
Exergaming 93
FITT 86
flexibility 81
force 81
functional fitness 81
HITT 93
hypertrophy 86
isokinetic 94
isometric 94
isotonic 94
muscular endurance 81, 94
muscular fitness 81
muscular strength 81, 94
one repetition maximum, or 1RM 94
osteoporosis 82
overloading 94
overload principle 84
overtrain 99
overuse injuries 99
physical activity 78
physical conditioning 81
physical fitness 80
plyometrics 81
PNF (proprioceptive neuromuscular facilitation) stretching 96
power 81
progressive overloading 86
rating of perceived exertion (RPE) 89
recovery principle 86
repetition (rep) 94
resting heart rate (RHR) 87
reversibility principle 86
set 94
specificity principle 86
speed 81
sport 81
static stretching 96
stretch receptors 96
target heart rate 89
tension 86
VO2 max 81

Answers to Chapter Summary Questions

1. c; 2. c; 3. b; 4. b; 5. b; 6. a; 7. d; 8. c; 9. b; 10. d

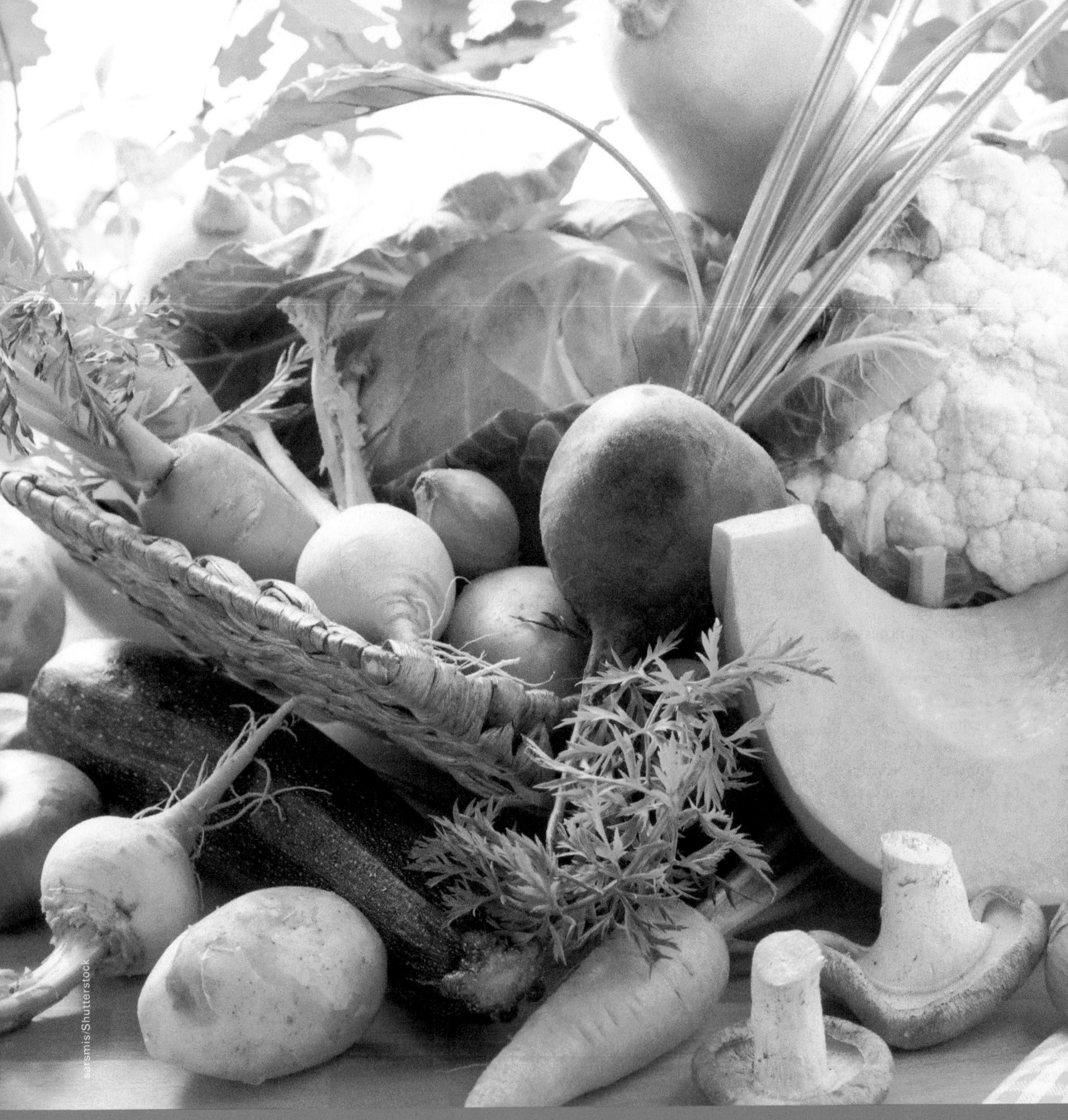

AFTER READING THIS CHAPTER, YOU WILL BE ABLE TO:

- **list** the basic macronutrients necessary for a healthy body and **describe** their functions
- **describe** *Eating Well with Canada's Food Guide* and **explain** its significance
- **explain** current recommendations for food portions and servings
- **compare** the advantages and disadvantages of various alternative diets and ethnic foods
- **list** the food-safety hazards and describe prevention measures

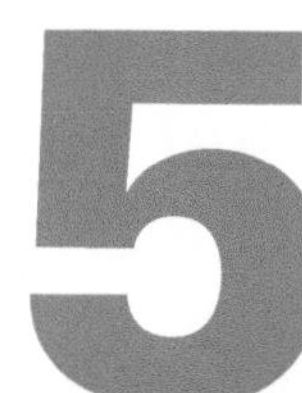

5

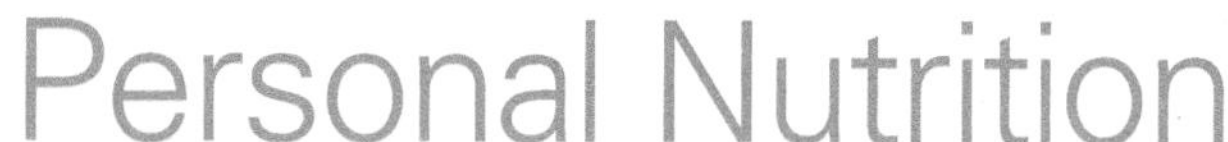

Personal Nutrition

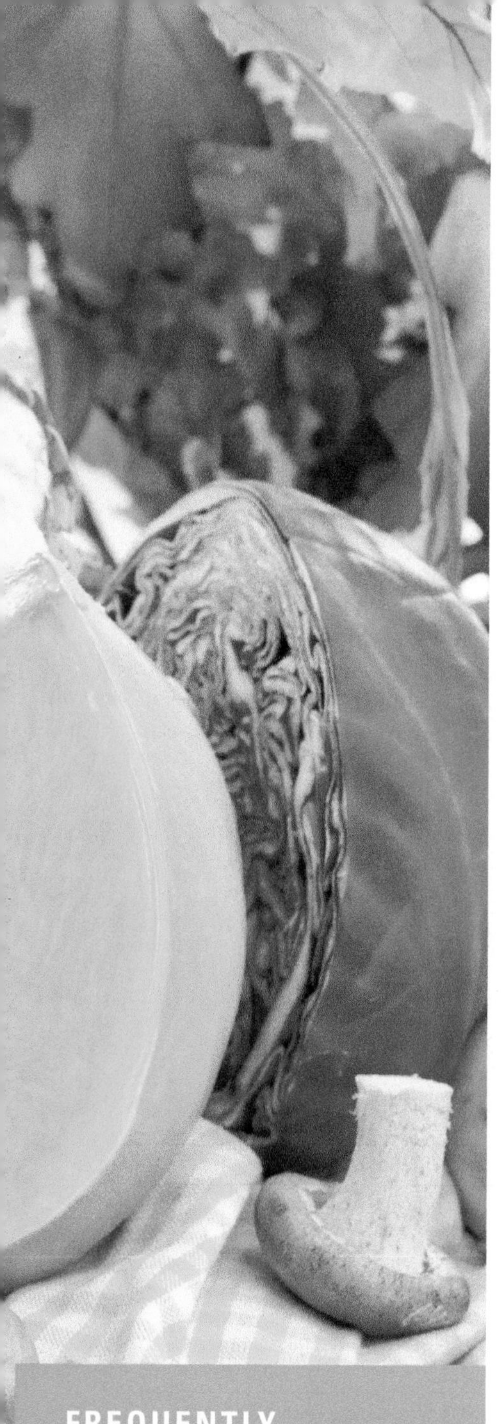

We are what we eat—and it shows in everything from our stamina and strength to the sheen in our hair and the health of our skin. Eating well helps us live and feel well. As demonstrated by the science of **nutrition**, the field that explores the connections between our bodies and the foods we eat, our daily diet affects how long and how well we live. Sensible eating can provide energy for our daily tasks, protect us from many chronic illnesses, and may even extend longevity.

Many foods can serve as the building blocks of a healthy lifestyle. However, making good food choices isn't easy. Faced with a bewildering array of food products and a blitz of advertising claims, you may well find it hard to select the foods that not only taste good but also are good for you. This chapter can help. It translates the latest information on good nutrition into specific advice that you can use to nourish yourself and enjoy eating well.

You will learn about macronutrients—carbohydrates, proteins, and fats. You will be reminded about the importance of vitamins. There is an introduction to the most recent *Canada's Food Guide* and the recommended number of food guide servings per day. We have included a variety of alternative food guides and culturally diverse diets. There is also information about nutrition labelling. The chapter will conclude with a section on food safety.

FREQUENTLY ASKED QUESTIONS

FAQ: How much fat is okay? p. 110

FAQ: What is a serving size? p. 111

FAQ: What should I look for on nutrition labels? p. 121

FAQ: What should I know about vegetarian diets? p. 126

FAQ: What causes food poisoning? p. 129

WHAT YOU NEED TO KNOW ABOUT NUTRIENTS

Every day your body needs certain **essential nutrients** that it cannot manufacture for itself. They provide energy, build and repair body tissues, and regulate body functions. The six classes of essential nutrients, which are discussed in this section, are water, protein, carbohydrates, fats, vitamins, and minerals (see Table 5-1).

Water makes up about 60 percent of our body and is essential for health and survival. Besides water, we also need energy to live, and we receive our energy from the carbohydrates, proteins, and fats in the foods we eat. These three essential nutrients are called **macronutrients** because they are the nutrients required by the human body in the greatest amounts. The amount of energy that can be derived from the macronutrients is measured in **calories**. There are nine calories in every gram of fat and four calories in every gram of protein or carbohydrate. The other two essential nutrients—the vitamins and minerals—are called **micronutrients** because our bodies need them in only very small amounts.

Your need for macronutrients depends on how much energy you expend. Because fats, carbohydrates, and protein can all serve as sources of energy, they can—to some extent—substitute for one another in providing calories. According to Health Canada,[1] the Acceptable Macronutrient Distribution Range (AMDR) for adults 19 and over is 45–65 percent of calories from carbohydrates, 25–35 percent from fat, and 10–30 percent from protein. Children's fat intake should be slightly higher: 25–40 percent of their caloric intake.

✓ CHECK-IN

How much water do you drink every day?

Water Water, which makes up between 50 and 60 percent of our body by weight—85 percent of blood, 70 percent of muscles, and about 75 percent of the brain—performs many essential functions. It carries nutrients, maintains temperature, lubricates joints, helps with digestion, rids the body of waste through urine, and contributes to the production of sweat, which evaporates from the skin to cool the body. Research has correlated high fluid intake with a lower risk of kidney stones, colon cancer, and bladder cancer.

You lose about 2–2.5 litres of water a day—the equivalent of 8–10 cups (250 millilitres equals one cup)—through perspiration, urination, bowel movements, and normal exhalation. You lose water more rapidly if you exercise, live in a dry climate or at a high altitude, drink a lot of caffeine or alcohol (which increase urination), skip a meal, or become ill. To ensure

TABLE 5-1

The Essential Nutrients

	Functions	Sources
Water	Carries nutrients and removes waste; dissolves amino acids, glucose, and minerals; cleans body by removing toxins; regulates body temperature	Liquids, fruits, and vegetables
Proteins	Help build new tissue to keep hair, skin, and eyesight healthy; build antibodies, enzymes, hormones, and other compounds; provide fuel for body	Meat, poultry, fish, eggs, beans, nuts, cheese, tofu, vegetables, some fruits, pasta, breads, cereal, and rice
Carbohydrates	Provide energy	Grains, cereal, pasta, fruits, vegetables, nuts, milk, and sugars
Fats		
Saturated Fats	Provide energy; trigger production of cholesterol	Red meat, dairy products, egg yolks, and coconut and palm oils (See Table 5-2)
Unsaturated Fats	Also provide energy, but trigger more "good" cholesterol production and less "bad" cholesterol production	Some fish; avocados; olive, canola, and peanut oils; shortening (not made with beef tallow or other animal sources); stick margarine; baked goods (See Table 5-2)
Vitamins	Facilitate use of other nutrients; involved in regulating growth, maintaining tissue, and manufacturing blood cells, hormones, and other body components	Fruits, vegetables, grains, some meat and dairy products (see Table 5-3)
Minerals	Help build bones and teeth; aid in muscle function and nervous system activity; assist in various body functions, including growth and energy production	Many foods (see Table 5-4)

adequate fluid intake, the Dietitians of Canada suggest that women 19 years and older need a minimum of approximately 2.2 litres (or nine cups) of fluid each day and men need 3 litres (or 12 cups).[2]

Water is the best beverage selection to prevent dehydration and to rehydrate, but sports drinks made up of 4–8 percent carbohydrates and unsweetened juices also help us to rehydrate. Alcoholic and caffeinated beverages (coffee, tea, cola) can contribute to total fluid consumption but are not recommended since they may have diuretic effects that can leave you less hydrated. We can survive only a few days without water, whereas deficiencies of other nutrients may take weeks, months, or possibly years to develop.

Calories Calories are the measure of the amount of energy that can be derived from food. Energy is expressed as the total calories you consume. **Estimated energy requirements (EER)**, or our daily caloric needs, depend on your sex, age, body-frame size, weight, height, percentage of body fat, and **basal metabolic rate (BMR)**—the number of calories needed to sustain your body at rest. Your activity level also affects your EER.[3] EER equations can help you determine and estimate your own personal energy requirements. We have included these equations in Chapter 6—see Table 6-2.

Health Canada suggests that we can also calculate the amount of calories we need by our activity level.[4] It is important to remember that the caloric requirements listed below are only guidelines because caloric expenditure depends on so many factors.

Following are caloric requirements for *females* aged 19–30 years:

- Sedentary level (participating in daily activities such as household tasks and walking to the bus)—1900 calories per day
- Low active level (daily living activities plus 30–60 minutes of daily moderate activity such as walking 5–7 km/hr)—2100 calories per day
- Active level (daily living activities plus at least 60 minutes of daily moderate activity)—2350 calories per day

Males aged 19–30 years have the following caloric requirements:

- Sedentary level—2500 calories per day
- Low active level—2700 calories per day
- Active level—3000 calories per day

If we compare the daily caloric needs of women and men to a fast-food meal, we can begin to understand why overweight and obese Canadians are becoming the norm. A double cheeseburger, large fries, and a large pop can add up to about 1800 calories. That is just one meal!

Protein Protein is critical for growth and repair; proteins form the basic framework for our muscles, bones, blood, hair, and fingernails. Supplying four calories per gram, they are made of combinations of 20 **amino acids**. Animal proteins—meat, fish, poultry, and dairy products—are **complete proteins** that provide the nine *essential amino acids*. We must get them from our diet because our body cannot produce them.

Grains, dry beans, and nuts are **incomplete proteins** that may have relatively low levels of one or two essential amino acids but fairly high levels of others. They may also be missing one or two essential amino acids. Combining incomplete proteins, such as beans and rice, ensures that the body gets sufficient protein or what is sometimes called a **complementary protein**.

Based on the latest data, the recommended level of protein intake for adults is 0.8 grams per kilogram of body weight.[5] The recommended intake of protein during pregnancy has been increased to provide an additional 25 grams a day above non-pregnant intake. Because of conflicting or inadequate data on the health risks of high-protein diets, the National Academy of Sciences has not set a tolerable upper intake level, although it does warn about this potential danger.

Carbohydrates **Carbohydrates** are organic compounds that provide our brain—our only truly carbohydrate-dependent organ—and body with **glucose**, their basic fuel. They supply us with four calories per gram. Carbohydrates can be classified according to the number and type of simple sugar units present. **Monosaccharides** (glucose, fructose, galactose), known as simple sugars or *simple carbohydrates*, consist of one simple sugar unit. **Disaccharides** (sucrose, lactose, maltose, table sugar) contain two sugar units linked by a chemical bond. They must be broken down into simple sugars before our body can use them. **Polysaccharides** (starches and glycogen), known as *complex carbohydrates*, have more than 10 units of sugar, and they must also be broken down to be used. **Fibre** and starches are the two major forms of complex carbohydrates.

Most digestible carbohydrates are broken down to monosaccharides in the intestine. Monosaccharides that are absorbed in the small intestine may be metabolized and stored as **glycogen** in the liver or muscle cells or oxidized to give metabolically usable energy. According to HealthLink BC, most adults need about 135–180 grams of carbohydrate per day.[6] That is about 45–60 grams of carbohydrate if you eat three meals per day. Pregnant women should consume 175 grams per day in order to ensure adequate glucose provision to the fetal brain in addition to meeting the needs of the mother. To ensure the replacement of the carbohydrate secreted in human milk, lactating women should consume 210 grams of carbohydrates each day. Recommended daily amounts depend on many aspects.

Simple Carbohydrates **Simple carbohydrates** include *natural sugars*, such as the lactose in milk and the fructose

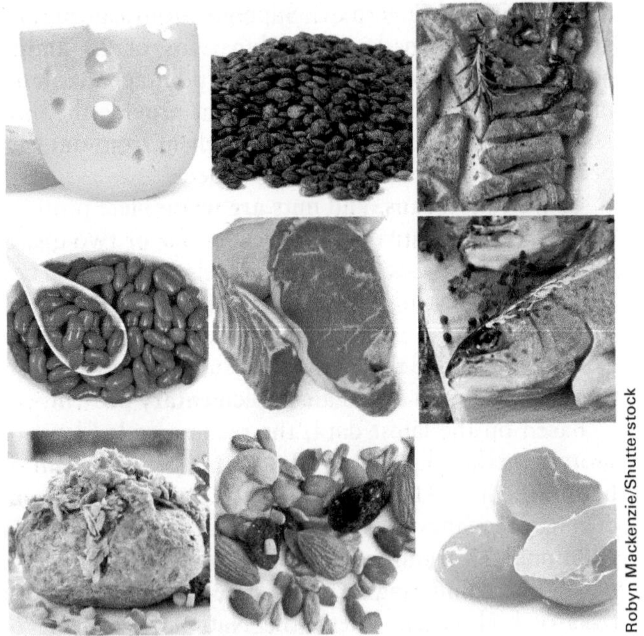
Robyn Mackenzie/Shutterstock

Protein comes in many different forms.

in fruits, and *added sugars*, including candy, pop, fruit drinks, pastries, and other sweets. Currently in Canada, there are no accepted scientific national or international limits on our sugar consumption. The Canadian Sugar Institute reports that the estimated added sugar consumption of Canadians is approximately 51–53 grams per day (about 13 teaspoons). This accounts for 11 percent of total energy intake.[7]

The Canadian Heart and Stroke Foundation recommends that Canadians decrease their consumption of added sugar to no more than 10 percent of their total daily calories. This does not include sugar that occurs naturally in fruit, vegetables, milk, grains, and other foods. If your diet consisted of 2000 calories in one day, 10 percent would equal about 48 grams or 12 teaspoons of sugar. To put this amount in perspective one can of pop can contain that much sugar.[8]

Complex Carbohydrates **Complex carbohydrates** are the foundation of a healthy diet. Dietary starches are where we get the most of our complex carbohydrates and include grains, cereals, vegetables, beans, and nuts. We store starch in our muscles and liver in the form of a polysaccharide called glycogen. Much like a starter in our car, when the body needs a sudden burst of energy, the glycogen is broken down into glucose. Unfortunately, many Canadians get most of their complex carbohydrates from refined grains, which have been stripped of fibre and many nutrients.

Far more nutritious are whole grains, which are made up of all components of the grain: the *bran* (or fibre-rich outer layer), the *endosperm* (middle layer), and the *germ* (the nutrient-packed inner layer).[9] Many health organizations are supporting *Canada's Food Guide* that recommends Canadians increase their consumption of whole-grain foods. Individuals who eat whole-grain products each day have about a 15–25 percent reduction in death from all causes, including heart disease and cancer.[10]

The popularity of diets that restrict carbohydrate intake prompted an explosion in products touted as "low-carb." Although many people may buy low-carb foods because they believe that they are healthier, that is not necessarily the case. A low-carb nutrition bar may be high in saturated fat and calories.[11] Some low-carb food products cause digestive problems because food companies often replace the carbohydrates in a cookie or cracker with substances such as the sweetener sorbitol, which can cause diarrhea or stomach cramps.

Fibre **Dietary fibre** is the non-digestible form of carbohydrates occurring naturally in plant foods, such as leaves, stems, skins, seeds, and hulls. **Functional fibre** consists of isolated, non-digestible carbohydrates that have been isolated and extracted from plants or animal sources and may be added to foods. **Total fibre** is the sum of both.

Fibre is described as either *soluble* or *insoluble*. Soluble fibre absorbs water. Then the fibres swell, form gels, and trap nutrients such as glucose. This slows the absorption process in the blood, keeping food longer in the small intestine. When you feel full, this is what has occurred in your digestive tract. Blood sugar regulation and weight management are the benefits of this process. Soluble fibre also interferes with absorption of dietary fat and cholesterol, which lowers the risk of heart disease and stroke. Good choices of soluble fibre in your diet are oatmeal and barley. Fruits and vegetables such as strawberries, oranges, apples, any type of legumes, and leafy greens are also recommended.

There are three main insoluble fibres: cellulose, lignin, and hemicelluloses. Insoluble fibres cling to water and help prevent constipation and diverticulosis (a painful inflammation of the bowel). The link between fibre and colon cancer is complex. Some studies have indicated that increased fibre intake reduces risk, but other studies found no such correlation.[12]

The Dietitians of Canada recommend daily intake levels of total fibre (dietary plus functional fibre): 38 grams of total fibre for men and 25 grams for women. For men and women over 50 years of age, who consume less food, the recommendations are, respectively, 30 and 21 grams.[13] Because sudden increases in fibre can cause symptoms like bloating and gas, experts recommend gradually adding more fibre to your diet with an additional serving or two of vegetables, fruits, or whole-wheat bread.[14]

Glycemic Index According to the Dietitians of Canada, the term **glycemic index (GI)** is a buzzword in many of the latest diet books.[15] Researchers developed the GI as a measure of how much a carbohydrate-containing food is likely to raise your blood sugar. According to the GI, foods can be divided into high-, medium-, and low-glycemic values. A food with a high GI will raise your blood sugar more than a food with a low GI.

Studies have found that low-glycemic index foods have health benefits such as the prevention of type 2 diabetes, control of blood sugar levels, and control of blood cholesterol levels. Use of the glycemic index is recommended in meal planning for people with diabetes or those at high risk of developing type 2 diabetes. Some studies have also found that including low-GI foods in your diet may result in short-term weight loss. However, there have been no studies to date that have determined whether or not low-GI foods can lead to long-term weight loss.

Foods that have a high GI are found in the grain products food group. They include bread, cereal, pasta, rice, and potatoes. There are some low-GI choices within this food group, and they include some types of bread such as pumpernickel, 100 percent stone-ground whole-wheat breads and cereals (such as oatmeal and bran), sweet potatoes, and converted rice.

Fats **Fats** (or lipids), although generally thought of as something to be avoided in our diet, are actually an important nutrient. Fats carry the fat-soluble Vitamins A, D, E, and K; aid in these vitamins' absorption in the intestine; protect organs from injury; regulate body temperature; and play an important role in growth and development. They provide nine calories per gram—more than twice the amount of calories in carbohydrates or proteins.

Forms of Fat From a scientific point of view, saturated and unsaturated fats are distinguished by the type of fatty acids in their chemical structures. They are both made up of chains of carbon and hydrogen atoms.

Saturated Fats Saturated fats are fats in which carbon atoms are *saturated* with hydrogen atoms.[16] Animal fats are saturated fats and are usually solid at room temperature. One example of this type of fat is butter. The problem with saturated fats is their link to cholesterol. When you eat a diet high in saturated fats, a rise in bad cholesterol (LDLs) occurs. This increases the risk of heart disease. There has been a lot of attention paid to coconut oil in the past few years. Coconut oil comes from the coconut "meat" inside the shell. It is a saturated fat. It is solid at room temperature and it can be kept unrefrigerated for many months. Coconut oil has become very popular and is readily available in grocery stores and health food stores. Claims of coconut oil preventing heart disease, helping with diabetic conditions, improving digestion, and strengthening the immune system are just a few of the current "amazing benefits" being advertised. To date, there has been very little scientific research on the saturated fats in coconut oil. Some research does suggest that because coconut oil's main saturated fatty acid is something called lauric acid, it may not affect blood cholesterol as much as other saturated fats. However, more research needs to be done. The nutrition experts caution on the use of too much coconut oil.[17] Caution by some nutrition experts with regard to palm oil and palm kernel oil continues too. Palm oil comes from the palm fruit. Palm kernel oil must be extracted from the palm seed. Palm oil is 50 percent saturated fat while palm kernel oil is 80 percent saturated fat. Using olive, canola, or other non-tropical oils daily in cooking and baking is encouraged.

Cholesterol Cholesterol is a form of fat manufactured by our bodies that circulates in our blood.[18] About 80 percent of cholesterol is made by our liver. The other 20 percent comes from the foods we eat. Cholesterol is made up of high-density lipoproteins (HDLs), low-density lipoproteins (LDLs), and very-low-density lipoproteins (VLDLs). The HDLs are considered to be a "good" type of cholesterol. They help to transport cholesterol to our livers for metabolism and elimination and remove the LDLs (sometimes labelled as bad cholesterol) that accumulate on the inner walls of our arteries. The LDL buildup is known as **plaque**. Plaque restricts blood flow, resulting in an increased risk in developing blood clots. If a blood clot lodges in a narrow part of the artery leading to the brain, it can cause a stroke. If it lodges in the arteries of the heart, it can cause a heart attack.

LDLs, while considered a "bad" type of cholesterol, are important for health and do help our bodies by transporting cholesterol to our body's cells. We may have to reconsider our understanding of dietary saturated fats and how they increase the risk of cardiovascular disease. Ongoing research by Dr. Ronald Krauss and his team has found that there are actually different types of LDL cholesterol. They range from small, dense particles to the larger "fluffy" type. The small, dense type shows a link to heart disease. Diets high in carbohydrates appear to be linked to this type of LDL cholesterol, whereas diets higher in fats are linked to the larger, fluffy type of cholesterol and at this time do not appear to increase the risk of heart disease.[19]

VLDLs are made by the liver, and they function as the body's internal transport highway for lipids. They enable fats and cholesterol to move within the water-based solution of the bloodstream. VLDLs also transport triglycerides. A more in-depth discussion of cholesterol and recommended target cholesterol ranges is included in Chapter 10, Lowering Your Risk of Major Diseases.

Unsaturated Fats Unsaturated fats are fats that have more than one double-bonded (unsaturated) carbon in the molecule. They are usually in liquid form at room temperature. They come in two forms: *monounsaturated* and *polyunsaturated*. Monounsaturated fats have been shown to improve our blood cholesterol levels. They include peanut and olive oils.[20] Polyunsaturated fats include omega-3 and omega-6 fatty acids.

Omega-3, found in cold-water fish such as salmon, sardines, herring, and rainbow trout as well as flaxseed and walnuts, helps prevent blood clots and lowers triglycerides (a type of blood fat linked to heart disease).[21] Omega-6, which helps to lower the LDL or bad cholesterol, might also lower HDLs so it is best to eat in moderation. Oils such as safflower, sunflower, and corn, and sunflower seeds are good sources.

In response to consumer and health professionals' demands for less saturated fat in the food supply, many manufacturers switched to partially hydrogenated oils. The process of hydrogenation creates unsaturated fatty acids called **trans fatty acids**. They are found in some margarine products and most foods made with partially hydrogenated oils, such as baked goods and fried foods. Even though trans fatty acids are unsaturated, they behave like saturated fats in terms of raising cholesterol levels. Epidemiological studies have suggested a possible link between cardiovascular-disease risk and high intakes of trans fatty acids, and researchers have concluded that they are, gram for gram, twice as damaging as saturated fat. They increase LDL levels and decrease HDL levels of cholesterol in our bloodstream. There is no safe level for trans fatty acids, which occur naturally in meats as well as in foods prepared with partially hydrogenated vegetable oils.[22]

How Much Fat Is Okay? For optimal health, total fat intake, based on a 2000-calorie intake, should be 25–35 percent of calories.[23] Try to keep the fat calories from saturated and trans fat below 10 percent of your daily calories. High-fat diets can lead to obesity and its related health dangers, which are discussed in Chapter 6.

Choose foods wisely (see Table 5-2). To reduce both saturated fats and trans fatty acids, choose soybean, canola, corn, olive, safflower, and sunflower oils, which are naturally free of trans fatty acids and lower in saturated fats. Olive oil is considered a good fat and one of the best vegetable oils for salads and cooking, and has been correlated with a lower incidence of heart disease, including strokes and heart attacks. Lower the amount of mayonnaise, butter, margarine, and regular sour cream. Look for reduced-fat, low-fat, fat-free, and trans fatty acid–free versions of baked goods, snacks, and other processed foods.

Choose lean meats and poultry. Remove all skin and visible fat and bake or broil instead of frying. Always drain the fat after cooking. Try to stay away from cold cuts, and go easy on the bacon and sausages. Just because these foods are readily available in the cafeteria lineup doesn't mean you should choose them on a daily basis.

TABLE 5-2

Major Sources of Various Fatty Acids

Healthful Fatty Acids		
Monounsaturated	**Polyunsaturated**	**Omega-3 Polyunsaturated**
Avocado	Margarine (non-hydrogenated)	Fatty fish (herring, mackerel, salmon, tuna)
Oils (canola, olive, peanut, sesame)	Oils (corn, cottonseed, safflower, soybean)	Flaxseed
Nuts (almonds, cashews, filberts/hazelnuts, macadamia nuts, peanuts, pecans, pistachios)	Nuts (pine nuts, walnuts)	Nuts (walnuts)
Olives	Mayonnaise	
Peanut butter	Salad dressing	
Seeds (sesame)	Seeds (pumpkin, sunflower)	

Unhealthy Fatty Acids	
Saturated	**Trans**
Bacon	Fried foods (hydrogenated shortening)
Butter	Margarine (hydrogenated or partially hydrogenated)
Chocolate	Non-dairy creamers
Coconut	Many fast foods
Cream cheese	Shortening
Cream, half-and-half	Commercial baked goods (including doughnuts, cakes, cookies)
Lard	Many snack foods (including microwave popcorn, chips, crackers)
Meat	
Milk and milk products (whole)	
Oils (coconut, palm, palm kernel)	
Shortening	
Sour cream	

That said, be careful of very-low-fat diets as they can be unhealthy, too. When people eat very low levels of fat and very high levels of carbohydrates, the level of high-density lipoproteins (HDLs) declines.

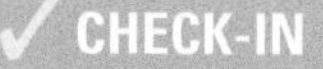

How healthful is your diet?

EATING FOR GOOD HEALTH

No one food can provide all the nutrients we need. To make sure you consume a healthful variety, Health Canada suggests that you follow *Eating Well with Canada's Food Guide* (see Figure 5-1).[24] A number of translated versions of the *Food Guide* have also been developed to celebrate our multicultural society and assist new immigrants to our country. The translated versions include French, Arabic, Chinese (simplified), Farsi (Persian), Korean, Punjabi, Russian, Spanish, Tagalong, Tamil, and Urdu. All versions are available at www.hc-sc.gc.ca/fn-an/food-guide-aliment/index-eng.php. Canada's first food guide, the *Official Food Rules*, was introduced in July 1942. This guide acknowledged war-time food rationing while endeavouring to prevent nutritional deficiencies and to improve the health of Canadians. Since 1942, the food guide has been changed many times. A document on the evolution of the food guide, titled *Canada's Food Guides from 1942 to 1992*, is available on the Health Canada website.[25]

What Is a Serving Size?

Food Portions and Servings In a study designed to determine if people knew the size of a serving and how many servings they should consume in one day, 68 percent of participants wrongly assumed they needed to increase their food consumption by more than 200 calories to meet the *Canada's Food Guide* recommendations.[26] This is not all that surprising considering that the average bagel has doubled in size in the last 10–15 years; the average size of a hamburger has increased from 42.5 grams (1.5 ounces) to 130 grams (4.5 ounces); and the average size of pop has increased from 236 millilitres (8 ounces) to 946 millilitres (32 ounces). See Figure 5-2 to compare serving sizes to common everyday items. See photograph of examples of "portion distortion" over the past 20 years.

Today's *Food Guide* has two parts. The rainbow side of the guide places foods into four groups: vegetables and fruits, grain products, milk and alternatives, and meat and alternatives. It also illustrates the kinds of foods to choose for healthy eating.

The bar side of the *Food Guide* provides the recommended number of servings per day for children, teens, and adults, and illustrates examples of what one serving looks like.

The *Food Guide* is based on guidelines from Health Canada that encourage us to enjoy a variety of foods and limit salt, alcohol, and caffeine. It also gives us advice on how to choose foods. You can create your own personal food guide using Health Canada's interactive website: My Food Guide Servings Tracker[27] or the Dietitians of Canada eaTracker.[28] There are many iPhone and Android apps available to help you track your food intake—Calorie Counter and Diet Track from My Fitness Pal; Pro by MyNetDiary; My Plate Caloric Tracker; and a specialty app, Food Intolerances.

- Choose lower-fat foods more often.
- Choose whole-grain and enriched products more often.
- Choose dark-green and orange vegetables and orange fruits more often.
- Choose lower-fat milk products more often.
- Choose leaner meats, poultry, and fish, as well as dried peas, beans, and lentils more often.

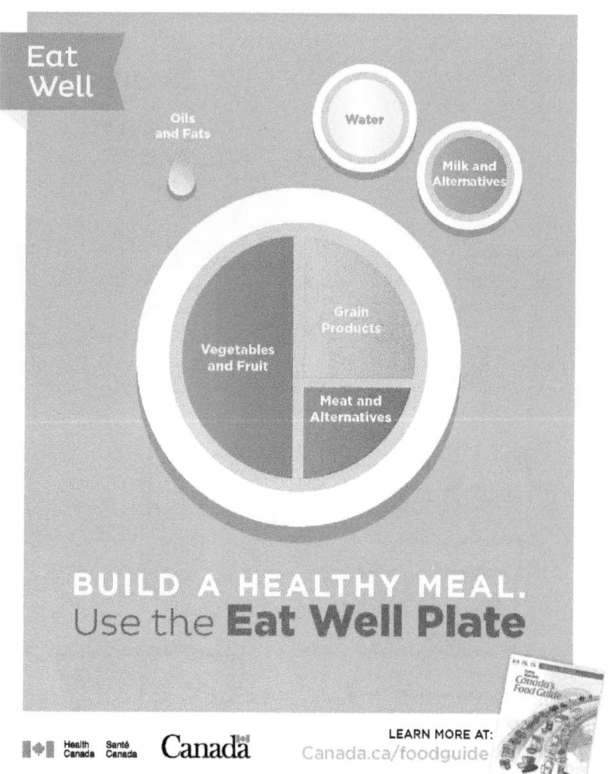

Eat Well Plate

You can also use the *Canada's Food Guide* Eat Well Plate to build a healthy meal. The plate illustrates the four food groups, as well as water, oils, and fats, in recommended proportions. Healthy eating tips are available for each image on the plate. Access this site at http://healthycanadians.gc.ca/eating-nutrition/healthy-eating-saine-alimentation/food-guide-aliment/index-eng.php. Enjoy a variety of foods from each group each day.

Source: *Eating Well with Canada's Food Guide*. Health Canada 2011. Adapted and reproduced with permission from the Minister of Health, 2016.

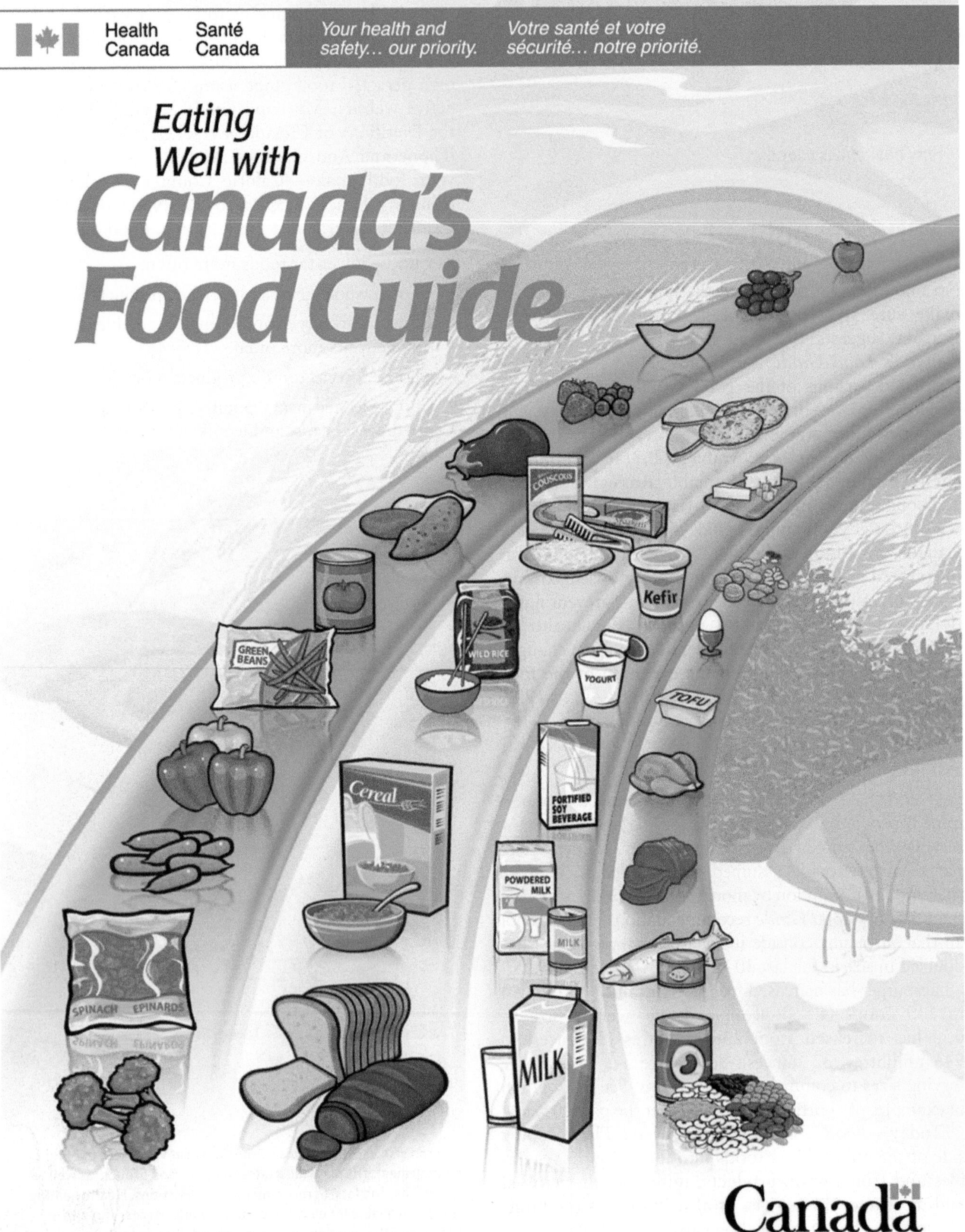

Figure 5-1 Eating Well with Canada's Food Guide

This graphic demonstrates the daily food choices that make up a healthy diet: modest amounts of meat, dairy products, and fats and a larger number of servings of foods containing grains, cereals, fruits, and vegetables.

Source: *Eating Well with Canada's Food Guide*. Health Canada, 2011. Adapted and reproduced with permission from the Minister of Health, 2016.

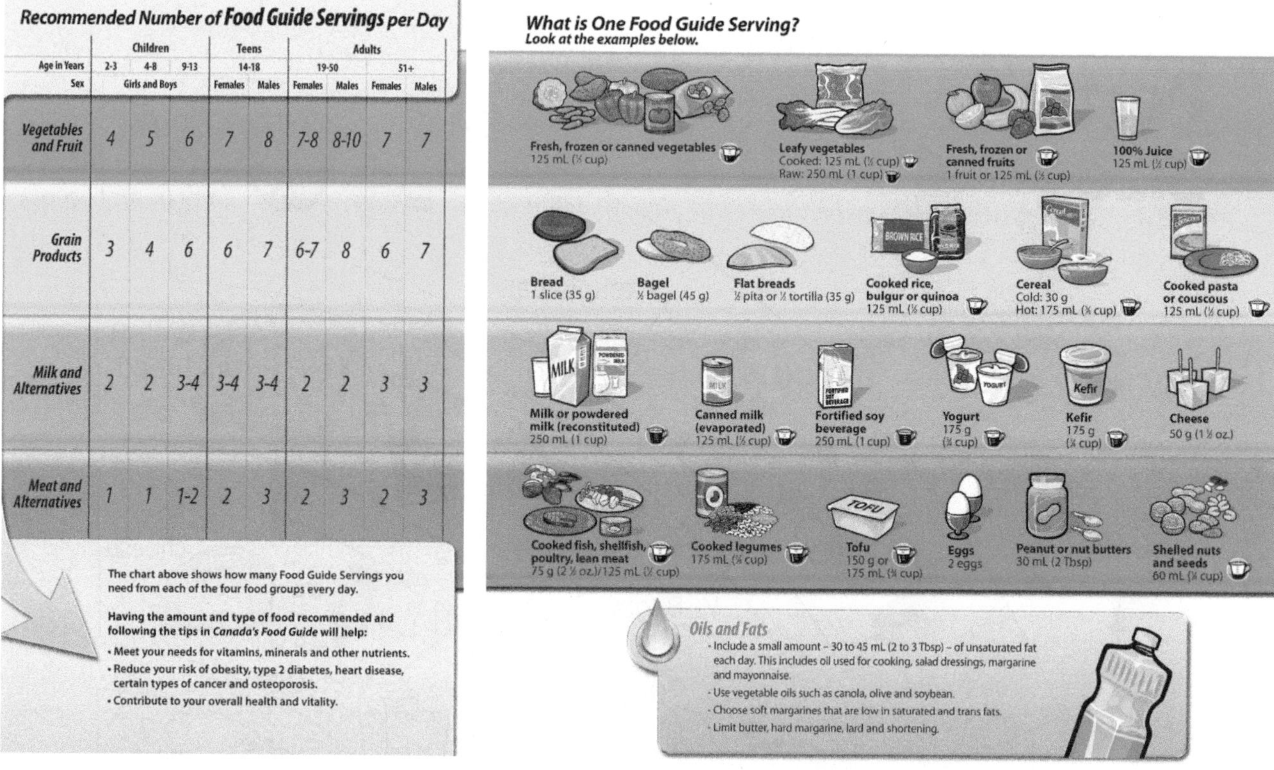

Recommended Number of Food Guide Servings per Day

	Children			Teens		Adults			
Age in Years	2-3	4-8	9-13	14-18		19-50		51+	
Sex	Girls and Boys			Females	Males	Females	Males	Females	Males
Vegetables and Fruit	4	5	6	7	8	7-8	8-10	7	7
Grain Products	3	4	6	6	7	6-7	8	6	7
Milk and Alternatives	2	2	3-4	3-4	3-4	2	2	3	3
Meat and Alternatives	1	1	1-2	2	3	2	3	2	3

The chart above shows how many Food Guide Servings you need from each of the four food groups every day.

Having the amount and type of food recommended and following the tips in *Canada's Food Guide* will help:

- Meet your needs for vitamins, minerals and other nutrients.
- Reduce your risk of obesity, type 2 diabetes, heart disease, certain types of cancer and osteoporosis.
- Contribute to your overall health and vitality.

Figure 5-1 *(Continued)*

Source: *Eating Well with Canada's Food Guide.* Health Canada, 2011. Adapted and reproduced with permission from the Minister of Health, 2016.

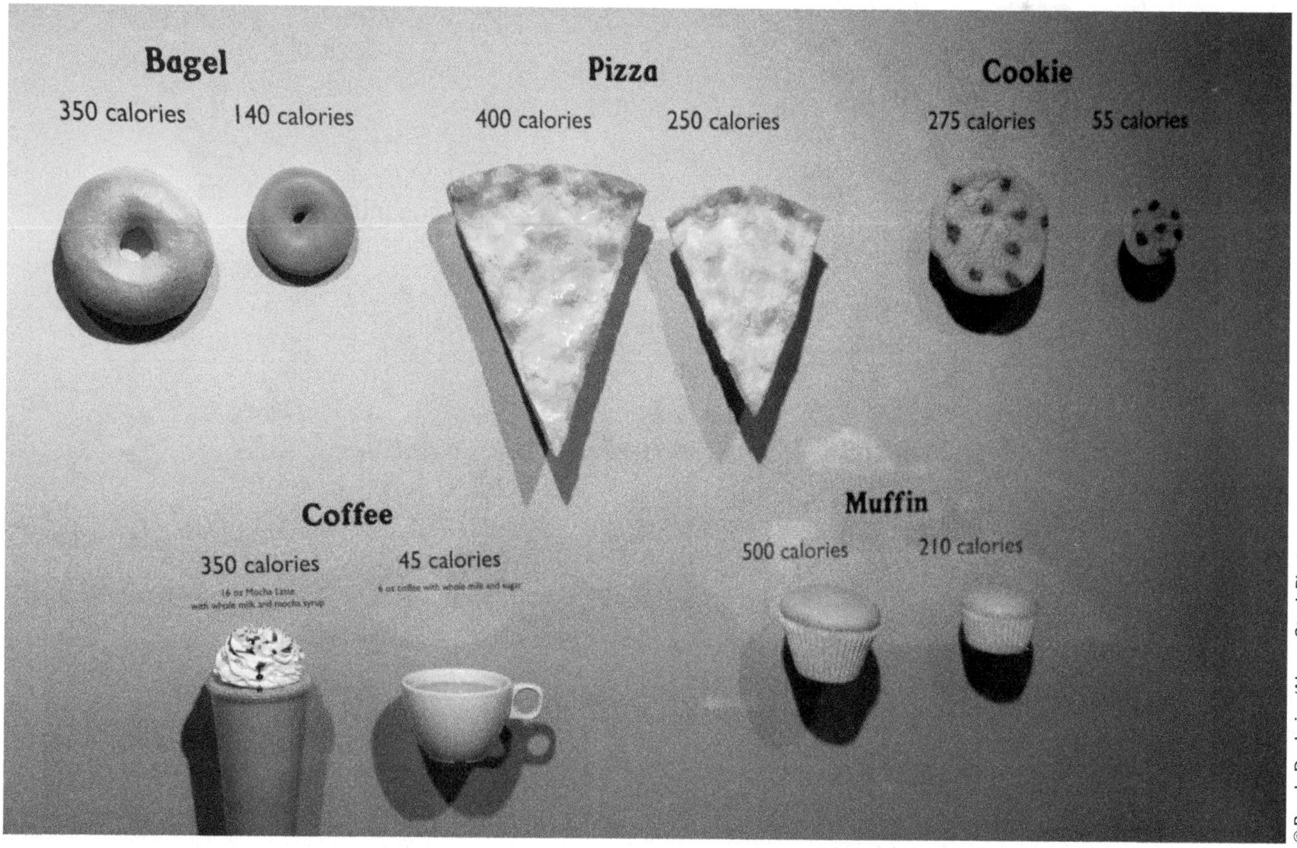

Bagel 350 calories 140 calories
Pizza 400 calories 250 calories
Cookie 275 calories 55 calories
Coffee 350 calories 45 calories
Muffin 500 calories 210 calories

© Randy Duchaine/Alamy Stock Photo

Examples of Portion Distortion.
On the left are examples of food portions today. On the right are examples of food portions 20 years ago.

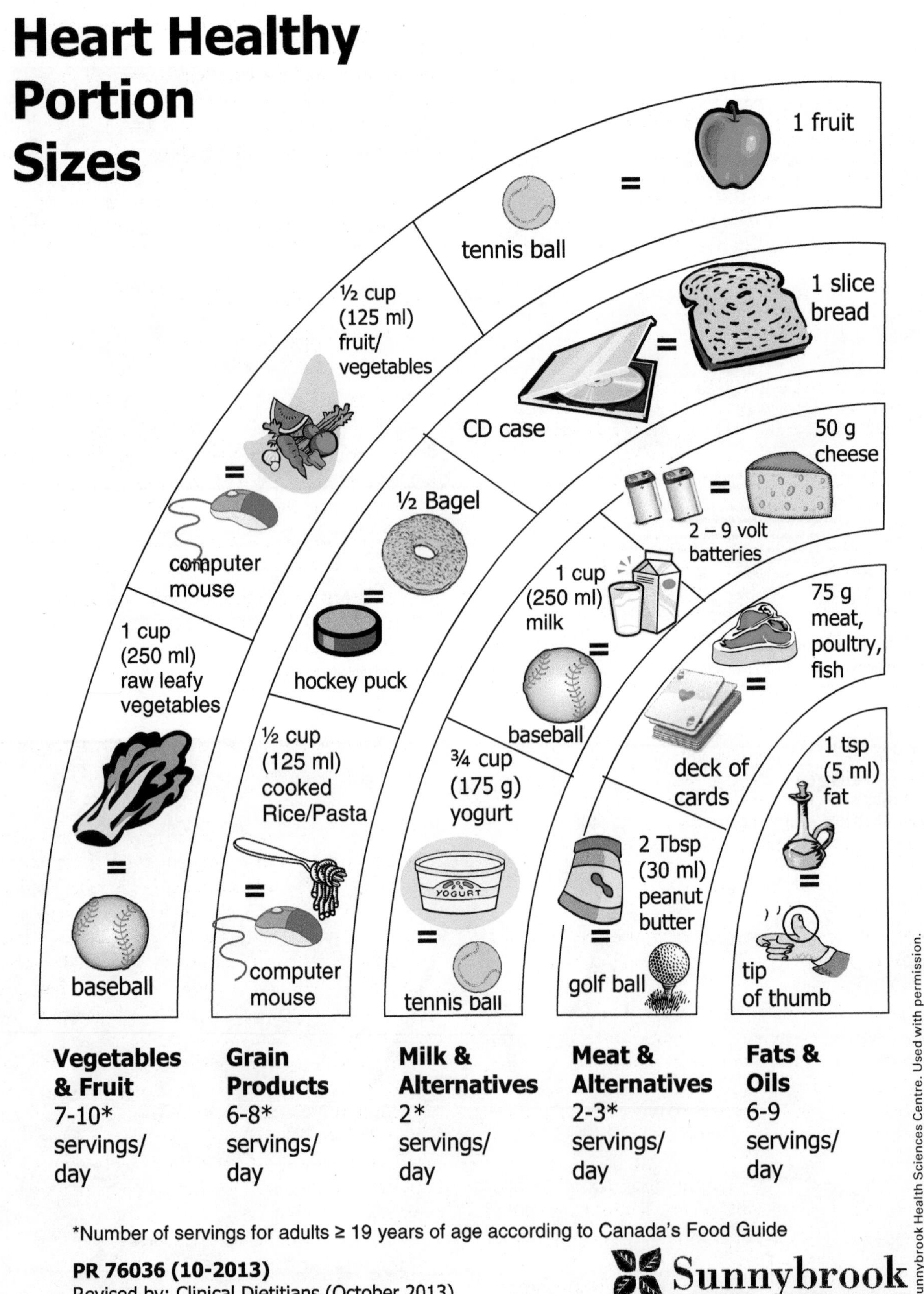

Figure 5-2 What Does a Serving from *Canada's Food Guide* Look Like?

X AND Y FILES

Do Men and Women Have Different Nutritional Needs?

Men and women do not need to eat different foods, but their nutritional needs are different. Because most men are bigger and taller than most women, they consume more calories. Eating more means it's easier for them to get the nutrients they need.

Women, particularly those who restrict their caloric intake or are chronically dieting, are more likely to develop specific deficiencies. Calcium is one example. Women drink less milk than men, and many do not consume the recommended 1000–1200 milligrams of calcium daily. This deficiency increases the risk of bone-weakening osteoporosis. Calcium supplementation can help individuals who are lactose intolerant.

Some women also get too little iron. Even in adolescence, girls are more prone to iron deficiency than boys; some suffer memory and learning impairments as a result. In adult women, menstrual blood loss and poor eating habits can lead to low iron stores, which puts them at risk for anemia. Women can increase their iron intake by eating meat (iron from animal sources is absorbed better than that from vegetable sources) or a combination of meat and vegetable iron sources together (e.g., a meat and bean burrito). Women who are low in iron should consult a physician. Because large doses of iron can be toxic, iron supplements should be taken only with medical supervision.

Women who could become pregnant should take a multivitamin with 0.4 milligrams of folic acid on a daily basis, which helps prevent neural-tube defects such as spina bifida. Folic acid is also useful to men because it may cut the risk of heart disease, stroke, and colon cancer.

Both men and women should increase their fruit and vegetable intake to ensure that they are getting adequate amounts of vitamins and fibre in their daily diet.

There is a range of servings recommended for each of the four food groups. The number of servings you need every day depends on your age, sex, body size, activity level, and whether you are pregnant or breast-feeding. People who need to have more than the lowest number of servings are pregnant and breast-feeding women, male teenagers, and highly active people. (See also X & Y Files: "Do Men and Women Have Different Nutritional Needs?")

Vegetables and Fruits Naturally low in fat and high in fibre, vegetables provide crucial vitamins (such as A and C) and minerals (such as iron and magnesium). Seven to eight servings per day are recommended for females aged 19–50. Eight to ten servings are recommended for men the same age. One serving of vegetables consists of 125 millilitres (½ cup) of fresh, frozen, or canned vegetables or fresh salad. It also equals one medium-sized carrot or potato. Dark-green vegetables are good sources of vitamins and minerals. Collards, kale, turnip, and mustard provide calcium and iron. Winter squash, carrots, broccoli, cabbage, kohlrabi, and cauliflower (the **crucifers**) are high in fibre and rich in vitamins, and are excellent sources of **indoles**, chemicals that help lower cancer risk.

Fruits are excellent sources of vitamins, minerals, and fibre. Along with vegetables, fruits may protect against cancer. One serving consists of a medium apple, banana, or orange; 125 millilitres (½ cup) of chopped, cooked, or canned fruit; or 125 millilitres (½ cup) of fruit juice.

Try the following suggestions to get more vegetables and fruits into your daily diet.

- Make or order sandwiches with extra tomatoes or other vegetable toppings.
- Add extra vegetables whenever you're preparing soups and sauces.
- Use raw vegetables for dipping, instead of chips.
- Carry a banana, apple, or package of dried fruit with you as a healthy snack.
- Start the day with a "daily double": a glass of juice and a banana or other fruit on cereal.
- Add citrus fruits (such as slices of grapefruit, oranges, or apples) to green salads, rice, or grains and to chicken, pork, or fish dishes.

✓ CHECK-IN

How many servings of vegetables and fruits do you eat every day?

Grain Products Breads, cereals, rice, and pasta are the foundation of a healthy diet because they are a good source of complex carbohydrates. For females aged 19–50, six to seven servings a day are recommended; for men, eight servings. Both simple and complex carbohydrates (starches) have four calories per gram. The sugars in simple carbohydrates provide little more than a quick spurt of energy, whereas complex carbohydrates are rich in vitamins, minerals, and other nutrients.

One serving in this category might be one slice of bread, 30 grams of cold cereal, or 175 millilitres (¾ cup) of hot cereal. Two servings would be one bagel, pita, or bun or 250 millilitres (1 cup) of pasta or rice. Although many people think of these foods as fattening, it's the butter on a roll or cream sauce on pasta that adds extra calories.

To get more grains in your diet,

- add brown rice or barley to soups;
- check labels of rolls and bread, and choose those with at least two to three grams of fibre per slice;
- choose pasta—it has 210 calories per cooked 250 millilitres (1 cup) and only nine calories from fat. Whole-grain pastas may provide more nutrients than those made with refined flour.

Milk and Alternatives Most milk products—milk, yogurt, and cheese—are high in calcium, riboflavin, protein, and Vitamins A and B_{12}. Dairy products, such as milk and yogurt, are the best calcium sources, but be sure you choose products that are low fat or, preferably, non-fat. Recommended daily amounts for both females and males aged 19–50 are two servings; pregnant and breast-feeding women, three to four servings. A serving in this category consists of 250 millilitres (1 cup) of milk, 185 millilitres (¾ cup) of plain yogurt, or 50 grams (2 ounces) of hard cheese.

A growing concern is the problem of lactose intolerance, or the inability to digest milk products. In people who do not produce adequate amounts of the intestinal enzyme lactase, milk products travel through the stomach undigested and ferment in the small bowel, causing gas, cramps, and diarrhea. Over-the-counter medicines such as oral lactase supplements can help, and many dairy products such as lactose-hydrolyzed milk are available for the lactose-intolerant. Some lactose-intolerance experts suggest that smaller quantities of milk, taken with meals or other foods spread throughout the day, or yogurt with active cultures, might help to slowly increase lactose tolerance.

To make sure you get more milk with less fat, try the following:

- Gradually switch from whole milk to 2 percent fat (reduced-fat) milk, to 1 percent fat (low-fat) milk, and then to skim (non-fat) milk.
- Substitute fat-free sour cream or non-fat plain yogurt for sour cream.
- Use part-skim or low-fat cheeses whenever possible.

Meat and Alternatives Foods in the meat and bean group include meat, poultry, fish, tofu, dry beans (lentils, soy, kidney, black, etc.), and nuts. Two servings a day are recommended for females aged 19–50, and three servings are recommended for men the same age. A serving in this category consists of 50–100 grams of lean, cooked meat, fish, or poultry (roughly the size of an average hamburger or the amount of meat on a chicken drumstick). An egg or 125–250 millilitres of cooked dry beans can substitute for one serving of lean meat. Thirty millilitres (2 tablespoons) of peanut butter count as one serving of meat. Thus, one day's total protein intake might include an egg at breakfast; a serving of beans, meat, or 30 millilitres of peanut butter in a sandwich at lunch; and 50–100 grams of fish for dinner.

To make healthy protein choices, follow these recommendations:

- Choose the leanest meats, such as beef round or sirloin, pork tenderloin, or veal. Broil or roast instead of fry. Trim fat before cooking, which can lower the fat content of the meat you eat by more than 10 percent.
- Cook stews, boiled meat, or soup stock ahead of time; refrigerate; and remove the hardened fat before using. Drain fat from ground beef after cooking.
- Watch out for processed chicken and turkey products; for example, bolognas and salamis made from turkey can contain 45–90 percent fat.
- Choose vegetables that have good protein sources—118 ml (½ cup) of soybeans for 15 grams of protein; 237 ml (1 cup) of peas for 18 grams; 118 ml (½ cup) of cooked black beans for 7.5 grams; 237 ml (1 cup) of broccoli for 4 grams; 237 ml (1 cup) of corn for 5 grams; and 237 ml (1 cup) of kale for 2.5 grams.[29]

Oils and Fats A small amount of unsaturated fat—30–45 millilitres (2–3 tablespoons)—can be included each day, such as oils for cooking, making salad dressing, or spreading on bread or food. Try to use vegetable oils such as olive, soybean, or canola oil. If you choose soft margarines, be sure to look for ones that are low in saturated and trans fats. Limit your intake of butter, hard margarine, lard, and shortening.

Nutritional Supplements Choosing foods according to *Eating Well with Canada's Food Guide* can provide all of the vitamins and minerals needed for good health for most Canadians. Yet many Canadians regularly use nutritional supplements—vitamins, minerals, and botanical and biological substances.

Natural health products (NHPs), defined as vitamins and minerals, herbal remedies, homeopathic medicines, traditional medicines, probiotics, and other products such as amino acids and essential fatty acids, used to be sold in Canada as either drugs or foods under the *Food and Drugs Act and Regulations* because there was no other category under which to classify them. As more Canadians began to use these products, it was felt that a new policy that would address the unique nature of NHPs was needed. As of January 1, 2004, the *Natural Health Product Regulations* in Canada came into force. Now all natural health products such as vitamins and minerals must have a special product licence before they are sold. Facilities that manufacture, package, label, and import these products must have site licences. The Natural and Non-prescription Health Products Directorate (NNHPD) oversees all NHPs as well as non-prescription and disinfectant drugs.[30]

Vitamins and Minerals **Vitamins**, which help put proteins, fats, and carbohydrates to use, are essential to regulating growth, maintaining tissue, and releasing energy from foods. Together with the enzymes in the body, they help produce the right chemical reactions at the right times. They're also involved in the manufacture of blood cells, hormones, and other compounds.

The body produces some vitamins, such as Vitamin D, which is manufactured in the skin after exposure to sunlight. Other vitamins must be ingested. Vitamins A,

D, E, and K are fat-soluble; they are absorbed through the intestinal membranes and stored in the body. The B vitamins and Vitamin C are water soluble; they are absorbed directly into the blood and then used up or washed out of the body in urine and sweat. They must be replaced daily. Table 5-3 summarizes key information about vitamins.

Many health experts feel that if you rely on vitamin/mineral pills and fortified foods to make up for poor nutrition, you may shortchange yourself. It's unlikely that changing any one nutrient will in itself produce great benefits; it may, by interfering with the complex balance of nutrients, do harm.

In particular, the fat-soluble vitamins, primarily A and D, can build up in our bodies and cause serious complications, such as damage to the kidneys, liver, or bones. Side effects of doses of Vitamin E greater than 400 units a day and long-term use can include blurred

TABLE 5-3

Key Information about Vitamins

Vitamin/ Recommended Intake Per Day	Significant Sources	Chief Functions	Signs of Severe, Prolonged Deficiency	Signs of Extreme Vitamin Excess
		Fat-Soluble		
Vitamin A Males 19–50: 900 μg RAE (Retinol Activity Equivalents) Females 19–50: 700 μg RAE	Fortified milk, cheese, cream, butter, fortified margarine, eggs, liver, spinach and other dark, leafy greens, broccoli, deep-orange fruits (apricots, cantaloupes) and vegetables (squash, carrots, sweet potatoes, pumpkins)	Antioxidant, needed for vision, health of cornea, epithelial cells, mucous membranes, skin health, bone and tooth growth, reproduction, immunity, regulation of gene expression, anemia	Cracks in teeth, tendency toward tooth decay, night blindness, keratinization, corneal degeneration	Overstimulated cell division, skin rashes, hair loss, hemorrhage, bone abnormalities, birth defects, fractures, liver failure, death
Vitamin D Males 19–50: 5 μg Females 19–50: 5 μg	Fortified milk or margarine, eggs, liver, sardines, exposure to sunlight	Mineralization of bones and teeth (promotes calcium and phosphorus absorption)	Abnormal growth, misshapen bones (bowing of legs), soft bones, joint pain, malformed teeth, muscle spasms	Raised blood calcium, excessive thirst, headaches, irritability, weakness, nausea, kidney stones, deposits in arteries
Vitamin E Males 19–50: 15 mg Females 19–50: 15 mg	Polyunsaturated plant oils (margarine, salad dressings, shortenings, green leafy vegetables, wheat germ, whole-grain products, nuts, seeds	Antioxidant; needed for stabilization of cell membranes, regulation of oxidation reactions	Red blood cell breakage, anemia, muscle degeneration, weakness, difficulty walking, leg cramps, nerve damage	Augments the effects of anti-clotting medication; general discomfort, blurred vision
Vitamin K Males 19–50: 120 μg Females 19–50: 90 μg	Green leafy vegetables, cabbage-type vegetables, soybeans, vegetable oils	Synthesis of blood—clotting proteins and proteins important in bone mineralization	Hemorrhage, abnormal bone formation	Interference with anti-clotting medication
		Water-Soluble		
Vitamin B_6 Males 19–50: 1.3 mg Females 19–50: 1.3 mg	Meats, fish, poultry, liver, legumes, fruits, whole grains, potatoes, soy products	Part of a coenzyme used in amino acid and fatty acid metabolism, helps make red blood cells	Anemia, depression, abnormal brain-wave pattern, convulsions, skin rashes	Impaired memory, depression, irritability, headaches, numbness, damage to nerves, difficulty walking, loss of reflexes
Vitamin B_{12} Males 19–50: 2.4 μg Females 19–50: 2.4 μg	Animal products (meat, fish, poultry, milk, cheese, eggs)	Part of a coenzyme used in new cell synthesis, helps maintain nerve cells	Anemia, nervous system degeneration progressing to paralysis, fatigue, memory loss, disorientation	None reported

(*Continued*)

TABLE 5-3

Key Information about Vitamins (*Continued*)

Vitamin/ Recommended Intake Per Day	Significant Sources	Chief Functions	Signs of Severe, Prolonged Deficiency	Signs of Extreme Vitamin Excess
Vitamin C Males 19–50: 90 mg Females 19–50: 75 mg Smokers: +35 mg	Citrus fruits, cabbage-type vegetables, dark-green vegetables, cantaloupe, strawberries, peppers, lettuce, tomatoes, potatoes, papayas, mangoes	Antioxidant, collagen synthesis (strengthens blood vessel walls, forms scar tissue, matrix for bone growth), amino acid metabolism, strengthens resistance to infection, aids iron absorption, restores Vitamin E to active form	Anemia, pinpoint hemorrhages, frequent infections, bleeding gums, loosened teeth, bone fragility, joint pain, rough skin, blotchy bruises, failure of wounds to heal	Nausea, abdominal cramps, diarrhea, excessive urination, headache, fatigue, rashes, interference with drug therapies and medical tests
Thiamin (B_1) Males 19–50: 1.2 mg Females 19–50: 1.1 mg	Pork, ham, bacon, liver, whole grains, legumes, nuts; occurs in all nutritious foods in moderate amounts	Part of a coenzyme used in energy metabolism, supports normal appetite and nervous function	Beriberi, edema, enlarged heart, nerve/muscular degeneration, difficulty walking, loss of reflexes, mental confusion	None reported
Riboflavin (B_2) Males 19–50: 1.3 mg Females 19–50: 1.1 mg	Milk, yogurt, cottage cheese, meat, leafy-vegetables, whole-grain or enriched breads and cereals	Part of a coenzyme used in energy metabolism, supports normal vision and skin health	Cracks at corner of mouth, magenta tongue, hypersensitivity to light, reddening of cornea, skin rash, sore throat	None reported
Niacin (B_3) Males 19–50: 16 mg NE (Niacin Equivalent) Females 19–50: 14 mg NE	Meat, poultry, fish, whole-grain and enriched breads and cereals, nuts, and all protein-containing foods	Part of a coenzyme used in energy metabolism	Diarrhea, black smooth tongue, irritability, loss of appetite, weakness, dizziness, mental confusion, flaky skin rash on areas exposed to sun	Nausea, vomiting, painful flush and rash, sweating, liver damage, blurred vision, impaired glucose tolerance
Folate (B_9) Males 19–50: 400 μg Females 19–50: 5 mg	Leafy green vegetables, legumes, seeds, liver, enriched bread, cereal, pasta, and grains	Part of a coenzyme needed for new cell synthesis	Anemia, heartburn, frequent infections, smooth red tongue, depression, mental confusion	Masks Vitamin B_{12} deficiency
Panothenic acid Males 19–50: 5 mg Females 19–50: 5 mg	Widespread in foods	Part of a coenzyme used in energy metabolism	Vomiting, intestinal distress, insomnia, fatigue, increased sensitivity to insulin	Water retention (rare)
Biotin Males 19–50: 30 μg Females 19–50: 30 μg	Widespread in foods	Used in energy metabolism, fat synthesis, amino acid metabolism, and glycogen synthesis	Abnormal heart action, loss of appetite, nausea, depression, muscle pain, drying of facial skin	None reported

Source: Adapted from From SIZER/WHITNEY. *Nutrition*, 11E. © 2008 Brooks/Cole, a part of Cengage Learning, Inc. Reproduced by permission. www.cengage.com/permissions.

vision, diarrhea, headaches, nausea, or stomach cramps, and unusual tiredness or weakness.

Large doses of water-soluble vitamins, including the B vitamins, may also be harmful. Excessive intake of Vitamin B_6 (pyridoxine), often used to relieve premenstrual bloating, can cause neurological damage, such as numbness in the mouth and tingling in the hands. High doses of Vitamin C can produce stomach aches and diarrhea. Niacin, often taken in high doses to lower cholesterol levels, can cause jaundice, liver damage, and irregular heartbeats as well as severe, uncomfortable flushing of the skin.

There are certain situations in which specific vitamin or mineral supplements are recommended. The evidence is clear that the use of supplements containing folic acid substantially reduces the risk of occurrence of birth defects known as neural-tube defects (NTDs). Women who are planning on getting pregnant should consider taking a supplement of 0.4 milligrams of folic acid each day, in addition to the amount of folate found in a healthy diet.

Neural tube defects can appear within the first month of a pregnancy so health experts recommend starting the supplement use as soon as birth control is stopped.

If you eat a balanced diet and get outside in the sunshine at least 1.5–2 hours a week, you should be getting all the Vitamin D you need. If you live in an area of Canada where the amount of sunshine is limited during specific times of the year, are over 50 years of age, or do not go outside very much, you might benefit from a supplement.[31]

If you are considering a multivitamin or multivitamin-mineral supplement, talk to your healthcare provider to find the best supplement for you. See Table 5-3 for the minimum and maximum daily dosages suggested by Health Canada.

Carbon, oxygen, hydrogen, and nitrogen make up 96 percent of our body weight. The other 4 percent consists of minerals that help build bones and teeth, aid in muscle function, and help our nervous system transmit messages. We also need **minerals** so vitamins can be absorbed. Every day we need about a 10th of a gram (100 milligrams) or more of the major minerals: sodium, potassium, chloride, calcium, phosphorus, and magnesium. We also need about a 100th of a gram (10 milligrams) or less of each of the trace minerals: iron (premenopausal women need more), zinc, selenium, molybdenum, iodine, copper, manganese, fluoride, and chromium. See Table 5-4 for a summary of mineral information.

Three minerals that deserve special attention are calcium, sodium, and iron. **Calcium**, the most abundant mineral in the body, builds strong bone tissue throughout life and plays a vital role in blood clotting and muscle and nerve functioning. One thousand milligrams of calcium per day are recommended for adults between 19 and 50. Twelve hundred milligrams are recommended for Canadians 50 years and over.[32] Calcium may also help control high blood pressure. National health

TABLE 5-4

Key Information about Minerals

Mineral	Significant Sources	Chief Functions	Signs of Severe, Prolonged Deficiency	Signs of Extreme Mineral Excess
		Major Minerals		
Sodium	Salt, soy sauce, processed foods	Needed to maintain fluid balance and acid-base balance in body cells; critical to nerve impulse transmission	Mental apathy, poor appetite, muscle cramps	High blood pressure
Potassium	All whole foods, meats, milk, fruits, vegetables, grains, legumes	Needed to maintain fluid balance and acid-base balance in body cells; needed for muscle and nerve activity	Muscle weakness, mental confusion, paralysis	Muscle weakness, irregular heartbeat, heart attacks, vomiting
Chloride	Salt, soy sauce, processed foods	Aids in digestion; needed to maintain fluid balance and acid-base balance in body cells	Does not occur under normal circumstances	Vomiting
Calcium	Milk and milk products, oysters, small fish (with bones), tofu, greens, legumes	Component of bones and teeth, needed for muscle and nerve activity, blood clotting	Stunted growth and weak bones in children, adult bone loss (osteoporosis)	Constipation; calcium deposits in kidneys, liver; decreased absorption of other minerals
Phosphorus	All animal tissues, milk and milk products, legumes	Component of bones and teeth, energy formation, needed to maintain cell membranes	Muscle weakness, impaired growth, bone pain	Calcification of soft tissue, particularly the kidneys
Magnesium	Nuts, legumes, whole grains, dark-green vegetables, seafood, chocolate, cocoa	Component of bones and teeth, nerve activity, energy and protein formation, immune function	Stunted growth in children, weakness, muscle spasms, personality changes, hallucinations	Diarrhea, dehydration, impaired nerve activity
Sulfate	All protein-containing foods	Component of certain amino acids; stabilizes–protein shape	None known; protein deficiency would occur first	None reported

(Continued)

TABLE 5-4

Key Information about Minerals *(Continued)*

Mineral	Significant Sources	Chief Functions	Signs of Severe, Prolonged Deficiency	Signs of Extreme Mineral Excess
		Trace Minerals		
Iron	Red meat, fish, poultry, shellfish, eggs, legumes, dried fruits	Aids in transport of oxygen, component of myoglobin, energy formation	Anemia, weakness, fatigue, pale appearance, reduced attention span, developmental delays in children	Vomiting, abdominal pain, blue coloration of skin, shock, organ damage
Zinc	Protein-containing foods: fish, shellfish, poultry, grains, vegetables	Protein reproduction, component of insulin, activates many enzymes, transport of Vitamin A	Growth failure, delayed sexual maturation, slow wound healing	Loss of appetite, impaired immunity, reduced copper and iron absorption, fatigue, metallic taste in mouth
Selenium	Meats and seafood, eggs, grains	Acts as an antioxidant in conjunction with Vitamin E, regulates thyroid hormone	Anemia, heart failure	Hair and fingernail loss, weakness, skin rash, garlic or metallic breath
Molybdenum	Dried beans, grains, dark-green vegetables, liver, milk and milk products	Aids in oxygen transfer from one molecule to another	Rapid heartbeat and breathing, nausea, vomiting, coma	Loss of copper from the body, joint pain, growth failure, anemia, gout
Iodine	Iodized salt, milk and milk products, seaweed, seafood, bread	Component of thyroid hormones that helps regulate energy production and growth	Goitre, cretinism in newborns (mental retardation, hearing loss, growth failure)	Pimples, goitre, decreased thyroid function
Copper	Organ meats, whole grains, nuts and seeds, seafood, drinking water	Helps to form hemoglobin and collagen, component of enzymes involved in the body's utilization of iron and oxygen	Anemia, nerve and bone abnormalities in children, growth retardation	From non-food sources: vomiting, diarrhea, liver disease
Manganese	Whole grains, coffee, tea, dried beans, nuts	Formation of body fat and bone	Weight loss, rash, nausea and vomiting	Infertility in men, disruptions in the nervous system, muscle spasms
Fluoride	Fluoridated water, foods, and beverages; tea; shrimp, crab	Component of bones and teeth (enamel), confers decay resistance on teeth	Tooth decay and other dental diseases	Fluorosis, brittle bones, mottled teeth, vomiting, diarrhea, chest pain
Chromium	Whole grains, liver, meat, beer, wine	Glucose utilization	Poor blood-glucose control, weight loss	Kidney and skin damage

Source: From SIZER/WHITNEY, *Nutrition Concepts and Controversies, MyPyramid Update (with Nutrition Connections CD-ROM and InfoTrac®)*, 10E. © 2006 Brooks/Cole, a part of Cengage Learning Inc. Reproduced by permission. www.cengage.com/permissions.

organizations are promoting greater calcium consumption among college students, particularly females, to increase bone density and safeguard against osteoporosis. Many students choose pop over milk and carbohydrates over vegetables such as broccoli and peas, pinto and soybeans, and sunflower or sesame seeds. Instead of pop, make healthy food choices that can support your calcium intake.

Sodium helps maintain proper fluid balance, regulates blood pressure, transmits muscle impulses, and relaxes muscles. The recommendation for Canadian adults is 1000–1500 milligrams per day of sodium. Excess sodium is not a problem for most healthy people, but for those who are sodium sensitive or who have high blood pressure and diseases related to hypertension such as stroke and kidney failure, it can be a health risk. Most fast-food options have high sodium content. Health Canada reports that the average Canadian consumes about 3400 milligrams of sodium per day, which is almost double the recommended amount.[33]

Getting enough **iron** is a common problem for many people, and iron deficiency can lead to **anemia**. Dietitians of Canada recommend that men 19 years and older plan for an intake of 8 milligrams per day and set a limit of 45 milligrams per day. Women aged 19–50 should aim for 18 milligrams per day and women 51 and older should try for 8 milligrams per day. Women of all ages should limit their daily iron intake to 45 milligrams per day.[34] More information on the benefits and health risks of toxicity of iron can be found in X & Y Files.

Other Substances in Food

Antioxidants **Antioxidants** are substances that prevent the harmful effects caused by oxidation within the body. They include Vitamins C, E, and beta carotene (a form of Vitamin A), as well as compounds such as carotenoids and flavonoids. All share a common enemy: renegade oxygen cells called *free radicals*, which are released by normal metabolism as well as by pollution, smoking, radiation, and stress.

Diets high in antioxidant-rich fruits and vegetables have been linked with lower rates of esophageal, lung, colon, and stomach cancers. But there continues to be conflicting findings in scientific studies. To date there is not conclusive evidence that any specific antioxidant, particularly in supplement form, can prevent cancer. Recent reports have shown that increased levels of Vitamin E (above the recommended 15–100 milligrams per day) might actually increase the risk of cardiovascular morbidity.[35]

Phytochemicals **Phytochemicals**, compounds that exist naturally in plants, serve many functions including helping a plant protect itself from bacteria and disease. Flavonoids, found in apples, strawberries, grapes, onions, green and black tea, and red wine, may decrease atherosclerotic plaque and DNA damage related to cancer developments. Phytochemicals are associated with a reduced risk of heart disease, certain cancers, age-related macular degeneration, adult-onset diabetes, stroke, and other diseases. However, research has yet to show a cause-and-effect relationship between consumption of phytochemicals and prevention of a specific disease.

Dietary Reference Intakes Since 1938, Health Canada has been reviewing nutrition research and defining nutrient needs for healthy people. Since 1995, scientists in Canada and the United States have worked together to develop nutrient recommendations based on current research. The joint recommendations are called **Dietary Reference Intakes (DRIs)**.[36] The DRIs replaced the 1990 Recommended Nutrient Intakes (RNIs) in Canada and the 1989 Recommended Dietary Allowances in the United States.

Dietary Reference Intakes is an umbrella term that describes reference values, which have different uses and are based on life stage and sex of individuals:

- *Estimated Average Requirement (EAR)*—the median usual intake value that is estimated to meet the requirement of half of healthy individuals.
- *Recommended Dietary Allowance (RDA)*—the average daily dietary intake level that is sufficient to meet the nutrient requirement of nearly all (97–98 percent of) healthy individuals. This is a goal for individuals and is calculated from the EAR.
- *Adequate Intake Level (AL)*—determined by the amount of a nutrient consumed by a group of healthy people, assuming that the amount they eat is adequate to promote health and when an EAR cannot be determined.
- *Tolerable Upper Intake Level (UL)*—the highest level of continuing daily nutrient intake that is likely to pose no risk in almost all individuals in the life-stage group for which it has been designed.
- *Acceptable Macronutrient Distribution Range (AMDR)*—the percentage range of protein, fat, and carbohydrate intakes that is associated with reduced risk of chronic disease while providing adequate intakes of essential nutrients.

It is important to note that DRIs are standards for apparently healthy people and are not meant to be applied for anyone who has an acute or chronic disease. The DRI approach has helped harmonize nutrient recommendations for Canada and the United States. A series of published reports are available, some of which outline DRIs for many vitamins and minerals. Another important finding in developing these nutrient-reference values was the importance of regular daily physical activity with regard to overall health levels.[37]

KNOWING WHAT YOU EAT

Canadian consumers now know much more about the food they eat because of nutrition-labelling requirements that were published on January 1, 2003. These regulations require most food labels on almost all prepackaged foods to carry a mandatory Nutrition Facts table listing calories and 13 key nutrients. They also contain science-based health claims and defined nutrient-content claims. The aim of these regulations is to give Canadians the information they need to make informed food choices and compare products. They are also designed to increase our understanding of the links between nutritional health and well-being.[38]

In evaluating food labels and product claims, keep in mind that while individual foods vary in their nutritional value, what matters is your total diet. If you eat too much of any one food—regardless of what its label states—you may not be getting the variety and balance of nutrients that you need.

What Should I Look for on Nutrition Labels? As Figure 5-3 shows, the Nutrition Facts on food labels present a wealth of information—if you know what to look for. The Nutrition Facts table[39] shows calories, the amount of fat including saturated and trans fats, cholesterol, sodium, carbohydrate, fibre, sugars, protein, calcium, iron, and Vitamins A and C in a specified amount of food. The nutrients chosen were those that consumers, health professionals, and scientists consider important to the health of Canadians.

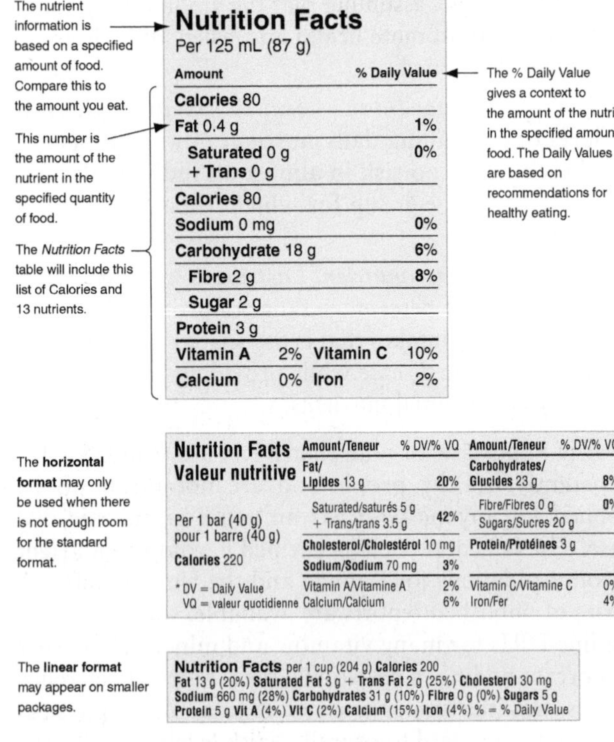

Figure 5-3 Understanding Nutrition Labels

The Nutrition Facts label lists the essential nutrient content of packaged food as well as the amount of potentially harmful substances such as fat and sodium.

- *Calories.* Calories are the measure of the amount of energy that can be derived from food. Science defines a *calorie* as the amount of energy required to raise the temperature of one gram of water by one degree Celsius. In the laboratory, the caloric content of food is measured in 1000-calorie units called *kilocalories*. The calorie referred to in everyday usage is actually the equivalent of the laboratory kilocalorie.

  The Nutrition Facts label lists two numbers for calories: calories per serving and calories from fat per serving. This allows consumers to calculate how many calories they'll consume and to determine the percentage of fat in an item.
- *Serving size.* You will find the specific amount of food listed under the Nutrition Facts title. All nutrient information is based on this amount of food and will be listed in common measures that you use at home. You will be able to compare this to the amount you eat and *Canada's Food Guide.*
- *Daily Values (DVs).* The Daily Values are based on recommendations for a healthy diet. The "% Daily Value" makes comparing foods easier because it puts all nutrients on the same scale. For example, a food that has a percent Daily Value of five or less for fat, sodium, or cholesterol would be low in these nutrients. A food that has a percent Daily Value of 15 or more for calcium, Vitamin A, or fibre would be high in these nutrients.

  Look for higher percent Daily Value next to nutrients you are trying to increase in your diet such as fibre, Vitamins A and C, calcium, and iron. Look for lower percent Daily Value for nutrients you are trying to decrease, such as saturated and trans fats, cholesterol, and sodium. If you eat double the amount that is listed, you must double the value for calories and nutrients.
- *Calories per gram.* The Nutrition Facts lists the number of calories per gram for fat, carbohydrates, and protein.
- *Calories from fat.* Get into the habit of calculating the percentage of fat calories in a food before buying or eating it.
- *Total fat.* It's easy to overload on fat. Saturated fat is a figure worthy of special attention because of its reported link to several diseases.
- *Cholesterol.* Cholesterol is made by and contained in products of animal origin only. Many high-fat products, such as potato chips, contain 0 percent cholesterol because they're made from plants and are cooked in vegetable fats. However, the vegetable fats they contain can be processed and made into saturated fats that are more harmful to the heart than cholesterol.
- *Fibre.* A high-fibre food has five or more grams of fibre per serving. A good source of fibre provides at least 2.5 grams.
- *Calcium.* High equals 200 milligrams or more per serving. Good means at least 100 milligrams per serving.
- *Sodium.* Since many foods contain sodium, most of us routinely get more than we need. Read labels carefully to avoid excess sodium, which can be a health threat.
- *Vitamins.* A Daily Value of 10 percent of any vitamin makes a food a good source; 20 percent qualifies it as high in a certain vitamin.

Although there is no implementation date as yet, the Government of Canada is intending on making changes to the Nutrition Facts table on food labels. The proposed food label changes are listed below:[40]*

- Make the information on serving size and calories easier to find and read.
- Add a percent daily value (percent DV) for sugars.
- Add a footnote at the bottom of the table about percent DV. This will help consumers understand

how much sugar and other nutrients (like sodium) are in their food. It would explain that

- 5 percent or less is a little
- 15 percent or more is a lot

- Add potassium because it is important for maintaining healthy blood pressure. Most Canadians are not getting enough of this nutrient.
- Remove Vitamin A and Vitamin C because most Canadians get enough of these nutrients in their diets.

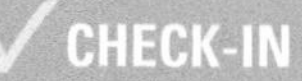

Do you read nutrition labels on the foods you buy?

HUMAN POTENTIAL

Dr. Stanley Zlotkin—Sprinkles Global Health Initiative: Creative Thought, Creative Purpose

As a college or university student, you may at times have wondered if research does make a difference. Our human potential story for this chapter suggests that it can. Dr. Stanley Zlotkin, M.D., Ph.D., FRCPC, the Chief of Global Child Health and a researcher at the Hospital for Sick Children, at the University of Toronto, used his academic knowledge and research skills to combat one of the most prevalent nutrition problems in the developing world today—iron-deficiency anemia in infants and young children.

The health issues linked to anemia during childhood and infancy include impaired mental and cognitive development and the capacity to learn. One common strategy used to prevent and treat iron deficiencies in young children is the use of iron drops. However, studies have demonstrated that because of the metallic taste of the drops, a strong odour, and gastric irritation, many children stop taking the drops. There are also cultural beliefs to honour and the expense of administering the iron drops to consider.

With creative thought and purpose, Dr. Zlotkin and his group of researchers developed an alternative micronutrient delivery system for infants and toddlers, called Sprinkles. Lipid-encapsulated iron (soy-lipid) and other essential micronutrients, including Vitamins A, B, C, and D, folic acid, and zinc, were packaged in powder form into individual packets as a single daily dose. The Sprinkles could be mixed into a bowl of any infant-weaning foods. There was no metallic aftertaste or change of colour, smell, or texture to the foods. No special measuring was required and the cost of this product was not prohibitively high.

The development of this product was admirable. Dr. Zlotkin could have stopped there. But what made his work special was his ongoing commitment to field test the Sprinkles through multi-country research studies in Afghanistan, Bangladesh, Bolivia, China, Cambodia, Indonesia, Guyana, Ghana, India, Mongolia, Pakistan, Vietnam, and Benin as well as First Nation and Inuit communities in Canada. This was no small task and took tenacity, commitment, and patience to deal with the many complex operational issues associated with the introduction of any new health intervention, especially when trying to reach some of the most at-risk people in the world.

He also determined that the distribution of Sprinkles would be better managed through international programs such as UNICEF, the World Food Program, the UN High Commission on Refugees, Save the Children, World Vision, and Care and Plan. To allow for worldwide distribution he gave the Sprinkles patent to the public domain, never personally profiting from it. Sprinkles is now being distributed in 62 countries and has reached approximately 20 million children.

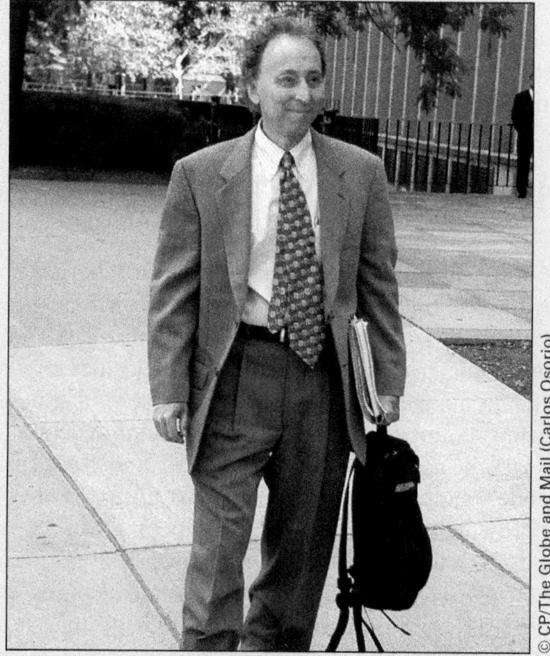

Dr. Stanley Zlotkin, creator of Sprinkles, is committed to reducing micronutrient deficiencies among infants and young children in developing countries.

There is not space in this story to describe all of the amazing work Dr. Zlotkin has done. Some examples include work with the French humanitarian relief agency Action Contre Le Faim (ACF) in regions in Afghanistan; the Helen Keller International (a large international NGO) in Cambodia and Indonesia; the Ministry of Health, Health Research Facility in Kintampo, Central Ghana; and Health Canada's First Nations, Inuit & Aboriginal Health branch in northern communities such as Attawapiskat, Fort Albany, and Igloolik. There *is* space, however, to report that Dr. Zlotkin continues to work on the Sprinkles Global Health Initiative. He has also been the recipient of many awards for his work—the *HJ Heinz Humanitarian Award* in 2001 for his international contribution to children's global health; the *Order of Canada* in 2007 for his contribution to improving children's lives on a global scale; the *International Ashoka Fellowship* in 2007; the *American Academy of Pediatrics (AAP) Samuel J. Fomon Nutrition Award*; and the *Mathile Institute Award for Career Achievement in Evidence Translation* in 2014.

If you are considering a research career, start asking yourself how you might use your knowledge and research skills to help others. Research can and does make a difference—as seen through the work and vision of people such as Dr. Zlotkin.

Nutrition labelling is not required for fresh fruits and vegetables, raw meat and poultry (except ground meat and poultry), raw fish and seafood, foods that are sold only in retail establishments where they are prepared or processed, and individual servings of food intended for immediate consumption.[41]

An investigation took place at the University of Saskatchewan to measure the reported use of nutrition information on food labels by university students. There were approximately equal numbers of label users and non-users among males, while label users outnumbered non-users by almost four to one among females. The only consistently observed difference between label users and non-users (male and female) was that users believed in the importance of nutrition information on food labels while non-users did not.[42]

THE WAY WE EAT

Dietary Diversity Whatever your cultural heritage, you may have sampled foods such as Chinese, Mexican, First Nations, Italian, or Japanese. If you belong to any of these ethnic groups, you may eat these cuisines regularly. Different images are used to represent food guides of different countries. The United Kingdom, Mexico, and the U.S.A. use a plate image. China and Korea use a pagoda image. Foods of the *Mediterranean Food Guide* are presented in a pyramid. Each type of ethnic cooking has its own nutritional benefits and potential drawbacks, yet food guides of all countries recommend eating a diet consisting of mainly carbohydrate-rich grains, vegetables, and fruits, and less high-protein meat and dairy.

Brazilian Diet In 2014, the Ministry of Health in Brazil published a new document titled *Dietary Guidelines for the Brazilian Population.*[43] The guidelines apply to anyone two years and over and emphasize social, cultural, economic, and environmental dimensions of healthy eating. The 10 main guidelines are based on three main themes—use fresh and minimally processed foods as the basis of each meal; use oils, fats, sugars, and salt in moderation; and limit intake of ready-to-eat food and drink products. The guidelines hope to inspire Brazilians to celebrate meals as an important part of family tradition.

Chinese Diet The Mainland Chinese diet—plant-based, high in carbohydrates, and low in fats and animal protein—is considered one of the healthiest in the world. The *Food Guide Pagoda* recommends plenty of cereals, vegetables, fruits, and beans, with physical activity balancing food intake.[44] However, Chinese food prepared in Canada contains more meat and sauces. According to laboratory tests of typical takeout dishes from Chinese restaurants, many have more fats and cholesterol than hamburger or egg dishes from fast-food outlets.

Try selecting boiled, steamed, or stir-fried dishes; mix entrées with steamed rice. If you are prone to high blood pressure, watch out for the high sodium content of soy and other sauces and the seasoning MSG (monosodium glutamate).

First Nations, Inuit, and Métis Food Guide To honour and reflect First Nations, Inuit, and Métis foods and traditions, Health Canada has modified *Canada's Food Guide*. This special guide, while recommending foods from each of the four food groups, shows examples of both traditional and store-bought foods that are commonly available in both rural and remote locations. Foods such as bannock, caribou, duck, and char are included in the guide and celebrate unique Aboriginal food choices (see Figure 5-4).[45] Researchers Receveur, Boulay, and Kuhnlein[46] evaluated the influence of traditional food on dietary intake for adult Dene-Métis in 16 communities of the Northwest Territories. Although there was an extensive consumption of traditional Dene-Métis foods, there appeared to be a trend in the younger generations toward eating less of these foods. The implications for health include higher levels of fat and saturated fat and lower intakes of calcium, Vitamin A, and dietary fibre.

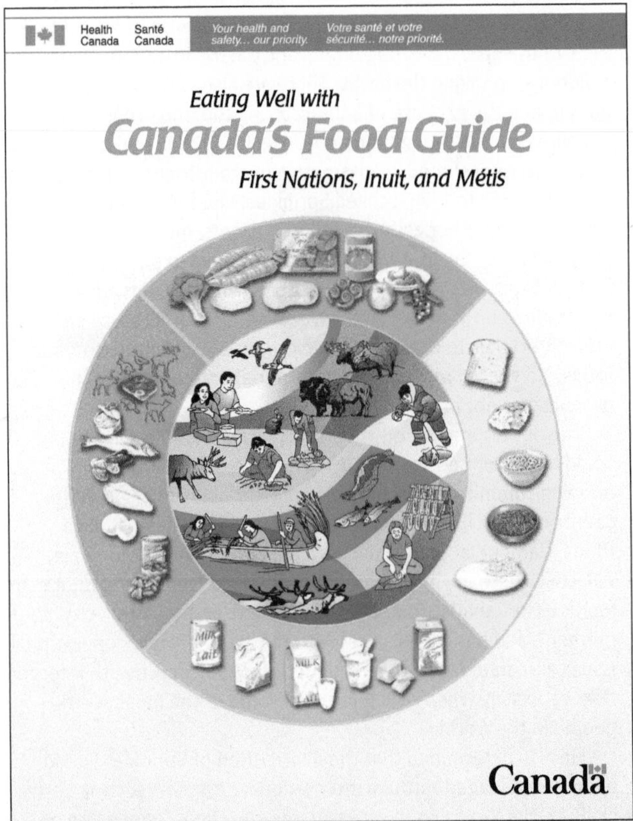

Figure 5-4 First Nations, Inuit, and Métis Food Guide

The First Nations, Inuit, and Métis Food Guide **illustrates how traditional foods such as bannock, caribou, duck, and char can be used in a healthy diet.**

Source: *Eating Well with Canada's Food Guide-First Nations, Inuit and Métis*. Health Canada, 2007. Adapted and reproduced with permission from the Minister of Health, 2016.

French Diet Traditional French cuisine, which includes rich, high-fat sauces and dishes, has never been considered healthful. Yet nutritionists have been stumped to explain the so-called French paradox. Despite a diet high in saturated fats, the French have had one of the lowest rates of coronary artery disease in the world.

However, fat consumption in France has risen as the French have begun eating more meat and fast foods, snacking more, eating fewer relaxed meals, exercising less, and drinking less wine.[47] They've also been getting fatter. The French diet increasingly resembles the Canadian and American diet, but French portions tend to be one-third to one-half the size of Canadian or American portions.

Indian Diet Many Indian dishes highlight healthful ingredients such as vegetables and legumes (beans and peas). However, many also use ghee (a form of butter) or coconut oil; both are rich in saturated fats. Good choices include daal or dal (lentils), *karbi* or *karni* (chickpea soup), and chapati (tortilla-like bread). Hold back on *bhatura* (fried bread), coconut milk, and samosas (fried meat or vegetables in dough).

Japanese Diet The traditional Japanese diet is very low in fat, which may account for the low incidence of heart disease in Japan. Dietary staples include soybean products, fish, vegetables, noodles, rice, and fruits. However, Japanese cuisine is high in salted, smoked, and pickled foods. Watch out for deep-fried dishes such as tempura and salty soups and sauces. Ask for broiled entrées or non-fried dishes made with tofu, which has no cholesterol.

Mediterranean Diet Research has confirmed that heart disease is much less common in countries along the Mediterranean than in other Western nations. No one knows exactly why. It could be that the plant-based Mediterranean diet, which is rich in fruits, vegetables, legumes, cereal, wine, and olive oil, may be the reason (see Figure 5-5).

Mexican Diet The cuisine served in Mexico features rice, corn, and beans, which are low in fat and high in nutrients. However, the dishes many Canadians think of as Mexican are far less healthful. Burritos, especially when topped with cheese and sour cream, are very high in fat. Nutritious choices include rice, beans, and shrimp or chicken tostadas on unfried cornmeal tortillas.

Southeast Asian Diet A rich variety of bamboo shoots, bok choy, cabbage, mangoes, papayas, and cucumbers provides a sound nutritional basis for this diet. In addition, most foods are broiled or stir-fried, which keeps fat low. However, coconut oil and milk, used in many sauces, are high in fat. The use of MSG and pickled foods means the sodium content is high. At Thai or Vietnamese restaurants, choose salads (*larb* is a chicken salad with mint) or seafood soup (*po tak*).

U.S. Diet Up until 2010, Americans followed a well-known food pyramid known as MyPyramid. In 2010 the MyPyramid was replaced with MyPlate, a new food guide that has been designed to encourage Americans to eat in a healthy way (see Figure 5-6). MyPlate illustrates five food groups—Fruits, Vegetables, Grains,

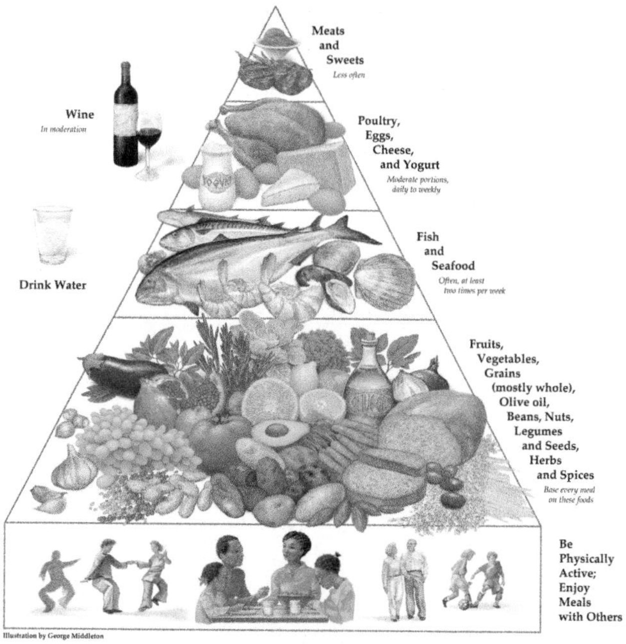

Figure 5-5 Mediterranean Food Pyramid

The Mediterranean diet relies heavily on fruits, vegetables, grains, and potatoes and includes considerable olive oil.

Source: © 2009 Oldways Preservation & Exchange Trust, www.oldwayspt.org.

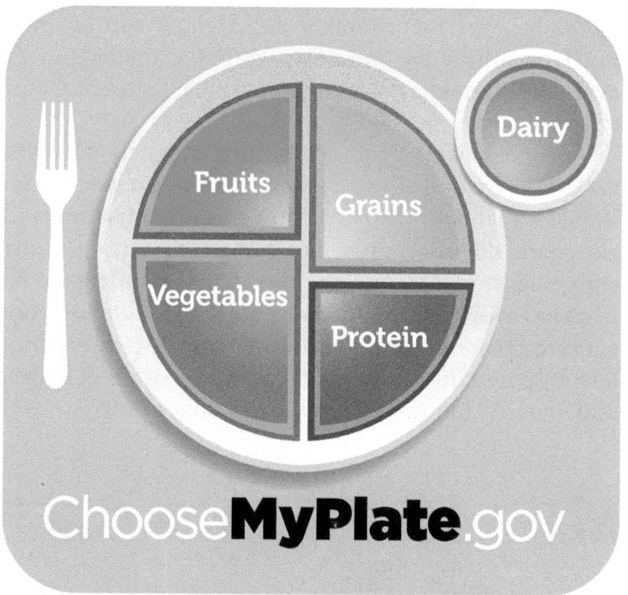

Figure 5-6 ChooseMyPlate

Source: United States Department of Agriculture.

Protein, and Dairy. It focuses on key eating behaviours. The new guidelines recommend that half the plate should be filled with fruits and vegetables; that half of the grains eaten should be whole grains; and that people should drink fat-free or low-fat (1 percent) milk. The plate image also discourages oversize portions.[48]

100-Mile Diet By now you have probably heard about the 100-mile diet.[49] Alisa Smith and J. B. McKinnon, long-time vegetarians, were moved to make a change in their own personal eating habits when they discovered that the food eaten by the average North American must travel over 1500 miles (2400 kilometres) from the farm to the grocery store. Their book, *The 100-Mile Diet: A Year of Local Eating,* is a story of their experience attempting to spend an entire year eating food grown within a 100-mile (160-kilometre) radius of their Vancouver apartment.

People are beginning to understand that supporting local food producers helps not only the local economy but also the world at large. Eating more seasonally, reducing greenhouse gases by reducing the distances food is shipped, and connecting with your own local community are all part of healthy living strategies.

Meal Exchange In every community, people are faced with rising food costs and feeding their families. Food banks are the norm in many cities and towns. Another innovative program called Meal Exchange, a national student-founded, student-driven, registered charity, is also assisting people in need.[50] Meal Exchange began in 1993, when Rahul Raj found he had money left over from his University of Wilfred Laurier meal plan. To honour his grandmother's commitment to the poor people in India, Rahul began donating and delivering food to local social service agencies. In 1998, Meal Exchange was incorporated and is now run on one-third of university campuses across Canada and in over 100 Canadian communities (see Figure 5-7 for charity logo).

This organization generates approximately 450 000 dollars in food and monetary donations for local food agencies each year. The vision of this organization is to eliminate the root causes of hunger and poverty by engaging students in volunteer work. Students who become involved in Meal Exchange help to donate food, educate others about the causes of hunger, create volunteer opportunities that address hunger-related issues, and identify and implement student solutions.

MEAL EXCHANGE

Hunger Problem. Student Solution.

Figure 5-7 Meal Exchange

Source: Meal Exchange.

Some of the Meal Exchange core successful programs include

- Trick or Eat®—a Halloween event where students collect non-perishable food items for local food assistance programs
- Skip-A-Meal®—a program that allows student meal-plan holders an opportunity to donate a meal from their campus meal plan to purchase food at wholesale prices for donation to a local food program
- Clear the Shelves—a program that encourages students to donate excess food, clothing, and furniture to local community members at the end of the academic year
- Meal Exchange All-Star—a recognition program for students who have made a tremendous effort to help the organization and promote social change

There may be a Meal Exchange program on your campus.

What Should I Know about Vegetarian Diets? A 2015 online survey suggests that approximately 12 million Canadians (33 percent) were eating less meat than previous years or described themselves as vegetarians. Thirteen percent of people living in British Columbia said they were vegetarians or mostly vegetarians. Twenty-six percent of British Columbians indicated that they were trying to eat less meat. Eight percent of people in Ontario reported they were vegetarian or mostly vegetarian while 23 percent were trying to eat less meat. Seven percent of people living in Quebec identified as vegetarian or mostly vegetarian. Thirty percent were trying to eat less meat. Twelve percent of younger Canadians (18–24 years of age) report that they are vegetarian or mostly vegetarian—more than older Canadians.[51]

Not all vegetarians avoid all meats. There are several types of vegetarian diets:

- **vegan** or total vegetarian diet—involves consuming only foods of plant origin, no animal products of any type

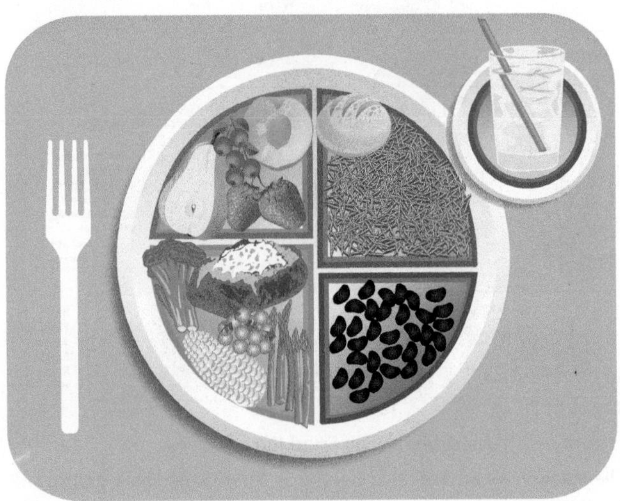

Basheera Designs/Shutterstock

Vegetarian Food Plate

- **lacto-vegetarian**—includes dairy products, grains, fruits, and vegetables, but no eggs or flesh animal foods
- **lacto-ovo-vegetarian**—includes both dairy products and eggs, grains, fruits, and vegetables
- **lacto-ovo-pesco-vegetarian**, also sometimes called semi-vegetarian—includes dairy products, eggs, and fish, but no red meat

The Dietitians of Canada have developed some excellent guidelines for vegetarian diets.[52,53] *Canada's Food Guide* can be adapted for vegetarians. Adequate nutrient intake can be made by choosing a variety of meat alternatives from the Meat and Alternatives food group, such as lentils, tofu, and soy-based meat substitutes.

Vegetarian diets have proven health benefits.[54] Studies show that vegetarians' cholesterol levels are low, they are seldom overweight, and they're less apt to be candidates for heart disease. They also have lower incidences of breast, colon, and prostate cancers; high blood pressure; and osteoporosis. When combined with exercise and stress reduction, vegetarian diets have helped reverse the buildup of harmful plaque within the blood vessels of the heart.

Pay special attention to the following:

- Protein—vary your sources of dietary protein. Soy protein has been shown to be equal in nutritional value to proteins of animal origin. By combining complementary protein sources, you can make sure that your body makes the most of the non-animal proteins you eat.
- Iron—dried beans, spinach, enriched products, brewer's yeast, and dried fruits are all good plant sources of iron.
- Vitamin B_{12}—comes naturally only from animal sources, so vegans should look for fortified breakfast cereals, fortified soy beverages, veggie meats, or Vitamin B_{12} supplement.
- Calcium and Vitamin D—dairy products provide calcium as do soy milk, rice milk, and orange juice. Certain green vegetables such as broccoli, kale, bok choy, and Chinese cabbage as well as almonds, figs, and blackstrap molasses are also good sources of calcium. Sunlight enables us to make our own Vitamin D, and cow's milk, fortified soy milk, and rice milk contain Vitamin D.

Fast Food: Nutrition on the Run "Burger and fries to go." Fast service and cheap prices keep consumers buying quick and easy meals. In 2014, the Canadian fast-food industry was led by Tim Horton's, which was ranked first in terms of value sales, outlets, and transaction volume. McDonald's was ranked second, followed by Subway in third place.[55] This is a 23 billion-dollar industry in Canada. However, it appears that a new trend is emerging among fast-food outlets due to stiff competition among casual dining restaurants and education about the health risks of consuming fast foods. McDonald's has reported the closing of more restaurants in the U.S.A. than it opened in 2014, something that the company has not done in 40 years. In an attempt to keep customers coming, McDonald's and other fast-food businesses are adding "health food" such as kale salads to their menus.[56] Even smartphone apps are now available for many fast-food chains and restaurants.[57]

Fast foods can contribute protein, carbohydrates, vitamins, and minerals. Some fast-food restaurants now offer healthier food options that are lower in fat and calories. There are even fruit and vegetable choices, too. But there are many problems with fast food.

- While many fast-food meals give you half of your daily energy requirements, they give you only one-quarter of your vitamin and mineral daily requirements.
- Almost half of the calories in typical fast-food meals come from fat. The fat content of many items is extremely high. A Burger King Whopper with Cheese contains 723 calories and 48 grams of fat, 18 grams from saturated fat. A McDonald's Sausage McMuffin with Egg has 517 calories and 33 grams of fat, 13 grams from saturated fat.[58]
- Recommended sodium intake is about 2000 milligrams per day. A typical fast-food meal with regular fries and a small shake gives you about 1500 milligrams of sodium.

If fast food is on your menu, choose food items wisely. Make the best of a fast-food meal by limiting the high-fat food choices or by making fast-food restaurant meals an option only occasionally.

Campus Cuisine Healthy food choices can sometimes be a challenge in college and university cafeterias and food outlets. Residence living does not always allow for individual meal preparation. Roommates may have different food likes and dislikes. Academic and financial pressures can also impact the way students eat. Two top influences on food choices are price and convenience. Cafeteria food plans almost always include hamburgers and fries, which can become a daily fare for many students. All-you-can-eat buffets are also tempting. Some students, on their own for the first time, have not been responsible for their own nutrition plan and do not know how to prepare nutritious food.

The good news is that many colleges and universities are addressing nutrition needs of students and are making changes to support healthy eating initiatives.[59] Menus are changing. They now include low-fat, low-sodium, less-processed foods. Vegetarian and vegan options have expanded, and organic food outlets or cafeteria options are becoming more readily available in both Canadian and American colleges and universities. Promotion of the intake of more fruits and vegetables for students has also resulted in an increase in consumption of this important food group.[60]

Residential life coordinators have been working with Housing and Food Services to welcome students from different cultures by adding ethnic cuisine from around the globe in cafeterias and special food outlets. Indian, Thai, Korean, Chinese, and Japanese meals are just a few examples of food being offered on campuses.

Nutrition education is another initiative evident in cafeterias and alternative food outlets. Fat, carbohydrate, and protein content and total calories for food items are being posted. Nutrition seminars are being offered. Some colleges and universities even have registered dietitians as part of their health team. Find out about nutrition options on your campus. There are many options available to students on campuses across the country. Making healthy food choices impacts overall health and wellness.

✓ CHECK-IN

Are nutritious food choices easily available at your college or university?

FOOD SAFETY

Increasingly, Canadians are concerned not just about whether the food they eat is nutritious but also whether it's safe. Many unsuspected safety hazards have been identified by **food toxicologists**—specialists who detect toxins (potentially harmful substances) in our food and treat the conditions they produce.

Pesticides, Irradiation, and Genetic Engineering

Plants and animals naturally produce compounds that act as pesticides to aid in their survival. The vast majority of the pesticides we consume are therefore natural—that is, not added by farmers or food processors. The problem lies with commercial pesticides, chemical wonders that save billions of dollars of valuable crops from pests, but endanger human health and life.

Many consumers are now purchasing **organic** foods. *Organic* refers to foods produced without the use of commercial chemicals at any stage. Independent groups now certify foods before they can be labelled organic. Foods that are truly organic have much lower levels of residues than standard commercial produce. There's no guarantee that the organic produce you buy at a grocery or health-food store is more nutritious than other produce. Organic food can also be more expensive. However, buying organic foods is one way in which you can work toward a healthier environment.

Irradiation is the use of radiation, either from radioactive substances or from devices that produce X-rays, on food. It doesn't make the food radioactive. Its primary benefit is to prolong the shelf life of food. Like the heat in canning, irradiation can kill all the microorganisms that might grow in a food, and the sterilized food can then be stored for years in sealed containers at room temperature without spoiling. Low-dose irradiation can inhibit the sprouting of vegetables such as potatoes and onions and delay the ripening of some fruits, such as bananas and tomatoes.

Nutritional studies have shown no significant decreases in the quality of the foods, but high-dose treatments may cause vitamin losses similar to those that occur during canning. It's also possible that the ionizing effect of radiation creates new compounds in foods that may be mutagenic or carcinogenic.

In Canada, several federal agencies are involved in regulating aspects of the food-irradiation process. The Health Products and Food Branch of Health Canada, through the *Food and Drugs Act*, is responsible for establishing standards related to the safety of foods sold to the Canadian consumer; the Canadian Food Inspection Agency (CFIA) is responsible for all enforcement and compliance issues relating to irradiated foods; and the Radiation Protection Bureau (RPB) of Health Canada is responsible for investigating, communicating, and reducing health risks to Canadians from exposure to ionizing and non-ionizing radiation. Food irradiation facilities must comply with these regulations.[61]

Genetically modified organisms (GMOs) describe plants, animals, or bacterium that have had their genetic material altered through traditional breeding techniques where an organism is mutated and desired traits are then selected and bred together. It can also describe **genetically engineered organisms (GE)**—organisms that are modified through the use of new technology, where genes are either transferred into or removed from the organism. Some GMO experts use the two terms interchangeably.[62]

Over the years, many plants have been genetically modified and are now accepted as common crops in Canada. Examples include corn, canola, soya, and sugar beets. Outside of Canada, examples include papaya, squash, and milk products. A new type of apple named the *Arctic Apple*, which has been modified and promises to be "non-browning" is waiting for approval from Health Canada at the time of writing this edition.[63] GMO crops were developed to increase hardiness and reduce toxic components. Some food experts thought modifying plants might make them more resistant to insects and diseases. The hope was that crop yields could be improved, and with a higher crop yield, world hunger issues might be addressed. Unfortunately the opposite has proven to be true. Weeds and bugs have adapted to the genetically modified crops, and reports indicate that in many circumstances this has led to the use of even more chemicals being applied to crops.[64] There are ethical concerns about introducing genetic material into organisms that would not naturally occur. Testing of genetically modified plants is ongoing, but the extent of long-term impact on human beings and the environment is not known. Questions about how genetically engineered plants move and interact with native species are being asked. Political and economic issues have also surfaced. Large, multinational companies own most of the GMO patents. For some people this is viewed as having an unfair advantage over developing countries who cannot afford the GMO seeds. The other important issue is the lack of knowledge about what foods have been genetically modified. As yet, Canada does not require labelling of all GMO foods so consumers do not know if the foods they are purchasing and eating have been modified unlike in many countries in Europe where labelling has been required.[65]

Additives: Risks versus Benefits **Additives** are substances added to foods to lengthen storage time, change taste in a way the manufacturer thinks is better, alter colour, or otherwise modify them to make them more appealing.

Additives provide numerous benefits. Sodium and calcium propionate, sodium benzoate, potassium sorbate, and sulfur dioxide prevent the growth of bacteria, yeast, and mould in baked goods. BHA (butylated hydroxyanisole), BHT (butylated hydroxytoluene), propyl gallate, and Vitamin E protect against the oxidation of fats (rancidity). Other additives include leavening agents, emulsifiers, stabilizers, thickeners, dough conditioners, and bleaching agents.

Some additives can pose a risk to eaters. Nitrites, used in bacon, sausages, and lunch meats to inhibit spoilage, prevent botulism, and add colour, can react with other substances in your body or in food to form potentially cancer-causing agents called *nitrosamines*. Sulfites, used to prevent browning, can produce severe, even fatal, allergic reactions in sensitive individuals. Labelling of sulfites in packaged foods is now mandatory.[66]

What Causes Food Poisoning? *Salmonella* is a bacterium that contaminates many foods, particularly undercooked chicken, eggs, and, sometimes, processed meat. Eating contaminated food can result in salmonella poisoning, which causes diarrhea and vomiting. Another bacterium, *Campylobacter jejuni*, may cause even more stomach infections than salmonella. Found in water, milk, and some foods, Campylobacter poisoning causes severe diarrhea and has been implicated in the growth of stomach ulcers.

Bacteria can also cause illness by producing toxins in food. *Staphylococcus aureus* is the most common culprit. When cooked foods are cross-contaminated with the bacteria from raw foods and not stored properly, staph infections can result, causing nausea and abdominal pain anywhere from 30 minutes to eight hours after ingestion.

An uncommon but sometimes fatal form of food poisoning is **botulism**, caused by the *Clostridium botulinum* organism. Improper home canning procedures are the most common cause of this potentially fatal problem.

✓ CHECK-IN

What can you do to improve your food safety?

Food Allergies Cow's milk, eggs, seafood, wheat, soybeans, nuts, seeds, and chocolate have all been identified as common triggers of food allergies. The symptoms they produce vary. One person might sneeze if exposed to an irritating food; another might vomit or develop diarrhea; and others might suffer headaches, dizziness, hives, or a rapid heartbeat. Symptoms may not develop for up to 72 hours, making it hard to pinpoint which food was responsible. If you suspect that you have a food allergy, see a physician with specialized training in allergy diagnosis.

STRATEGIES FOR PREVENTION

Protecting Yourself from Food Poisoning

- Clean food thoroughly. Wash produce thoroughly. Wash utensils, plates, cutting boards, knives, blenders, and other cooking equipment with very hot water and soap after preparing raw meat, poultry, or fish to avoid contaminating other foods or the cooked meat.
- Drink only pasteurized milk.
- Don't eat raw eggs—they can be contaminated with salmonella.
- Cook chicken thoroughly. About one-third of all poultry sold contains harmful organisms.
- Cook pork thoroughly to kill a parasite called *trichina* occasionally found in the muscles of pigs.
- Know how to store foods. Don't leave food out for more than two hours in the temperature danger zone—between 4° Celsius (40° Fahrenheit) and 50° Celsius (140° Fahrenheit). After that time, throw the food away.
- Stored food doesn't last forever. Refrigerate leftovers as soon as possible and use them within three days. Use frozen leftovers within two to three months.

SELF-SURVEY

How Healthful Is Your Diet?

STEP 1

Keep a food diary for a week. Write down everything you eat and drink for meals and snacks. Include the approximate number of Food Guide Servings as recommended by *Eating Well with Canada's Food Guide* (see below and also Figure 5.1). If you are very active and need more food, choose extra Food Guide Servings from the four food groups.

	Mon	Tues	Wed	Thurs	Fri	Sat	Sun
Vegetables & Fruits							
Grain Products							
Milk and Alternatives							
Meat and Alternatives							
Oils and Fats							

Recommended Number of Food Guide Servings per Day

	Children			Teens		Adults			
	2–3	4–8	9–13	14–18 Years		19–50 Years		51+ Years	
	Girls and Boys			Female	Male	Female	Male	Female	Male
Vegetables & Fruits	4	5	6	7	8	7–8	8–10	7	7
Grain Products	3	4	6	6	7	6–7	8	6	7
Milk and Alternatives	2	2	3–4	3–4	3–4	2	2	3	3
Meat and Alternatives	1	1	1–2	2	3	2	3	2	3

Examples of one Food Guide Serving are:

Vegetables and Fruit

- 125 mL (½ cup) fresh, frozen, or canned vegetable or fruit or 100% juice
- 250 mL (1 cup) leafy raw vegetables or salad
- 1 piece of fruit

Grain Products

- 1 slice (35 g) bread or ½ bagel (45 g)
- ½ pita (35 g) or ½ tortilla (35 g)
- 125 mL (½ cup) cooked rice, pasta, or couscous
- 30 g cold cereal or 175 mL (¾ cup) hot cereal

Milk and Alternatives

- 250 mL (1 cup) milk or fortified soy beverage
- 175 g (¾ cup) yogurt
- 50 g (1½ oz.) cheese

Meat and Alternatives

- 75 g (2½ oz.) or 125 mL (½ cup) cooked fish, shellfish, poultry, or lean meat
- 175 mL (¾ cup) cooked beans
- 2 eggs
- 30 mL (2 Tbsp) peanut butter

Oils and Fats

Include a small amount—30–45 mL (2 to 3 Tbsp)—of unsaturated fat each day to get the fat you need. This amount includes oil used for cooking, salad dressings, margarine, and mayonnaise.

Unsaturated vegetable oils include the following:

- Canola
- Corn
- Flaxseed
- Olive
- Peanut
- Soybean
- Sunflower

Limit butter, hard margarine, lard, and shortening.

Here's what 30 mL (2 Tbsp) of unsaturated fat looks like in a sample day of eating:

Breakfast

- 5 mL (1 tsp) of soft non-hydrogenated margarine on your toast or bread

- 5 mL (1 tsp) of canola oil in your pan to make scrambled eggs

Lunch

- 15 mL (1 Tbsp) of vinegar and oil-type salad dressing (e.g., Balsamic, Italian, raspberry vinaigrette) on your salad

Dinner

- 5 mL (1 tsp) of canola or olive oil used to cook your stir-fry

Source: Health Canada. (2007, February 05). What is a food guide serving? Food and Nutrition. http://www.hc-sc.gc.ca/fn-an/food-guide-aliment/basics-base/serving-portion-eng.php; Health Canada. (2015, July 17). What type and amount of fat do I need? Food and Nutrition. http://www.hc-sc.gc.ca/fn-an/food-guide-aliment/choose-choix/oil-huile/oil-huile-eng.php

STEP 2

Are You Getting Too Much Sodium?

How often do you eat:	Seldom/ Never	1–2 times a week	3–5 times a week	Almost daily
Cured or processed meats, such as ham, sausage, frankfurters, or luncheon meats?				
Canned vegetables or frozen vegetables with sauce?				
Frozen TV dinners or entrées, or canned or dehydrated soups?				
Salted nuts, popcorn, pretzels, corn chips, or potato chips?				
Seasoning mixes or sauces containing salt?				
Processed cheese?				
Salt added to table foods before you taste them?				

Ideally, you should be eating these high-sodium items no more than one or two times a week. If your food diary indicates that you're eating them more frequently, your sodium intake may well be too high.

Source: *Eating Well with Canada's Food Guide.* Health Canada, 2011. Adapted and reproduced with permission from the Minister of Health, 2016.

Chapter Summary

1. Which of the following are classes of essential nutrients?
   a. amino acids, antioxidants, fibre, and cholesterol
   b. proteins, calcium, calories, and folic acid
   c. carbohydrates, protein, vitamins, minerals, fat, and water
   d. iron, whole grains, fruits, and vegetables
2. Which type of fat is NOT considered a threat to heart health?
   a. omega-3 fatty acids
   b. trans fatty acids
   c. cholesterol
   d. saturated fats
3. What are antioxidants?
   a. Antioxidants are nutrients important in the production of hemoglobin.
   b. Antioxidants are substances added to foods to make them more flavourful or physically appealing.
   c. Antioxidants are suspected triggers of food allergies.
   d. Antioxidants are substances that prevent the harmful effects of free radicals.
4. Which of the following is a recommendation from *Eating Well with Canada's Food Guide?*
   a. On a daily basis, people should eat the same amounts of food from each of the food groups represented in the guide.
   b. Oils and fats should be a major part of a healthy diet.
   c. People should eat 6–11 servings of meat and alternatives every week.
   d. Males aged 19–50 should eat eight servings of grain products and 8–10 servings of vegetables and fruits daily.
5. Which statement about essential nutrients is false?
   a. Carbohydrates provide body cells with glucose.
   b. Fats are necessary for the growth and repair of body cells.
   c. Water is an essential nutrient but doesn't provide any energy.
   d. Vitamins are necessary for the body to manufacture blood cells and hormones.
6. Which of the following is NOT included on food labels for packaged food?
   a. total recommended servings
   b. total amount of nutrients contained in the food

c. the percentage of nutrient Daily Values provided in the food
d. serving size

7. Which of the following statements is true?
   a. The Chinese diet, which is high in fats and low in carbohydrates, leads to a high incidence of obesity and heart disease.
   b. The French diet is considered to be healthful because the food is high in saturated fats.
   c. The Mediterranean diet is rich in fruits, vegetables, wine, and olive oil and may help prevent heart disease.
   d. Mexican recipes often include MSG, which is unhealthy for people with high blood pressure.

8. Which statement is true for some vegetarians?
   a. They include chicken and fish in their diets.
   b. They avoid Vitamin B_{12} supplements if they eat only plant foods.
   c. They eat only legumes or nuts because these provide complete proteins.
   d. They have high cholesterol levels because of the saturated fats in fruits and vegetables.

9. Which of the following is NOT a food hazard?
   a. nitrites
   b. raw eggs
   c. pesticides
   d. refrigerated leftovers used within three days

10. Which of the following are common causes of food-borne infections?
   a. influenza virus
   b. salmonella and E. coli bacteria
   c. additives
   d. irradiation

Answers to these questions can be found on page 133.

SELF-RESPONSIBILITY—SOCIAL RESPONSIBILITY

SELF-RESPONSIBILITY

Fresh food for a fresh attitude.

Julie Patterson

Many of us want to change the way we eat, but are stuck in the contemplation stage—thinking about making changes, but not doing much about it. How might you get started? Think about the type of diet you would like to try. You can lower the fat content in your diet, try a vegetarian approach to eating, find out more about ethnic food, or simply eat more fruits and vegetables. You could try the 100-mile diet. Check out your local library or bookstore or find a reputable website to learn more about healthy nutrition. What can you do to move from contemplation to preparation and then to action?

SOCIAL RESPONSIBILITY

There is hunger for ordinary bread, and there is hunger for love, for kindness, for thoughtfulness; and this is the great poverty that makes people suffer so much.

Mother Teresa

Find out more about food bank programs on your campus. Many colleges and universities are setting up student food banks. There are many opportunities to help out through your academic year.

CRITICAL THINKING

1. Which alternative or ethnic diet do you think has the best-tasting food? Which is the most healthy? Why?
2. Is it possible to meet nutritional requirements on a limited budget? Have you ever been in this situation? What would you recommend to someone who wants to eat healthfully on $75 a week?
3. Consider the number of times a week you eat fast food. How much money would you have saved if you had eaten home-prepared meals? Which fast foods could you have selected that would have provided more nutritional value?

WEB LINKS

Dietitians of Canada

www.dietitians.ca

The Dietitians of Canada website is an excellent source for comprehensive information that includes dietary guidelines, *Canada's Food Guide to Healthy Eating*, information about nutritional supplements, healthy diets, and current nutrition news.

Dietitians of Canada—Assess Yourself

www.dietitians.ca/Your-Health/Assess-Yourself.aspx

You can assess your current lifestyle and eating habits by using the tools available on this website. Check out the BMI assessment for health status based on your height and weight. Use eaTracker to check your food and activity choices and find new recipes for healthy eating with the Recipe Analyzer.

Food Guide Serving Sizes for 13–18 years

http://www.albertahealthservices.ca/assets/info/nutrition/if-nfs-food-guide-serving-sizes-13-to-18-years.pdf

Did you know that 125 millilitres (1/2 cup) of fresh or soft vegetable slices equals the size of one small computer mouse? If you have ever wondered just what a food guide serving looks like, you can access this report from Healthy Alberta to find out more.

Health Canada

www.hc-sc.gc.ca/fn-an/food-guide-aliment/index-eng.php

Eating Well with Canada's Food Guide (2007)

Access this site for downloadable *Canada's Food Guides*. Many translated guides are available, including a First Nations, Inuit, and Métis guide.

Please note that links are subject to change. If you find a broken link, use a search engine such as www.google.ca and search for the website by typing in keywords.

Key Terms

The terms listed here are used within the chapter on the page indicated. Definitions of the terms are in the Glossary at the end of this book.

Answers to Chapter Summary Questions

1. c; 2. a; 3. d; 4. d; 5. b; 6. a; 7. c; 8. a; 9. d; 10. b

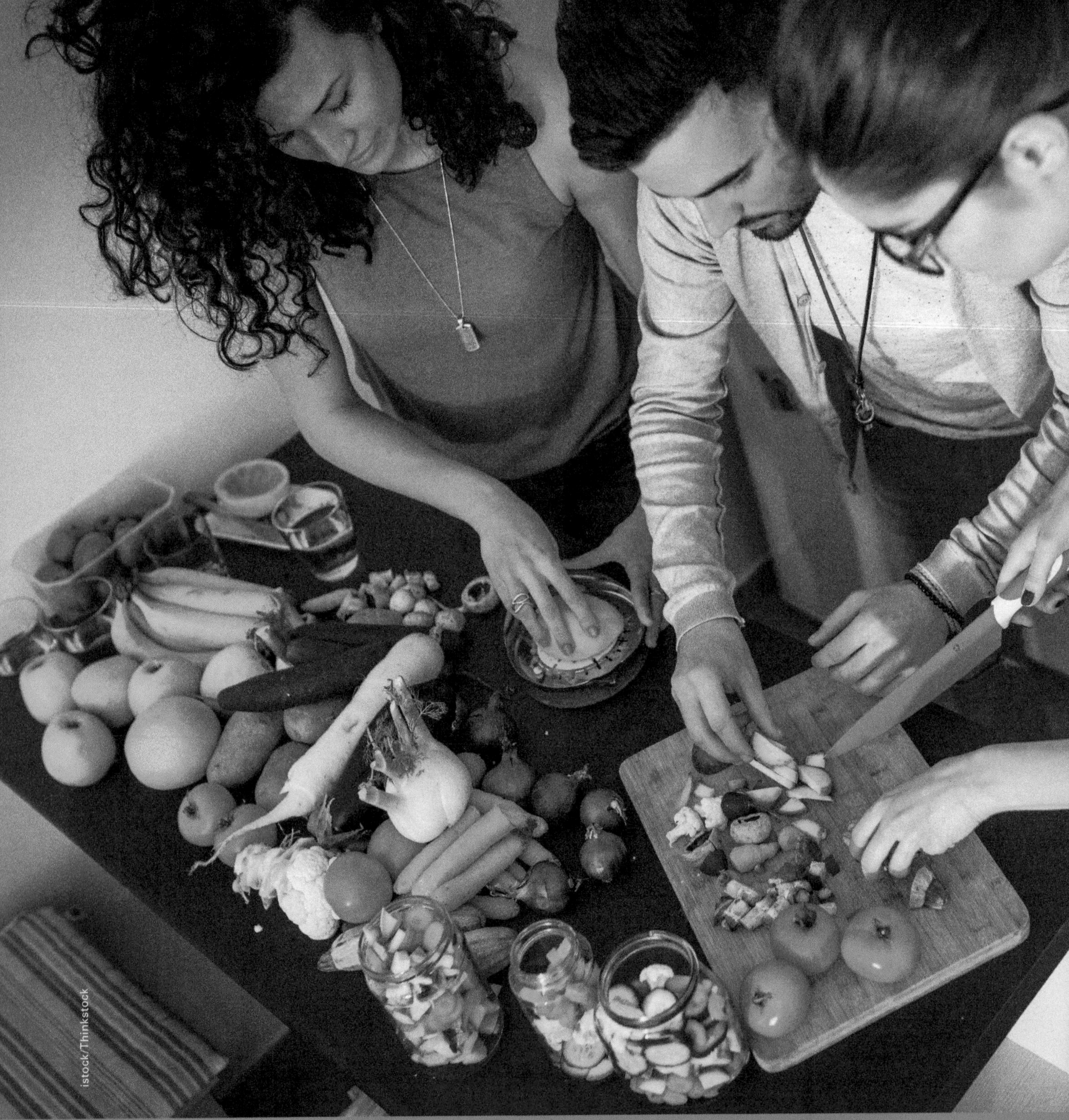
istock/Thinkstock

AFTER READING THIS CHAPTER, YOU WILL BE ABLE TO:

- **identify** a variety of factors that cause obesity
- **describe** body mass index (BMI), waist circumference, and waist-to-hip ratio
- **identify** the health dangers of excess weight
- **understand** how to avoid diet traps
- **assess** various approaches to weight management
- **identify** and **describe** the symptoms and dangers associated with eating disorders

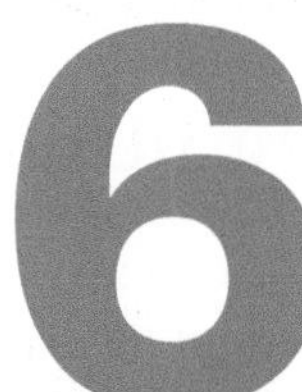

6

Managing Your Weight

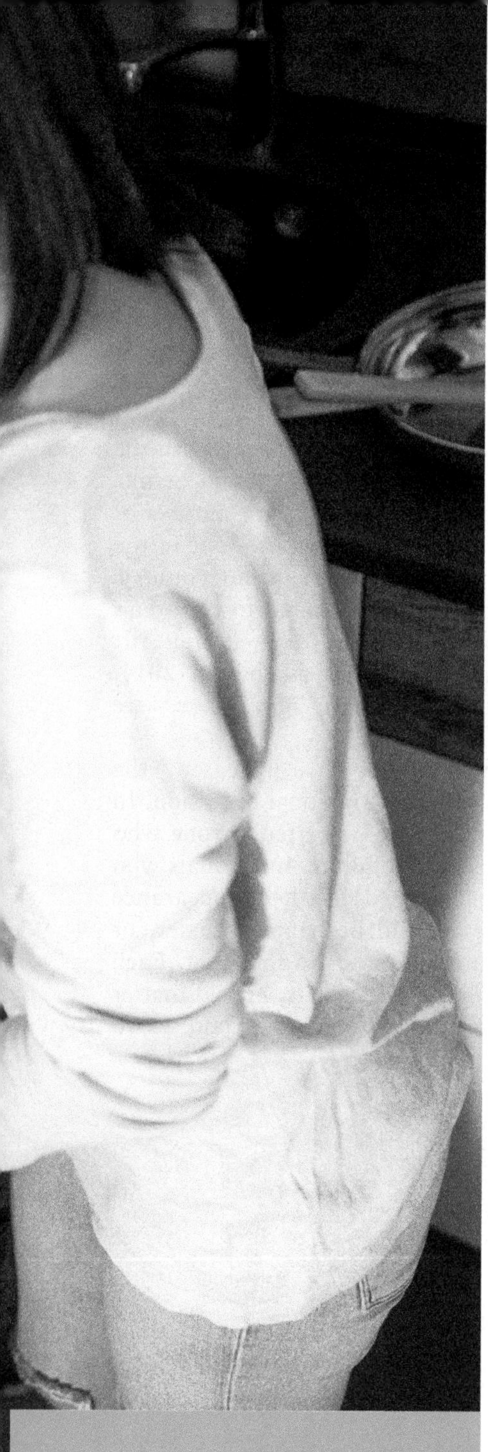

Healthy eating is essential for healthy living. It is one of the most important things we can do to improve and maintain our overall health. The question is—if we know better why don't we do better? Why is it so difficult to make healthy food choices? Why is there an obesity epidemic in Canada? Why do so many college and university students struggle with unhealthy eating behaviours? The answers are complex. Fast food is available 24 hours a day. Academic pressures sometimes take precedence over care and attention to nutrition habits. Many people have not been well educated about healthy eating practices. Learning about nutrition issues, accepting responsibility for your own food choices, and planning for a lifetime of healthy eating can be both empowering and exciting.

This chapter examines the global epidemic of obesity and how we can take control and manage our weight. It explains body mass index (BMI), waist circumference, and waist-to-hip ratio as they link to our understanding of healthy weights. Helpful tips on how to avoid diet traps, diet food, and the ever popular fad diets are presented. Psychosocial aspects to being overweight and obesity are shared. There is also a discussion of unhealthy eating and an exploration of body image and eating disorders.

FREQUENTLY ASKED QUESTIONS

THE GLOBAL OBESITY EPIDEMIC

Since 1980, obesity rates have more than doubled around the world. About 1.9 billion (39 percent) adults 18 years and over were considered overweight in 2014. Of the 1.9 billion, 600 million (13 percent) were considered obese. Most of the world's population live in countries where more people die of complications from being overweight and obese than they do from being underweight.[1] According to Statistics Canada, in 2014, 20.2 percent of Canadians aged 18 and older, or about 5.3 million adults, were classified as obese from self-reported data on their height and weight. Obesity rates for men increased from 20.1 percent in 2013 to 21.8 percent in 2014. This is the highest rate of obesity for men reported since 2003. Obesity rates for women increased from 17.4 percent in 2013 to 18.7 percent in 2014[2] (see Figure 6-1).

Self-reported data also indicates that 40 percent of men and 27.5 percent of women were classified as being overweight in 2014. This was a decrease of overweight levels for men from 41.9 percent in 2013. The rate for women has stayed stable since 2003. If we combine the numbers of Canadian men and women who self-reported being overweight with those who self-reported being obese, we see 61.8 percent of men (8.2 million) and 46.2 percent of women (6.1 million) had increased health risks due to excess weight[3] (see Figure 6-1).

Statistics Canada also reports provincial differences in obesity rates. Both British Columbia and Quebec report a lower-than-national-average level of obesity, with 16 percent of citizens of British Columbia and 18.2 percent of Quebec citizens considered obese. Ontario, Alberta, Prince Edward Island, Nunavut, and the Yukon record obesity levels about the same as the national average. All other provinces are significantly above the national average with the top three being Newfoundland and Labrador at 30.4 percent, Nova Scotia at 27.8 percent, and New Brunswick at 26.4 percent[4] (see Figure 6-2).

Health and education professionals concur with the dire warnings being made by the Heart and Stroke Foundation of Canada[5]—that the increasing number of overweight and obese Canadians now poses one of the greatest threats ever to public health in our country. The growing body of research dedicated to children's health and nutrition patterns is also setting off alarm bells. What is disconcerting is that in 2014, nearly 42 million children under the ages of five were overweight.[6]

Ironically, as average weights have increased,[7] the quest for thinness has become a national obsession. In a society where slimmer is seen as better, anyone who is less than lean may feel like a failure. Individuals who are overweight or embarrassed by their appearance often assume that they would be happier, sexier, or more successful in thinner bodies.[8] So they diet. Each year millions of Canadians go on diets, but no matter how much they lose, 90–95 percent regain extra pounds within five years.

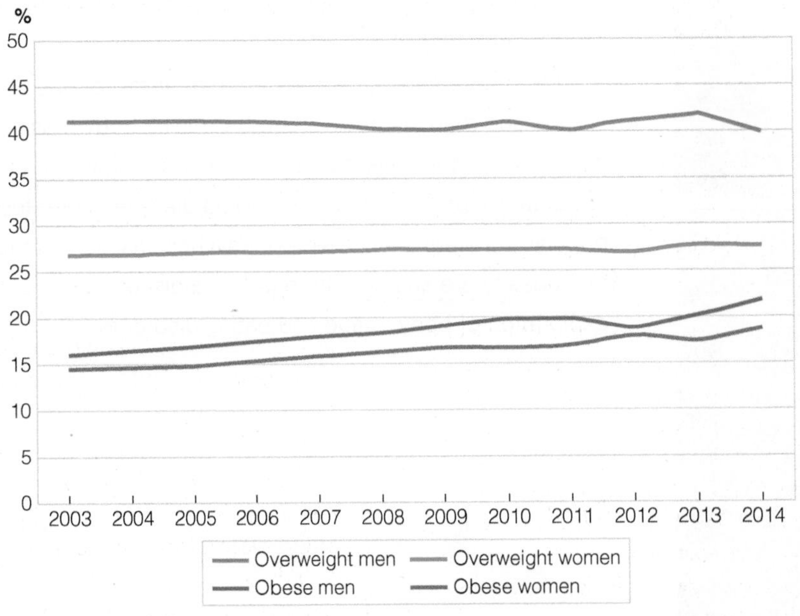

Figure 6-1 Percentage Who Were Obese and Overweight (Self-reported), by Sex, Household Population Aged 18 and Older. Canada, 2003–2014.

Source: Statistics Canada. (2015, November 27). *Overweight and obese adults (self-reported), 2014*. Health Fact Sheets. Publications. Catalogue no. 82-625-X. http://www.statcan.gc.ca/pub/82-625-x/2015001/article/14185-eng.htm.

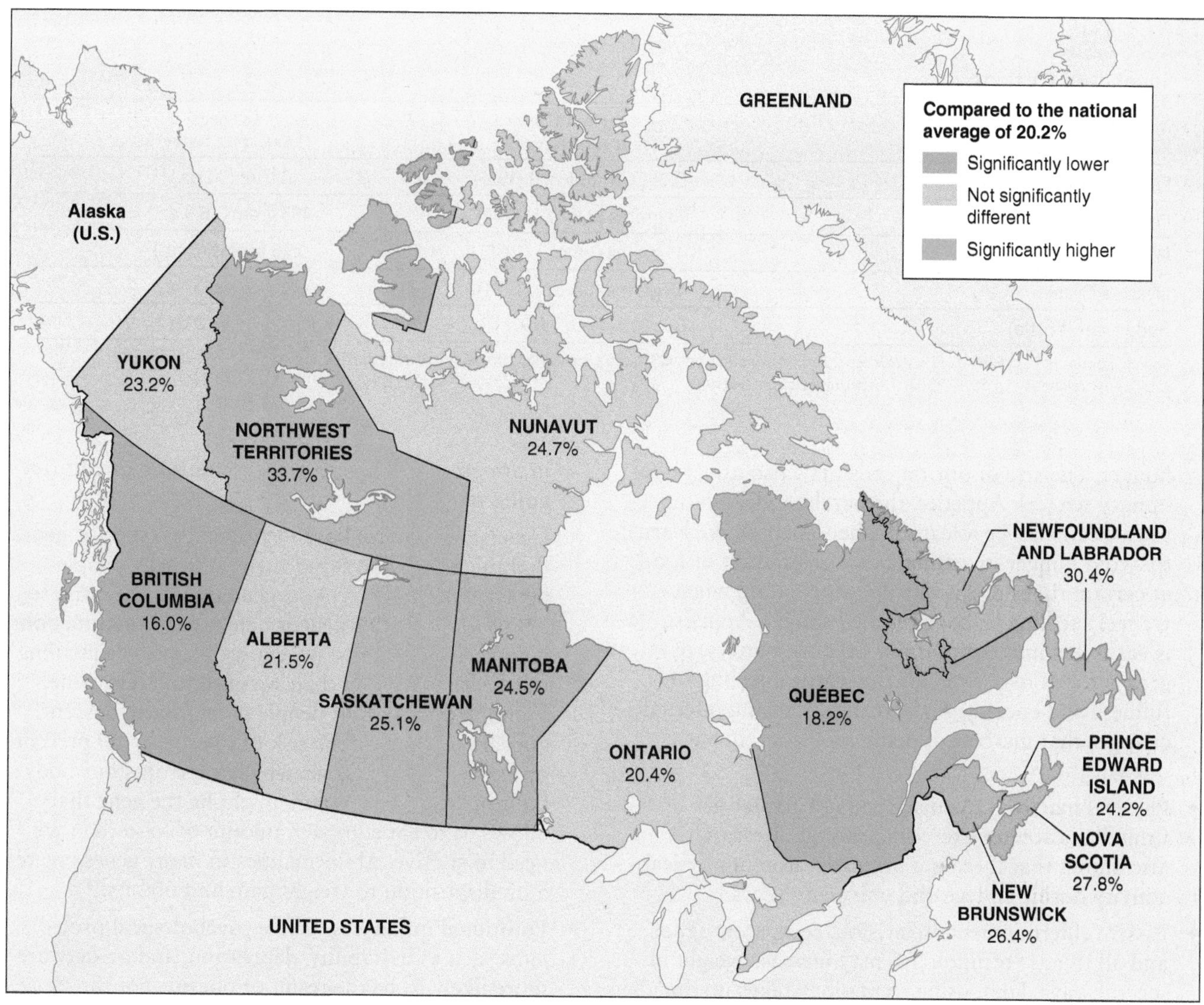

Figure 6-2 **Adults Who Are Obese in 2014 by Province and Territory (Population Aged 18 and Over Who Reported Height and Weight That Classified Them as Obese)**

Source: Statistics Canada. (2015, November 27). *Overweight and obese adults (self-reported), 2014*. Health Fact Sheets. Publications. Catalogue no. 82-625-X. http://www.statcan.gc.ca/pub/82-625-x/2015001/article/14185-eng.htm.

What Causes Obesity? A variety of factors, ranging from behaviour to environment to genetics, have played a role in the increase in individuals becoming overweight and obese. They include the following:

- **More calories.** Bombarded by non-stop commercials for tasty treats, tempted by foods in every form to munch and crunch, many people are consuming more calories per day than they need. Chapter 5 recommended caloric intake ranges between 1900 for sedentary lifestyles and 2350 for active lifestyles for women and between 2500 and 3000 for men. Internationally, Austria reported an average of 3769 calories served per person per day in 2013, while Canada reported 3419. In 1961 Canada reported an average of 2807 calories served per person.[9] Many of these extra calories come from refined carbohydrates.
- **Bigger portions.** The size of many popular restaurant and packaged foods has increased two to five times during the past 20 years. Some foods, like chocolate bars, have grown more than 10 times in size since they were first introduced. A 1.8 litre pop can has approximately 800 calories. Studies also show that with larger portion sizes people eat many more calories than they would otherwise (see Table 6-1).[10]
- **Fast food.** People who eat frequently at fast-food restaurants gain more weight and develop metabolic abnormalities that increase their risk of type 2 diabetes.[11]
- **Hunger and satiety.** In addition to genes, there are other signals that can influence our **hunger**. Hormones, including insulin and stress-related epinephrine (adrenaline), may stimulate or suppress

TABLE 6-1

Supersized Portions

Food/Beverage	Original Size (Year Introduced)	Largest Available Today
Pop (Coca-Cola)	0.19 litres (6.5 oz.) (1916)	1 litre (34 oz.)
French fries (Burger King)	73 grams (2.6 oz.) (1954)	195 grams (6.9 oz.)
Hamburger (McDonald's; beef only)	45 grams (1.6 oz.) (1955)	226 grams (8 oz.)
Nestlé's Crunch	45 grams (1.6 oz.) (1938)	141 grams (5 oz.)
Budweiser (bottle)	0.2 litres (7 oz.) (1976)	1.1 litres (40 oz.)

Source: Reprinted from *Journal of the American Dietetic Association*, Vol. 103, Issue 1, by Marion Nestle, "Increasing portion sizes in American diets: More calories, more obesity," p. 39, © 2003, with permission from Elsevier.

hunger. The size of our fat cells may also affect how hungry we feel. **Appetite**, the psychological desire to eat, can also be a learned phenomenon. We learn to avoid hunger by eating a certain amount of food at certain times of the day. We stop eating when we feel satisfied or have reached **satiety**. Appetite is easily led into temptation. Creamy, buttery, or greasy foods may override our natural feeling of fullness and encourage overeating, causing internal changes that increase appetite and, consequently, our weight.

- **Physical inactivity.** As discussed in Chapter 4, Canadians are not exercising enough. Research also shows that there is a dramatic drop in physical activity during college and university years.[12]
- **Passive entertainment.** Television, computers, iPads, and all things "technology" may increase weight in several ways. First, using technology takes up time that otherwise might be spent in physical activities. Secondly, it increases food intake since people tend to eat more while watching TV or sitting at a computer.
- **Prenatal factors.** A woman's weight before conception and weight gain during pregnancy influences her child's weight. A substantial number of children are prone to gaining weight because their mothers developed gestational diabetes during their pregnancies. Children born to obese women are more than twice as likely to become overweight.
- **Developmental factors.** Some obese people have a high number of fat cells, others have large fat cells, and the most severely obese have both a high number and large fat cells. **Hyperplasia** describes a point in time where the number of fat cells increases. Usually this only occurs during infancy and puberty. However, it does appear that fat cells can also increase in numbers when a person consumes more calories than they burn on a regular basis over a period of time. **Hypertrophy** is a process whereby the fat cells increase in size and this can happen at any time in life if calories taken in are greater than caloric expenditure, or calories going out.
- **Genetics.** Scientists have identified two specific genes that might provide some answers to why people become obese. The GAD2 gene signals the brain to tell us to eat. If this gene is defective or malfunctions, it could contribute to weight problems by signalling us to eat more often than we need to.[13] The gene, found in one-sixth of people of European descent, appears to increase the risk of obesity by 30 percent or more.[14] The Ob gene, which interrupts our body's built-in "feel full" system, might be the gene that allows us to eat a greater amount of food than we need to survive. Abnormalities in many genes create a predisposition to weight gain and obesity.[15]
- **Emotional influences.** While psychological problems such as irritability, depression, and anxiety are more likely to be the result of obesity, not the cause, some people who are emotionally fragile do cope by overeating.
- **Social networks.** Friends might have a significant effect on a person's risk of obesity. Researchers cannot fully explain why this happens, but it may be that friends alter your perception of fatness: when a close friend is obese, obesity might seem normal and acceptable.[16]
- **Social determinants.** In affluent countries, more people in lower socio-economic classes tend to be obese. For reasons unknown, those in the upper classes, who can afford as much food as they want, tend to be leaner. Education may be a factor.

WHAT SHOULD I WEIGH?

For any individual of a given height, there is no single best weight, but a range of healthy weights. Health Canada has developed guidelines that have changed the definition of what it means to be overweight or obese by focusing on body composition. The guidelines shift focus away from body weight—the numbers on the scale—to body mass index (BMI), waist circumference, waist-to-hip ratio, and individual risk factors for diseases and conditions associated with obesity.

Body Mass Index **Body mass index (BMI),**[17] a ratio between weight and height, is a mathematical formula that correlates with body fat. The BMI numbers apply to both men and women (see Figure 6-3). You can calculate your body mass index by dividing your weight (in kilograms) by your height (in metres) squared. The formula is BMI = weight(kg)/height(m^2). An interactive body mass index calculator is available at Dietitians of Canada.[18]

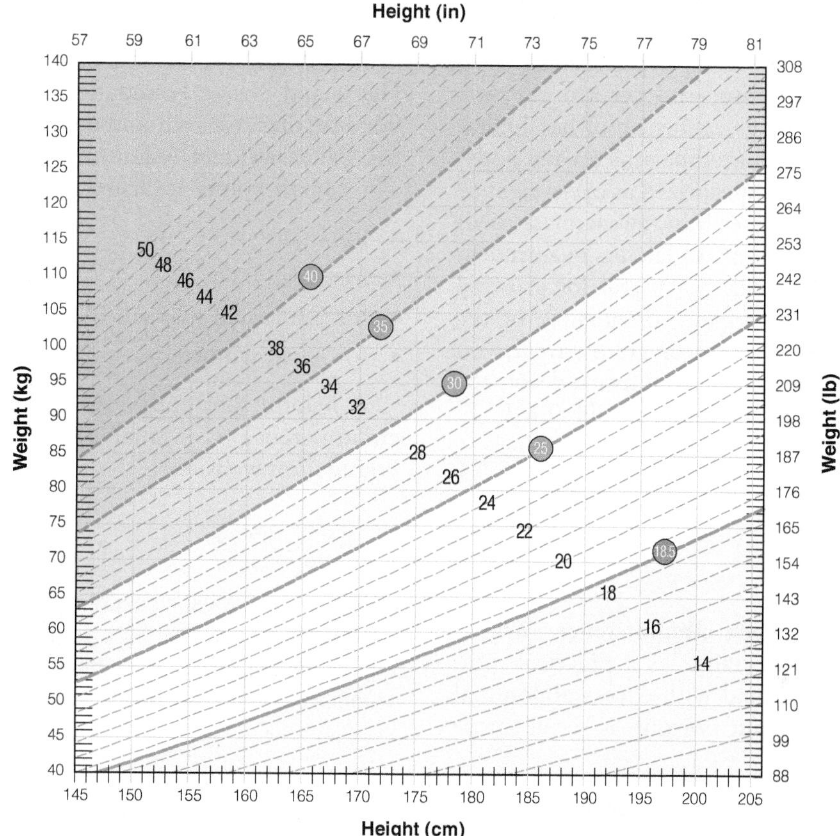

For a quick determination of BMI (kg/m^2), use a straightedge to help locate the point on the chart where height (in or cm) and weight (lb or kg) intersect. **Read the number on the dashed line closest to this point.** For example, an individual who weighs 69 kg and is 173 cm tall has a BMI of approximately 23.

This BMI nomogram is not intended for use with those under 18 years of age; and pregnant and lactating women. You can calculate your BMI using this formula: BMI = weight (kg)/height (m^2).

Refer to the table below to identify the level of health risk associated with a particular BMI.

Health Risk Classification According to Body Mass Index (BMI)

Classification	BMI Category (kg/m^2)	Risk of Developing Health Problems
Underweight	<18.5	Increased
Normal weight	18.5–24.9	Least
Overweight	25.0–29.9	Increased
Obese class I	30.0–34.9	High
Obese class II	35.0–39.9	Very high
Obese class III	≥40.0	Extremely high

Note: For persons 65 years and older the "normal" range may begin slightly above BMI 18.5 and extend into the "overweight" range. To clarify risk for each individual, other factors such as lifestyle habits, fitness level, and presence or absence of other health risk conditions also need to be considered.

Body Mass Index (BMI) Nomogram. Office of Nutrition Policy and Promotion. Health Products and Food Branch, Health Canada. Available at www.hc-sc.gc.ca/fn-an/ nutrition/weights-poids/ guide-ld-adult/bmi_chart_java-graph_imc_java-eng.php. Reproduced with permission of the Minister of Public Works and Government Services, 2008.

Figure 6-3 Body Mass Index Nomogram

Source: © All rights reserved. *Canadian Guidelines for Body Weight Classification in Adult–Quick Reference Tool for Professionals.* Health Canada, 2003. Adapted and reproduced with permission from the Minister of Health, 2016.

Doctors, health professionals, and personal trainers use BMI to identify weight-related health risks in populations and individuals. It is intended for use among Canadian adults age 18 and older. Health risks associated with the underweight category, or a BMI under 18.5, include malnutrition, osteoporosis, and infertility.

The guidelines define **overweight** as a BMI of 25–29.9 and **obesity** as a BMI of 30 and above. Health risks associated with overweight and obesity, or a BMI of 25 or higher, include type 2 diabetes, hypertension, sleep apnea, cardiovascular disease, and certain cancers. However, using BMI as an assessment tool has limitations. Muscular individuals, including athletes and bodybuilders, may be incorrectly categorized as overweight or obese because they have greater lean muscle mass. BMI also does not reliably reflect body fat, an independent predictor of health risk, and is not useful for growing children, women who are pregnant or nursing, or the elderly. If you work with children or are a parent, you might want to use an interactive tool available on the HealthLinkBC[19] website, to determine a child's BMI.

✓ CHECK-IN

Do you know your BMI?

Waist Circumference **Waist circumference** (WC) is used along with body mass index as a practical indicator of risk that is associated with excess abdominal fat. Where you carry your weight is even more important than how much weight you carry. People who have apple-shaped bodies (weight around the waist) are more likely than those with pear-shaped bodies (weight on hips and thighs) to have high cholesterol levels, high blood pressure, and an increased risk of diabetes (see Figure 6-4). Cut-off points for both men and women have been established by Health Canada. A waist circumference above these cut-off points is associated with increased risk of coronary heart disease, type 2 diabetes, and hypertension. The Heart and Stroke Foundation BC Yukon Division has done further research and determined that healthy WC for Caucasian and Asian men and women does differ. The cut-off points are listed below.

- for Caucasian men: WC ≥ 102 cm (40.2 inches)
- for Asian men: WC ≥ 90 cm (35.4 inches)
- for Caucasian women: WC ≥ 88 cm (34.6 inches)
- for Asian women: WC ≥ 80 cm (31.5 inches)

A helpful tool and video clip for calculating waist circumference is available at the Heart & Stroke Foundation website.[20]

✓ CHECK-IN

What is your waist measurement? Place a tape measure around your bare abdomen just above your hip bone. Be sure that the tape is snug but does not compress your skin. Relax, exhale, and measure.

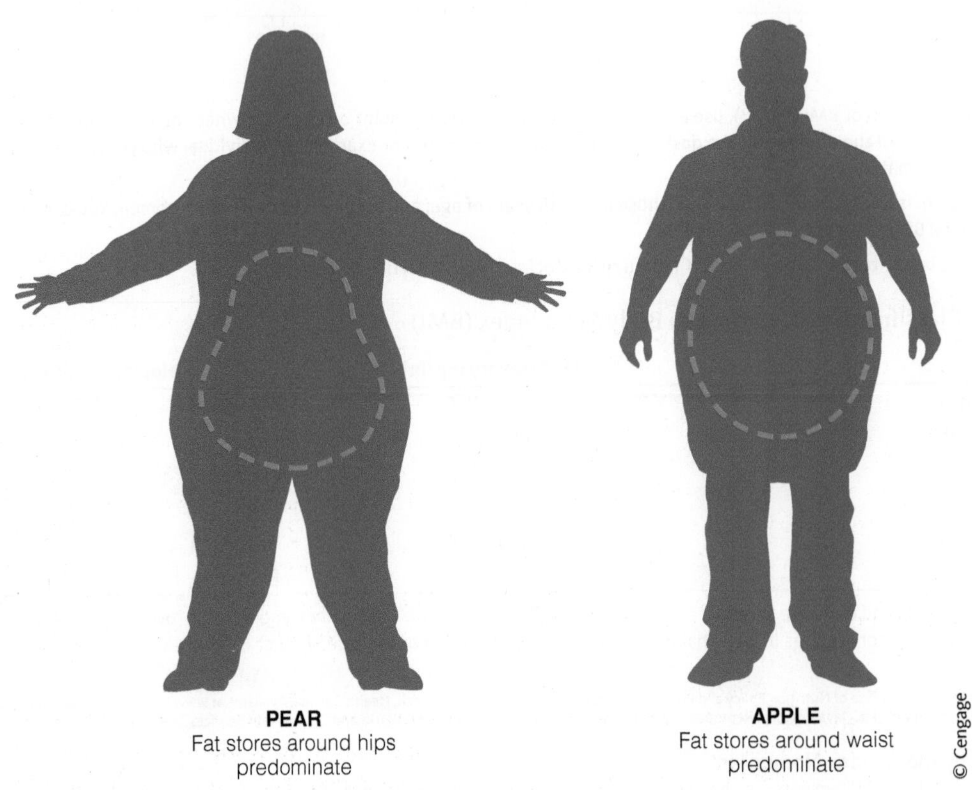

Figure 6-4 Pear-shaped versus Apple-shaped Bodies

Waist-to-Hip Ratio The **waist-to-hip ratio (WHR)** is yet another tool that can be used to measure the health of an individual. It is not used as a health measurement as extensively as it once was, but there is research that suggests WHR can be a good predictor of mortality in older people because it takes into account the differences in body structure.[21] While the waist is technically measured midway between the lowest rib and the iliac crest, practically it is measured at the smallest circumference of the natural waist, usually just above the belly button. The hip circumference is measured at the widest part of the buttocks or hips.

To determine your WHR, divide your waist circumference by your hip circumference.[22] A WHR greater than 1.0 for men or 0.85 for women is considered a signal of high risk for disease; a WHR of 0.90–1.0 for men or 0.80–0.85 for women indicates moderately high risk; and a WHR less than 0.90 for men or less than 0.80 for women indicates lower risk.

Assessing Body Fat There are two types of body fat. One type is essential fat, which makes up about 3–7 percent of body fat in men and 10–15 percent in women and helps with physiological function such as nerve conduction. It is stored in small amounts in our organs and muscles. The second type is storage fat, which for healthy adults is somewhere between 5 and 25 percent. It helps keep us warm by insulating our bodies. Overall ideal body-fat percentages for men range from 7–25 percent and for women from 16–35 percent.

Women have a higher percentage of overall body fat compared to men due to genetic differences that include the size of bones, muscle mass, and fat fluctuation during menstruation, pregnancy, and menopause.

Methods of assessing body composition include the following:

Skinfold Fat Measurement Trained fitness assessors use skinfold measurements to calculate body fat. They grasp folds of skin with their thumb and index finger and then measure the skinfold with a tool called a calliper. Various sites on the body are measured, depending on the skinfold test used. The sum of five skinfolds or the sum of eight skinfolds are two common skinfold tests. The skinfold sites can include triceps (back of the upper arm), biceps (front of the upper arm), subscapular (two centimetres below the tip of the shoulder blade on the back), chest (between the nipple and the arm pit), abdomen (a vertical or horizontal fold is taken 2 centimetres to the right of the umbilicus or bellybutton), suprailiac, or iliac, (two centimetres right above the iliac crest), thigh (halfway from the upper part of the knee to top of leg), and medial calf (middle inside of the lower leg). To get the most consistent measurements all skinfolds are usually taken on the same side and by the same fitness assessor. A minimum of two measurements at each location is recommended. If the measurements differ by more than two millimetres, a third measurement is recommended and the average of the three measurements used when calculating the total sum of the skinfolds. The sum is then compared to body fat percentage norms that have been developed through equations that take into account age, sex, race, and other factors. Limitations include lack of precision in taking skinfold measurements at exact sites.[23]

Bioelectrical Impedance Analysis (BIA) This rapid, noninvasive method of calculating body fat percentage uses a BIA analyzer. Electrodes are attached to various parts of a person's body. A low-level electrical current is then passed through the body and the resistance or impedance (Z) to the flow of current that travels through the water that is found in muscle and fat is measured. The more muscle a person has, the more water their body can hold. The greater the amount of water a person holds in their body, the easier it is for the current to pass through. If a person has more fat tissue, there will be more resistance to the current because adipose tissue is a poor conductor of electrical current. In addition to measurement of resistance, information about the individual's age, sex, height, weight, body type, and physical activity levels is also used in the calculations. This tool is considered a reliable method of measuring body fat percentage. Limitations include following strict pre-test protocols such as not exercising or drinking water prior to the test.[24]

Dual-Energy X-Ray Absorptiometry (Dxa) X-rays are used to quantify the skeletal and soft-tissue components of body mass. The test requires 10–20 minutes, and radiation dosage is low (800–2000 times lower than a typical chest X-ray). Some researchers believe that DXA will supplant hydrostatic testing as the standard for body composition assessment. Limitations are the expense and availability of equipment, few trained technicians, and concern about radiation.

Hydrostatic (Underwater) Weighing This method, also known as hydrodensitometry, measures the weight of displaced fluid. Muscle has a higher density than water, and fat has a lower density. Thus fat people tend to displace less water than lean people. The limitations include expensive and complex testing methods and the inability for some people to be lowered under the water and exhale fully.

Air Displacement Plethysmography In this method of determining an estimate of body fat, total body volume is measured from air displacement. To determine this measurement the following equation is used: formula density = mass ÷ volume.[25]

How Many Calories Do I Need? In Chapter 5, we defined calories and **basal metabolic rate (BMR)**, the amount of energy our bodies use when at complete rest, and discussed briefly how many calories men and women need on a daily basis.

Table 6-2 provides details on the **estimated energy requirement (EER)**, which is defined as the dietary energy intake that is predicted to maintain energy balance in a healthy adult of a defined age, sex, weight, height, and level of physical activity consistent with good health.

It is also important to understand that most of our daily caloric expenditure—almost 90 percent—occurs because of our **resting metabolic rate (RMR)**.

TABLE 6-2

Estimated Energy Requirements (EER) for Different Ages and Activity Levels

	Males			Females*		
Age—Years	**Sedentary[1]**	**Low Active[2]**	**Active[3]**	**Sedentary[1]**	**Low Active[2]**	**Active[3]**
2–3	1100	1350	1500	1100	1250	1400
4–5	1250	1450	1650	1200	1350	1500
6–7	1400	1600	1800	1300	1500	1700
8–9	1500	1750	2000	1400	1600	1850
10–11	1700	2000	2300	1500	1800	2050
12–13	1900	2250	2600	1700	2000	2250
14–16	2300	2700	3100	1750	2100	2350
17–18	2450	2900	3300	1750	2100	2400
19–30	2500	2700	3000	1900	2100	2350
31–50	2350	2600	2900	1800	2000	2250
51–70	2150	2350	2650	1650	1850	2100
71 +	2000	2200	2500	1550	1750	2000

Source: *Eating Well with Canada's Food Guide*. Health Canada, 2011. Adapted and reproduced with permission from the Minister of Health, 2016.

These values are approximations calculated using Canadian median heights and weights that were derived from the median normal BMI for different levels of physical activity.

Your individual values may be different. The requirement for energy varies between individuals due to factors such as genetics, body size, and body composition.

*These values are not for women who are pregnant or breastfeeding.

[1] Sedentary: Typical daily living activities (e.g., household tasks, walking to the bus)

[2] Low Active: Typical daily living activities PLUS 30–60 minutes of daily moderate activity (e.g., walking at 5–7 km/h)

[3] Active: Typical daily living activities PLUS at least 60 minutes of daily moderate activity

To calculate your individual estimated energy requirement, use the following formula:

Adults 19 years and older

Estimated Energy Requirement (kcal/day) = Total Energy Expenditure

Men

EER = 662 − (9.53 × age [y]) + PA*× { (15.91 × weight [kg]) + (539.6 × height [m]) }

Women

EER = 354 − (6.91 × age [y]) + PA*× { (9.36 × weight [kg]) + (726 × height [m]) }

* Physical Activity Coefficents (PA values) for use in the EER equations are as follows:

Physical Activity Coefficients (PA Values)	**Sedentary**	**Low Active**	**Active**
Men			
19 years+	1.00	1.11	1.25
Women			
19 years+	1.00	1.12	1.27

Source: *Estimated Energy Requirements*. Health Canada, 2011. Reproduced with permission from the Minister of Health, 2013.

RMR can be defined as the largest component of our daily energy budget.[26] It includes our BMR and any extra energy we expend through the day in sedentary activities such as sitting, standing, and even food digestion. The remaining 10 percent of energy expenditure is defined as **exercise metabolic rate (EMR)**, which comes from all types of daily physical activities such as walking, climbing stairs, and running for the bus.[27] To increase your EMR, follow the principles of exercise described in Chapter 4—FITT.

How many calories you will utilize when you are physically active depends on how much you weigh, how intense the exercise activity or session is, and how much time you take part in the activity. The more you weigh, the more calories you burn during activity. Intense levels of exercise require more energy, thus more calorie usage. The longer you are active the more calories you will burn. Based on 63 kilograms (140 pounds) for females and 79 kilograms (175 pounds) for males, the following activities and caloric expenditures might inspire you to use physical activity as part of a weight management plan.

- **Light activity**—cleaning house, playing golf, or playing baseball

  Female = 240 calories/hour

  Male = 300 calories/hour
- **Moderate activity**—walking briskly or cyling (5.5 km/hour), gardening

  Female = 370 calories/hour

  Male = 460 calories/hour
- **Strenuous activity**—running (1.6 km/7 min), racquetball, skiing

  Female = 740 calories/hour

  Male = 920 calories/hour

Other activities you might consider are raking leaves for 30 minutes, shovelling snow for 15 minutes, pushing a stroller 2.4 kilometres in 30 minutes, and washing and waxing a car for 45–60 minutes.[28] As discussed briefly in Chapter 4, high intensity interval training (HITT) is showing notable results with regard to weight loss too. A study on active recreational women who participated in a six-week high-intensity sprint interval training (SIT) program found a significant decrease in body fat mass and waist circumference. The authors of this study suggest that sprint interval training could be considered a time-efficient option for decreasing body fat while improving cardio-respiratory fitness.[29] Shiraev and Barclay[30] report that HITT has proven to significantly reduce abdominal fat and total body mass. Compared to continuous moderate aerobic exercise (CME), HITT also burned more calories and increased post-exercise energy expenditure.

HEALTH DANGERS OF EXCESS WEIGHT

If you have put on weight, you might be most concerned about looking fat or not fitting into your clothes. But the younger individuals are when they gain weight, the more health risks they may face over their lifetimes, including

- A higher chance of becoming overweight or obese throughout life.
- Greater likelihood of high total cholesterol levels and other cardiovascular diseases risk factors such as elevated blood pressure.
- Higher prevalence of type 2 diabetes.
- Increased risk of premature death. In a recent study, the first to focus on risk factors and mortality among adolescents and young adults (aged 12–39) in a national representative sample, obesity, smoking, and high blood sugar levels significantly increased the risk of dying before age 55.[31]
- Physiological changes that are the equivalent to 20 years of aging, including increased risk of cardiovascular disease, diabetes, cancer, rheumatoid arthritis, sleep apnea, gout, and liver disease, as well as difficulties in walking, balance, and rising from a chair.

The Impact on the Body Major diseases linked to obesity include

- **Type 2 diabetes:** More than 80 percent of people with type 2 diabetes are overweight. Although the reasons are not known, being overweight may make cells less efficient at using sugar from the blood. This then puts stress on the cells that produce insulin (a hormone that carries sugar from the blood to cells) and makes them gradually fail. Those with BMIs of 35 or more are approximately 20 times more likely to develop diabetes. Excess weight also increases the risk of premature death among people with type 2 diabetes.[32]
  - You can lower your risk for developing type 2 diabetes by losing weight and increasing the amount of physical activity you do.
  - If you have type 2 diabetes, losing weight and becoming more active can help you control your blood sugar levels and might allow you to reduce the amount of diabetes medication you take.
- **Heart disease and stroke:** People who are overweight are more likely to suffer from high blood pressure, high levels of triglycerides (blood fats) and harmful low-density lipoprotein (LDL) cholesterol, and low levels of beneficial high-density lipoprotein (HDL) cholesterol. Even relatively small amounts of excess fat—as little as 2.2 kilograms (5 pounds)—can add to the dangers to those already at risk for hypertension. People with more body fat have higher blood levels of substances that cause inflammation, which may raise heart disease risk. Obese men face a much

greater risk of dying from a heart attack, regardless of whether they have other risk factors.
  - Losing 5–15 percent of your weight can lower your chances for developing heat disease or having a stroke.
- **Cancer:** Obesity contributes to a variety of types of cancer—among them cancers of the endometrium, esophagus, pancreas, gallbladder, kidney, breast, ovaries, and colon. Excess weight also contributes to cancer deaths in both men and women.
  - Losing weight, researchers estimate, could prevent as many as one in every six cancer deaths.
- **Other health problems:** Overweight men and women are also more likely to develop
  - knee injuries that require surgery to repair;
  - spinal disc degeneration, a common cause of low back pain;
  - alterations in various measures of immune function;
  - greater risk of gall stones, kidney stones, and kidney disease;
  - less responsiveness to flu vaccination;
  - cognitive problems and dementia;
  - worsened symptoms of fibromyalgia, a musculoskeletal disorder; and
  - poor sleep, which could add to the risk of medical problems.
- **Premature death:** Obese adults die an average of almost four years earlier than those with normal weight, and middle-aged obese adults face the highest risk of early death. According to recent research, obesity is associated with at least 20 percent increased risk of death from all causes. Overall, obese adults died 3.7 years earlier from all causes and 1.7 years earlier from heart disease, compared with normal-weight adults.[33]

The Emotional Toll In our calorie-conscious and thinness-obsessed society, obesity also affects quality of life, including sense of vitality and physical pain. Many see excess weight as a psychological burden, a sign of failure, laziness, or inadequate willpower. Overweight men and women often blame themselves for becoming heavy and feel guilty and depressed as a result. In fact, the psychological problems once considered to be the cause of obesity may be its consequence.

PRACTICAL GUIDE TO WEIGHT MANAGEMENT

No diet—high protein, low fat, or high carbohydrate—can produce permanent weight loss or weight gain. Successful weight management requires a lifelong commitment to healthy lifestyle behaviours emphasizing sustainable and enjoyable eating practices and daily physical activity.[34] Studies have shown that individuals who maintained a healthy weight were highly motivated, were educated about nutrition, monitored their food, were physically active, set realistic goals, and received social support from others. Another key to long-term success is tailoring any weight-management program to an individual's sex, lifestyle, and cultural, racial, and ethnic values.

Overcoming a Serious Weight Problem Each year an estimated 70 percent of women and 35 percent of men are dieting at any given time, but no matter how much weight they lose, 95 percent gain it back within five years. Most dieters cut back on food not because they want to feel better, but because they want to look better. Those who drastically reduce their food intake and make weight loss a major part of their lives may be jeopardizing their physical and psychological well-being.

The best approach to a weight problem depends on how overweight a person is. For extreme obesity—a BMI higher than 40 (or higher than 35 for those with other conditions)—medical treatments such as gastric bypass surgery or laparoscopic gastric banding surgery[35] to reduce the volume of the stomach and to tighten the passageway from the stomach to the intestine are sometimes performed. Others opt for a gastric bubble, a soft, polyurethane sac placed in the stomach to make the person feel full while following a low-calorie diet. It is important to note that these medical procedures have inherent risks. There are many reports of injury to the stomach, intestines, and other organs during surgery. Leaking through the staples in the stomach after surgery sometimes requires a second operation. There can also be an increased risk for blood clots in your legs that can travel to your heart or lungs and cause a heart attack, stroke, lung problems, gastritis, or even death.

For people who are moderately or mildly obese—individuals with a BMI of 30–39—doctors recommend a six-month trial of lifestyle therapy, including a supervised diet and exercise. The initial goal should be a 10 percent reduction in weight, an amount that reduces obesity-related risks. With success and if warranted, individuals can attempt to lose more weight.[36] The keys to overcoming obesity are addressing individual differences, altering unrealistic expectations, setting limits, and learning coping skills to provide self-nurturing without relying on food.

Rather than going on a low-calorie diet, people who are overweight—with BMIs of 25–29—should cut back moderately on their food intake and concentrate on developing healthy eating and exercise habits. Support for healthy eating can be found in many communities across Canada. The Dietitians of Canada[37] offer information about finding nutrition professionals.

✓ CHECK-IN

What steps do you take to maintain a healthy weight?

Customizing a Weight-Loss Plan Whether you want to lose some weight or need to lose a lot of weight, there are many things you can do to reach your goals. "If there's one thing we've learned in decades of research into weight management, it's that the one-diet-fits-all approach doesn't work," says clinical psychologist David Schlundt.[38] The key is recognizing the ways you tend to put on weight and developing strategies to overcome them. Here are some examples.

- Do you simply like food and consume lots of it? If so, keep a diary of everything you put in your mouth and tally up your daily total in calories and fat grams. Look for the source of most of the calories—probably high-fat foods such as whole milk, cookies, fried foods, potato chips, steaks—and cut down on how much and how often you eat them. Also watch portion sizes.
- Do you eat when you're bored, sad, frustrated, or worried? "People get in the habit of using food to soothe bad feelings or cope with boredom," says Schlundt. "Sometimes the real issue is a self-esteem or body-image problem." Dealing with these concerns is generally more helpful in the long run than dieting.
- Do you graze, nibbling on snacks rather than eating regular meals? If so, limit yourself to low-calorie, low-fat foods, such as carrots, celery, or grapes. Drink water regularly. Try to eat in the same place, preferably while seated. This helps you break the habit of putting food in your mouth without thinking.
- Move more often. As you have heard before, physical activity can help you burn calories and get fit at the same time. Choose aerobic activities. Start slowly, then build up your walking, jogging, running, or swimming program. Get to the gym. Find a workout partner.

There are many diet and exercise tracking tools available. As mentioned in Chapter 5, the Dietitians of Canada have a free online nutrition tracking tool called eaTracker.[39] You can track your day's food and activity choices. eaTracker assesses your food choices and provides personalized feedback on your total intake of energy (calories) and essential nutrients and compares this to what is recommended for your age, sex, and activity level. It also determines your BMI and provides information to help you achieve and maintain a healthy weight. As with all food tracking tools, not all foods that are available to us in Canada are listed, but the majority of foods that we consume are. And, as mentioned in Chapter 5, there are also many nutrition apps available that can help you track your daily food intake.

How Do I Avoid Diet Traps? There are many diet plans and diet products that promise quick, easy results. These almost invariably turn into dietary dead ends. If the diet seems too good to be true, it probably is. Five common traps to avoid are diet foods, the yo-yo diet, the very low-calorie diet, fad diets, and diet pills.

Diet Foods When choosing "diet foods," don't be fooled. Many companies advertise their food products as "lite" or "low calorie." What some people don't realize is that many foods that are low in fat are still high in sugar and calories. Refined carbohydrates, rapidly absorbed into the bloodstream, raise blood glucose levels. As they fall, appetite increases.

Nutritionists caution us about the use of artificial sweeteners and fake fats that appear in many products in moderation. One such product is Olestra, originally created in 1968 by Proctor and Gamble researchers as sucrose polyester, a synthetic product to help increase premature babies' intake of fat. When it was discovered that it didn't work very well, Olestra was then offered as a fat substitute. It tastes like fat, but the molecules are so large they cannot be digested, so they pass through the digestive tract without leaving any calories behind.[40] This product seemed ideal for diet foods and has been used in snack foods such as chips, crackers, and tortilla chips in the United States. However, Health Canada has rejected Olestra as a food additive based on its own research and the fact that the U.S. Food and Drug Administration (FDA) received more than 18 000 adverse-reactions reports of gastrointestinal distress.[41] Products that contain Olestra must still carry a warning label.

Foods made with fat substitutes might have fewer grams of fat, but they don't necessarily have significantly fewer calories. Many people who eat more of the low- or no-fat foods actually end up with higher daily-calorie intake, while forgoing nutritious foods such as fresh fruits and vegetables.

The Yo-Yo Syndrome On-and-off-again dieting, especially by means of very low-calorie diets (under 800 calories a day), can be self-defeating and dangerous. Some studies have shown that weight cycling may make it more difficult to lose weight or keep it off (see Figure 6-5). Repeated cycles of rapid weight loss followed by weight gain may even change food preferences. Chronic crash dieters often come to prefer foods that combine sugar and fat.

You can avoid the yo-yo syndrome and overcome its negative effects by exercising. Some researchers have found that when overweight women who also exercised went off a very low-calorie diet, their metabolism did not stay at a low level but bounced back to the

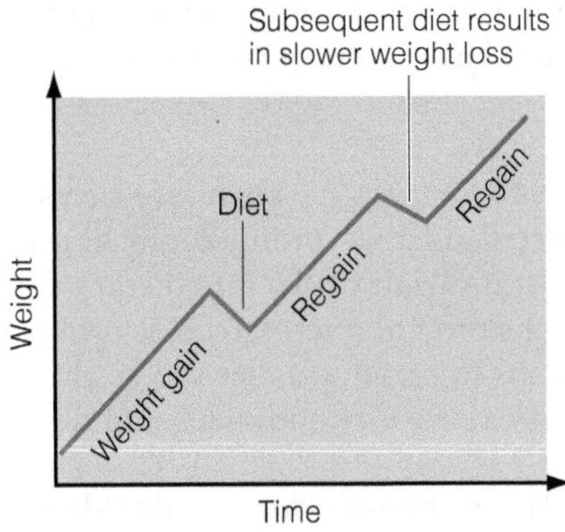

Figure 6-5 Weight-Cycling Effect of Repeated Dieting

Each round of dieting is typically followed by a rebound leading to a greater weight gain.

Source: *An Invitation to Health*, 8E. © 2014 Brooks/Cole, a part of Cengage Learning, Inc. Reproduced by permission. www.cengage.com/permissions.

appropriate level for their new, lower body weight. The reason may be exercise's ability to preserve muscle tissue. The more muscle tissue you have, the higher your metabolic rate.

If you have been losing and regaining the same two to five kilograms for years, try the following suggestions for long-term success:

- Set a danger zone. Once you've reached your desired weight, don't let your weight climb more than two kilograms higher. Take into account normal daily weight fluctuations, but watch out for an upward trend. Once you hit your upper weight limit, take action immediately instead of waiting until you gain five kilograms.
- Be patient. Give yourself time to lose weight safely and steadily.
- Try, try again. You can always start over. First-time weight management plans don't always work. The people who eventually succeed in maintaining a healthy weight find a plan that works for them over time.

Very Low-Calorie Diets Any diet that promises to take pounds off fast can be dangerous. For reasons that scientists don't fully understand, rapid weight loss is linked with increased mortality. Most risky are very low-calorie diets that provide fewer than 800 calories a day. Whenever people cut back drastically on calories, they immediately lose several pounds because of a loss of fluid. As soon as they return to a more normal way of eating, they regain this weight.

On a very low-calorie diet, as much as 50 percent of the weight you lose may be muscle (so you'll actually look flabbier). Because your heart is a muscle, it may become so weak that it no longer can pump blood through your body. Your blood pressure may plummet, causing dizziness, light-headedness, and fatigue. You may develop nausea and abdominal pain. You may lose hair. If you're a woman, your menstrual cycle may become irregular, or you may stop menstruating altogether. As you lose more water, you also lose essential vitamins, and your metabolism slows down. Even reaction time slows, and crash dieters may not be able to respond as quickly as usual. These metabolic changes may make it harder for people to maintain a reduced body weight after dieting.

Fad Diets It seems as if every week there is a new fad diet on the market promising quick and easy weight loss with no effort and usually no physical activity as part of the plan. High-protein, low-carbohydrate diets, such as the Atkins diet, emerged as a diet fad of the 21st century. This diet appealed to many people because they could eat as much protein as they wanted, including steaks, eggs, and fatty foods they had long been told to shun, as long as they strictly limited their carbohydrates. Protein is more satiating than carbohydrates and fat so these dieters complain less of hunger.

The Dietitians of Canada, the American College of Sports Medicine, the American Dietetic Association, and other professional groups have challenged diets that are high in protein and fat and low in carbohydrates. As they note, no scientific evidence proves that a diet providing more than the 10–15 percent protein recommended by federal guidelines enhances health or athletic performance. Scientific advisory warnings that high-protein diets are potentially dangerous because they may increase the risk of heart diseases, diabetes, stroke, kidney and liver disease, and cancer have been made too. However, some research has shown no increased risk of diabetes from following the low-carbohydrate diets.[42] Other studies are showing that high-protein diets are effective in reducing body fat, maintaining lean body mass, and improving blood pressure and other health biomarkers.[43] Ongoing studies are assessing their long-term impact on weight and well-being. And, while it is possible to lose weight on a high-protein, high-fat, low-carbohydrate diet, the reason may just be the same as for all other diets—a low calorie count.

Low-carbohydrate, low-fat diets are also popular. They are based on the premise that the correct proportions of various nutrients, particularly carbohydrates, fats, and proteins, lead to hormonal balance, weight loss, and greater vitality. They also promise additional health benefits including lower blood pressure and cholesterol. While dieters may eat just as much or even more food than usual, they ingest fewer calories and much less fat. This can be so unsatisfying that many people cannot stay on these diets for a sustained period. While nutrition experts do not recommend diets that are too low in any macronutrient, over the past decade we have been encouraged to lower the amount of fat in our diets. Dr. Ronald Krauss is encouraging another look at this recommendation. His research is showing that it may not be the saturated fat in our diets that creates an increased risk for cardiovascular disease, which is often linked to being overweight or obese; it may be the high level of carbohydrates in our diets.[44]

Current research is also suggesting that it may be more complicated than lowering both fat and carbohydrates in our body when we are hoping for fat loss. Kevin Hall and his team of researchers[45] determined that dietary fat restriction resulted in much more body fat loss than carbohydrate restriction in obese participants. However this research does not suggest a return to low-fat diets only. The message is that moderation seems to be the key to healthy eating and that more research is necessary to determine the optimal balance of carbohydrates, fats, and proteins.

The acai berry diet, cabbage soup diet, zone diet, South Beach diet, grapefruit diet, Beverley Hills diet, and apple cider diet are just a few of the fad diets that have come and gone and, in some cases, come again. The latest crazes include the green tea extract diet, the engine 2 diet, the military diet, the whole 30 diet, the paleo diet, and the bulletproof diet.

Remember, if you are promised a quick fix, the claims sound too good to be true, recommendations for the diet come from paid celebrity endorsements, you are encouraged to limit specific foods such as fruits and vegetables, or the diet comes complete with a product line, the fad diet may be just that—a fad.

Over-the-Counter Diet Pills In their search for a quick fix to weight problems, millions of people have tried often-risky remedies. An estimated 15 percent of adults—21 percent of women and 10 percent of men—have used weight-loss supplements. Women between ages 18 and 34 are the highest users.[46] In the 1920s, some women swallowed patented weight-loss capsules that turned out to be tapeworm eggs. In the 1960s and 1970s, addictive amphetamines were common diet aids. In the 1990s, fen-phen (fen referring to fenfluramine [Pon-dimin] or dexfenfluramine [Redux]—appetite depressants, and phen referring to phentermine—a type of amphetamine) became popular. They were taken off the market after being linked to heart-valve problems.

More weight-loss drugs, including Meridia® (sibutramine) and Xenical® (orlistat), both intended only for people with a BMI of at least 30 or a BMI of 27 with additional risk factors and available only by prescription, are now being marketed over the Internet to anyone who fills out a computerized form reviewed by a company doctor. As a result, many people are taking this medication without medical supervision. Such misuse could cause health risks. The search for the perfect diet drug continues—with plenty of economic incentives for drug makers.

Physical Activity—A Helpful Approach A combination of exercise and cutting back on calories may be the most effective way of taking weight off and keeping it off. According to a number of research studies, most successful weight losers restrict how much they eat and increase their physical activity.

Exercise has other benefits: it increases energy expenditure, builds up muscle tissue, burns off fat stores, and stimulates the immune system. Exercise also may reprogram metabolism so that more calories are burned during and after a workout, as mentioned in Chapter 4. Everyday activities, such as walking, gardening, and heavy household chores, are effective as a way of maintaining or losing weight. Once you start an exercise program, keep it up. People who have started an exercise program during or after a weight-loss program are consistently more successful in keeping off most of the pounds they have shed.

Unplanned daily activities, such as fidgeting and pacing, can also make a difference in preventing weight gain. Scientists use the acronym **NEAT**—for **non-exercise activity thermogenesis**—to describe such non-volitional movement and have verified that it can be an effective way of burning calories. In a study of ten lean and ten mildly obese people—all self-confessed couch potatoes—the thinner ones sat an average of two hours less per day and moved and stood more often than the heavier individuals.[47]

HOW TO GAIN WEIGHT

Being underweight is not an uncommon problem either, particularly among adolescent and young adult men as well as among those who diet excessively or suffer from an eating disorder (discussed later in this chapter). If you lose weight suddenly and don't know the reason, talk to a doctor. Rapid weight loss can be an early symptom of a health problem.

If you are trying to gain weight, you need to do the opposite of those attempting to lose weight. Consume more calories than you burn. But, as with losing weight, you should try to gain weight in healthy ways. Here are some suggestions:

- **Eat more of a variety of foods** rather than more high-fat, high-calorie foods. Get no more than 30 percent of your daily calories from fat. A higher percentage poses a threat to your heart and your health.
- **If your appetite is small, eat more frequently.** Try for five or six smaller meals rather than a big lunch and dinner. Always eat breakfast.
- **Drink juice or milk** rather than regular or diet soda.
- **Manage your stress levels.** People who are highly stressed often have higher levels of NEAT—-non-exercise activity thermogenesis—as described earlier in this chapter. This type of activity does burn calories. Meditate, breathe deeply, take time out to relax.
- **Exercise regularly** to build up both your appetite and your muscle mass. But monitor your physical activity levels to make sure you are eating enough calories to compensate for your caloric expenditure.

PSYCHOSOCIAL VIEWS ON WEIGHT MANAGEMENT

We are designed to move, but modern living and technology has changed the way we "do business" each and every day. Foraging for food often means heading to the closest fast-food outlet, daily work habits include many hours of sitting, and food quality has changed immensely. Katzmarzyk, a research specialist in the area of obesity, suggests that we might just have to rethink the current model of physical activity and health. He reasons that what might be in order is a paradigm shift where "we must begin to explore novel approaches to reduce the widespread exposure to sedentary behaviours, as the potential health benefits to be gained could be substantial."[48]

There is no doubt that genetic factors and personal motivation play a role in weight gain, obesity, and physical inactivity. However, new research is showing that social determinants (introduced in Chapter 1), such as the social and physical environments we live in, the food that is sold at our local grocery stores, and socio-economic factors, are critical contributors to the rise of overweight and obesity levels.

Weight Discrimination To address obesity issues in our society, we must be cognizant of the need for sensitive and caring approaches. There are many different methods being used to educate citizens about the benefits of making healthy food choices and participating in regular physical activity to deal with weight issues. In 2012 in New York City, an Obesity Task Force was formed to address obesity issues. Members of this task force worked to address the social determinants that create disparities within the city. Health education programs and initiatives were offered and implemented that encouraged citizens to become more physically active and make healthy food choices. City planners also changed their practices to incorporate healthy physical spaces into design proposals.[49] The plan included education, alternative options, and healthy community policy, but was not biased against individuals who were overweight.

There are other examples where government agencies that attempt to improve the health status of their city, municipality, or county end up proposing programs that discriminate against overweight and obese people. In one U.S. state, a program proposal was discussed in which obese individuals would have to enrol in a Medicaid program and would be required to develop a weight-loss plan under a doctor's supervision. They were to pay a 50-dollar fee if they were unable to meet specific weight-loss goals.[50] This last example is what Rebecca Puhl, the Center Director of Research and Weight Stigma Initiatives at the Rudd Center for Food Policy and Obesity, calls **weight discrimination.**

Puhl's research shows that stigma and discrimination toward people who are obese is pervasive and impacts both psychological and physical health. Society is condoning weight stigmatization as a way of motivating obese persons to lose weight. According to Puhl, discrimination is not beneficial in reducing obesity rates; instead, it generates health disparities and interferes with effective obesity intervention.[51]

In another study, Heuer, McClure, and Puhl[52] analyzed over 400 images of overweight and obese individuals associated with news reports about obesity from five major news websites. Their findings are disconcerting:

- 72 percent of the images depicted overweight or obese persons in a negative and stigmatizing way.
- Obese individuals were often portrayed without clothing (bare stomachs) and from unflattering side or rear views compared to thin individuals who were depicted in flattering manners.
- Obese individuals were more likely to be portrayed in clothing that would not be considered professional, and they were not portrayed as experts compared to thinner individuals. Heurer concludes that the news media can help to reduce pervasive society weight stigma by shifting the visual content of their news reports.

Economics and Obesity We have all heard that healthcare dollars are diminishing and health costs are rising. The increased costs can be directly attributed, in a number of ways, to the health issues linked to the high prevalence of overweight or obese Canadians. However, a new area of study has emerged—that of economics and obesity where economic frameworks are now helping to explain some of the psychosocial aspects of obesity. Mavromaras,[53] from the Melbourne Institute of Applied Economic and Social Research, says that in some cases, people now have more discretionary funds; therefore they have the option of purchasing and consuming things they value. He defines this as *income effect.* Since one of the things we value is food, purchase of food has increased, which has resulted in higher caloric intakes. Whereas a bagged lunch from home might have consisted of one sandwich, an apple, a juice, and a small dessert item, we now have hundreds of choices that we deem affordable at all times of the day.

Secondly, technology has improved both food production and preparation, reducing the cost of many food items. Options for food purchase have also increased, from corner coffee stores to bakeries to fast-food restaurants. We are consuming foods and drinks that were previously never readily available. Many of them are high in fat calories and low in food quality. He defines this as the *substitution effect.* Based on this economic model, an emerging economic recovery, and further technological advances, the prediction is an inevitable rise in obesity levels. Further economic modelling research is needed to help us understand lifestyle interventions that lower obesity levels and improve overall well-being.

Provincial and National Initiatives Changes are being made. Our provincial and national governments are attempting to address nutrition, overweight, and obesity issues by developing nutrition initiatives and programs. They include basic nutrition education and legislative changes such as setting policies that have seen vending machines taken out of schools or changes in the type of beverages for sale in school and community settings, and an encouragement to industry and businesses to do their part in workplace health programs that support healthy eating. Health Canada has also come on board with an extensive nutrition Web-based presence (see Table 6-3).

TABLE 6-3

Provincial, National, and Territorial Nutrition Strategies and Programs

Program	Website
BC Healthy Living Alliance (BCHLA) *Healthy Eating*	http://www.bchealthyliving.ca/healthy-living/healthy-eating
Government of Alberta, Health and Wellness *Nutrition Eat Healthy*	http://www.health.alberta.ca/health-info/nutrition.html
Government of Saskatchewan *Healthy Living—Nutrition and Exercise*	https://www.saskatchewan.ca/residents/health/wellness-and-prevention/nutrition-and-exercise
Government of Manitoba *Healthy Living and Healthy Populations—Healthy Eating*	http://www.gov.mb.ca/cgi-bin/print_hit_bold.pl/healthyliving/hlp/nutrition/index.html
Government of Ontario, Ministry of Health Promotion and Sport *Eat Right Ontario*	https://www.eatrightontario.ca/en/aboutero.aspx
Foundation Lucie et André Chagnon *Foundation Prevention*	http://www.fondationchagnon.org/en/what-we-do/partnerships/quebec-en-forme-healthy-lifestyle.aspx
Healthy Eating Physical Activity Coalition of New Brunswick (HEPAC) *Resources—Healthy Eating and Physical Activity*	http://hepac.ca/
Prince Edward Island, Healthy Eating Alliance *Resources*	http://www.healthyeatingpei.ca/
Nova Scotia Canada *Healthy Eating Nova Scotia*	http://novascotia.ca/dhw/healthy-communities/healthy-eating.asp
Newfoundland Labrador Department of Health and Community Services *Healthy Eating*	http://www.swsd.gov.nl.ca/healthyliving/healthyeating.html
Government of Yukon, Yukon Health and Social Services *Nutrition*	http://www.hss.gov.yk.ca/nutrition.php
Northwest Territories, Health and Social Services *Healthy Eating/Active Living*	http://www.hss.gov.nt.ca/health/healthy-eating
Government of Nunavut, Health and Social Services *Nunavut Nutrition*	http://www.livehealthy.gov.nu.ca/en/food-0
Health Canada *Food and Nutrition*	http://www.hc-sc.gc.ca/fn-an/index-eng.php

One thing is for sure. This needs to be a shared responsibility. Embracing the concept of self-responsibility for self-care is one step. Another is government-level interventions. Diller and Graff,[54] in a study about retail food regulation, show how important local, provincial, and national governments are in the fight against obesity. Enacting innovative policies and strategies to improve access to quality food and decreasing the availability of unhealthy food is an important next step. Some strategies include

- improving serving size and nutritional labelling;
- banning certain foods and ingredients;
- regulating sodium consumption;
- limiting access to junk food in schools and community centres;
- designing "walkable" communities, towns, and cities; and
- building partnerships between nutrition, physical activity, health, economic, medical school, and community leaders.

CAMPUS EATING

College and university students often find that their eating habits change immensely when they begin their studies. The most common weight-related problem on campuses might be gaining weight, particularly in the first year. Weight gain can occur for many reasons. Moving away from home, settling into residence or off-campus living, academic responsibilities, and a lack of space to cook are some examples. Cafeterias serve up hearty and sometimes fat- and calorie-laden meals; fast-food outlets and vending machines in every building provide many food options, sometimes 24 hours a day.

Many students find themselves snacking on high-fat, high-calorie, low-nutrient foods as they attempt to balance academic studies and social lives. Other college and university students find themselves eating at restaurants on a regular basis. A study done to measure the effect of social pressures on eating habits of college students in restaurant environments found that students consumed significantly more second servings of a main course and dessert when they were aware that others at the table opted for second servings.[55] Several studies have documented changes in both weight and body fat. In one study, the average weight gain of female college students was 1.4 kilograms (3.1 pounds) over a twelve-month period.[56] Researchers Vella-Zarb and Egler found that the overall mean weight gain among first-year Canadian university students was 0.89 kilograms (1.96 pounds), with weight gain of 1.65 kilograms (3.64 pounds) among students who were living in residences on campus. This weight was gained within the first eleven weeks of beginning university.[57] The average Canadian adult gains 0.5–1 kilogram every two years, so the weight gain of the university students is worrisome if this level of weight gain were to continue each year throughout university.

In a study of Canadian undergraduate university students where researchers examined the relationships between students who were living at home (having the same living arrangements since high school) and students who were not living at home (defined as having changed living arrangements at least once since high school) and campus eating behaviours, some interesting conclusions were found:[58]

- Eating behaviour was related to lifestyle factors: hours spent on campus, commute time to campus, and weekly budget for food.
- Students who walked to campus packed a lunch significantly fewer times than those who drove to campus or took public transit.
- Students who lived at home packed a lunch 4.1 times per week, compared to students who were not living at home, at 2.8 times per week.
- Students who purchased breakfast on campus were more likely to purchase dinner on campus.
- Students who reported to be highly active most days of the week consumed significantly less fast food than those who reported that they rarely or never participated in physical activity.
- When food is brought to campus, less fast food is purchased and consumed on campus.

Nutrition choices are also affecting students from different cultures. Self-reports from Hawaiian students, recruited via email from colleges in Oregon and Hawaii for a study looking at intention and perceived control in eating a healthy diet, indicate that more Hawaiian students who attended university in Hawaii than Hawaiian students who studied in the state of Oregon had intended to eat a relatively low-fat diet. The researchers[59] concluded that interventions might need to be put in place to increase social support for healthier diets for students relocating from different cultural areas.

Nutrition Initiatives on College and University Campuses To address the unique nutritional needs of college and university students, administrators, faculty, student services, recreation departments, and students themselves are making inroads to improve nutrition alternatives on campuses. At York University there has been a substantial effort made so students can access healthy food options. A Nutrition Team organizes campaigns such as Bring Your Lunch to School Day, has demonstration cooking classes for students living in residences, keeps a Nutrition for YU blog that is updated on a regular basis, and has developed an *Eat Smart Guide* that provides students with information about healthy eating options.[60] At the University of Saskatchewan, the Health and Counselling department maintains a Staying Healthy on Campus Web page with a specific page dedicated to eating well on campus. There students can find healthy nutrition tips and descriptions of where to eat on campus.[61]

At one college campus in the U.S.A., food services personnel helped students monitor the amount of food they were eating by removing plastic dinner trays from the cafeterias. University officials noticed that students were eating less. Instead of filling trays with numerous plates, bowls, and several glasses, students took one plate of food and a drink. Other positive outcomes of the tray-take-away initiatives were a decrease in food waste and conserving water and energy used in cleaning the trays. Aramark, a food-service provider at 500 colleges in the United States, predicts that 50–60 percent of the campuses it serves will eventually go tray-less. It also predicts that food waste will be reduced by 34–51 grams (1.2–1.8 ounces) per person at each meal.[62]

Other campus initiatives include

- education on allergies and alternative diets;[63]
- nutrition education in dining halls on topics such as portion sizes, plate piling, and fat calories;[64]
- menu changes that offer Indian and Thai cuisine and other ethnic entrées from around the globe;[65]
- low-sodium foods, less-processed foods, vegetarian and vegan options, gluten-free options, sushi and organic salad bars;[66] and
- online weight management credit courses. Students wear accelerometers, keep food logs, watch video tutorials in nutrition and exercise science, write nutrition blogs, and participate in student online discussions.[67]

If you are a student who is noticing a small weight gain or have made plans to lose some weight but have not been successful in the past, check out nutrition and exercise options available to you on your campus. There is support for students at many Canadian college and university campuses. The sooner you take charge, the better.

✓ CHECK-IN

What healthy initiatives are promoted and offered at your college or university?

UNHEALTHY EATING BEHAVIOUR

Unhealthy eating behaviour takes many forms, ranging from not eating enough to eating too much too quickly. Its roots are complex. In addition to media and external pressures, family history can play a role, as can stress and culture.[68] At certain times in life or in certain situations, many people don't eat the way they should. They may skip meals, thereby increasing the likelihood that they'll end up with more body fat, a higher weight, and a higher blood cholesterol level. They may live on diet foods but consume so much of them that they gain weight anyway. Some people engage in more extreme eating behaviour. Dissatisfied with almost all aspects of their appearance, they continuously go on and off diets or eat compulsively.[69] Such behaviours can be warning signs of potentially serious eating disorders that should not be ignored.

In this section, you will learn about body image, and eating disorders such as anorexia nervosa, anorexia athletica, bulimia nervosa, binge eating disorder (BED), disordered eating, extreme dieting, and compulsive overeating.

Body Image Throughout most of history, bigger was better. The great beauties of centuries past, as painted by such artistic masters as Rubens and Renoir, were soft and fleshy, with rounded bellies and dimpled thighs. Culture often shapes views of beauty and health. Many developing countries still regard a full figure, rather than a thin one, as the ideal.

Not so in North America where, influenced by the media and the need to belong or conform, many young women are attempting to become slimmer while young men are attempting to become more muscular. In a study of high-school girls, those who regularly read women's health and fitness magazines, which may present unrealistic physical ideals, were more likely to go on low-calorie diets, take pills to suppress their appetites, use laxatives, or force themselves to vomit after eating.[70] In other research, girls who watched a lot of television and expressed concern about slimness and popularity were more dissatisfied with their bodies than girls involved in sports.[71] Boys' body images also are influenced by media images depicting super-strong, highly muscular males.[72,73]

Other studies have shown that college students of different ethnic and racial backgrounds, including Asians, express as much—and sometimes more—concern about their body shape and weight as whites.[74] As shown in X & Y Files (page 152), men and women are prone to different distortions in body image.

Eating Disorders **Eating disorders** involve a serious disturbance in eating behaviour. In addition to either eating too much or too little, individuals who suffer from eating disorders have great concerns over body size and shape. For some people, the concern develops into a compulsion of unhealthy eating behaviours and lifestyles.

Individuals with eating disorders display a broad range of symptoms that occur along a continuum. Those with anorexia nervosa refuse to maintain a minimally normal body weight and have an intense fear of gaining weight and a distorted perception of the shape or size of their body. Those with bulimia nervosa binge eat and then use vomiting, excessive exercise, or laxatives to purge the food eaten. A diagnosis of binge eating disorder (BED) is made when binge eating is not followed by purging. This disorder is often associated with obesity.

Who Develops Eating Disorders? Most people with eating disorders are young (ages 14–25), white, female, and affluent, with perfectionist personalities. However, despite past evidence that eating disorders were primarily problems for white women, they are increasing among men and members of different ethnic and racial groups[75] (for major risk factors, see X & Y Files: "Men, Women, and Weight").

In a survey at a large, public, rural university, eating disorders did not discriminate, equally affecting women of different races, religions, athletic involvement, and living arrangements. Although the students viewed eating disorders as both mental and physical problems and felt that individual therapy would be most helpful, all said that they would first turn to a friend for help.[76]

In a study of Australian male undergraduates, one in four men worried about shape and weight; one in five displayed attitudes and behaviours characteristic of disordered eating and eating disorders. None ever sought treatment, even if the students recognized they had a problem. The reason, the researchers theorized, may be that the young men hesitated to seek treatment for an illness stigmatized as a problem that affects only women.[77]

One study that followed more than 100 undergraduate women through their first year found that those who reported the most body dissatisfaction and unhealthy eating patterns at the beginning of the first semester were most likely to experience more eating problems, such as losing control of their eating when feeling strong emotions. The strongest predictor that eating symptoms would get worse over the first year was not BMI or weight, but body dissatisfaction.[78] Research has also shown that foreign students, who have a high level of exposure to Western cultural norms, are more likely to be susceptible to eating disorders.[79]

Male and female athletes are also vulnerable to eating disorders because of the pressure to maintain ideal body weight or to achieve a weight that might enhance their performance.[80,81] Many athletes, particularly those participating in sports or activities that emphasize leanness (such as gymnastics, distance running, diving, figure skating, and classical ballet), have subclinical eating disorders that could undermine their nutritional status and energy levels. However, there is often little awareness or recognition of their disordered eating. Athletes competing in weight-class sports such as rowing or boxing are also under pressure to lose weight to "make class."[82]

If you have an eating disorder please ask for help. Campus counselling centres, peer helpers, and medical professionals can assist you. If someone you know has an eating disorder, let him or her know you're concerned and that you care. Don't criticize or make fun of eating habits. Encourage discussion about other problems and feelings and suggest that he or she see a counsellor or someone at the mental health centre, the family doctor, or another trusted adult. Offer to go along if you think that will make a difference. See Table 6-4 for the physiological and psychological repercussions of eating disorders.

Anorexia Nervosa Although *anorexia* means "loss of appetite," most individuals with **anorexia nervosa** are, in fact, hungry all the time. For them, food is an enemy—a threat to their sense of self, identity, and autonomy. In the distorted mirror of their mind's eye, they see themselves as fat or flabby even at a normal or below-normal body weight. Some simply feel fat; others think that they are thin in some places and too fat in others, such as the abdomen, buttocks, or thighs.

The incidence of anorexia nervosa has increased in the last three decades in most developed countries. An estimated 0.5–4 percent of women in Canada develop anorexia nervosa.[83] Not everyone who has a low weight

X AND Y FILES

Men, Women, and Weight

Women have long been bombarded by the media with idealized images of female bodies that bear little resemblance to the way most women look. Increasingly, more advertisements and men's magazines are featuring idealized male bodies. Sleek, strong, and sculpted, they too do not resemble the bodies most men inhabit. The gap between reality and ideal is getting bigger for both genders.

Women are more prone to unhealthy eating and eating disorders than men, but the incidence among men is increasing. About 90 percent of people diagnosed with anorexia and bulimia are women; however, binge eating disorder affects women and men more equally.[84] In many cases, BED starts during adolescence or young adulthood.

Men and women with eating disorders share many psychological similarities and experience similar symptoms. However, men are more likely to have other psychiatric disorders and are less likely to seek professional treatment. Some feel that eating disorders fall under the category of "women's diseases." Others may not recognize the symptoms because eating disorders have long been assumed to plague only women.

TABLE 6-4

Physiological and Psychological Repercussions from Eating Disorders

Sufferers may not have all symptoms
Physiological Repercussions
Excessive facial or body hair because of inadequate protein in diet
Abnormal weight loss
Sensitivity to cold
Absent or irregular menstruation
Hair loss
Intestinal ulcers
Dehydration
Ruptured stomach
Serious heart, kidney, and liver damage
Tooth and gum erosion
Tears of the esophagus
Shortness of breath
Chest pain
Stunted bone growth
Toxicity to heart with use of laxatives, diuretics, or emetics
Reduced bone strength
Psychological Repercussions
Depression
Low self-esteem
Shame and guilt
Impaired family and social relationships
Mood swings
Perfectionism
"All or nothing" thinking
Listlessness
Difficulty concentrating

Source: National Association of Anorexia Nervosa and Associated Disorders. www.anad.org.

is anorexic, but there is a risk of anorexia nervosa when anyone is 15 percent below their ideal weight or under 18.5 BMI.

Anorexia nervosa is a complex disorder. Treatment usually requires medical, nutritional, and behavioural therapies. In the restricting type of anorexia, individuals lose weight by avoiding any fatty foods and by dieting and fasting. They may eat only a couple hundred calories per day or just drink water. Many of them start exercising as well as fasting. Others start smoking as a way of controlling their weight; it is difficult when you are starving not to eat. Some anorexics, although eating very little, feel that even a cookie or a normal meal is too much food. When they eat something they feel they should not have, they may purge, similar to bulimics.

Obsessed with an intense fear of fatness, anorexics may weigh themselves several times a day, measure various parts of their body, check mirrors to see if they look fat, and try on different items of clothing to see if they feel tight.[85]

Anorexia Athletica and Muscle Dysmorphia While not clinically defined as an eating disorder, **anorexia athletica** is a condition similar to that of anorexia nervosa in that individuals deal with body image issues by overcompensating, except when dealing with this condition it is by over-exercising. Exercising to the extreme gives people a sense of control and power over their bodies. Signs of anorexia athletica include exercising compulsively and being fanatical about exercise sessions to the detriment of other healthy lifestyle habits such as regular eating, socializing, and sleeping. Individuals who suffer from this condition also believe that their self-worth depends on their physical activity levels and often rationalize their obsessive exercise sessions by insisting that exercise is good for them. People who suffer from this condition often are meticulous about their eating habits and may restrict calories too.[86]

Some men suffer from **muscle dysmorphia** where they engage in excessive strength training sessions because they have an obsessive desire to appear more muscular and lean. They see themselves as small and frail. In addition to exercising compulsively, they may also take steroids or muscle-building drugs. This condition is sometimes described as bigorexia—the opposite of anorexia.

Bulimia Nervosa Individuals with **bulimia nervosa** go on repeated eating binges and rapidly consume large amounts of food. Those with purging bulimia induce vomiting or take large doses of laxatives to relieve guilt and control their weight. In nonpurging bulimia, individuals use other means, such as fasting or excessive exercise, to compensate for binges.

An estimated 1–3 percent of women develop bulimia. Some experiment with bingeing and purging for a few months and then stop when they change their social or living situation. Others develop longer-term bulimia. Among males, this disorder is about one-tenth as common. The average age for developing bulimia is 18.[87]

Binge Eating Disorder Binge eating disorder (BED)—the rapid consumption of an abnormally large amount of food in a relatively short time—often occurs in compulsive eaters. Individuals who binge eat may feel a lack of control over eating and binge at least twice a week for at least a six-month period.[88] During most of these episodes they often eat alone because they are embarrassed by how much they eat and by their eating habits.

As their weight climbs, they become depressed, anxious, or troubled by other psychological symptoms to a much greater extent than others of comparable weight. Treatment includes education, behavioural approaches, cognitive therapy, and psychotherapy.[89]

Extreme Dieting Extreme dieters go beyond cutting back on calories or increasing physical activity. They become preoccupied with what they eat and weigh. Although their weight never falls below 85 percent of normal, their weight loss is severe enough to cause uncomfortable physical consequences, such as weakness and sensitivity to cold, and they are at increased risk for anorexia nervosa.

Extreme dieters may think they know a great deal about nutrition, yet many of their beliefs about food and weight are misconceptions or myths. They may eat only protein because they believe complex carbohydrates, including fruits and breads, are fattening. When they're anxious, angry, or bored, they focus on food and their fear of fatness. Dieting and exercise become ways of coping with any stress in their lives.

Sometimes nutritional education alone can help change this eating pattern. However, many avid dieters who deny that they have a problem with food may need counselling to correct dangerous eating behaviours and prevent further complications.

Compulsive Overeating Compulsive overeaters eat compulsively and cannot stop putting food in their mouths. They eat fast, and they eat a lot. They eat even when they're full. They may eat around the clock rather than at set meal times, often in private because of embarrassment over how much they consume.

Some mental health professionals describe compulsive eating as a food addiction that is much more likely to develop in women. According to Overeaters Anonymous (OA), an international 12-step program, many women who eat compulsively view food as a source of comfort against feelings of inner emptiness, low self-esteem, and fear of abandonment.[90]

The following behaviours may signal a potential problem with compulsive overeating:

- turning to food when depressed or lonely, when feeling rejected, or as a reward
- a history of failed diets and anxiety when dieting
- thinking about food throughout the day
- eating quickly and without pleasure
- continuing to eat even when no longer hungry
- frequent talking about food or refusing to talk about food
- fear of not being able to stop eating once started

Recovery from compulsive eating can be challenging because people with this problem cannot give up entirely the substance they abuse. However, they can learn new eating habits and ways of dealing with underlying emotional problems.

HUMAN POTENTIAL

Théa Pheasey—A Message of Hope

Théa Pheasey, a graduate of a recreation and health education program at the University of Victoria, is now living in Houston, Texas, with her husband and children. She has explored many career opportunities in her travels around the world, from real estate in Calgary, Alberta, and Dubai, United Arab Emirates; to media sales in Dubai; and, most recently, to starting her own business as a makeup artist in Houston. Currently she spends her days running after her four- and two-year-old daughters, which has proved to be her most challenging and rewarding job yet. Théa always has had a sense of hope about what the future holds for her; however, it took a lot of emotional work and time to get to this frame of mind. The story she would like to share is one that began just over 14 years ago, in high school.

Théa was very active in sports and dance. There was also musical theatre, the leadership club, and community youth groups. She is convinced that the pressure to "do everything" came from within. "My achievements and success began to form my identity."

One year she also grew nine inches. She comes from a family that is genetically tall and thin; however, she did not think of family genes when she heard comments such as "Do you have a hollow leg?" and "You are a human coat hanger!" said in joking ways by people of all ages. As Théa says, when you grow that fast no amount of healthy eating is going to prevent you from being "skinny." Then there were the mixed messages. While attending a professional ballet school, she was told she had the perfect body type to be a ballerina but was asked to withdraw for growing too tall as there was no partner available for someone her height. That is when she began drinking Coca-Cola to stunt her growth.

Quitting dancing, attending an outdoor education school, and physically maturing during her Grade 11 and 12 years resulted in major changes in her outward body appearance. With the changes came comments such as "You are finally filling out" and "You look so different—not a skinny Théa anymore."

"It was a loss of identity. It had a huge impact on me. If I wasn't skinny Théa, then who was I?"

She remembers the day when she read about a diet in a magazine—a diet that would soon go wrong. Théa is convinced that the media played a role in her eating disorder. The models were people she looked up to. She began restricting food and

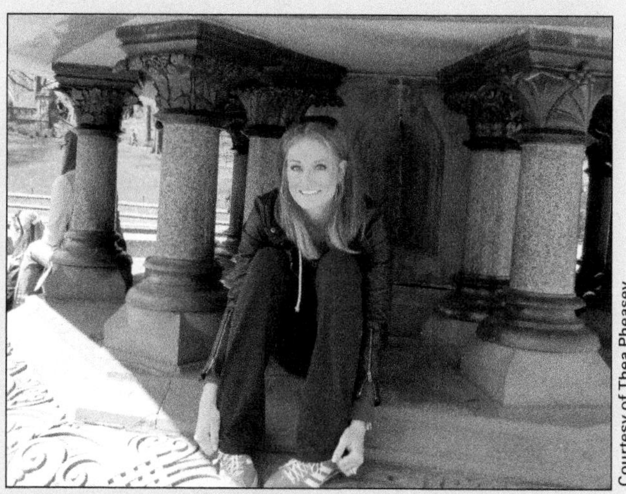

Courtesy of Thea Pheasey

Théa Pheasey, a young woman who faced the despair of eating disorders, now encourages others with a message of hope.

over-exercising. New comments started right away—"You're so thin again." "Skinny Théa is back."

Théa's parents were concerned and sent her to a nutritionist. She went to "get them off my back." She was thin but managed to convince them she was recovering. She also graduated at the top of her class. After graduation she took a summer job away from home. She clung to her eating disorder, losing 13 more kilograms (30 pounds). At her lowest weight, she was 45 kilograms (100 pounds) and 183 centimetres (6 feet) tall. She lost control of her emotions and began crying all of the time. "Lying was my survival. Much of the deceit is meant for you so you can continue to stay in deep denial. You don't even realize that you are lying. Anorexia became my life, all consuming. I did not care about anything except how much I ate and how much I exercised."

It was a visit from her brother—his shock at seeing her, his care and compassion—that helped Théa realize, for the first time, that something was very wrong. She returned home and started on the road of recovery. Initially, the recovery began for her family. Then it shifted to being for her. Théa says that "ultimately the recovery has to be for yourself." It was a two-steps-forward, one-step-back process. She feels that for some individuals, this is the way it will be, no matter what interventions are used. "You must reprogram your brain to think outside the disorder's reality, and separate yourself from the disorder. It can be a very long and painful process."

During her recovery, there was still much deceit at first. She credits an amazing team of professionals—a pediatrician, a nutritionist, a psychiatrist, family, and friends—for helping her in her recovery process. "You can't expect help from just one person, and you can't expect all the healing to come from yourself." She is in her 14th year of recovery now, and her life is completely different. Dealing with an eating disorder has changed her life. She discovered that she has strength and power that can be used in positive ways. She has found her experience to be humbling and healing. She has developed a much greater understanding of herself and others. Recovering from anorexia nervosa required a huge leap of faith on Théa's part. It required letting go of a control mechanism that made her feel safe, whereas in reality it was killing her slowly.

Her advice for students with an eating disorder: "Know that you are not alone. Do what you can to convince yourself that you can ask for help. This is about you, and you have the power to be sick or to get better." Her advice for parents and friends: "Know your role—you are not their doctor. Your job is to be honest, find professional help, and be there for support. Know that you will be met with great resistance. Find strength to do what you know needs to be done." Her advice for teachers: "Be brave. Be honest. Be interested in your students. You might save a life."

Although there are times when she struggles with her body image, she has found a deep appreciation for what her body is capable of; health and contentment are the focus, not calories and fat content. She feels that there is a protective mechanism inside her that will never let her starve herself again. She has a deep trust in herself, and a respect for her body and her own strength and resilience. She no longer relies solely on the opinions of others for validation, but has learned to recognize her accomplishments and failures for what they are: the highs and lows of life are not the defining things that make her who she is.

STRATEGIES FOR PREVENTION

Do You Have an Eating Disorder?

Physicians have developed a simple screening test for eating disorders, consisting of the following questions:

- Do you make yourself sick because you feel uncomfortably full?
- Do you worry you have lost control over how much you eat?
- Do you believe yourself to be fat when others say you are too thin?
- Would you say that food dominates your life?

Score one point for every "yes." A score of two or more is a likely indication of anorexia nervosa or bulimia nervosa.

STRATEGIES FOR CHANGE

Working Off Weight

- Get moving. Take the stairs instead of the elevator. Get off the bus a few blocks from your home and walk the rest of the way.
- Walk. Most people find it hard to make excuses for not walking 15 minutes every day. Once you start, increase gradually so that you go farther and faster.
- Exercise daily. You're more likely to lose and keep weight off if you exercise regularly. Try to burn 1800–2000 calories a week through exercise.
- Get physical. There are more ways to burn calories than traditional exercise activities. Dancing, hiking, and gardening can all help you get in shape. Check your campus bulletin boards and newspapers for information on rock climbing, kayaking, skiing, and other fun forms of working out.

SELF-SURVEY

Are You Ready to Lose Weight?

As discussed in Chapter 1, people change the way they behave stage by stage and step by step. The same is true for changing behaviours related to weight. If you need to lose excess pounds, knowing your stage of readiness for change is a crucial first step. Here is a guide to identifying where you are right now.

If you are still in the *precontemplation* stage, you don't think of yourself as having a weight problem, even though others might. If you can't fit into some of your clothes, you might think that they have shrunk in the dryer. Or you look around and think, "I'm no bigger than anyone else in this class." Unconsciously, you may feel helpless to do anything about your weight. So you deny or dismiss its importance.

In the *contemplation* stage, you would prefer not to have to change, but you can't avoid reality. Your coach or doctor may comment on your weight. You wince at the vacation photos of you in a swimsuit. You look in the mirror, try to suck in your stomach, and say, "I've got to do something about my weight."

In the *preparation* stage, you're gearing up by taking small but necessary steps. You may buy athletic shoes or check out several diet books from the library. Maybe you experiment with some minor changes, such as having fruit instead of cookies for an afternoon snack. Internally, you are getting accustomed to the idea of change.

In the *action* stage of change, you are deliberately working to lose weight. You no longer snack all evening long. You stick to a specific diet and track your daily calories. You hop on a treadmill or stationary bike for 30 minutes a day or you start a walking program. Your resolve is strong, and you know you're on your way to a healthier you.

In the *maintenance* stage, you strengthen, enhance, and extend the changes you've made. Whether or not you have lost all the weight you want, you've made significant progress. As you continue to watch what you eat and to be physically active, you lock in healthy new habits.

In the *termination stage*, you have reached your goal weight and have learned how to make healthy food choices. You have discovered ways in which to maintain a healthy weight by combining healthy eating and participating in regular physical activity.

Where are you right now? Read each of the following statements and decide which best applies to you.

Precontemplation Stage

1. I never think about my weight.

Contemplation Stage

2. I'm trying to zip up a pair of jeans and wondering when was the last time they fit.

Preparation Stage

3. I'm downloading a food diary to keep track of what I eat. (Try using eaTracker from Dieititians of Canada, available at http://www.eatracker.ca/.).

Action Stage

4. I have been following a diet for three weeks and have started working out.

Maintenance Stage

5. I have incorporated better eating habits and regular physical activity into my lifestyle for the past six months.

Termination Stage

6. I am able to maintain a healthy weight through wise food choices and regular physical activity. I have maintained my goal weight for the past two years.

Chapter Summary

1. What is the best way to determine whether you are at a healthy weight?
   a. stand on a scale
   b. calculate your body-fat percentage
   c. check ideal weight tables
   d. calculate your body mass index
2. Which method can be used to obtain body fat assessments?
   a. weighing yourself using a scale
   b. skinfold measurement
   c. height-weight charts
   d. basal metabolic rate measurement
3. Requiring people who are overweight or obese to register in weight-loss programs under a doctor's supervision and pay a fee if they are unable to meet a certain weight target is an example of
   a. economics and obesity—income effect
   b. economics and obesity—substitution effect
   c. weight discrimination
   d. genetic health factors

4. Which statement about body weight is NOT true?
   a. BMI is a mathematical formula that correlates with body fat.
   b. Daily energy requirements depend on your activity level.
   c. Only women have body weight and shape concerns.
   d. If your BMI is high, you may be at increased risk of heart disease.
5. Which of the following may be a warning sign of a serious eating disorder?
   a. vegetarianism
   b. compulsive food washing
   c. binge eating
   d. weight gain during the first year of college or university
6. Which statement about individuals with anorexia nervosa is true?
   a. They believe they are overweight even if they are extremely thin.
   b. They typically feel full all the time, which limits their food intake.
   c. They usually look overweight even though their body mass index is normal.
   d. They have a reduced risk for heart-related abnormalities.
7. Which statement about bulimia nervosa is true?
   a. It is characterized by excessive sleeping followed by periods of insomnia.
   b. It is found primarily in older women who are concerned with the aging process.
   c. It is associated with the use of laxatives or vomiting to control weight.
   d. It does not have serious health consequences.
8. Which of the following statements is NOT true?
   a. Obesity is a greater threat to heart health than smoking.
   b. Men who accumulate fat around their waist are at increased risk for cardiovascular disease.
   c. Individuals who are obese are neither more nor less psychologically troubled than people of normal weight.
   d. Children with an obese parent are more likely to be thin because of their embarrassment about the parent's appearance.
9. Which of the following is a weight-management strategy that works?
   a. Increase your activity level and eat less, aiming for a weekly weight loss of about 0.7 kilograms.
   b. Ask friends for recommendations for methods that helped them lose weight quickly.
   c. Practise good eating habits about 50 percent of the time so that you can balance your cravings with healthy food.
   d. Try a number of weight-loss diets to find the one that works best for you.
10. Which of the following statements is true?
   a. Very low-calorie diets increase metabolism, which helps burn calories more quickly.
   b. An individual eating low-calorie or fat-free foods can increase the serving sizes.
   c. High-protein, low-carbohydrate diets may increase the risk of heart disease.
   d. Yo-yo dieting works best for long-term weight loss.

Answers to these questions can be found on page 159.

SELF-RESPONSIBILITY—SOCIAL RESPONSIBILITY

SELF-RESPONSIBILITY

Believe in yourself! Have faith in your abilities! Without a humble but reasonable confidence in your own powers, you cannot be successful or happy.

Norman Vincent Peale

Changing eating habits is not an easy thing to do. Recognizing that change takes time is helpful. Knowing that people follow certain stages—such as Prochaska's Stages of Change—can help. What would it take to move you from contemplation to preparation? From preparation to action? From action to maintenance? Friends, family, books, websites, and professional health experts can all be part of your change process. You have to start with the belief that you can make a change.

SOCIAL RESPONSIBILITY

The wise man (woman) should consider that health is the greatest of human blessings. Let food be your medicine.

Hippocrates

Making healthy food choices can also be considered part of social responsibility. The more people eat in a healthy way, the less we will be paying for healthcare costs later.

CRITICAL THINKING

1. Do you think you have a weight problem? If so, what makes you think so? Is your perception based on your actual BMI measurement or on how you believe you look? If you found out that your BMI was within the ideal range, would that change your opinion about your body? Why or why not?
2. You have noticed that many of your friends are eating out at the fast-food outlets on campus. You are also starting to hear complaints about weight gain. You have also experienced an increase in weight since you started your studies. As an active health advocate, what could you do to change not only your eating habits and physical activity levels, but your friends' lifestyle habits too?
3. Suppose one of your roommates appears to have symptoms of an eating disorder. You have told him or her of your concerns, but your roommate has denied having a problem and brushed off your fears. What can you do to help this individual? Should you contact his or her parents? Why or why not?

WEB LINKS

Heart and Stroke Foundation

http://www.heartandstroke.com/site/c.iklQLcMWJtE/b.3484281/k.10E/Healthy_living__Healthy_weight_and_waist.htm

Check out this site for a video clip on how to measure your waist circumference.

Canadian Obesity Network

www.obesitynetwork.ca/

Access Canada's largest professional obesity association for many reports, presentations, and links to many resources such as the 5As of Obesity Management—a special tool kit for practitioners working in the area of obesity management. You can also join this association as a Student and New Professional Member (SNP). This association aims to address the social stigma associated with obesity and work with stakeholders to prevent and treat obesity.

Health Canada, Food and Nutrition, Healthy Weights

www.hc-sc.gc.ca/fn-an/nutrition/weights-poids/index-eng.php

Calculate your body mass index (BMI) using this interactive BMI nomogram. Find out more about BMI by accessing the Question and Answer section on weight classification and weight and health.

National Eating Disorders Association

www.nedic.ca

The National Eating Disorder Information Centre (NEDIC) is a Toronto-based, nonprofit organization that provides information and resources on eating disorders and weight preoccupation.

A Report on Mental Illnesses in Canada—Chapter 6, Eating Disorders

www.cmha.ca/bins/content_page.asp?cid=4-42-215

This comprehensive report includes a special chapter on eating disorders and information on the impact, causes, and treatment of eating disorders.

Please note that links are subject to change. If you find a broken link, use a search engine such as www.google.ca and search for the website by typing in keywords.

Key Terms

The terms listed here are used within the chapter on the page indicated. Definitions of the terms are in the Glossary at the end of the book.

anorexia athletica 153
anorexia nervosa 152
appetite 138
basal metabolic rate (BMR) 142
binge eating disorder (BED) 153
body mass index (BMI) 139
bulimia nervosa 153
compulsive overeaters 154
eating disorders 151
estimated energy requirement (EER) 142
exercise metabolic rate (EMR) 143
extreme dieters 154
hunger 137
hyperplasia 138
hypertrophy 138
muscle dysmorphia 153
non-exercise activity thermogenesis (NEAT) 147
obesity 140
overweight 140
resting metabolic rate (RMR) 142
satiety 138
waist circumference (WC) 140
waist-to-hip ratio (WHR) 141
weight discrimination 148

Answers to Chapter Summary Questions

1. d; 2. b; 3. c; 4. c; 5. c; 6. a; 7. c; 8. d; 9. a; 10. c

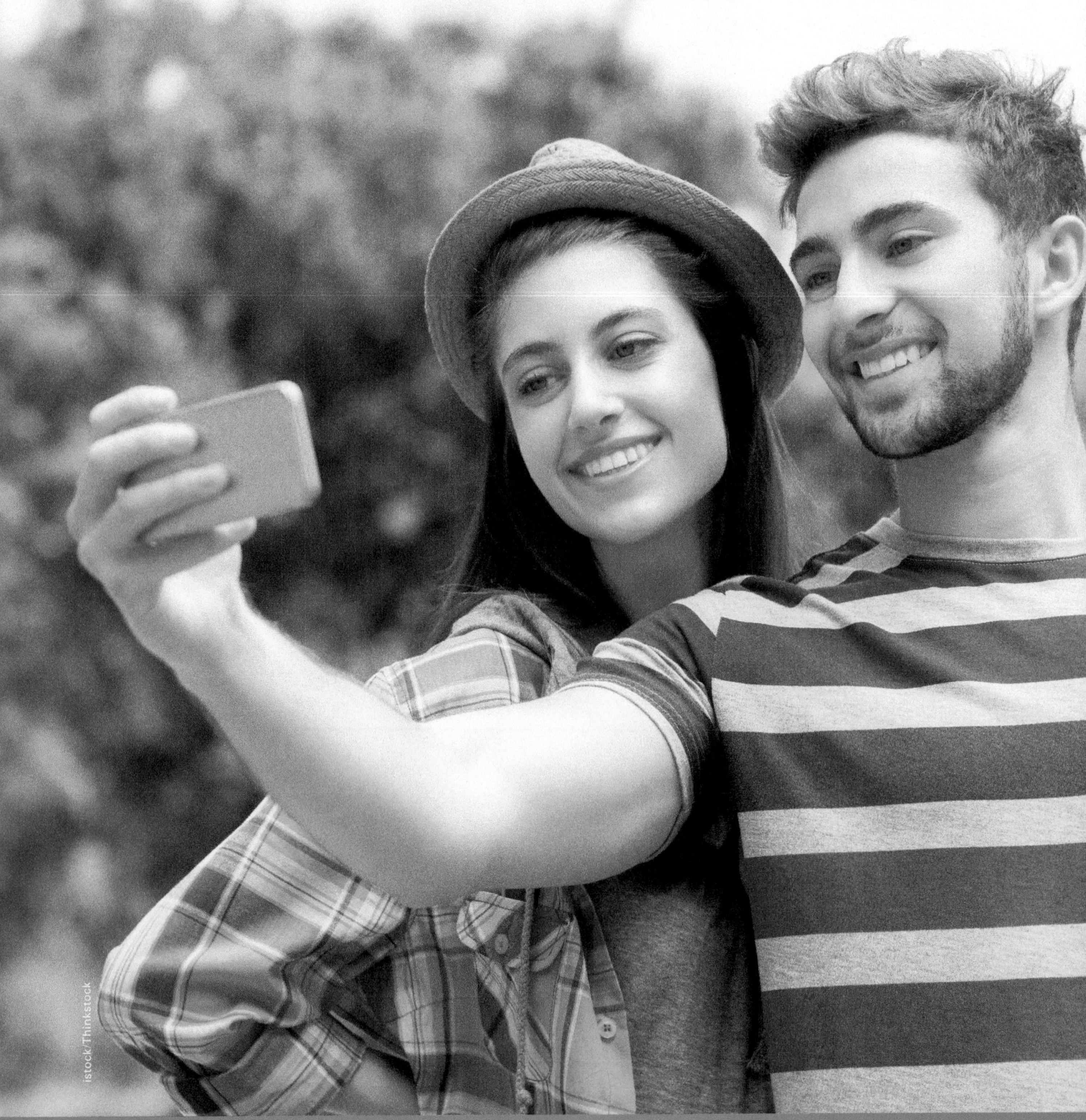

AFTER READING THIS CHAPTER, YOU WILL BE ABLE TO:

- **describe** the role verbal and nonverbal communication plays in forming and maintaining relationships
- **define** friendship and **explain** how friendship grows
- **discuss** the behaviour and emotional expectations for friendship, dating, and intimate relationships
- **compare** and **contrast** romantic, companionate, fatuous, and consummate love
- **list** and **describe** the five love languages
- **describe** dysfunctional relationships
- **define** sexual and gender identity and sexual orientation
- **list** a range of sexual behaviours
- **describe** the male and female reproductive systems and the functions of the individual structures of each system
- **describe** conditions or issues unique to women's and men's sexual health

7

Personal Relationships and Sexuality

Humans are social beings. From our first days of life, we reach out to others, struggle to express ourselves, and strive to forge connections. People make us smile, laugh, cry, hope, and dream. Our lives become richer as others share their experiences with us. We grow and develop through our connectedness to others. It is through this connectedness that many of us discover who we are. Our need for connection also lasts a lifetime. Relationships, whether they are friendships or long-term committed partnerships, need nurturing, patience, caring, and compassion. They also need an authentic voice—being in touch with our "best selves" so that we share our true values and beliefs with others.

We are also sexual beings. Physical closeness or sexual intimacy can be both rewarding and challenging. Although sexual expression and experience can provide intense joy, they also can involve great emotional turmoil. You make decisions that affect how you relate to others, how you express your sexuality, and how you respond sexually. Yet most sexual activity involves another person so decisions about sex affect other people. Sexual responsibility means learning about your relationships, your body, your partner's body, your sexual development and preferences, and the health risks associated with sexual activity.

This chapter will help you explore different types of relationships and sexuality because, ultimately, we are responsible for our personal relationships and sexual health and behaviour.

FREQUENTLY ASKED QUESTIONS

COMMUNICATING WITH OTHERS

Getting to know someone is one of life's greatest challenges and pleasures. When you find another person intriguing—as a friend, a teacher, a colleague, or a possible partner—you want to find out more about him or her. Roommates may talk for hours. Friends may spend years getting to know each other. Partners in committed relationships may get great satisfaction in learning new things about each other throughout their lifetime together.

Building relationships means learning about how to communicate with others. Communication stems from a desire to know and a decision to tell. Each of us chooses what information about ourselves we want to disclose and what we want to conceal or keep private. But in opening up to others, we increase our own self-knowledge and understanding. Good communication skills and building relationships support the social health dimension of health and wellness.

Talking and Listening A great deal of daily communication focuses on facts: on who, what, where, when, and how. Information is easy to convey and comprehend. Emotions are not. Some people have great difficulty saying "I appreciate you" or "I care about you," even though they are genuinely appreciative and caring. Others find it hard to know what to say in response and how to accept such expressions of affection.

Some people feel relationships shouldn't require any effort, that there's no need to talk of responsibility between people who care about each other. Yet responsibility is implicit in our dealings with anyone or anything we value—and what can be more valuable than those with whom we share our lives? Friendships and other intimate relationships always demand an emotional investment, but the rewards they yield are great.

Sometimes people convey strong emotions with a kiss or a hug, a pat or a punch, but such actions aren't precise enough to communicate exact thoughts. Stalking out of a room and slamming the door may be clear signs of anger, but they don't explain what caused the anger or suggest what to do about it. As two people build a relationship, it is important to sharpen communication skills so discussions about various issues can be had. We must all learn how to communicate anger as well as affection, sadness as well as joy.

One study, completed at the University of Florida, found that self-revelation within a relationship is especially important for female students when dating the opposite sex. Male and female heterosexual students were asked how their partner's authenticity affected the quality of their relationship and their personal well-being. Female students were more likely than male students to report greater happiness when their partner presented himself as he "really was," rather than presenting "false" behaviours to try and please his partner.[1] The study also found that when female students revealed their real selves, they tended to function better in the relationship, which then improved their partner's satisfaction.

Listening is also an integral part of communicating in a healthy and mature way. Listening involves more than waiting for the other person to stop talking. It is an active process of trying to understand the other person's feelings and motivation. Effective listeners ask questions when they're not sure they understand what the other person is trying to say. They also prompt the other person to continue once their questions have been answered. Next time you are having a conversation with someone, ask yourself two questions to determine whether or not you are a good listener:

- When someone is talking to me, am I really listening to them or do I interrupt them or ignore what they are saying because I can't wait to jump into the conversation?
- When someone is talking to me, am I jumping to conclusions or judging what they are saying instead of "just listening" and letting them "be heard"?

Nonverbal Communication More than 90 percent of communication may be nonverbal. The most common elements of nonverbal communication include the use of space or proximity, touch, eye contact, facial expressions, gestures, posture, physical appearance, and paraverbal language—sounds made by people that are not distinguishable by words, such as um, uh, or uh huh.[2]

Learning to interpret what people *don't* say can reveal more than what they *do* say. "Understanding nonverbal communication is probably the best tool there is for a good life of communicating, be it personally or professionally," says Marilyn Maple, a university educator. "It's one of the most practical skills you can develop. When you can consciously read what others are saying unconsciously, you can deal with issues before they become problems."[3]

Culture has a great deal of influence over body language. In some cultures, establishing eye contact is considered hostile or challenging; in others, it conveys friendliness. A person's sense of personal space—the distance from others at which he or she feels most comfortable—also varies in different societies.

Nonverbal messages also reveal something important about the individual. "Nonverbal messages come from deep inside of you, from your own sense of self-esteem," says Maple. "To improve your body language, you have to start from the inside and work out. If you're comfortable with yourself, it shows. People who have good self-esteem, who give themselves status and respect, who know who they are, have a relaxed way of talking and moving."[4]

STRATEGIES FOR CHANGE

How to Enhance Communication

- Use "I" statements. Describe what's going on with you. Say "I worry about being liked" or "I get frustrated when I can't put my feelings into words." Avoid generalities such as "You never think about my feelings" or "Nobody understands me."
- Gently ask how the other person feels. If your friend or partner describes thoughts rather than feelings, ask for more adjectives. Was he or she sad, excited, angry, hurt?
- Become a good listener. When another person talks, don't interrupt, ask why, judge, or challenge. Nod your head. Use your body language and facial expression to show you're eager to hear more.
- Respect confidences. Treat a friend or partner's secrets with the discretion they deserve. Consider them a special gift entrusted to your care.

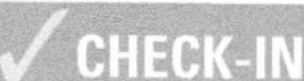

How would you assess your communication skills?

FORMING RELATIONSHIPS

As children we first learn how to relate in our families. Our relationships with parents and siblings change dramatically as we grow toward independence. In college or university, students can choose to spend their leisure time socializing or engaging in solitary activities. Relationships between friends also change as they move or develop different interests; between lovers, as they come to know more about each other; between spouses or partners, as they pass through life together; and between parents and children, as youngsters develop and mature and parents age. Close relationships are tested and strengthened by time. They allow a deep exploration of "self" and what one hopes for in that relationship.

Understanding Ourselves The way each of us perceives ourselves affects all the ways we reach out and relate to others. If we feel unworthy of love, others may share that opinion. Self-esteem provides a positive foundation for our relationships with others. Self-esteem doesn't mean vanity or preoccupation with our own needs; rather, it is a genuine concern and respect for ourselves so that we remain true to our own feelings and beliefs. We can't know or love or accept others until we know and love and accept ourselves, however imperfect we may be.

If we're lacking in self-esteem, our relationships may suffer. Sometimes, individuals with negative views of themselves seek out partners (friends, roommates, dates) who are critical and rejecting—and who confirm their low opinion of their own worth. Gullette and Lyons, who studied sensation-seeking, self-esteem, and unprotected sex in college students, found that students with low self-esteem had higher levels of alcohol consumption, had more sexual partners, and had more risk-taking behaviours linked to HIV transmission than other students.[5]

Lack of self-esteem can also sabotage a relationship as self-doubting individuals may read non-existent meaning into their partners' ambiguous cues. The misreading of cues occurs not just in dating couples but also in long-term partnerships or marriages where one of the partners may develop an irrational fear that he or she is not loved.

Findings by Khanchandani and Durham, who examined jealousy in relationships among college women, show that women who scored higher in self-esteem and lower in neuroticism reported less jealousy in a dating relationship than women scoring lower in self-esteem and higher in neuroticism.[6]

✓ CHECK-IN

Do you put effort into maintaining and strengthening your close relationships?

What Is Friendship? Friendship has been described as the bond of society. Every culture values the ties of respect, tolerance, and loyalty that friendship builds and nurtures. Friends can be a basic source of happiness, a connection to a larger world, a source of solace in times of trouble. Although we have different friends throughout life, often the friendships of adolescence and young adulthood are the closest we ever form. They ease the normal break from parents and the transition from childhood to independence.

In the past, many people believed that men and women couldn't become close friends without getting romantically involved. But as the genders have worked together and come to share more interests, this belief has changed. Yet, unique obstacles arise in male–female friendships, such as distinguishing between friendship and romantic attraction and dealing with sexual tension. When men and women overcome such barriers and become friends, they can benefit from their relationship—but in different ways. For men, a friendship with a woman offers support and nurturance. What they report liking most is talking and relating to women, something they don't do with their male buddies. Women view their friendships with men as more light-hearted and casual, with more joking and less fear of hurt feelings. They especially like gaining insight into what men really think.

Bisson and Levine investigated the prevalence of **friends with benefits (FWB)**, which refers to relationships between friends who have sex. They found that 60 percent of the individuals surveyed had had this type of relationship. These relationships were desirable because while there was no commitment for romance and the benefits included trust and comfort. However, a common concern was that the sex might complicate the friendship if one of the friends began wanting a committed relationship. They also discovered that people involved in a FWB relationship sidestepped clear relational rules. While this supported the concept of friendship instead of romantic relationship, it was at times challenging and difficult to cope when a romantic attraction began with one of the friends.[7]

Friendship transcends all boundaries of distance and differences and enhances feelings of warmth, trust, love, and affection between two people. It is a common denominator of human existence that cuts across major social categories—in every country, culture, and language, human beings make friends. Friendship is both a universal and a deeply satisfying experience.

The qualities that make a good friend include honesty, acceptance, dependability, empathy, and loyalty. To sustain a close friendship, both people must be able to see the other's perspective, anticipate each other's needs, and take each other's viewpoint into account. More than anything else, good friends are there when we need them. They see us at our worst but never lose sight of our best. They share our laughter and tears, our triumphs and tragedies.

Hooking Up **Hooking up** is loosely defined as sexual activity with a casual partner who may be a friend or a stranger.[8] College and university students use the term to describe a variety of sexual interactions, including kissing, fondling, oral sex, and sexual intercourse. A common aspect to hooking up is an agreement that there is no commitment or exclusivity in the "hookup." Some studies have found that hooking up is a common practice on college campuses.[9] Other studies show that overall sexual activity of college students is actually less frequent than what is perceived. Holman and Sillars[10] studied how college social networks promoted high-risk sexual relationships such as hooking up. While peer approval was a predictor for the hookup behaviour and attitudes of the students, their research also showed that students misjudged how often their colleagues were actually hooking up. Students who frequently talked about hooking up often inflated the estimates of how many times they did hook up.

Authors Kooyman, Pierce, and Zavadil explore hooking up from a feminist developmental perspective and propose female participation in this form of sexual experience may be viewed by students as an expression of sexual freedom and equality.[11] However, they point out that hooking up can present problems for some young women because they differ with regard to their psychosocial development compared to young men. According to their research, not all, but many adult young women find comfort and solace in connection and feel fearful of separation, whereas many, but not all young men value independence and are hesitant to become attached.

Following are results of some significant studies on the psychosocial and physiological health of college and university students and casual sex, including hooking up:

- Persistent depressive symptoms among young women engaged in casual sex.[12]
- Sex differences with regard to regret and hooking up. Females often felt shame and self-blame because they did not know their partner and there was no discussion on past sexual history so potential health risks were not addressed. Regret for females was also compounded because of lack of future contact, which resulted in anger at themselves. Regret for males was linked to disappointment at having chosen an unattractive or undesirable hookup or a partner who was labelled as being promiscuous.[13]
- Men reported more positive and fewer negative emotional reactions to hooking up. Women reported that condom use was associated with fewer positive and more negative emotional reactions.[14]
- Eighty percent of students surveyed reported that alcohol use was involved in hooking up.[15]
- Of the sexually active female students, only 36.8 percent reported using condoms and only 41.6 percent reported using birth control pills.[16]

Bogle suggests that hooking up might be best described as a culture of casual sex, not as a social problem.[17] We must be careful that we are not too quick to judge hooking up as a moral or ethical issue. However, looking forward, young adults might take heed of the increasing levels of chlamydia, gonorrhea, human papillomavirus, syphilis, and HIV/AIDS in the 15–24 age group. Untreated STIs are estimated to cause many women to become infertile each year.[18]

Wentland and Reissing explored other casual sexual relationships (CSRs) among Canadian students—One Night Stands (ONS), Booty Calls (BC), and Fuck Buddies (FB), in addition to Friends with Benefits (FWB). Participants in their study identified both implicit and explicit rules that influenced how these relationships were initiated, maintained, and terminated. The findings suggest that some young adults are open to different ways of engaging in non-committed sexual relationships. The study also found that there were minimal differences between male and female participants with regard to their understanding of the rules that linked to expected behaviours of these CSRs.[19]

College and university is a critical stage for the development of identity. Sexual behaviour is part of that identity. Consider the benefits and challenges of this type of relationship and recognize that choices made during the college and university years do impact you after graduation.

✓ CHECK-IN

Do you think sexual "benefits" affect a friendship?

Dating A date is any occasion during which two people share their time. It can be dancing at a club, a bicycle ride, a dinner for two, or a walk in the park. Friends and lovers go on dates; so do complete strangers. Some men date other men, some women date other women, and some people date both men and women. We don't expect to love, or even like, everyone we date.

While in school, you may go out with people you meet in class or on campus. Some students form close relationships; others connect only for a one-time sexual encounter that might involve anything from kissing to intercourse. With more people remaining single longer, the search for a date has become more complex. While bars and clubs are still popular places for college and university students to meet, cafés, health clubs, and bookstores have become acceptable as places to meet new people, too. Many people now meet dates through online dating websites.

In a study on the dynamics of Internet dating, authors Lawson and Leck explored the motivations of Internet daters, their styles of courtship, and also how they coped with problems of trust and deception.[20] Some of their findings were as follows:

- Internet dating raises issues of negotiation and trust.
- Risks include physical danger, possible rejection, and humiliation.
- Internet dating allows women to behave more assertively and men to be more open.
- This method of dating demands the development of skills in reading user profiles to understand and develop trust and future compatibility. The use of telephone conversations becomes an "in-between space" prior to meeting in person for many Internet daters.
- Dating problems exist in Internet dating that are similar to traditional dating—people lie, appearance issues become problematic, and personality characteristics such as shyness do not disappear once people meet in person.
- Emotional pain and rejection are part of Internet dating, just as they are part of traditional dating.

Dating can do more than help you meet people. Dating helps you learn how to converse with others, helps you get to know more about others, and provides you with an opportunity to share feelings, opinions, and interests. In adolescence and young adulthood, dating also provides an opportunity for exploring sexual identity. Some people date for months and never share more than a kiss. Others have sex before they fall in love or even "like."

Scheleicher and Gilbert[21] investigated contemporary dating practices and whether or not traditional dating protocol and beliefs are still prevalent among heterosexual college students. The students reported that

- sexual expression for both males and females was perceived as positive,
- sex brought couples closer together,
- sex did not have to be the central reason to date,
- it was normal for men to initiate sex,
- it was normal for women to wait for men to initiate dates,
- pressure to have sex when one partner was not ready was seen in a negative way,
- both male and female students saw women or men conveying their sexual desires as positive, and
- both male and female students also indicated that a person's desirability was not in question if a partner was not interested in sexual activity.

Bartoli and Clark studied the perceptions of college students and their understanding of the "first date."[22] They found, as was consistent with other studies, males had greater expectations for sexual activities on a date. They also found that the responsibility for limiting sexual activities was still the female's.

Long-distance dating relationships (LDDR) are something that many college and university students have to find their way through too. Knox et al. surveyed undergraduates at a large southeastern university in the United States about their attitudes and previous experiences with long-distance relationships.[23] The definition of LDDR was living apart for not less than three months and being 321 kilometres (200 miles) away from their partner. The findings of this study indicate that long-distance dating relationships are not easy and that one in five relationships end. Another 20 percent reported that their relationships became more difficult. Many students stayed in touch with each other on a weekly or daily basis. Eighteen percent of the students reported that the separation helped to improve their relationship.

Infidelity in dating relationships can be difficult to deal with. College students, when surveyed, define infidelity in a broad way. According to an extensive review of literature by McAnulty and Brineman, students suggest that any form of emotional or sexual intimacy with a person other than a primary dating partner meets the criteria of infidelity.[24] It could mean flirtation, passionate kissing, or sexual intercourse. The majority of students also reported that they disapproved of infidelity, although it appears they thought it was more excusable if the primary relationship was in trouble or there was an irresistible attraction to another person. The most common reaction to infidelity was jealousy. The ending of a relationship often resulted from infidelity.

Harris measured reactions of perceived infidelity and actual infidelity across four samples: gay men, lesbians, and heterosexual men and women.[25] For perceived infidelity, emotional infidelity was the most upsetting for all groups. However, heterosexual men (74 percent) were more likely than all other groups to report that emotional infidelity was more upsetting than sexual infidelity.

When the participants were asked about their reactions to actual infidelity of a partner, all groups were more distressed by emotional infidelity. Over half of the students surveyed reported that their relationships had ended because of this type of infidelity.

Separating your emotional feelings about someone you're dating from your sexual desire is often difficult. The first step to making responsible sexual decisions is respecting your sexual values and those of your partner. If you care about the other person—not just his or her body—and the relationship you are creating, sex will be an important, but not the all-important, factor. You will also be responsible with regard to the health risks of a sexual relationship. Disclosure about your sexual health history and a willingness to have sexual health medical tests prior to engaging in a sexual relationship can alleviate stress and tension as you become more involved at an intimate level. You will also practise safe sex.

Dating does have potential dangers. Authors of a review of literature examining dating violence among college students found that physical and sexual dating violence are common on college campuses; psychological dating violence appears to be more common than physical and sexual dating violence; individual risk factors for dating violence include family history, peer influences, personal beliefs, alcohol use and abuse, and psychological factors; college students who experience dating violence often tell their friends about the experience, but are reluctant to report the violence to counsellors or law enforcement officers.[26]

With all the ups and downs of dating, studies on dating relationships have shown that love has been found to increase for individuals who advance to a deeper, more long-lasting commitment.

✓ CHECK-IN

How do you define infidelity?

What Causes Romantic Attraction? What draws two people to each other and keeps them together: chemistry, fate, survival instincts, or sexual longings?

Scientists have tried to analyze the combination of factors that attracts two people to each other. In several studies, predictors ranked as the most important reasons for attraction were warmth and kindness, desirable personality, something specific about the person, and reciprocal liking.[27]

The reason for romantic attraction could be evolutionary. Dr. Susan Johnson, a clinical psychologist and the developer of Emotionally Focused Therapy (EFT), suggests that love is "the pinnacle of evolution, the most compelling survival mechanism of the human species. Not because it induces us to mate and reproduce. We do manage to mate without love! But because love drives us to bond emotionally with a precious few others who offer us safe haven from the storms of life. Love is our bulwark, designed to provide emotional protection so we can cope with the ups and downs of existence."[28]

Through her research, the application of Bowlby's attachment theory in children to adult love, and the work of other relationship experts, she determined that this drive to emotionally attach—"to find someone to whom we can turn and say 'Hold me tight'—is wired into our genes and our bodies. . . . We need emotional attachments with a few irreplaceable others to be physically and mentally healthy—to survive."[29]

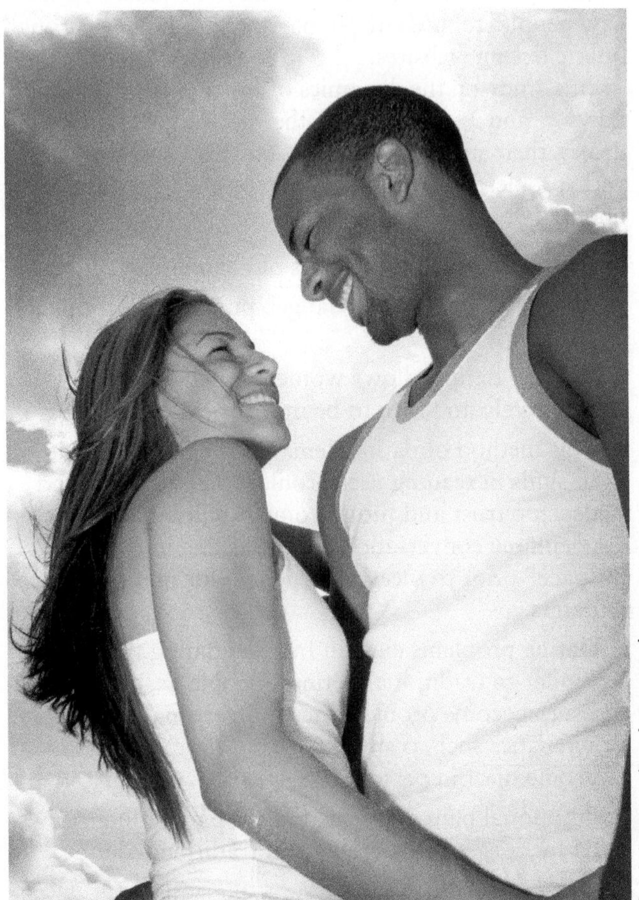

iStockphoto.com/martin purmensky

Romantic attraction is characterized by a high level of emotional arousal, reciprocal liking, and mutual sexual desire.

However, research also shows that the romantic attraction stage is just that—a stage. Telltale signs of romantic love are an acute longing for attention from the love object, fear of rejection, drastic mood swings, the growth of passion through difficult times or challenges, and intrusive thinking. According to the late psychologist, Dr. Dorothy Tennov, during the first wave of passion in the "in-love" stage, the person thinks of his/her love object about 30 percent of the time. During the second wave of passion, which can come months later, an individual can become nearly obsessed and think of the other person almost 100 percent of the time.[30] The upside is a feeling of euphoria—that everything is perfect in the world, that nothing else really matters. The downside is a lack of productivity at work or school, isolation from family and friends, daydreaming, and an unrealistic view of the future of the relationship.

Tennov's research also showed that the average life span of a romantic attraction or love is about two years. If it is a secretive affair, it may last a little longer.[31] While charisma might be the attraction for dating in the first place, it is good to remember that personal character is often an even more important aspect to any long-term committed relationship.

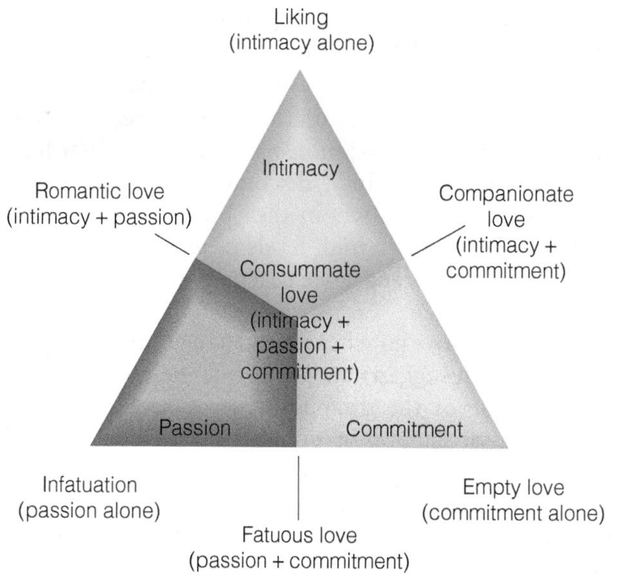

Figure 7-1 Sternberg's Love Triangle

The three components of love are intimacy, passion, and commitment. The various kinds of love are composed of different combinations of the three components.

INTIMATE RELATIONSHIPS

The term **intimacy**—the open, trusting sharing of close, confidential thoughts and feelings—comes from the Latin word for *within*. Intimacy doesn't happen at first sight or in a day or a week or a number of weeks. Intimacy requires time and nurturing; it is a process of revealing rather than hiding, of wanting to know another and to be known by that other. Although intimacy doesn't require sex, an intimate relationship often includes a sexual relationship.

All of our close relationships, whether they're with parents or friends, have a great deal in common. We feel we can count on these people in times of need. We feel they understand us and we understand them. We give and receive loving emotional support. We care about their happiness and welfare. However, when we choose one person above all others, there is something even deeper and richer—something we call *mature love*.

Mature Love Relationships can begin with *liking* (characterized by intimacy alone) and evolve into various kinds of love. Social scientists have distinguished between *romantic love* (a combination of intimacy and passion), *companionate love* (described as a combination of intimacy and commitment), *fatuous love* (passion and commitment), and *consummate love* (symbolized by a blend of intimacy, passion, and commitment). (See Figure 7-1 for the elements of love).

A romantic relationship shows promise if

- you feel at ease with your new partner;
- you feel good about your new partner when you're together and when you're not;
- your partner is open with you about his or her life—past, present, and future;
- you can say no to each other without feeling guilty;
- you feel cared for, appreciated, and accepted as you are; and
- your partner really listens to what you have to say.

Mature love is a complex combination of intimacy, passion, and commitment—or consummate love, as Sternberg describes it. The intimacy is unique between the two lovers, the passion is not simply a matter of orgasm but also entails a crossing of the psychological boundaries between oneself and one's lover, and the commitment is based on personal values and ethics. There is a sense of "oneness," while simultaneously retaining a sense of yourself. Reality and awareness that the partner is not "perfect" develops. Personality traits and characteristics are understood and accepted.

✓ CHECK-IN

How do you nurture your relationships?

Breaking Up—Staying Together Breaking up is indeed hard to do. Sometimes two people gradually grow apart, and both of them realize that they must go their separate ways. More often, one person falls out of love first. It hurts to be rejected; it also hurts to inflict pain on someone who once meant a great deal to you. In surveys, college and university students say it's more difficult to initiate a breakup than to be rejected. Those who decided to end a relationship reported greater feelings of guilt, uncertainty, discomfort, and awkwardness than those with whom they broke up. However, rejected students with high levels of jealousy are likely to feel a desire for vengeance that can lead to aggressive behaviour.[32]

Where does love go when an end to a relationship feels near? Research suggests people do not end their relationships because of the disappearance of love. Rather, a sense of dissatisfaction or unhappiness develops, which may then cause love to stop growing. Dr. Gary Chapman, an internationally known author, speaker, and expert on relationships and marriage, believes that instead of love disappearing from a relationship, we become confused because we think our partner or spouse does not understand or appreciate us.

After 30 years of marriage counselling he feels he has uncovered five primary or basic love languages—five ways that we speak and understand emotional love. When we learn about our own way of expressing love and the preferred way that our partner expresses and appreciates love, we can be better at sustaining the love we once experienced in the romantic love stage. One example is when one partner provides many acts of service—housecleaning, grocery shopping, and doing errands, a primary love language for some—but feels unappreciated and unloved. Discussion with the other partner might reveal that his or her primary love language is quality time; this person might feel unappreciated and unloved because of the lack of time spent together due to the time taken up by household chores.

Dr. Chapman also says that our own emotional love language and the language of our partner may be as "different as Chinese from English. No matter how hard you try to express love in English, if your spouse understands only Chinese, you will never understand how to love each other."[33] Disappointment, nagging, judgment, lack of connection and understanding, separateness, and injury can happen within a relationship over time because we are not speaking the same primary love languages—because we usually speak in our own preferred language.

Following are the five love languages:[34]

- **Words of affirmation**—verbal compliments, words of appreciation, words that build others up, straightforward or indirect statements that help someone feel worthy, wanted, or loved
- **Quality time**—focused and full attention, quality conversation, quality activities done together
- **Giving gifts**—inexpensive or expensive, purchased or handmade, a gift of presence—being available for a special event, a lasting tribute, a living gift
- **Acts of service**—housework, yard work, organizing a room, cooking dinner, buying the groceries, anything your partner has asked you to do in the past month
- **Physical touch**—as simple as a touch on the shoulder or a hug; handholding or massage; passionate sex

If breaking up is on your list of things to do, you might take a step back and attempt to determine what love language your partner might need you to speak. You might also attempt to determine what love language you might need from your partner. It takes time and energy to learn a new love language. It takes patience and commitment to enter into a new way of relating to your partner. If you don't know your love language or that of your partner's, try them all out and see if changes within the relationship start developing.

Love and Stonsny, relationship therapists, encourage nurturing small moments of connection every day. While romantic getaways and vacations can bring fun and excitement to a relationship, they suggest that long-term relationships last because there is a loving routine. When people know and feel that they are cared for and loved deeply, they are more likely to care and love back. As Love and Stonsny worked with clients, they discovered that when couples were having difficulty, women often went to a place of fear and men went to a place of shame. If the circle of fear and shame continued, a breakup was often the result. They are convinced that the best way to sustain a long-term relationship is to honour the basic law of human interaction—that of giving what we expect. Showing appreciation, cooperation, compassion, integrity, and love each day will help you and your partner develop a deep connection that can lead to a healthy and happy long-term relationship.[35]

There are certainly times when the decision to end a relationship is the best decision. If relationships involve alcohol or drug misuse and abuse, there is physical or emotional violence, or, for some couples, infidelity, saying goodbye and starting over is the next step. Individuals might also begin to realize that while the romantic love stage made the relationship exciting and adventurous, a common commitment to basic values and ethics is missing. Admitting that "I don't feel the way I once did about you; I don't want to continue our relationship" is hard, but it's also honest and direct.

The fact that love does not dissipate completely may be one reason why breakups are so painful. While the pain does ease over time, ending a relationship in a way that shows kindness and respect can help both parties. Your basic guideline should be to think of how you would like to be treated if someone were breaking up with you. Would it hurt more to find out from someone else? Would it be more painful if the person you cared for lied to you or deceived you, rather than admitted the truth?

X AND Y FILES

Men, Women, and Online Dating

Online dating has transformed the dating process. Numerous studies have investigated the similarities and differences between male and female use of the Internet for dating purposes. While the findings of the studies are not generalizable among all heterosexual males and females, nor do they apply to all transgendered, lesbian, gay, bisexual, transgender, two-spirit, intersex, asexual, queer, or questioning individuals, they do provide some interesting information that might guide you should you decide to participate in online dating.

Misrepresentation of personal characteristics was a major finding. Explanations for gender differences in misrepresentation based on evolutionary psychology suggest that men and women will vary their self-presentation to emphasize traits that are desirable to the opposite sex.

- The strongest predictor of strategic misrepresentation was self-monitoring, which can be defined as the extent that someone is aware of social demands on his or her behaviour and then modifies it for that reason.
- Men were more likely to misrepresent themselves in general.
- Men were more likely to misrepresent personal assets.
- Women were more likely to misrepresent their weight.
- Older daters were more likely to misrepresent their age than younger daters, and men between the ages of 20 and 40 years were more likely to misrepresent their age than were women.
- After 50 years of age, men and women did not differ in the likelihood of misrepresenting their age.
- During the online courtship, men were more willing to, and were perceived to, lie more than women to achieve a short-term mating goal.

Sources: H.M. Lawson & M. Leck, "Dynamics of Internet Dating," *Social Science Computer Review*, Vol. 24 (2), Pg. 189–208, 2006; M.T. Whitty, "Revealing the "real" me, searching for the "actual" you: Presentations of self on an internet dating site," *Computers in Human Behavior*, Vol. 24 (4), Pg. 1707–1723, 2006; J.A. Hall, N. Park, H. Song, & M.J. Cody, "Strategic misrepresentation in online dating: The effects of gender, self-monitoring, and personality traits," *Journal of Social and Personal Relationships*, Vol. 27(1), Pg. 117–135, 2010.

For anyone who has struggled with betrayal or experiences a breakup they were not expecting, Dr. Janis Spring has some helpful advice and wise counsel about forgiveness and moving forward.[36] She describes *cheap forgiveness* as superficial and undeserved. Many of us give cheap forgiveness out of desperation to preserve a relationship. Be careful of giving this type of forgiveness. It often results in a cycle of more hurt and pain. *Refusing to forgive* might make you feel in control of the situation, but often deepens the feelings of regret and increases the feelings of revenge. It does not lead to reconciliation.

Acceptance is a form of forgiveness when the person who hurt you is not able to or will not attempt to participate in the healing process. You do not need to ask anything of the offender. It is a form of self-care, a way of restoring and integrating yourself. It is a way of opting for an incomplete and imperfect relationship or no future relationship at all with the person who hurt you or decided to leave the relationship. *Genuine forgiveness* is an exchange between two people. There are conditions. The person who has been hurt must allow for forgiveness. The person who changed the course of the relationship must either earn forgiveness or help the "hurt party" deal with the situation in a caring way.

Dysfunctional Relationships Relationships that do not promote healthy communication, honesty, and intimacy are sometimes called **dysfunctional.** Individuals with addictive behaviours or dependence on drugs or alcohol and the children or partners of those who had addictions sometimes find themselves in dysfunctional relationships. They occur in all economic and social groups.

At times, people have magical, unrealistic expectations that a relationship with the *right* person will make their life all right. They use their partners almost as if they were mood-altering drugs. The partner may compulsively try to get the other person to act the way they want them to. Both partners may end up deceiving or mistrusting the other. They begin to isolate themselves not only from each other but also from friends and other family members.

Physical symptoms, such as headaches, digestive troubles, and an inability to sleep, can be signs of a destructive relationship. It can be difficult to change the unhealthy dynamic of a relationship when one person may repeatedly attack, demean, dominate, abandon, betray, criticize, or bully the other person. Sociologist Jan Yager encourages us to ask ourselves if we want or have to keep the relationship going. If our answer is yes, we have to determine why we want the relationship to continue and how, and if we are willing to invest time and energy to turn it around."[37] Getting out of a dysfunctional relationship is difficult, but is sometimes the best thing to do.

Emotional Abuse Abuse consists of any behaviour that uses fear, humiliation, or verbal or physical assaults to control another human being. **Emotional abuse** often takes the form of constant berating, belittling, and criticism. Aggressive verbal abuse includes calling names, blaming, threatening, accusing, demeaning, and judging. Trivializing, minimizing, or denying what a person says or feels is a more subtle but equally destructive type of abuse. Sometimes done to teach or help another person, emotional abuse wears away at our self-confidence, sense of self-worth, and trust and belief in ourselves. Emotional abuse can leave deep, long-lasting scars.

In a survey of more than 1500 never-married undergraduate students, 25 percent reported that they had experienced at least two acts of physical abuse in a dating relationship, whereas only 12 percent believed they had ever physically abused their current or past dating partner. This discrepancy may be because of denial, ignorance, or acceptance of physical violence as a norm in a dating relationship.[38]

Among the signs of emotional abuse are

- attempting to control various aspects of your life—what you say or wear,
- frequently humiliating you—making you feel bad about yourself,
- wanting to know where you are—and who you are with—at all times,
- becoming jealous or angry—when you spend time with friends,
- threatening to harm you—if you have other interests or you are attempting to break off the relationship, and
- trying to coerce you—into doing anything that does not feel comfortable to you such as unwanted sexual activity.

If you find yourself in such a relationship, take steps to ensure your safety. Find a trusted friend who can help. Seek professional counselling.

COMMITTED RELATIONSHIPS

Even though men and women today may have more sexual partners than in the past, and may cohabit with a number of partners prior to committing to a lifelong relationship, many of them still yearn for an intense, supportive, exclusive relationship, based on mutual commitment that endures over time. In our society, many such relationships take the form of heterosexual or homosexual marriages, or long-lasting, deeply committed cohabitation relationships.

Partners who are in committed relationships and agree upon exclusive sexual involvement only with their partner practise **monogamy.** *Physical monogamy* can be defined as an exclusive physical sexual experience with one's partner and can include kissing, vaginal intercourse, oral sex, and anal sex. However, some men and women who desire to be thought of as monogamous do not necessarily practise monogamy. Kissing another person outside their primary relationship may not be considered by some as a violation of their monogamous relationship. In a study by Anderson on undergraduate heterosexual men, the definition of monogamous varied greatly among the subjects. Some of the participants in the study had oral sex, extradyadic intercourse, or threesomes with other females outside of their primary relationship without their partner's knowledge or permission, but still considered themselves to be monogamous.[39]

Emotional monogamy sets boundaries around emotional connections and affairs with others outside the primary relationship. This category is complex because it can include relationships at work, with friends, and online. For some, *social monogamy*—the perception of being monogamous by others—is more important than actually practising monogamous behaviour.[40]

A common practice among college and university students is **serial monogamy,** where a committed monogamous relationship is entered into until the relationship ends and another monogamous relationship begins. In an **open relationship,** partners agree to sexual involvement with others outside of their primary relationship. Open relationships are sometimes labelled as **polyamory,** where there is an acceptance of having intimate relationships with more than one person at a time, with both the knowledge and consent of everyone involved.

✓ CHECK-IN

How do you define commitment in a dating relationship?

Cohabitation Although couples have always shared homes in informal relationships without any official ties, "living together," or **cohabitation,** has become more customary in the last two decades. Cohabitation is also known as a common-law relationship.

For many young adults living together seems like a good way to get to know each other and find out if they are suited to each other. Other reasons are convenience, economics, and not wanting to live alone.

In Canada, the courts determine whether or not people are cohabiting by referring to seven factors:[41]

- **Shelter**—do the unmarried parties share accommodation?
- **Sexual and personal behaviour**—do the unmarried parties maintain an intimate interdependent relationship, and are they perceived by others to do so?
- **Services**—do the unmarried couple share the traditional functions of a family?
- **Social**—do the unmarried couple portray themselves as a couple to the outside world?
- **Societal**—how are the unmarried partners treated by their community?
- **Children**—do the unmarried couple see children as part of their home and interact parentally with each other's children, if there are any?

If you are considering cohabitation, you might want to learn about federal and provincial laws that guide common-law relationships. If your relationship discontinues there are legal issues you might be surprised you have to contend with.

If you and your partner have been working and have been contributing to the federal Canada Pension Plan, each partner can request a division of CPP benefits if you have lived together for 12 consecutive months. The same income-tax rules also apply to married and unmarried couples after 12 months. This may affect your income-tax deductions and possible returns.[42]

Provincial law determines many other issues. For example, in British Columbia, if you cohabit for two years in a marriage-like relationship and you decide to split up, child support and child custody is assessed the same way that married couples are assessed. Changes in B.C. law also mean that cohabiting couples will be able to claim for spousal support and a share of any common property. They will also divide equally the debts and assets that they share. Any pre-relationship property, inheritances, or gifts are excluded from the division.[43]

In Ontario, family law says that you must cohabit for three years for common-law relationship status. However, even if you have cohabited for this length of time, the division of property does not follow the same laws as if you were legally married. The legal concept known as "unjust enrichment" might force both parties in the relationship to document all property that was brought into the relationship and property acquired throughout the relationship. You might get out of the property division what you brought into the relationship if you have a legally signed cohabitation agreement in place. Even then, it may be difficult to have your rights enforced.[44] Before you decide to cohabit, check out the provincial and federal laws that are in place in Canada so there are fewer surprises should a breakup of your relationship occur.

Of course, laws governing the legal aspect of cohabitation are just one consideration. Personal values, long-term goals, and future family plans are just a few of the other things you will want to reflect upon as you prepare to share your life with another person.

Marriage As of 2011, Statistics Canada stopped collecting data on marriage, common-law relationships, divorce rates, and family household information.[45] However, using data from two different sources[46, 47] we can estimate that of the total population of Canada (35 589 809 people) at the end of 2015, 38.8 percent were married and approximately 9.2 percent were living in common-law relationships. Approximately 5.2 percent were divorced.

Not too long ago, marriage was often a business deal, a contract made by parents for economic or political reasons when the spouses-to-be were still very young. In some countries, arranged marriages are still culturally acceptable. Even in Canada, certain ethnic groups continue to plan marriages for their children. However, personal choice of marriage partners in Canada tends to be the norm. Generally, men and women marry people from the geographical area they grew up in and from the same social background. However, in our culturally diverse society, interracial, cross-cultural, and same-sex marriages are becoming more common and accepted. Although there have been studies that show the odds of failure are greater for long-term relationships that blend race and culture, many couples say these differences enrich their relationship.

Some of the traits that appeal to us when we are dating become less important when we select a mate; others become key ingredients in the emotional cement holding two people together in a relationship such as a marriage. According to psychologist Robert Sternberg, the crucial ingredients for commitment are the following:

- shared values
- a willingness to change in response to each other
- a willingness to tolerate flaws
- a match in religious beliefs
- the ability to communicate effectively

The single best predictor of how satisfied one will be in a relationship, according to Sternberg, is not how one feels toward a lover, but the difference between how one would like the lover to feel and how the lover actually feels. Feeling that the partner you have chosen loves too little or too much is, as he puts it, "the best predictor of failure."[48]

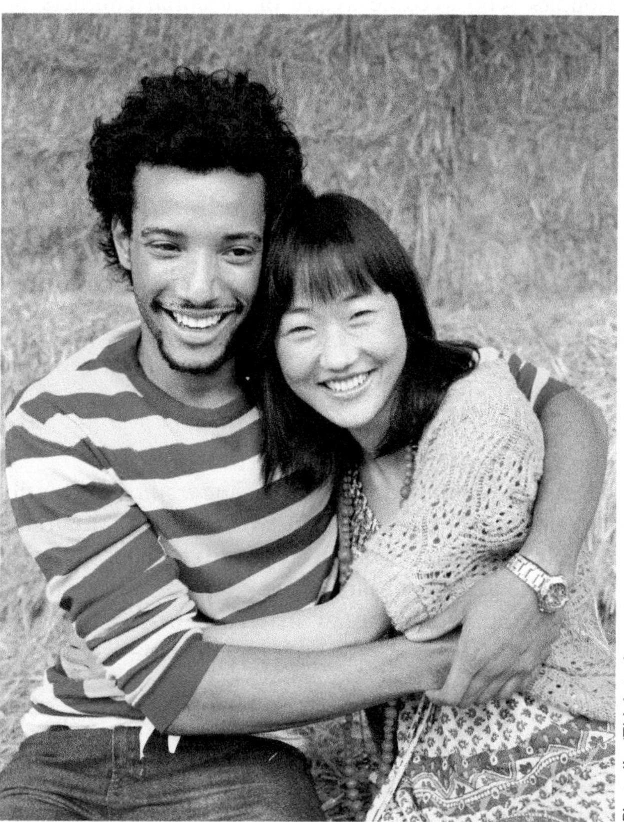

Photodisc/Thinkstock

STRATEGIES FOR PREVENTION

Things to Consider: When to Think Twice about Cohabiting or Getting Married

Don't rush into cohabitation or marriage if

- you or your partner is constantly asking the other such questions as "Are you sure you love me?";
- you spend most of your time together disagreeing and quarrelling;
- you're both still very young (under the age of 20);
- your boyfriend or girlfriend has behaviours (such as lack of responsibility), traits (such as bossiness), or problems (such as drinking too much or doing drugs) that affect the health of the relationship and that you hope will change after you live together or are married; or
- your partner wants you to stop seeing your friends, quit a job you enjoy, or change your life in some other way that diminishes your overall satisfaction.

Pre-cohabitation and Marital Assessments There are scientific ways of predicting marital happiness. Some pre-cohabitation and marital assessment inventories identify strengths and weaknesses in many aspects of a relationship: realistic expectations, personality issues, communication, conflict resolution, financial management, leisure activities, sex, children, family and friends, egalitarian roles, and religious orientation. Couples who become aware of potential conflicts by means of such inventories can sometimes resolve them through discussion or professional counselling. In other cases, reflection and reconsideration about the relationship occurs.

Other common predictors of relationship discord, unhappiness, and separation are

- a high level of arousal during a discussion, and
- defensive behaviours such as making excuses and denying responsibility for disagreements.

FAMILY TIES

Canadian families are changing. The traditional family structure that once included two heterosexual parents and children has shifted into a more complex variation of married couples that include families with or without children, common-law marriages or relationships, same-sex marriages, re-marriages, stepfamilies, empty-nesters, lone-parent families, multiple generations living together, and Canadians living alone. However, research commissioned by the Vanier Institute of the Family suggests that even though the traditional family structure is a minority in Canada today, many people still define family in a traditional sense.[49]

Our multicultural population is also redefining the changing face of the Canadian family. Immigrant Services Societies working with the Canadian government to resettle Syrian refugees in 2016 found that the families needing assistance were much larger than the average Canadian family. Many families had four or five children. Some had as many as eleven children. Housing families this large proved to be challenging.[50] Welcoming immigrant and refugee families to Canada has made many people reflect on their understanding of "family."

One of the major changes within a family setting in the past 10 years has been an increase in the number of young adults who continue to live with their parents throughout their 20s. Young adults in their early 20s are more likely to live with their parents than those in their late 20s. Young men are more likely to live at home than young women.

There has also been a decrease of young adults aged 20–29 living as couples. The latest data we can access from Statistics Canada in this regard is from a 2011 report where 30.8 percent were living as couples compared to 32.8 percent in 2006. If we look back to 1981, we discover that 51.8 percent of young adults in this age group were living as couples.[51]

Diversity within Families The 2001 Census[52] was the first to provide data on same-sex partnerships. The number of same-sex common-law couples was 34 200. The latest data available from Statistics Canada from the 2011 census showed that there were 64 575 same-sex couples, which included both married and common-law couples.[53]

Legalization of gay and lesbian marriage in Canada occurred with Parliament passing Bill C-38 on June 28, 2005.[54] Its passing ended a long, controversial debate, and Canada joined Belgium, the Netherlands, Spain, and the United States as countries granting same-sex couples the same benefits as heterosexual couples. The controversy surrounding this issue has been ongoing for many years. In 1967, then–Justice Minister Pierre Trudeau proposed amendments be made to the Criminal Code that would relax the laws against homosexuality. The amendments did pass in 1969, and homosexuality was decriminalized. Quebec became the first province to include sexual orientation in its Human Rights Code, in 1977. In 1979, the Human Rights Commission in Canada recommended that sexual orientation be added to the Canadian Human Rights Act.

It would not be until 2000, with the passing of Bill C-23, that same-sex couples who had lived together for more than a year would gain the same benefits and obligations as common-law couples. Yet the definition of marriage would still include the "lawful union of one man and one woman to the exclusion of all others." Two same-sex couples were married in Ontario in 2001, but the government refused to register them. At the same time, the B.C. NDP government issued legal proceedings against the federal government, seeking the right to marry same-sex couples.

In 2002, the Ontario Superior Court ruled that prohibiting gay couples from marrying was unconstitutional and violated the Charter of Rights and Freedoms. It gave Ontario two years to extend marriage rights to same-sex couples. In June 2003, Toronto began issuing marriage licences to same-sex couples after a ruling by the Court of Appeal for Ontario, whereby couples from anywhere could now marry—no residency limitations were required. In 2004, Quebec's appellate court ruled that same-sex marriage would be legal in the province.

On June 26, 2013, the Supreme Court in the United States struck down the Defense of Marriage Act (DOMA) in a five-to-four ruling that the federal law passed in 1996 violated the Fifth Amendment's equal-protection provision. The message became clear that same-sex marriages should be equal with all other marriages.[55]

WHAT IS SEXUAL AND GENDER IDENTITY?

Sexual Identity Sexual identity can be defined in two ways. When we define **sexual identity** based on *biology*, sexual identity begins at the moment of conception. All ova (eggs) carry an X chromosome. The sperm carry either an X or a Y chromosome. When a sperm carrying an X chromosome fertilizes an egg, the combination of the two (XX) chromosomes creates a female. When a sperm carrying a Y chromosome combines with an egg, the (XY) chromosome combination creates a male. The sex chromosomes then guide the development of the male and female **gonads** approximately eight days after conception. The job of the male gonads or testes and the female gonads or ovaries is the production of the sex hormones. These hormones support ongoing sexual development. The primary female hormones are estrogen and progesterone. The primary male hormone is testosterone. As the fetus begins to develop, female genitals form if there is no testosterone released. If testosterone is released the development of a penis begins.

When we reach **puberty**, sex hormones continue their work in sexual development. The **pituitary gland** releases hormones called gonadotropins that stimulate the testes and ovaries to increase production of the female and male sex hormones. This begins the development of **secondary sex characteristics**. For females this includes the development of breasts, menarche, widening of the hips, and the growth of pubic and underarm hair. For males, the voice changes, facial and body hair appear, and the penis and testes continue to develop.

Sexual identity can also be defined from a *personal self-identification perspective* and be based on how someone interprets who they are sexually attracted to. This sexual attraction could be to a member of the same sex or the opposite sex. Sexual identity may or may not be the same as sexual orientation as some individuals may be primarily attracted to the same sex but not think of themselves as gay, lesbian, or bisexual.[56]

Gender Identity and Gender Roles The term **gender**[57] is primarily based on the role we play or are expected to play by the society in which we live. It can be built on a sense of femininity or masculinity. Different from biological sex, gender is often based on cultural associations. Physical characteristics do not necessarily define one's gender. **Gender identity**[58] refers to a person's internal sense of themselves where they may identify as being male, female, or transgender. **Gender expression**[59] influences the way individuals manage their appearance, dress, behave, and present their gender identity. Gender expression can change. A drag king may present as a male during a public performance, but present as a female in daily life.

Gender roles are socially determined behavioural rules and standards assigned to men and women in our society. They have evolved and changed over the past century. For the first half of the 20th century, the primary role for women was to care for their family and home. While men were assigned the role of head of the household, most men worked outside of the home. Women who worked in the home were not viewed as being gainfully employed. Before 1931, in Canada, women were considered to have no occupation at all. Even when they did work in an unusual or non-traditional occupation, they were not included in the Canadian census.[60] Generalizations about male and female gender roles still exist today, but there has been a shift in understanding and acceptance of a blending of the roles of men and women. Now we must begin to understand and accept gender presentation and expression.

A person may identify his or her gender in a wide number of ways, such as the following:

- Male.
- Female.
- **Androgynous**—refers to people who identify as neither male nor female.
- **Intersex**—refers to people who were born with both male and female anatomy, or ambiguous genitalia. This term can also refer to an individual who physically falls between what is defined as male or female based on gender, hormones, internal organs, and chromosomal differences. For some this is seen as

a medical condition and for others it is seen as an identity. In some cases a doctor may decide on the sex of the newborn. For many intersex persons an awareness of being intersex occurs later in life.[61]

- **Transgender/trans person/trans folk**—an umbrella term for people whose gender identity or gender expression differs from the sex they were assigned at birth. This term is not indicative of sexual orientation, hormonal makeup, or physical anatomy. Transgender persons may feel themselves to be neither gender, to be both genders, or to be a gender other than their sex assigned at birth.[62]

Many other definitions of gender identity are possible, and some individuals choose to not label their gender at all.

Sexual Diversity Human beings are diverse in all ways—including sexual preferences and practices. Physiological, psychological, and social factors determine whom we are attracted to. This attraction is our **sexual orientation.** It can be defined as a socially constructed pattern of emotional, romantic, or sexual fantasies, desires, behaviours, and attractions to others. The sexual excitement for others can include an attraction to women, men, multiple genders, neither gender, or another gender.[63] Sigmund Freud argued that we all start off **bisexual**, or attracted to both sexes. As we reach adulthood we determine our preference for our sexual partners and discover our sexual orientation.

Heterosexual is the term used for individuals whose primary sexual orientation is toward members of the opposite sex.[64] Heterosexuality in our society is also broader than a form of sexual expression. It is an understanding of both sexual and non-sexual aspects of life. When one is heterosexual there is sometimes an assumption that a person will act in a specific way, that they will live their lives with a specific set of rules.[65] Some Canadians believe that heterosexuality is and should be the norm, and homosexuality and bisexuality are not normal. In reality, these orientations are opposite ends of a spectrum of sexual preferences. Sex researcher Alfred Kinsey devised a seven-point continuum representing sexual orientation. At one end of the continuum are those exclusively attracted to members of the other sex; at the opposite end are people exclusively attracted to members of the same sex. In between are varying degrees of homosexual, bisexual, and heterosexual orientation.[66]

A **homosexual** is defined as a person who is sexually or romantically attracted to or involved with individuals of the same sex.[67] Homosexuality exists in almost all cultures. Homosexual men and women are commonly referred to as *gay*; female homosexuals are also called *lesbians*. For decades, behavioural and medical specialists have debated whether homosexuality is biologically or socially determined. Some say that sexual orientation is genetically determined. Others contend that prenatal hormones influence sexual preference. Some recent studies suggest there is indeed a genetic link to homosexuality. However, the general consensus at this time is that there is not a clear specific determinant, but instead a number of factors that interact to make same-sex attraction and interaction more likely.[68]

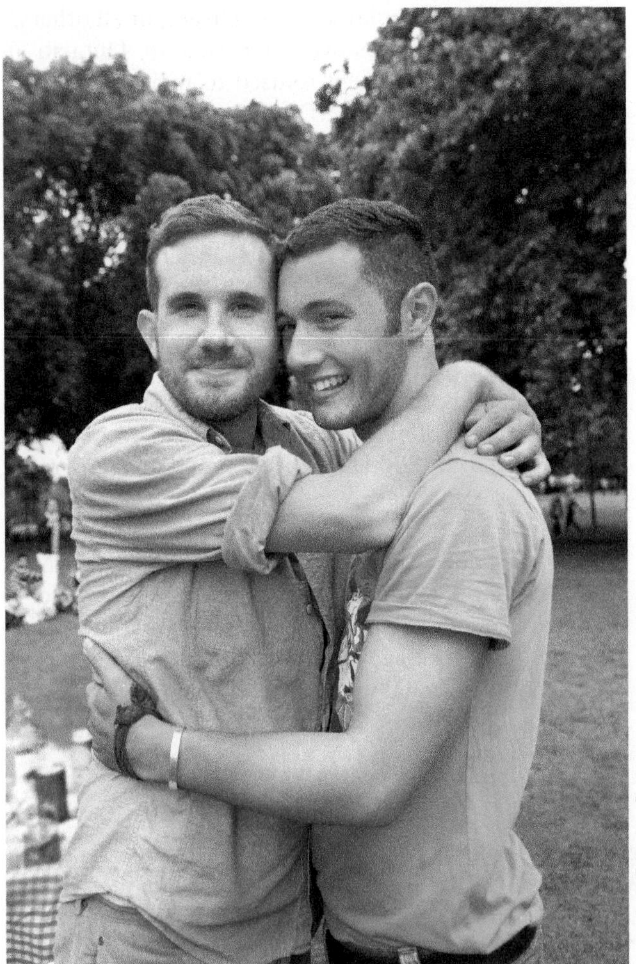

Paper Boat Creative/Getty

More gay couples are forming and celebrating committed and long-term relationships. Same-sex marriages are now legal in Canada and many states in the United States.

Homosexuality threatens some people. **Homophobia,**[69] the irrational fear and hatred of someone who is a homosexual, is evident in a number of ways in our society. Reactions range from subtle demeaning comments to an increase in *gay bashing* (attacking homosexuals) in many communities, including college and university campuses. Some blame the emergence of AIDS as a societal danger. However, researchers have found that fear of AIDS has not created new hostility but has simply given bigots an excuse to act out their hatred.

Gays and lesbians have conceived children in heterosexual relationships; others have become parents through adoption or artificial insemination. Their families are much like any other, and studies of lesbian mothers have found that their children are essentially no different from children of heterosexual couples in self-esteem, gender-related issues and roles, sexual orientation, and general development.[70]

> *In First Nations culture, some of the Elders taught that "**two-spirited**" people—gays and lesbians—were special, to be respected and honoured. They had specific duties and responsibilities to perform, including counselling, healing, and being visionaries. After colonization, many two-spirited First Nations peoples came to be ostracized from their own communities. There is a movement to reclaim traditions and a rightful place in the Aboriginal community. The 2 Spirited People of the 1st Nations is a nonprofit social service organization located in Toronto. This agency is attempting to provide a space where Aboriginal two-spirited people can come together as a community. A 2 Spirited People of the 1st Nations information guide provides educators culturally sensitive information on the history, teachings, and spirituality of two-spirited people.*[71]

Someone who is bisexual is physically, emotionally, or sexually attracted to individuals of both sexes.[72] Bisexuality can develop at any point in one's life. Some people identify themselves even if they do not behave bisexually. Individuals can be serial bisexuals—they are sexually involved with same-sex partners for a time and then with partners of the opposite sex at other times.

✓ CHECK-IN

How would you describe your attitudes toward sexual orientation and gender expression?

SEXUAL ACTIVITY

Part of learning about your own sexuality is learning about your own preferences for sexual satisfaction. Meeting your own sexual needs helps you understand how to meet others' sexual needs. Enjoying your sexuality is a life-long discovery process.

Sexual Intercourse There are four basic types of **sexual intercourse.** *Manual intercourse* occurs when the sex organs of one partner are in contact with the hand or hands of the other partner. *Oral intercourse* takes place when the sex organs of one partner are in contact with the mouth of the other partner. *Genital intercourse* happens when the sex organs of one partner are in contact with the sex organs of the other partner. *Anal intercourse*, as described below, is when the sex organs of one partner are in contact with the anus of the other partner.

We will describe one type of genital intercourse, vaginal intercourse, also known as coitus, here. Vaginal intercourse refers to the penetration of the vagina by the penis. This is a common form of sexual intimacy for many heterosexual couples, who may use a wide variety of positions. The most familiar position is the missionary position, with the man on top, facing the woman. An alternative is the woman on top, either lying down or sitting upright. Other positions include lying side by side, lying with the man on top of the woman in a rear-entry position, kneeling, or standing. Many couples move into several different positions for intercourse during a single episode of lovemaking; others may have a personal favourite or may choose different positions at different times.

Vaginal intercourse, like other forms of sexual activity involving an exchange of bodily fluids, carries a risk of sexually transmitted infections, including HIV. In many other parts of the world, in fact, heterosexual intercourse is the most common means of HIV transmission.

Anal Stimulation and Intercourse Because the anus has many nerve endings, it can produce intense erotic responses. Stimulation of the anus by the fingers or mouth can be a source of sexual arousal; anal intercourse involves penile penetration of the anus. As with oral-genital sex, not everyone feels comfortable with anal stimulation and anal intercourse. An estimated 25 percent of adults have experienced anal intercourse at least once. However, anal sex involves important health risks, such as damage to sensitive rectal tissues and the transmission of various intestinal infections, hepatitis, and STIs, including HIV.

Celibacy A celibate person does not engage in sexual activity. Complete **celibacy** means that the person doesn't masturbate (stimulate himself or herself sexually) or engage in sexual activity with a partner. In partial celibacy, the person masturbates but doesn't have sexual contact with others. Just as every person has the right to decide for themselves what degree of sexual activity they are comfortable with, a person's choice to not be sexually active at all must be respected. For some people, choosing to be celibate is an important part of their identity, faith, or belief system. People also make the decision to be celibate at certain times of their lives. Some don't have sex because of concerns about pregnancy or STIs; others haven't found a partner for a permanent, monogamous relationship. Many simply have other priorities, such as finishing school or starting a career, and believe that sex outside of a committed relationship does not support their physical and psychological well-being.

Kissing and Touching Many couples use kissing and touching as a way of arousing their partners in a sexual way. Areas of the human body that respond to kissing and touching are known as **erogenous zones.** These zones include both non-genital and genital areas. Some couples use massage as a way of sexually stimulating their partners.

Masturbation **Masturbation**, self-stimulation of the genitals, produces similar physical responses to those of sexual activity with a partner and can be an enjoyable form of sexual release.

Masturbation has been described as immature, unsocial, tiring, frustrating, and a cause of hairy palms, warts, blemishes, and blindness. None of these myths are true. Throughout adolescence and adulthood,

HUMAN POTENTIAL

Niki Hodgkinson—Redefining "Normal"

If asked to describe myself, I would say that I'm an athletic, kind, passionate, easygoing, and confident 30-year-old. I hope that when people spend time with me, they experience the above qualities. I am also Queer, and as much as I wish I lived in a world where such a descriptor was as neutral as "kind" or "athletic," I acknowledge that homophobia exists and such a label not only describes a part of me, but for many people triggers assumptions and judgments. I believe that in order to move towards a world free of discrimination, there must be a combination of visibility and education; this belief developed from my journey through my own homophobia, and has motivated my community involvement. Growing up in the 90s, I considered myself to be a "normal" kid; I had friends, played sports, had crushes on boys, and enjoyed games with gender-specific and gender-neutral toys. My friends and I would pass notes and cut out pictures from popular culture teen magazines of our favorite celebrities. I was consistently taught that it was normal and ideal for men to date woman, women to compete for handsome men, women to look pretty, and men to be stronger and more intelligent than women. Since I believed I was "normal," I also believed that those were expectations of me.

My first definition of the word "gay" came from a common use of the word by my friends and me to mean "weird," "undesirable," and "abnormal." We would use the word often as an expression of something or someone we didn't like; we would say, "That's so Gay!" The use of the phrase in that negative way became normalized, and at no point did we have any idea that it was homophobic. I cognitively understood that the word "gay" also meant people who dated other people of the same gender; however, that too seemed "abnormal," considering my education of the world around me. I knew that the word "gay" made adults around me uncomfortable and that our high school had a secret support group for gay kids at an undisclosed location. I also knew that adults whom I had assumed or guessed were gay had never actually expressed to me that they were, or talked about their life openly the way that straight adults did. So, even though my family raised me to respect all people and appreciate differences, I was inadvertently taught that being "gay" should be a big secret.

Denial kicked in when I began having feelings for a girl in high school; I thought that I just wanted to be her best friend. This denial was fuelled by my belief that I was "normal" and continued even after we began a relationship. Our relationship remained a secret because of my heteronormative upbringing until my desire for the relationship far outweighed my original expectations, so I "came out." The process of sharing with friends and family that I was in love with someone of the same gender appeared to mean much more than a difference in pronouns—girlfriend instead of boyfriend. It seemed as though people saw me differently and expected me to

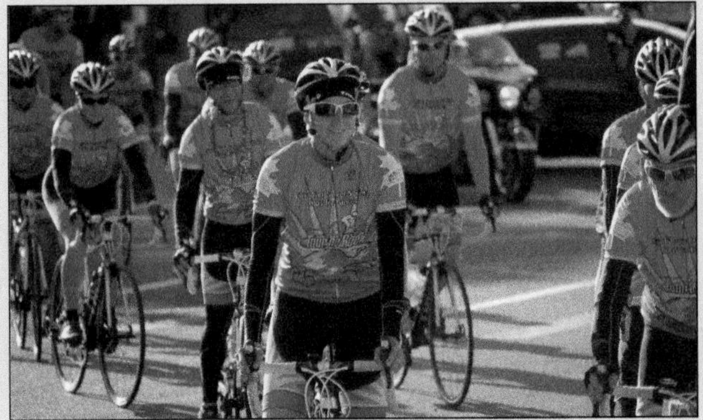

Jodi Lang

Niki Hodgkinson—athlete, police officer, and advocate for living in transparent ways.

know facts about queer history and homosexuality. My choice to be visible brought an expectation of an ability to advocate.

I educated myself in order to redefine my "normal" and became equipped with a knowledge base to advocate. I immersed myself in the queer community and began building a collection of queer role models. I vowed that I would combat the heteronormative environment I grew up in by sharing aspects of my life with people in the same way I would if I were in a heterosexual relationship; I would never avoid talking about my partner if the conversation was geared to it, and would tell the story as naturally as anyone would, without highlighting the fact that I was in a same-sex relationship. I joined the local school district's LGBTQ committee and coordinated a "'that's so gay' is not ok" campaign. I assisted with the Pride office on my University campus. I designed an anti-homophobia merchandising window at Lululemon, and initiated a local municipal police agency's involvement in the Pride parade.

I currently live as transparently as possibly, and apply my belief that visibility and education are required in order to move towards a world free of homophobia and transphobia. I have been a police officer for five years, and am currently in the Mountain Bike Section; prior to that, I was a youth worker for court-ordered programs and a specialized care home. I coach youth basketball and am on the Board of Directors for the Victoria Child Abuse Prevention and Counselling Center. I have fundraised for the Sexual Assault Center, and volunteered at community events for different causes. I was co-captain of the Canadian Cancer Society's Cops for Cancer Tour de Rock team in 2012, and have delivered numerous presentations on the topic of leadership. I have been engaged in my community while being honest about who I am, and have sought out learning about others. I am not an expert of Queer studies or diversity; however, I have lived through discrimination and hope that my future children will have a new definition of "normal" because they will have been educated inclusively and every person they meet will feel safe enough to be visible.

Source: Niki Hodgkinson

masturbation often is the primary sexual activity of individuals not involved in a sexual relationship, or when a partner is absent. It can also be useful when illness, divorce, and death deprive a person of a partner.

In a survey of college students, nearly all learned about masturbation through the media or through peers rather than from parents or teachers. Most of the female students reported struggling with feelings of stigma and taboo about enjoying masturbation. Most of the men saw masturbation as a part of healthy sexual development.[73]

Oral–Genital Sex Our mouths and genitals give us some of our most intense pleasures. Though it might seem logical to combine the two, some people are very uncomfortable with oral–genital sex. Some even consider it a perversion; it is a sin in some religions. However, others find it normal and acceptable.

The formal terms for oral sex are **cunnilingus**, which refers to oral stimulation of the woman's genitals, and **fellatio**, oral stimulation of the man's genitals. For many couples, oral–genital sex is a regular part of their lovemaking. For others, it's an occasional experiment. Oral sex with a partner carrying a sexually transmitted infection, such as herpes or HIV, can lead to infection, so a condom should be used. (With cunnilingus, a condom cut in half to lay flat can be used.)

Sexual Fantasies **Sexual fantasies** are also known as a form of autoerotic sexual behaviour. They are sexually arousing thoughts or dreams where individuals fantasize about sexual experiences. They can be used with masturbation.

Variant Sexual Behaviour **Variant sexual behaviour** is sometimes defined as unconventional behaviour. Other descriptions include non-conforming or divergent sexual behaviour. Some behaviours enhance the sexual experience. Some provide different options for a sexual experience. They can include bondage, exhibitionism, group sex, and the use of sex toys.

SEXUAL BEHAVIOUR

From birth to death, we are sexual beings. Our sexual identities, needs, likes, and dislikes emerge in adolescence and become clearer as we enter adulthood, but we continue to change and evolve throughout our lives. In men, sexual interest is most intense at age 18; in women, it reaches a peak in the 30s. Although age brings changes in sexual responsiveness, we never outgrow our sexuality.

How Sexually Active Are College and University Students? Many college and university students are concerned about their sexual health. They also report wanting more information about sexual health and relationships. While some students turn to their parents, guardians, and friends for sexual health education, Toews and Yazedjian, in a study of 1004 college students, discovered that the students were limited in their knowledge about contraceptives and sexually transmitted infections. They also found that (1) there was no difference in the age at which females and males became sexually active; (2) females had a more positive view about contraceptives and; (3) males had more permissive attitudes about sex.[74]

One of the largest surveys of Canadian postsecondary students was conducted during the spring of 2013. A total of 34 039 students from 32 different universities and colleges across Canada participated in the National College Health Assessment II. In addition to a number of health-related questions, students were also asked about their sexual behaviour. Following are the findings from this survey:[75]

- Overall, 45.3 percent of students had had one sexual partner in the previous 12 months. Males were somewhat higher at 47.5 percent compared to females at 30.4 percent. Only 8 percent had had four or more partners. Almost one-third of the students had had no sexual partners during that time.
- Forty-five percent of students indicated that they had had oral sex within the past 30 days. Almost 26 percent reported that they had had oral sex, but not within the past 30 days. Almost 30 percent had never had oral sex.
- Within the past 30 days, 49.5 percent of students had had vaginal sex; 19.3 percent had vaginal sex, but not in the past 30 days; and 31.2 percent of students had never had vaginal sex.
- Only 4.9 percent of students had had anal sex within the past 30 days; 19.4 students had had anal sex, but not within the last 30 days; and 75.7 percent had never had anal sex.
- Only 50.3 percent of students had used a condom or other protective barrier most of the time or always within the past 30 days when having vaginal intercourse.
- The most common form of contraception by the student or their partner was the use of birth control pills (monthly or extended cycle), reported by 64.3 percent of students.
- The use of male condoms and one other contraceptive method at the same time was used by 46.2 percent overall.

Another study done in partnership between the Sex Information and Education Council of Canada (SIECCAN) and Trojan, by an online survey of 1500 young people aged 18–24 years, as reported by Schwartz, found the following:[76]

- Sixty percent of men and 70 percent of women indicated that their last sex partner was either a spouse, fiancé, or committed romantic partner. Thirty percent of men and 23 percent of women disclosed that the last time they had had sex it was with a casual sex partner.

- When asked about current relationship status, just over 50 percent of men and 40 percent of women revealed that they were not dating. Thirty-four percent of men and 46 percent of women were either in a committed dating relationship, married, or living together.
- The data collected from this study also found that condoms and the birth control pill were the two top choices used for contraceptive methods.
- Generally, the majority of the respondents of the survey also implied that they were happy with their sex lives.

Students' sexual activity, particularly unsafe practices, often correlates with other risky behaviours. Researchers have found that students who misuse alcohol, are heavy drinkers, or use drugs are less likely to use condoms or other forms of protection or contraception.[77]

A substantial proportion of college students, both male and female, report that they engage in unwanted sexual activity. Sometimes this is the result of sexual coercion or alcohol use.[78] However, some students admit to feigning desire and consenting to an unwanted sexual activity for various reasons, including satisfying a partner's needs, promoting intimacy, and avoiding relationship tension.

College and university students do not always take precautions to reduce the risk of sexually transmitted infections (STIs). Often they believe that HIV and other infections could not happen to them, or they use misleading criteria in assessing risk. Men especially rely too much on a potential partner's physical attractiveness and give less consideration to sexual history. Women tend to insist on safe-sex practices with a new partner, but as they become more seriously involved, they use protection less often—a potentially dangerous practice since knowing someone better doesn't make sex safer.[79]

Research has also revealed that students who have a history of sexual trauma are at an increased risk of a number of harmful consequences linked to risky sexual behaviour. Victims of past sexual trauma often report more problems with substance abuse and the contraction of HIV.[80]

Some research has also been done to explore potential differences between cultures and their attitudes about sex. First-generation Asian-American university students were more tolerant and more accepting of sexual harassment.[81]

Sex and the Internet The Internet has become a new medium for relationships, including sexual relationships. In chat rooms, individuals can share explicit sexual fantasies or engage in the equivalent of mutual fantasizing. Individuals can assume any name, gender, race, or personality and can pretend to lead lives entirely different from their actual existences. Many see online sexual connection as a harmless way of adding an extra erotic charge to their daily lives. In some cases, individuals who meet online develop what they come to think of as a meaningful relationship and arrange to meet in person. Sometimes these meetings are awkward; sometimes they do lead to a real-life romance. Flirting and erotic activities on the Internet can build unrealistic expectations in the real world. When couples do meet in person, they often discover they are not physically or emotionally attracted to each other, and the relationship comes to an end.[82] While there is research that suggests we should be somewhat cautious about online dating, there is also research that suggests the many dating apps and online dating sites have proven to be very beneficial for many people. Relationships that begin online can be the beginning of a lifetime partnership.

The use of the Internet for sexual exploration can also lead, for some, to online sexual affairs, or cyber affairs. These romantic or sexual relationships, maintained through virtual contact, can be intrusive and detrimental to a primary relationship with a partner or spouse.[83] Researchers have discovered that both men and women consider online sexual interactions, whether sexual or emotional infidelity, a form of betrayal.[84, 85]

In other cases, the Internet can help to kindle new romances because people feel more comfortable expressing themselves. The anonymity factor provides a sense of personal space while allowing intimate communication. This effect is especially important for individuals who are shy, inhibited, or socially anxious in person, as it gives them a chance to get to know someone and share information about themselves with that person before actually meeting.[86]

If you take part in Internet dating, remember to protect yourself; people you meet online may not always be who they appear. In one study of Internet intimacy, 77 percent of men and 46 percent of women reported lying about themselves online, mostly about their age and physical appearance.[87] In another study, individuals who had sexual intercourse with partners they met through the Internet had a greater risk of sexually transmitted infections.[88]

Don't give out personal information over the Internet, such as your address or home phone number, and if you decide to meet someone in person, make sure you meet in public and let a friend know who you are going out with, what your plans are, and when you plan to return. Sexting—sending, receiving, or forwarding nude or semi-nude photos or videos and/or sexually explicit text messages via cellphones—can also have serious consequences. A survey sent to 1652 undergraduate college students showed that 65 percent of them had sent sexually explicit text messages or photographs to partners they were dating or hoped to date. Sixty-nine percent had received these types of messages and photographs. Thirty-one percent had actually shared these texts and images with a third-party friend. The majority of the students surveyed did think there could be negative consequences when sexting although some of the students had positive thoughts about sharing nude photographs. The survey results also showed significant differences between male and female students. The female students felt much more pressured to send text messages compared to the male students.[89] There are many news reports of cyberbullying that began with sexting messages. Some situations have resulted in serious mental health issues and suicides.

Safer Sex Having sex is never completely safe. Talking to a potential partner is the first step toward safer sex. Professionals offer advice on how to discuss a topic that makes many people uncomfortable: choose a time and place that is relaxed and comfortable. Arm yourself with facts so you can answer any questions or objections your partner raises. If you have had or still carry any STIs or are HIV-positive, this is the time for you to be honest. Give your partner time to take in what you have disclosed.

If you choose to be sexually active, you can reduce your risk of contracting sexually transmitted infections by undergoing and asking your partner to undergo medical examinations and testing for STIs and HIV/AIDs. Restricting sexual activity to a mutually exclusive, monogamous relationship is also a way of practising safe sex. Sober sex, in which both partners are not under the influence of drugs or alcohol, is more likely to be safer sex.

Sexual Concerns Many sexual concerns stem from myths and misinformation. There is no truth behind these misconceptions: men are always capable of erection, sex always involves intercourse, partners should experience simultaneous orgasms, and people who truly love each other always have satisfying sex lives.

Cultural and childhood influences can affect our attitudes toward sex. Even though Canadians' traditionally puritanical values have eased, our society continues to convey mixed messages about sex. Some children, repeatedly warned of the evils of sex, never accept the sexual dimensions of their identity. Young boys may be exposed to macho attitudes toward sex and feel a need to prove their virility. Young girls may feel confused by media messages that encourage them to look and act provocatively and a double standard that blames them for leading boys on. In addition, virtually everyone has individual worries. A woman may feel self-conscious about the shape of her breasts, a man may worry about the size of his penis, or both partners may fear not pleasing the other.

The concept of sexual normalcy differs greatly in different times, cultures, or racial and ethnic groups. In certain times and places, only sex between a husband and wife has been deemed normal. In other circumstances, "normal" has been applied to any sexual behaviour that does not harm others or produce great anxiety and guilt.

Sexual dysfunction is a broad term for a number of physical, psychological, or emotional problems that can interfere with healthy sexual functioning. Sexual dysfunction can occur for many reasons and throughout your lifetime. However, with medical assistance, healthy lifestyle choices, and a commitment from both partners, many sexual dysfunctions can be resolved.

A common sexual arousal disorder for men is **erectile dysfunction** or impotence. This term describes a condition where a man has difficulty maintaining a penile erection long enough for sexual intercourse. Erectile dysfunction can be caused by fatigue, diabetes, prostate problems, stress, alcohol, and depression. It can also be caused

STRATEGIES FOR CHANGE

How to Be Clear about Sexual Initiation and Consent

Understanding sexual initiation and consent requires communication between partners in heterosexual or same-sex relationships. Findings from two studies might provide some insights into sexual initiation and consent behaviours.[90,91]

- In general, nonverbal behaviours were used more frequently than verbal behaviours when initiating and responding to a partner's initiation for sex.
- Examples of nonverbal sexual initiation behaviours included hugging and caressing a partner, getting physically close, touching and kissing, smiling, rubbing and fondling a partner, and undressing a partner.
- Examples of nonverbal consent behaviours included hugging and caressing a partner in return, getting physically close to a partner, touching and kissing a partner in return, and smiling and letting the partner take off clothing.
- Examples of verbal initiation included talking about having positive feelings about having sex with the partner, saying that they wanted to have sex with their partner, and asking if it was okay to have sex with the partner.
- Examples of verbal consent included saying yes, responding in an affirmative way to comments about wanting to have sex with the partner, and asking if the partner did want to have sex.
- In heterosexual relationships women stressed the importance of asking for consent before initiating sex and that consent was necessary on an ongoing basis.
- In heterosexual relationships women more than men preferred that a verbal "yes" be asked for prior to any sexual advances even though the study indicated more nonverbal signals and cues were used during sexual encounters than verbal ones.

Remember that if saying no to sex puts an end to a relationship, it wasn't much of a relationship in the first place. If you are unsure you want to have sex with someone, give yourself time to think. It is all right to wait until you determine what your feelings are for that person. If your date wants to have sex and you are not sure you want to, it is all right to end the date without having sex. You can make plans for sex another time if you decide to see that person again.

by prescription medication. As men age, it also becomes more common. Treatment can include lifestyle changes, or medical treatments such as Viagra, Levitra, and Cialis.

Another orgasm disorder for males is **premature ejaculation**, where ejaculation occurs very quickly after the penis is inserted into the vagina. **Retarded ejaculation** is the inability to ejaculate once a man has an erect penis. Physical examinations, lifestyle changes, and sex therapy can assist men who are affected.

Sometimes women have a difficult time achieving an orgasm. The term used for this condition is **preorgasmic.** The causes can include fatigue, stress, depression, alcohol, lifestyle choices, and physical issues. Physical examinations and therapy can help. Masturbation is sometimes the first step in helping a woman achieve an orgasm. Then help from a partner can assist a woman in achieving an orgasm during a sexual encounter.

SEXUAL ANATOMY AND PHYSIOLOGY

This section will be a review for some and provide more detailed information for others. Knowing about both the female and male reproductive systems is another aspect of sexual health.

Female Sexual Anatomy and Physiology As illustrated in Figure 7-2(a), the **mons pubis** is the rounded, fleshy area over the junction of the pubic bones. The

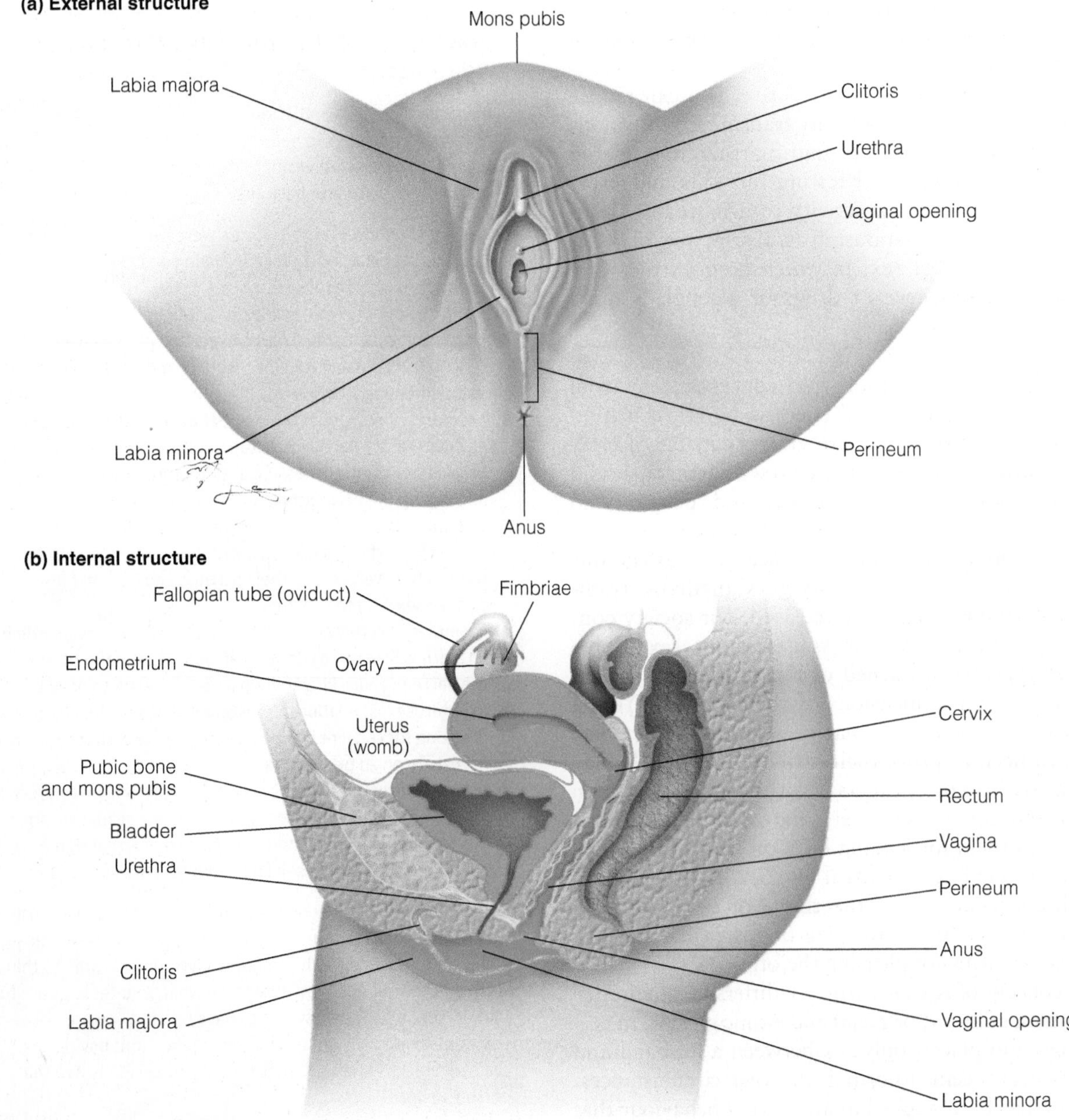

Figure 7-2 Female Sex Organs and Reproductive Structures

folds of skin that form the outer lips of a woman's genital area are called the **labia majora.** They cover soft flaps of skin (inner lips) called the **labia minora.** The inner lips join at the top to form a hood over the **clitoris,** a small elongated erectile organ and the most sensitive spot in the entire female genital area. Below the clitoris is the **urethral opening,** the outer opening of the thin tube that carries urine from the bladder. Below that is a larger opening, the mouth of the **vagina,** the canal that leads to the primary internal organs of reproduction. The **perineum** is the area between the vagina and the anus (the opening to the rectum and large intestine).

At the back of the vagina is the **cervix,** the opening to the womb, and **uterus** (see Figure 7-2(b)). The uterine walls are lined by a layer of tissue called the **endometrium.** Two **ovaries**—about the size and shape of almonds, with one on the left of the uterus and one on the right—contain egg cells called **ova** (singular, **ovum**). Extending outward and back from the upper uterus are the **fallopian tubes,** the canals that transport ova from the ovaries to the uterus. When an egg is released from an ovary, the finger-like ends of the adjacent fallopian tube catch the egg and direct it into the tube.

The Menstrual Cycle As shown in Figure 7-3, the hypothalamus monitors hormone levels in the blood and sends messages to the pituitary gland to release follicle-stimulating hormone (FSH) and luteinizing hormone (LH). In the ovaries, these hormones stimulate the growth of a few of the immature eggs stored in every woman's body. Usually, only one ovum matures completely during each monthly cycle. As it does, the ovaries increase production of the female sex hormone **estrogen,** which in turn triggers the release of a larger surge of LH.

At mid-cycle, the increased LH levels trigger **ovulation,** the release of the ovum from the ovary. Estrogen levels drop, and the remaining cells of the follicle then enlarge, change character, and form the **corpus luteum,** or yellow body. In the second half of the menstrual cycle, the corpus luteum secretes estrogen and larger amounts of **progesterone.** The endometrium (uterine lining) is stimulated by progesterone to thicken and become more engorged with blood in preparation for nourishing an implanted, fertilized ovum.

If the ovum is not fertilized, the corpus luteum disintegrates. As the level of progesterone drops, **menstruation** occurs—the uterine lining is shed during the course of a menstrual period. If the egg is fertilized and pregnancy occurs, the cells that eventually develop into the placenta secrete *human chorionic gonadotropin* (HCG), a messenger hormone that signals the pituitary not to start a new cycle. The corpus luteum then steps up its production of progesterone. It is important to note that the visual representation of a woman's menstrual cycle in Figure 7-3 uses 28 days as the average duration. Many women have cycles that vary and can be as short as 21 days or as long as 32 days. Some women also ovulate more than once a month.

Many women experience physical or psychological changes, or both, during their monthly cycles. Usually the changes are minor, but more serious problems can occur.

Premenstrual Syndrome Women with **premenstrual syndrome (PMS)** experience bodily discomfort and emotional distress for up to two weeks, from ovulation until the onset of menstruation. Some women develop very severe symptoms. In some studies, as many as 40–45 percent of women have reported at least one PMS symptom.

Once dismissed as a psychological problem, PMS has been recognized as a very real physiological disorder that may be caused by a hormonal deficiency: abnormal levels of thyroid hormone, an imbalance of estrogen and progesterone, and changes in brain chemicals. Social and environmental factors, particularly stress, also play a part. The most common symptoms of PMS are mood changes, anxiety, irritability, difficulty concentrating, forgetfulness, impaired judgment, tearfulness, digestive symptoms (diarrhea, bloating, constipation), hot flashes, palpitations, dizziness, headache, fatigue, changes in appetite, cravings (usually for sweets or salt), water retention, breast tenderness, and insomnia.

Treatments for PMS depend on specific symptoms. Diuretics (drugs that speed up fluid elimination) can relieve water retention and bloating. Relaxation techniques have led to a 60 percent reduction in anxiety symptoms. The use of bright lights to adjust a woman's circadian, or daily, rhythm also has proven beneficial. Behavioural approaches, such as regular physical activity, have helped. Charting cycles helps by letting women know when they're vulnerable.

Low doses of medications known as *selective serotonin-reuptake inhibitors* (SSRIs), such as fluoxetine (marketed as Prozac, Sarafem, or generic forms), provide relief for symptoms such as tension, depression, irritability, and mood swings.[92] Calcium supplements also may be beneficial.[93] Other treatments with some reported success include vitamins; less caffeine, alcohol, salt, and sugar; acupuncture; and stress-management techniques such as meditation or relaxation training.[94]

Premenstrual Dysphoric Disorder **Premenstrual dysphoric disorder (PMDD)**, which is not related to PMS, occurs in an estimated 3–8 percent of all menstruating women.[95] It is characterized by regular symptoms of depression (depressed mood, anxiety, mood swings, diminished interest or pleasure) during the last week of the menstrual cycle. Women with PMDD cannot function as usual at work, school, or home. They feel better a few days after menstruation begins. Medications used to treat PMS also are effective in relieving symptoms of PMDD.[96]

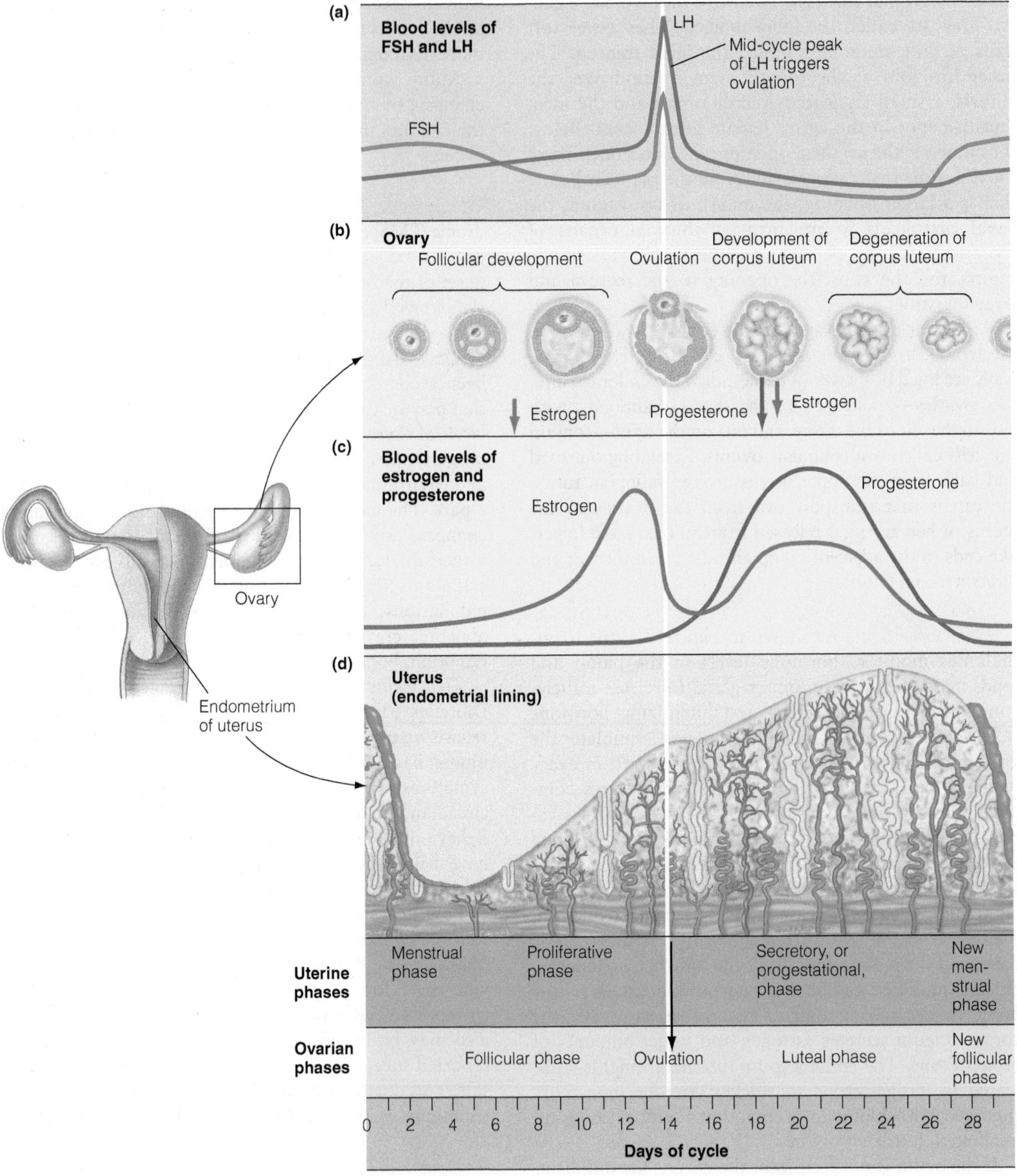

Figure 7-3 Menstrual Cycle

(a) In response to the hypothalamus, the pituitary gland releases the gonadotropins FSH and LH. Levels of FSH and LH stimulate the cycle (and in turn are affected by production of estrogen and progesterone).

(b) FSH does what its name says—it stimulates follicle development in the ovary. The follicle matures and ruptures, releasing an ovum (egg) into the fallopian tube.

(c) The follicle produces estrogen, and the corpus luteum produces estrogen and progesterone. The high level of estrogen at the middle of the cycle produces a surge of LH, which triggers ovulation.

(d) Estrogen and progesterone stimulate the endometrium, which becomes thicker and prepares to receive an implanted, fertilized egg. If a fertilized egg is deposited in the uterus, pregnancy begins. If the egg is not fertilized, progesterone decreases, and the endometrium is shed (menstruation). At this point, both estrogen and progesterone levels have dropped, so the pituitary responds by producing FSH, and the cycle begins again.

Menstrual Cramps **Dysmenorrhea** is the medical name for the discomforts—abdominal cramps and pain, back and leg pain, diarrhea, tension, water retention, fatigue, and depression—that can occur during menstruation. About half of all menstruating women suffer from dysmenorrhea. The cause seems to be an overproduction of bodily substances called *prostaglandins*, which typically rise during menstruation.

Women who produce excessive prostaglandins have more severe menstrual cramps. During a cramp, the uterine muscles may contract too strongly or frequently and temporarily deprive the uterus of oxygen, causing pain. Medications that inhibit prostaglandins can reduce menstrual pain, and exercise can also relieve cramps.

Amenorrhea Women may stop menstruating—a condition called **amenorrhea**—for a variety of reasons, including a hormonal disorder, drastic weight loss, or a change in the environment. Distance running and strenuous exercise also can lead to amenorrhea. The reason may be a drop in body fat from the normal range of 18–22 percent to a range of 9–12 percent. A woman is considered to have amenorrhea if her menstrual cycle is typically absent for three or more consecutive months. Prolonged amenorrhea can have serious health consequences, including a loss of bone density that may lead to stress fractures or osteoporosis.

In recent years, scientists have discovered that the menstrual cycle actually begins in the brain with the production of gonadotropin-releasing hormone (GnRH). Each month a surge of GnRH sets into motion the sequence of steps that lead to ovulation, the potential for conception, and, if conception doesn't occur, menstruation. This understanding has led to the development of chemical mimics, or analogues, of GnRH—usually administered by nasal spray—that trigger ovulation in women who don't ovulate or menstruate normally.

Toxic Shock Syndrome This rare, potentially deadly bacterial infection primarily strikes menstruating women under the age of 30 who use tampons. Both *Staphylococcus* aureus and group A *Streptococcus pyogenes* can produce **toxic shock syndrome (TSS)**. Symptoms include a high fever; a rash that leads to peeling of the skin on the fingers, toes, palms, and soles; dizziness; dangerously low blood pressure; and abnormalities in several organ systems (the digestive tract and the kidneys) and in the muscles and blood. Treatment usually consists of antibiotics and intense supportive care; intravenous administration of immunoglobulins that attack the toxins produced by these bacteria also may be beneficial.

To reduce the risk of TSS, menstruating women should use sanitary napkins instead of tampons. If tampons are used, they should be changed every four to eight hours and a switch to less-absorbent tampons should be made as the menstrual flow decreases.[97]

Male Sexual Anatomy and Physiology The visible parts of the male sexual anatomy are the **penis** and the **scrotum**, the pouch that contains the **testis or testes (testicles)** (see Figure 7-4). The testes manufacture **testosterone**, the hormone that stimulates the development

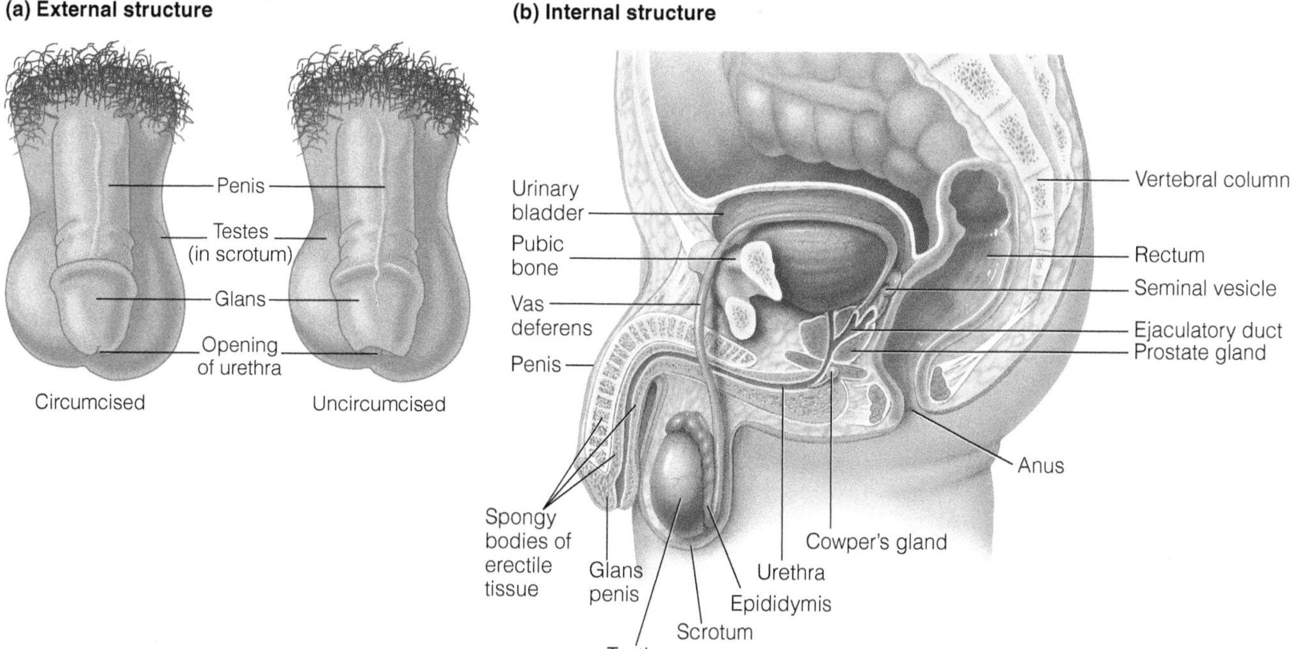

Figure 7-4 Male Sex Organs and Reproductive Structures

STRATEGIES FOR PREVENTION

Preventing Premenstrual Problems

- Get plenty of exercise. Physically fit women usually have fewer problems both before and during their periods.
- Eat frequently and nutritiously. In the week before your period, your body doesn't regulate the levels of sugar, or glucose, in your blood as well as it usually does.
- Swear off salt. If you stop using salt at the table and while cooking, you may gain less weight premenstrually, feel less bloated, and suffer less from headaches and irritability.
- Cut back on caffeine. Coffee, colas, diet colas, chocolate, and tea can increase breast tenderness and other symptoms.
- Don't drink or smoke. Some women become so sensitive to alcohol's effects before their periods that a glass of wine hits with the impact of several stiff drinks. Nicotine worsens low blood-sugar problems.
- Watch out for sweets. Premenstrual cravings for sweets are common. Sugar may pick you up, but later you'll feel worse than before.

of a male's secondary characteristics, and **sperm**, the male reproductive cells. Immature sperm are stored in the **epididymis**, a collection of coiled tubes adjacent to each testis.

The penis contains three hollow cylinders loosely covered with skin. The two major cylinders, the *corpora cavernosa*, extend side by side through the length of the penis. The third cylinder, the *corpus spongiosum*, surrounds the **urethra**, the channel for both seminal fluid and urine (see Figure 7-4).

When hanging down loosely, the average penis is about 9 centimetres long. During erection, its internal cylinders fill with so much blood that they become rigid, and the penis stretches to an average length of 15 centimetres. About 90 percent of all men have erect penises measuring between 12 and 18 centimetres in length. A woman's vagina naturally adjusts during intercourse to the size of her partner's penis.

Inside the body are several structures involved in the production of seminal fluid, or **semen**, the liquid in which sperm cells are carried out of the body during ejaculation. The **vas deferens** are two tubes that carry sperm from the epididymis into the urethra. The **seminal vesicles**, which make some of the seminal fluid, join with the vas deferens to form the **ejaculatory ducts**. The **prostate gland** produces some of the seminal fluid, which it secretes into the urethra during ejaculation. The **Cowper's glands** are two pea-sized structures on either side of the urethra (just below where it emerges from the prostate gland) and connected to it via tiny ducts. When a man is sexually aroused, the Cowper's glands often secrete a fluid that appears as a droplet at the tip of the penis. This fluid is not semen, although it occasionally contains sperm.

Circumcision In its natural state, the tip of the penis is covered by a fold of skin called the *foreskin*. In some instances this foreskin is removed. The procedure is called **circumcision**. In Canada in 1996–1997, circumcision was performed as common procedure on about 20 percent of newborn Canadian male babies. The latest data shows that the current circumcision rate in Canada is about 32 percent depending on provincial and territorial fluctuations.[98] In the United States the rate of circumcision currently stands at about 58 percent of males.[99] Reasons vary from religious traditions to preventive health measures.

Until the last half century, scientific evidence to support or repudiate routine circumcision was limited. A review of 40 years of data concluded that although there are potential medical benefits, the data are not strong enough to recommend routine neonatal circumcision.[100] However, other experts, challenging this view, argue that lack of circumcision increases the risk of sexually transmitted infections, including HIV and syphilis. The Canadian Paediatric Society is working on a new policy that will attempt to put forward a balanced position that takes into the consideration the risks, benefits, and religious issues. This will continue to be a difficult decision for some parents.[101]

SELF-SURVEY

Healthy Relationship Quiz

Everyone deserves to be in a safe and healthy relationship. Do you know if your relationship is healthy? Answer Yes or No to the following questions to find out. Make sure to write down your responses. At the end, you'll find out how to score your answers.

The person I'm with

1. is very supportive of things that I do. ❑ YES ❑ NO
2. encourages me to try new things. ❑ YES ❑ NO
3. likes to listen when I have something on my mind. ❑ YES ❑ NO
4. understands that I have my own life too. ❑ YES ❑ NO
5. is not liked very well by my friends. ❑ YES ❑ NO
6. says I'm too involved in different activities. ❑ YES ❑ NO
7. texts me or calls me all the time. ❑ YES ❑ NO
8. thinks I spend too much time trying to look nice. ❑ YES ❑ NO
9. gets extremely jealous or possessive. ❑ YES ❑ NO
10. accuses me of flirting or cheating. ❑ YES ❑ NO
11. constantly checks up on me or makes me check in. ❑ YES ❑ NO
12. controls what I wear or how I look. ❑ YES ❑ NO
13. tries to control what I do and who I see. ❑ YES ❑ NO
14. tries to keep me from seeing or talking to my family and friends. ❑ YES ❑ NO
15. has big mood swings, getting angry and yelling at me one minute but being sweet and apologetic the next. ❑ YES ❑ NO
16. makes me feel nervous or like I'm "walking on eggshells." ❑ YES ❑ NO
17. puts me down, calls me names, or criticizes me. ❑ YES ❑ NO
18. makes me feel like I can't do anything right or blames me for problems. ❑ YES ❑ NO
19. makes me feel like no one else would want me. ❑ YES ❑ NO
20. threatens to hurt me, my friends, or my family. ❑ YES ❑ NO
21. threatens to hurt him or herself because of me. ❑ YES ❑ NO
22. threatens to destroy my things. ❑ YES ❑ NO
23. grabs, pushes, shoves, chokes, punches, slaps, holds me down, throws things, or hurts me in some way. ❑ YES ❑ NO
24. breaks or throws things to intimidate me. ❑ YES ❑ NO
25. yells, screams, or humiliates me in front of other people. ❑ YES ❑ NO
26. pressures or forces me into having sex or going farther than I want to. ❑ YES ❑ NO

Scoring

Give yourself one point for every No you answered to numbers one through four, one point for every Yes response to numbers five through eight, and five points for every Yes to numbers nine and above.

Now that you're finished and have your score, the next step is to find out what it means. Simply take your total score and see which of the categories below apply to you.

Score: 0 Points

You got a score of zero? Don't worry—it's a good thing! It sounds like your relationship is on a pretty healthy track. Maintaining healthy relationships takes some work—keep it up! Remember that while you may have a healthy relationship, it's possible that a friend of yours does not. If you know someone who is in an abusive relationship, find out how you can help them.

Score: 1–2 Points

If you scored one or two points, you might be noticing a couple of things in your relationship that are unhealthy, but it doesn't necessarily mean they are warning signs. It's still a good idea to keep an eye out and make sure there isn't an unhealthy pattern developing.

The best thing to do is to talk to your partner and let him or her know what you like and don't like. Encourage your partner to do the same. Remember, communication is always important when building a healthy relationship. It's also good to be informed so you can recognize the different types of abuse.

Score: 3–4 Points

If you scored three or four points, it sounds like you may be seeing some warning signs of an abusive relationship. Don't ignore these red flags. Something that starts small can grow much worse over time. No relationship is perfect—it takes work! But in a healthy relationship you won't find abusive behaviours.

Score: 5 or More Points

If you scored five or more points, you are definitely seeing warning signs and may be in an abusive relationship. Remember the most important thing is your safety—consider making a safety plan right now.

Source: Courtesy loveisrespect.org. Healthy Relationship Quiz. Found at: http://www.loveisrespect.org/dating-basics/healthy-relationships/healthy-relationships-text-only-quiz

Chapter Summary

1. Which statement about friendships and other intimate relationships is NOT true?
   a. Friends can communicate feelings as well as facts.
   b. Listening is just as important as talking.
   c. Emotional investment is required but the rewards are great.
   d. There is no need to pay attention to nonverbal communication.
2. Which of the following is a characteristic of a good relationship?
   a. trust
   b. financial stability
   c. identical interests
   d. physical attractiveness
3. When looking for a mate, what is one of the crucial ingredients for commitment?
   a. shared values and a willingness to tolerate flaws
   b. desire to make the relationship work and a financial plan
   c. cohabitation and happiness
   d. a verbal commitment and discussion
4. Which statement about partners in successful marital relationships is true?
   a. They are generally from the same social and ethnic background.
   b. They usually lived together before marrying.
   c. They were usually very young at the time of their marriage.
   d. They have premarital agreements.
5. Hooking up is loosely defined as
   a. a committed relationship
   b. an exclusive relationship
   c. sexual activity with a casual partner who may be a friend or a stranger
   d. a long distance relationship
6. Which statement about menstruation and the menstrual cycle is true?
   a. Prolonged amenorrhea is not a concern.
   b. Premenstrual syndrome is a physiological disorder that usually results in amenorrhea.
   c. Ovulation occurs at the end of the menstrual cycle.
   d. Distance running can lead to amenorrhea.
7. Which statement about male anatomy is NOT correct?
   a. The testes manufacture testosterone and sperm.
   b. Sperm cells are carried in the liquid semen.
   c. Cowper's glands secrete semen.
   d. Circumcision is the surgical removal of the foreskin of the penis.
8. From which of the following do young Canadians primarily learn about relationships and sexuality?
   a. their parents, friends, and sex-education classes
   b. the Internet
   c. the media
   d. books
9. Which statement about sexual orientation is true?
   a. Most individuals who identify themselves as bisexual are really homosexual.
   b. Homosexuality is caused by a poor family environment.
   c. Homosexual behaviour is found only in affluent and well-educated cultures.
   d. Homosexuality exists in almost all cultures.
10. Which of the following is the best definition of abstinence?
    a. refraining from oral sex
    b. refraining from all sexual activities that involve vaginal, anal, and oral intercourse
    c. having sexual intercourse with only one partner
    d. refraining from drinking alcohol before sexual activity

Answers to these questions can be found on page 188.

SELF-RESPONSIBILITY—SOCIAL RESPONSIBILITY

SELF-RESPONSIBILITY

The Law of Giving—

Every relationship is one of give and take; if you stop the flow of either, you interfere with nature's intelligence.

Deepak Chopra

Building relationships takes time, energy, and commitment. In Prochaska's Stages of Change model, maintenance also demands care and attention to avoid a relapse. If you are in a relationship that is lacking in enthusiasm and energy, commitment and caring, it may be time to reevaluate why this is so. What can you do to rejuvenate this relationship? Spend more time together? Seek out new adventures? Make a change in lifestyle habits that encourage healthy lifelong living? Take time to give and take.

SOCIAL RESPONSIBILITY

Go out into the world today and love the people you meet. Let your presence light new light in the hearts of people.

Mother Teresa

CRITICAL THINKING

1. While our society has become more tolerant, marriages between people of different religious and racial groups still face special pressures. What issues might arise if you marry someone from another culture? How could these issues be resolved? What are your own feelings about mixed marriages? Would you date someone of a different religion or race? Why or why not?
2. What are your personal criteria for a successful relationship? Develop a brief list of factors you consider important, and support your choices with examples or experiences from your own life.
3. Bill told his girlfriend, Anita, that he has never taken any sexual risks. But when she suggested that they get tested for STIs, he became furious and refused. Anita doesn't want to take any risks, but she doesn't want to lose him either. What would you advise her to say or do? What would you advise Bill to say or do?

WEB LINKS

The Canadian Sex Research Forum
www.canadiansexresearchforum.com
The Canadian Sex Research Forum is a valuable website that provides up-to-date information for teachers, researchers, and clinical practitioners who are involved in the area of human sexuality and sexual behaviour. You can access newsletters, annual conference information, and a special student page.

International Association for Relationship Research
www.iarr.org
This site contains links to professional organizations and publications that support research about relationships.

Sex Information and Education Council of Canada
www.sieccan.org
SIECCAN, a national nonprofit educational organization, provides both the public and professionals with human sexuality education.

SexualityandU
www.sexualityandu.ca
This site provides up-to-date information and education on sexual and gender orientation, STIs, and contraception FAQs.

The Vanier Institute of the Family
www.vifamily.ca
This site has many interesting articles on family facts and family issues. Lists of publications and links to other professional organizations are also available.

Please note that links are subject to change. If you find a broken link, use a search engine such as www.google.ca and search for the website by typing in keywords.

Key Terms

The terms listed here are used within the chapter on the page indicated. Definitions of the terms are in the Glossary at the end of the book.

amenorrhea 183
androgynous 173
bisexual 174
celibacy 175
cervix 181
circumcision 184
clitoris 181
cohabitation 170
corpus luteum 181
Cowper's glands 184
cunnilingus 177
dysfunctional 169
dysmenorrhea 183
ejaculatory ducts 184
emotional abuse 169
endometrium 181
epididymis 184
erectile dysfunction 179
erogenous zones 175
estrogen 181
fallopian tubes 181
fellatio 177
friends with benefits (FWB) 163
gender 173
gender expression 173
gender identity 173
gender roles 173
gonads 173
heterosexual 174
homophobia 174
homosexual 174
hooking up 164

infidelity 165
intersex 173
intimacy 167
labia majora 181
labia minora 181
masturbation 176
menstruation 181
monogamy 170
mons pubis 180
open relationship 170
ovaries 181
ovulation 181
ovum (ova) 181
penis 183
perineum 181
pituitary gland 173
polyamory 170
premature ejaculation 180
premenstrual dysphoric disorder (PMDD) 181
premenstrual syndrome (PMS) 181
preorgasmic 180
progesterone 181
prostate gland 184
puberty 173
retarded ejaculation 180
scrotum 183
secondary sex characteristics 173
semen 184
seminal vesicles 184
serial monogamy 170
sexual dysfunction 179
sexual fantasies 177
sexual identity 173
sexual intercourse 175
sexual orientation 174
sperm 184
testis (testes, testicles) 183
testosterone 183
toxic shock syndrome (TSS) 183
transgender/trans person/trans folk 174
two-spirited 175
urethra 184
urethral opening 181
uterus 181
vagina 181
variant sexual behaviour 177
vas deferens 184

Answers to Chapter Summary Questions

1. d; 2. a; 3. a; 4. a; 5. c; 6. d; 7. c; 8. a; 9. d; 10. b

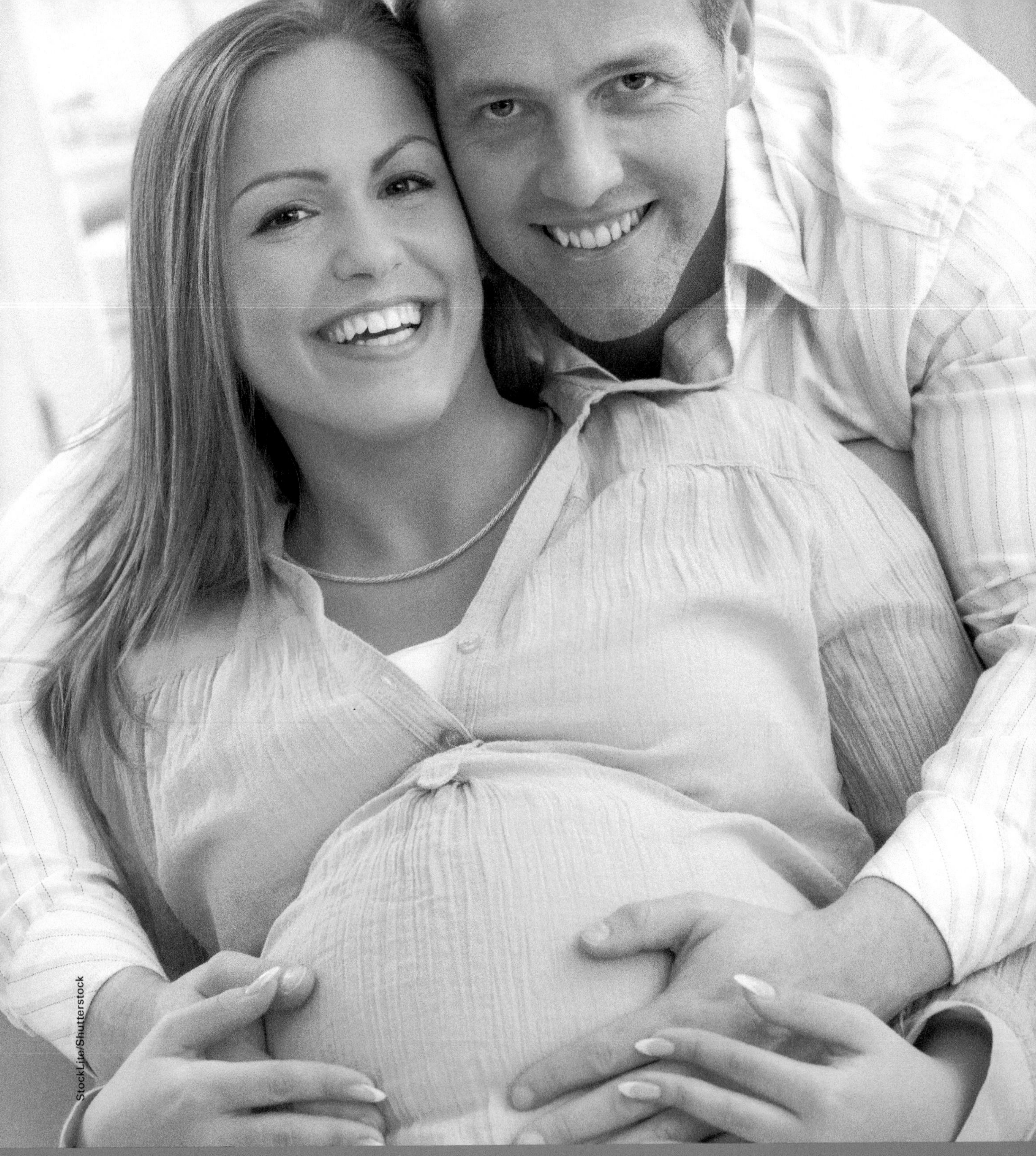
StockLite/Shutterstock

AFTER READING THIS CHAPTER, YOU WILL BE ABLE TO:

- **describe** the process of human conception
- **list** the major options available for contraception and **identify** the advantages and risks of each
- **describe** the commonly used abortion methods
- **discuss** the physiological effects of pregnancy on a woman and **describe** fetal development
- **describe** the three stages of labour and the birth process
- **give examples** of infertility treatments

8

Birth Control Choices and Pregnancy

As human beings, we have a unique power—the ability to choose to conceive or not to conceive. No other species on Earth can separate sexual activity and pleasure from reproduction. However, simply not wanting to get pregnant is never enough to prevent conception nor is planning to have a child always enough to get pregnant. Both require individual decisions and actions.

Mature sexual relationships include the ability to discuss, with your partner, past sexual history, STI (sexually transmitted infections) testing, STI protection, birth control options, and personal attitudes and values with regard to the possibility of pregnancy and responsibility for the child who might be conceived. Conscientious sexual relationships also demand ongoing education about the benefits and risks of different types of birth control available or how to plan for a healthy pregnancy.

While some people are concerned about the risks associated with contraception, medical professionals suggest that using birth control can be a safe and healthy option for most people. According to Peipert et al.,[1] the use of contraceptives, including oral contraceptives, saves lives each year, prevents unplanned pregnancies, can increase the enjoyment of sexual pleasure by reducing stress levels with regard to pregnancy, and can lower the risk of sexually transmitted infections.

This chapter provides information on conception, birth control options, and abortion. It also includes a section on the pro-life viewpoint. The chapter ends with an overview of pregnancy, childbirth, and infertility issues.

FREQUENTLY ASKED QUESTIONS

CONCEPTION

The equation for making a baby is quite simple: one sperm plus one egg equals one fertilized egg, which can develop into an infant. But the processes that affect or permit **conception** are quite complicated. The creation of sperm, or **spermatogenesis**, starts in the male at puberty, and the production of sperm is regulated by hormones (see Figure 8-1). Sperm cells form in the seminiferous tubules of the testes and are passed into the epididymis, where they are stored until ejaculation; a single male ejaculation may contain 500 million sperm. Each sperm released into the vagina during intercourse moves on its own, propelling itself toward its target: an ovum.

To reach its goal, the sperm must move through the acidic secretions of the vagina, enter the uterus, travel up the fallopian tube containing the ovum, then fuse with the nucleus of the egg (**fertilization**). Just about every sperm produced by a man in his lifetime fails to accomplish its mission.

There are far fewer human egg cells than there are sperm cells. Each woman is born with her lifetime supply of ova, and between 300 and 500 eggs eventually mature and leave her ovaries during ovulation. Every month, one or the other of the woman's ovaries releases an ovum to the nearby fallopian tube. It travels through the fallopian tube until it reaches the uterus, a journey that takes three to four days. An unfertilized egg lives for about 24–36 hours, disintegrates, and, during menstruation, is expelled along with the uterine lining.

Even if a sperm, which can survive in the female reproductive tract for two to five days, meets a ripe egg in a fallopian tube, its success is not assured. It must penetrate the layer of cells and a jellylike substance that surrounds each egg. Every sperm that touches the egg deposits an enzyme that dissolves part of this barrier. When a sperm bumps into a bare spot, it can penetrate the egg membrane and merge with the egg (see Figure 8-2). The fertilized egg travels down the fallopian tube, dividing to form a tiny clump of cells called a **zygote**. When it reaches the uterus, about a week after fertilization, it burrows into the endometrium, the lining of the uterus. This process is called **implantation.**

Conception can be prevented by **contraception.** Some contraceptive methods prevent ovulation or implantation, and others block the sperm from reaching the egg. Some methods are temporary; others permanently alter one's fertility.

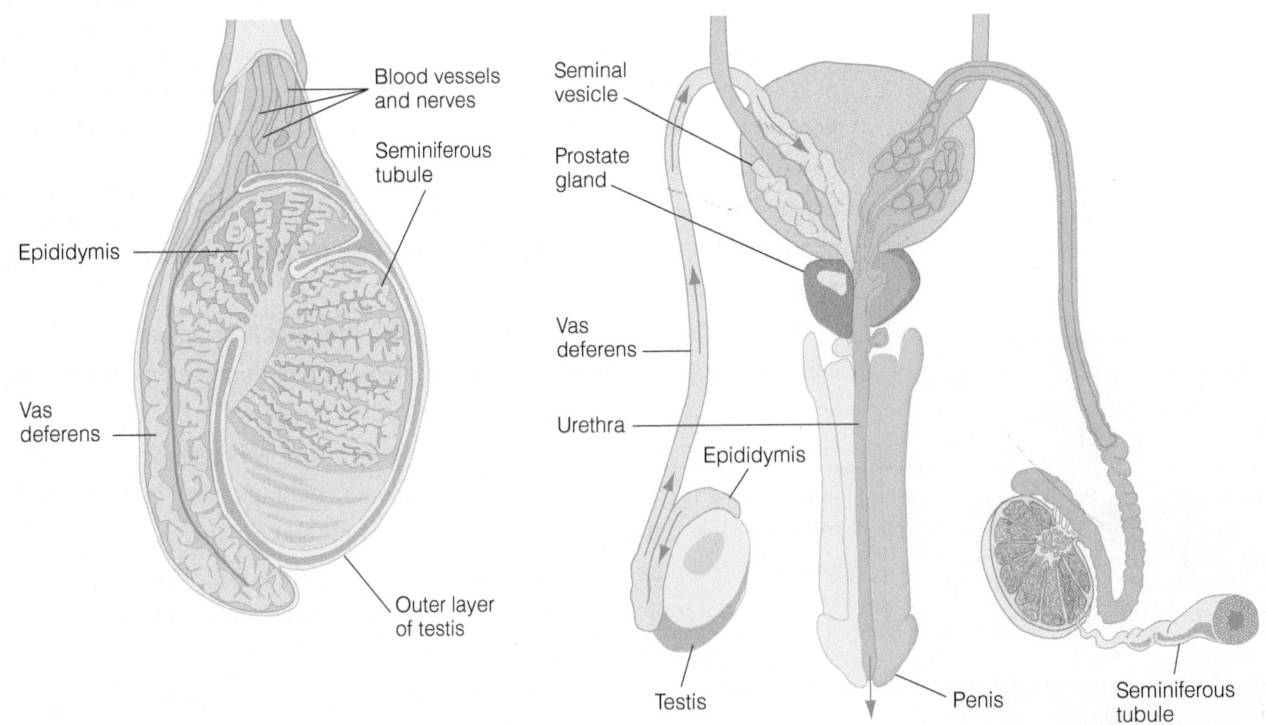

Figure 8-1 The Testes

Spermatogenesis takes place in the testes. Sperm cells form in the seminiferous tubules and are stored in the coils of the epididymis. Eventually, the sperm drain into the vas deferens, ready for ejaculation.

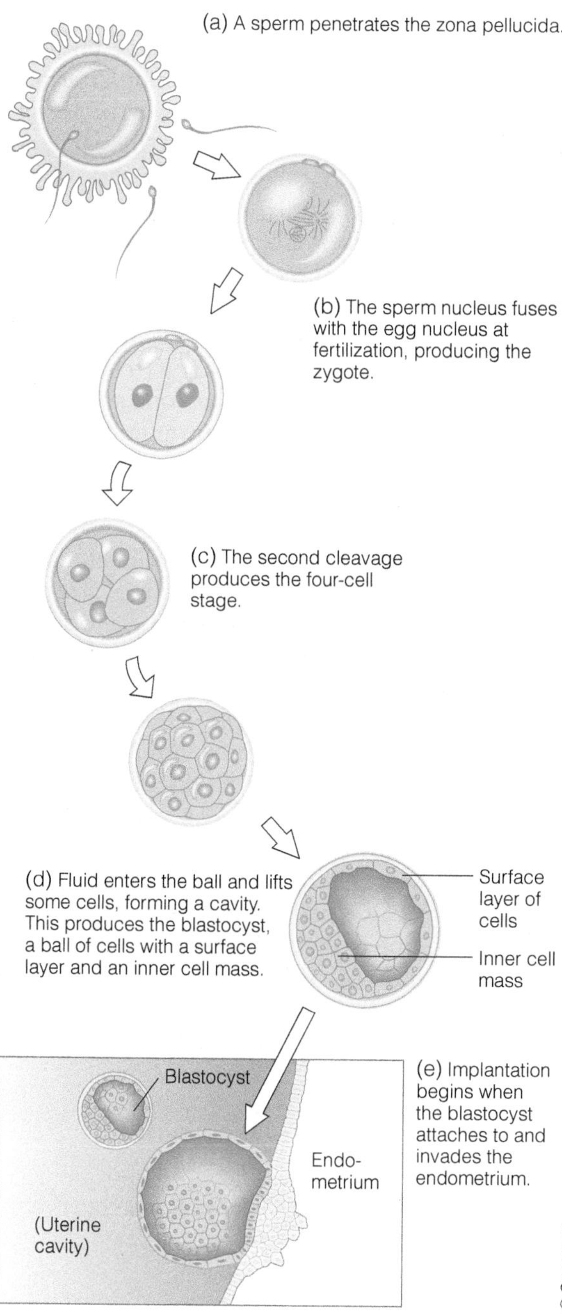

Figure 8-2 Fertilization

(a) The efforts of hundreds of sperm allow one to penetrate the ovum's corona radiata, an outer layer of cells, and then the zona pellucida, a thick inner membrane. (b) The nuclei of the sperm and the egg cells merge, and the male and female chromosomes in the nuclei come together, forming a zygote. (c) The zygote divides into two cells, then four cells, and so on. (d) At first, the zygote becomes a solid ball of cells. Then fluid enters the ball and forms a cavity. Now the ball has a surface layer and inner cell mass. It becomes known as a blastocyst. (e) The blastocyst then makes its way to the uterine cavity and burrows itself in a site in the endometrium (uterine lining). About 10 days following fertilization, the blastocyst is firmly embedded in the endometrium. The blastocyst becomes the embryo. The placenta is formed.

BIRTH CONTROL BASICS

A heterosexual woman in a Western country spends 90 percent of her reproductive years trying to prevent pregnancy and 10 percent of these years trying to become or being pregnant. Today birth control is safer, more effective, and more convenient than in the past—yet none of today's contraceptives is 100 percent safe, 100 percent effective, or 100 percent convenient.

Ideally, two partners should decide together which form of birth control to use. However, female methods account for 63 percent of all contraceptive methods reported by women between the ages of 15 and 44.[2] Another barrier to birth control is cost. In some provinces, health insurers have not covered the cost of reversible methods of birth control. However, even when birth control is affordable and available, many college and university students do not use it consistently. Huber and Ersek found in a study of sexually active female university students that the most common reason for non-use of contraceptives was related to the perceived cost.[3]

If you are engaging in sexual activity that could lead to conception, you have to be realistic about your situation. This may mean assuming full responsibility for your reproductive ability, whether you're a man or a woman. The more you know about contraception, the more likely you are to use birth control. As it turns out, college and university health courses help in this regard.[4] Using birth control can also alleviate stress that accompanies the risks of not using it. In one study, researchers found that 25.5 percent of undergraduate university students expressed regret at engaging in sexual activity and not using condoms.[5]

You also have to recognize the risks associated with various methods of contraception. If you're a woman, the risks are chiefly yours. Although many women never experience any serious complications, it is important to be aware of the potential for long-term risks of using oral contraceptives, as just one example. Risks that are acceptable to others may not be acceptable to you.

How Do I Choose a Birth Control Method? When it comes to deciding which form of birth control to use, there's no one "right" decision. Good decisions are based on sound information. You should consult a physician if you have questions or want to know how certain methods might affect existing or familial medical conditions, such as high blood pressure or diabetes. Table 8-1 presents some contraceptive choices. As the table indicates, contraception doesn't always work. When you evaluate any contraceptive, always consider its *effectiveness* (the likelihood that it will indeed prevent pregnancy). The **failure rate** refers to the

TABLE 8-1

Contraceptive Choices

Type of Birth Control	Success Rate
Permanent (also called sterilization)	
Tubal ligation (female)	99.9%
Vasectomy (male)	99.9%
Available with a prescription	
"The pill" (oral contraceptive)	99.0%
Intrauterine device (IUD)	95.0%
Contraceptive patch	99.0%
Vaginal ring (NuvaRing)	98.0%
Diaphragm with spermicide (foam or jelly)*	81.0%
Available without a prescription	
Condom with spermicide	95.0%
Condom alone	90.0%
Contraceptive sponge	90.0%
Emergency contraceptive pill (ECP)	98.0%
Natural family planning	
Withdrawal	77.0%
Rhythm method	76.0%

*** The only diaphragm currently available in Canada is a non-latex silicone diaphragm. As of August 2009, purchasing the necessary spermicidal jelly to use with the diaphragm remains a challenge.[6]**

Source: sexualityandU.ca. Contraception. Contraception methods. June 12, 2007. Found at www.sexualityandu.ca/adults/contraception-2.aspx

number of pregnancies that occur per year for every 100 women using a particular method of birth control. It is important to remember, though, that the reliability of contraceptives in actual, real-life use is much lower than that reported in surveys or clinical trials.

Some couples use withdrawal or **coitus interruptus**, removal of the penis from the vagina before ejaculation, to prevent pregnancy, even though this is not a reliable form of birth control. About half the men who have tried coitus interruptus find it unsatisfactory, either because they don't know when they're going to ejaculate or because they can't withdraw quickly enough. Also, the Cowper's glands, two pea-sized structures located on each side of the urethra, often produce a fluid that appears as drops at the tip of the penis any time from arousal and erection to orgasm. This fluid can contain active sperm and, in infected men, the human immunodeficiency virus (HIV).

Millions of unintentional pregnancies each year in Canada are the result of contraceptive failure, either from problems with the drug or device itself or from improper use. Partners can lower the risk of unwanted pregnancy by using backup methods—that is, more than one form of contraception simultaneously. Emergency contraception (EC), discussed in more detail further on in this chapter, is an option. Known as Plan B, or the emergency contraceptive pill (ECP), and sometimes referred to as the morning-after pill, it has proven to be a safe and effective way to prevent a pregnancy in an emergency situation. Research findings have shown that it can reduce the risk of pregnancy within five days after failed contraception or unprotected intercourse.[7] The sooner you take it, the better it works. If seven days have passed since you had unprotected sex and you do not get your menstrual period on time, you should take a pregnancy test or see your family physician. It is important to remember that ECP is not a replacement for regular contraception, nor does it protect against sexually transmitted infections. It does have some side effects for some women. Once a pregnancy has occurred, ECP will not work.

Often college and university students aware of the risks associated with unprotected sexual intercourse do not practise safe-sex behaviours. There are many reasons, ranging from the influence of alcohol and drugs to embarrassment about buying condoms. A survey of college students found that a significant percentage of both men and women either tried to dissuade a potential partner from condom use or had a sexual partner who had tried to discourage condom use. Both men and women generally used the same arguments against condoms: that sex felt better without them, that the woman wouldn't get pregnant, and that neither would get a sexually transmitted infection.[8]

The bottom line is that it takes two people to conceive a baby, and two people should be involved in deciding *not* to conceive a baby. In the process, they can also enhance their skills in communication, critical thinking, and negotiating.

✓ CHECK-IN

How do you take responsibility for your reproductive ability?

Abstinence and Outercourse For many individuals, **abstinence** represents a deliberate choice regarding their bodies, minds, spirits, and sexuality. People choose abstinence for various reasons, including waiting until they are ready for a sexual relationship or until they find the "right" partner, respecting religious or moral values, enjoying friendships without sexual involvement, recovering from a breakup, or preventing pregnancy and sexually transmitted infections.

Abstinence is the only form of birth control that is 100 percent effective and risk-free. It is also an important, increasingly valued lifestyle choice. A growing number of individuals, including some who have been sexually active in the past, are choosing abstinence until they establish a relationship with a long-term partner. There are even student-led abstinence groups on college

STRATEGIES FOR PREVENTION

Choosing a Contraceptive

Your contraceptive needs may change throughout your life. To decide which method to use now, you need to know the following:

- How well will it fit into your lifestyle?
- How convenient will it be?
- How effective will it be?
- How safe will it be?
- How affordable will it be?
- How reversible will it be?
- Will it protect against sexually transmitted infections?

Source: Courtesy of Planned Parenthood Federation of America, Inc.

and university campuses such as Harvard University—the True Love Revolution undergraduate group, Arizona State University—the New Sexual Revolution group, and Princeton University and the Massachusetts Institute of Technology—the Anscombe Society.[9]

Abstinence offers health benefits. Those who abstain until their 20s and engage in sex with fewer partners during their lifetime are less likely to get sexually transmitted infections, to suffer infertility, or to develop cervical cancer.[10]

Individuals who choose abstinence from vaginal intercourse often engage in activities sometimes called **outercourse**, such as kissing, hugging, sensual touching, and mutual masturbation. Outercourse is nearly 100 percent effective as a contraceptive measure, but pregnancy is possible if there is genital contact. If the man ejaculates near the vaginal opening, sperm can swim up into the vagina and fallopian tubes to fertilize an egg. Except for oral–genital and anal sex, outercourse also may lower the risk of contracting sexually transmitted infections. However, because some STIs, such as herpes and human papillomavirus (HPV, or genital warts), can be transmitted through skin-to-skin contact even when no bodily fluids are exchanged, outercourse cannot be considered "safe" sex.

Prescription Contraceptives The most effective and most widely used methods of birth control in Canada include oral contraceptives, the intrauterine device, the diaphragm, and the cervical cap. The newest prescription contraceptives are the contraceptive ring and the contraceptive patch. All are available only from health-care professionals by prescription. All are reversible.

Birth Control Pill *The pill*—the popular term for **oral contraceptives**—is the method of birth control used by about 100 million women all over the world.[11] It is also the preferred method of birth control by unmarried women and by those under age 30, including college and university students. Women 18–24 years old are most likely to choose oral contraceptives. In use for 40 years, the pill is one of the most researched, tested, and carefully followed medications in medical history—and one of the most controversial.[12] The impact of the pill has been enormous. By virtually eliminating the risk of pregnancy, the introduction of the pill encouraged women's careers. It also altered the marriage market by enabling young men and women to delay marriage while not having to delay sex.[13]

Although many women think that the risks of the pill are greater than those of pregnancy and childbirth, long-term studies show that oral contraceptive use does not increase mortality rates. For some time there was concern that oral contraceptives increased the risk of breast cancer. Some research suggests that in some women there is an increased risk; however, other studies show that oral contraceptives can be used for contraception safely by healthy women at low baseline risk for cardiovascular disease and breast cancer. The risk of ovarian and endometrial cancers was actually reduced in some women taking the pill.[14] There is concern, though, about an increased risk of blood clots and venous thromboembolism (VTE), especially in the first year of use, although these conditions are rare in younger women. There is a higher risk from oral contraceptives containing desogesterl, gestodene, or norgestimate, known as the third-generation pills, than oral contraceptives from the second generation that contain levonorgestrel or the progestogen-only pill. Women who smoke are also at an increased risk for VTE when they use oral contraceptives.[15]

Three types of oral contraceptives are widely used in Canada: the constant-dose combination pill, the multiphasic pill, and the progestin-only pill. The **constant-dose combination** or **monophasic pill** releases two hormones, synthetic estrogen and progestin, which play important roles in controlling ovulation and the menstrual cycle, at constant levels throughout the menstrual cycle.

The **multiphasic pill** mimics normal hormonal fluctuations of the natural menstrual cycle by providing different levels of estrogen and progestin at different times of the month. Multiphasic pills reduce total hormonal dose and side effects. Both constant-dose combination and multiphasic pills block the release of hormones that would stimulate the process leading to ovulation. They also thicken and alter the cervical mucus, making it more hostile to sperm, and they make implantation of a fertilized egg in the uterine lining more difficult. Multiphasic pills may heighten a woman's sex drive.

The **progestin-only pill**, or **minipill**, contains a small amount of progestin and no estrogen. Unlike women who take constant-dose combination pills, those using minipills probably ovulate at least occasionally. The minipills make the mucus in the cervix so thick and tacky, however, that sperm can't enter the uterus. Minipills also may interfere with implantation by altering the uterine lining.

Advantages Birth control pills have several advantages: They are extremely effective. Among women who do not miss any pills, only one in 1000 becomes pregnant in the first year of use. They are reversible, so a woman can easily stop using them. They do not interrupt sexual activity. Women on the pill have more regular periods, less cramping, and fewer tubal, or ectopic, pregnancies. After five years of use, the pill halves the risk of endometrial and ovarian cancer.

In a major study, scientists at the Centers for Disease Control and Prevention and the National Institutes of Health in the United States looked at more than 9200 women aged 35–64 and found that the pill does not raise the risk of breast cancer, even among women who started taking it early or who have close relatives with the disease.[16] This held true regardless of a woman's race or weight or whether she had started taking contraceptives before 20 years of age, took the early higher-dose oral contraceptives, or had a family history of breast cancer.[17] A similar study suggests that among women aged 36–64, there was no significant risk for breast cancer taking different formulations of oral contraceptives.[18] However, it is important here to say that while there are many advantages of using oral contraceptives, current research does continues to show somewhat conflicting data with regard to health risks. Another study found that long- term use of oral contraceptives for five years and more was associated with an increased risk of breast cancer among 20- to 44-year-old women.[19]

The pill also reduces the risk of benign breast lumps, ovarian cysts, iron-deficiency anemia, and pelvic inflammatory disease (PID). In actual use, the failure rate is 1–5 percent for estrogen/progesterone pills and 3–10 percent for minipills. Some physicians also prescribe the pill to assist women with a number of menstrual disorders and menstrual cycle regulation.[20]

Disadvantages The pill does not protect against HIV infection and other sexually transmitted infections, so condoms should also be used.[21] Some pills are time-sensitive, and pregnancy can result if the pills are not taken at the same time each day.[22] In addition, the hormones in oral contraceptives may cause various side effects, including spotting between periods, weight gain or loss, nausea and vomiting, breast tenderness, and decreased sex drive. Some women using the pill report emotional changes, such as mood swings and depression. Oral contraceptives can interact with other medications, which can make the birth control pill less effective or alter the effect of the other medication. Women should inform any physician providing medical treatment that they are taking the pill.[23]

Current birth control pills contain much lower levels of estrogen than early pills. As a result, the risk of heart disease and stroke among users is much lower than it once was; the danger may be lowest with the minipill. Yet a risk of cardiovascular problems is still associated with use of the pill, primarily for women over 35 who smoke and those with other health problems, such as high blood pressure.[24] For women 40–45 years of age, risk of ischemic stroke appears to be higher with estrogen dose oral contraceptives. Combined oral contraceptive (COC) use shows a substantial increase in the risk of ischemic stroke when associated with hypertension, cigarette smoking, and migraine headaches. Research also revealed that COC use was associated with an increased risk of myocardial infarction (MI) as well as other forms of ischemic heart disease, especially among women over 35 years of age who smoke and who have current risk factors for coronary-artery disease.[25]

Before Using Oral Contraceptives

- Before starting on the pill, you should undergo a thorough physical examination that includes the following tests:
- routine blood pressure test
- pelvic exam, including a Pap smear
- breast exam
- blood test
- urine sample

Let your doctor know about any personal or family incidence of high blood pressure or heart disease; diabetes; liver dysfunction; hepatitis; unusual menstrual history; severe depression; sickle-cell anemia; cancer of the breast, ovaries, or uterus; high cholesterol levels; or migraine headaches.

How to Use Oral Contraceptives Many women worldwide become unintentionally pregnant every year because they do not use the pill as directed.[26] The pill usually comes in 28-day packets: 21 of the pills contain the hormones, and 7 are "blanks," included so that the woman can take a pill every day, even during her menstrual period. If a woman forgets to take one pill, she should take it as soon as she remembers. However, if she forgets during the first week of her cycle or misses more than one pill, she should rely on another form of birth control until her next menstrual period.

Even if you experience no discomfort or side effects while on the pill, see a physician at least once a year for an examination, which should include a blood pressure test, a pelvic exam, and a breast exam. Notify your doctor at once if you develop severe abdominal pain, chest pain, coughing, shortness of breath, pain or tenderness in the calf or thigh, severe headaches, dizziness, faintness, muscle weakness or numbness, speech disturbance, blurred vision, a sensation of flashing lights, a breast lump, severe depression, or yellowing of your skin.

Generally, when you stop taking the pill, your menstrual cycle resumes the next month, but it may be irregular for the next couple of months. However, 2–4 percent of pill users experience prolonged delays.

Women who become pregnant during the first or second cycle after discontinuing use of the pill may be at greater risk of miscarriage; they also are more likely to conceive twins. Most physicians advise women who want to conceive to change to another method of contraception for three months after they stop taking the pill.

The Male Pill Research is beginning to focus on male hormonal contraception.[27] Scientists are attempting to find a way to block the effects of testosterone so the testicles do not produce healthy sperm cells. This has proven to be tricky because lowering testosterone can result in the loss of sexual desire. One possibility is the administration of a synthetic version of testosterone in combination with progestogen, a hormone used in female contraceptives. This prevents normal sperm production, but keeps a certain amount of testosterone in the blood and lowers the risk of side effects.

Studies have shown this is a viable form of male birth control; however, in some men, the production of sperm continues at a level that can result in a pregnancy. Research is also showing that men of different ethnic origins produce sperm at different rates when they use synthetic testosterone. Further studies are necessary before this form of birth control can be approved.

Contraceptive Ring The first contraceptive vaginal ring, the **NuvaRing®**, became available in 2002 in the United States. It is now available in Canada.[28] Once in place, the NuvaRing® releases a low dose of estrogen and progestin into the surrounding tissue. The ring contains a lower amount of hormones than birth control pills.

The flexible plastic two-inch ring compresses so a woman can easily insert it. Each ring stays in place for three weeks, then it is removed for the fourth week of the menstrual cycle. Like the pill and the patch, the ring works by preventing ovulation.

Advantages Women have no need for a daily pill, a fitting by a doctor, or the use of a spermicide. A woman's ability to become pregnant returns quickly once she stops using the ring.

Disadvantages There were increased complaints of vaginal discharge, irritation, and infection. Women cannot use oil-based vaginal medicine to treat yeast infections while the ring is in place or a diaphragm or cervical cap for a backup method of birth control. Women who cannot take the birth control pill for medical reasons cannot use the ring either. This includes women who have had a blood clot, heart attack, stroke, or breast cancer, as well as women with active liver disease or women over 35 who smoke.

Contraceptive Patch The **contraceptive patch** (Evra®) was a method of birth control that was introduced in Canada in January 2004.[29] Ortho Evra is no longer available in the United States, although it is still available in Europe and Canada, in a generic birth control patch form called Xulane. After the U.S. Food and Drug Administration approved the generic option, Janssen Pharmaceuticals discontinued their production of the of Ortho Evra patch.[30] The beige patch sticks to the skin and continuously releases estrogen and a progestin (two female hormones) into the bloodstream. It can be applied to the skin of the upper arm, abdomen, back, or buttocks.

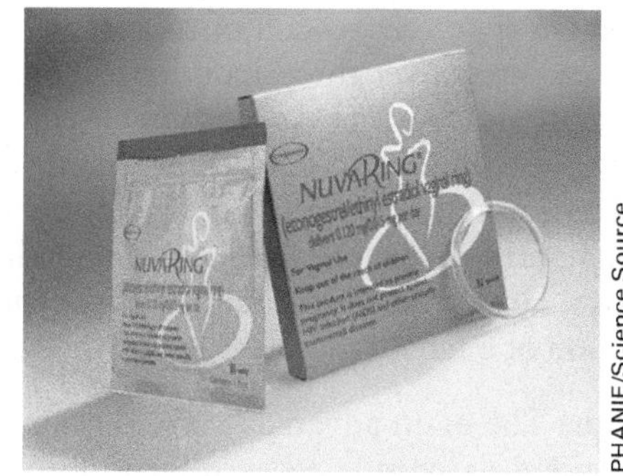

PHANIE/Science Source

The NuvaRing® releases estrogen and progestin, preventing ovulation.

Rather than taking a daily pill, a woman replaces the patch every seven days for three consecutive weeks. The fourth week is patch-free.

In clinical studies, it was found that most contraceptive patch detachments occurred during the first cycle of use. As women became more experienced at applying the patches, detachment decreased. The rates of complete detachment ranged from 0.5 to 2.4 percent. Partial detachments ranged from 1.4 to 2.9 percent. Reattaching the patch with some other type of adhesive decreases the effectiveness of this type of contraceptive.[31]

Clinical studies have shown that the patch is as effective as the low-dose birth control pill in preventing pregnancy and less likely to cause breakthrough bleeding or spotting.[32]

Advantages Like the pill, the patch is also more than 99 percent effective at preventing pregnancy when used perfectly, with about a 3 percent failure rate for typical users. A woman does not have to remember to take a daily pill and can become pregnant quickly once she stops its use.

Disadvantages Users have an increased risk of heart attacks and strokes. Because the birth control patch may increase a woman's estrogen levels there can also be a higher risk of estrogen-related issues such as blood clots. A study by Phelps and Kelver suggests that there is a growing concern over possible legal risks of prescribing the contraceptive patch.[33] Smoking increases the risk of serious cardiovascular side effects. The patch may be less effective in women who weigh more than 89.8 kilograms or 198 pounds.[34] Wearers of contact lenses may experience a change in vision or be unable to continue to wear lenses.

Contraceptive Injectables One injection of **Depo-Provera®**—hormonal birth control method that contains a progestin, a synthetic version of the natural hormone progesterone—provides three months of contraceptive protection. This long-acting hormonal contraceptive raises levels of progesterone, thereby simulating pregnancy. The pituitary gland doesn't produce FSH and LH, which normally cause egg ripening and release. The endometrial lining of the uterus thins, preventing implantation of a fertilized egg.

Advantages The main advantage is that women do not need to take a daily pill. Because Depo-Provera® contains only progestin, it can be used by women who cannot take oral contraceptives containing estrogen (such as those who have had breast cancer). Depo-Provera® also may have some protective action against endometrial and ovarian cancer.

Disadvantages Injectable contraceptives provide no protection against HIV and other STIs. Depo-Provera® causes menstrual irregularities in most users, and in a small percentage of users, it causes a delayed return of fertility, excessive endometrial bleeding, and other side effects, including decreased libido, depression, headaches, dizziness, weight gain, frequent urination, and allergic reactions. Weight gain was another concern. The average weight gain in the first year of use is approximately 2.26 kilograms (5 pounds).[35]

In June 2005, safety information was released by Pfizer Canada, in consultation with Health Canada, stating that new clinical studies with premenopausal adult women (25–35 years of age) and with adolescent women (12–18 years of age) indicated that women who used Depo-Provera™ for conception control might lose significant bone-mineral density. These studies also showed that the longer the contraceptive was used, the more bone-mineral density was lost. Of special concern was the finding that bone-mineral density might not return completely once the use of Depo-Provera® had been discontinued and that cases of osteoporosis and fracture were associated with the use of the product.[36]

Intrauterine Device The **intrauterine device (IUD)** is a small T-shaped device with a nylon string attached that is inserted into the uterus through the cervix. It prevents pregnancy by interfering with implantation. Once widely used, IUDs became less popular after most brands were removed from the market because of serious complications such as pelvic infection and infertility. The currently available IUDs have not been shown to increase the risk of such problems for women in mutually monogamous relationships (see Figure 8-3).

The IUD is effective and cost-efficient for preventing pregnancy, although some women may expel the device. The IUD does not offer protection against STIs.

In Canada, there are two types of IUDs available, the Nova-T and the Mirena®.[37] The Nova-T is a polyethylene T-shaped frame with a coil of copper wire on the outside. A thin string attached to the IUD hangs down through the cervix into the top of the vagina to allow you to check to see that it is in place. Copper acts as an effective spermicide to destroy sperm. It is suggested that women change this IUD after 30 months, but the effective lifespan is five years.[38] It fails in only one out of 100 users per year.

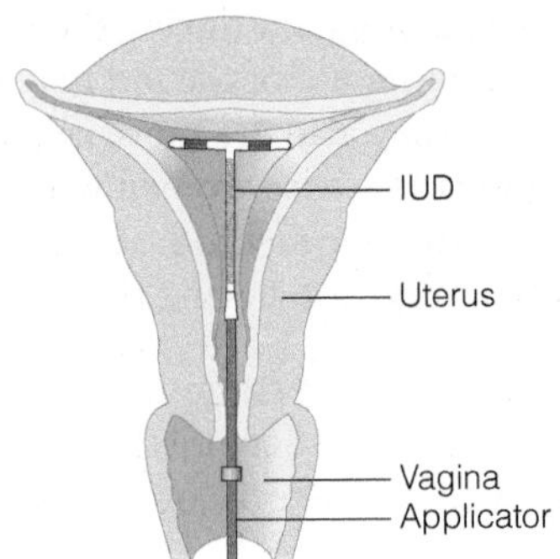

Figure 8-3 **Intrauterine Device (IUD)**
The IUD is placed in the uterus.

The Mirena® IUD, launched in Canada in 2001, also consists of a polyethylene T-shaped device, but it is surrounded by a sleeve containing the progestin levonorgestrel, which is released directly to the lining of the uterus. Mirena® contains no estrogen and is 99 percent effective in preventing pregnancy for up to five years.[39]

Advantages The advantages of IUDs are many—they are safe, highly effective, estrogen-free, rapidly reversible, convenient, and practical and have a long duration of use. The IUD should not alter the timing of a woman's period, and women who use an IUD have a lower rate of ectopic pregnancy than women who do not use any birth control. The hormonal IUD Mirena® decreases the amount of menstrual bleeding and may decrease menstrual cramping.

IUDs were long believed to increase the risk of pelvic inflammatory disease (PID), which can lead to scarring and infertility. More recent research has shown that although IUD users are more likely to develop PID than non-users, it is an uncommon complication. The greatest risk of PID occurs during the first two weeks following insertion; it falls at about 20 days.[40]

Disadvantages Many gynecologists recommend other forms of birth control for childless women who someday may want to start a family. Women who have never given birth and have used an IUD for an extended period of time may find it more difficult to conceive after discontinuing its use.[41] In addition, women with many sexual partners, who are at highest risk of PID, are not good candidates for this method.[42] Some women are allergic to copper or have adverse effects from hormones. Other disadvantages include the possibility of weight gain and the development of acne.

During insertion of an IUD, women may experience discomfort, cramping, bleeding, or pain, which may continue for a few days or longer. Women using the Nova-T IUD may find that their periods are heavier and that they experience more menstrual cramping, while users of the Mirena® IUD often find that their periods become quite light and sometimes disappear entirely. For either type, an estimated 5–10 percent of users expel an IUD within a year of insertion.

If a woman using an IUD does become pregnant, the IUD is removed to reduce the risk of miscarriage (which can be as high as 50 percent).

How to Use an IUD A physician inserts an IUD into a woman's uterus through the cervix and trims the IUD strings so that they can be felt at the entrance to the cervix. An IUD can be inserted during a woman's period or at other times in her menstrual cycle. An IUD can be removed by a doctor at any point if a woman no longer wants to use it. The strings should be checked regularly, particularly after each menstrual cycle, since IUDs can be expelled. Antibiotics may be prescribed to lower any risk of infection.

Diaphragm The **diaphragm** is a bowl-like rubber cup with a flexible rim that is inserted into the vagina to cover the cervix and prevent the passage of sperm into the uterus during sexual intercourse (see Figure 8-4). When used with a spermicide, the diaphragm is both a physical and a chemical barrier to sperm.[43] Access to diaphragms has become limited in Canada. Currently, the only diaphragm available in Canada is a non-latex silicone type. As well, since 2009, finding the right spermicidal jelly to use with the diaphragm has become a difficult challenge.[44] Without a spermicide, the diaphragm is not effective. The use of spermicide nonoxynol-9 with the diaphragm, while effective as a

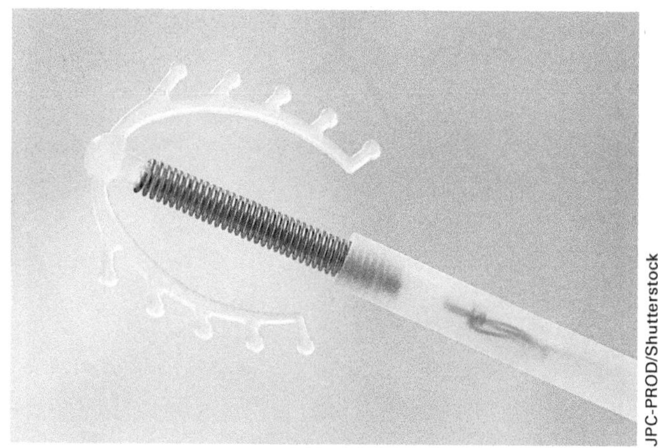

JPC-PROD/Shutterstock

Copper T

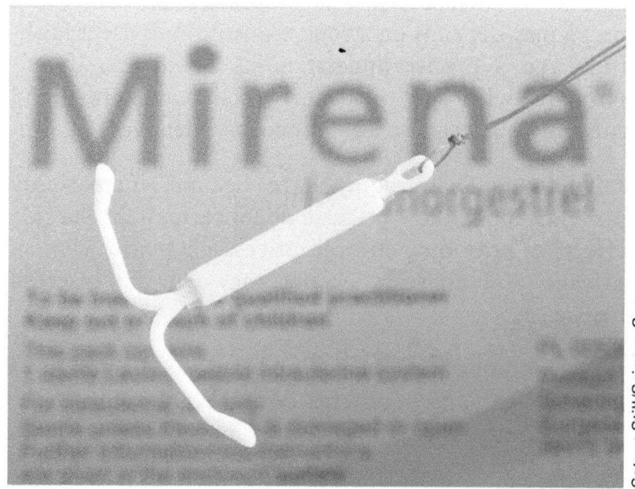

Saturn Still/Science Source

IUD Mirena®

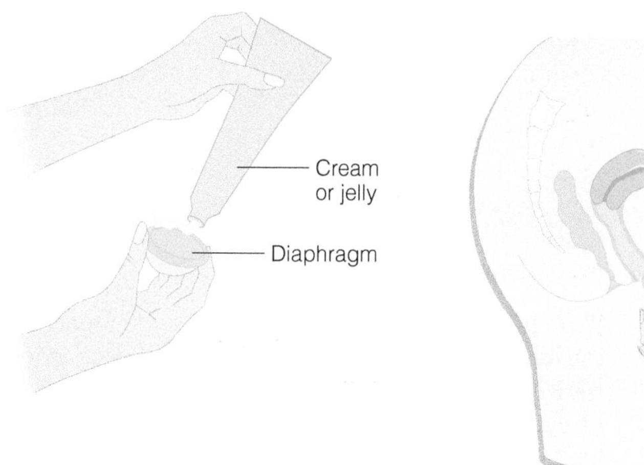

Squeeze spermicide into dome of diaphragm and around the rim.

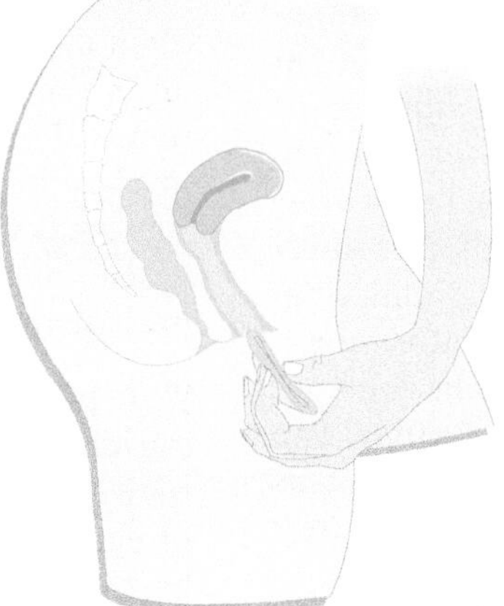

Squeeze rim together; insert jelly-side up.

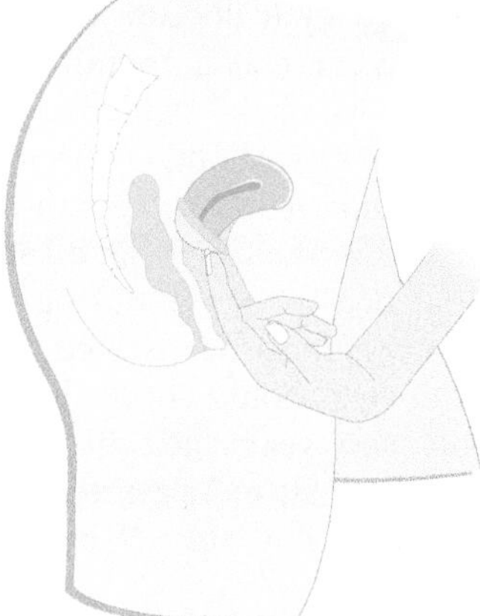

Check placement to make certain cervix is covered.

© Cengage

Figure 8-4 **Diaphragm**

When used correctly and consistently and with a spermicide, the diaphragm is effective in preventing pregnancy and STIs. It must be fitted by a healthcare professional.

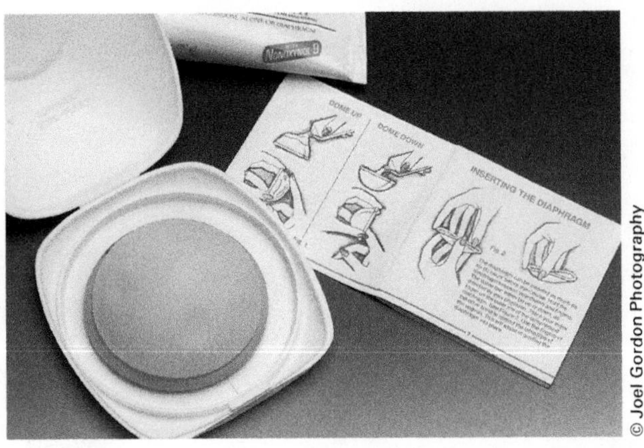
© Joel Gordon Photography

microbicide, has been questioned and research indicates that it may actually increase the risk of STI and HIV transmission.[45]

The effectiveness of the diaphragm in preventing pregnancy depends on strong motivation to use it faithfully and a precise understanding of its use. If diaphragms with spermicide are used consistently and carefully, they can be 84–94 percent effective.[46]

Advantages Diaphragms have become increasingly popular, most likely because of concern about the side effects of hormonal contraceptives. They offer women privacy and control because they can be inserted before sex.

Disadvantages Some people find that the diaphragm is inconvenient and interferes with sexual spontaneity. The spermicidal cream or jelly is messy, detracts from oral–genital sex, and can cause irritation. A poorly fitted diaphragm may cause discomfort during sex; some women report bladder discomfort, urethral irritation, or recurrent cystitis as a result of diaphragm use.

How to Use a Diaphragm Diaphragms are fitted and prescribed by a doctor. The diaphragm's main function is to serve as a container for a spermicidal foam or jelly, which is available at a limited number of pharmacies without a prescription. A diaphragm should remain in the vagina for at least six hours after intercourse to ensure that all sperm are killed. If intercourse occurs again during this period, additional spermicide must be inserted with an applicator tube.

A doctor should check the diaphragm's fit and condition every year when the woman has her annual Pap smear. It needs to be refitted if a woman loses or gains up to 4.5 kilograms (9 pounds, 14 ounces) or after pregnancy.

The key to proper use of the diaphragm is having it available. A sexually active woman should keep it in the most accessible place—her purse, bedroom, or bathroom. Before every use, a diaphragm should be checked for tiny leaks (hold up to the light or place water in the dome). Oil-based lubricants will deteriorate the latex of the diaphragm and should not be used.

Cervical Cap Like the diaphragm, the **cervical cap**, combined with spermicide, serves as both a chemical and physical barrier blocking the path of the sperm to the uterus. The rubber or plastic cap is smaller and thicker than a diaphragm and resembles a large thimble that fits snugly around the cervix. It is about 84–91 percent effective, but the failure rate is higher in women who have already had a baby.[47] At this time, the only cervical cap available in Canada is called FemCap. It is now distributed only through some private and community health agencies. Contragel, the contraceptive gel that is recommended for use with the FemCap, has become difficult to access.[48]

Advantages Women who cannot use a diaphragm because of pelvic-structure problems or loss of vaginal muscle tone can often use the cap. Also, the cervical cap is less messy and does not require additional applications of spermicide if intercourse occurs more than once within several hours.

Disadvantages A cervical cap is more difficult to insert and remove than a diaphragm, and using it requires a woman to be comfortable with touching her vagina and cervix. Users of the cervical cap also need to plan ahead, since the cap must be inserted at least half an hour prior to intercourse. Some women find it uncomfortable to wear or cannot get the right fit, or their partners are able to feel the cervical cap during sex. The cervical cap does not protect against STIs, and an allergy to latex can prevent some women from using the cap.

How to Use a Cervical Cap Like the diaphragm, the cervical cap must be fitted by a doctor. For use, the woman fills it one-third to two-thirds full with spermicide and inserts it by holding its edges together and sliding it into the vagina. The cup is then pressed onto the cervix. (Most women find it easiest to do so while squatting or in an upright sitting position.) The cap can be inserted up to six hours prior to intercourse and should not be removed for at least six hours afterward. It can be left in place for up to 24 hours. Pulling on one side of the rim breaks the suction and allows easy removal. Oil-based lubricants should not be used with the cap because they can deteriorate the latex.

Non-prescription Contraceptives

Condoms, spermicides, and contraceptive sponges are also known as **barrier contraceptives** because they block the meeting of egg and sperm by means of a physical or chemical barrier. Some of these forms of birth control, such as condoms, have become increasingly popular because they can do more than prevent conception—they can also help reduce the risk of STIs.

Male Condom The male **condom** covers the erect penis and catches the ejaculate, thus preventing sperm from entering the woman's reproductive tract (see Figure 8-5).

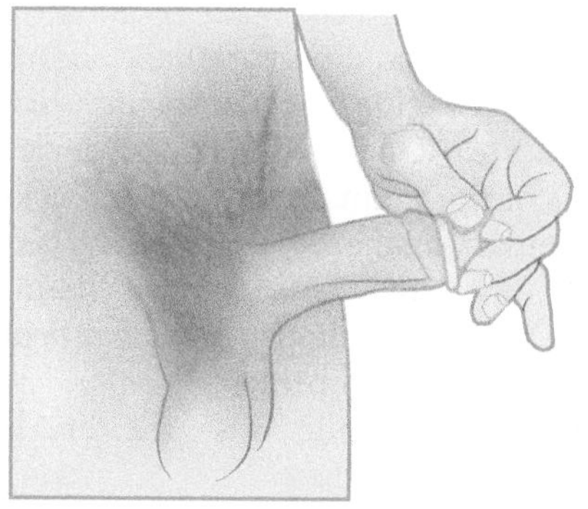
Pinch or twist the tip of the condom, leaving one-half inch at the tip to catch the semen.

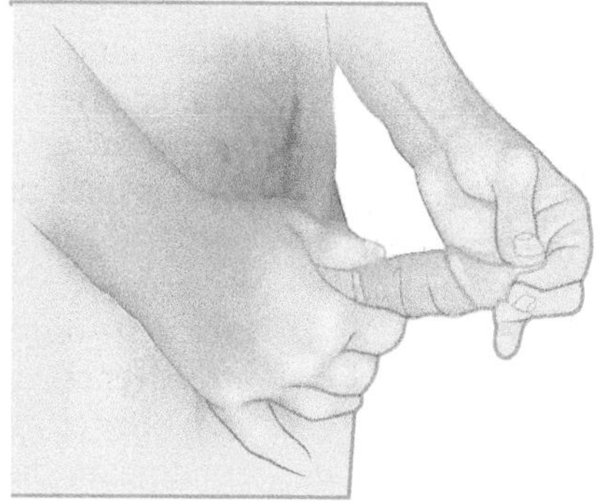
Holding the tip, unroll the condom.

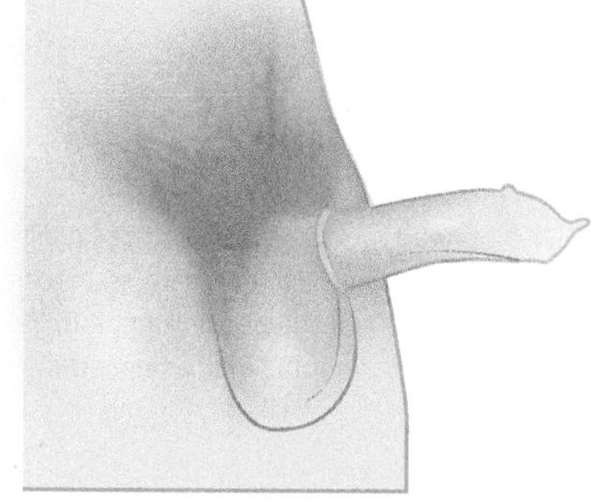
Unroll the condom until it reaches the pubic hairs.

Figure 8-5 Male Condom

Condoms effectively reduce the risk of pregnancy as well as STIs. Using them consistently and correctly are important factors.

There are three types of condoms and they come in different types, sizes, colours, and flavours:[49]

- Latex condoms—the most commonly available. They protect against pregnancy and STIs.
- Polyurethane condoms—used by people who have latex allergies. They are made of plastic. They protect against pregnancy and STIs.
- Natural condoms—made from animal membranes. They protect against pregnancy, but do not offer protection from STIs.

Condoms are 85–98 percent effective.[50] The condom can be torn during the manufacturing process or during its use. Careless removal can also decrease the effectiveness of condoms. However, the major reason that condoms have such a low actual effectiveness rate is that couples don't use them each and every time they have sex.

Condoms are second only to the pill in popularity among college- and university-age adults. Condom use has increased in the last decade. In one study by researchers Tolani and Yen, 1399 university students were surveyed. Sixty-nine percent of all sexually active participants in this study reported using condoms the last time they had heterosexual intercourse. Seven percent of the sexually active students used both a condom and withdrawal, while 24 percent used birth control pills and a condom.[51]

Research also shows that for girls, being from an intact family and having a mother with higher educational achievement are associated with greater condom use at first intercourse. Teens with more educated parents and teens who were older at first intercourse also had greater condom use. The less similar adolescents are to their partners—whether because of a difference in age, grade, or school—the less likely adolescents are to use condoms and other contraceptive methods.[52]

Advantages Condoms made of latex or polyurethane can help reduce the risk of certain STIs, including syphilis, gonorrhea, chlamydia, and herpes. They appear to lower a woman's risk of pelvic inflammatory disease (PID) and may protect against some parasites that cause urinary tract and genital infections. Public health officials view condoms as the best available defence against HIV infection. They are available without a prescription or medical appointment, and their use does not cause harmful side effects. Some men appreciate the slight blunting of sensation they experience when using a condom because it helps prolong the duration of intercourse before ejaculation.

Disadvantages Condoms are not 100 percent effective in preventing pregnancy or STIs, including infection with HIV. Condoms can reduce the risks of sexual involvement, but they cannot eliminate them. Condoms may have manufacturing defects, such as pin-size holes, or they may break or slip off during intercourse. As mentioned above, Health Canada has put out a warning about the use of condoms with the spermicidal lubricant nonoxynol-9. The best STI and HIV barrier is a latex condom without nonoxynol-9.

The main objections to condoms include odour, lubrication (too much or too little), rips or breaks, access, disposal, feel, taste, and difficulty opening the packages. Some couples feel that putting on a condom interferes with sexual spontaneity; others incorporate it into their sex play. Some men dislike the reduced penile sensitivity or will not use them because they believe they interfere with sexual pleasure. Others cannot sustain an erection while putting on a condom. A small number are allergic to latex condoms.

How to Use a Condom Most physicians recommend prelubricated, latex, or polyurethane condoms, not membrane condoms ("natural" or "sheepskin"). Before using a condom, check the expiration date, and make sure it's soft and pliable. If it's yellow or sticky, throw it out. Don't check for leaks by blowing up a condom before using it; you may weaken or tear it.

X AND Y FILES

Males, Females, and Condom Use

In a series of focus groups with sexually active, young, ethnically and racially diverse individuals, researchers discovered that both males and females found it difficult to believe that any young people used condoms every single time they had sex. Although they acknowledged that everyone is at risk for sexually transmitted infections, the young people saw their own risk as minimal.

The genders had different motives both for engaging in sex and for using condoms. In the interviews, young women said they engaged in sexual relations because of a desire for physical intimacy and a committed relationship. They generally reported having sex only with men they cared for and deeply trusted and expected that these men would be honest and forthright about their sexual history. This trust played a significant role in their decision whether to insist on condom use.

In contrast, few of the young men said relationships were an important dimension of their sexual involvements. Their primary motivation was a desire for physical and sexual satisfaction. Most said they were not interested in commitment and viewed emotional expectations as a complication of becoming sexually involved with a woman. The young men also admitted to making judgments about women.

Which partner determined whether a couple would use a condom? In these interviews, the answer was the women. Regardless of race or ethnicity, many of the young women were adamant in demanding that their partners use condoms—and many young men said they would not challenge such a demand out of fear of losing the opportunity for sex. Men often expected potential partners to want to use condoms and described themselves as "suspicious" of women who did not.

The young people were most strongly motivated to use condoms when they did not know a potential sexual partner well or were at the earliest stages of sexual involvement with others. Nearly all said they solicited information about a potential partner's sexual history from this person or from friends. Rather than directly asking about the number of past partners, they more often relied on feelings and visual observations. Some admitted to lying when asked about their own sexual experience in order to avoid being seen as promiscuous. Once a couple had sex without a condom, both partners—but especially women—found it awkward to resume condom use because doing so would imply a lack of trust.

The condom should be put on at the beginning of sexual activity, before genital contact occurs (see Figure 8-5). There should be a little space at the top of the condom to catch the semen. Any vaginal lubricant should be water-based. Petroleum-based creams or jellies (such as Vaseline®, baby oil, massage oil, vegetable oils, or oil-based hand lotions) can deteriorate the latex. After ejaculation, the condom should be held firmly against the penis so that it doesn't slip off or leak during withdrawal. Couples engaging in anal intercourse should use a water-based lubricant as well as a condom, but should never assume the condom will protect them from HIV infection or other STIs.

Female Condom The female condom, made of polyurethane, consists of two rings and a polyurethane sheath and is inserted into the vagina with a tampon-like applicator (see Figure 8-6). Once in place, the device loosely lines the walls of the vagina. Internally, a thickened rubber ring keeps it anchored near the cervix. Externally, another rubber ring, two inches in diameter, rests on the labia and resists slippage.[53] The rate of effectiveness is between 79 and 95 percent.[54]

Although not widely used in the West, the female condom is gaining acceptance in Africa, Asia, and Latin America. Properly used, it is believed to be as good as or better than the male condom for preventing infections, including HIV, because it is stronger and covers a slightly larger area. However, it is slightly less effective at preventing pregnancy.

Advantages The female condom gives women more control in reducing their risk of pregnancy and STIs. It does not require a prescription or medical appointment. One size fits all.

Disadvantages The failure rate for the female condom is higher than for other contraceptives. Women have complained that the condom is difficult to use.

How to Use a Female Condom As illustrated in Figure 8-6, a woman removes the condom and applicator from the wrapper and inserts the condom slowly by gently pushing the applicator toward the small of the back. When properly inserted, the outer ring should rest on the folds of skin around the vaginal opening, and the inner ring (the closed end) should fit against the cervix. The condom should be used with a water-based lubricant.

Vaginal Spermicide The various forms of **vaginal spermicide** include chemical foams, creams, jellies, vaginal suppositories, and gels. Some creams and jellies are made for use with a diaphragm or cervical cap; others can be used alone. Vaginal contraceptive film (VCF) is a small, thin piece of solid gel.[55]

Advantages Conscientious use of a spermicide together with another method of contraception, such as a condom, can provide safe and effective birth control and reduce the risk of some vaginal infections, pelvic inflammatory disease, and STIs. The side effects of vaginal spermicides are minimal. Again, remember Health Canada's caution about products that have the spermicide nonoxynol-9 in them.

Disadvantages Even though spermicides can be applied in less than a minute, couples may feel that they interfere with sexual spontaneity. Some people are irritated by the chemicals in spermicides, but often a change of brand solves this problem. Others find foam spermicides messy or feel they interfere with oral–genital contact.

How to Use a Vaginal Spermicide The various types of spermicide come with instructions that should be

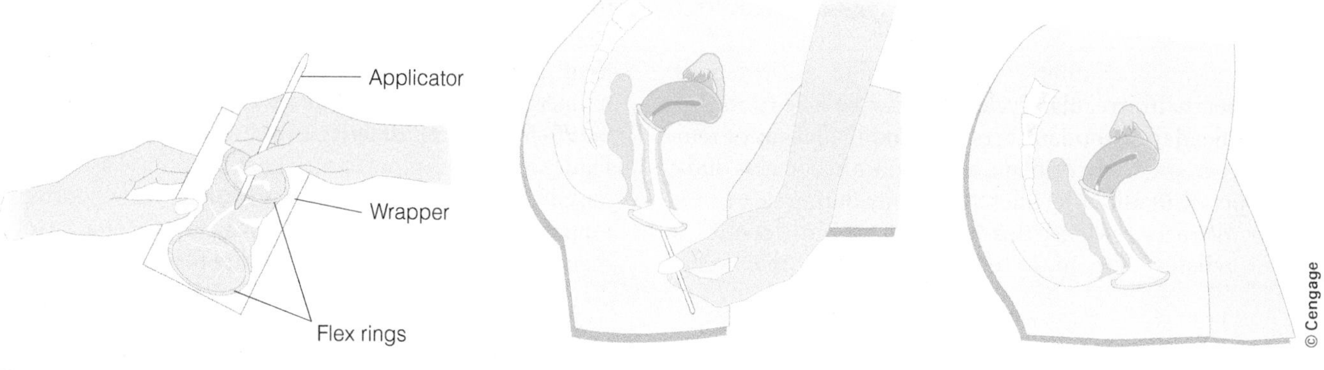

Figure 8-6 **Female Condom**

This device is less effective than the male condom for preventing pregnancy and STIs (since no spermicide is used). Like the male condom, this method does not require a prescription.

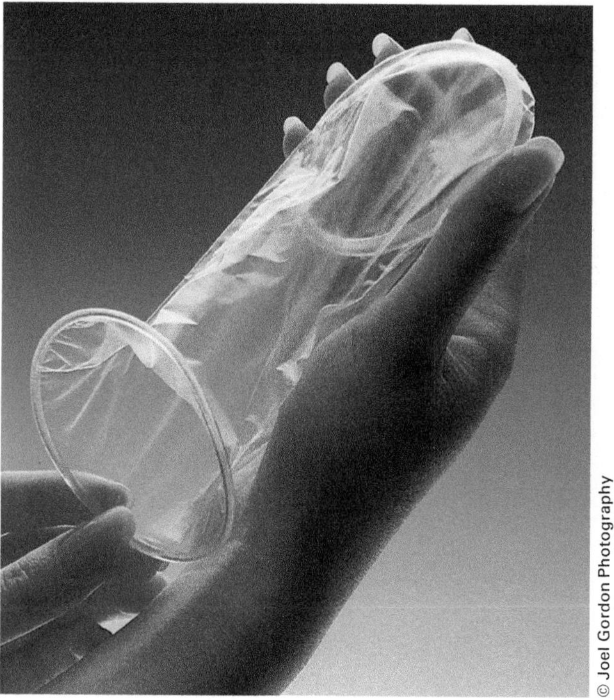

followed carefully for maximum protection. Contraceptive vaginal suppositories take about 20 minutes to dissolve and cover the vaginal walls. Foam, inserted with an applicator, goes into place much more rapidly. You must apply additional spermicide before each additional intercourse. Vaginal contraceptive film is inserted into the vagina using your fingers 15 minutes to one hour prior to intercourse so that the gel can soften and coat both the vagina and cervix.

After sex, women should shower rather than bathe to prevent the spermicide from being rinsed out of the vagina, and they should not douche for at least six hours.

> **✓ CHECK-IN**
>
> If you are sexually active, do you use condoms every time you engage in sex?

Contraceptive Sponge The soft, disposable polyurethane sponge is a one-size-fits-all, non-prescription barrier method containing spermicide. It is inserted through the vagina and placed at the cervix. A small perforation in the sponge allows the woman to remove the sponge six hours or more after intercourse.[56]

Advantages This barrier method provides 12-hour protection, and it is not necessary to change the sponge if sex is repeated during this time.

Disadvantages Some women find it difficult to remove the sponge, or forget to take it out, or are allergic to the spermicide. The sponge should also be used with a condom to ensure maximum protection from pregnancy and STIs.

> **✓ CHECK-IN**
>
> How well informed are you about contraceptive options?

Periodic Abstinence and Fertility Awareness Method Awareness of a woman's cyclic fertility can help in both conception and contraception. The different methods of birth control based on a woman's menstrual cycle are sometimes referred to as *natural family planning* or *fertility awareness methods*. They include the cervical-mucus method, the calendar method, and the basal body temperature method.[57] Fertility monitors that use saliva for testing can improve the accuracy of these methods.

Advantages Birth-control methods based on the menstrual cycle involve no expense, no side effects, and no need for prescriptions or fittings. On the days when the couple can have intercourse, there is nothing to insert, swallow, or check. In addition, abstinence during fertile periods complies with the teachings of some religions.

Disadvantages During times of possible fertility (usually eight or nine days a month), couples must abstain from vaginal intercourse or use some form of contraception. Conscientious planning and scheduling are essential. Women with irregular cycles may not be able to rely on the calendar method. Others may find the mucus or temperature methods difficult to use. Both partners must cooperate in initiating intercourse only during safe times. For all these reasons, this approach to birth control is less reliable than many others. In theory, the overall effectiveness rate for the various fertility awareness methods is 80 percent. In practice, of every 100 women using one of these methods for a year, 24 become pregnant. However, using a combination of the basal body temperature method and the cervical-mucus method may be 90–95 percent effective in preventing pregnancy (see Figure 8-7). It is important to note here that Figure 8-7 is based on a 28-day cycle. Many women have shorter or longer cycles; therefore, this visual representation of a menstrual cycle may not be accurate for all women.

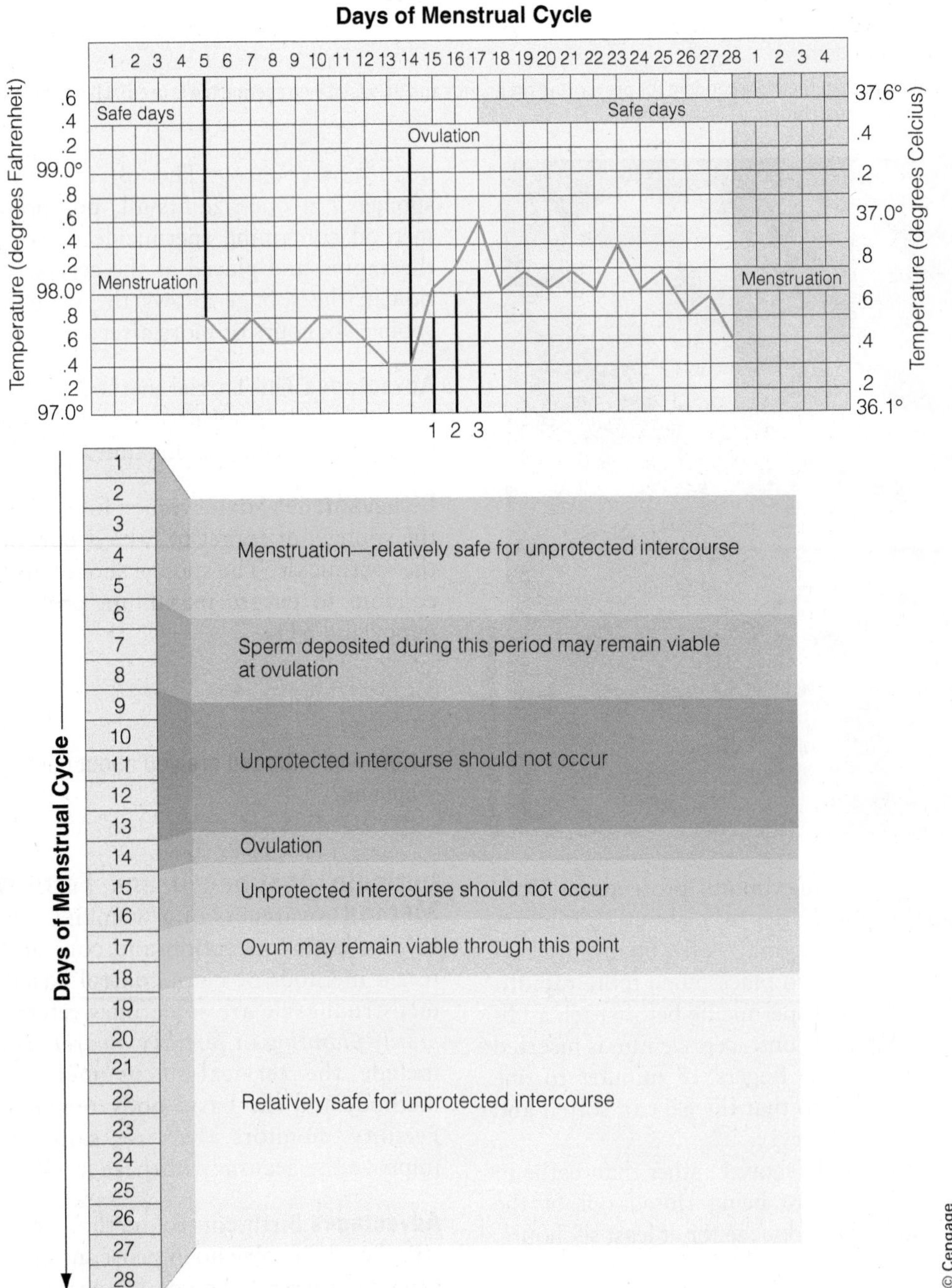

Figure 8-7 Fertility Awareness Methods

These methods are based on a woman's menstrual cycle and involve charting basal body temperature (top), careful calculation of the menstrual cycle (bottom), or careful observations of cervical mucus. Use of other contraceptive methods during fertile days or periods of abstinence are a necessary part of these methods. Figure is based on a 28-day cycle. Note that cycles can vary from 21 to 32 days.

Basal Body Temperature Method In this method the woman measures her **basal body temperature**, the body temperature upon waking in the morning, using a specially calibrated rectal thermometer, which is more precise than an oral one. She records her temperature on a chart (see Figure 8-7). The basal body temperature remains relatively constant from the beginning of the menstrual cycle to ovulation. After ovulation, however, the basal body temperature rises by more than 1.75 degrees Celsius (approximately 0.5 degrees Fahrenheit). The woman knows that her safe period has begun when her temperature has been elevated for three consecutive days. After 8–10 months, she should have a sense of her ovulatory pattern, in addition to knowing her daily readings.

Calendar Method This approach, often called the **rhythm method**, involves counting the days after menstruation begins to calculate the estimated day of ovulation. The first day of menstruation is day one. A woman counts the number of days until the last day of her cycle, which is the day before menstrual flow begins. To determine the starting point of the period during which she should avoid unprotected intercourse, she subtracts 18 from the number of days in her shortest cycle. For instance, if her shortest cycle was 28 days, day 10 would be her first high-risk day. To calculate when she can again have unprotected intercourse, she subtracts 10 from the number of days in her longest cycle. If her longest cycle is 31 days, she could resume intercourse on day 21. Other forms of sexual activity can continue from day 10–day 21. This method requires careful timing to avoid the possible meeting of a ripe egg and active sperm in the woman's fallopian tube.

Cervical-Mucus Method This method, also called the **ovulation method**, is based on the observation of changes in the consistency of the mucus in the vagina. In the first days after menstruation, the vagina feels dry because of a decline in hormone production, indicating a safe period for unprotected intercourse. Within a few days, estrogen levels rise, and the mucus begins to thin out and becomes less cloudy: the fertile period begins. At peak estrogen levels, the mucus is smooth, stretchable, and slippery (like raw egg white) and very clear. Mucus with these characteristics is usually observed within 24 hours of ovulation and lasts one to two days, signalling maximum fertility. The mucus becomes sticky and cloudy again three days thereafter, and the second safe period begins. Most women using this method have to refrain from unprotected intercourse for about nine days of each 28-day menstrual cycle.

What Is Emergency Contraception? **Emergency contraception (EC)** is the use of a method of contraception to prevent unintended pregnancy after unprotected intercourse or the failure of another form of contraception, such as a condom breaking or slipping off. As briefly discussed in the section How Do I Choose a Birth Control Method? there are different options for emergency contraception. The four types of emergency contraceptive pills available now in Canada are *Next Choice*, *Norlevo*, *Option 2*, and *Plan B*.[58] Medical researchers do not fully understand how ECPs work. They may inhibit or delay ovulation, prevent union of sperm and ovum, or alter the endometrium so a fertilized ovum cannot implant itself.

The copper-bearing intrauterine device (IUD) is also an EC option.[59]

It is not necessary to wait until the morning after to take ECPs. A woman can start right away or up to five days after unprotected sex. Therapy is more effective the earlier it is initiated. If taken within 24 hours of having unprotected sex, it can be 95 percent effective in preventing an unintended pregnancy. If taken within 72 hours, it is 85 percent effective; however, it will not have an impact if the pregnancy is already established. Most women can safely use them, even if they cannot use birth control pills as their regular method of birth control. (Although ECPs use the same hormones as birth control pills, not all brands of birth control pills can be used for emergency contraception.) Some women may experience spotting or a full menstrual period a few days after taking ECPs, depending on where they were in their cycle when they began therapy. Most women have their next period at the expected time.

As of April 2005, in Canada, ECPs became available without a doctor's prescription. New warnings have been added to the labels of ECPs indicating that the effectiveness of the pills decreases in women weighing 75–80 kilograms (165–176 pounds) and that they are not effective for women who weigh over 80 kilograms (176 pounds).[60]

The other option, the copper IUD, can be inserted by a physician up to five days after ovulation to prevent pregnancy. IUDs are more effective at preventing pregnancy than hormonal ECPs and reduce the risk of pregnancy by 99 percent. However, they are not used as commonly as hormonal methods for EC.

✓ CHECK-IN

Have you or your partner ever used emergency contraception?

Sterilization Another method of birth control is **sterilization** (surgery to end a person's reproductive capability).[61]

Advantages Sterilization has no effect on sex drive in either men or women. Many couples report that their sexual activity increases after sterilization because they are free from the fear of pregnancy or the need to deal with contraceptives.

Disadvantages Sterilization should be considered permanent and should be used only if both individuals are sure they do not want any more children.

Male Sterilization In men, the cutting of the vas deferens, the tube that carries sperm from one of the testes into the urethra for ejaculation, is called **vasectomy.** During the 15- to 20-minute office procedure, done under a local anesthetic, the doctor makes small incisions in the scrotum, lifts up each vas deferens, cuts them, and ties off the ends to block the flow of sperm (see Figure 8-8). Sperm continue to form, but they are broken down and absorbed by the body.

The man usually experiences some local pain, swelling, and discoloration for about a week after the procedure. More serious complications, including the formation of a blood clot in the scrotum (which usually disappears without treatment), infection, and an inflammatory reaction, occur in a small percentage of cases. After a vasectomy the male must monitor his sperm count for about three months or 20 ejaculations. When there is no sperm in the ejaculate the procedure is considered to be effective.

Although anyone who chooses to have a vasectomy should consider it permanent, surgical reversal (*vasovasostomy*) is sometimes successful. New microsurgical techniques have led to annual pregnancy rates for the wives of men undergoing vasovasostomies of about 50 percent, depending on such factors as the doctor's expertise and the time elapsed since the vasectomy.

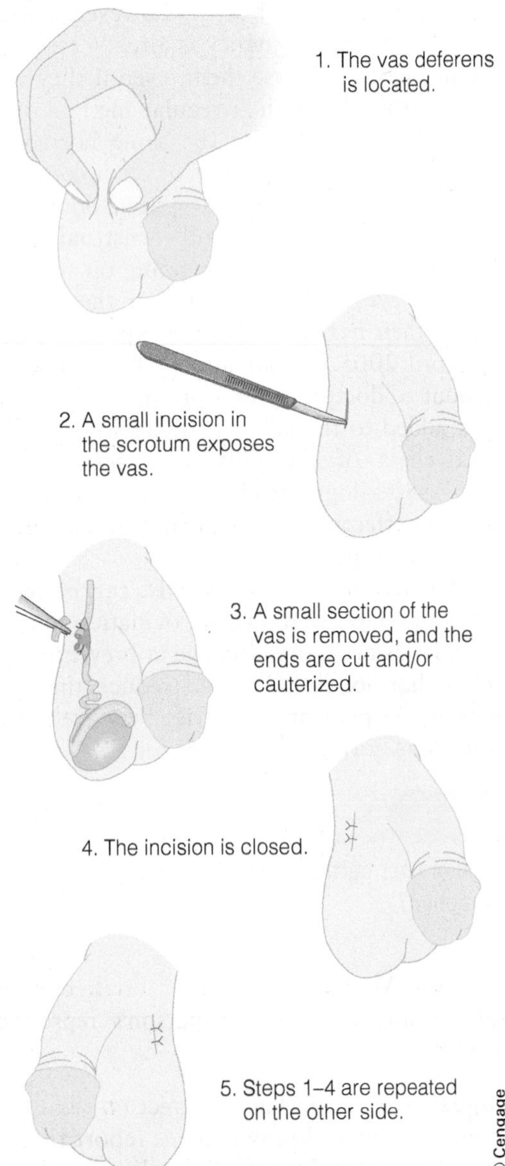

Figure 8-8 Male Sterilization, or Vasectomy

Female Sterilization Female sterilization procedures modify the fallopian tubes, which each month normally carry an egg from the ovaries to the uterus. The two terms used to describe female sterilization are **tubal ligation** (the cutting or tying of the fallopian tubes) and **tubal occlusion** (the blocking of the tubes). The tubes may be cut or sealed with thread, a clamp, or a clip, or by coagulation (burning) to prevent the passage of eggs from the ovaries (see Figure 8-9). They can also be blocked with bands of silicone.

The procedures used for sterilization are laparotomy, laparoscopy, and colpotomy. **Laparotomy** involves making an abdominal incision about two inches long and cutting the tubes. A laparotomy usually requires a hospital stay and up to several weeks of recovery. It leaves a scar and carries the same risks as all major surgical procedures: the side effects of anesthesia, potential infection, and internal scars. In a **minilaparotomy,** an incision about an inch long is made just above the pubic hairline. The tubes may be tied, cut, plugged, or sealed by electrical coagulation. The

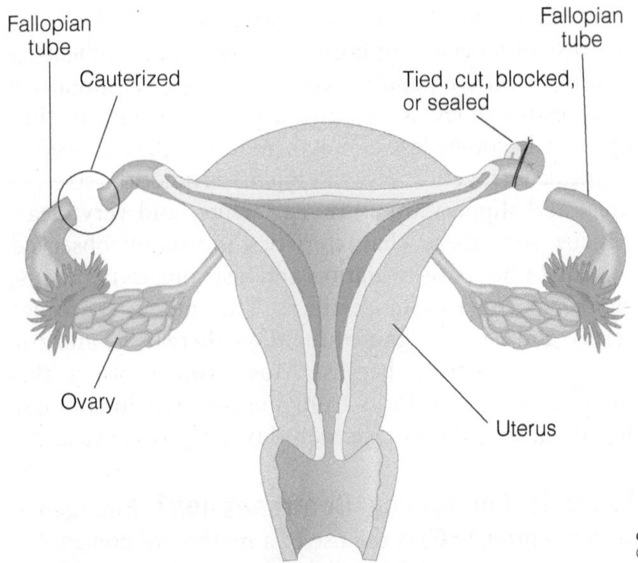

Figure 8-9 Female Sterilization, or Tubal Ligation

operation can be performed by a skilled physician in 10–30 minutes, usually under local anesthesia, and the woman can generally go home the same day. The failure (pregnancy) rate is only one in 1000.

Tubal ligation or occlusion can also be performed with the use of **laparoscopy**, commonly called *belly-button* or *Band-aid surgery*. This procedure is done on an outpatient basis and takes 15–30 minutes. A lighted tube called a *laparoscope* is inserted through an approximately one-centimetre incision made right below the navel, giving the doctor a view of the fallopian tubes. Using surgical instruments that may be inserted through the laparoscope or through other tiny incisions, the doctor then cuts or seals the tubes, most commonly by electrical coagulation. The possible complications are similar to those of minilaparotomy, as is the failure rate.

In a **colpotomy**, the fallopian tubes are reached through the vagina and cervix. This procedure leaves no external scar but is somewhat more hazardous and less effective. A **hysterectomy** (removal of the uterus) is a major surgical procedure that is not commonly used as a method of sterilization, unless there are other medically urgent reasons for removing the uterus.

ABORTION

More than half of unintended pregnancies end in induced abortions. Abortion rates vary greatly around the world. In many nations with fewer unwanted pregnancies and lower abortion rates, contraceptives are generally easier and cheaper to obtain, and early sex education strongly emphasizes their importance.

Abortion Rights Coalition of Canada reports that there were a total of 81 897 abortions in 2014; hospital abortions totalled 33 931 and clinic abortions totalled 47 966. The highest rates of abortions recorded were in Quebec at 25 083, followed by Ontario at 23 746, Alberta at 13 815, and British Columbia at 9196. Abortions in other provinces ranged from 85 to 2061.[62]

Induced abortions have not been performed in hospitals or clinics in Prince Edward Island since the 1980s. Women had to travel off the island to obtain abortion services. However, on March 31, 2016, the Liberal provincial government announced that abortions would become available in Prince Edward Island. The announcement came as a pro-choice group called Abortion Access Now PEI Inc. was set to mount a legal court challenge against the government. With this announcement, abortions will now be available in every province. Yet not all women will have equal access to an abortion in Canada as they are difficult to obtain in many small communities or in rural areas.[63]

No woman ever elects to be in a situation where she has to consider abortion. But if faced with an unwanted pregnancy, many women consider elective abortion as an option.

> *Women who have abortions do not fit neatly into any particular category. About 80 percent are unmarried. Most—70 percent—intend to have children, but not at this point in time. Many cannot afford a baby. Some feel unready for the responsibility; others fear that another child would jeopardize the happiness and security of their existing family.*

Thinking through the Options A woman faced with an unwanted pregnancy can find it extremely difficult to decide what to do. There is the political debate over the right to life. There are also practical and emotional matters, such as the quality of the woman's relationship with the baby's father, her capacity to provide for the child, the impact on any children she already has, and other important life issues.

Giving up a child for adoption is an option for women who do not feel abortion is right for them. Advocates of adoption reform are pressing for mandatory counselling for all pregnant women considering abortion and for extending the period of time during which a new mother can change her mind about giving up her child for adoption.

What Do I Do about an Unplanned Pregnancy? If you are a woman who has an unplanned pregnancy and you either have to make the decision on your own or with a partner willing to help you make the decision, and you are not sure what to do, start by asking yourself the following questions:

- How do I feel about the man with whom I conceived this baby? Do I love him? Does he love me? Is this man committed to staying with me?
- What sort of relationship, if any, have we had or might we have in the future?
- Who can help me gain perspective on this problem?
- Do I want to continue the pregnancy and raise the child?
- If I keep my child, can I properly care for him or her?
- Do I have marketable skills, an education, an adequate income? Would I be able to go to school or keep my job if I have a child? Who would help me?
- Have I thought about adoption? If I continue the pregnancy, do I think I could surrender custody of my baby? Would it make a difference if there was an open adoption process and I could know the adoptive parents?
- Do I want to end the pregnancy with an abortion?
- How does abortion fit with what I believe is morally correct? Could I emotionally handle this option?

Answering these questions honestly and objectively may help you think through the realities of your situation.

Medical Abortion The term **medical abortion** describes the use of drugs, also called *abortifacients*, to terminate a pregnancy.[64] Methotrexate is given first. It stops the implantation of the embryo. Sometimes there is bleeding after the medication is given. Two days after taking this compound, misoprostol is administered. Misoprostol causes the uterus to contract, which helps expel a fertilized egg. The uterine lining is expelled along with the fertilized egg. Women have compared the discomfort of this experience to severe menstrual cramps. Common side effects include excessive bleeding, nausea, fatigue, abdominal pain, and dizziness. About one woman in 100 requires a blood transfusion.

Medical abortion does not require anesthesia, can be performed very early in pregnancy, and may feel more private. However, women experience more cramping and bleeding during medical abortion than during surgical abortion, and bleeding lasts for a longer period.

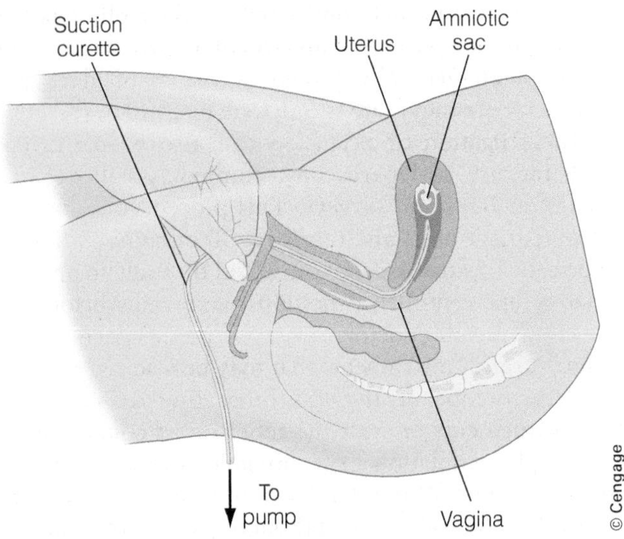

Figure 8-10 Suction Curettage

The contents of the uterus are extracted through the cervix with a vacuum apparatus.

Other Abortion Methods More than half of all abortions are performed within the first eight weeks of pregnancy. Medically, first-trimester abortion is less risky than childbirth. However, the likelihood of complications increases when abortions are performed in the second trimester (the second three-month period) of pregnancy.

The vast majority of abortions performed are **surgical abortions** where the contents of the uterus are emptied.[65] Surgical abortions are usually performed within 12–14 weeks from the last normal menstrual period in the first trimester of the pregnancy. This type of abortion can be performed on women as early as 6 weeks pregnant up until 20 weeks. **Suction curettage,** usually done from 6 to 14 weeks after the last menstrual period, involves the gradual dilation (opening) of the cervix by inserting and removing a dilator (tapered rods of increasing diameter) into the cervix. Some women feel pressure or cramping at this time. Once the cervix has dilated, the physician inserts a suction tip into the cervix, and the uterine contents are drawn out via a vacuum system (see Figure 8-10). A *curette* (a spoon-shaped surgical instrument used for scraping) is used to check for complete removal of the contents of the uterus. This procedure is called *dilation and curettage* (D&C). With suction curettage, the risks of complication are low. Major complications, such as perforation of the uterus, occur in less than one in 100 cases.

For early second-trimester abortions, physicians generally use a technique called **dilation and evacuation (D&E)**, in which they open the cervix and use medical instruments to remove the fetus from the uterus. D&E procedures are performed under local or general anesthesia.

To induce abortion from week 15 to week 19, prostaglandins (natural substances found in most body tissues) are administered as vaginal suppositories or injected into the amniotic sac by inserting a needle through the abdominal wall. They induce uterine contractions, and the fetus and placenta are expelled within 24 hours. Injecting saline or urea solutions into the amniotic sac can also terminate the pregnancy by triggering contractions that expel the fetus and placenta. Vaginal suppositories or drugs that help the uterus contract can also be used. Sometimes the physician will use suction as in first-trimester abortions, as well as forceps to remove additional fetal tissue. Complications from abortion techniques that induce labour include nausea, vomiting, diarrhea, tearing of the cervix, excessive bleeding, and possible shock and death.

Hysterotomy involves surgically opening the uterus and removing the fetus. This is generally done from week 16 to week 24 of the pregnancy, primarily in emergency situations when the woman's life is in danger or when other methods of abortion are considered too risky. However, late-pregnancy abortions increase the risk of spontaneous abortion or premature labour in subsequent pregnancies and should be avoided if possible.

What Is the Psychological Impact of Abortion?

Many people assume that abortion must be psychologically devastating and that women who abort a fetus will likely experience *post-abortion trauma syndrome.* Some studies suggest otherwise. Following a widespread review of the research, a group of researchers who updated a report of the American Psychological Association's Task Force on Mental Health and

Abortion determined that there were no greater mental health problems if a woman elected to have an abortion in the first trimester than if she had delivered a baby. It was not the abortion itself that increased the risk of mental health problems. Instead, lack of self-esteem, belonging to a religion that was against abortion, a perception of being stigmatized, or the necessity of keeping the abortion a secret reduced a woman's ability to cope.[66] At the highest risk were women who had a psychiatric illness, such as an anxiety disorder or clinical depression, prior to an abortion and those whose abortions occurred among complicated circumstances such as a rape or coercion by parents or a partner. However, findings from a study on 151 female university students who had abortions determined that they all suffered from varying levels of post-traumatic stress disorder (PTSD). Their grief also lasted approximately three years.[67]

The best predictor of psychological well-being after an abortion is a woman's emotional well-being prior to the pregnancy. Green Foster, Gould, and Kimport[68] found that most women believe that they will cope well after an abortion. The most common emotions that the women in their study anticipated feeling were relieved (63 percent) and confident (52 percent).

Politics of Abortion Abortion is one of the most controversial political, religious, and ethical issues of our time. The issues of when life begins, a woman's right to choose, and an unborn child's right to survival are divisive.

Pressure to liberalize Canada's abortion law began in the 1960s and came from medical and legal associations and various women's and social justice groups such as the Humanist Fellowship of Montreal, headed at that time by Dr. Henry Morgentaler. In 1969, a law was passed in Canada to regulate abortion under the Criminal Code. Abortion would still be illegal, but women could apply for special permission from a therapeutic abortion committee (TAC). Ongoing problems resulted from this new law. Many hospitals did not set up TACs since they were not required to do so by law. Where abortions were available, the application process sometimes took six to eight weeks. Some hospitals imposed a quota system. A 1988 Supreme Court of Canada decision found this process unconstitutional. The 1969 law was rendered unenforceable and found to violate Section Seven of the Charter of Rights and Freedoms. Abortion was decriminalized.[69]

As of March 1998, women could obtain an abortion in all provinces and territories in Canada except, as mentioned in the previous section, Prince Edward Island, where the government did not provide any abortion services whatsoever, although it did pay for hospital abortions in other provinces for women willing to travel. In British Columbia, Alberta, Ontario, Newfoundland, and most facilities in Quebec, the province pays for hospital fees or clinic fees. In the remaining provinces and territories, only abortions performed in hospitals are funded; abortion clinics require private payment. First Nations women have the highest rates of abortion in Canada, but many of them must travel to access abortion services.

The debate over abortion continues to stir passionate emotions, with pro-life supporters arguing that life begins at conception and that abortion is therefore immoral and pro-choice advocates countering that an individual woman should have the right to make decisions about her body and health. The controversy over abortion has at times become violent: physicians who performed abortions have been shot in British Columbia, Ontario, and Manitoba.

✓ CHECK-IN

Which alternatives would you consider if faced with an unplanned pregnancy?

Pro-Life **Pro-life** is a term that is used to refer to the opposition to abortion and support of the inherent right to life of every human being. This term is based on the scientific and ethical understanding that human life begins at the moment of conception and should therefore be valued from that point until one's natural death. Individuals working on behalf of the pro-life movement are committed to upholding the legal protection of human beings at all levels of development, including embryos in the womb.[70] Certain forms of birth control, such as birth control pills or the emergency contraceptive pill (EPC), are sometimes opposed due to their potential to prevent the human being at the embryonic stage from surviving.

Pro-life students are challenging those working in academe to be fair and accurate when lecturing on pro-life issues. Planned Parenthood groups on college and university campuses support students who do not choose abortion as a way to deal with an unexpected pregnancy. Many Canadian college and university students support the pro-life viewpoint. There are right-to-life campus clubs such as Youth Protecting Youth,[71] and groups such as the National Campus Life Network (NCLN),[72] an umbrella organization that has members at various universities, colleges, and cities across the country. These clubs and organizations host debates, run educational booths, and provide educational pro-life materials to students. There is also a movement by some students to encourage health centres to refer students to crisis pregnancy centres instead of abortion facilities.

Anastasia Pearse—Past Western Campus Coordinator for NCLN, and presently working for Life Canada—says that the goal of these organizations is to encourage dialogue among young people about the

HUMAN POTENTIAL

*Alison Chamberlain—Extraordinary Balance**

Eager to please others, it has taken Alison years to learn that doing something extraordinary is not necessarily doing something outside of oneself.

I have always been driven to be "helpful and caring." Unfortunately I spent most of my 20s being focused on others and I lost my own sense of self. Although I was pursuing a university education, the classes I chose to take did not resonate with me. The jobs I took to pay for my education only helped to sustain unhealthy relationships and leisure-time choices where I was not true to myself. I was a mess. I also became pregnant in a volatile relationship, and I made the extremely difficult, personal decision to not carry through with that pregnancy. Although a controversial decision for many, this decision helped me recognize that I needed to make some major changes in my life.

I stopped giving fuel to things that did not lead to the future I ultimately wanted— a healthy self, and a healthy family. I began taking care of myself, in tandem with caring for others. I enrolled in coursework in the health and wellness field. It seemed as if I had learned all the lessons I needed to put my happiness first, but it turned out that I was about to test my ability to put into practice what I had learned. A year and a half later, in a better relationship, on a path to a career and a triathlon under my belt, I became pregnant a second time.

My daughter was seven months old when I returned to university determined to finish my education. I completed both an undergraduate and master's degree. However, this decision created challenges. I was worried about the workload and how I was going to complete group projects. I was also concerned with timing. Being a mother often meant I was half an hour late for classes or meetings. I had to face trade-offs with my class schedule so that it fit well with my daughter's morning schedule and nap times. I traded jogging with her in the stroller for riding the bus back and forth to school daily. At 11 months old my daughter was so active she took every ounce of energy I had. I took online courses for two semesters so that I could "attend" sessions at night after she went to bed at 8:30 p.m. I had to consider my own self-doubts arising from comments made by people who cared about me suggesting that I was hurting my daughter because I was spending time studying during her formative years. And, unfortunately, the relationship with my daughter's father ended. I found myself a single mom, moving homes, finding part-time work and trying to complete school work during the first semester into my master's degree. There was no time for down-time.

Continually I had to reach out to others more than give to them. With no campus daycare spots available I had to depend on my sister, who was taking courses at the same time. She was amazing! We would coordinate schedules and class choices together at registration time each semester. It took extraordinary balance and compromise on her part to help me out. Peers offered to babysit, and some professors provided space for me to have my daughter in class.

Overall, my university life and full-time motherhood helped me to develop organizational skills. Procrastination was not possible anymore! I became efficient at preparing for the next day and being proactive using time available to concentrate on my studies when my daughter went down for a nap or to bed at night.

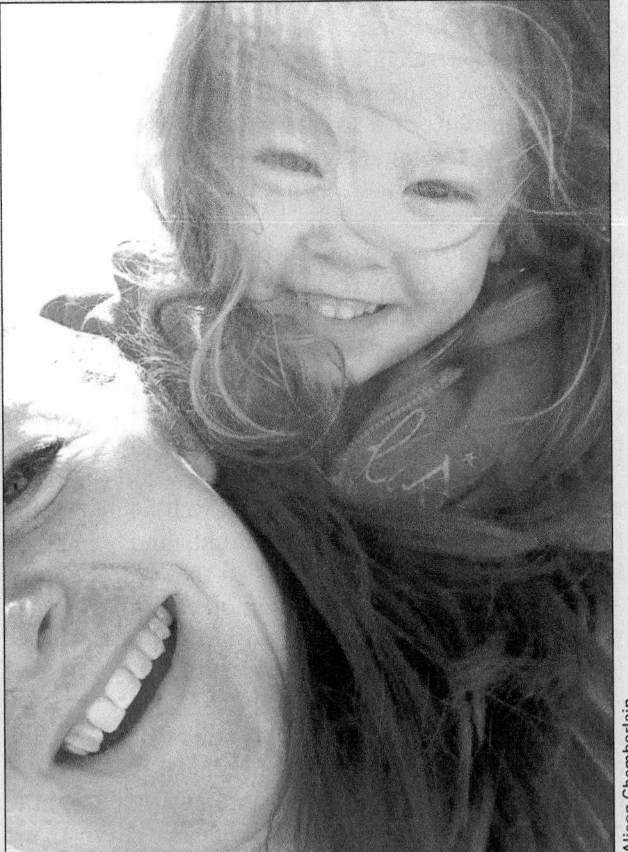

Alison Chamberlain

Alison Chamberlain and her daughter Yoshimi. Alison is finding ways to balance motherhood, postgraduate student life, and healthy living.

I also learned how to be "super-hero flexible" and had to ask that of others as well. I continue to be touched and surprised at how people reacted to me and my daughter on campus, in classes, and in the community when I was completing out-of-class assignments. I am additionally grateful for the amount of work I did. It showed me how tenacious and resilient I could be when necessary.

I am now a Recreation Coordinator and love my job. I have a fantastic group of clients and my workplace has a full-time daycare for which I receive a subsidy. This has helped make my transition to working full time and balancing motherhood somewhat easier. I am currently blending families with a new wonderful partner and his daughter. I am finally getting a glimpse at what a healthy family life looks like. I am so glad I have had these lessons in extraordinary balance and giving to myself before entering into this relationship. I, once again, face the ultimate challenge and rewards of balancing my integrity, sense of wellness, and caring for others at work, home, and play, but I finally feel like I have the foundation of self-care to take it all on.

*Alison Chamberlain

pro-life viewpoint. While many college and university campuses have groups dedicated to promoting the views of pro-choice students, other students promote the pro-life position. She suggests that society needs to provide more support for women who want to keep their children. She would like to see "baby-friendly" universities. She also feels that men need to accept more responsibility for unplanned pregnancies.

Abortion, for some, becomes a birth control method. The perspective the YPY and the NCLN take is that when another life is at stake, we need to step back and think through the consequences of our actions. Anastasia thinks the arguments that a child might not be loved enough, or will be impoverished in the future, are not truly predictable and do not justify killing an innocent human life through abortion. She does not deny that for women who despair because of the pressures of abortion and a lack of support and information, decisions about the life of their child can be confusing and difficult. She is encouraged that groups such as the one she has been involved with are making a difference by educating all students and assisting students who choose not to abort. She respects alternative viewpoints but believes she and other members of pro-life organizations must be willing to stand up for those who cannot stand up for themselves.[73]

What is important to remember about the pro-choice/pro-life debate is that every individual has certain values and beliefs. Honouring and celebrating "differences" is important when it comes to making healthy lifestyle choices.

PREGNANCY

Between 2010–2011 and 2014–2015, Canada has seen a growth in the number of births (see Table 8-2). Overall births during the year 2010–2011 totalled 376 951. In 2014–2015, overall births totalled 388 729.[74]

The average age of first-time mothers has changed as well. In 1983 young women were on average 26.9 years old when they had their first child. In 2012 the average age of first-time mothers was just over 29 years old. Mothers are now averaging slightly fewer than two children each. It is important to remember, though, that not all married or unmarried couples choose parenthood.[75]

Of course, you do not have to be part of a couple to want or to conceive a child. The number of never-married college- and university-educated career women who are becoming single parents has risen considerably. They

TABLE 8-2

Births, Estimates, by Province and Territory

	2010/2011	2011/2012	2012/2013	2013/2014	2014/2015
			Number		
Canada	376 951	377 897	382 980	386 044	388 729
Newfoundland and Labrador	4 775	4 552	4 533	4 484	4 409
Prince Edward Island	1 428	1 426	1 431	1 429	1 428
Nova Scotia	8 818	8 727	8 687	8 613	8 588
New Brunswick	7 140	7 028	6 933	6 827	6 715
Quebec	88 611	88 311	89 000	88 250	86 950
Ontario	139 448	139 658	141 248	142 970	144 395
Manitoba	15 614	15 702	15 979	16 248	16 540
Saskatchewan	14 438	14 498	14 951	15 345	15 676
Alberta	50 853	52 230	54 054	56 078	57 677
British Columbia	43 908	43 774	44 153	43 781	44 323
Yukon	404	440	445	439	443
Northwest Territories	676	692	697	695	687
Nunavut	838	859	869	885	898

Notes: Period from July 1 to June 30.
The numbers for births are final up to 2011/2012, updated for 2013/2014, and preliminary for 2014/2015.
Preliminary and updated estimates of births were produced by Demography Division, Statistics Canada. Final data were produced by Health Statistics Division, Statistics Canada. However, the final estimates included in this table may differ from data released by the Health Statistics Division, due to distribution of unknown province.

Source: Statistics Canada. CANSIM, Table 051-0004 and Catalogue no. 91-215-X. http://www.statcan.gc.ca/tables-tableaux/sum-som/l01/cst01/demo04a-eng.htm.

want children—with or without an ongoing relationship with a partner—and may feel that, because of their age, they cannot delay getting pregnant any longer. Waiting to have children does have some inherent risks. Miscarriage is higher among older expectant mothers. Down Syndrome, a condition where the baby is born with an extra chromosome that results in varying levels of physical abnormalities and cognitive disabilities, is a common birth defect among babies born of older mothers.

Preconception Care: A Preventive Approach The time *before* a child is conceived can be crucial in ensuring that an infant is born healthy, full size, and full term. Women who smoke, drink alcohol, take drugs, eat poorly, are too thin or too heavy, suffer from unrecognized infections or illnesses, or are exposed to toxins at work or home may start pregnancy with one or more strikes against them and their unborn babies. **Preconception care**—the enhancement of a woman's health and well-being prior to conception in order to ensure a healthy pregnancy and baby—includes risk assessment (evaluation of medical, genetic, and lifestyle risks), health promotion (such as good nutrition and regular physical activity), and interventions to reduce risk (such as treatment of infections and other diseases and assistance in quitting smoking or drug use). More information on the use of drugs, alcohol, and tobacco products during pregnancy is available in Chapters 11 and 12.

How a Woman's Body Changes during Pregnancy The 40 weeks of pregnancy transform a woman's body. At the beginning of pregnancy, the woman's uterus becomes slightly larger, and the cervix becomes softer and bluish due to increased blood flow. Progesterone and estrogen trigger changes in the milk glands and ducts in the breasts, which increase in size and feel somewhat tender. The pressure of the growing uterus against the bladder causes a more frequent need to urinate. As the pregnancy progresses, the woman's skin stretches as her body shape changes, her centre of gravity changes as her abdomen protrudes, and her internal organs shift as the baby grows (see Figure 8-11). Pregnancy is typically divided into three-month periods called trimesters.

How a Baby Grows Silently and invisibly, over a nine-month period, a fertilized egg develops into a human being. When the zygote reaches the uterus, it's still smaller than the head of a pin. Once nestled into the spongy uterine lining, it becomes an **embryo**. The embryo takes on an elongated shape, rounded at one end. A sac called the **amnion** envelops it (see photo, Figure 8-11). As water and other small molecules cross the amniotic membrane, the embryo floats freely in the absorbed fluid, cushioned from shocks and bumps. At nine weeks the embryo is called a **fetus**.

A special organ, the **placenta**, forms. Attached to the embryo by the umbilical cord, it supplies the growing baby with fluid and nutrients from the maternal bloodstream and carries waste back to the mother's body for disposal.

Emotional Aspects of Pregnancy Almost all prospective parents worry about their ability to care for a newborn. By talking openly about their feelings and fears, however, they can strengthen the bonds between them, so that they can work together as parents as well as partners. Psychological problems, such as depression, can occur during pregnancy. Social support and other resources for coping with stress can make a great difference in the potential impact of emotional difficulties.

The physiological changes of pregnancy can affect a woman's mood. In early pregnancy, she may feel weepy, irritable, or emotional. As the pregnancy continues, she may become calmer and more energetic. Men, too, feel a range of intense emotions about the prospect of having a child: pride, anxiety, hope, and fears for their unseen child and for the woman they love. The more involved fathers become in preparing for birth, the closer they feel to their partners and babies afterward.

Complications of Pregnancy In about 10–15 percent of all pregnancies, there is increased risk of some problem, such as a baby's failure to grow normally. **Perinatology**, or maternal–fetal medicine, focuses on the special needs of high-risk mothers and their unborn babies. Several of the most frequent potential complications of pregnancy are discussed following.

Ectopic Pregnancy In an **ectopic pregnancy**, the fertilized egg remains in the fallopian tube instead of travelling to the uterus. Ectopic, or tubal, pregnancies have increased dramatically in recent years. STIs, particularly chlamydia infections, have become a major cause of ectopic pregnancy. Other risk factors include previous pelvic surgery, particularly involving the fallopian tubes; pelvic inflammatory disease; infertility; and use of an IUD.

Miscarriage About 10–20 percent of pregnancies end in **miscarriage**, or spontaneous abortion, before the 20th week of gestation. Major genetic disorders may be responsible for 33–50 percent of pregnancy losses. Up to 60 percent of first-trimester miscarriages are associated with abnormal chromosomes.[76] About 0.5–1 percent of women suffer three or more miscarriages, possibly because of genetic, anatomic, hormonal, infectious, or autoimmune factors.[77] An estimated 70–90 percent of women who miscarry eventually become pregnant again.

Infections The infectious disease most clearly linked to birth defects is **rubella** (German measles). All women should be vaccinated against this disease at least three

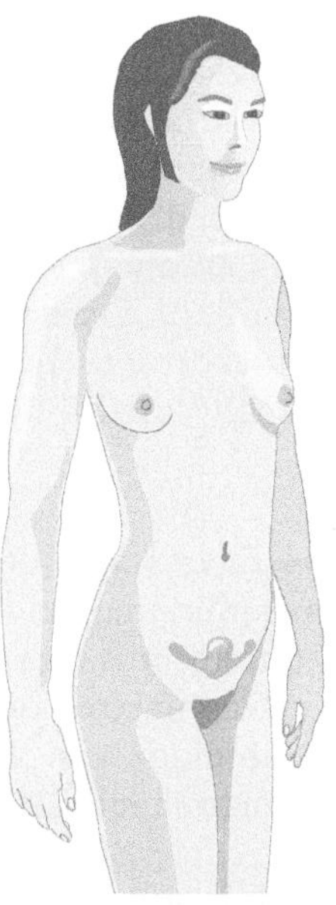

Before conception

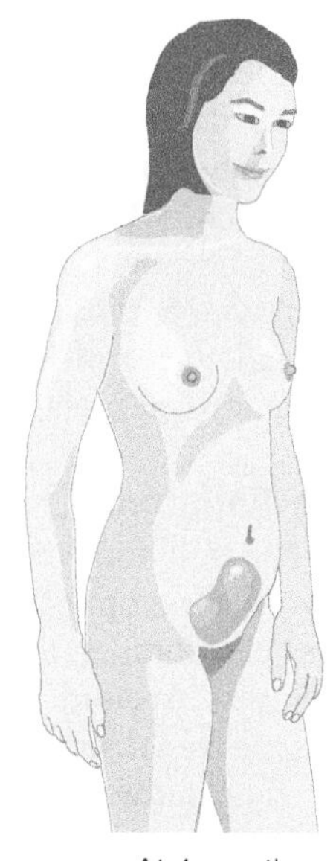

At 4 months

First Trimester

Increased urination because of hormonal changes and the pressure of the enlarging uterus on the bladder.

Enlarged breasts as milk glands develop.

Darkening of the nipples and the area around them.

Nausea or vomiting, particularly in the morning.

Fatigue.

Increased vaginal secretions.

Pinching of the sciatic nerve, which runs from the buttocks down through the back of the legs, as the pelvic bones widen and begin to separate.

Irregular bowel movements.

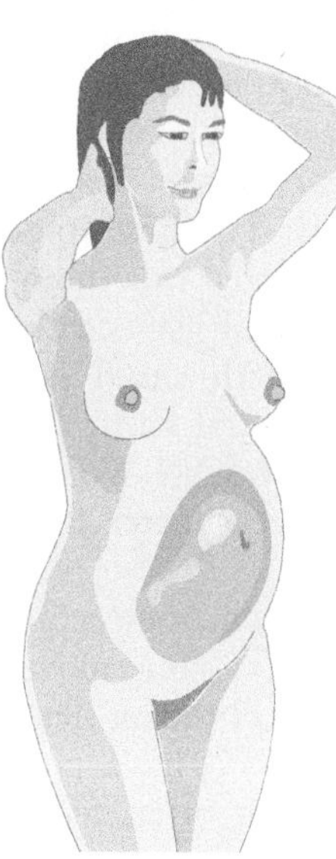

At 7 months

Second Trimester

Thickening of the waist as the uterus grows.

Weight gain.

Increase in total blood volume.

Slight increase in size and change in position of the heart.

Darkening of the pigment around the nipple and from the navel to the pubic region.

Darkening of the face.

Increased salivation and perspiration.

Secretion of colostrum from the breasts.

Indigestion, constipation, and hemorrhoids.

Varicose veins.

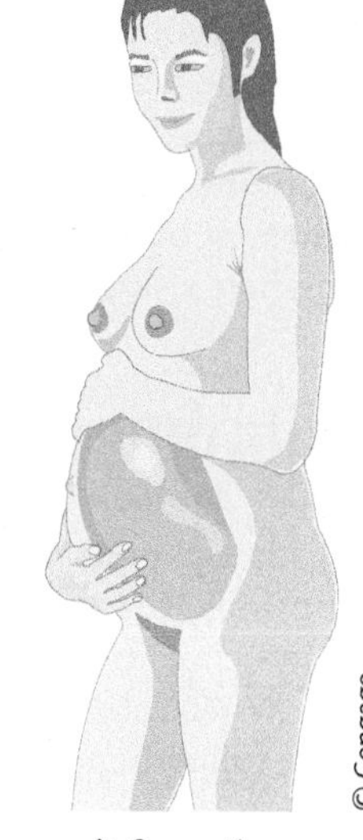

At 9 months

© Cengage

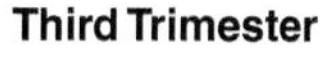

Third Trimester

Increased urination because of pressure from the uterus.

Tightening of the uterine muscles (called Braxton-Hicks contractions).

Shortness of breath because of increased pressure by the uterus on the lungs and diaphragm.

Heartburn and indigestion.

Trouble sleeping because of the baby's movements or the need to urinate.

Descending ("dropping") of the baby's head into the pelvis about two to four weeks before birth.

Navel pushed out.

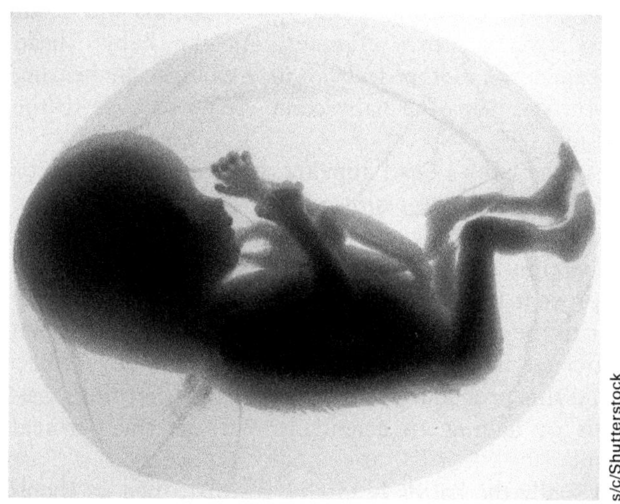

s/c/Shutterstock

Figure 8-11 Physiological Changes of Pregnancy

months prior to conception to protect themselves and any children they may bear. The most common prenatal infection today is *cytomegalovirus*. This infection produces mild flu-like symptoms in adults but can cause brain damage, retardation, liver disease, cerebral palsy, hearing problems, and other malformations in unborn babies.

STIs, such as syphilis, gonorrhea, and genital herpes, can be particularly dangerous during pregnancy if not recognized and treated. If a woman has a herpes outbreak around the date her baby is due, her physician will deliver the baby by Caesarean section to prevent infecting the baby. HIV infection endangers both a pregnant woman and her unborn baby, and all pregnant women and new mothers should be aware of the risks to themselves and their babies.

Premature Labour Approximately 10 percent of all babies are born too soon (before the 37th week of pregnancy). Prematurity is the main underlying cause of stillbirth and infant deaths within the first few weeks after birth. Bed rest, close monitoring, and, if necessary, medications for at-risk women can buy more time in the womb for their babies. But women must recognize the warning signs of **premature labour**—dull, low backache; a feeling of tightness or pressure on the lower abdomen; and intestinal cramps, sometimes with diarrhea. Low-birth-weight premature babies face the highest risks.

CHILDBIRTH

Today parents can choose from an array of birthing options that include hospital births attended by a physician and possibly a midwife, to home births.

When interviewing physicians or midwives, look for the following:

- experience in handling various complications
- extensive prenatal care
- a commitment to be at the mother's side for the entire labour in order to quickly spot complications and provide assistance
- a compatible philosophy toward childbirth and medical interventions

Preparing for Childbirth The most widespread method of childbirth preparation is **psychoprophylaxis**, or the **Lamaze method**. Fernand Lamaze, a French doctor, instructed women to respond to labour contractions with pre-learned, controlled breathing techniques. As the intensity of each contraction increases, the labouring woman concentrates on increasing her breathing rate in a prescribed way. Her partner coaches her during each contraction and helps her cope with discomfort.

Women who have had childbirth-preparation training tend to have fewer complications and require fewer medications. However, painkillers or anesthesia are options if labour is longer or more painful than expected. The lower body can be numbed with an **epidural block**, which involves injecting an anesthetic into the membrane around the spinal cord, or a **spinal block**, in which the injection goes directly into the spinal canal. General anesthesia is usually used only for emergency Caesarean births.

What Is Childbirth Like? There are three stages of **labour**. The first starts with *effacement* (thinning) and *dilation* (opening up) of the cervix. Effacement is measured in percentages and dilation in centimetres or finger-widths. Around this time, the amniotic sac of fluids usually breaks, a sign that the woman should call her doctor or midwife.

The first contractions of the early, or *latent*, phase of labour are usually not uncomfortable; they last 15–30 seconds, occur every 15–30 minutes, and gradually increase in intensity and frequency. The most difficult contractions come after the cervix is dilated to about eight centimetres, as the woman feels greater pressure from the fetus. The first stage ends when the cervix is completely dilated to a diameter of 10 centimetres (or five finger-widths) and the baby is ready to come down the birth canal (see Figure 8-12). For women having their first baby, this first stage of labour averages 12–13 hours. Women having another child often experience shorter first-stage labour.

When the cervix is completely dilated, the second stage of labour occurs, during which the baby moves into the vagina, or birth canal, and out of the mother's body. As this stage begins, women who have gone through childbirth-preparation training often feel a sense of relief from the acute pain of the transition phase and at the prospect of giving birth.

This second stage can take up to an hour or more. Strong contractions may last 60–90 seconds and occur every two to three minutes. As the baby's head descends, the mother feels an urge to push. By bearing down, she helps the baby complete its passage to the outside.

As the baby's head appears, or *crowns*, the doctor may perform an *episiotomy*—an incision from the lower end of the vagina toward the anus to enlarge the vaginal opening. The purpose of the episiotomy is to prevent the baby's head from causing an irregular tear in the vagina, but routine episiotomies have been criticized as unnecessary. Women may be able to avoid this procedure by trying different birthing positions or having an attendant massage the perineal tissue.

Usually the baby's head emerges first, then its shoulders, then its body. With each contraction, a new part is

1. The cervix is partially dilated, and the baby's head has entered the birth canal.

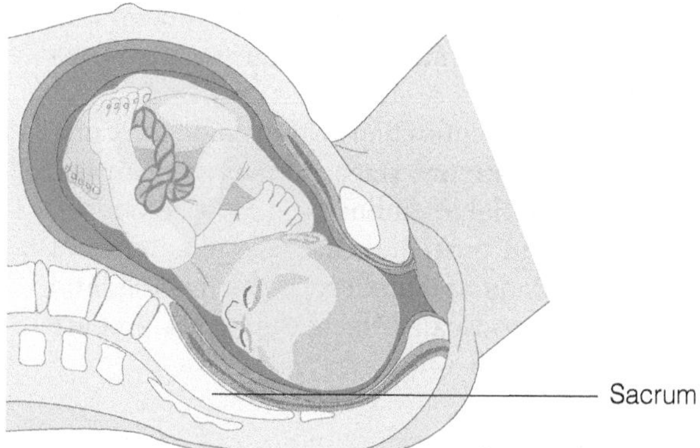

2. The cervix is nearly completely dilated. The baby's head rotates so that it can move through the birth canal.

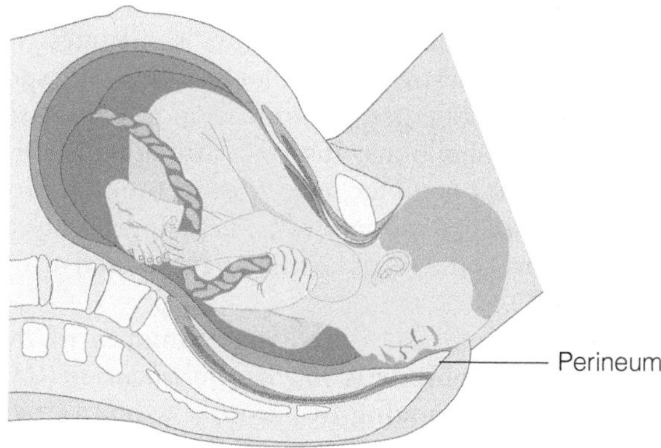

3. The baby's head extends as it reaches the vaginal opening, and the head and the rest of the body pass through the birth canal.

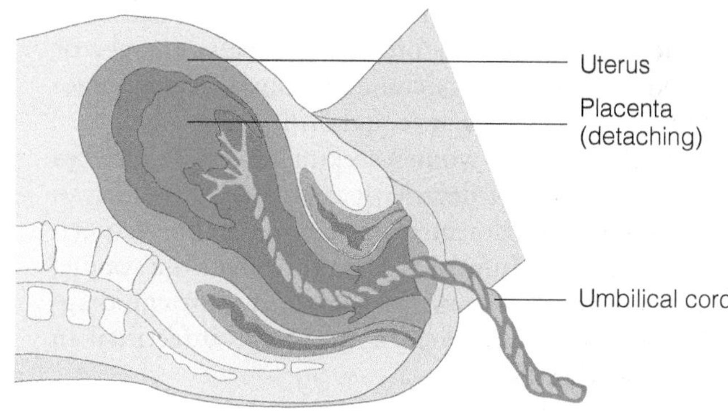

4. After the baby is born, the placenta detaches from the uterus and is expelled from the woman's body.

Figure 8-12 **Birth**

born. However, the baby can be in a more difficult position, facing up rather than down, or with the feet or buttocks first (a **breech birth**), and a Caesarean birth may then be necessary.

In the third stage of labour, the uterus contracts firmly after the birth of the baby and, usually within five minutes, the placenta separates from the uterine wall. The woman may bear down to help expel the placenta, or the doctor may exert gentle external pressure. If an episiotomy has been performed, the doctor sews up the incision. To help the uterus contract and return to its normal size, it may be massaged manually, or the baby may be put to the mother's breast to stimulate contraction of the uterus.

Caesarean Birth In a **Caesarean delivery** (also referred to as a *Caesarean section*), the doctor lifts the baby out of the woman's body through an incision made in the lower abdomen and uterus. The most common reason for Caesarean birth is *failure to progress*, a vague term indicating that labour has gone on too long and may put the baby or mother at risk. Other reasons include the baby's position (if feet or buttocks are first) and signs that the fetus is in danger.

About 36 percent of Caesarean sections are performed because the woman has had a previous Caesarean birth. However, four of every five women who have had Caesarean births *can* have successful vaginal deliveries in subsequent pregnancies.

Caesarean birth involves abdominal surgery, so many women feel more physical discomfort after a Caesarean than a vaginal birth, including nausea, pain, and abdominal gas. Women who have had a Caesarean section must refrain from strenuous activity, such as heavy lifting, for several weeks.

After the Birth Hospital stay for new mothers are shorter than in the past. In some provinces, the average length of stay is now one day after vaginal delivery and four days after a Caesarean birth. A primary reason has been the pressure to reduce medical costs. Obstetricians have voiced concern that the rush to release new mothers may jeopardize their well-being and the health of their babies, who are more likely to require emergency care for problems such as jaundice.

There is not room in this chapter to include information about the postpartum stage. However there are many resources available online and in bookstores. Learning more about postnatal care, the possibility of postpartum depression and anxiety, breastfeeding, and celebrating parenthood can help new parents prepare for this next stage in life.

INFERTILITY

The World Health Organization defines **infertility** as the failure to conceive after one year of unprotected intercourse. Western societies regard infertility as a medical rather than social problem. The main causes of infertility are ovulation problems, tubal damage, or sperm dysfunction. Less common causes are endometriosis, cervical factors, or coital difficulties.

The percentage of women seeking infertility services has risen in the past decade. It is estimated that up to one in six or 16 percent of Canadian couples experiences infertility.[78] Infertility is a problem of the couple, not of the individual man or woman. A thorough diagnostic workup can reveal a cause for infertility in 90 percent of cases.

In women, the most common causes of infertility are age, abnormal menstrual patterns, suppression of ovulation, and blocked fallopian tubes. A woman's fertility peaks between ages 20 and 30 and then drops quickly: by 20 percent after 30, by 50 percent after 35, and by 95 percent after 40.

Male infertility is usually linked to either the quantity or the quality of sperm, which may be inactive, misshapen, or insufficient (less than 20 million sperm per millilitre of semen in an ejaculation of three to five millilitres). Sometimes the problem is hormonal or a blockage of a sperm duct. Some men suffer from the inability to ejaculate normally or from retrograde ejaculation, in which some of the semen travels in the wrong direction, back into the body of the male.

Infertility can have an enormous emotional impact. For some women the ability to become pregnant touches on a core aspect of femininity. Some feel a great loss if they cannot conceive. Women in their 30s and 40s fear that their biological clock is running out of time. Men may be confused and surprised by the intensity of their partner's emotions.

The treatment of infertility has become a multi-billion-dollar-a-year enterprise. The odds of achieving a successful pregnancy range from 30 to 70 percent, depending on the specific cause of infertility.[79] One result of successful infertility treatments has been a boom in multiple births, including quintuplets and sextuplets. Some obstetricians have urged less aggressive treatment for infertility to avoid such high-risk multiple births.

Artificial Insemination **Artificial insemination** is the introduction of viable sperm into the vagina by artificial means. There are variations of artificial insemination. One is intrauterine insemination (IUI), which usually includes ovarian stimulation and preparation of the semen. Another variation is donor insemination (DI). Sperm from a donor is used to achieve pregnancy when the husband or partner has few or no sperm, has sperm of poor quality, or might risk passing on an inherited disease.[80]

Assisted Reproductive Technology New approaches to infertility include microsurgery, sometimes with lasers, to open destroyed or blocked egg and sperm ducts; new hormone preparations to induce ovulation; and the use of balloons, inserted through the cervix and inflated, to open blocked fallopian tubes (a procedure called *balloon tuboplasty*). These approaches and techniques are known as **artificial reproductive technology (ART)**.

Among the most well-known techniques to overcome fertility problems is *in vitro fertilization (IVF)*, which involves removing ova from a woman's ovary and placing the woman's egg and a man's sperm in a laboratory dish for fertilization. If the fertilized egg cell shows signs of development, within several days it is returned to the woman's uterus, the egg cell implants itself in the lining of the uterus, and the pregnancy continues as normal. The Canadian Fertility and Andrology Society (CFAS) reports that complication rates for IVF are low. In 2012, the overall clinical pregnancy rates per cycle started were 31 percent for women under 35 years old, 23 percent for women aged 35–39, and 10 percent for women who were 40 years and older.[81]

In Canada, there is much debate about assisted human reproduction (AHR). In March 2004 the *Assisted Human Reproduction Act* became law. The act ensured that Canada had one of the most comprehensive legislative frameworks in the world. It prohibited human cloning and protected the health and safety of Canadians who used AHR. As of April 2012, amendments to the AHR were approved as part of Bill C-38, the *Jobs, Growth and Long-term Prosperity Act*. This resulted in the dissolution of the AHR agency; all responsibilities of the AHR were transferred to the federal Ministry of Health. There is concern among some health professionals that there will no longer be a standardized health reporting process in reproductive technology. Another concern is the inconsistency of AHR methods across Canada.[82]

SELF-SURVEY

Which Contraceptive Method Is Best for You?

Answer Yes or No to each statement as it applies to you and, if appropriate, your partner.

1. You have high blood pressure or cardiovascular disease. _______
2. You smoke cigarettes. _______
3. You have a new sexual partner. _______
4. An unwanted pregnancy would be devastating to you. _______
5. You have a good memory. _______
6. You or your partner has multiple sexual partners. _______
7. You prefer a method with little or no bother. _______
8. You have heavy, crampy periods. _______
9. You need protection against STIs. _______
10. You are concerned about endometrial and ovarian cancer. _______
11. You are forgetful. _______
12. You need a method right away. _______
13. You're comfortable touching your own and your partner's genitals. _______
14. You have a cooperative partner. _______
15. You like a little extra vaginal lubrication. _______
16. You have sex at unpredictable times and places. _______
17. You are in a monogamous relationship and have at least one child. _______

Answers to Self-Survey

Scoring:
Recommendations are based on Yes answers to the following numbered statements:
The combination pill: 4, 5, 6, 8, 10, 16
The progestin-only pill: 1, 2, 5, 7, 16
The patch: 4, 7, 8, 11, 16
The NuvaRing: 4, 7, 8, 11, 13, 16
Condoms: 1, 2, 3, 6, 9, 12, 13, 14
Depo-Provera: 1, 2, 4, 7, 11, 16A
Diaphragm, cervical cap, or FemCap: 1, 2, 13, 14
Mirena® IUD: 1, 2, 7, 8, 11, 13, 16, 17
Spermicides: 1, 2, 12, 13, 14, 15B
Sponge: 1, 2, 12, 13

Source:
1 According to Pfizer Canada, Inc., data from some clinical studies suggest that women who use Depo-Provera may lose significant Bone Mineral Density (BMD). The bone loss appears to be greater the longer the use. Health Canada is evaluating Depo-Provera. (Sexual Health Centre Saskatoon. March 21, 2012) 2012 Sexual Health Centre Saskatoon—Updated March 21, 2012. Found at: http://www.sexualhealthcentresaskatoon.ca/bc/depo.php
2 Researchers have found that Nonoxynol-9 (N-9), a common chemical ingredient in spermicides, may increase the risk of HIV and STI transmission due to causing skin irritations in users. (Spermicides. Canadian Federation for Sexual Health. September 1, 2009. Found at:www.cfsh.ca/Your_Sexual_Health/Contraception-and-Safer-Sex/Contraception-and-Birth-Control/Spermicides.aspx

Chapter Summary

1. When does conception occur?
   a. when a fertilized egg implants in the lining of the uterus
   b. when sperm is blocked from reaching the egg
   c. when a sperm fertilizes the egg
   d. after the uterine lining is discharged during the menstrual cycle

2. Which of the following is NOT a factor to consider when choosing a contraceptive method?
   a. cost
   b. failure rate
   c. effectiveness in preventing sexually transmitted infections
   d. preferred sexual position

3. When used correctly, which of the following contraceptives is 85–98 percent effective?
   a. Nova-T intrauterine device (IUD)
   b. condom
   c. spermicide
   d. diaphragm

4. Which of the following choices is the only form of birth control that is 100 percent effective?
   a. condom
   b. IUD
   c. abstinence
   d. withdrawal

5. Which statement about prescription contraceptives is false?
   a. Prescription contraceptives do not offer protection against STIs.
   b. Some prescription contraceptives contain estrogen and progestin, and some contain only progestin.
   c. The contraceptive ring must be changed every week.
   d. IUDs prevent pregnancy by preventing or interfering with implantation.

6. Which statement about sterilization is true?
   a. In women, the most frequently performed sterilization technique is hysterectomy.

b. Many couples experience an increase in sexual encounters after sterilization.
c. Vasectomies are easily reversed with surgery.
d. Sterilization is recommended for single men and women who are unsure about whether they want children.

7. Which statement about many nations with fewer unwanted pregnancies and lower abortion rates is true?
a. The population of women older than 30 is high.
b. The majority of women are affluent.
c. The majority of women are poor.
d. Birth control education begins early and contraceptives are generally easier and cheaper to obtain.

8. Which statement about the third trimester of pregnancy is true?
a. The woman experiences shortness of breath as the enlarged uterus presses on the lungs and diaphragm.
b. The embryo is now called a fetus.
c. The woman should begin regular prenatal checkups.
d. The woman should increase her activity level to ensure that she is fit for childbirth.

9. Which statement about childbirth is true?
a. Breech birth can be prevented by practising the Lamaze method.
b. The cervix thins and dilates so that the baby can exit the uterus.
c. The intensity of contractions decreases during the second stage of labour.
d. The placenta is expelled immediately before the baby's head appears.

10. Which statement about in vitro fertilization is true?
a. Infertility is most often caused by female problems.
b. In men, infertility is usually caused by a combination of excess sperm production and an ejaculation problem.
c. In vitro fertilization involves removing ova from a woman's ovary and placing the woman's egg and a man's sperm in a laboratory dish for fertilization.
d. Less than 1 percent of live births are the result of artificial reproductive technology.

Answers to these questions can be found on page 219.

SELF-RESPONSIBILITY—SOCIAL RESPONSIBILITY

SELF-RESPONSIBILITY

Knowing is not enough; we must apply. Willing is not enough; we must do.
Goethe

When we have reproductive choices, we also have the responsibility to contemplate and prepare for those choices. Self-responsibility becomes responsibility between two people. On the Stages of Change model continuum, where are you? Are you prepared for both the joys of positive sexual relations as well as the inherent risks of having sex? If you are not ready to have sex with your partner, do you have an action plan in place so you are not pressured to do so? If you are not ready to have children, are you using birth control? Do you protect yourself and your partner against STIs? Planning and protecting yourself now can prevent many unnecessary problems in the future.

SOCIAL RESPONSIBILITY

Making the decision to have a child is momentous. It is to decide forever to have your heart go walking around outside your body.
Elizabeth Stone

CRITICAL THINKING

1. After reading about the various methods of contraception, which do you think would be most effective for you? What factors enter into your decision (convenience, risks, effectiveness, etc.)?
2. As the debate over abortion continues, with pro-life supporters on one side and pro-choice advocates on the other, what is your opinion about a woman's right to make decisions about her own body? What about a man's right to participate in the decision-making process along with his partner if an unexpected pregnancy happened?
3. Suppose that you and your partner were told that your only chance of having a child is by using fertility drugs. After taking the drugs, you and your partner are informed that there are seven fetuses. Would you carry them all to term? What if you knew that the chances of them all surviving were very slim and that eliminating some of them would improve the odds for the others? What ethical issues do cases like this raise?

WEB LINKS

National Campus Life Network
www.ncln.ca/
This national student organization provides support for pro-life students on Canadian college and university campuses. Check out resources, articles and news, information on a national symposium, and training opportunities.

Options for Sexual Health.org
www.optionsforsexualhealth.org/
Information on sexual health issues, birth control options, and education services and resources are all available at this comprehensive and up-to-date site.

Sexuality and U
www.sexualityandu.ca
This site has an excellent section on the different types of contraception.

Please note that links are subject to change. If you find a broken link, use a search engine such as www.google.ca and search for the website by typing in keywords.

Key Terms

The terms listed here are used within the chapter on the page indicated. Definitions of the terms are in the Glossary at the end of the book.

Answers to Chapter Summary Questions

1. c; 2. d; 3. b; 4. c; 5. c; 6. b; 7. d; 8. a; 9. b; 10; d

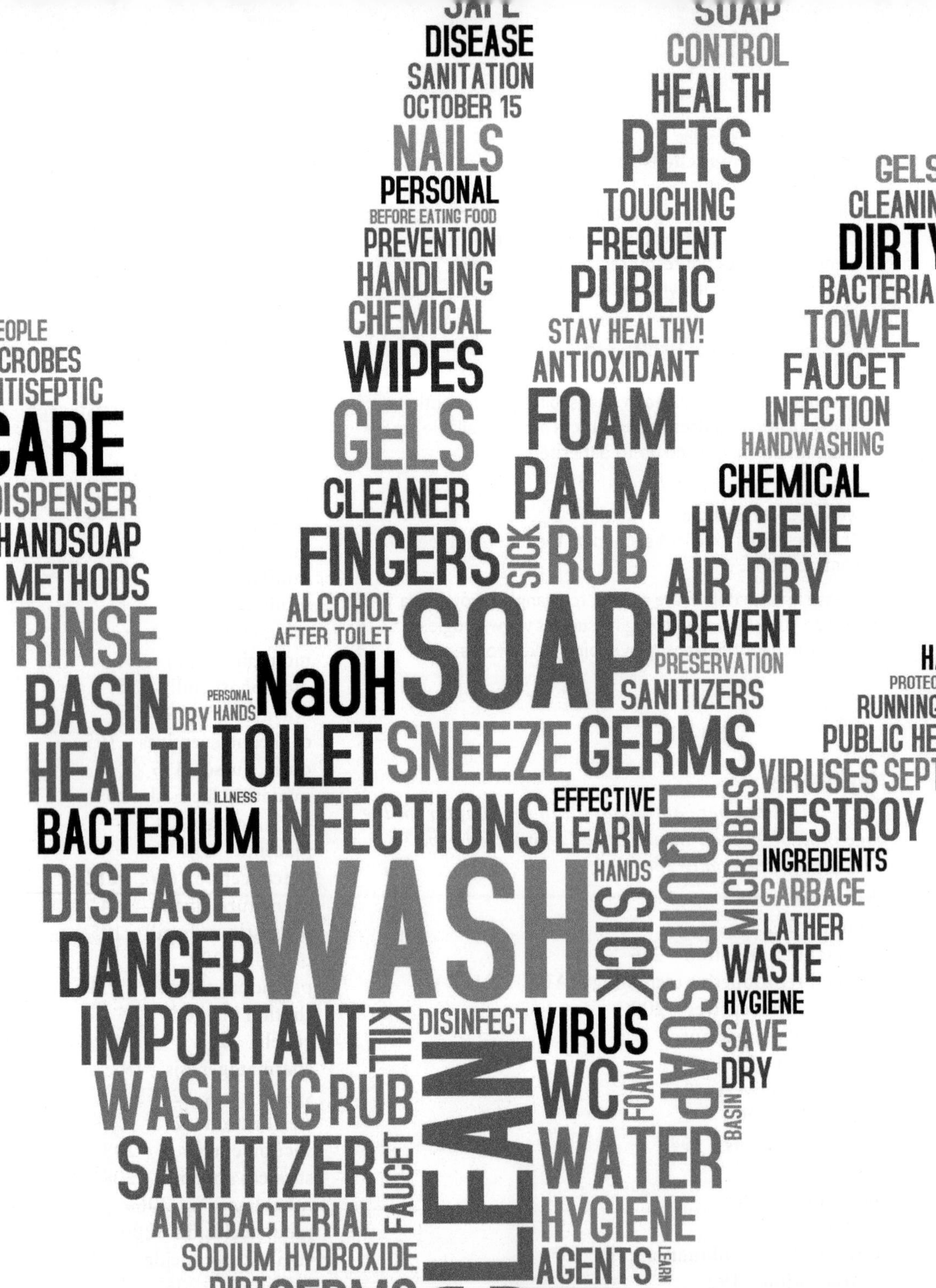

alpimages/Shutterstock

AFTER READING THIS CHAPTER, YOU WILL BE ABLE TO:

- **explain** how the different agents of infection spread disease
- **describe** how your body protects itself from infectious disease
- **list** and **describe** some common infectious diseases, such as the common cold, hepatitis, meningitis, SARS, and influenza
- **identify** some sexually transmitted diseases and the symptoms and treatments for each
- **define** HIV infection and **describe** its symptoms
- **list** the methods of HIV transmission
- **explain** some practical methods for preventing HIV infection and other sexually transmitted infections

9

Protecting Yourself from Infectious Diseases

Throughout history, infectious diseases have claimed more lives than any military conflict or natural disaster. Although modern medicine has won many victories against the agents of infection, we remain vulnerable to a host of infectious illnesses. Drug-resistant strains of tuberculosis and *Staphylococcus aureus* bacteria challenge current therapies. Scientists are also warning of the potential danger of new emerging viruses.

As well, some of today's most common and dangerous infectious illnesses are spread primarily through sexual contact, and their incidence has skyrocketed. However, we can, by our behaviour, prevent and control many of them. Learning about the ways in which infections are acquired and spread can support the process of self-care and care of others. Education about sexual health can help reduce anxiety about sexually transmitted infections and how they can be avoided.

This chapter is a lesson in self-defence against many forms of infection. There is a short review section on the infection triangle. You will find information about agents of infection such as bacteria, viruses, and fungi. You will learn how infections are passed on to humans through animals and insects, and other people, through food sources and water. There is a section on how our immune system works and how our body protects itself. Some common bacterial and viral infections are described. The chapter ends with a comprehensive section on sexually transmitted infections—what they are, how you can prevent them, and how you can manage them.

FREQUENTLY ASKED QUESTIONS

FAQ: Where do microorganisms live, grow, and multiply? p. 224

FAQ: Who is at highest risk of infectious diseases? p. 231

FAQ: What is human papillomavirus? p. 243

FAQ: What progress has been made in treating HIV? p. 248

UNDERSTANDING INFECTION

We live in a sea of microbes. Most of them do not threaten our health or survival; some, such as the bacteria that inhabit our intestines, are actually beneficial. Yet in the course of history, disease-causing microorganisms have claimed millions of lives. Infection is a complex process. The six links in the **chain of infection,**[1] (see Figure 9-1) sometimes described as a series of infection events, must be connected for any infection to develop. When any link of the chain is broken, the transmission of an infection can be stopped. The six links are the **infectious agents,** also known as **pathogens,** reservoirs, portals of exit, modes of transmission, portals of entry, and a susceptible host. We will discuss three of the links in detail—infectious agents, reservoirs, and modes of transmission. We will define portals of exit and entry and susceptible hosts briefly.

Infectious Agents or Pathogens The types of microbes that can cause infections are viruses, bacteria, fungi, protozoa, and helminths (parasitic worms).

Viruses **Viruses** are tough, tiny pathogens (see Figure 9-2(a)). These small infectious organisms, 10–100 times smaller than bacteria and much smaller than fungi, consist of a bit of nucleic acid (DNA or RNA, but never both) with a protein coat. A virus may or may not have an outermost spiky layer called the *envelope.*[2] Unlike bacteria, which can grow on non-living surfaces, a virus is unable to reproduce on its own, so it must invade a living cell (plant or animal) to reproduce. It then instructs the cell to produce new viral particles. Usually the infected cell dies because it can no longer perform its normal functions. But before it dies, the cell releases new viruses, which are then released to enter other cells.

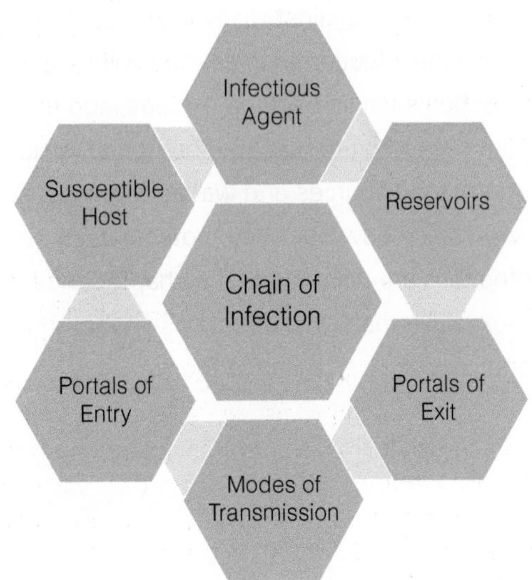

Figure 9-1 Chain of Infection

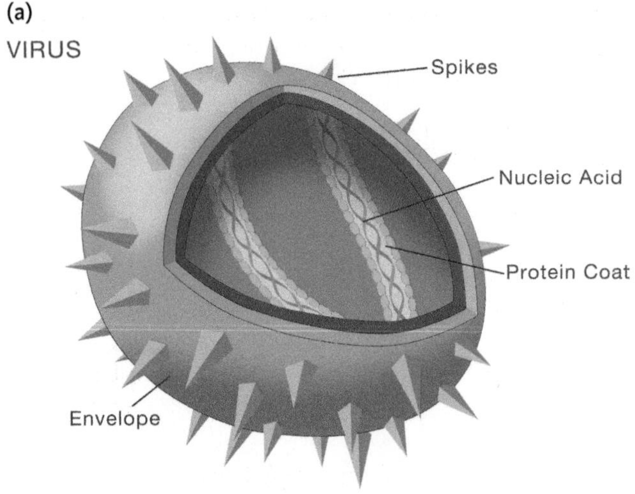

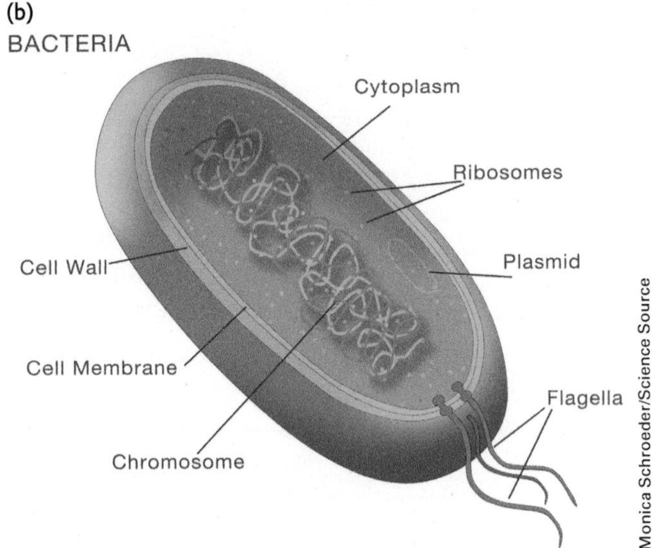

Monica Schroeder/Science Source

Figure 9-2 Virus and Bacterium

(a) A virus consists of a bit of nucleic acid (DNA or RNA, but never both) with a protein coat. A virus may or may not have an outermost spiky layer called the envelope. (b) Bacteria have a rigid cell wall and a thin, rubbery cell membrane that surrounds fluid (cytoplasm) inside the cell. They contain genetic information they need to make copies of themselves (DNA) in a structure called a chromosome.

Some viruses do not kill the cells that they infect. Instead, they alter the cell's functions. If the cell loses control over normal cell division, it can become cancerous. Other viruses leave their genetic material in a host cell where it can remain dormant for an extended period of time. When the cell is disturbed, the virus sometimes begins growing again and causes disease.

Usually, viruses infect one particular type of cell. A cold virus would infect the cells of the upper respiratory tract. Some viruses only infect a few species of plants or animals, whereas some only infect people. They are transmitted in a number of ways. Sometimes we swallow viruses or sometimes we inhale them. Some viruses are transmitted by the bites of insects or other parasites—mosquitoes and ticks are two examples. Human viruses don't grow on food, but food can act as a method of transportation, moving a virus from one host to another and causing food-borne illnesses.[3]

The most common viruses are

- *filoviruses,* which resemble threads and are extremely lethal;
- *hepatitis viruses,* which cause several forms of liver infection, ranging from mild to life-threatening;
- *herpes viruses,* which take up permanent residence in the cells and periodically flare up;
- *influenza viruses,* which cause the flu, and can change their outer protein coats so dramatically that individuals resistant to one strain cannot fight off a new one;
- *noroviruses,* part of a family called *caliciviruses,* which cause gastroenteritis in people;
- *papillomaviruses,* which cause few symptoms in women and almost none in men, but may be responsible, at least in part, for a rise in the incidence of cervical cancer among younger women;
- *retroviruses,* which are named for their backward (*retro*) sequence of genetic replication compared to other viruses. One retrovirus, human immunodeficiency virus (HIV), causes acquired immune deficiency syndrome (AIDS);
- *rhinoviruses* and *adenoviruses,* which get into the mucous membranes and cause upper respiratory tract infections and colds; and
- *slow viruses,* which give no early indication of their presence but can produce fatal illnesses within a few years.

The problem in fighting viruses is that it's difficult to find drugs that will harm the virus but not the cell it has commandeered. **Antibiotics** (drugs that inhibit or kill bacteria) have no effect on viruses. **Antiviral drugs** don't completely eradicate a viral infection, although they can decrease its severity and duration. Because viruses multiply very quickly, antiviral drugs are most effective when taken before an infection develops or in its early stages.

Bacteria Simple one-celled organisms, **bacteria,** have a rigid cell wall and a thin, rubbery cell membrane that surrounds fluid (cytoplasm) inside the cell (see Figure 9-2(b)). Bacteria are complex compared to viruses because they contain all of the genetic information they need to make copies of themselves (DNA) in a structure called a *chromosome.* They also have *ribosomes,* which are tools necessary for copying the DNA so they can reproduce.[4] Some even have *flagella*—threadlike structures that they use to move. Bacteria are the most plentiful microorganisms as well as the most pathogenic.

Most kinds of bacteria don't cause disease. Some aid in digestion or play other important roles within our bodies. However, even friendly bacteria can get out of hand and cause acne, urinary tract infections, vaginal infections, and other problems.[5]

Bacteria that harm the body do so by releasing either enzymes that digest body cells or toxins that produce the specific effects of such diseases as diphtheria or toxic shock syndrome. In self-defence, the body produces specific proteins (called *antibodies*) that attack and inactivate the invaders. Tuberculosis, tetanus, gonorrhea, scarlet fever, and diphtheria are examples of bacterial diseases.

Because bacteria are sufficiently different from the cells that make up our bodies, antibiotics can kill them without harming our cells. Antibiotics work only against specific types of bacteria. Tests of your blood, pus, sputum, urine, or stool can identify particular bacterial strains.[6]

Fungi **Fungi** are eukaryotic organisms that come in a variety of shapes and sizes. They can be single-celled (yeasts) or consist of long chains of cells that can stretch for miles (moulds or mushrooms). Fungi are basically static, but they can spread by reproductive spores or by growing threadlike fibres. They do not make their own food from the sunlight because they lack chlorophyll. Instead, they absorb nutrients from organic material, which may include human tissue.[7]

Fungi can be helpful to us. Many antibiotics are made from natural compounds that fungi produce. Yeast makes bread rise and helps to brew beer. Fungi break down dead plants and animals.[8] They can also be a nuisance to humans. Fungi release enzymes that digest cells and can attack hair-covered areas of the body, including the scalp, beard, groin, and external ear canals. They also cause athlete's foot. Treatment consists of antifungal drugs. Fungi also affect fruits and vegetables.

Protozoa These single-celled, microscopic animals release enzymes and toxins that destroy cells or interfere with their function. Diseases caused by **protozoa** are not a major health problem in our country, primarily because of public-health measures. Around the world, however, millions of people are at risk for acquiring malaria—a protozoan-caused disease. According to the World Health Organization (WHO), there were approximately 214 million new cases of malaria in 2015 worldwide. There were an estimated 438 000 deaths overall, with the majority of these deaths—306 000—being children under five. Children who live in the African region were the most affected at 292 000 estimated deaths.[9] Many more come down with amoebic dysentery. Treatment for protozoa-caused diseases consists of general medical care to relieve the symptoms, replacement of lost blood or fluids, and drugs that kill the specific protozoan.

The most common disease caused by protozoa in Canada is *giardiasis,* an intestinal infection caused by microorganisms in human and animal feces. It has become a threat at daycare centres, as well as among campers and hikers who drink contaminated water.

Symptoms include nausea, lack of appetite, gas, diarrhea, fatigue, abdominal cramps, and bloating. Many people recover in a month or two without treatment. However, in some cases the microbe causes recurring attacks over many years. Giardiasis can be life-threatening in small children and the elderly, who are especially prone to severe dehydration from diarrhea. Treatment usually consists of antibiotics.

Helminths (Parasitic Worms) Small parasitic worms that attack specific tissues or organs and compete with the host for nutrients are called **helminths.** One major worldwide health problem is *schistosomiasis*, a disease caused by a parasitic worm, the fluke, which burrows through the skin and enters the circulatory system. Infection with another helminth, the tapeworm, may be contracted from eating undercooked beef, pork, or fish containing larval forms of the tapeworm. Helminthic diseases are treated with appropriate medications.

✓ CHECK-IN

Which of the above agents do you see as the greatest threat to your health?

Reservoirs—Where Do Microorganisms Live, Grow, and Multiply? A **reservoir** is a place where any infectious agent can live, grow, and multiply. A reservoir can be an animal or insect, a person, food, or water.

Animals and Insects House pets, livestock, and wild animals can transmit disease. Insects also spread a variety of diseases. The housefly may spread dysentery, diarrhea, typhoid fever, or trachoma (an eye disease rare in Canada, but common in other parts of the world). Other insects, including mosquitoes, ticks, mites, fleas, and lice, can transmit such diseases as malaria, yellow fever, encephalitis, dengue fever, and Lyme disease.

A threat in Canada is West Nile virus (WNV), a virus mainly transmitted to people through the bite of an infected mosquito.[10] Mosquitoes transmit the virus after becoming infected themselves by feeding on the blood of birds that carry the virus. Canada had its first confirmed cases of West Nile virus in 2002.[11] Transmission of WNV also occurs through transplanted organs and possibly from blood products.

While WNV interferes with normal central nervous system functioning and causes inflammation of brain tissue, many people infected with WNV do not have any symptoms and do not get sick. Others experience mild to severe symptoms. Symptoms, which usually appear within 2–15 days, include fever, body aches, brain swelling, coma, and paralysis. Less than 1 percent of those infected with WNV develop severe illness. Among these, 3–15 percent die, with the highest mortality rate among the elderly. People with chronic diseases such as cancer, diabetes, alcoholism, or heart disease are also at a higher risk for serious health issues from WNV.[12]

Presently, there is no specific vaccine, treatment, medication, or cure for West Nile virus. The Government of Canada has coordinated a national surveillance plan and is working closely with Health Canada, the Pest Management Regulatory Agency, and other government departments on a national response to WNV.[13]

Another virus transmitted through a bite from an infected mosquito is the Zika virus (ZIKV). This virus was identified in 1947 in Uganda in Asian monkeys known as macaques. In 1952 the virus was reported in humans who lived in Africa and Asia. In 2015 there was a large outbreak of this virus in Central and South America—especially in Brazil. Outbreaks were also reported in the Caribbean and Mexico.[14] There are reports of possible transmission through semen from infected men and blood transfusions from infected donors in addition to mosquito bites.[15] The symptoms of the Zika virus include a low-grade fever, a red rash, muscle or joint pain, red eyes, weakness, lack of energy, and headaches. The symptoms are usually mild and last between 2 and 7 days.[16] While the majority of people who are infected with the virus do not suffer from severe complications, reports of many babies being born with abnormally small heads and incomplete brain development (microcephaly) have been linked to mothers who were infected during their pregnancy. A link between the Zika virus and microcephaly in newborns was being considered at the time of this textbook revision.[17]

People The people you are closest to can transmit pathogens through the air, touch, or sexual contact. To avoid infection, stay out of range of anyone who is coughing, sniffling, or sneezing, and don't share food or dishes. Carefully wash your dishes, utensils, and hands, and abstain from sex or make self-protective decisions about sexual partners.

✓ CHECK-IN

What precautions do you take to avoid being infected by others?

Food Every year food-borne illnesses strike many Canadians, sometimes with fatal consequences. Bacteria account for two-thirds of food-borne infections. Thousands of suspected cases of infection with ***Escherichia coli* (*E. coli*)** bacteria in undercooked or inadequately washed food are reported annually. *E. coli* infections are now a public-health problem worldwide. Symptoms include mild to severe diarrhea with no blood to high levels of blood in the stools.[18] Most people recover without antibiotic treatment within 5–10 days after exposure; however, young children under five years of age and older adults are susceptible to HUS—hemolytic uremic syndrome. This is a condition where the red blood cells are destroyed and the kidneys fail. HUS can be life-threatening and often requires intensive care, blood transfusions, and kidney dialysis.

Adults are capable of transmitting the infection for one week or less (as long as the bacteria are present in stools). In 33 percent of infected children, transmission can occur for up to three weeks.

In the summer of 2011, an *E. coli* outbreak in Germany seriously affected thousands of people and left 49 people dead. The European Food Safety Authority determined that the bacteria likely came from bean sprouts on an organic farm. Raw sprouts are one of the highest-risk foods for food poisoning. In our increasingly globalized food marketplace, we have to be diligent with food contamination and inspection services.[19]

Another group of bacteria—salmonella—is found in the intestines of birds and animals, raw or undercooked meat and poultry, milk and eggs, and also fruits and vegetables. It is the second most frequently reported food-related illness in Canada.[20] Diarrhea, fever, and abdominal cramps are typical symptoms, which occur 12–72 hours after being infected. These usually last four to seven days, and many people recover without specific treatment. However, these infections can be serious enough to require hospitalization and can lead to arthritis, neurological problems, and even death. You can greatly reduce your risk of salmonella infections by proper handling, cooking, and refrigeration of food.[21] Proper washing of fresh fruits and vegetables is also important. Exotic pets are also another source—so wash your hands after contact.

A deadly food disease, *botulism,* is caused by certain bacteria that grow in improperly canned foods. Although its occurrence is rare in commercial products, botulism is a danger in home canning.[22] Infant botulism can affect healthy children who are under one year old. Sources of the bacterium, called *Clostridium botulinum*, are soil, dust, and honey. Parents and caregivers can help to prevent infant botulism by not adding honey to baby food or using honey on a soother.[23]

Another threat, though not as common, is *trichinosis*, caused by the larvae of a parasitic roundworm in uncooked meat. This infection, which causes nausea, vomiting, diarrhea, fever, thirst, profuse sweating, weakness, and pain, can be avoided by thoroughly cooking meat.[24]

In the summer of 2008, an outbreak of *Listeria monocytogenes*, commonly known as **listeria**, occurred in Canada. Although a relatively rare disease in Canada, at least 18 people died of this disease, and many more were taken ill. Health officials confirmed that the outbreak began at the Maple Leaf Foods plant in Ontario, a result of contaminated slicing equipment. Listeria is a type of bacterium found in food, soil, vegetation, water, sewage, and the feces of humans and animals.[25] Listeria is unlike most other bacteria in that it can survive and sometimes even grow on foods that are stored in your refrigerator, although it can be killed if you properly cook your food. Many people carry listeria, but not many actually develop listeriosis, a serious and sometimes life-threatening disease. Pregnant women, the elderly, and people with weakened immune systems are at risk. The mild form of listeriosis begins as soon as one day after eating contaminated food, whereas the incubation period of the more serious form of the disease can be up to 90 days.

BSE (bovine spongiform encephalopathy), often called mad cow disease, has become a concern in the past two decades in places such as the United Kingdom, Canada, the United States, and Japan. It is a disease that affects the central nervous system, especially in cows. Infected animals become aggressive, sometimes lack coordination, and find it difficult to stand. You can only determine if an animal has BSE by examining its brain after it dies. The brains of animals afflicted with this disease look spongy because holes have developed in the nerve cells. As well, a deposit of fibrous protein is also apparent in the brain tissue.[26]

There is still much mystery surrounding this disease. It has been suggested that a human form of BSE, variant Creutzfeldt-Jakob disease (vCJD), has been linked to eating beef products that have come from animals infected with BSE. Presently, there is no proof as to how BSE is transmitted, but scientists believe that **prions**, infectious self-reproducing protein structures, might be the cause. What is known for sure is that prions are not viruses, bacteria, fungi, or parasites. What is unclear is how prions seem to have the ability to reproduce themselves by changing the shape of an apparently normal protein found within a cell—a change that results in the clogging up of infected brain cells that don't work properly or die. Scientists are even more concerned that prions might have the ability to jump from one species to another, causing deadly diseases such as vCJD in humans. Scientists have also discovered that there is a standard type of prion, unlike the infectious type. These prions appear to help the brain develop and maintain the myelin sheath in the cells that protect our nerves. They may also be involved in a process known as developmental plasticity, in which the structure and function in our maturing brain is shaped by our learning.[27]

Water Water is a scarce commodity worldwide. According to the World Health Organization (WHO), there are approximately 842 000 deaths every year because of a lack of access to safe drinking water. About 1.9 billion people are without proper sanitation facilities and in need of safer water sources. Safe drinking water and basic sanitation means that water can be used for drinking, personal hygiene, and cooking. It also means that the source for safe drinking water needs to be less than one kilometre away from where it will be used and that people can access at least 20 litres per member of their household per day.[28] We are fortunate in Canada to have the distinction of having 7 percent of the world's supply of renewable fresh water. However, more than half of our renewable fresh water actually drains into the Hudson Bay and the Arctic Ocean. This water resource is not available to 85 percent of Canadians because they live along the USA border.[29] Guidelines for treating water so it is safe to drink have been developed by experts working for the Canadian federal, provincial, and territorial governments. The guidelines set specific criteria for measuring potential contaminants and provide information about treatment goals.[30]

In Canada, we have been reminded that water quality and safety and *E. coli* are not just developing-country or food-related issues. An *E. coli* outbreak in Walkerton, Ontario, from a community water supply, in May 2000, caused seven deaths, made more than 2000 people ill, and had an estimated direct economic impact of more than 64.5 million dollars.[31] A combination of a lack of training and expertise of the Walkerton Public Utilities Commission (PUC) operators, years of improper operating practices, and the discontinuation of government-laboratory water testing for municipalities in 1996 were just some of the reasons this tragedy occurred.[32] Public health depends on reliable systems and integrity in monitoring those systems.

Health Canada reported 1838 drinking water advisories in 2015. One hundred and sixty-nine of the advisories were for First Nations communities for their public and semi-public water systems. Some of these advisories have been in place for over 20 years. They include advisories for water contamination, unacceptable turbidity, inadequate disinfection or treatment, and unacceptable microbiological quality.[33] The federal government is responsible for drinking water on all First Nations reserves except for those in British Columbia, where water quality is now monitored by the First Nations Health Authority (FNHA).[34]

Modes of Transmission Microorganisms are not able to travel by themselves. They need a **mode of transmission** to move from the reservoir to the host. Direct and indirect human contact presents an opportunity for disease-producing organisms to be transmitted. When an insect or an animal transmits disease to a human it is known as a **vector-borne transmission.**[35] There are five ways that a pathogen can be transmitted.[36]

- Direct contact—body surface to body surface. Examples include blood-borne and sexual contact.
- Indirect contact—contact of a susceptible host with hands or objects that are contaminated. This is a common transmission route. Examples include a TV remote, computer keyboards, and eating utensils.
- Droplet transmission—often spread by nasal, oral, or conjunctival mucosa that comes into contact with large droplets containing germs from another infected person that is close by. Examples include someone sneezing, coughing, or even talking within about three feet.
- Airborne transmission—very small droplets containing germs that are suspended in the air or dust. They are spread by air currents and enter into the respiratory tract. Examples include measles, chickenpox, and tuberculosis.
- Common vehicle transmission—contact with contaminated equipment, food, water, or medications. Examples include contaminated leftover food and polluted water supply.

The Process of Infection Once a pathogen is transmitted to a **susceptible host** through any of the five routes of transmission, the infection process begins. Anyone can be a susceptible host. The susceptibility level depends on a person's health condition and the level of exposure to the infectious agent or a pathogen. If someone does not have antibodies to protect them through immunizations or having had a previous infection, they can become ill. Other factors to consider are the age of an individual and current or underlying medical conditions. During the **incubation period,** the time between invasion and the first symptom, you're unaware of the pathogen multiplying inside you. Incubation may go on for months, even years; for most diseases, it lasts several days or weeks.

The early stage of the battle between your body and the invaders is called the *prodromal period.* As infected cells die, they release chemicals that help block the invasion. Other chemicals, such as *histamines,* cause blood vessels to dilate, thus allowing more blood to reach the battleground. During all of this, you feel mild, generalized symptoms, such as headache, irritability, and discomfort. You're also highly contagious. At the height of the battle—the typical illness period—you cough, sneeze, sniffle, ache, feel feverish, and lose your appetite.

Recovery begins when the body's forces gain the advantage. With time, the body destroys the last of the invaders and heals itself. However, the body is not able to develop long-lasting immunity to certain viruses, such as colds, flu, or HIV.

How Your Body Protects Itself Various parts of your body safeguard you against infectious diseases by providing **immunity,** or protection, from these health threats. Your skin, when unbroken, keeps out most potential invaders. Your tears, sweat, skin oils, saliva, and mucus contain chemicals that can kill bacteria. Cilia, the tiny hairs lining your respiratory passages, move mucus, which traps inhaled bacteria, viruses, dust, and foreign matter, to the back of the throat, where it is swallowed; the digestive system then destroys the invaders. However, it is important to remember that parts of our body and

STRATEGIES FOR PREVENTION

Protecting Yourself from Insect-Borne Diseases

- Consider staying indoors at dawn, dusk, and in the early evening, which are peak mosquito-biting times.
- When outdoors, apply insect repellent containing DEET (N, N-diethyl-meta-toluamide), which provides the longest-lasting protection against bites.
- Follow all of the label directions, including restrictions for use on young children and the maximum number of applications allowed per day.
- Wear long-sleeved clothes and long pants treated with repellents containing permethrin or DEET, since mosquitoes may bite through thin clothing. Do not apply repellents containing permethrin directly to exposed skin. If you spray your clothing, there is no need to spray repellent containing DEET on the skin under your clothing.
- Avoid breathing spray mists and never apply sprays inside a tent. Use only in well-ventilated areas. Do not use near food.
- Limit the number of places available for mosquitoes to lay their eggs by eliminating standing water sources from around your home.

Source: Government of Canada. (2016) Healthy Canadians. Pests and Source: Pests and pesticides. http://healthycanadians.gc.ca/product-safety-securite-produits/pest-control-products-produits-antiparasitaires/pesticides/about-au-sujet/insect_repellents-insectifuges-eng.php#s1

tears, sweat, and mucus can also act as both a **portal of exit** and a **portal of entry** for infection. If a bacteria or virus has been harboured in a reservoir (another person, for example) in an excretion, open wound, respiratory or gastrointestinal tract, or any mucous membrane in an eye, nose, or mouth, it can exit from this reservoir through skin contact or sneezing, coughing, or even talking. The infectious agent can then enter a new susceptible host the same way.

When these protective mechanisms can't keep you infection free, your body's immune system, which is on constant alert for foreign substances that might threaten the body, swings into action. The immune system includes structures of the lymphatic system—the spleen, thymus gland, lymph nodes, and lymph vessels—that help filter impurities from the body (see Figure 9-3). More than a dozen different types of white blood cells are concentrated in the organs of the lymphatic system or patrol the entire body by way of the blood and lymph vessels. The two basic types of immune mechanisms are humoral and cell-mediated.

Humoral immunity refers to the protection provided by antibodies—proteins derived from white blood cells called *B lymphocytes* or B cells. Humoral immunity is most effective during bacterial or viral infections. An *antigen* is any substance that enters the body and triggers production of an antibody. Once the body produces antibodies against a specific antigen—the mumps

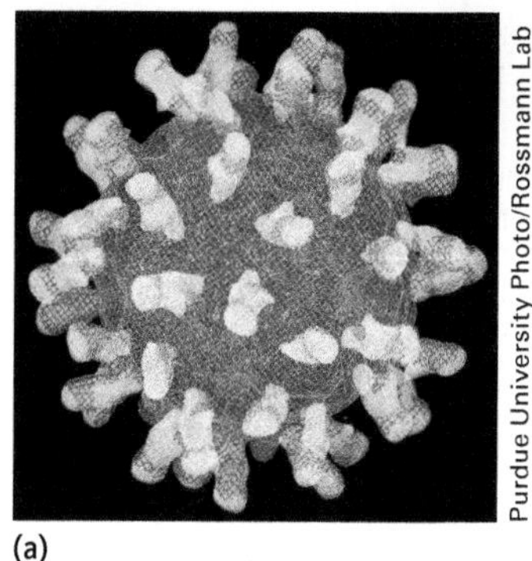

Purdue University Photo/Rossmann Lab

(a)

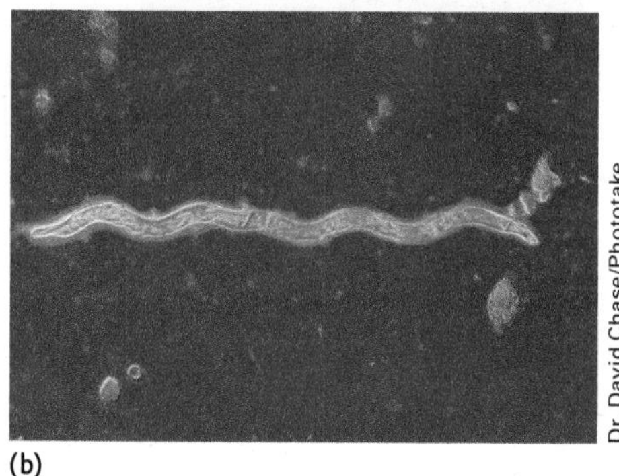

Dr. David Chase/Phototake

(b)

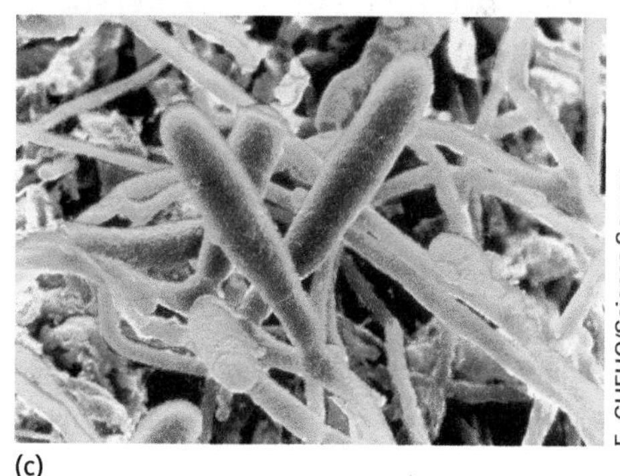

E. GUEHO/Science Source

(c)

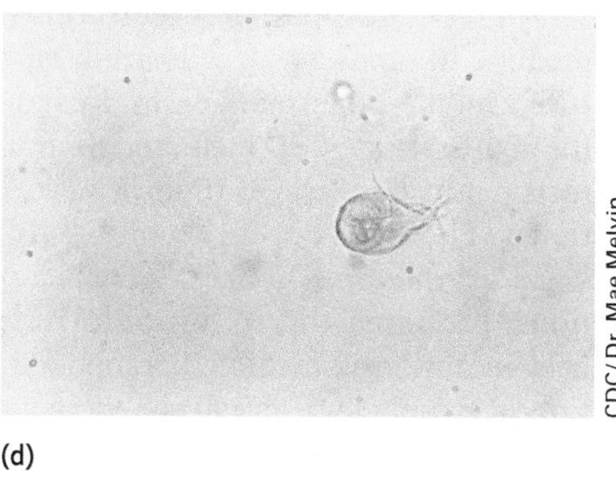

CDC/ Dr. Mae Melvin

(d)

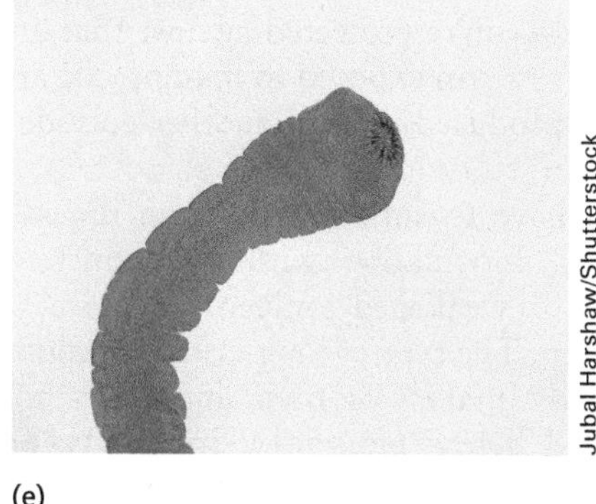

Jubal Harshaw/Shutterstock

(e)

Examples of the major categories of organisms that cause disease in humans. Except for the helminths (parasitic worms), pathogens are microorganisms that can be seen only with the aid of a microscope. (a) Viruses: common cold, (b) Bacteria: syphilis, (c) Fungi: athlete's foot/fungus, (d) Protozoa: *Giardia lamblia*, (e) Helminths: tapeworm.

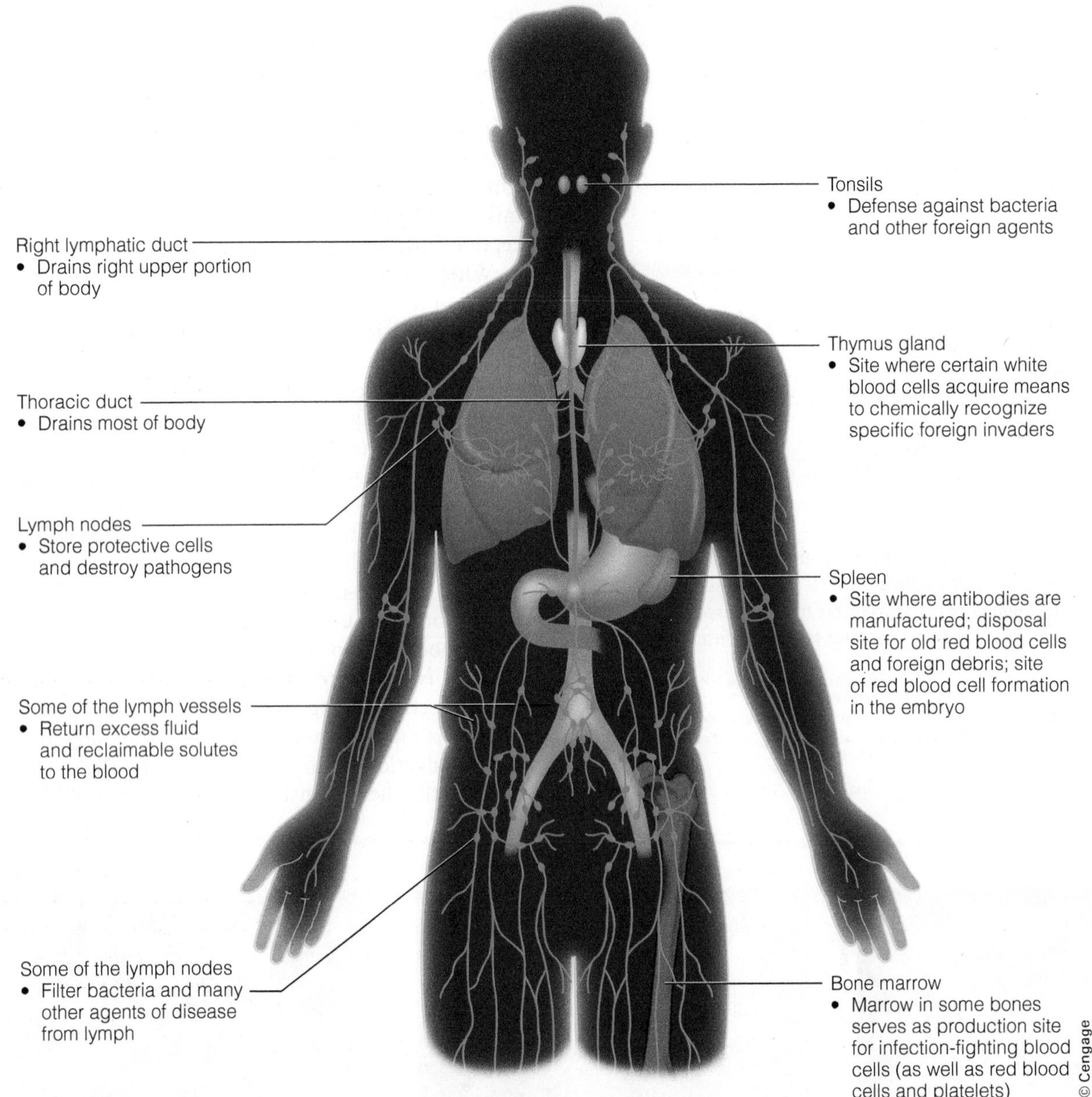

Figure 9-3 The Human Lymphatic System and Its Functions
The lymphatic system helps filter impurities from the body.

virus, for instance—you're protected against that antigen for life. If you're again exposed to mumps, the antibodies previously produced prevent another episode of the disease.

But you don't have to suffer through an illness to acquire immunity. Inoculation with a vaccine containing synthetic or weakened antigens can give you the same protection. The type of long-lasting immunity in which the body makes its own antibodies to a pathogen is called *active immunity*. Immunity produced by the injection of **gamma globulin**, the antibody-containing part of the blood from another person or animal that has developed antibodies to a disease, is called *passive immunity*.

The various types of T cells are responsible for **cell-mediated immunity**. T cells are lymphocytes manufactured in the bone marrow and carried to the thymus for maturation. Cell-mediated immunity mainly protects against parasites, fungi, cancer cells, and foreign tissue. Thousands of different T cells work together to ward off disease. Different T cells have differing functions, including the activation of other immune cells, help in antibody-mediated responses, and the suppression of lymphocyte activity.

Immune Response Attacked by pathogens, the body musters its forces and fights. Together, the immune cells work like an internal police force. When an antigen

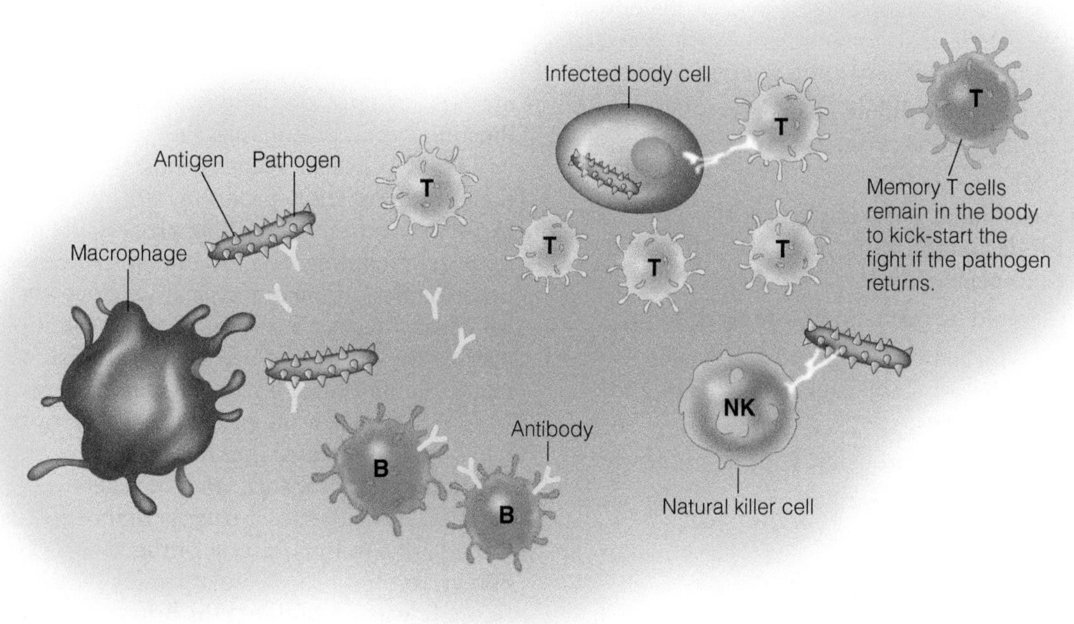

Figure 9-4 The Immune Response

Some T cells can kill infected body cells. B cells churn out antibodies to tag pathogens for destruction by macrophages and other white blood cells.

enters the body, the T cells, aided by *macrophages* (large scavenger cells with insatiable appetites for foreign cells, diseased and run-down red blood cells, and other biological debris), engage in combat with the invader. Meanwhile, the B cells churn out antibodies, which rush to the scene and join in the fray. Also busy at surveillance are natural killer cells that, like the elite forces of a SWAT team, seek out and destroy viruses and cancer cells (see Figure 9-4).

The **lymph nodes**, or glands, are small tissue masses in which some protective cells are stored. If pathogens invade your body, many of them are carried to the lymph nodes to be destroyed. This is why your lymph nodes often feel swollen when you have a cold or the flu.

If the microbes establish a foothold, the blood supply to the area increases, bringing oxygen and nutrients to the fighting cells. Tissue fluids, as well as antibacterial and antitoxic proteins, accumulate. You may develop redness, swelling, local warmth, and pain—the signs of **inflammation**. As more tissue is destroyed, a cavity, or **abscess**, forms and fills with fluid, battling cells and dead white blood cells (pus). If the invaders aren't killed or inactivated, the pathogens are able to spread into the bloodstream and cause what is known as **systemic disease**. The toxins released by the pathogens cause fever, and the infection becomes more dangerous.

Immunity and Stress Stress affects the body's immune system in different ways, depending on two factors: the controllability or uncontrollability of the stressor and the mental effort required to cope with the stress. An uncontrollable stressor that lasts longer than 15 minutes may interfere with *cytokine interleukin-6*, which plays an essential role in activating the immune defences. Uncontrollable stressors also produce a high level of the hormone *cortisol*, which suppresses immune system functioning. The mental efforts required to cope with high-level stressors produce only brief immune changes that appear to have little consequence for health. However, stress has been shown to slow pro-inflammatory cytokine production, which is essential for wound healing.

THE KEY TO PREVENTION

Breaking the Chain of Infection The Canadian Centre for Occupational Health and Safety (CCOHS) has taken the stance that the single, most effective, and simplest way to prevent the spread of communicable diseases and infections is hand hygiene.[37] Hand hygiene is defined as removing or killing microorganisms (germs) on the hands. Using soap and running water or alcohol-based hand gel or rubs are recommended. The following tips can help you break the link of infection.

- Any type of soap and running water should be used for handwashing any time the hands have come into contact with other people, their body substances, or items contaminated by them; before preparing, handling, serving, or eating food, or feeding someone else; after any personal function such as blowing your nose or going to the washroom; when hands come into contact with secretions, excretions, blood, and body fluids; when hands are soiled; or when hands have touched items that harbour germs such as cellphones, computer keyboards, and steering wheels.

- If bar soap is used, it should be kept on a self-draining holder that is cleaned thoroughly on a regular basis.
- Alcohol-based hand gels and rubs are the preferred method for decontaminating hands if they contain more that 60 percent alcohol.
- Jewellery should be taken off before washing.
- Rub hands with soap lather for 15 seconds or longer. Wash the front and back of the hands and between the fingers.
- After rinsing hands thoroughly, wipe hands gently.
- If you are using a public facility, use a piece of paper towel to turn the taps on and off.

Immunization A success story of modern medicine has been the development of vaccines that provide protection against many infectious diseases. **Immunization** is a process that helps your body fight off diseases caused by certain viruses and bacteria by exposing your body to vaccines. These are usually in the form of injections or shots. The vaccines contain tiny amounts of material that make your immune system produce certain substances called *antibodies*. These antibodies attack and destroy viruses and bacteria.

Your immune system stores this information on how to make these antibodies. Even many years later when your body is exposed to the same virus or bacteria, it remembers how to make these antibodies. Your body then produces those antibodies again, stopping the virus or bacteria from making you sick.[38]

Immunization has reduced cases of measles, mumps, tetanus, whooping cough, and other life-threatening illnesses by more than 95 percent. Shen, Fields, and McQuestion suggest that immunization should be an important public health initiative in which we should invest. Research has shown that the cost-effectiveness of vaccinations—the cost to prevent just one undesired incident such as death, hospitalization, infection, or complications from infections—is relatively low.[39]

The position of the World Health Organization (WHO) on vaccines is that by inducing immunity, suffering, disability, and death are avoided. It also helps health organizations to care for the most vulnerable members of society. Global access to safe vaccines for diseases such as measles, Haemophilus Influenza B (HIB), rotavirus, and pneumococcal could help to reduce worldwide child mortality and address poverty and inequities.[40] Less strain on the healthcare system results in savings that can be used for other health services.

A comprehensive document, the *Canadian Immunization Guide*, contains changes that have been made in the immunization field.[41] The National Advisory Committee on Immunization (NACI) recommends that children be immunized against diphtheria, tetanus, acellular Peruses (whooping cough), polio, HIB infection, measles, mumps, German measles (rubella), hepatitis B, Pneumococcal, pneumonia, and meningococcal C.

The NACI also recommends that adults continue their immunization program. Prevention of infection by immunization is a lifelong process. What immunizations are recommended for adults? Tetanus, diphtheria, hepatitis B, and pneumococcal vaccines are on the list. Influenza vaccines are recommended for anyone 65 and over or for those who are at greatest risk of influenza-related complications, such as healthcare workers.[42]

A second dose of measles (MMR) vaccine is also highly recommended for health-care workers, college and university students, and travellers to areas where measles is epidemic. Measles outbreaks continue in Canada due to importation of the virus in communities known to object to vaccinations for their children. One example was an outbreak in British Columbia in 2014 in the Fraser Valley region. Due to religious beliefs, almost all the students at an elementary school were not vaccinated. A total of 433 cases of measles (325 cases were confirmed and 108 were listed as probable) were identified. Ninety-nine percent of the cases were among unvaccinated children.[43]

Mumps vaccine (given as MMR) is recommended for young adults with no history of mumps. Rubella vaccine is recommended for all female adolescents and women of childbearing age unless they have documented evidence of vaccination.[44]

If you're uncertain about your past immunizations, check with family members or your doctor. If you can't find answers, a blood test can show whether you carry antibodies to specific illnesses.

If you're pregnant or planning to get pregnant within the next three months, do not get a measles, mumps, rubella, or oral polio vaccination. If you're allergic to neomycin, consult your doctor before getting a measles, mumps, rubella, or intramuscular polio vaccination. Those with egg allergies should also check with a doctor before getting a measles, mumps, or flu vaccination. Also, never get a vaccination when you have a high fever.

Although statistics show that minor side effects such as mild fevers or soreness at the injection site are common, severe allergic reactions from vaccinations are very rare. However, some people are concerned about getting their children or themselves vaccinated. Reports that vaccines are linked to chronic diseases, sudden infant death syndrome (SIDS), autism, inflammatory bowel disease, brain damage, or asthma have not been proven through rigorous scientific studies according to the Public Health Agency of Canada.[45] The use of the preservative thimerosal, which contains mercury and was used in some vaccines, has been reduced or discontinued in most vaccines. In Canada, the only routine vaccine for children that contained thimerosal was the Hepatitis B vaccine. A new formula for this vaccine that does not include thimerosal is now available.[46]

✓ CHECK-IN

Do you get the vaccines recommended by health experts?

INFECTIOUS DISEASES

An estimated 500 microorganisms cause disease; no effective treatment exists for about 200 of these illnesses. Although infections can be unavoidable at times, the more you know about their causes, the more you can do to protect yourself.

Who Is at Highest Risk of Infectious Diseases?

Among the most vulnerable are the following groups:

- **Children and their families.** Youngsters get up to a dozen colds annually; adults average two a year. When a flu epidemic hits a community, about 40 percent of school-aged boys and girls get sick, compared with only 5–10 percent of adults. Parents get up to six times as many colds as other adults.
- **The elderly.** People over 65 who get the flu have a 1 in 10 chance of being hospitalized for pneumonia or other respiratory problems and a one in 50 chance of dying from the disease.
- **The chronically ill.** Lifelong diseases, such as diabetes, kidney disease, or sickle-cell anemia, decrease an individual's ability to fend off infections. Individuals taking medications that suppress the immune system, such as steroids, are more vulnerable to infections, as are those with medical conditions that impair immunity, such as infection with HIV.
- **Smokers and those with respiratory problems.** Smokers are a high-risk group for respiratory infections and serious complications, such as pneumonia. Chronic breathing disorders, such as asthma and emphysema, also greatly increase the risk of respiratory infections.
- **Those who live or work in close contact with someone who is sick.** Healthcare workers who treat high-risk patients, nursing-home residents, and others living in close quarters—such as students in dormitories—face greater odds of catching others' colds and flus.
- **Residents or workers in poorly ventilated buildings.** Building technology has helped spread certain airborne illnesses, such as tuberculosis, via recirculated air. Indoor air quality can be closely linked with disease transmission in winter, when people spend a great deal of time in tightly sealed rooms.

Common Cold There are more than 200 distinct cold viruses, or rhinoviruses. Although in a single season you may develop a temporary immunity to one or two, you may then be hit by a third. Colds can strike in any season, but different cold viruses are more common at different times of the year. Rhinoviruses cause most spring, summer, and early fall colds and tend to cause more symptoms above the neck (stuffy nose, headache, runny eyes). Adenoviruses, parainfluenza viruses, coronaviruses, influenza viruses, and others that strike in the winter are more likely to get into the bronchi and trachea (the breathing passages) and cause more fever and bronchitis.

Cold viruses are spread by coughs, sneezes, and touch. Cold sufferers who sneeze and then touch a doorknob or countertop leave a trail of highly contagious viruses behind them. The best preventive tactics are frequent handwashing, replacing toothbrushes regularly, and avoiding stress overload. New research shows that people who feel unable to deal with everyday stresses have an exaggerated immune reaction that may intensify cold or flu symptoms once they've contracted a virus.

Until scientists develop truly effective treatments, experts advise against taking acetylsalicylic acid (Aspirin®) and acetaminophen (Tylenol®), which may suppress the antibodies the body produces to fight cold viruses and increase symptoms such as nasal stuffiness. A better alternative for cold "aches" is ibuprofen (brand names include Motrin®, Advil®, and Nuprin®), which doesn't seem to affect immune response. Children, teenagers, and young adults should never take Aspirin® for a cold or flu because of the danger of Reye's syndrome, a potentially deadly disorder that can cause convulsions, coma, swelling of the brain, and kidney damage.

The main drawback of *antihistamines*, the most widely used cold remedy, is drowsiness, which can impair a person's ability to safely drive or operate machinery. Another ingredient, *pseudoephedrine*, can open and drain sinus passages without drowsiness but can speed up heart rate and cause complications for individuals with high blood pressure, diabetes, heart disease, or thyroid disorders. Decongestant nasal sprays can clear a stuffy nose, but they invariably cause a rebound effect. The use of a saline nasal spray is not addictive and can be used to loosen mucus in the nose and help to wash it out. It is also helpful during dry weather to keep the mucous membranes moist.

Fluids (especially chicken soup) help, but dairy products can contribute to congestion. Mild exercise boosts immunity, but once you're sick, it's better not to work out strenuously. In general, doctors recommend treating specific symptoms—headache, cough, chest congestion, sore throat—rather than taking a multi-symptom medication.

X AND Y FILES

Male and Female Differences in Susceptibility

The female immune system responds more vigorously than the male's immune system to common infections, offering extra protection against viruses, bacteria, and parasites. But this enhanced immunity doesn't apply to sexually transmitted infections (STIs). A woman who has unprotected sex with an infected man is more likely to contract an STI than a man who has sex with an infected woman. Symptoms of STIs also tend to be more "silent" in women, so they often go undetected and untreated, leading to potentially serious complications.

The sexes also differ in their vulnerability to allergies and **autoimmune disorders.** Although both men and women frequently develop allergies, allergic women are twice as likely to experience potentially fatal anaphylactic shock. A woman's robust immune system also is more likely to overreact and turn on her own organs and tissues. On average, three of four people with autoimmune disorders, such as multiple sclerosis, Hashimoto's thyroiditis, and scleroderma, are women. Another autoimmune disease, lupus, affects nine times as many women as men.

Autoimmune disorders often follow a different course in men and women. Women with multiple sclerosis develop symptoms earlier than men, but the disease tends to progress more quickly and be more severe in men. In lupus, women first show symptoms during their childbearing years, while men develop the illness later in life.

Scientists believe that the sex hormones have a great impact on immunity. Through a woman's childbearing years, estrogen, which protects heart, bone, brain, and blood vessels, also bolsters the immune system's response to certain infectious agents. Women produce greater numbers of antibodies when exposed to an antigen; after immunization, they show increased cell-mediated immunity.

In contrast, testosterone may dampen this response—possibly to prevent attacks on sperm cells, which might otherwise be mistaken as alien invaders. When the testes are removed from mice and guinea pigs, their immune systems become more active.

Pregnancy dampens a woman's immune response, probably to ensure that her natural protectors don't attack the fetus as a foreign invader. This impact is so great that pregnant women with transplanted kidneys may require lower doses of drugs to prevent organ rejection. Pregnant women with multiple sclerosis and rheumatoid arthritis typically experience decreased symptoms during the nine months of gestation, then return to their pre-pregnancy state after giving birth. Oral contraceptives also can diminish symptoms of multiple sclerosis and rheumatoid arthritis. Neither pregnancy nor birth control pills has such an impact on lupus.

Other hormones, such as prolactin and growth hormones, may affect autoimmune diseases. Women have higher levels of these hormones, which may act directly on immune cells through interactions with receptors on the surface of cells. These hormones also may affect the complex inter-workings of the hypothalamus, pituitary, and adrenal glands.

For a cough, the ingredient to look for in any suppressant is *dextromethorphan*, which turns down the brain's cough reflex. In expectorants, the only medicine deemed effective is *guaifenesin*, which helps liquefy secretions so you can bring up mucus from the chest. Unless you're coughing up green or foul yellow mucus (signs of a secondary bacterial infection), antibiotics won't help. They have no effect against viruses and may make your body more resistant to such medications when you develop a bacterial infection in the future.

Many Canadians try alternative remedies for colds. One of the most popular herbal remedies is an extract of the echinacea plant. Echinacea is believed to increase the number and efficiency of white blood cells, components of the immune system that battle infection. Some evidence indicates that taking echinacea several times a day at the first sign of sniffles diminishes the symptoms or shortens the duration of an oncoming cold. Most experts recommend only limited use of echinacea, since long-term use can actually suppress the immune system.[47]

Zinc lozenges, although a popular alternative treatment, do not have consistent research results indicating their effectiveness. Eby reports that 14 double-blind, placebo-controlled, randomized clinical trials over a 25-year period resulted in a reduction of cold symptoms for about one-half of those taking zinc lozenges. He also determined that very few of the more than 40 different brands of zinc lozenges studied had an adequate level of iZn, the active ingredient that shortens common colds.[48]

Although sore throats are caused by viruses, many people seek treatment with antibiotics, which are effective only against bacteria. An estimated 85–90 percent of sore throats in adults are caused by viruses. Seventy percent of sore throats in children aged 5–16 and 95 percent in children younger than five years are also caused by viruses.[49]

Your own immune system can do something modern science cannot: cure a cold. All it needs is time, rest, and plenty of fluids. Warmth also is important because the aptly named "cold" viruses replicate at lower temperatures. Hot soups and drinks (particularly those with a touch of something pungent, such as lemon or ginger) raise body temperature and help clear the nose. Taking it easy reduces demands on the body, which helps speed recovery.

✓ CHECK-IN

Which of the following steps do you take to prevent colds? Frequent handwashing? Replacing toothbrushes often? Exercising regularly? Avoiding stress overload?

Influenza Although similar to a cold, **influenza**—the flu—causes more severe symptoms that last longer.

The Public Health Agency of Canada reports that there are approximately 12 200 people hospitalized per year due to seasonal flu cases. There are approximately 3500 deaths in Canada due to complications from the flu. Many more deaths occur due to complications of influenza, such as pneumonia.[50]

Flu viruses, transmitted by coughs, sneezes, laughs, and even normal conversation, are extraordinarily contagious, particularly in the first three days of the disease. The usual incubation period is two days, but symptoms can hit hard and fast. Two varieties of viruses—influenza A and influenza B—cause most flus.

The Public Health Agency of Canada recommends that all Canadians over the age of six months get the flu shot. New vaccines are available each year to protect us from new strains of the influenza virus. The flu shot is effective throughout the year, but the best time to get the vaccine is October or November. The flu shot gives you full protection about two weeks after the immunization. The only individuals who should steer clear are those allergic to eggs, since the inactivated flu viruses are grown in chick embryos.[51]

Many health service units in colleges and universities recommend that students get flu shots.[52] Influenza disrupts academic progress for significant numbers of students each year.

A new alternative to flu shots is an intranasal spray containing a live, attenuated influenza virus (LAIV) vaccine. Researchers have found that the aerosol vaccine significantly reduces flu severity, days lost from work, healthcare visits, and the use of over-the-counter medication. The approval by the U.S. Food and Drug Administration allows for the use of this nasal spray in the United States in healthy children and adolescents aged 2–49 years.[53] Health Canada has also approved this vaccine for individuals 2–59 years of age. Studies have demonstrated significantly superior effectiveness of the LAIV vaccine compared to the injectable inactive influenza vaccine.[54]

Concerns about the vaccine have surfaced from a study by Mutsch et al.,[55] where researchers discovered that the inactivated intranasal vaccine significantly increased the risk of Bell's palsy in adults. As with many medical interventions, we must take note of the risks as well as the benefits.

Antiviral drugs such as zanamivir (Relenza™) and oseltamivir (Tamiflu™) are the next best line of defence.[56] These *neuraminidase inhibitors* are designed to block a protein (neuraminidase) that allows the flu virus to escape from one cell and infect others. A small handheld oral inhaler, used twice a day for five days, delivers zanamivivir (Relenza™) to the surface of the lungs, the primary site of flu infection. Oral oseltamivir (Tamiflu™), taken twice a day for five days, comes in pill form. These agents act against both influenza A and influenza B viruses and cause few side effects. In research trials, they shortened the duration of flu by up to two days and decreased the likelihood of complications such as bronchitis, sinusitis, and ear infections. However, to be effective, treatment with either medication must begin within 36–48 hours of the first flu symptom. Although approved only for use as a treatment, antiviral drugs also can prevent flu from spreading through a family, workplace, or school.

STRATEGIES FOR PREVENTION

Protecting Yourself from Colds and Flus

- Wash your hands frequently with hot water and soap. In a public restroom, use a paper towel to turn off the faucet after you wash your hands, and avoid touching the doorknob.
- Make sure you're getting adequate sleep. Eat a balanced diet. Exercise regularly.
- Don't share food or drinks.
- Don't touch your eyes, mouth, and nose after being with someone who has cold symptoms.
- Use tissues rather than cloth handkerchiefs, which may harbour viruses for hours or days.
- Don't smoke. Smoking destroys protective cells in the airways and worsens any cough.
- Limit your intake of alcohol, which depresses white blood cells and increases the risk of bacterial pneumonia in flu sufferers.

Avian Influenza **Avian influenza**, or bird flu, is caused by viruses that occur naturally among wild birds. Most strains of bird flu virus cannot affect humans, but a few can, usually with great difficulty.[57] Influenza viruses jumped from birds to humans three times in the 20th century. In each case a mutation in the genes of the virus allowed it to infect humans. Wild waterfowl act as a natural reservoir for the virus and may be spreading it to domestic poultry flocks, which are especially vulnerable. Pigs might also become infected because of outdoor breeding programs, such as exist in the United Kingdom. Migrating wild birds could possibly bring avian influenza from other parts of the world, although researchers now suggest that this risk is low.

The H5N1 strain—isolated in 1996 with human infections being reported in Hong Kong in 1997, has caused serious sickness and death in humans, especially in people under the age of 40 years. This strain changes quickly or mutates by borrowing genes from other viruses. The outbreaks were unprecedented in their scope and geographic and economic impact.[58] It is anticipated that human cases of avian influenza will continue to be detected in countries where outbreaks in poultry are occurring. Research continues to learn more about the avian–human connection.

H1N1 The H1N1 flu virus began as a strain of influenza that primarily affected pigs. However, in the spring of 2009 it showed up in people in North America and then spread to other countries around the world. It proved to be highly contagious and the World Health Organization (WHO) declared it a pandemic in June of 2009.[59] It differed from the seasonal flu. Humans had no natural immunity to protect themselves from this particular influenza strain. Another concern was that it affected more healthy young people than the regular seasonal flu.

Currently, there is a vaccine available in Canada for H1N1 called Influenza A (H1N1) 2009 Pandemic Monovalent Vaccine (without adjuvant). Health Canada recommends this vaccine for anyone travelling in areas where H1N1 is circulating.[60]

The Threat of a Pandemic **Pandemic flu** is any virulent human flu that causes a global outbreak, or pandemic, of serious illness. Influenza pandemics tend to occur when disease-causing organisms that typically affect only animals adapt and infect humans, then further adapt so they can pass easily from human to human. Concern about the spread of both the avian flu and H1N1 has led to the development of a Canadian Pandemic Influenza Plan. A number of provinces have also developed provincial influenza plans.[61]

Suggestions from health officials include the following:

- **Stay informed.** Check reliable sources of information such as Health Canada or the World Health Organization (WHO).
- **Get an annual flu shot.** It will not protect you from a pandemic flu virus, but it can prevent simultaneous infections.
- **See your doctor.** Make an appointment within two days of developing flu symptoms.
- **Wash your hands frequently.** Do so at home and in public places.
- **Stay healthy.** Eating right, exercising, and getting enough sleep helps to keep your immune system strong.
- **Think carefully about travel in flu seasons.** Viruses are easily transmitted in confined spaces such as airplanes, trains, and buses. If possible, try not to travel to places with outbreaks of deadly viruses.

Coronavirus Coronaviruses are common viruses that most people get some time throughout their life. Human coronaviruses usually cause mild to moderate upper-respiratory tract illnesses. Some strains cause the common cold. However, other strains have been known to cause two serious coronaviruses—severe acute respiratory syndrome (SARS) and the Middle East respiratory syndrome coronavirus (MERS-CoV).

Severe acute respiratory syndrome (SARS) is a respiratory illness caused by a previously unknown type of coronavirus. SARS can progress from a cough, shortness of breath, difficulty in breathing, and a fever higher than 38°C to severe pneumonia or respiratory failure.[62] Presently, the known risk factors for developing SARS are recent travel to an area where SARS is spreading locally and recent close contact with someone who is ill and either has SARS or has been to an area where SARS is spreading locally. It does appear that people with SARS are not contagious until they develop symptoms, which may take up to 10 days from the time they were in close contact with someone affected by SARS.

SARS became a new global health threat in 2003, with major outbreaks in several Asian countries, including China and Hong Kong, as well as Toronto, Canada. Another outbreak occurred in China in 2004. There are no specific treatments for SARS. Patients receive supportive care, fluids to prevent dehydration, and ventilators to aid breathing. Scientists are working on the development of a possible vaccine and antiviral agents.

Middle East respiratory syndrome coronavirus (MERS-CoV) has been identified in many countries in the Middle East such as Jordan, Saudi Arabia, Qatar, Lebanon, and Iran. Other countries such as France, Italy, and the United Kingdom have reported MERS-CoV in citizens who have travelled to the Middle East.[63] Since 2012, medical experts have been monitoring this disease. In May of 2012 there was a large outbreak in South Korea. However, no new cases have been reported since July 2015.[64]

While the symptoms of MERS-CoV are similar to the symptoms of SARS—and include fever, cough, and shortness of breath—the virus is different than SARS. Illness tends to be less severe in younger people, but has caused death in older individuals and those who have other medical conditions. An investigation of the source of this virus and how it is spread is ongoing. Research that has been done on MERS-CoV is pointing toward contact with live camels or camel meat or milk. No cases have been reported in Canada as yet.

Meningitis **Meningitis**, or invasive meningococcal disease, is an infection of the fluid and membranes around the brain and spinal cord. It can be caused by three kinds of germs: bacteria, viruses, or fungi. The two most common forms of bacteria are *Neisseria meningitidis*, which causes meningococcal meningitis, and *Streptococcus pneumoniae*, which causes pneumococcal meningitis. The symptoms, which are similar in all types of meningitis, include fever, drowsiness or confusion, severe headache, stiff neck, nausea, and vomiting. Meningitis progresses rapidly, often in as little as 12 hours. If untreated, it can lead to permanent hearing loss, brain damage, seizures, or death. If it is caught early and treated with antibiotics, it is usually curable.[65]

Most common in the first year of life, the incidence of bacterial meningitis rises again in young people between the ages of 15 and 24.[66] College and university students are generally not at greater risk, except when they live in dormitories.[67]

Viral meningitis is more common, but usually less serious. Fungal meningitis is quite rare. It can occur in premature babies with very low birth weights or in people with disorders of the immune system such as AIDS, cancer, or diabetes. Antifungal drugs are used in treatment.[68]

Meningitis Vaccination The National Advisory Committee on Immunization (NACI) recommends that all children under the age of five be vaccinated against meningococcal and Pneumococcal infection.[69] Meningitec®, a vaccine that protects against meningococcus, is now available in Canada. It is a conjugate vaccine approved for children under two years of age.[70] Prevnar® is a conjugate vaccine that protects infants and young children from pneumococcal disease. It was approved by Health Canada in June 2001.

Research into the success of meningococcal vaccination programs on college campuses has shown that women are more likely than men to be vaccinated. Students majoring in science-oriented fields have higher vaccination rates than those majoring in the humanities. More younger students living on campus than older ones get vaccinations, possibly because of greater parental influence or because they see themselves as being at higher risk.[71] Public acceptance is also an important factor. A study done in the Sherbrooke region of Quebec found that although the effectiveness of meningitis vaccines was agreed upon, 35.9 percent of college students surveyed doubted the safety of the vaccine.[72]

Hepatitis In Canada, May is Hepatitis Awareness Month, a campaign that advises Canadians of the potential for hepatitis outbreaks. At least five different viruses, referred to as hepatitis A, B, C, Delta, and E, target the liver, the body's largest internal organ. Newly identified viruses also may be responsible for some cases of what is called "non-A, non-B" hepatitis.

Symptoms of **hepatitis** include headaches, fever, fatigue, stiff or aching joints, nausea, vomiting, and diarrhea. The liver becomes enlarged and tender to the touch; sometimes the yellowish tinge of jaundice develops. Treatment consists of rest, a high-protein diet, and the avoidance of alcohol and drugs that may stress the liver. Alpha interferon, a protein that boosts immunity and prevents viruses from replicating, may be used for some forms.[73]

As many as 10 percent of those infected with hepatitis B and up to two-thirds of those with hepatitis C become carriers of the virus for several years or even life.[74] Some have persistent inflammation of the liver, which may cause mild or severe symptoms and increase the risk of liver cancer. Fatigue and other symptoms can also linger.

Hepatitis A virus (HAV), a less serious form, is the most frequently reported vaccine-preventable disease in North America.[75] The low prevalence of hepatitis A in Western countries has resulted in an overall decrease in population immunity. The result is a low prevalence of hepatitis A antibodies (HAV antibody seroprevalence) in many Canadians. A study by a group of researchers on Canadian and immigrant university students in Toronto supports other Canadian HAV seroprevalence studies.[76] HAV seroprevalence was significantly lower in the young, urban, Canadian-born students than the immigrant students. This was true in each age group. The findings suggest that there is the potential for outbreaks of HAV infection.

Hepatitis A is generally transmitted by poor sanitation, primarily fecal contamination of food or water. Among those at highest risk in Canada are children and staff at daycare centres, residents of institutions, sanitation workers, and workers who handle primates such as monkeys. In Canada, hepatitis A vaccine is currently recommended by the NACI for individuals at increased risk.[77]

Hepatitis B is a potentially fatal disease transmitted through the blood and other bodily fluids. People aged 30–39 are at most risk, followed by those aged 15–29. The major risk factors include injection-drug use, having multiple heterosexual partners, sex with HBV-infected individuals, drug snorting, blood transfusions, and male homosexual activity.[78]

Vaccination can prevent hepatitis B and is recommended for children, teens, and adults at high risk. Since the early 1990s, a school-based, universal hepatitis B vaccination program, which targets 9- to 13-year-olds, has been implemented in all provinces and territories. Some provinces also have an infant vaccination program.

Hepatitis C virus (HCV) is four times as widespread as HIV. However, many people do not realize they are infected.[79] Hepatitis C, which can lead to chronic liver disease, cirrhosis, and liver cancer, is the leading reason for liver transplantation.

Tattooing and body piercing are creating a new concern for medical professionals. A review of the literature shows that these forms of body art are playing a role in transmitting various infections, including hepatitis.[80]

✓ CHECK-IN

Do you have a tattoo or piercing? Did you make sure the tattoo or piercing was done by a professional?

Mononucleosis You can get **mononucleosis** through kissing—or any other form of close contact. "Mono" is a viral disease that's most common among people 15–24 years old; its symptoms include a sore throat, headache, fever, nausea, and prolonged weakness. The spleen is swollen and the lymph nodes are enlarged. You may also develop jaundice or a skin rash similar to German measles.

The major symptoms usually disappear within two to three weeks, but weakness, fatigue, and often depression may linger for at least two more weeks. The greatest danger is from physical activity that might rupture the spleen, resulting in internal bleeding. The liver may also become inflamed. A blood test can determine whether you have mono. In a study conducted at Edinburgh University in the United Kingdom, researchers found that students who had infectious mononucleosis reported a decrease in their study time, social activities, and physical exercise. They also reported an increase in the number of hours they slept. Female students reported a higher level of fatigue and were also more likely to discontinue their academic work after contracting mononucleosis.[81] Health professionals say that there is no specific treatment other than rest.

CURRENT GLOBAL CONCERNS

While medical professionals continue their research and work in keeping our population healthy, there is growing concern about the emergence of superbugs and bioterrorism.

The Superbug Threat: MRSA For decades most strains of the bacterium *Staphylococcus aureus* responded to treatment with penicillin. When the bacterium became resistant to penicillin, physicians switched to a new antibiotic, methicillin. Within a year the first case of **methicillin-resistant *S. aureus* (MRSA)** was detected. This "superbug," which fights off traditional antibiotics, has become a major health threat.[82]

One in three healthy people carry *S. aureus* on their skin. Of these, as many as one in 100 may be carrying MRSA. In medical terms, these individuals are "colonized" but not infected. For infection to occur, MRSA must enter the body through an accidental injury such as a scrape or burn or via a deliberate break in the skin such as a surgical incision. The rate of MRSA infections is highest in hospitals and healthcare facilities, but MRSA also can develop among sports teams, child-care attendees, and prison inmates. Rates of MRSA infection among hospital patients are quite high.[83]

MRSA spreads by touch. In healthcare settings, it can spread from patient to patient through contact with doctors and nurses with unwashed hands or contaminated gloves, or contact with unsterile medical equipment. Health advocates are calling for increased screening of patients for MRSA, isolating and treating MRSA carriers, more conscientious handwashing, and more diligent use of gowns, gloves, and masks to prevent transmission of MRSA.[84]

Outside hospitals, community-associated MRSA (CA-MRSA) is also a growing threat that can occur in people without any established risks, including college and university students. Living in close quarters, participating in contact sports, and sharing housing and personal items such as bath towels, balms, and lubricants increases the chance of transmission. People with cuts or abrasions are at the highest risk.

MRSA poses the greatest danger to individuals who

- have a weakened immune system;
- have a preexisting infection;
- have open wounds, cuts, or burns;
- have other types of wounds, such as skin breaks from an intravenous drug line;
- have undergone surgery;
- have taken antibiotics recently or for a long period;
- are athletes in contact sports;
- are elderly; or
- are premature or newborn babies.

Bioterror Threats In the past decade, we have learned first-hand that certain infectious agents can be used as weapons of terrorism and war. **Bioterror agents**, such as anthrax and, potentially, smallpox, botulism, and tularaemia, have been added to the ranks of emerging infectious diseases.[85]

- **Anthrax**—Anthrax, which is found naturally in wild and farm animals, can also be produced in a laboratory. The disease is spread through exposure to anthrax spores, not through exposure to an infected person.
- **Smallpox**—Smallpox is a serious, contagious, and sometimes fatal infectious disease. The last naturally occurring case in the world was in Somalia in 1977. There is no treatment, and up to 30 percent of those infected with smallpox die. There is fear that terrorists might use smallpox as a biological weapon.
- **Botulism**—Botulism is a muscle-paralyzing disease caused by a toxin made by the bacterium *Clostridium botulinum*. Botulinum toxin is among the most lethal substances known, and it can kill within 24 hours. Botulism causes muscle weaknesses and eventual paralysis that starts at the top of the body and works its way down. The disease kills by paralyzing muscles used to breathe. Treatment includes taking the antidote and possibly using a ventilator for breathing until the toxin works its way out of the system.

- **Tularaemia**—Tularaemia is an illness that normally infects wild animals, such as rabbits and squirrels. Humans can acquire the illness by coming in contact with the blood or bodily fluids of infected animals, from the bite of a fly or tick that carries blood from an infected animal, or from contaminated food or water. As a biological weapon, tularaemia-causing bacteria could be dispersed through the air to be inhaled.

REPRODUCTIVE AND URINARY TRACT INFECTIONS

Reproductive and urinary tract infections are very common. Many are not spread exclusively by sexual contact, so they are not classified as sexually transmitted infections.

Vaginal Infections The most common vaginal infections are trichomoniasis, candidiasis, and bacterial vaginosis.[86]

Protozoa (*Trichomonas vaginalis*) that live in the vagina can multiply rapidly, causing itching, burning, and discharge—all symptoms of **trichomoniasis.** Male carriers usually have no symptoms, although some may develop urethritis or an inflammation of the prostate and seminal vesicles. Anyone with this infection should be screened for syphilis, gonorrhea, chlamydia, and HIV. Sexual partners must be treated with oral medication (metronidazole, known as Flagyl™), even if they have no symptoms, to prevent reinfection.

Populations of a yeast called *Candida albicans*—normal inhabitants of the mouth, digestive tract, and vagina—are usually held in check. Under certain conditions, however, the microbes multiply, causing burning, itching, and a whitish discharge and producing what is commonly known as a yeast infection. Common sites for **candidiasis** are the vagina, vulva, penis, and mouth. The women most likely to test positive for candidiasis have never been pregnant, use condoms for birth control, have sexual intercourse more than four times a month, and have taken antibiotics in the previous 15–30 days. Stress can also be a factor. Vaginal medications, such as GyneLotrimin and Monistat, are non-prescription drugs that provide effective treatment. Male sexual partners may be advised to wear condoms during outbreaks of candidiasis. Women should keep the genital area dry and wear cotton underwear.

Bacterial vaginosis (BV) is characterized by alterations in the microorganisms that live in the vagina, including depletion of certain bacteria and overgrowth of others. It typically causes a white or grey vaginal discharge with a strong odour similar to that of trichomoniasis. Its underlying cause is unknown, although it occurs most frequently in women with multiple sex partners. Long-term dangers include pelvic inflammatory disease and pregnancy complications. BV is diagnosed based on symptoms, a pelvic examination, and sometimes a whiff test, where drops of a potassium hydroxide (KOH) solution are added to a sample of vaginal discharge. A fishy odour on the whiff test suggests BV. Metronidazole (Flagyl™), either in the form of a pill or a vaginal gel, is the primary treatment. Treatment for male sex partners appears to be of little benefit, but some health practitioners recommend treatment for both partners in cases of recurrent infections.

Urinary Tract Infections A urinary tract infection (UTI) can be present in any of the three parts of the urinary tract: the urethra, the bladder, or the kidneys. An infection involving the urethra is known as **urethritis.** If the bladder is also infected, it's called **cystitis.** If it reaches the kidneys, it's called **pyelonephritis.**[87]

More women than men develop UTIs. Bacteria, the major cause of UTIs, have a shorter distance to travel up the urethra to infect a woman's bladder and kidneys. Conditions that can set the stage for UTIs include irritation and swelling of the urethra or bladder as a result of pregnancy, bike riding, irritants (such as bubble bath, douches, or a diaphragm), urinary stones, enlargement of the prostate gland in men, vaginitis, and stress. Early diagnosis is critical because infection can spread to the kidneys and, if unchecked, result in kidney failure. Symptoms include frequent burning, painful urination, chills, fever, fatigue, and blood in the urine.

Recurrent UTIs, a frequent problem among young women, have been linked with a genetic predisposition, sexual intercourse, and the use of diaphragms. Frequent recurrence of symptoms may not be caused by infection but by interstitial cystitis, a little-understood bladder inflammation that affects mostly women.

SEXUALLY TRANSMITTED INFECTIONS

Venereal diseases (from the Latin *venus,* meaning *love* or *lust*) are more accurately called **sexually transmitted infections (STIs)** or sexually transmitted diseases (STDs).[88] The highest rates of sexually transmitted infections occur among 16- to 24-year-olds, particularly older teenagers.[89] STIs are much more widespread in developing nations because of the lack of adequate health standards, prevention practices, and access to treatment.

STIs are the major cause of preventable sterility. STIs have tripled the rate of ectopic (tubal) pregnancies, which can be fatal if not detected early. STI complications include miscarriage, premature delivery, and uterine infections after delivery. Moreover, infection

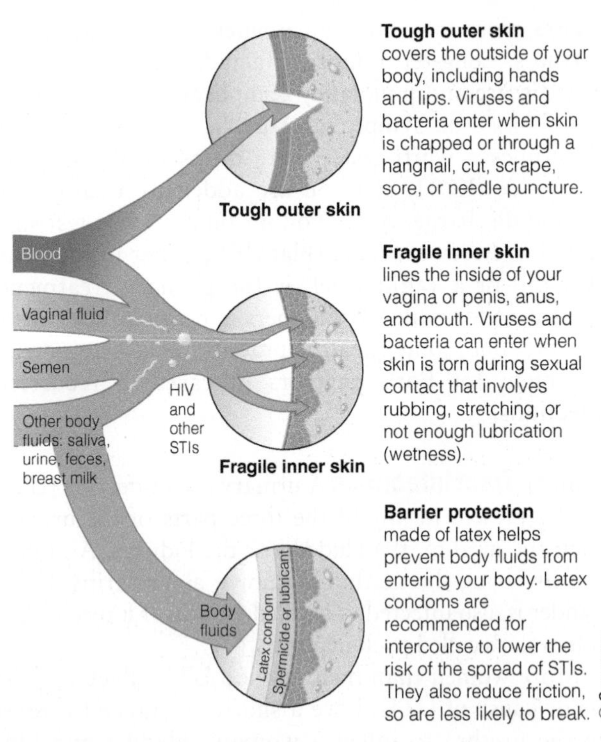

Figure 9-5 How HIV Infection and Other STIs Are Spread
Most STIs are spread by viruses or bacteria carried in certain body fluids.

with an STI greatly increases the risk of HIV transmission. Unborn and newborn children can be affected by STIs in the womb or during birth.[90]

Although each STI is a distinct disease, all STI pathogens like dark, warm, moist body surfaces, particularly the mucous membranes that line the reproductive organs (see Figure 9-5); they hate light, cold, and dryness. It is possible to catch or have more than one STI at a time. Curing one doesn't necessarily cure another, and treatments don't prevent another bout with the same STI (see Table 9-1).

Many STIs, including early HIV infection and gonorrhea in women, may not cause any symptoms. As a result, infected individuals may continue their usual sexual activity without realizing that they're jeopardizing others' well-being.

STIs in Adolescents and Young Adults The college and university years are a prime time for contracting STIs. College-age women are at increased risk for human papillomavirus (HPV) infections.[91] Contracting STIs may increase the risk of being infected with HIV, and half of new HIV infections occur in people under age 25. Because college and university students have more opportunities to have different sexual partners and may use drugs and alcohol more often before sex, they are at greater risk.[92]

Even when high-school and college students have generally accurate knowledge about STIs, they don't necessarily practise safe sex. According to research, those students with the greatest number of sexual partners are least likely to use condoms.[93] While college and university students admit to engaging in behaviours that put them at risk of HIV and other STIs, they believe that other students do so much more often.[94]

Various factors put young people at risk of STIs, including the following:

- **Feelings of invulnerability.** These lead to risk-taking behaviour. Even though well informed of the risks, adolescents may remain unconvinced that anything bad can or will happen to them.
- **Multiple partners.** In surveys of students, a significant minority report having had four or more sexual partners during their lifetime.
- **Failure to use condoms.** Among those who reported having had sexual intercourse in the previous three months, fewer than half reported condom use. Students who had had four or more sexual partners were significantly less likely to use condoms than those who had fewer partners.
- **Substance abuse.** Teenagers who drink or use drugs are more likely to engage in sexually risky behaviours, including sex with partners whose health status and history they do not know and unprotected intercourse.[95]

Prevention and Protection Abstinence is the only guarantee of sexual safety—and an option that some people are choosing as a way to safeguard their physical health, their fertility, and their future.

For men and women who are sexually active, a mutually faithful sexual relationship with just one healthy partner is the safest option. For those not in such relationships, safer-sex practices are essential for reducing risks. However, no protection is 100 percent safe. You can't tell if someone you're dating or hope to date has been exposed to an STI. Ideally, before engaging in any

STRATEGIES FOR CHANGE

What to Do if You Have an STI

- If you suspect that you have an STI, put your embarrassment aside and get help through a physician's office or a clinic. Treatment relieves discomfort, prevents complications, and halts the spread of the disease.
- Following diagnosis, take oral medication (which may be given instead of or in addition to shots) exactly as prescribed.
- Try to figure out from whom you got the STI. Be sure to inform that person, who may not be aware of the problem.
- If you have an STI, never deceive a prospective partner about it. Tell the truth—simply and clearly. Be sure your partner understands exactly what you have and what the risks are.

TABLE 9-1

Common Sexually Transmitted Infections (STIs): Mode of Transmission, Symptoms, and Treatment

STI	Transmission	Symptoms	Treatments
Chlamydia	The *Chlamydia trachomatis* bacterium is transmitted primarily through sexual contact. It can also be spread by fingers from one body site to another.	In women, PID (pelvic inflammatory disease) as a result of chlamydia may cause disrupted menstrual periods, pelvic pain, elevated temperature, nausea, vomiting, headache, infertility, and ectopic pregnancy. In men, chlamydia infection of the urethra may cause a discharge and burning during urination. Chlamydia-caused epididymitis may produce a sense of heaviness in the affected testicle(s), inflammation of the scrotal skin, and painful swelling at the bottom of the testicle.	Doxycycline, azithromycin, or ofloxacin
Gonorrhea ("clap")	The *Neisseria gonnorheae* bacterium ("gonococcus") is spread through genital, oral–genital, or genital–anal contact.	Common symptoms in men are a cloudy discharge from the penis and burning sensations during urination. If disease is untreated, complications may include inflammation of scrotal skin and swelling at base of the testicle. In women, some green or yellowish discharge is produced but often remains undetected. Later, PID may develop.	Dual therapy of a single dose of ceftriaxone, cefixime, ciprofloxacin, or ofloxacin plus doxycycline for seven days or a single dose of azithromycin
Non-gonococcal urethritis (NGU)	Primary causes are believed to be the bacteria *Chlamydia trachomatis* and *Ureaplasma urealyticum*, most commonly transmitted through coitus. Some NGU may result from allergic reactions or from Trichomonas infection.	Inflammation of the urethral tube. A man has a discharge from the penis and irritation during urination. A woman may have a mild discharge of pus from the vagina but often shows no symptoms.	A single dose of azithromycin or doxycycline for seven days
Syphilis	The *Treponema pallidum* bacterium ("spirochete") is transmitted from open lesions during genital, oral–genital, or genital–anal contact.	Primary stage: A painless chancre appears at the site where the spirochetes entered the body. Secondary stage: The chancre disappears, and a generalized skin rash develops. Latent stage: There may be no visible symptoms. Tertiary stage: Heart failure, blindness, mental disturbance, and many other symptoms occur. Death may result.	Benzathine penicillin G, doxycycline, erythromycin, or ceftriaxone
Herpes simplex	The genital herpes virus (HSV–2) seems to be transmitted primarily by vaginal, anal, or oral–genital intercourse. The oral herpes virus (HSV–1) is transmitted primarily by kissing.	Small, painful red bumps (papules) appear in the genital region (genital herpes) or mouth (oral herpes). The papules become painful blisters that eventually rupture to form wet, open sores.	No known cure. A variety of treatments may reduce symptoms; oral or intravenous acyclovir (Zovirax) promotes healing and suppresses recurrent outbreaks.
Chancroid	The *Haemophilus ducrevi* bacterium is usually transmitted by sexual interaction.	Small bumps (papules) in genital regions eventually rupture and form painful, soft, crater-like ulcers that emit a foul-smelling discharge.	Single doses of either ceftriaxone or azithromycin, or seven days of erythromycin

(Continued)

TABLE 9-1

Common Sexually Transmitted Infections (STIs): Mode of Transmission, Symptoms, and Treatment *(Continued)*

STI	Transmission	Symptoms	Treatments
Human papilloma-virus (HPV) (genital warts)	The virus is spread primarily through vaginal, anal, or oral–genital sexual interaction.	Hard and yellow-grey on dry skin areas; soft, pinkish-red, and cauliflower-like on moist areas	Freezing; application of topical agents such as trichloroacetic acid or podofilox; cauterization, surgical removal, or vaporization by carbon dioxide laser
Pubic lice ("crabs")	*Phthirus pubis*, the pubic louse, is spread easily through body contact or through shared clothing or bedding.	Persistent itching. Lice are visible and may often be located in pubic hair or other body hair.	1% permethrin cream for body areas; 1% Lindane shampoo for hair
Scabies	*Sarcoptes scabiei* is highly contagious and may be transmitted by close physical contact, sexual and nonsexual.	Small bumps and a red rash that itch intensely, especially at night.	5% permethrin lotion or cream
Acquired immune deficiency syndrome (AIDS)	Blood and semen are the major vehicles for transmitting HIV, which attacks the immune system. It appears to be passed primarily through sexual contact or needle sharing among—injection-drug users.	Vary with the type of cancer or opportunistic infections that afflict an infected person. Common symptoms include fevers, night sweats, weight loss, chronic fatigue, swollen lymph nodes, diarrhea and/or bloody stools, atypical bruising or bleeding, skin rashes,—headache, chronic cough, and a whitish coating on the tongue or throat.	Commence treatment early after a positive HIV test with a combination of three or more antiretroviral drugs (HAART) plus other specific treatment(s), if necessary, of opportunistic infections and tumours.
Viral hepatitis	Hepatitis A seems to be primarily spread via the fecal–oral route, but oral–anal sexual contact is a common mode for transmission. The hepatitis B virus can be transmitted in blood, semen, vaginal secretions, and saliva. Manual, oral, or penile stimulation of the anus is strongly associated with the spread of this virus.	Varies from non-existent to mild, flu-like symptoms, to an incapacitating illness characterized by high fever, vomiting, and severe abdominal pain.	No specific therapy for A and B types; treatment generally consists of bed rest and adequate fluid intake. Combination therapy with interferon and ribavarin may be effective for hepatitis C infections.
Bacterial vaginosis	The most common causative agent, the *Gardnerella vaginalis* bacterium, is sometimes transmitted through coitus.	In women, a fishy or musty-smelling thin discharge, like flour paste in consistency and usually grey. Most men are asymptomatic.	Metronidazole (Flagyl) by mouth or intravaginal applications of topical metronidazole gel or clindamycin cream
Candidiasis (yeast infection)	The *Candida albicans* fungus may accelerate growth when the chemical balance of the vagina is disturbed; it may also be transmitted through sexual interaction.	White, "cheesy" discharge; irritation of vaginal and vulval tissues	Vaginal suppositories or topical cream, such as clotrimazole and miconazole, or oral fluconazole
Trichomoniasis	The protozoan parasite *Trichomonas vaginalis* is usually passed through genital sexual contact.	White or yellow vaginal discharge with an unpleasant odour; vulva is sore and irritated.	Metronidazole (Flagyl™) for both women and men

Source: Robert L. Crooks and Karla Baur, *Our Sexuality*, 8th ed. Pacific Grove, CA: Wadsworth, 2002; Canadian Guidelines on Sexually Transmitted Infections. 2010 update. Found at: http://www.phac-aspc.gc.ca/std-mts/sti-its/guide-lignesdir-eng.php

such behaviour, both of you should talk about your prior sexual history (including number of partners and sexually transmitted diseases) and other high-risk behaviour, such as the use of injection drugs. If you know someone well enough to consider having sex with that person, you should be able to talk about STIs. If the person is unwilling to talk, you shouldn't have sex.

✓ CHECK-IN

How are you protecting yourself and your partner from sexually transmitted infections?

Chlamydia The most widespread sexually transmitted infection in Canada is *Chlamydia trachomatis*—**chlamydia**. Those at greatest risk of chlamydial infection are individuals 25 years old or younger who engage in sex with more than one new partner within a two-month period and women who use birth control pills or other non-barrier contraceptive methods.[96]

As many as 75 percent of women and 50 percent of men with chlamydia have no symptoms or symptoms so mild that they don't seek medical attention. Without treatment, up to 40 percent of cases of chlamydia can lead to pelvic inflammatory disease, a serious infection of the woman's fallopian tubes that can also damage the ovaries and uterus. Also, women infected with chlamydia may have three to five times the risk of getting infected with HIV if exposed. Babies exposed to chlamydia in the birth canal during delivery can be born with pneumonia or with an eye infection called conjunctivitis, both of which can be dangerous unless treated early with antibiotics. Men can develop scarring of the urethra, making urination difficult.

Pelvic Inflammatory Disease Infection of a woman's fallopian tubes or uterus, called **pelvic inflammatory disease (PID)**, is not actually an STI, but rather a complication of STIs. The Public Health Agency of Canada reports that 10–15 percent of women who are of reproductive age have had one episode of PID. It is also estimated that up to two-thirds of cases of PID are not identified and many women do not report PID to their health professionals.[97]

Ten to 20 percent of initial episodes of PID lead to scarring and obstruction of the fallopian tubes severe enough to cause infertility. Other long-term complications are ectopic pregnancy and chronic pelvic pain. Smoking also may increase the likelihood of PID. Two bacteria—gonococcus (the culprit in gonorrhea)—and chlamydia are responsible for one-half to one-third of all cases of PID.

Women may learn that they have PID only after discovering that they cannot conceive or after they develop an ectopic pregnancy. PID causes an estimated 15–30 percent of all cases of infertility every year and about half of all cases of ectopic pregnancy. Most women do not experience any symptoms, but some may develop abdominal pain, tenderness in certain sites during pelvic exams, or vaginal discharge.

Gonorrhea **Gonorrhea** (sometimes called "the clap") is another common STI. The incidence is highest among teenagers and young adults. Sexual contact, including oral–genital sex, is the primary means of transmission.[98]

Most men who have gonorrhea know it. Thick, yellow-white pus oozes from the penis and urination causes a burning sensation. These symptoms usually develop two to nine days after the sexual contact that infected them. Men have a good reason to seek help: it hurts too much not to. Women also may experience discharge and burning on urination. However, as many as eight out of ten infected women have no symptoms.

Gonococcus, the bacterium that causes gonorrhea, can live in the vagina, cervix, and fallopian tubes for months, even years, and continue to infect the woman's sexual partners.

If left untreated in men or women, gonorrhea spreads through the urinary–genital tract. In women, the inflammation travels from the vagina and cervix, through the uterus, to the fallopian tubes and ovaries. The pain and fever are similar to those caused by stomach upset, so a woman may dismiss the symptoms. Eventually these symptoms diminish, even though the disease spreads to the entire pelvis. Pus may ooze from the fallopian tubes or ovaries into the peritoneum (the lining of the abdominal cavity), sometimes causing serious inflammation. However, this, too, can subside in a few weeks. Gonorrhea, the leading cause of sterility in women, can cause PID. In pregnant women, gonorrhea becomes a threat to the newborn. It can infect the infant's external genitals and cause a serious form of conjunctivitis, an inflammation of the eye that may lead to blindness. As a preventive step, newborns may have penicillin dropped into their eyes at birth.

In men, untreated gonorrhea can spread to the prostate gland, testicles, bladder, and kidneys. Among the

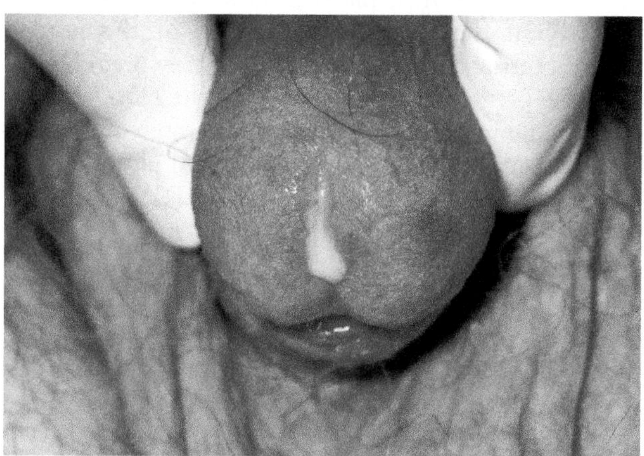

Dr. P. Marazzi/Science Source

A cloudy discharge is symptomatic of gonorrhea.

serious complications are urinary obstruction and sterility caused by blockage of the vas deferens (the excretory duct of the testis). In both sexes, gonorrhea can develop into a serious, even fatal, blood-borne infection that can cause arthritis in the joints and meningitis, attack the heart muscle and lining, and attack the skin and other organs.

Although a blood test has been developed for detecting gonorrhea, the tried-and-true method of diagnosis is still a microscopic analysis of cultures from the male's urethra, the female's cervix, and the throat and anus of both sexes.

Nongonococcal Urethritis The term **nongonococcal urethritis (NGU)** refers to any inflammation of the urethra that is not caused by gonorrhea.[99] NGU is the most common STI in men. Three microorganisms—*Chlamydia trachomatis*, *Ureaplasma urealyticum*, and *Mycoplasma genitalium*—are the primary causes; the usual means of transmission is sexual intercourse. Other infectious agents, such as fungi or bacteria, allergic reactions to vaginal secretions, or irritation by soaps or contraceptive foams or gels may also lead to NGU.

NGU is more common in men than gonococcal urethritis. The symptoms in men are similar to those of gonorrhea, including discharge from the penis (usually less than with gonorrhea) and mild burning during urination. Women frequently develop no symptoms or very mild itching, burning during urination, or discharge. Symptoms usually disappear after two or three weeks, but the infection may persist and cause cervicitis or PID in women and in men may spread to the prostate, epididymis, or both. Treatment usually consists of doxycycline and should be given to both sexual partners after testing. For men, a single oral dose of azithromycin has proven as effective as a standard seven-day course of doxycycline.

Syphilis A corkscrew-shaped, spiral bacterium called *Treponema pallidum* causes **syphilis.**[100] This frail microbe dies in seconds if dried or chilled but grows quickly in the warm, moist tissues of the body, particularly in the mucous membranes of the genital tract. Entering the body through any tiny break in the skin, the germ burrows its way into the bloodstream. Sexual contact, including oral sex or intercourse, is a primary means of transmission. Genital ulcers caused by syphilis may increase the risk of HIV infection, while individuals with HIV may be more likely to develop syphilis.

Infectious syphilis is the least commonly reported bacterial sexually transmitted infection. The rate of infectious syphilis is increasing in both males and females in Canada—more so in males, however.[101]

Syphilis has clearly identifiable stages: primary, secondary, early latent (asymptomatic syphilis, within the first year), late latent (asymptomatic syphilis, after one year), and tertiary syphilis.[102] During the latent stage, highly contagious lesions of the skin or mucous membranes become evident. They may recur for two to four years. After four years, there is a loss of infectiousness. Until this stage of the disease, however, a pregnant woman can pass syphilis to her unborn child. If the fetus is infected in its fourth month or earlier, it may be disfigured or even die. If infected late in pregnancy, the child may show no signs of infection for months or years after birth but may then become disabled with the symptoms of tertiary syphilis.

In the tertiary stage, 10–20 years after the beginning of the latent stage, the most serious symptoms of syphilis emerge, generally in the organs in which the bacteria settled during latency. Syphilis that has progressed to this stage has become increasingly rare. Victims of tertiary syphilis may die of a ruptured aorta or of other heart damage or may have progressive brain or spinal cord damage, eventually leading to blindness, insanity, or paralysis.

Early diagnosis of syphilis can lead to a complete cure. Penicillin is the drug of choice for treating primary, secondary, and latent syphilis. The earlier treatment begins, the more effective it is. Those allergic to penicillin may be treated with doxycycline, ceftriaxone, or erythromycin. An added danger of not getting treatment for syphilis is an increased risk of HIV transmission.

Herpes Herpes (from the Greek word that means *to creep*) collectively describes some of the most common viral infections in humans. **Herpes simplex virus (HSV)** transmission occurs through close contact with mucous membranes or abraded skin. Herpes simplex exists in several varieties. *Herpes simplex virus 1* (*HSV-1*) generally causes cold sores and fever blisters around the mouth. *Herpes simplex virus 2* (*HSV-2*) may cause blisters and lesions on the penis, inside the vagina, on the cervix, in the pubic area, on the buttocks, or on the thighs.[103] However, both forms of the virus can infect any of these areas. With the increase of oral–genital sex, some doctors report finding type 2 herpes lesions in the mouth and throat.

Many individuals do not realize they carry the virus because they never develop genital lesions, or they experience only very subtle symptoms. Men and women aged 20–29 have higher rates of infection than other age groups. Most people with herpes contract it from partners who were not aware of any symptoms or of their own contagiousness. Standard methods of diagnosing genital herpes in women, which rely primarily on physical examination and viral cultures, may miss as many as two-thirds of all cases. Newly developed blood tests are more effective in detecting unrecognized infections with HSV-2.[104]

In the past, patients and most doctors thought people with herpes could not pass on the infection when they did not have any symptoms. Research shows, however, that the herpes virus is present in genital secretions and can also be transmitted from skin-to-skin contact even when no bodily fluids are exchanged. This means that even when individuals do not show any signs of infection, they are still at risk for spreading HSV to a sex partner. There is also growing evidence that genital herpes promotes the spread of HIV.[105]

When herpes sores are present, the infected person is highly contagious and should avoid bringing the lesions into contact with someone else's body through touching, sexual interaction, or kissing.

A newborn can be infected with genital herpes while passing through the birth canal, and the frequency of mother-to-infant transmission seems to be increasing. Most infected infants develop typical skin sores, which should be cultured to confirm a herpes diagnosis. Because of the risk of severe damage and possible death, Caesarean delivery may be advised for a woman with active herpes lesions.

The virus that causes herpes never entirely goes away; it retreats to nerves near the lower spinal cord, where it remains for the life of the host. Herpes sores can return without warning weeks, months, or even years after their first occurrence, often during menstruation or times of stress or with sudden changes in body temperature.

Antiviral drugs, such as acyclovir (Zovirax), have proven effective in treating and controlling herpes. Infection with herpes viruses resistant to acyclovir is a growing problem, especially in individuals with immune-suppressing disorders. Clinical trials of an experimental vaccine to protect people from HSV-2 infections are underway, but to date, there is no effective and safe vaccine available for HSV-2.[106]

What is Human Papillomavirus? Infection with **human papillomavirus (HPV)**, a pathogen that can cause *genital warts*, is the most common viral STI. There are over 150 different strains of the HPV virus, and some of these viral strains can lead to cervical cancer in women.[107] Health Canada has approved three HPV vaccines—Gardasil®, Cervarix®, and Gardasil 9.

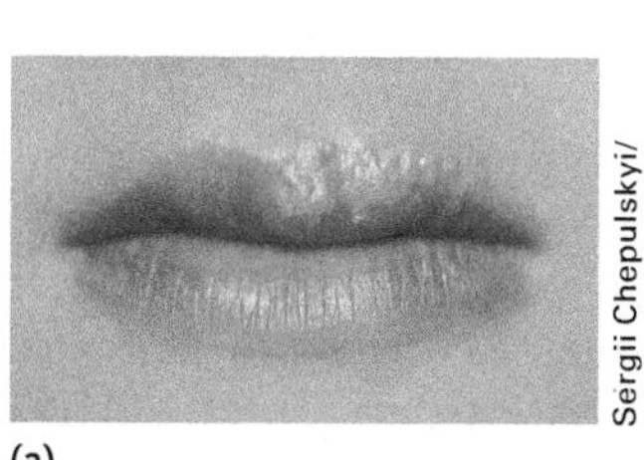
Sergii Chepulskyi/ Shutterstock
(a)

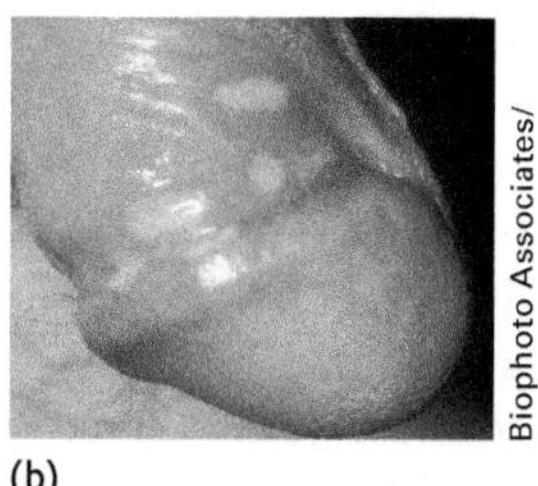
Biophoto Associates/ Science Source
(b)

(a) Herpes simplex virus (HSV-1) as a mouth sore, (b) Herpes simplex virus (HSV-2) as a genital sore

Gardasil® was the first HPV vaccine approved in Canada. It provides protection against HPV-16 and HPV-18, two types of HPV that cause approximately 70 percent of all cervical cancers, and against HPV-6 and HPV-11, which cause approximately 90 percent of all anogenital warts in both males and females. The vaccine is given three times over six months (zero, two, and six months) and helps protect females aged 9–45 years and males aged 9–26.

Cervarix® provides protection against the HPV-16 and HPV-18 types. It has been approved for use only in females aged 10–25 so far. Gardasil 9 provides protection against nine types of HPV: HPV-6, HPV-11, HPV-16, HPV-18, HPV-31, HPV-33, HPV-45, HPV-52, and HPV-58. This newest HPV vaccine is available for females between the ages of nine and 45 years and males between 9 and 26 years.[108]

The Society of Obstetricians and Gynaecologists of Canada (SOGC) supports the HPV vaccine use as "safe and effective."[109] All provinces and territories have launched HPV immunization initiatives for pre-adolescent and adolescent girls. Some Canadian colleges and universities are encouraging students to get the vaccine.

The HPV vaccine is not without controversy, however. Canadian researchers have raised many questions about the efficacy of the vaccine and the value of focusing on widespread vaccination for HPV as a routine part of sexual health treatment. Because the HPV vaccine is relatively new, it's not clear for how long the vaccine will be effective or if a booster shot will be required in later years. Research results are also not yet available on the effectiveness of the HPV vaccine when given at the same time as other immunizations. Finally, because cervical cancer is relatively rare, some sexual health experts are concerned that focus on and funding for HPV immunizations may take resources away from preventing other, more widespread, sexually transmitted infections.[110]

Regardless of whether or not you or your partner have had the HPV vaccine, it is vital to remember that a vaccine is just one step in the actions necessary to prevent genital warts or cervical cancer. The HPV vaccination should not be used as a replacement for cervical cancer screening such as a Pap test, nor a replacement for prevention strategies such as condom use.

Young women who engage in sexual intercourse at an early age are more likely to become infected with HPV. Their risk also increases if they have multiple sexual partners or a history of a sexually transmitted disease, use drugs, smoke, use oral contraceptives, or have sex with partners with a history of HPV.

HPV is transmitted primarily through vaginal, anal, and oral–genital sex. More than half of HPV-infected individuals do not develop any symptoms. After contact with an infected individual, genital warts may

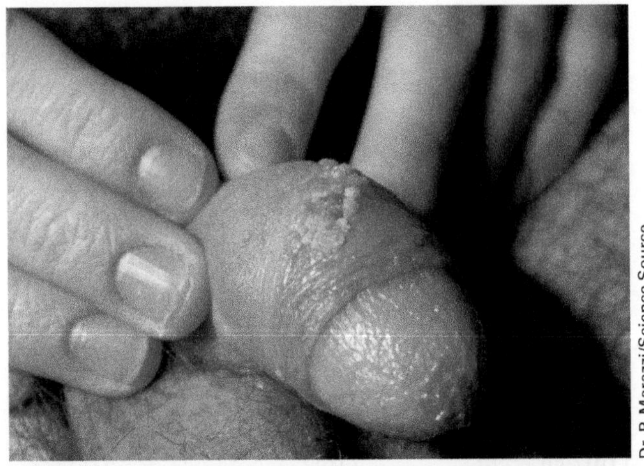

Dr. P. Marazzi/Science Source

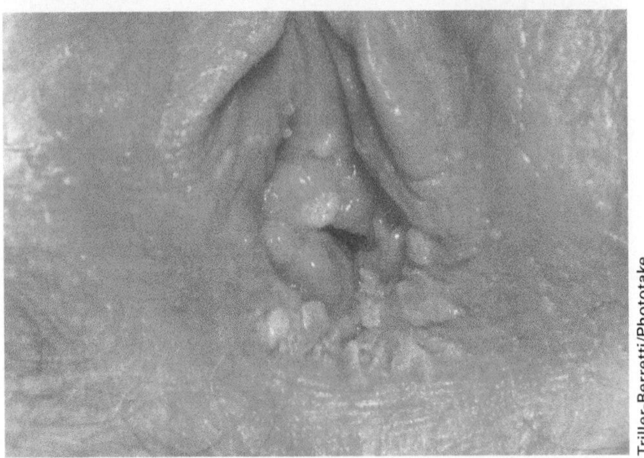

Triller-Berretti/Phototake

Human papillomavirus, which causes genital warts, is the most common viral STI.

appear from three weeks to 18 months, with an average period of about three months. The warts are treated by freezing, cauterization, chemicals, or surgical removal. Recurrences are common because the virus remains in the body.

HPV infection may invade the urethra and cause urinary obstruction and bleeding. It greatly increases a woman's risk of developing a precancerous condition called *cervical intraepithelial neoplasia*, which can lead to cervical cancer. There also is a strong association between HPV infections and cancer of the vagina, vulva, urethra, penis, and anus.

Women who have had an HPV infection should examine their genitals regularly and get an annual Pap smear. However, this diagnostic test for cervical cancer doesn't identify HPV infection. A newer, more specific test can recognize HPV soon after it enters the body. Women who test positive should undergo checkups for cervical changes every 6–12 months. If precancerous cells develop, surgery or laser treatment can prevent further growth.

HPV may also cause genital warts in men and increase the risk of cancer of the penis. HPV-infected men, who may not develop any symptoms, can spread the infection to their partners. People with visible genital warts also may have asymptomatic or subclinical HPV infections that are extremely difficult to treat.

No form of therapy has been shown to completely eradicate HPV, nor has any single treatment been uniformly effective in removing warts or preventing their recurrence.

✓ CHECK-IN

Have you considered getting an HPV vaccination? If not, why not?

Chancroid A **chancroid** is a soft, painful sore or localized infection caused by the bacterium *Haemophilus ducrevi* and usually acquired through sexual contact.[111] Half of the cases heal by themselves. In other cases, the infection may spread to the lymph glands near the chancroid, where large amounts of pus can accumulate and destroy much of the local tissue. Chancroids, which may increase susceptibility to HIV infection, are believed to be a major factor in the heterosexual spread of HIV. This infection is treated with antibiotics (ceftriaxone, azithromycin, or erythromycin) and can be prevented by keeping the genitals clean and washing them with soap and water in case of possible exposure.

Pubic Lice and Scabies These infections are sometimes, but not always, transmitted sexually. *Pubic lice* (or "crabs") are usually found in the pubic hair, although they can migrate to any hairy areas of the body. Lice lay eggs called *nits* that attach to the base of the hair shaft. Irritation from the lice may produce intense itching. Scratching to relieve the itching can produce sores. *Scabies* is caused by a mite that burrows under the skin, where they lay eggs that hatch and undergo many changes in the course of their life cycle, producing great discomfort, including intense itching.[112]

Lice and scabies are treated with applications of permethrin cream and Lindane shampoo to all the areas of the body where there are concentrations of body hair (genitals, armpits, scalp). You must repeat treatment in seven days to kill any newly developed adults. Wash or dry clean clothing and bedding.

HIV/AIDS Once seen as an epidemic affecting primarily gay men and injection-drug users, **human immunodeficiency virus (HIV)** and **acquired immune deficiency syndrome (AIDS)** have taken on very different forms today. Heterosexuals in developing countries have the highest rates of infection and mortality. According to estimates from the Joint United Nations Program on HIV/AIDS (UNAIDS), 36.9 million people in 2014 were living with HIV infection worldwide.[113] The region that has been most affected is sub-Saharan Africa where nearly one in every 20 adults now lives with HIV. Reports also show that approximately five million people are living with HIV in South, Southeast, and East Asia.

It is important to note that the number of new HIV infections has decreased around the world with 2 million adults and children infected in 2014, compared to 3.1 million in 2001. That is a decrease of 30 percent. Deaths from AIDS-related causes are also down, with 1.2 million worldwide in 2014 compared to 2 million in 2005.[114]

Prevention strategies have included reducing the incidence of unprotected sex and the number of sex partners, delaying sexual initiation, decreasing the incidence of other STIs, directing injection-drug users into drug treatment programs, and reducing needle sharing. Screening the blood supply has reduced the rate of transfusion-associated HIV transmission. Work at eliminating mother-to-child transmission of HIV during the perinatal and breastfeeding periods has also resulted in a decrease of new infections.[115] HIV antiretroviral therapy (ART) has increased worldwide too. About 15.8 million people living with HIV received ART as of June 2015. Forty-one percent were adults and 32 percent were children.[116]

In Canada the number of people living with HIV decreased from an estimated 2076 cases reported in 2013–2044 in 2014, a 1.5 percent decrease. Also, HIV cases in 2014 was the lowest rate since 1985 when a reporting structure was started in Canada.[117] People aged 30–39 years were the largest group diagnosed with HIV in Canada in 2014 at 31.6 percent. Almost 23 percent of people diagnosed with HIV were aged 40–49. That was followed by 21.9 percent of adults 50 and older. This age group surpassed the 20- to 29-year-old age group at 21.4 percent.[118]

The Spread of HIV/AIDS HIV/AIDS is characterized by a relatively long gap between the HIV infection and the onset of AIDS. Several factors—including frequent sexual activity with multiple, anonymous partners and high-risk sexual practices, such as anal intercourse—may have caused its quick spread through homosexual communities in the 1980s. When HIV reporting began in Canada, over 80 percent of all cases of HIV exposure were in men who had sex with men (MSM). HIV also spread among injection-drug users who, by sharing contaminated needles, injected the virus directly into their bloodstream as well as through heterosexual contact.[119]

A report by the Government of Canada[120] indicates that in 2014, the greatest proportion of reported HIV cases among adult males, 15 years or older, at 63.3 percent, was due to the exposure category of MSM. For females, aged 15 and older, the greatest proportion of reported HIV cases, at 25.5 percent, was due to heterosexual (Het-Endemic) contact compared to 5.4 percent among males. The injection drug use (IDU) exposure category accounted for approximately one-quarter of adult female HIV cases (24.5%), compared to 9.6 percent of adult male HIV cases. (see Figures 9-6 and 9-7).

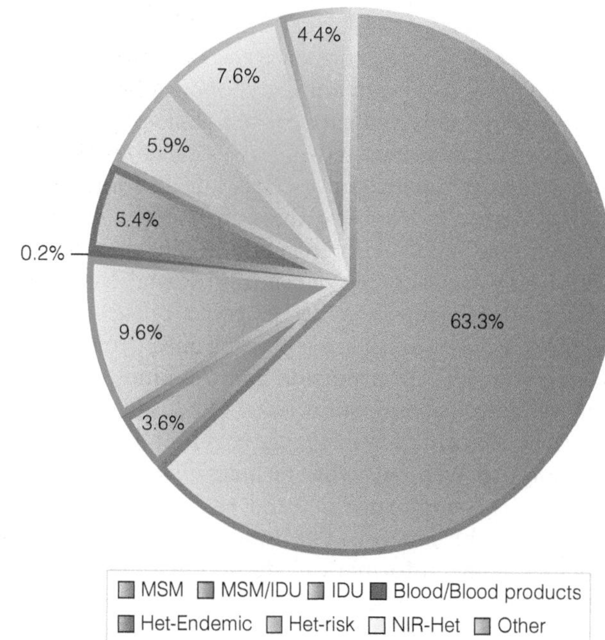

Figure 9-6 **Proportion of Reported HIV Cases among Adult Males (> 15 years old) by Exposure Category—Canada, 2014**

Source: © All rights reserved. *HIV and AIDS in Canada. Surveillance Report to December 31, 2014.* Public Health Agency of Canada, 2015. Adapted and reproduced with permission from the Minister of Health, 2016.

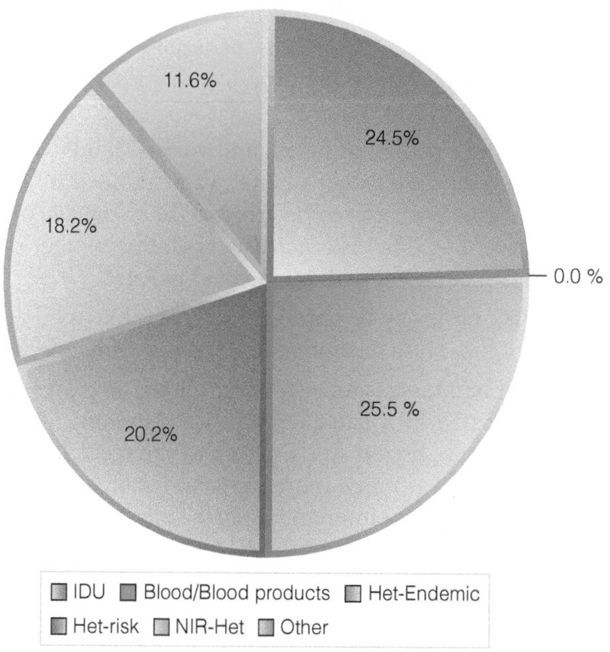

Figure 9-7 **Proportion of Reported HIV Cases among Adult Females (> 15 years old) by Exposure Category—Canada, 2014**

Source: © All rights reserved. *HIV and AIDS in Canada. Surveillance Report to December 31, 2014.* Public Health Agency of Canada, 2015. Adapted and reproduced with permission from the Minister of Health, 2016.

Youth are at risk because many young people perceive that HIV is not a threat to them and do not adopt and maintain behaviours that protect them against infection.[121]

Reducing the Risk of HIV Transmission Although no one is immune to HIV, you can reduce the risk if you abstain from sexual activity, remain in a monogamous relationship with an uninfected partner, and do not inject drugs. If you're not in a long-term monogamous relationship with a partner you are convinced is safe and you are not willing to abstain from sex, there are things you can do to lower your risk of HIV infection. Remember that the risk of HIV transmission depends on sexual behaviour, not sexual orientation. Whether you are heterosexual, lesbian, gay, bisexual, transgender, or queer, you need to know about HIV transmission and the kinds of sexual activity that increase your risk. The Canadian Aids Treatment Information Exchange (CATIE) has an extensive resource Web page that includes links to websites, research, client information, and evaluation reports,[122] which may be helpful. The following checklist also provides some information about reducing the risk of HIV.[123]

- Casual contact does *not* spread HIV infection. You cannot get HIV infection from drinking from a water fountain, contact with a toilet seat, or touching an infected person. Compared to other viruses, HIV is extremely difficult to get.
- HIV can live in blood, semen, vaginal fluids, and breast milk.
- You cannot tell visually whether a potential sexual partner has HIV. A blood test is needed to detect the antibodies that the body produces to fight HIV, thus indicating infection.
- HIV can be spread in semen and vaginal fluids during a single instance of anal, vaginal, or oral sexual contact between heterosexuals, bisexuals, or homosexuals. The risk increases with the number of sexual encounters with an infected partner.
- Teenage girls may be particularly vulnerable to HIV infection because the immature cervix is easily infected.
- Anal intercourse is an extremely high-risk behaviour because HIV can enter the bloodstream through tiny breaks in the lining of the rectum. HIV transmission is much more likely to occur during unprotected anal intercourse than during vaginal intercourse.
- Other behaviours that increase the risk of HIV infection include having multiple sexual partners, engaging in sex without condoms, sexual contact with persons known to be at high risk (for example, prostitutes or injection-drug users), and sharing injection equipment for drugs.
- Individuals are at greater risk if they have an active sexual infection. Sexually transmitted diseases, such as herpes, gonorrhea, and syphilis, facilitate transmission of HIV during vaginal or rectal intercourse.
- Oral sex can lead to HIV transmission. The virus in any semen that enters the mouth could make its way into the bloodstream through tiny nicks or sores in the mouth. A man's risk in performing oral sex on a woman is smaller because an infected woman's genital fluids have much lower concentrations of HIV than does semen.
- HIV infection is not widespread among lesbians, although there have been documented cases of possible female-to-female HIV transmission. In each instance, one partner had had sex with a bisexual man or male injection-drug user or had injected drugs herself.

Helping college and university students understand that HIV/AIDS is not just a risk in developing countries but also a risk in Canada is an important part of sexual health education. Findings from a study by Graffingna and Olson[124] show that HIV/AIDS was not considered a danger to the 18- to 25-year-old adults who participated in focus group sessions. Instead, the students suggested HIV/AIDS was a disease linked to gay men, drug users, and homeless people—not them. The authors also discovered that mass media was the main source of information about HIV/AIDS for the participants of the study but that it did not always provide correct or meaningful information. They recommend that interpersonal exchange of information and specific media initiatives geared to young adults about the risk of HIV/AIDS might help to change attitudes and behaviour.

HIV Infection **Human immunodeficiency virus (HIV)** infection refers to a spectrum of health problems that result from immunologic abnormalities caused by the virus when it enters the bloodstream. In theory, the body may be able to resist infection by HIV. In reality, in almost all cases, HIV destroys the cell-mediated immune system, particularly the CD41 T-lymphocytes (also called *T4 helper cells*). The result is greatly increased susceptibility to various cancers and opportunistic infections (infections that take hold because of the reduced effectiveness of the immune system).[125]

Researchers now know that HIV triggers a state of all-out war within the immune system. Almost immediately following infection with HIV, the immune system responds aggressively by manufacturing enormous numbers of CD41 cells. It eventually is overwhelmed, however, as the viral particles continue to replicate, or multiply. The intense war between HIV and the immune system indicates that the virus itself, not a breakdown in the immune system, is responsible for disease progression.

Shortly after becoming infected with HIV, individuals may experience a few days of flu-like symptoms, which most ignore or attribute to other viruses. Some people develop a more severe mononucleosis-type syndrome. After this stage, individuals may not develop any signs or symptoms of disease for a period ranging from weeks to more than 12 years.

HIV symptoms, which tend to increase in severity and number the longer the virus is in the body, may include any of the following:

- swollen lymph nodes
- fever, chills, and night sweats
- diarrhea
- weight loss
- coughing and shortness of breath
- persistent tiredness
- skin sores
- blurred vision and headaches
- development of other infections, such as certain kinds of pneumonia

HIV infection is associated with a variety of HIV-related diseases, including different cancers and dangerous infections. HIV-infected individuals may develop persistent generalized lymphadenopathy, enlargement of the lymph nodes at two or more different sites in the body. This condition typically persists for more than three months without any other illness to explain its occurrence. Diminished mental function may appear before other symptoms. Tests conducted on infected but apparently healthy men have revealed impaired coordination, problems in thinking, or abnormal brain scans. However, people on antiretroviral therapy are finding success with current treatments and are living much longer.[126]

HIV Testing As of May 1, 2003, HIV infection became legally notifiable in all provinces and territories.[127] In most testing situations, laboratories and physicians are responsible for reporting HIV infection; however, this varies in each province or territory. Notification to the Centre for Infectious Disease Prevention at the national level is still voluntary, but all provinces and territories have been reporting positive HIV and AIDS cases. This information is considered important for designing and targeting intervention programs.

All HIV tests measure antibodies, cells produced by the body to fight HIV infection. A negative test indicates no exposure to HIV. It can take three to six months for the body to produce the telltale antibodies, however, so a negative result may not be accurate, depending on the timing of the test.

There are three types of HIV testing available in Canada:[128]

- Nominal/name-based HIV testing:
  - Available at health clinics or the office of a healthcare provider.
  - The person ordering the tests knows the identity of the person being tested for HIV, and the HIV test is ordered using the name of the person being tested.
  - Patient information such as age, sex, city of residence, name of diagnosing healthcare provider, country of birth, HIV-related risk factors, and laboratory data is collected.
  - If the HIV test result is positive, the person ordering the test is legally obligated to notify public-health officials.
  - The test result is recorded in the healthcare record of the person being tested.
- Non-nominal/non-identifying HIV testing:
  - As above, but the HIV test is ordered using a code name or the initials of the person being tested.
- Anonymous testing:
  - The HIV test is carried out using a code. The person ordering the HIV test and the laboratory carrying out the testing on the blood sample does not know to whom the code belongs.
  - Test results are not recorded on the healthcare record of the person being tested.
  - If someone tests positive for HIV infection through anonymous testing, that person may subsequently decide to give his or her name and include the HIV test result in the medical record.

Newly developed blood tests can determine how recently a person was infected with HIV and distinguish between longstanding infections and those contracted within the previous four to six months. Health officials recommend HIV testing for the following individuals:

- Men who have had sex with other men, regardless of whether they consider themselves homosexual.
- Anyone who uses injection drugs or has shared needles.
- Anyone who has had sex with someone who uses injection drugs or has shared needles.
- Women who have had sex with bisexual men.
- Anyone who has had sex with someone from an area with a high incidence of HIV infection.

- Individuals who have had sex with people they do not know well.
- Anyone who received blood transfusions or blood products between 1978 and 1985, their sexual partners, and, if they are new mothers, their infants.

> **✓ CHECK-IN**
>
> How are you minimizing your risk of becoming infected with HIV?

AIDS In Canada a person is diagnosed with **acquired immune deficiency syndrome (AIDS)** if (1) they have undergone testing for HIV and received a positive result, and (2) they have one or more of the clinical illnesses or indicator diseases that characterize AIDS. All provinces and territories in Canada have adopted this definition.[129] Forty-eight countries of the WHO European Region, Australia, and New Zealand also follow this definition of AIDS diagnosis. In the United States, individuals must also have a CD4T–lymphocyte count of less than 200 cells per cubic millimetre of blood in order to meet the definition of AIDS.[130] The median time from HIV infection to AIDS diagnosis now exceeds 10 years.

People with AIDS also may experience persistent fever, diarrhea that persists for more than one month, or involuntary weight loss of more than 10 percent of normal body weight. Generalized lymphadenopathy may persist. Neurological disease—including dementia (confusion and impaired thinking) and other problems with thinking, speaking, movement, or sensation—may occur. Secondary infectious diseases that may develop in people who have had AIDS for a long time include *Pneumocystis carinii* pneumonia, tuberculosis, or oral candidiasis (thrush). Secondary cancers associated with HIV infection include Kaposi's sarcoma and cancer of the cervix. For individuals diagnosed in the last ten years, prophylactic medications have lowered the incidence of these diseases.

In Canada, 188 cases of AIDS were reported in 2014 (see Figure 9-8). This is a decrease from 226 reported cases in 2013. Males comprised the majority of reported AIDS cases at 75.4 percent (15 years and older).[131]

What Progress Has Been Made in Treating HIV?

New forms of therapy have been remarkably effective in boosting levels of protective T cells and reducing *viral load*—the amount of HIV in the bloodstream. People with high viral loads are more likely to progress rapidly to AIDS than people with low levels of the virus.

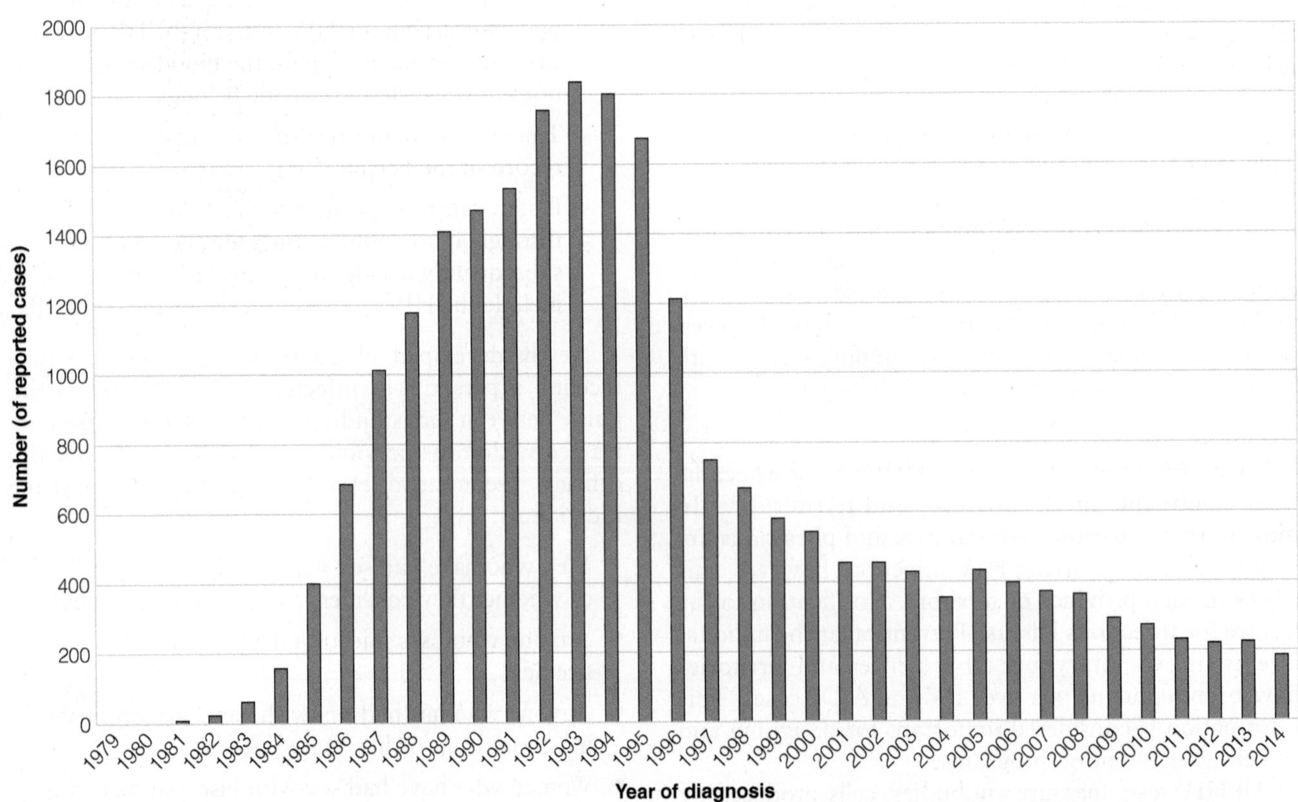

Figure 9-8 Number of Reported AIDS Cases by Year of Diagnosis—Canada, 1979–2014

Source: © All rights reserved. *HIV and AIDS in Canada. Surveillance Report to December 31, 2014*. Public Health Agency of Canada, 2015. Adapted and reproduced with permission from the Minister of Health, 2016.

The current "gold-standard" approach to combating HIV is known as HAART (Highly Active AntiRetroviral Therapies), which dramatically reduces viral load even though it does not eradicate the virus. This complex regimen uses one of 250 different combinations of three or more antiretroviral drugs. Since the development of HAART, the number of deaths among persons with AIDS has declined substantially, and the number of those living with AIDS has risen.

A drawback to the treatment is serious side effects, including anemia, mouth ulcers, diarrhea, respiratory difficulties, digestive problems, liver damage, and skin rashes. There also is concern about emerging resistance to some antiretroviral medications. Some Canadian medical experts suggest that drug resistance among individuals receiving treatment is on the rise. Currently there are studies on new treatment and prevention.

The Canadian HIV Vaccine Initiative (CHVI), a collaboration between a private funder—the Bill & Melinda Gates Foundation—and the Government of Canada, is bringing together leading research and medical experts to develop a safe and effective vaccine that would be affordable and globally available. The Foundation is funding this initiative until 2017. A vaccine that could slow the HIV infection rate on a global basis could save lives and healthcare costs.[132]

HUMAN POTENTIAL

Saleema Noon—The Best Job in the World

Our human potential story for this chapter is about Saleema Noon, a sexual health educator. Her job is to make sexual health easy to talk about. This can be a difficult task, but Saleema finds her work to be both meaningful and challenging. Her story is unique, one that might inspire you to not only take care with regard to your own sexual health but also encourage you to find ways to include sexual health education in the work you might do in the future.

Her entry into this field came by way of a master's degree at the University of British Columbia in an area called Family Studies. Her work as a teaching assistant for a course called Human Sexuality 316 taught her that many university students had not been educated about sexual health. Findings from her graduate research with Grade 10 students supported what she had discovered in her university classes—that students wanted more sexual education, they wanted it earlier, and they wanted it to be more relevant to their lives.

After graduation she had many jobs while she was building her business. They included house-sitter, bank teller, daycare worker, and dog-sitter. She laughs and says, "Unfortunately, there are not many want ads for sexual health educators!" She also worked as a family support worker with pregnant and parenting teens. The girls taught her about the value of accurate information in making smart decisions about sex.

A turning point for Saleema with regard to her career choice was a conversation she had with a Grade 8 student upon returning from a doctor's appointment where the young girl's pregnancy had been confirmed. The conversation went something like this: "Saleema, I don't get it, how could this be happening?" Saleema responded, "Well, did you have sex?" The young woman replied, "Yes." Saleema asked, "Then why are you surprised?" The young woman replied, "But I had it on a Tuesday." Saleema was to learn later that this young girl had been told by a friend that as long as she didn't have sex on the weekend, she didn't need to worry about getting pregnant.

Saleema knew then that she had to do whatever she could to help young people get the information they needed about sex education. She now works in schools, workplaces, and recreation centres. She speaks enthusiastically about seeing the excited

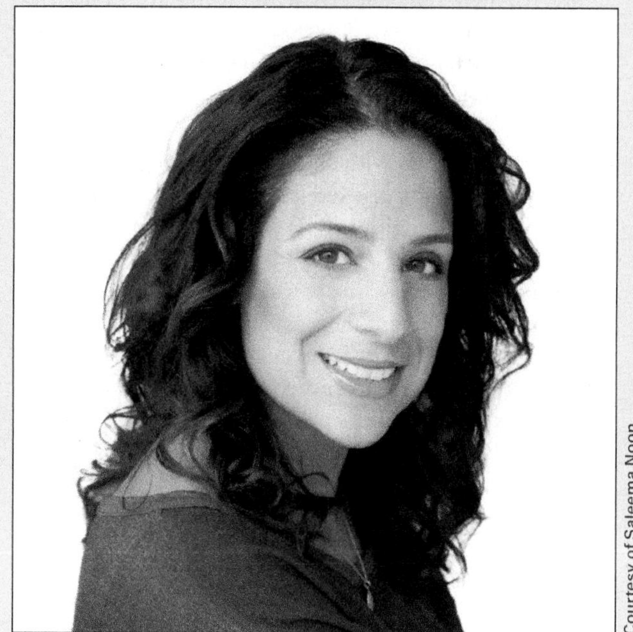

Courtesy of Saleema Noon

Saleema Noon, a sexual health educator and workshop leader

faces of kindergarten children as they learn to be body scientists and the "grossed out" faces of Grade 4 children who are beginning to learn about sex. She provides workshops and seminars for educators, healthcare professionals, counsellors, and social workers. She also runs iGirl and iGuy Empowerment Programs for 9- to 12-year-old girls and boys. An iMatter workshop helps Grade 8 students learn about bullying and online social media and how their decisions impact not only themselves but also others.

Is this work easy? Not at all, but Saleema says she takes a moment each day to be grateful for a job she loves. She travels a lot. She must be enthusiastic when she is educating and performing for an entire school day. Spare moments find her replying to requests that come in through her website, www.saleemanoon.com. She must also deal with some parents who are convinced that sexual education might harm their children. However, the pros outweigh

(Continued)

the cons, and she continues to enjoy work that is rewarding, fun, and inspirational—"the best job in the world!"

Her success did not come easily. She volunteered for many years. She thanks her mentor, Meg Hickling, a renowned sexual health educator, for teaching her so much. She has become a respected sexual health educator and has appeared as a regular guest on Global News, CKNW Radio, CityTV Breakfast Television, and a CBC Doc Zone documentary—*Sext Up Kids*. She is the recipient of the Options for Sexual Health's Educator of the Year Award and a 2011 YWCA Vancouver's Women of Distinction Award.

Advice she gives students about sexual health: "get informed, be aware, love your body, and be proud of the smart decisions you make." Advice on career choices: "ask yourself what you are passionate about, what motivates you, and what type of job you see yourself doing. Be realistic, but be creative, too." She also suggests volunteering because "the experience you gain through volunteering will be invaluable in any work you do."

SELF-SURVEY

What's Your Infection IQ?

Check the items that apply to you.

___ I wash my hands with soap and water after I use the restroom.
___ I wash my hands with soap and water before I eat.
___ Before and after using exercise equipment, I wipe the handles.
___ I wash my hands with soap and water after working out with weights or exercise equipment at a gym.
___ I avoid contact with people who are coughing and sneezing.
___ I wash my hands with soap and water more often during the cold and flu season.
___ All of my vaccinations are current.
___ I eat at least three balanced meals a day.
___ I get six to eight hours of sleep at night.
___ I use relaxation techniques to lower my stress level.
___ I do not smoke.
___ I do not drink or I keep alcohol consumption to a minimum.
___ I do not use illicit drugs of any kind, including steroids.
___ I use prescription drugs as prescribed.
___ I throw leftovers out after three days.
___ I wash fruits and vegetables before eating.
___ I check expiration dates on food items.
___ I apply insect spray (containing DEET) when I am outdoors.
___ I wear long-sleeved clothing and long pants when hiking.
___ I check myself for ticks after a hike.

Answers to Self-Survey

Scoring

Add up your checkmarks, and look for patterns in your protective behaviours. Are you conscientious about exercise and sleep, but careless about washing your hands or wiping down gym equipment? Do you protect yourself against food infections (discussed in Chapter 5) but not against sexually transmitted infections (discussed in Chapter 9)? Identify the aspects of infection protection that need the most work, and start practising the defensive behaviours that will lower your risk.

Chapter Summary

1. Which statement about disease-causing microbes is false?
   a. Helminths cause malaria, one of the major worldwide diseases.
   b. AIDS is caused by a retrovirus.
   c. In Canada, the most common protozoan disease is giardiasis.
   d. Salmonella and botulism are food-borne illnesses caused by bacteria.
2. Which statement about the immune system is false?
   a. The immune system has two types of white blood cells: B cells, which produce antibodies that fight bacteria and viruses, and T cells, which protect against parasites, fungi, and cancer cells.
   b. Immune-system structures include the spleen, tonsils, thymus gland, and lymph nodes located throughout the body.
   c. Inoculation with a vaccine confers active immunity.
   d. The effect of stress on the human immune system depends on whether you can control the stressor and on the mental effort required to cope.
3. Before you have a vaccination it is NOT important that you consider which of the following?
   a. if you are pregnant
   b. if you are allergic to eggs
   c. if you have a fever
   d. if you hate needles

4. Which statement about the common cold and influenza is true?
   a. Influenza is just a more severe form of the common cold.
   b. Aspirin should be avoided by children and young adults who have a cold or influenza.
   c. The flu vaccine is also effective against most of the viruses that cause the common cold.
   d. Antibiotics are appropriate treatments for colds but not for influenza.
5. Which statement about specific infectious diseases is false?
   a. Yeast infections can be treated with non-prescription drugs.
   b. Symptoms of UTIs include burning urination, chills, fever, and blood in the urine.
   c. Hepatitis A is usually transmitted through contaminated needles, transfusions, and sexual contact.
   d. College freshmen are at higher risk for contracting meningitis than the general population of young people between the ages of 18 and 23.
6. Which statement about sexually transmitted infections is true?
   a. They are the major cause of preventable sterility in Canada.
   b. They can result in a severe kidney disease called pylonephritis.
   c. They have declined in incidence in developing nations due to improving health standards.
   d. They do not increase the risk of being infected with HIV.
7. Which STI is NOT caused by bacterial agents?
   a. genital warts
   b. syphilis
   c. chlamydia
   d. gonorrhea
8. Which STI is NOT caused by viral agents?
   a. herpes
   b. genital warts
   c. hepatitis B
   d. candidiasis
9. Which statement about HIV transmission is true?
   a. Individuals are not at risk for HIV if they are being treated for chlamydia or gonorrhea.
   b. HIV can be transmitted between heterosexual couples.
   c. Heterosexual men who do not practise safe sex are at less risk for contracting HIV than homosexual men who do practise safe sex.
   d. HIV cannot be spread in a single instance of sexual intercourse.
10. Which statement about people with AIDS is true?
   a. They have a low viral load and a high number of T4 helper cells.
   b. They can no longer pass HIV to a sexual partner.
   c. They may suffer from secondary infectious diseases and cancers.
   d. They will not respond to treatment.

Answers to these questions can be found on page 253.

SELF-RESPONSIBILITY—SOCIAL RESPONSIBILITY

SELF-RESPONSIBILITY

As to diseases, make a habit of two things—to help, or at least, to do no harm.

Hippocrates

Becoming more aware of the ways you can protect yourself from infectious diseases is a step toward becoming self-responsible. It is also a way of supporting a healthy lifestyle. What stage are you at according to Prochaska's Stages of Change model? Did reading this chapter move you from pre-contemplation to contemplation? How might you prepare for the flu season or sexual relationships? What does the maintenance stage mean to you when you think about infectious diseases? How does protecting yourself from infectious diseases support your "human potential"?

SOCIAL RESPONSIBILITY

The global HIV/AIDS epidemic is an unprecedented crisis that requires an unprecedented response. In particular it requires solidarity—between the healthy and the sick, between rich and poor, and above all, between richer and poorer nations. We have 30 million orphans already. How many more do we have to get, to wake up?

Kofi Annan

What can you do to help educate others about sexual health? Volunteer at a sexual health centre? Join a movement such as Stephen Lewis Foundation? Reach out if you can.

CRITICAL THINKING

1. Before you read this chapter, describe what you did to avoid contracting an infectious disease. Now that you have read the chapter, will you be making any changes in your practices? Briefly explain the convenience, advantages, and disadvantages of each practice that you have been using and/or will be using to prevent infection.
2. Some employers are now screening personnel for HIV. Some insurance companies test for HIV before selling a policy. Do you believe that an individual has the right to refuse to be tested for HIV? Should a physician be able to order an HIV test without a patient's consent? Can a surgeon refuse to operate on an HIV-infected patient or one who refuses HIV testing? Do patients have the right to know if their doctors, dentists, or nurses are HIV-positive?
3. A man who developed herpes sued his former girlfriend. A woman who became sterile as a result of pelvic inflammatory disease (PID) took her ex-husband to court. A woman who contracted HIV infection from her dentist, who died of AIDS, filed suit against his estate. Do you think that anyone who knowingly transmits an STI should be held legally responsible? Do you think such an act should be a criminal offence?

WEB LINKS

The Canadian AIDS Treatment Information Exchange (CATIE)
www.catie.ca
CATIE is a leading source of HIV/AIDS treatment information for Canadians living with the virus and their caregivers. At this site you can also access information about AIDS service organizations.

Canadian Immunization Guide
http://www.phac-aspc.gc.ca/publicat/cig-gci/index-eng.php
Recommendations by the National Advisory Committee on Immunization (NACI) on the use of vaccines in Canada are contained in this guide.

Sexuality and U
www.sexualityandu.ca
This comprehensive site has information about many sexually transmitted infections, contraception, sexuality, and reproductive health issues.

Travel Health
http://www.phac-aspc.gc.ca/tmp-pmv/index-eng.php
If you are travelling outside Canada, this site is a must. Find up-to-date information on international disease outbreaks, immunization recommendations for international travel, and general health advice for travelling.

UNAIDS—Joint United Nations Programme on HIV/AIDS
http://www.unaids.org/
Access this site to find information about the goals and countries this organization is reaching and numerous resources that include documents, campaigns, and videos. Please note that links are subject to change. If you find a broken link, use a search engine such as www.google.ca and search for the website by typing keywords.

Key Terms

The terms listed here are used within the chapter on the page indicated. Definitions of the terms are in the Glossary at the end of this book.

Answers to Chapter Summary Questions

1. a; 2. c; 3. d; 4. b; 5. c; 6. a; 7. a; 8. d; 9. b; 10. c

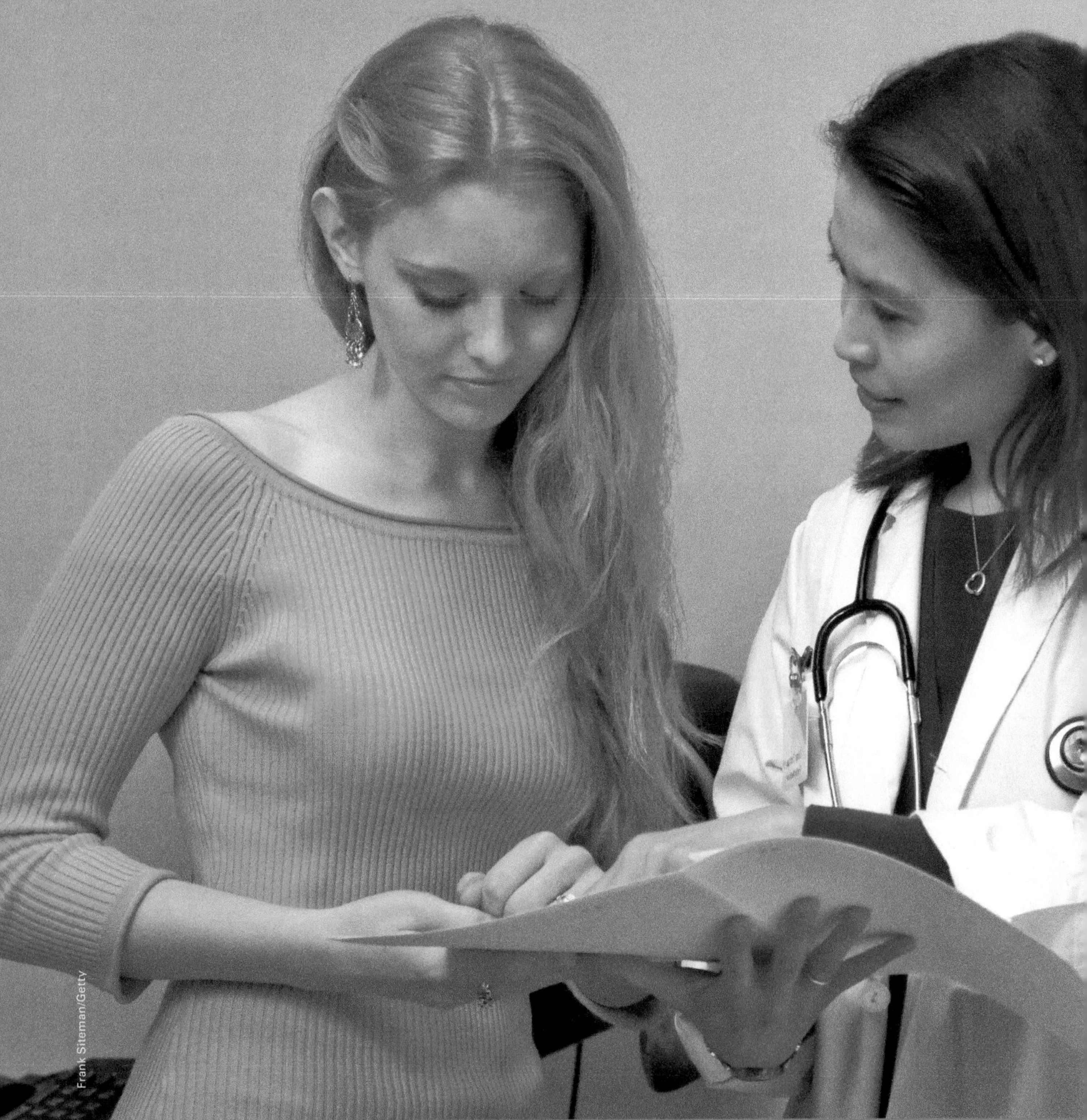
Frank Siteman/Getty

AFTER READING THIS CHAPTER, YOU WILL BE ABLE TO:

- **explain** how the heart functions
- **describe** the four main types of cardiovascular diseases
- **identify** the risk factors for cardiovascular disease that you can control and those you cannot control
- **list** the risk factors for cancer and **describe** practical ways to reduce the risk
- **identify** the risk factors for diabetes (type 1 and type 2)

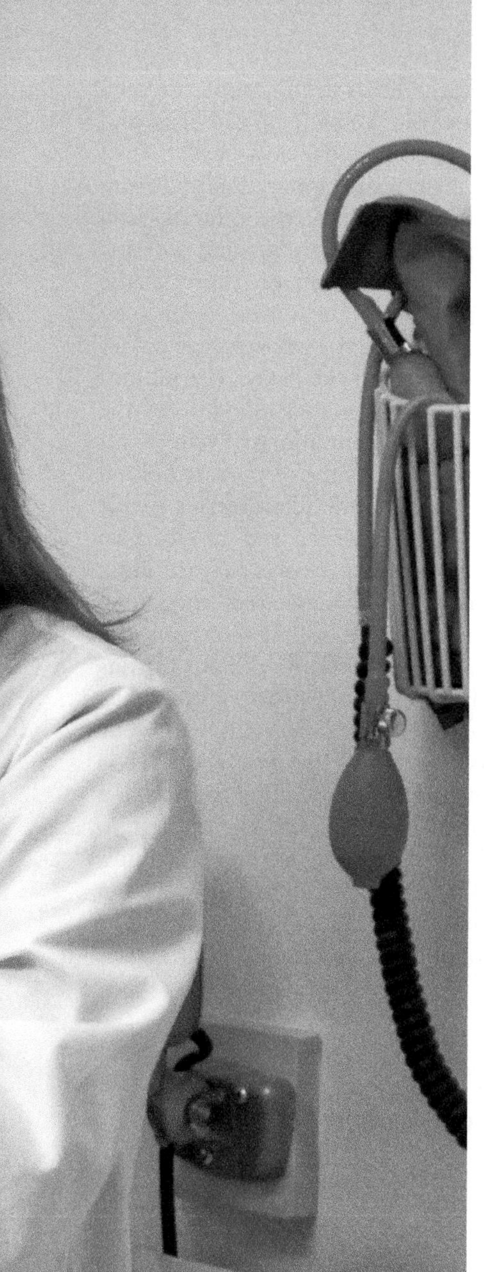

10

Lowering Your Risk of Major Diseases

Whether or not you will get a serious disease at some time in your life may seem to be a matter of odds. Genetic tendencies, environmental factors, and luck affect your chances of having to face many health threats. However, you do have some control over such risks, and even if a major disease or illness may be inevitable, you can often prevent or delay it for years, even decades.

Cancer is the leading cause of death in Canada, claiming the lives of 30.2 percent of Canadians, followed by heart disease at 19.7 percent, and stroke at 5.3 percent.[1] These diseases cost the Canadian economy millions of dollars every year in physician services, hospital costs, lost wages, and decreased productivity. Nevertheless, lifestyle changes, such as making dietary modifications that lower blood pressure and cholesterol levels, increasing your physical activity levels, and quitting smoking can make a positive difference.

Some people mistakenly think of heart disease, cancer, and other disorders as illnesses of middle and old age. But the events leading up to these diseases often begin in childhood, develop in adolescence, and become a health threat to men and women sometimes as early as in their 20s, 30s, or 40s.

This chapter provides information about cardiovascular disease, cancer, and diabetes. It outlines the risk factors you can't control and those you can. There is also a section on the newest medical advances that can improve your chances of leading a healthier, longer life.

FREQUENTLY ASKED QUESTIONS

CARDIOVASCULAR DISEASE

Cardiovascular disease (CVD) refers to any disease that affects the structure and function of the heart and cardiovascular system. This includes disease and injury to the heart, the **coronary arteries** and **veins**, and the arteries and veins throughout the body and within the brain.[2] According to the World Health Organization (WHO), cardiovascular diseases are the number one cause of death around the world. An estimated 17.5 million people died from CVDs in 2012.[3] Heart disease and stroke are the second- and third-leading causes of death in Canada (see Table 10-1). There are about 1.6 million Canadians who are living with heart disease and the consequences of stroke.[4]

There are many types of cardiovascular disease. An overview of the four most common types—atherosclerosis, coronary heart disease (also known as coronary artery disease or ischemic heart disease), hypertension, and stroke—will be presented. Arrhythmia, as well as congenital and rheumatic heart disease, some of the other less common types of CVDs, will also be noted. First, it is a good idea to review how the cardiovascular system works.

How the Heart Works **Arteries** and **veins** supply blood to the heart muscle and all other organs of the body. The two major veins that bring deoxygenated blood from the body to the heart are the **superior vena cava** and **inferior vena cava.**[5] Veins from the head and upper body feed the superior vena cava, which then empties into the right atrium of the heart. Blood from the lower torso and legs feeds into the inferior vena cava, which also empties into the right atrium.

The largest single blood vessel in our body is the **aorta.**[6] In size, it compares to the diameter of your thumb. Oxygen-rich blood from the left ventricle passes through the aorta to all parts of the body. The **pulmonary artery**[7] transports deoxygenated blood from the right ventricle to the lungs. The **pulmonary vein**[8] is yet another special vessel that carries the oxygenated blood from the lungs to the left atrium. The *arteries* divide into smaller and smaller branches, and finally into **capillaries,**[9] the smallest blood vessels of all (only slightly larger in diameter than a single red blood cell). The blood within the capillaries supplies oxygen and nutrients to the cells of the tissues and takes up various waste products. Blood returns to the heart via the veins.

The heart is a hollow, muscular organ with four chambers that serve as two pumps (see Figure 10-1). It is about the size of a clenched fist. Each pump consists of a pair of chambers formed from muscles. The upper two chambers are called the atrium. The **right atrium**[10] receives deoxygenated blood, as mentioned above, from the superior vena cava and inferior vena cava. The **sinoatrial node (SA node)**[11] sends an impulse that causes

TABLE 10-1

Ranking, Number, and Percentage of Deaths for the 10 Leading Causes, Canada, 2000 and 2012

	2000			2012		
	Rank	**Number**	**%**	**Rank**	**Number**	**%**
All causes of death	...	218 062	100.0	...	246 596	100.0
Total, 10 leading causes of death	...	175 149	80.3	...	184 869	75.0
Malignant neoplasms (cancer)	1	62 672	28.7	1	74 361	30.2
Diseases of the heart (heart disease)	2	55 070	25.3	2	48 681	19.7
Cerebrovascular diseases (stroke)	3	15 576	7.1	3	13 174	5.3
Chronic lower respiratory diseases	4	9 813	4.5	5	11 130	4.5
Accidents (unintentional injuries)	5	8 589	3.9	4	11 290	4.6
Diabetes mellitus (diabetes)	6	6 714	3.1	6	6 993	2.8
Alzheimer's disease	7	5 007	2.3	7	6 293	2.6
Influenza and pneumonia	8	4 966	2.3	8	5 694	2.3
Intentional self-harm (suicide)	9	3 606	1.7	9	3 926	1.6
Nephritis, nephritic syndrome, and nephrosis (kidney disease)	10	3 136	1.4	10	3 327	1.4
All other causes	...	42 913	19.7	...	61 727	25.0

... Not applicable

Source: Statistics Canada. (2015, December 10). The 10 leading causes of death, 2012. Health Fact Sheets. Publications. 82-625-X. Available at http://www.statcan.gc.ca/pub/82-625-x/2015001/article/14296-eng.htm.

Figure 10-1 The Healthy Heart

(a) The heart muscle is nourished by blood from the coronary arteries, which arise from the aorta.

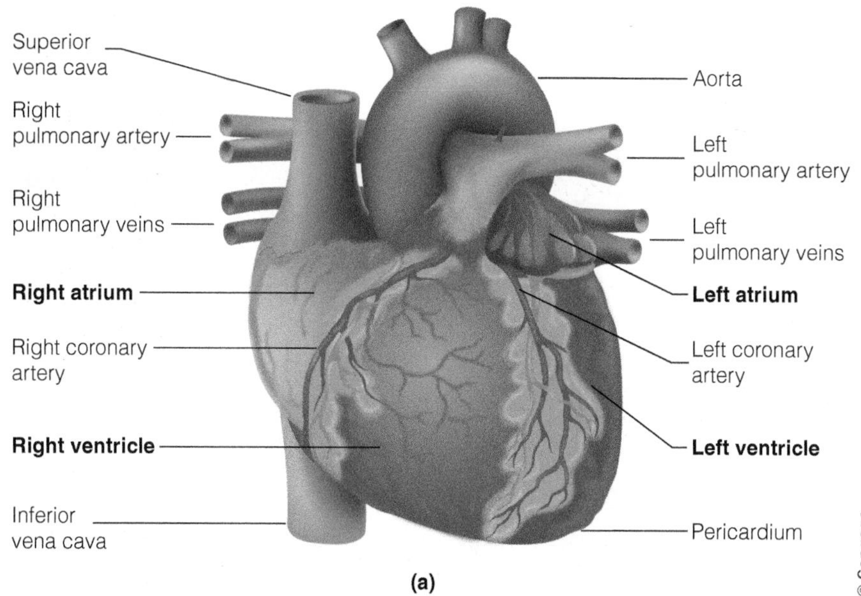

(b) The cross-section shows the four chambers and the myocardium, the muscle that does the heart's work. The pericardium is the outer covering of the heart.

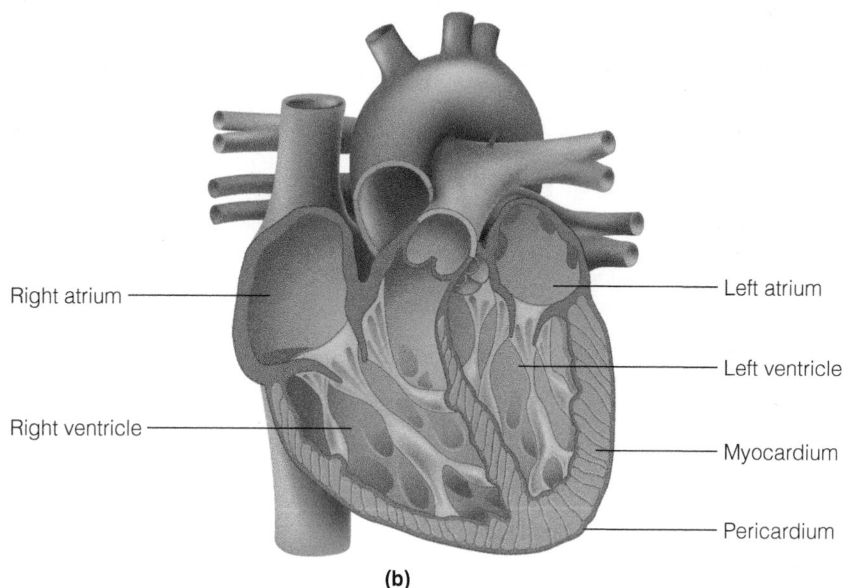

the cardiac muscle tissue of the atrium to contract. When this contraction occurs, the **tricuspid valve,**[12] whose job is to separate the right atrium from the right ventricle, opens and allow deoxygenated blood collected in the right atrium to flow into the right ventricle.

Once the **right ventricle**[13] has collected the deoxygenated blood in its chamber, it contracts. The tricuspid valve closes to prevent blood from back-flowing into the right atrium while the **pulmonary valve,**[14] which separates the right ventricle from the pulmonary artery, opens to allow the deoxygenated blood to flow through the pulmonary artery toward the lungs. As the ventricles relax, it closes so that the blood does not back-flow into the heart.

The blood is then oxygenated in the lungs and flows into one of the upper chambers of the heart, the **left atrium,**[15] through the pulmonary vein. It then must pass through the **mitral valve**[16] into the **left ventricle.**[17] The mitral valve is important because it separates the left atrium from the left ventricle. Its job is to open to allow the oxygenated blood collected in the left atrium to flow into the left ventricle. Then it must close when the left ventricle contracts to prevent a back-flow of blood into the left atrium. By closing, it forces the blood to move through the **aortic valve** and into the aorta. Then the cycle begins again (Figure 10-2 shows the path of blood flow).

A thick wall divides the right side of the heart from the left side; even though the two sides are separated, they contract at almost the same time. Contraction of the ventricles is called **systole;** the period of relaxation between contractions is called **diastole.**[18] The heart valves, all located at the entrance and exit of the ventricular chambers, are designed with flaps that open and close to allow blood to flow through the chambers of the heart.

Figure 10-2 The Path of Blood Flow

Blood is pumped from the right ventricle through the pulmonic valve into the pulmonary arteries, which lead to the lungs, where gas exchange (O_2 for CO_2) occurs. Oxygenated blood returning from the lungs drains into the left atrium and is pumped into the left ventricle through the mitral valve. It then passes through the aortic valve to the aorta and its branches. The oxygenated blood flows through the arteries, which extend to all parts of the body. Gas exchange occurs in the body tissues; oxygen is "dropped off" and carbon dioxide "picked up." Deoxygenated blood enters the right atrium through the inferior and superior vena cava, then flows to the right ventricle through the tricuspid valve.

Another important anatomical structure of the heart is the **papillary muscles**, which attach to the lower portion of the interior wall of the ventricles. They, in turn, attach to the **chordae tendineae**, which attach directly to the tricuspid valve in the right ventricle and also the mitral valve in the left ventricle. When the papillary muscles contract, the valves open. When they relax, the valves close.[19]

The *myocardium* (heart muscle) consists of branching fibres that enable the heart to contract or beat. The average adult heart beats between 70 and 80 times per minute. A "fit" or well-conditioned heart

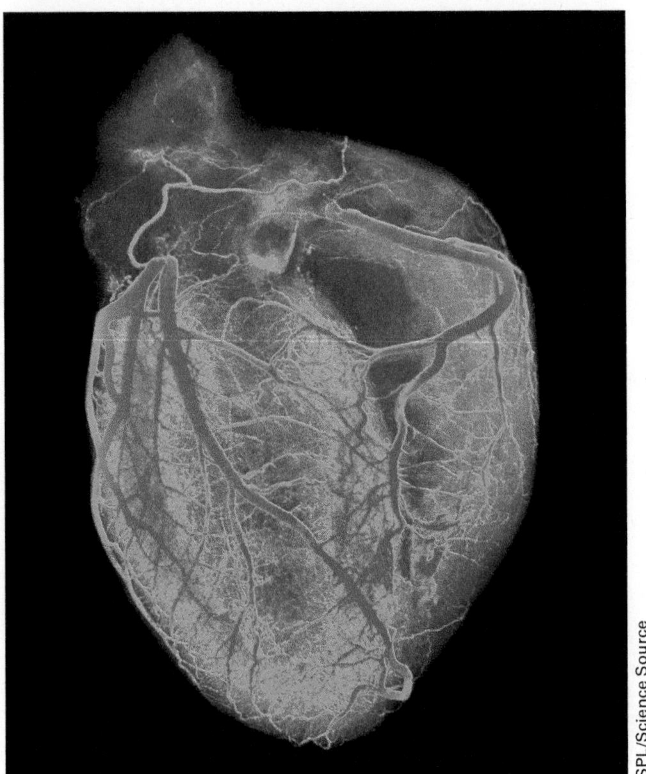
SPL/Science Source

A computer-enhanced image of a healthy heart.

may beat between 50 and 60 beats per minute. With each beat, the heart pumps about 56 millilitres of blood. This may not sound like much, but it adds up to approximately 4.72 litres of blood pumped by the heart in one minute, or about 283 litres per hour.[20]

The heart is surrounded by the *pericardium*, which consists of two layers of a tough membrane. The space between the two contains a lubricating fluid that allows the heart muscle to move freely. The *endocardium* is a smooth membrane lining the inside of the heart and its valves.[21]

The workings of this remarkable pump affect your entire body. If the flow of blood to or through the heart or to the rest of the body is reduced or if a disturbance occurs in the small bundle of highly specialized cells in the heart that generate electrical impulses to control heartbeats, the result may at first be too subtle to notice. However, without diagnosis and treatment, these changes could develop into a life-threatening problem.

Perhaps the biggest breakthrough in the field of cardiology has not been a test or a treatment, but a realization: *Heart disease is not inevitable.* We can keep our hearts healthy for as long as we live, but the process of doing so must start early and continue throughout life.

Types of Cardiovascular Disease

Atherosclerosis Arteries are blood vessels that carry both oxygen and nutrients from our heart to the rest of our body. Healthy arteries are strong and flexible. Arteries that have had too much pressure put upon them over time become thick and stiff. This can reduce and restrict blood flow to the organs and body tissue. The general term for the impairment of blood flow through the blood vessels, often referred to as "hardening of the arteries," is **arteriosclerosis.**[22]

Atherosclerosis,[23] a specific type of arteriosclerosis, is a disease of the lining of the arteries in which **plaque**—deposits of fat, fibrin (a clotting material), cholesterol, other cell parts, and calcium—builds up on the artery walls, which narrows the artery channels and restricts blood flow (see following photos).

Plaques can burst, causing a blood clot or thrombus to form on the plaque's surface. The blood clot can block the supply of blood at the site of the plaque. Or it can flow through the body and get lodged in a smaller blood vessel. If a blood clot reduces the blood flow in the coronary artery, which supplies blood to the heart, a person might experience chest pain, known as angina. This is the beginning of coronary heart disease. If the blood flow is cut off completely, a heart attack occurs. If the blockage happens in the brain, a stroke is the result. Bleeding or hemorrhaging into the plaque can also take place.[24]

Atherosclerosis is the leading cause of heart attacks and strokes. The major risks for atherosclerosis are high blood pressure, high blood fats and cholesterol, cigarette smoking, diabetes, and family history.[25]

What is Coronary Heart Disease? Coronary heart disease (CHD), also known as coronary artery disease (CAD) or **ischemic heart disease** (IHD), is the most common heart condition in Canada. **Coronary heart disease (CHD)** refers specifically to problems with coronary arteries, which provide blood circulation to the heart muscle.[26] As described in the How the Heart Works section, the *myocardium* is the cardiac muscle layer of the wall of the heart. It receives its blood supply, and thus its oxygen and other nutrients, from the coronary arteries. If a coronary artery is blocked by a clot or plaque or by a spasm, the myocardial cells do not get sufficient oxygen, and the portion of the myocardium deprived of its blood supply begins to die (see Figure 10-3). Although such an attack may seem sudden, usually it has been building up for years, particularly if the person has ignored risk factors and early warning signs.[27] The medical name for a heart attack, or coronary, is **myocardial infarction (MI).**[28]

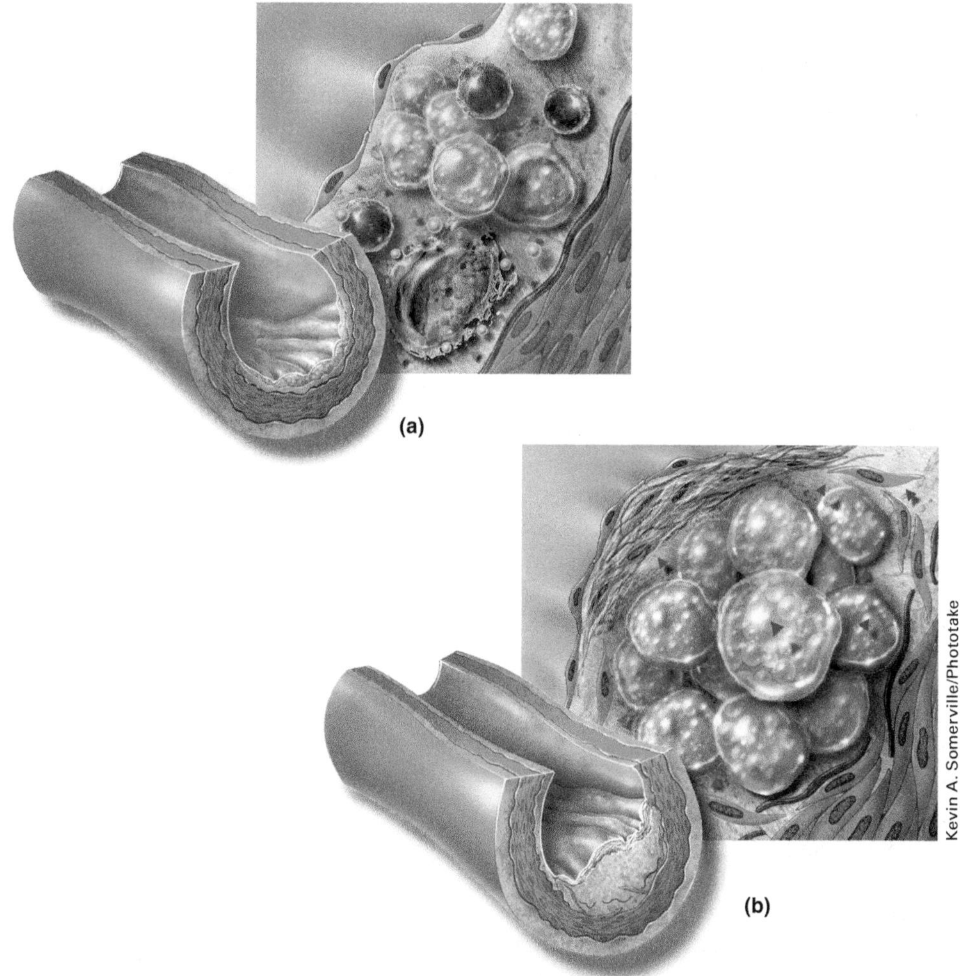

(a) A healthy coronary artery, (b) An artery partially blocked by the buildup of atherosclerotic plaque

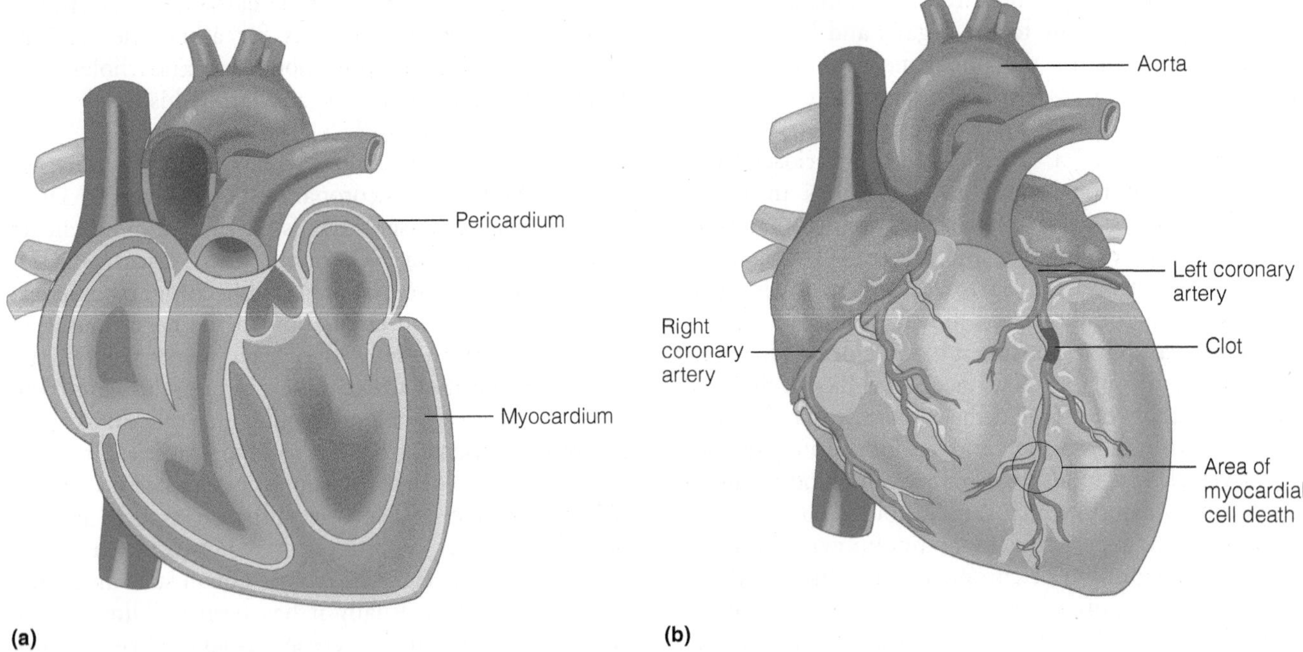

Figure 10-3 The Making of a Heart Attack

(a) The bulk of the heart is composed mainly of the myocardium, the muscle layer that contracts. (b) A clot in one of the arteries that feeds into the myocardium can cut off the blood supply to part of the myocardium, causing cells in that area to die. This is called a myocardial infarction, or heart attack.

Individuals should seek immediate medical care if they experience the following symptoms:

- a tight ache; heavy, squeezing pain; or discomfort in the centre of the chest, which may last for 30 minutes or more and is not relieved by rest
- chest pain that radiates to the shoulder, arm, neck, back, or jaw
- anxiety
- sweating or cold, clammy skin
- nausea and vomiting
- shortness of breath
- dizziness, fainting, or loss of consciousness

The two hours immediately following the onset of such symptoms are the most crucial. About 40 percent of those who suffer an MI die within this time. According to the Heart and Stroke Foundation of Canada, Canadians, on average, wait almost five hours before deciding to get help. This greatly reduces the chance of surviving a heart attack. Thousands of Canadians die of heart attacks because they do not seek medical help fast enough.[29]

Women tend to wait hours longer after a heart attack before going to the hospital compared to men and then are treated less aggressively than men. This delay, which allows further damage to the oxygen-starved heart, occurs because women tend to experience less painful heart attack symptoms. Sometimes they feel only pressure or a burning feeling, not crushing pain.[30]

Clot-dissolving drugs called thrombolytic agents are the treatment of choice for acute myocardial infarction in most clinical settings. Administered through a *catheter* (flexible tube) threaded through the arteries to the site of the blockage (the more effective method of delivery) or injected intravenously (the faster, cheaper method of delivery), these agents can save lives and dissolve clots but don't remove the underlying atherosclerotic plaque.

Patients receiving such therapy may require further procedures such as **angioplasty** or **coronary bypass** surgery, which can reduce their risk of another heart attack or death. Angioplasty is a surgical repair of an artery that has been clogged or obstructed. A surgeon inserts a flexible tube, called a catheter, through a person's groin area and guides it up to the blocked artery. Two common places where arteries are blocked are the carotid artery in the neck area and the coronary artery in the heart. A wire is then moved through the catheter to the blocked area. Another catheter with a tiny balloon on it is then pushed over the wire into the blocked area. The balloon is inflated and the pressure against the wall of the artery allows for an opening of the artery. Sometimes a wire mesh tube, called a stent, is placed in the area of the damaged artery. The stent helps to keep the artery open. The balloon is removed but the stent stays in place. Coronary bypass surgery is another procedure that helps restore blood flow to the heart muscle. A healthy piece of artery from a patient's leg, chest, arm, or abdomen is grafted onto a coronary artery to detour blood around the blocked area.

✓ CHECK-IN

Would you recognize the symptoms of a heart attack?

High Blood Pressure (Hypertension) Blood pressure is a result of the contractions of the heart muscle, which pumps blood through your body, and the resistance of the walls of the vessels through which the blood flows. Each time your heart beats, your blood pressure goes up and down within a certain range. It's highest when the heart contracts; this is called **systolic blood pressure.** It's lowest between contractions; this is called **diastolic blood pressure.** A blood pressure reading consists of the systolic measurement "over" the diastolic measurement, recorded in millimetres of mercury (mm Hg) by a sphygmomanometer.[31]

High blood pressure, or **hypertension,** occurs when the artery walls become constricted and the force exerted as the blood flows through them is greater than it should be. Hypertension can accelerate the development of plaque buildup within the arteries. When the heart must force blood into arteries that are offering increased resistance to blood flow, the left side of the heart often becomes enlarged. The term *essential hypertension* indicates that the cause is unknown.[32] Occasionally, abnormalities of the kidneys or the blood vessels feeding them or certain substances in the bloodstream are identified as the culprits. As a result of the increased work in pumping blood, the heart muscle of a person with hypertension can also become stiffer. This stiffness increases resistance to filling up with blood between beats, which can cause shortness of breath with exertion.

Often called the silent killer, hypertension is a major risk factor for stroke and coronary heart disease because excessive pressure can wear out arteries, leading to serious CVD, vision problems, and kidney

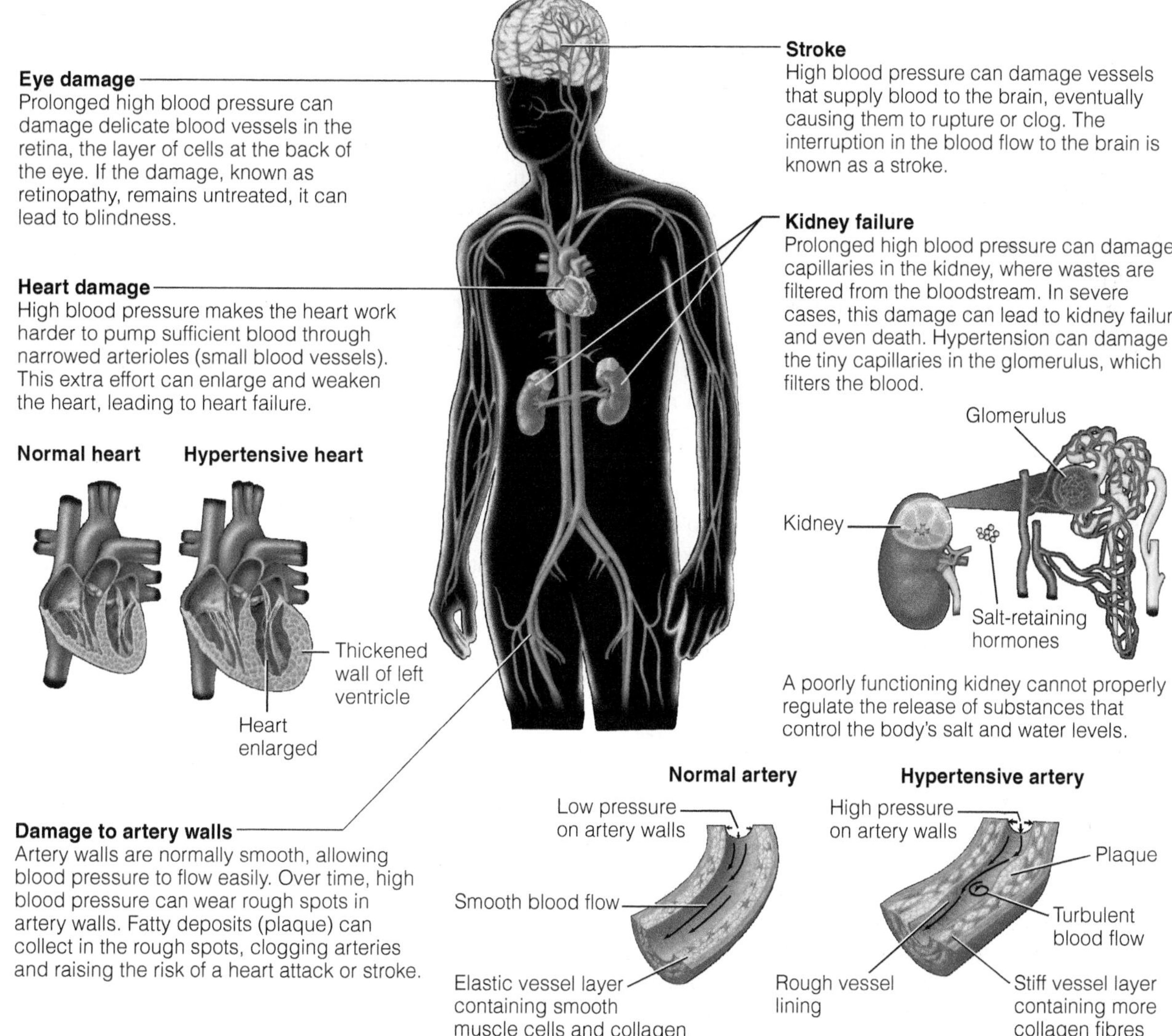

Figure 10-4 Consequences of High Blood Pressure

If left untreated, elevated blood pressure can damage blood vessels in several areas of the body and lead to serious health problems.

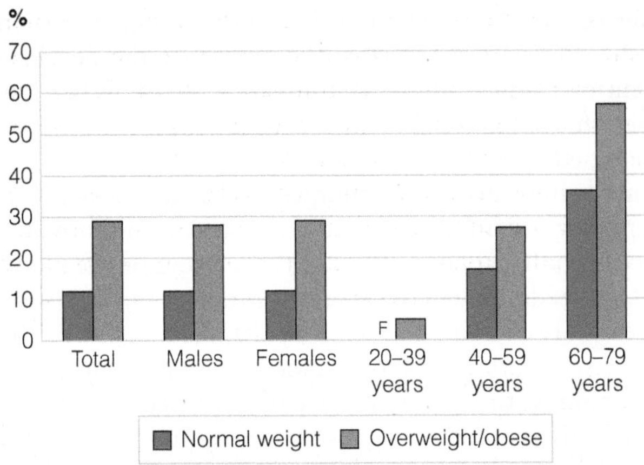

F too unreliable to be published (data with a coefficient of variation [CV] greater than 33.3%; suppressed due to extreme sampling variability)
1. The body mass index (BMI) classification is based on the "Canadian guidelines for body weight classification in adults" (Health Canada, 2003)

Figure 10-5 Distribution of adults aged 20–79 with hypertension, by sex, age group, and body mass index (BMI),[1] household population, Canada, 2012–2013

Source: Statistics Canada. Catalogue no. 82-625-X. Blood pressure of adults, 2012–2013. http://www.statcan.gc.ca/pub/82-625-x/2014001/article/14101-eng.htm.

disease (see Figure 10-4). When combined with obesity, smoking, high cholesterol levels, or diabetes, hypertension increases the risks of cardiovascular problems even more. Approximately 5.3 million Canadians aged 12 and older in 2013 reported that they were living with hypertension.[33] Figure 10-5 shows that the proportion of Canadians with high blood pressure increases as we age.

Physicians see blood pressure as a continuum: the higher the reading, the greater the risk of stroke and heart disease. Physicians urge all adults to have their blood pressure checked at least once a year. A blood pressure reading that's slightly above normal isn't necessarily proof of a blood pressure problem. Due to nervousness, blood pressure may shoot up when anxious individuals enter a medical office. Other factors, such as warm weather or variations in how healthcare practitioners do the test, also can result in elevated readings.

What Is a Healthy Blood Pressure? Ideal blood pressure is 120/80 mm Hg (120 systolic pressure, 80 diastolic pressure). High blood pressure or hypertension is diagnosed when blood pressure rises above 140/90 mm Hg (see Table 10-2). In the past, physicians relied mainly on the diastolic reading—the lower of the two blood pressure numbers—in diagnosing hypertension. In young people, diastolic pressure, a reflection of the constriction of the small blood vessels, continues to be a good indicator of cardiovascular risk. However, a rise in systolic blood pressure—the first and higher of the numbers in a blood pressure reading—also can be dangerous.

TABLE 10-2

Blood Pressure Ranges

Category	Systolic/Diastolic
• Normal	120–129/80–84
• High-normal	130–139/85–89
• High blood pressure (measured in a doctor's office)	140/90
• High blood pressure (measured at home with home monitoring device)	135/85
• High blood pressure for people with diabetes	140/90

Source: © 2013, Heart and Stroke Foundation of Canada Reproduced with the permission of the Heart and Stroke Foundation of Canada. www.heartandstroke.ca.

Systolic hypertension, a reading of 140 mm Hg or higher, reflects stiffening or hardening of the large arteries.[34] Systolic blood pressure typically rises with age and poses the greatest risk for those middle-aged and older. However, the ideal time to start caring about blood pressure is in your 20s and 30s. In a young person, even mild hypertension can cause organs such as the heart, brain, and kidneys to start to deteriorate. By age 50 or 60, the damage may be irreversible.

✓ CHECK-IN

What is your blood pressure reading?

Stroke When the blood supply to a portion of the brain is blocked, a cerebrovascular accident, or **stroke**, occurs.[35] The result is a sudden loss of brain function. In Canada, about 5.3 percent of deaths each year can be attributed to strokes—it is the third leading cause of death in our country.[36] The financial burden of stroke is high—it costs the Canadian economy over $3.6 billion per year in physician services, hospital costs, lost wages, and decreased productivity.[37]

Yet strokes can be prevented, and key risk factors can be modified through either lifestyle changes or drugs. The most important steps are treating hypertension, not smoking, managing diabetes, lowering cholesterol, and taking aspirin.

✓ CHECK-IN

Do you have any risk factors for stroke?

What Causes a Stroke? There are two types of stroke: *ischemic stroke*, which is the result of a blockage that disrupts blood flow to the brain, and *hemorrhagic*

STRATEGIES FOR PREVENTION

How to Prevent a Stroke

- Quit smoking. Smokers have twice the risk of stroke that non-smokers have. When they quit, their risk drops 50 percent in two years. Five years after quitting, their risk is nearly the same as that of non-smokers.
- Keep blood pressure under control. Treating hypertension with medication can lead to a 40 percent reduction in fatal and non-fatal strokes.
- Eat a low-saturated-fat, low-cholesterol diet. This will reduce your risk of fatty buildup in blood vessels. Be sure to include fruits and vegetables in your diet.
- Avoid obesity. Extra weight burdens the blood vessels as well as the heart.
- Exercise. Moderate amounts of exercise improve circulation and may help dissolve deposits in the blood vessels that can lead to stroke.
- Get enough Vitamin B_{12}—2.4 mg/day.

stroke, which occurs when a blood vessel ruptures. About 80 percent of strokes are ischemic,[38] and one of the most common causes of ischemic stroke is the blockage of a brain artery by a thrombus, or blood clot—a *cerebral thrombosis* or thrombotic stroke. Clots generally form around deposits sticking out from the arterial wall. Sometimes a wandering blood clot (embolus), carried in the bloodstream, becomes wedged in one of the cerebral arteries. This is called a *cerebral embolism* or embolic stroke, and it can completely plug up a cerebral artery.

A **transient ischemic attack**, or **TIA**, is known as a mini-stroke and is caused by a temporary interruption of blood flow to the brain. Most TIAs last from 30 seconds to 10 minutes, but they can last up to 24 hours. Minor damage to the brain often goes unnoticed because healthy brain cells that are left carry out the normal brain functions. The symptoms are similar to an ischemic stroke, but they disappear quite quickly. It is a warning sign, though, of a higher risk of ischemic stroke.

About 20 percent of strokes are hemorrhagic.[39] In a hemorrhagic stroke, a diseased artery in the brain floods the surrounding tissue with blood. The cells nourished by the artery are deprived of blood and can't function, and the blood from the artery forms a clot that may interfere with brain function. This is most likely to occur if the patient suffers from a combination of hypertension and atherosclerosis. Hemorrhaging (bleeding) may also be caused by a head injury or by the bursting of an aneurysm, a blood-filled pouch that balloons out from a weak spot in the wall of an artery.

Brain tissue, like heart muscle, begins to die if deprived of oxygen, which may then cause difficulty speaking and walking and loss of memory. These effects may be slight or severe, temporary or permanent, depending on how widespread the damage is and whether other areas of the brain can take over the function of the damaged area. About 30 percent of stroke survivors develop dementia, a disorder that robs a person of memory and other intellectual abilities.

The following stroke warning signs listed by the Heart and Stroke Foundation should be recognized and responded to quickly:[40]

- **Face**—Is it drooping? Are you having sudden trouble with vision: dimness of vision or double vision in one eye?
- **Arms**—Can you raise both? Do you have a sudden loss of strength?
- **Speech**—Is it slurred or jumbled? Do you have sudden difficulty speaking or understanding? Are you experiencing sudden confusion, even if temporary?
- **Time**—Call 911 right away. Do not drive yourself or the person having the stroke to the hospital. Call for an ambulance.

Cardiovascular Disease—Risk Factors You Can Control While we cannot control all risk factors for cardiovascular disease, we can control some. Many people don't realize that they are at risk of cardiovascular disease; one-quarter of heart-attack victims have no prior symptoms. To identify individuals in potential danger, health professionals look for risk factors such as lack of fruit and vegetable consumption, lack of physical activity, obesity levels, smoking, and hypertension. Ninety percent of Canadians have at least one risk factor. Four in ten Canadians have three or more of these risk factors.[41] While the percentage of deaths due to heart disease and stroke has declined slightly since 2000, the authors of the *2014 Heart and Stroke Foundation Report on Canadians' Health* remind us that it is not time to celebrate yet.[42] We must not be complacent. The best way to protect your heart is by making positive changes in your lifestyle behaviours. You can start by completing the Heart & Stroke Risk Assessment at http://www.heartandstroke.com/site/c.ikIQLcMWJtE/b.5374487/k.91C2/Health_eTools.htm.

Alcohol Consumption Research about the benefits of alcohol consumption and cardiovascular disease has been ongoing for many decades. There are thousands of studies about this complex topic. Presently, there are still questions that need answering. Research in many countries does show that excessive alcohol intake has been associated with an elevated risk of heart failure.[43] A study by Zhou et al. further supports past research with regard to the negative effects of heavy alcohol consumption and the risk for coronary artery disease.[44] However, his research also showed that even moderate drinking might increase the risk of heart disease. His findings do not support the many studies over the past decade that suggest otherwise—that light to moderate alcohol consumption can help to increase the level of HDL, the good cholesterol, and decrease LDL, the bad cholesterol; can decrease thrombosis (blood clotting); can increase coronary blood flow; and can reduce blood pressure.[45]

Researchers Smyth et al.[46] support Zhou's findings based on their comprehensive review of the current literature, and suggest that drinking alcohol is "not associated with a net health benefit" as a way to lower the risks for coronary artery disease.

Research has shown that consumption of alcohol does increase the risk of hemorrhagic stroke.[47] So, what should you do about alcohol consumption with regard to lowering your risk of heart disease? If you do not drink alcohol, some health experts suggest that there are many other ways to take care of your cardiovascular system such as getting regular physical activity and eating a healthy diet. If you do drink alcohol, consider being a light to moderate drinker.

Blood Fats **Cholesterol** is a fatty substance found in certain foods and also manufactured by the body. The measurement of cholesterol in the blood is one of the most reliable indicators of the formation of plaque, the sludge-like substance that builds up on the inner walls of arteries. You can lower blood cholesterol levels by cutting back on foods high in saturated fats and exercising more, thereby reducing the risk of a heart attack. Several studies have shown that for every 1 percent drop in blood cholesterol, there is a 2 percent decrease in the likelihood of a heart attack.[48]

What Is a Healthy Cholesterol Reading? Lipoproteins are compounds in the blood that are made up of proteins and fat. The different types are classified by their size or density. Medical science has changed the way it views and targets the blood fats that endanger the healthy heart. In the past, the focus was primarily on total cholesterol in the blood. The higher this number was, the greater the risk of heart disease. New guidelines and recommendations now call for more comprehensive testing, called a lipoprotein profile.

A blood test, which should be performed after a 9- to 12-hour fast, provides readings of

- HDL (good) cholesterol, which helps prevent cholesterol buildup
- LDL (bad) cholesterol, the main culprit in the buildup of plaque within the arteries
- total cholesterol
- triglycerides, which are blood fats released into the bloodstream after a meal

The heaviest are *high-density lipoproteins*, or HDLs, which have the highest portion of protein. These "good guys" pick up excess cholesterol in the blood and carry it back to the liver for removal from the body. An HDL level of higher than 1.0 mmol/L for men and 1.3 mmol/L for women substantially decreases the risk of heart disease (cholesterol levels are measured in millimole of cholesterol per litre of blood). Low-density lipoproteins, or LDLs, and very low-density lipoproteins (VLDLs) carry more cholesterol than HDLs and deposit it on the walls of arteries—they are the "bad guys." The higher your LDL cholesterol, the greater your risk for heart disease. The recommended level of LDLs is less than 3.5 mmol/L.[49] The recommended ratio of total cholesterol to HDL cholesterol (TC/HDL-C) is < 5.0 (see Table 10-3 to determine the healthy level of lipids in blood).

The body contains another type of fat called **triglyceride.** It is the most common form of fat found within our body. Triglycerides do not adhere to the walls of our blood vessels. They are more like thick cream that flows through our blood after meals. They have been linked to an increased risk of coronary artery disease, especially in women, since they increase the tendency of the blood to clot. Triglyceride levels tend to be highest in those whose diets are high in calories, sugar, alcohol, and refined starches. High levels of these fats may increase the risk of obesity, and cutting back on these foods can reduce high triglyceride levels. The recommended level of triglycerides is less than 1.7 mmol/L.

While some studies show that people with high triglyceride levels do not show signs of plaque buildup in

TABLE 10-3

Healthy Levels of Lipids in Blood

Total Cholesterol	<4.5 mmol/L (6–19 years)[1] <5.2 mmol/L (20–79 years)[1]
Triglycerides	<1.7 mmol/L[1]
Low density lipoprotein-cholesterol, LDL ("bad" cholesterol)	<3.5 mmol/L[2]
High density lipoprotein-cholesterol, HDL ("good" cholesterol)	>1.0 mmol/L men[1] >1.3 mmol/L women[1]
Ratio of total cholesterol to HDL cholesterol (TC/HDL-C)	<5[2]

[1] Based on recommendations from the CHMS Physician Advisory Committee.

[2] Based on recommendations from the US National Cholesterol Education Program.

Source: Statistics Canada. (2010). *Healthy levels of lipids in blood* (table). Heart health and cholesterol levels of Canadians, 2007–2009. Catalogue no. 82-625-XWE. Ottawa, Ontario. Statistics Canada. http://www.statcan.gc.ca/pub/82-625-x/2010001/article/11136-eng.htm; Statistics Canada. (2015, November 27). Cholesterol levels of adults, 2012–2013. Catalogue no. 82-625-X. http://www.statcan.gc.ca/pub/82-625-x/2014001/article/14122-eng.htm.

their blood, many people who have heart disease also have high triglyceride levels.[50]

A lipoprotein profile also measures triglycerides, the free-floating molecules that transport fats in the bloodstream. Ideally, this should be less than 1.7 mmol/L.

Lowering Cholesterol Depending on your lipoprotein profile and an assessment of other risk factors, your physician may recommend that you take steps to lower your LDL cholesterol. For some people, therapeutic life changes can make a difference. Lowering your fat intake, especially saturated fat, may help.[51] Simply eating more often may have an effect on cholesterol. According to several small studies, "grazers" who eat small meals six or more times a day tend to have lower cholesterol levels than "gorgers" who eat three times a day.[52] There is also growing evidence that increasing the amount of fibre you eat is beneficial for lowering cholesterol levels.

Drug therapy is another option, but this is only recommended when a high cholesterol level does not respond to dietary intervention. Bile acid sequestrants, fibric acids, and statins are categories of cholesterol-lowering drugs that your doctor can prescribe. Each of them has advantages and disadvantages. Sometimes combined drug therapy is suggested.[53]

✓ CHECK-IN

Have you ever had your lipoproteins measured?

Healthy Blood Pressure Prevention pays off when it comes to high blood pressure. The most effective preventive measures involve lifestyle changes. The best approach for individuals who are overweight and who have high blood pressure values is weight loss. Exercise may be effective in lowering mildly elevated blood pressure.

Restriction of sodium intake also helps. Salt is sodium chloride, and it is the major source of sodium in our diets. Canadians are encouraged to limit their salt intake. Although the body requires only about 2300 mg (1 teaspoon) of salt each day to function, most Canadians eat an average of 3400 mg (1 ½ teaspoons) of salt each day. Much of the salt consumed in our diet comes from hidden salt added in the processing of many foods. Approximately 35 percent of Canadians are salt-sensitive. This means that excess dietary salt has the ability to raise their blood pressure, which in turn can increase their risk of heart disease.[54]

Healthy eating is also a key factor, and foods that are rich in potassium, such as dried and fresh fruits and vegetables, appear to help maintain the normal function of the heart and lower blood pressure.[55, 56] Adults should consume at least 4.7 grams of potassium per day. Presently, Canadian men consume between 3.2 and 3.4 grams, and women eat 2.4–2.6 grams. Once again, fruits and vegetables are recommended since they are both low in sodium and high in potassium. Foods with the highest amount of potassium per calorie are spinach, cantaloupes, almonds, Brussels sprouts, mushrooms, bananas, oranges, grapefruits, and potatoes.

Treating Hypertension For some people, particularly those with mild hypertension, lifestyle changes alone can bring blood pressure down. For other people, diet and exercise are not enough. Medications called beta-blockers and diuretics are recommended as the first-line treatment for hypertension, but newer drugs such as angiotensin-converting enzyme (ACE) inhibitors and calcium channel blockers are becoming increasingly popular. No single drug works well for everyone, so physicians have to rely on clinical judgment and trial and error to find the best possible medication for an individual patient.[57]

Diabetes Mellitus **Diabetes mellitus**, a disorder of the endocrine system, increases the likelihood of hypertension and atherosclerosis, thereby increasing the risk of heart attack and stroke.[58] Even before developing diabetes, individuals at high risk for this disease—those who are overweight, have a family history of the disease, have mildly elevated blood pressure and blood sugar levels, and have above ideal levels of harmful blood cholesterol—may already be at increased risk of heart disease. Up to one-half of diabetics also have hypertension, another risk factor. Cardiovascular disease is the most prevalent complication of diabetes mellitus.[59] More than 80 percent of people with diabetes die from some form of heart or blood vessel disease. (More information on diabetes is presented later in the chapter.)

Metabolic Syndrome **Metabolic syndrome**, also known as Syndrome X or insulin-resistant syndrome, is a cluster of medical abnormalities that increases the risk of heart disease and diabetes. Genetics, lack of exercise, and overeating are its probable causes. According to the National Institutes of Health, three or more of the following symptoms indicate metabolic syndrome:

- Waist measurement of more than 102 centimetres (40.2 inches) for Caucasian men, 90 centimetres (35.4 inches) for Asian men, 88 centimetres (34.6 inches) for Caucasian women, or 80 centimetres (31.5 inches) for Asian women.
  (In one recent study, waist circumference proved the best indicator of increased heart disease risk.)[60]
- Levels of triglycerides of more than 1.7 mmol/L.
- Levels of high-density lipoprotein—"good" cholesterol—lower than 1.0 mmol/L in men or 1.3 mmol/L in women.

- Blood pressure of 130 mm Hg systole over 85 mm Hg diastole (130/85) or higher.
- Fasting blood sugar of 5.6 mmol/L or higher.

Keown et al. studied the risk of metabolic dysfunction in a sample of U.S. college students. They measured blood pressure, triglyceride and high-density lipoprotein (HDL) levels, blood glucose, and waist circumference. They discovered that the overall occurrence of metabolic syndrome in their participant sample was only 10 percent, but the rate of having at least one metabolic risk was 43 percent, and 14.3 percent of the students had two elements of metabolic syndrome.[61]

✓ CHECK-IN

Do you have any risk factors for metabolic syndrome?

Nutrition for a Healthy Heart There is so much nutritional information available through many sources—the media, Internet, brochures, pamphlets, and books—that it is sometimes a challenge to plan a heart-healthy diet. A balanced, low-saturated-fat diet that includes a variety of foods is still the best recipe for a healthy heart. In addition to regular physical activity, you can lower your risk of heart disease and stroke by eating well. An introduction to healthy eating was presented in Chapter 5. The following information will provide a nutrition review with specific emphasis on heart health.

B Vitamins B_6, B_{12}, and folic acid help to regulate blood levels of homocysteine, an amino acid produced by the body and believed to damage the lining of the artery walls, which can lead to a buildup of plaque, which in turn increases your risk of heart attack or stroke.[62] You can find B_6 in whole-grain cereals, potatoes, bananas, chicken, milk, and tuna. Vitamin B_{12} is found in meat, fish, poultry, dairy products, eggs, and some fortified cereals. Sources of folate include dark leafy green vegetables such as lettuce and broccoli.

Fat—Good and Bad Saturated fats can raise our levels of blood cholesterol or low-density lipoproteins (LDLs). As mentioned in the blood fat section, this is the type of cholesterol that leaves plaque deposits on the artery walls. Foods containing saturated fats come from animal sources. They include fatty meat, poultry with skin, higher-fat dairy products, and butter. Palm and coconut oils also contain saturated fats. Fast foods are notorious for saturated fats as are many ready-made or prepared foods. You should also watch for foods made with hydrogenated vegetable oil.[63] As discussed in Chapter 5, a low-fat eating plan means about 30 percent of one day's calories come from fat. For a woman this means about 65 grams of fat; for men, about 90 grams of fat. To put this amount in perspective, one jelly doughnut provides 15–20 grams of fat.[64] However, new research mentioned in Chapter 5 also suggests that saturated fats may not be the dietary villain that we have come to know it for.

Not all fats are bad for us. Monounsaturated and polyunsaturated fats, found in vegetable oils, nuts, and fish, can help to reduce LDL cholesterol levels. Unfortunately, they are high in calories, so it is important to consume in moderation. Safflower, sunflower, canola, corn, and olive oil, and non-hydrogenated margarines are good choices. Dry roasted and raw nuts are also recommended because they contain mainly monounsaturated fats. Almonds are high in vegetable protein, whereas walnuts are a good source of omega-3 fatty acids, believed to have heart-healthy benefits.

Research has shown that the most damaging kind of fat is trans fat. Found in foods made with shortening, partially hydrogenated vegetable oil, snack foods, baked goods, fast foods, and many prepared foods, these fats raise LDL cholesterol while lowering HDL, the "good" cholesterol that takes away excess "bad" cholesterol from the body.[65]

Fibre and Whole Grains A daily intake of 25 grams for women and 38 grams for men of soluble fibre each day has been shown to lower blood cholesterol levels. You can find this type of fibre in oatmeal, oat bran, lentils, legumes, and fruits such as apples and strawberries. Flax, a healthy-heart food, has been shown to be rich in omega-3 fatty acids. Flax can also significantly lower cholesterol blood levels and reduce the development of blood clots.[66] When increasing your fibre intake, try to drink up to two litres of water per day. Whole grains are a better choice than refined carbohydrates when it comes to heart health.

Fish Eating fish improves cardiovascular health in a number of ways. All fish, but especially salmon, mackerel, herring, trout, and sardines, contain omega-3 fatty acids, which help reduce the stickiness of your blood. Fish may also prevent erratic heart rhythms, a common cause of sudden cardiac death.[67] The recommendation for eating fish is two to three times per week.

Vegetables and Fruits When it comes to vegetables and fruits, more is good. They are an excellent source of Vitamins C and A, beta carotene, fibre, folic acid, potassium, and plant chemicals called phytochemicals, all of which reduce your risk of developing heart disease and stroke.[68]

DASH Diet and Portfolio Diet In Chapter 5, *Eating Well with Canada's Food Guide* was introduced as a way of encouraging healthy food choices. The Heart and Stroke Foundation of Canada does recommend following the food guide. They are also endorsing the *DASH Diet—Dietary Approaches to Stopping*

Hypertension. Research studies by the National Heart, Lung, and Blood Institute (NHLBI) in the United States found that the DASH eating plan lowered blood pressure. The DASH Diet recommends fruits, vegetables, and fat-free or low-fat dairy products. Whole grains, fish, poultry, legumes, and nuts are also an important part of the diet. This diet is lower in sodium than the typical American or Canadian diet. It is also low in saturated fat, cholesterol, and total fat.[69] See Table 10-4 for a comparison between *Canada's Food Guide* and the DASH Diet.

Canadian researchers offer one more approach to healthy eating to lower risks for heart disease. It is called the *Portfolio Diet.* In addition to eating a heart-healthy diet that is low in saturated fats and includes lots of fruits, vegetables, beans, and whole grains, people are encouraged to add cholesterol-lowering foods to their daily diet. Examples include a handful of nuts every day, two servings of soy-based food, two teaspoons of sterol-enriched margarine, and two servings a day of foods rich in soluble fibre such as oatmeal or barley.[70]

Physical Activity For years we have known that regular exercise reduces the risk of heart attack, helps maintain a healthy body weight, lowers blood pressure, and improves metabolism. If rigorous and frequent enough, it also may increase longevity.[71,72] But you don't have to head to a gym or hit the bike path to keep your heart healthy. Studies have confirmed that lifestyle activities, such as walking and gardening, are also effective in improving heart function, lowering blood pressure, and maintaining or losing weight.[73] (See Chapter 4 for a more comprehensive discussion of the benefits of regular physical activity.)

For heart health, aerobic endurance activities are the most important. The Canadian Society of Exercise Physiology recommends accumulating 150 minutes of moderate aerobic physical activity per week to stay healthy. You can add up activities in periods of at least 10 minutes each.[74]

People who are not physically active face a much greater risk of fatal heart attack than those who engage in some form of exercise or activity. Women who are active have lower coronary heart disease rates than those who are inactive. Even walking for a minimum of half an hour a day reduces women's risk of coronary heart disease.[75] However, studies have found that in men, more rigorous exercise produced greater protection against heart disease. Those who ran for an hour or more per week reduced their risk of heart disease by 42 percent, compared with an 18 percent reduction for those who walked briskly for a half-hour per day or more. With walking, pace, not duration, was linked with lower danger of heart disease.[76]

Psychosocial Factors Various psychological and social influences may affect vulnerability to heart disease. Anger and hostility, depression and anxiety, stress levels, work characteristics, and social supports are all factors that may act alone or combine and exert different effects at different ages and stages of life.

New research is linking emotional health to heart health. Emerging studies on depression and heart disease suggest that the two are linked. Heart-disease patients are more likely to become depressed. This has been known for a long time.[77] However, some research suggests that depression might actually trigger heart disease. A large study done on post-menopausal women found that women who become depressed are 50 percent more likely to develop heart disease.[78]

Stress levels also impact heart health. One of the reasons that some students are stressed is their lack of preparation for college. Zeindenberg found that substantial numbers of students were just not equipped for the level of academic work expected in basic first-year courses such as mathematics and English. While remedial courses are offered at many college and universities, students tend to be reluctant to take them because they believe they are academically prepared.[79]

Smith[80] suggests that heart-health education could be put in place at colleges and universities. Students might benefit in many ways if primary health education about cardiovascular disease was included as part of the primary healthcare system. Many students are not yet aware of the risk of high stress levels, depression, anxiety, and unhealthy lifestyle habits on heart health.

Even students who indicate that they are aware of cardiovascular risks often behave in ways that do not reflect their knowledge. In one recent study of 226 students at a college, half or more ate a high-saturated-fat diet or reported moderate to severe stress. Many did not exercise frequently; some already had high cholesterol or high blood pressure.[81]

Tobacco Smoke Two more important preventable risk factors for cardiovascular disease are use of tobacco and exposure to second-hand smoke. The major cause of preventable death in Canada is tobacco use.[82] Canadians who smoke cigarettes increase their risk of developing lung cancer, chronic obstructive pulmonary disease (COPD), and asthma. Smokers who have heart attacks are more likely to die from them than are non-smokers. Smoking is the major risk factor for *peripheral vascular disease*, in which the vessels that carry blood to the leg and arm muscles become hardened and clogged.

Both active and passive smoking accelerate the process by which arteries become clogged and increase the risk of heart attacks and strokes. Health Canada estimates that approximately 37 000 people die each year from smoking-related causes.[83] It is estimated that exposure to second-hand smoke causes over 1000 deaths per year in Canada with 700 of those deaths from coronary heart disease.[84] Overall, non-smokers exposed to

TABLE 10-4

A Comparison of the DASH—Dietary Approaches to Stopping Hypertension—Eating Plan and *Canada's Food Guide*

DASH Food Groups	DASH Daily Servings (except as noted)	DASH Serving Sizes	*Canada's Food Guide* (CFG) Groups	CFG Daily Servings	CFG Serving Sizes	CFG Recommendations
Vegetables	4–5	250 mL (1 cup) raw leafy vegetables 125 mL (½ cup) cooked vegetables 170 mL (6 oz) juice	Vegetables and fruit	Females (age 19–50)—7–8 Males (age 19–50)—8–10 Females & Males (age 51+)—7	1 medium vegetable or fruit 125 mL (1/2 cup) cut up 250 mL (1 cup) salad or raw leafy greens 125 mL (1/2 cup) cooked vegetable 125 mL (1/2 cup) juice	Eat at least one dark green and one orange vegetable each day. Choose vegetables and fruit prepared with little or no added fat, sugar, or salt. Have vegetables and fruit more often than juice.
Fruit	4–5	1 medium piece of fruit 63 mL (¼ cup) dried fruit 125 mL (½ cup) fresh, frozen, or canned fruit				
Grains (mainly whole grains)	7–8	1 slice bread 250 mL (1 cup) ready to eat cereal 125 mL (½ cup) cooked rice, pasta, or cereal	Grain products	Females (age 19–50)—6–7 Males (age 19–50)—8 Females (age 51+)—6 Males (age 51+)—7	1 slice bread (35 g) ½ a bagel (45 g) ½ a flatbread or tortilla (35 g) 125 mL (1/2 cup) cooked rice or pasta 30 g of cereal (see box for cup equivalent)	Make at least half of your grain products whole grain each day. Choose grain products that are low in fat, sugar, or salt.
Low-fat or no-fat dairy foods	2–3	250 mL (1 cup) milk 250 mL (1 cup) yogurt 50 g (1½ oz) cheese	Milk and alternatives	Females & Males (age 19–50)—2 Females & Males (age 51+)—3	250 mL (1 cup) milk 175 g (3/4 cup) yogurt or kefir 50 g (1½ oz) cheese 125 mL (1/2 cup) evaporated milk	Drink skim, 1%, or 2% milk each day. Select lower-fat milk alternatives, such as fortified soy beverages, if you do not drink milk.
Lean meats, poultry, and fish	2 or less	85 g (3 ounces) cooked lean meats, skinless poultry, or fish	Meat and alternatives	Females (age 19–50)—2 Males (age 19–50)—3 Females (age 51+)—2 Males (age 51+)—3	175 mL (3/4 cup) beans or tofu 75 g (2 ½ ounces) cooked fish, chicken, beef, pork, or game meat 60 mL (1/4 cup) of nuts or seeds 30 mL (2 tbsp) nut butter	Have meat alternatives such as beans, lentils, and tofu often. Eat at least two *Food Guide* servings of fish each week. Select lean meat and alternatives prepared with little or no added fat or salt.
Nuts, seeds, and dry beans	4–5 per week	42 g (1½ oz.) nuts 30 mL (2 tbsp) peanut butter 14 g (2 tbsp) seeds 118 mL (1/2 cup) cooked dry beans or peas				
Fats and oils	2–3	5 mL (1 tsp) soft margarine 15 mL (1 tbsp) low-fat mayonnaise 30 mL (2 tbsp) light salad dressing 5 mL (1 tsp) vegetable oil	Oils and fats	For all age groups and genders	30–45 mL (2–3 tablespoons)	Include a small amount of unsaturated fat each day. This includes oil used for cooking, salad dressings, soft non-hydrogenated margarine, and mayonnaise.

Source: © 2013, Heart and Stroke Foundation of Canada Reproduced with the permission of the Heart and Stroke Foundation of Canada. www.heartandstroke.ca.

second-hand smoke are at a 25 percent higher relative risk of developing coronary heart disease than non-smokers not exposed to second-hand tobacco smoke.

Cigarette smoking and second-hand smoke can damage the heart in several ways:

- The nicotine may repeatedly overstimulate the heart.
- Carbon monoxide may take the place of some of the oxygen in the blood, which reduces the oxygen supply to the heart muscle.
- Tars and other smoke residues may damage the lining of the coronary arteries, making it easier for cholesterol to build up and narrow the passageways.
- Smoking increases blood clotting, leading to a higher incidence of clotting in the coronary arteries and subsequent heart attack. Clotting in the peripheral arteries is also increased, which can cause leg pain with walking and, ultimately, stroke.
- Even ex-smokers may have irreversible damage to their arteries.

Body Mass Index and Waist Circumference If you are between the ages of 18 and 64 and have a body mass index (BMI) of 25.0–29.9 (overweight) or a BMI greater than 30.0 (obesity)—you could be at risk of developing high blood pressure and diabetes. Some research suggests that the greater the BMI, the greater the risk of heart disease and stroke.[85] Loss of visceral body fat mass can reduce high blood pressure too, another risk factor for heart disease. As discussed in Chapter 6, Managing Your Weight, weight circumference above cut-off points is also associated with increased risk of cardiovascular disease.

There is also cause for alarm about the growing obesity epidemic among Canadian children. Young people who are obese over a long period of time are more likely to become overweight adults, putting them at risk for heart disease, juvenile diabetes, and adult-onset diabetes. A landmark study on overweight and obese children in China[86] (some as young as nine years old) found that the carotid arteries—arteries that feed blood to the brain—were thickening and that large blood vessels in their arms were not functioning properly. The results matched those of adults who had been smoking for more than 10 years. The good news is that dietary changes and increased physical activity can reverse the trend.

Cardiovascular Disease—Risk Factors You Can't Control

Age and Sex By the age of 70, one in five women and one in four men have been told by a physician that they have heart problems. As we get older our risk of heart disease increases. A person's risk of stroke more than doubles every decade after age 55.[87]

More men (of all ages) than women die of heart disease and stroke, but the male to female ratio decreases from 5 to 1 among those 40–49 years of age to 1.2–1 among those aged 90 years and older.[88] While more men than women die from coronary heart disease and heart attack, more women than men die from congestive heart failure. Heart disease and stroke combined are the leading cause of hospitalization for women (excluding childbirth and pregnancy).[89]

Seven times as many women die every year from these two diseases than die from breast cancer, making heart disease and stroke a major cause of death for women. The Canadian Heart and Stroke Foundation's *Heart Smart™ Women: A Guide to Living with and Preventing Heart Disease and Stroke* is designed to teach women about how heart disease and stroke can affect their lives and what they can do to reduce risk factors for these conditions.[90]

Heredity Anyone whose parents, siblings, or other close relatives suffered heart attacks before age 50 is at increased risk of developing heart disease. Certain risk factors, such as abnormally high blood levels of lipids, can be passed down from generation to generation. All is not lost, however. You may not be able to rewrite your family history, but you can change your lifestyle behaviours, including the decisions you make about the foods you eat, the amount of exercise you do, or whether to smoke. These changes can help to lessen the impact of inherited risk factors. As an added preventive step, some cardiologists are prescribing a small daily dose of aspirin to individuals with a history of coronary artery disease who are at risk of clots forming that could block blood supplies to the heart, brain, and other organs. (Daily aspirin is not advised for individuals who are not at risk because of their age or health history.)

Male Pattern Baldness **Male pattern baldness** (the loss of hair at the vertex, or top, of the head) is associated with an increased risk of heart attack in men. A long-term study of 10 885 men and women over a 35-year period showed an increased risk of ischemic heart disease and myocardial infarction for men who presented frontoparietal or crown-top baldness. The results also showed this increased risk for heart disease was independent of chronological age or other cardiovascular risk factors.[91] Scientists speculate that men with male pattern baldness who lose their hair quickly may metabolize male sex hormones differently than others, thereby increasing the likelihood of heart disease. Health experts advise bald men to follow basic guidelines, such as not smoking and controlling their cholesterol levels, to lower any possible risk.

Race and Ethnicity Aboriginal peoples, South Asians, and Eastern Europeans are particularly vulnerable to heart disease. Aboriginal adults 20 years of age and older are more likely to be overweight and to smoke compared to the Canadian population as a whole. Some studies have also found that Aboriginal peoples have a higher incidence of diabetes. In part, the increase in cardiovascular disease and mortality among Aboriginal peoples in Canada is linked to the changes in their way of living. The lack of access to traditional hunting and fishing opportunities has resulted in a change of diet that now includes processed foods and lack of physical activity. This has contributed to the increase of CVD. All of these factors are risk conditions for heart disease.[92]

Research also shows that new immigrants develop increased rates of cardiovascular disease as they become long-term Canadian residents. White, South Asian, Chinese, and black immigrants who had resided in Canada for 15 years or longer had a higher percentage of major cardiovascular risk factors that included diabetes, hypertension, and obesity than new immigrants.[93]

UNDERSTANDING CANCER

Cancer is the uncontrolled growth and spread of abnormal cells. Normal cells follow the code of instructions embedded in DNA (the body's genetic material); cancer cells do not. Think of the DNA within the nucleus of a cell as a computer program that controls the cell's functioning, including its ability to grow and reproduce itself. If this program or its operation is altered, the cell goes out of control. The nucleus no longer regulates growth. The abnormal cell divides to create other abnormal cells, which again divide, eventually forming **neoplasms** (new formations), or tumours.

Tumours can be either *benign* (slightly abnormal, not considered life-threatening) or *malignant* (cancerous). The only way to determine whether a tumour is benign is by microscopic examination of its cells. Cancer cells have larger nuclei than the cells in benign tumours, they vary more in shape and size, and they divide more often.

At one time cancer was thought to be a single disease that attacked different parts of the body. Now scientists believe that cancer comes in countless forms, each with a genetically determined molecular "fingerprint" that indicates how deadly it is. With this understanding, doctors can identify how aggressively a tumour should be treated.

Without treatment, cancer cells continue to grow, crowding out and replacing healthy cells. This process is called **infiltration**, or invasion. Cancer cells may also **metastasize**, or spread to other parts of the body via the bloodstream or lymphatic system (see Figure 10-6). For many cancers, as many as 60 percent of patients may have metastases (which may be too small to be felt or seen without a microscope) at the time of diagnosis.

Although all cancers have similar characteristics, each is distinct. Some cancers are relatively simple to cure, whereas others are more threatening and mysterious. The earlier any cancer is found, the easier it is to treat and the better the patient's chances of survival.

CLASSIFICATIONS OF CANCER

Cancers are classified according to the type of cell and the organ in which they originate, such as the following:

- *Carcinoma*, the most common kind, which starts in the epithelium, the layers of cells that cover the body's surface or line internal organs and glands
- *Sarcoma*, which forms in the supporting or connective tissues of the body: bones, muscles, blood vessels
- *Leukemia*, which begins in the blood-forming tissues (bone marrow, lymph nodes, and the spleen)
- *Lymphoma*, which arises in the cells of the lymph system, the network that filters out impurities

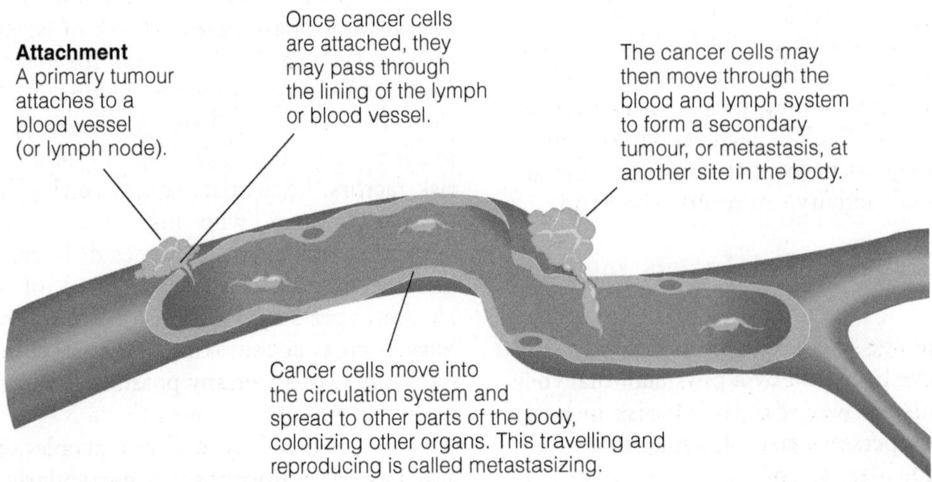

Figure 10-6 Metastasis, or Spread of Cancer

Cancer cells can travel through the blood vessels to spread to other organs or through the lymphatic system to form secondary tumours.

HUMAN POTENTIAL

Darbi Aitchison—Life Relearnt

Have you ever thought about living your life as someone else? What you would do if things changed in your life in a moment? Those were questions that Darby Aitchison, a past Kinesiology student of mine, posed when I asked her to share her story of challenge and recovery from Guillain-Barré Syndrome, a rare disorder in which the body's immune system attacks a part of the peripheral nervous system.

It was mid-term time. Darbi was studying for exams and also playing soccer. Her identity can be summed up in two words—student and athlete. During a game her feet began to tingle. She knew it wasn't because she had tied her cleats too tightly. That was a task she had performed countless times, the same way, each time. Later that day she experienced spasms in her head and back. "Too much mid-term chocolate," she said to herself. Her mid-terms came and went, but her symptoms continued. She called her mother, a 25-year emergency-room nurse, who encouraged Darbi to seek medical attention. Darbi went to her local hospital in Cowichan Valley on Vancouver Island. Two visits in three days and still no answers. Despite four competent doctors, two lumbar punctures, 57 needle pokes, a CT scan, x-rays, and urine tests, there continued to be more questions than answers.

Six days after the tingling in her feet began, she couldn't walk on her own or swallow; she had double vision and significant Bell's palsy on the left side of her face. One possible diagnosis was viral meningitis. Her health continued to deteriorate. She went from being able to sit up, talk, and wiggle her ankles to being admitted to the intensive care unit (ICU) with only the ability to move part of her arms, intubated on a ventilator, and finally diagnosed with Guillain-Barré Syndrome, a condition that strikes about one person in 100 000. This disorder can cause a variety of symptoms. For Darbi it turned out to be paralysis—complete paralysis. By April—on her 22nd birthday—she hit rock bottom. There was nothing she could do except blink her eyes. She had to be flown to a larger hospital near Victoria, B.C., where her long journey of rebuilding and rehabilitation began.

She tells me that the days were always painful and the nights were always long. She had to learn how to breathe, swallow, stand, and move again. However, she had an amazing support team that included family members, friends, and strangers who became friends. She discovered that no one knows what causes this disorder and there is no known cure. Recovery is possible. It just takes time, sometimes weeks or years. She made a decision to not let anything stand in her way on her road to recovery, including a comment from a psychiatrist, a member of her medical team, who suggested she might never walk again. She had her identity as a strong athlete and she knew that being a disgruntled patient was not going to help. She says, "We can choose to be happy and I knew I didn't deserve special treatment. And I'm not one to ever give up on a challenge."

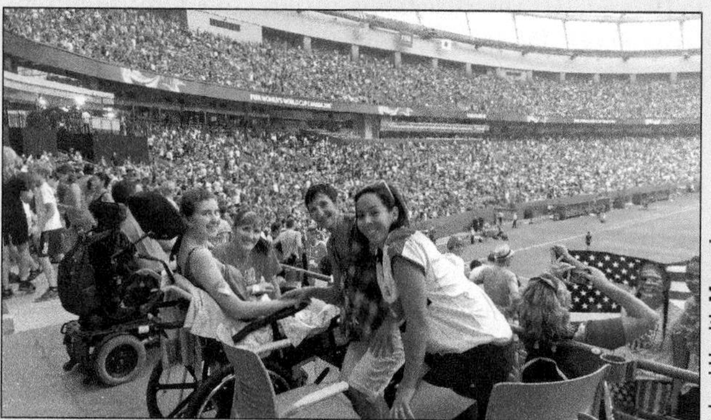

Island Health Magazine

L-R: Darby Aitchison, Libby McMullen, RN, Debbie Aitchison (Darby's mother), and Sarah Yager, RN

Two-hundred and thirty days came and went in the hospital. One hundred of those days were spent in the ICU. Ninety days were spent on a ventilator. What she remembers the most was that 200 of those days she had the opportunity to get outside and breathe fresh air. She is convinced that it made a difference. She also noticed that the effort she put into her own recovery was directly proportional to the effort others put into her recovery too.

The last three months of her hospital stay were the most difficult. She had been transferred to neuro-rehab, a specialized unit for patients with nervous system issues. The shift from being doted on and cared for in an individual way shifted to care to encourage independence. She rose to the challenge and credits this type of care to helping her prepare for her homecoming where she would also be expected to continue her own rehabilitation.

There is not room here to tell Darbi's entire story, but I want to share that the medical teams at both the Victoria General Hospital (VGH) and the Royal Jubilee Hospital (RJH) were so inspired by Darbi's strong will, indomitable spirit, and positive attitude during her rehabilitation period they set up a GoFundMe website raising enough money to help Darbi get to Vancouver, B.C., to watch a Women's World Cup Final soccer game, for which she had tickets. The logistics were difficult, but a Medi-Van with two attendants was offered up for free, medications and extra equipment booked, ferry and taxi reservations made, and personal vacation days taken so two nurses could join the attendants and make a 12-hour return trip possible. Darbi's mother says, "Getting her to that World Cup final, watching her in the stadium, laughing with her friends, it was overwhelming."

I can also report that she is walking and back at university, completing her Kinesiology degree. Everyone in our School of Exercise Science, Physical and Health Education continues to be inspired by Darbi. Her story is truly one of Health + Wellness = Potential.

Stages of Cancer When health professionals talk about the **stages or staging of cancer** they are talking about the extent or the seriousness of the cancer. Each type of cancer has specific factors that determine stages. However, not all cancers are diagnosed with the staging process.[94] The most common staging system used is TNM, where T stands for the size of the primary tumour; N links to whether or not the cancer cells have spread to lymph nodes or other tissues or organs close to the location of the primary tumour; and M stands for metastasis, which means that cancer has spread to other parts of the body.

For a number of different types of cancer, the TNM system corresponds to one of four stages. Again, it is important to remember that the staging system can vary for different types of cancer. Stage 0 can mean that there are atypical cells present but that they are localized and there are no signs that these cells have spread to the lymph nodes. In each of stages I, II, and III, the disease is progressively more extensive. Stage IV means that the cancer has spread to other tissues or organs that are located farther away from the original site.[95]

Who Is at Risk for Developing Cancer? According to the *2015 Canadian Cancer Statistics* report, about two in five Canadians will develop cancer in their lifetime and about one in four will die of cancer.[96] Four types of cancer account for the majority of new cases—lung, breast, colorectal, and prostate.[97] Lung cancer remains the leading cause of cancer death for both men (26.6 percent) and women (27 percent). The second-leading cause of death from cancer for men is colorectal cancer and for women, breast cancer.[98]

Common Types of Cancer Cancer refers to a group of more than a hundred diseases characterized by abnormal cell growth. Figures 10-7 and 10-8 show the estimated new cases and deaths from cancer by type for males and females in Canada. The following section will describe some of the more common types of cancer.

Breast Cancer In Canada, breast cancer is the most commonly diagnosed cancer in Canadian women. Women have a one in nine chance of developing breast cancer in their lifetime.

Risk factors include the following:

- **Age.** Breast cancer can occur in women of any age, but each woman's risk increases as she ages.
- **Age at menarche.** Women who had their first period before age 12 are at greater risk than women who began menstruating later. The reason is that the more menstrual cycles a woman has, the longer her exposure to estrogen, a hormone known to increase breast cancer danger. For similar reasons, childless women, who menstruate continuously for several decades, are also at greater risk.
- **Age at birth of first child.** An early pregnancy—in a woman's teens or 20s—changes the actual maturation of breast cells and decreases risk. But if a woman has her first child in her 40s, precancerous cells may actually flourish with the high hormone levels of the pregnancy.
- **Breast biopsies.** Even if laboratory analysis finds no precancerous abnormalities, women who require such tests are more likely to develop breast cancer. Fibrocystic breast disease, a term often used for "lumpy" breasts, is not a risk factor.
- **Estrogen.** The role of estrogen replacement as a cancer risk factor remains controversial. Some

Males 100 500 New cases		Females 96 400 New cases	
Prostate	23.9%	Breast	25.9%
Colorectal	13.9%	Lung	13.5%
Lung	13.5%	Colorectal	11.5%
Bladder	6.1%	Body of uterus	6.5%
Non-Hodgkin lymphoma	4.5%	Thyroid	5.0%
Kidney	3.9%	Non-Hodgkin lymphoma	3.8%
Melanoma	3.6%	Melanoma	3.2%
Leukemia	3.5%	Ovary	2.9%
Oral	2.9%	Leukemia	2.8%
Pancreas	2.4%	Pancreas	2.5%
Stomach	2.1%	Kidney	2.4%
Brain/CNS	1.7%	Bladder	2.1%
Esophagus	1.7%	Cervix	1.5%
Liver	1.7%	Oral	1.5%
Multiple myeloma	1.5%	Brain/CNS	1.3%
Thyroid	1.4%	Stomach	1.3%
Testis	1.0%	Multiple myeloma	1.2%
Larynx	0.9%	Liver	0.6%
Hodgkin lymphoma	0.5%	Esophagus	0.5%
Breast	0.2%	Hodgkin lymphoma	0.5%
All other cancers	9.0%	Larynx	0.2%
		All other cancers	9.3%

CNS=central nervous system

Figure 10-7 Percentage Distribution of Estimated New Cancer Cases, by Sex, Canada, 2015

Source: Cancer Statistics 2015. Special topic: Predictions of the future burden of cancer in Canada. Toronto, Ontario. https://www.cancer.ca/~/media/cancer.ca/CW/cancer%20information/cancer%20101/Canadian%20cancer%20statistics/Canadian-Cancer-Statistics-2015-EN.pdf (Chapter 1, p. 17).

Males 41 000 Deaths		Females 37 000 Deaths	
Lung	26.6%	Lung	27.0%
Colorectal	12.4%	Breast	13.6%
Prostate	10.1%	Colorectal	11.5%
Pancreas	5.6%	Pancreas	6.2%
Bladder	4.0%	Ovary	4.7%
Esophagus	3.9%	Non-Hodgkin lymphoma	3.3%
Leukemia	3.8%	Leukemia	3.1%
Non-Hodgkin lymphoma	3.5%	Body of uterus	2.8%
Stomach	3.1%	Brain/CNS	2.3%
Brain/CNS	3.0%	Stomach	2.1%
Kidney	2.7%	Bladder	1.8%
Liver	2.1%	Kidney	1.8%
Oral	2.0%	Multiple myeloma	1.7%
Melanoma	1.8%	Esophagus	1.2%
Multiple myeloma	1.8%	Melanoma	1.1%
Larynx	0.8%	Oral	1.1%
Breast	0.1%	Cervix	1.0%
All other cancers	12.5%	Liver	0.7%
		Larynx	0.2%
		All other cancers	12.8%

CNS=central nervous system

Figure 10-8 Percentage Distribution of Estimated Cancer Deaths, by Sex, Canada, 2015

Source: Canadian Cancer Society's Advisory Committee. (2015, June). Canadian Cancer Statistics 2015. Special topic: Predictions of the future burden of cancer in Canada. Toronto, Ontario. https://www.cancer.ca/~/media/cancer.ca/CW/cancer%20information/cancer%20101/Canadian%20cancer%20statistics/Canadian-Cancer-Statistics-2015-EN.pdf (p. 39).

studies have documented an increase in certain types of breast cancer in women who have used hormone replacement therapy (HRT) for more than five years.

- **Family history.** Having a first-degree relative—mother, sister, or daughter—with breast cancer does increase risk, and if the relative developed breast cancer before menopause, the cancer is more likely to be hereditary.

Detection The Canadian Cancer Society suggests that *mammograms* offer women the best defence against breast cancer. Routine breast self-examinations (BSE) are no longer recommended; however, women are encouraged to be familiar with their breasts and to look and feel for any changes. Clinical breast examinations done by a trained professional are no longer routinely recommended for women.

A **mammography** exam is a low-dose X-ray. The breast is placed between two plastic plates, which are pressed together to flatten the breast. The compression of the breast assists in providing a clear image. Detailed images of the breast are taken from a number of different angles. While uncomfortable, the screening only takes a few seconds for each image.[99] Figure 10-9 shows the sizes of lumps found by having a clinical breast exam, mammogram, and breast self-exam. Research has shown that breast cancers found in women who have regular mammograms are smaller and more easily treatable or operable and result in a better chance of survival. However, there are risks too. False positive results indicating there is cancer present when it is not can cause stress and unnecessary medical interventions. False negative results can mean lack of or delay in treatment that is necessary.

Cancer calcifications of this size and smaller can be seen on mammograms.

Average-size lump found by mammogram.

Average-size lump found by women practising frequent breast self-exam.

Smallest-size cancer that can be felt by physician's palpation exam.

Average-size lump found by women practising occasional breast self-exam.

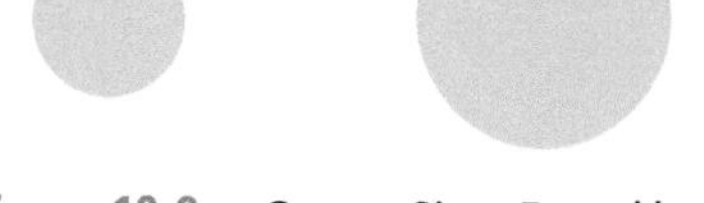

Figure 10-9 Cancer Sizes Found by Breast Cancer Detection Methods

Based on current research and evaluation, the Canadian Cancer Society recommends the following:[100]

- **40–49 years of age**—Talk to your doctor about your risk of breast cancer, along with the benefits and risks of mammography.
- **50–69 years of age**—Have a mammogram every two years.
- **70 or older**—Talk to your doctor about how often you should have a mammogram.

Treatment Breast cancer can be treated with surgery, radiation, and drugs (chemotherapy and hormonal therapy). Doctors may use one of these options or a combination, depending on the type and location of the cancer and whether the disease has spread.

Most women undergo some type of surgery. **Lumpectomy** or breast-conserving surgery removes only the cancerous tissue and a surrounding margin of normal tissue. A modified radical **mastectomy** includes the entire breast and some of the underarm lymph nodes. Radical mastectomy, in which the breast, lymph nodes, and chest wall muscles under the breast are removed, is rarely performed today because modified radical mastectomy has proven just as effective. Removing underarm lymph nodes is important to determine if the cancer has spread, but a new method, sentinel node biopsy, allows physicians to pinpoint the first lymph node into which a tumour drains (the sentinel node) and remove only the nodes most likely to contain cancer cells.

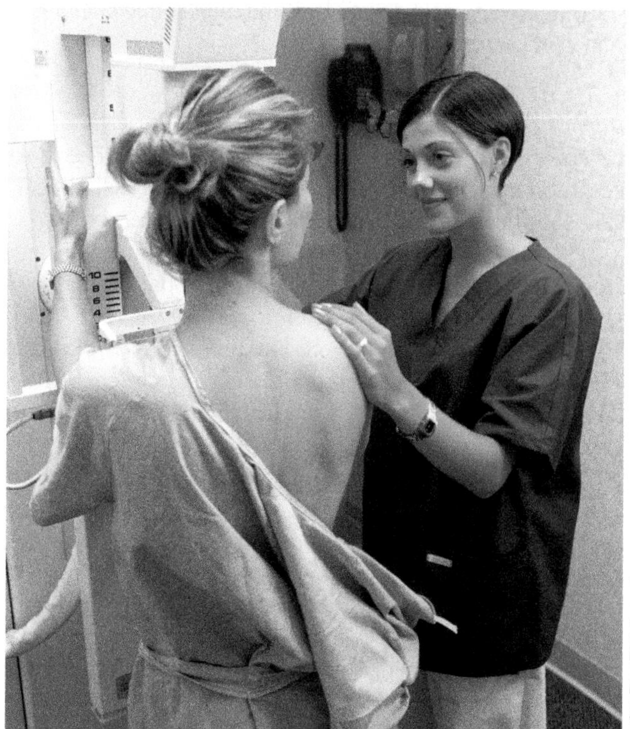

John Fox/Thinkstock

Mammography has been shown to be a reliable method of finding breast cancer.

Radiation therapy is treatment with high-energy rays or particles to destroy cancer. In almost all cases, lumpectomy is followed by six to seven weeks of radiation. Chemotherapy is used to reach cancer cells that may have spread beyond the breast—in many cases even if no cancer is detected in the lymph nodes after surgery.

In March 2005, a major clinical trial looking at new ways to prevent breast cancer in women who were at risk of developing the disease was launched. Risk factors included a woman's age, a family history of breast cancer, the age of the first menstrual period, and the age at the birth of a first child. The study tested the drug *exemestane*—a member of a class of drugs called aromatase inhibitors. Exemestane suppresses estrogen production, which has been found to be a factor in the development of some types of breast cancer.

Forty-five thousand post-menopausal women from Canada, the United States, and Spain were followed over a five-year period. Researchers found that exemestane reduces the risk by 65 percent compared to the use of a placebo. They also found that women in the experimental group using exemestane had fewer cases of pre-cancerous lesions. Exemestane was approved by Health Canada in 2000 for the treatment of advanced breast cancer in post-menopausal women whose tumours had stopped responding to *tamoxifen*, another drug used in breast cancer therapy.[101]

✓ CHECK-IN

If you are a female do you look and feel for any changes in your breasts on a regular basis?

Cervical Cancer Cervical cancer starts in the cells of the cervix—the lower portion of a woman's uterus. The most common type of cervical cancer (squamous cell cancer) starts in the cells that line the surface of the cervix.[102]

The primary risk factor for cervical cancer is infection with certain types of the human papillomavirus (HPV), discussed in Chapter 9. However, not every HPV infection becomes cervical cancer, and while HPV infection is very common, cervical cancer is not. The National Advisory Committee on Immunization (NACI) has recommended that girls and women who have not already been exposed to the HPV virus get an HPV vaccine to lower the risk of cervical cancer. Three vaccines are available in Canada. It is important to note that getting the vaccine does not guarantee prevention of cervical cancer.[103] Other risk factors for cervical cancer include early age of first intercourse, multiple sex partners, genital herpes, and significant exposure to second-hand smoke.

Regular Pap tests are an excellent way to find cervical cancer at an early stage when it can be treated successfully.

Colon and Rectal Cancer Colorectal cancer is a common cancer for both men and women; it is the second most common cause of cancer death for men and third for women.[104] There is no single cause of colorectal cancer, but some factors do appear to increase the risk of developing it. They include age (especially those over 50), polyps (small growths on the inner wall of the colon and rectum), a family history, diet, obesity, physical inactivity, heavy alcohol consumption, smoking, and living with inflammatory bowel disease.

Colon polyps are fleshy growths that usually begin growing in the epithelium lining of the bowel. These polyps are very common, especially in older adults. Many polyps are benign. However, when some polyps are left untreated, they can grow into the muscle layers underneath the epithelium lining, go through the bowel wall, and develop into an adenoma, a special type of polyp that is likely to become cancerous. When they do become cancerous the term "adenocarcinoma" is used. The definition for adenocarcinoma is a malignant tumour in the epithelial tissue. Early signs of colorectal cancer are bleeding from the rectum, blood in the stool, or a change in bowel habits. Treatment may involve surgery, radiation therapy, and chemotherapy.

Regular colorectal screening is advised for everyone over age 50, or younger if you have a family history of this type of cancer. The simplest test, the fecal occult blood test, detects blood in a person's stool. Another test, the flexible sigmoidoscopy, can detect between 50 and 65 percent of colon rectal cancers (CRC). This test examines the sigmoid colon, where 60 percent of colorectal cancers are found. A colonoscopy examines the entire colon. During this procedure, lesions or polyps can be removed. This screening method is advised for people who are at a high risk for CRC.

Lung Cancer Lung cancer begins with the development of abnormal cells in the lungs. The cells form lumps and can grow into tumours.[105] Tumours can be benign or malignant. Benign tumours, while a serious health threat, are more easily dealt with. Malignant tumours are very harmful and often fatal.

There are two main types of lung cancer:[106]

- non–small cell lung cancer (NSCLC), which is the most common type and grows slowly
- small cell lung cancer (SCLC), which grows quickly and can spread to other parts of the body

As stated in the opening section about cancer, lung cancer remains the leading cause of cancer death for both men and women. It is also the second-leading estimated new cancer diagnosis for women (13.5 percent) and third for men (13.5 percent).[107] The main risk for lung cancer is smoking. Cigarette smoking damages the lungs by destroying the cleansing layer in the lungs. The cancer-causing chemicals combine to form a sticky tar. The tar sticks to the cilia or tiny hairs that line the lungs. This causes a buildup of mucus, which results in a "smoker's cough"—the lungs' way of attempting to clean themselves. All of the harmful cancer-causing agents in cigarette smoke become lodged in the mucus and can develop into cancerous tumours.[108]

There has been a long debate in the past couple of decades as to the link between smoking marijuana and lung cancer. Some studies suggest that there is no statistically significant link between the two. More recent studies are beginning to suggest the opposite. McGuinness presents an overview of the use of cannabis and the link to health and says that cannabis smoke delivers 50–70 percent more carcinogenic hydrocarbons compared to tobacco smoke. Individuals who smoke cannabis experience similar symptoms as cigarette smokers—frequent coughing, respiratory infections, higher rates of asthma, and an increased risk of lung cancer.[109] Callaghan, Allebeck, and Sidorchuk tracked a group of young Swedish men (18–20 years old) for over 40 years attempting to assess the link between smoking marijuana and lung cancer.[110] Their findings raise concern that smoking marijuana at a young age may result in a modest increase in the risk of lung cancer due to the specific period of lung development during young adulthood. Heavy marijuana smoking was significantly associated with more than double the risk of developing lung cancer over the 40-year follow-up. This remains a controversial issue. The safe way to reduce your risk of lung cancer is to quit smoking any substance or to not start in the first place.

Other factors that can increase your risk of lung cancer include air pollution, a family history of lung cancer, previous diagnosis of lung cancer, and exposure to asbestos, arsenic, chromium, nickel, or radon gas.

Detection Lung cancer often does not cause any symptoms in its early stages. As the cancer grows, symptoms may include[111]

- a cough that just will not go away;
- shortness of breath or wheezing;
- constant chest pain, especially when you cough;
- frequent chest infections such as pneumonia;
- coughing up blood;
- a deep sense of fatigue; and
- loss of appetite or unexplained weight loss.

Diagnosing lung cancer is done by a number of tests. X-rays, ultrasounds, low-dose spiral CT (computed tomography) scans, and MRIs (medical resonance imaging) are some of them. Others include a sputum cytology, biopsies of the tumour site, and blood tests.

Treatment Surgery is the most common method of treatment for non-small cell lung cancers that have not grown to a large size and have not spread to other tissues. The surgeon can remove a wedge section, the lobe of the lung containing the tumour, or the entire lung.

Radiation treatment is used to treat a tumour. Radiation damages the cancerous cells. Unfortunately, the beam of radiation can also damage any cells in the path of the external beam. Other side effects include fatigue and skin damage where the treatment was given. Chemotherapy may also be used as a treatment option. Pills or injection are the two most common chemotherapy options.[112]

Ovarian Cancer Ovarian cancer is the leading cause of death from gynecological cancers. There are three main types of ovarian cancer: [113]

- **Epithelial cell cancer**, the most common type of ovarian cancer, begins in the cells that cover the outer surface of the ovary.
- **Germ cell tumours**, which being in the egg cells within the ovary. This type is more common in young women and can even develop in young children.
- **Sex chord stromal tumours**, which start in the connective tissue cells that hold the ovary together.

Risk factors include a family history of ovarian cancer; personal history of breast cancer; obesity; infertility (because the abnormality that interferes with conception may also play a role in cancer development); and low levels of transferase, an enzyme involved in the metabolism of dairy foods.

Often women do not develop obvious symptoms until the advanced stages, although they may experience painless swelling of the abdomen, irregular bleeding, lower abdominal pain, digestive and urinary abnormalities, fatigue, backache, bloating, and weight gain.

Skin Cancer Skin cancer is a very common cancer in Canada. Sunlight is the primary culprit. Once scientists thought exposure to the B range of ultraviolet light (UVB), the wavelength of light responsible for sunburn, posed the greatest danger. However, longer-wavelength UVA, which penetrates deeper into the skin, also plays

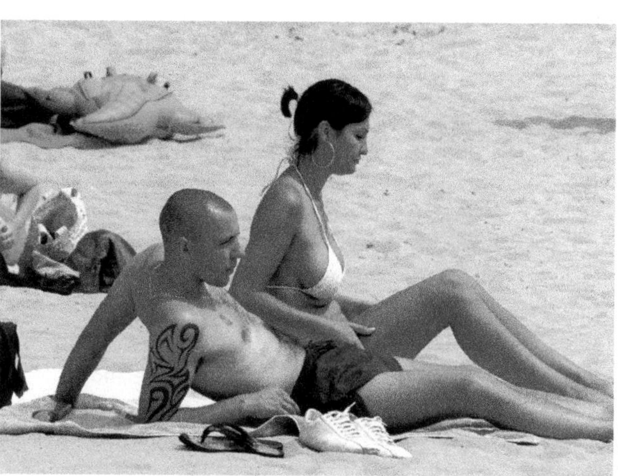
chris fotoman/Alamy

a major role in skin cancers.[114] An estimated 80 percent of total lifetime sun exposure occurs during childhood, so sun protection is especially important in youngsters.

Tanning salons and sunlamps also increase the risk of skin cancer because they produce ultraviolet radiation. A half-hour dose of radiation from a sunlamp can be equivalent to the amount you would get from an entire day in the sun.

Research does suggest that adequate levels of Vitamin D may protect against some types of cancer. The Canadian Cancer Society recommends 1000 IU/day for adults during the fall and winter months or year-round for anyone at a high risk for low Vitamin D levels.[115] There have been reports on the benefits of unprotected sun exposure for the production of Vitamin D—a vitamin the skin naturally produces when exposed to solar UVB rays. This message contradicts the health message of protecting our skin from the sun to reduce the risk of skin cancer. A few minutes a day of unprotected sun exposure is all that we really need to get enough Vitamin D.

The most common skin cancers are *basal cell* (involving the base of the epidermis, the top level of the skin) and *squamous cell* (involving cells in the epidermis).[116]

Smoking and exposure to certain hydrocarbons in asphalt, coal tar, and pitch may increase the risk of squamous cell skin cancer. Other risk factors include occupational exposure to carcinogens and inherited skin disorders, such as xeroderma pigmentosum and familial atypical multiple-mole melanoma.

Malignant *melanoma*, the deadliest type of skin cancer, starts in the melanocytes, which are the cells that produce brown pigment and colour our skin. When the skin is exposed to the sun, the melanocytes make more melanin and cause the skin to get even darker. When melanocytes cluster together they form moles. While not usually cancerous, moles can be a site for melanoma.

Melanoma can start in any part of the body where melanocytes are found, such as the eyes, mouth, vagina, or under the fingernails. Melanoma often metastasizes to other parts of the body and is very difficult to treat once that has occurred. Melanoma occurs more often among people over 40 years old but is increasing in younger people, particularly those who had severe sunburns in childhood.[117] Early diagnosis is the key for successful treatment.

Individuals with any of the following characteristics are at increased risk:[118]

- fair skin, light eyes, or fair hair
- a tendency to develop freckles and to burn instead of tan
- a personal or family history of melanoma
- a large number of *nevi*, or moles (200 or more, or 50 or more if under age 20) or dysplastic (atypical) moles

Detection Non-melanoma symptoms to watch for are skin lesions known as actinic keratoses (AKs). They are rough red or brown scaly patches that develop in the upper layer of the skin, usually on the face, lower lip, bald scalp, neck, and back of the hands and forearms. Forty percent of squamous cell carcinomas begin as AKs.

The most common predictor for melanoma is a change in an existing mole or development of a new and changing pigmented mole. The most important early indicators are change in colour, an increase in diameter, and changes in the borders of a mole (see Figure 10-10). An increase in height signals a corresponding growth in depth under the skin. Itching in a new or long-standing mole also should not be ignored.

STRATEGIES FOR PREVENTION

Seven Warning Signs of Cancer

If you note any of the following seven warning signs, immediately schedule an appointment with your doctor:

- change in bowel or bladder habits
- a sore that doesn't heal
- unusual bleeding or discharge
- thickening or lump in the breast, testis, or elsewhere
- indigestion or difficulty swallowing
- obvious change in a wart or mole
- nagging cough or hoarseness

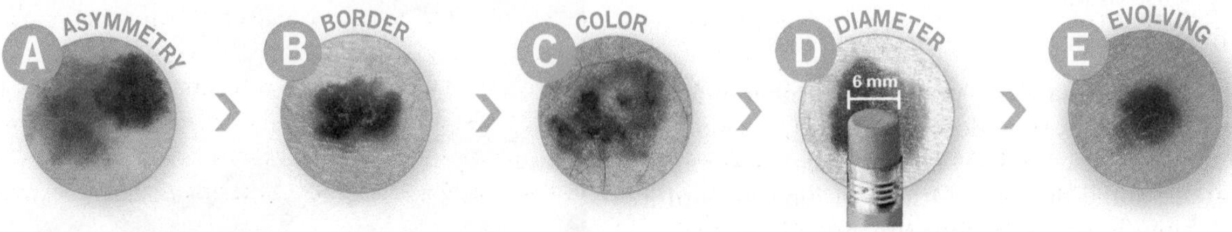

Figure 10-10 **ABCDE: The Warning Signs of Melanoma**

An estimated 95 percent of cases of melanoma arise from an existing mole. A normal mole is usually round or oval, less than six millimetres (about 1/4 inch) in diameter, and evenly coloured (black, brown, or tan). Seek prompt evaluation of any moles that change in ways shown in the photos.

Source: Reprinted with permission from the American Academy of Dermatology. All Rights Reserved.

Treatment Treatments for non-melanoma include surgical removal; cryosurgery (freezing the skin); electrodesiccation (heat generated by an electric current); topical chemotherapy; and removal with lasers, chemical peels, or dermabrasion.

If melanoma is suspected, biopsies of the site are usually taken and a microscopic exam will be done. The treatment plan is based on the type of melanoma and the size, location, and depth of the tumour. If caught early, melanoma is highly curable, usually with surgery alone. Once it has spread, chemotherapy with a single drug or a combination can temporarily shrink tumours in some people. However, the five-year survival rate for metastatic melanoma is less than 10 percent.

Prostate Cancer Prostate cancer is a commonly diagnosed cancer in Canadian men. It is the third most common cause of cancer death in men, although the death rates are falling.[119] The risk of prostate cancer increases with age, family history, exposure to the heavy metal cadmium, high number of sexual partners, and history of frequent sexually transmitted infections. An inherited predisposition may account for 5–10 percent of cases.

The development of a simple screening test that measures levels of a protein called prostate-specific antigen (PSA) in the blood has revolutionized the diagnosis of prostate cancer. However, the Canadian Cancer Society reminds us that a PSA test cannot diagnose cancer. However, it can help to detect a problem with the prostate. If the PSA levels are high, follow-up tests are usually needed. Follow-up testing can help find the cancer before it spreads beyond the prostate.[120]

The downside to a PSA test is that it does not discriminate between cancers that require treatment and those that do not. Sometimes individuals may undergo unnecessary treatment that carries the risk of severe side effects such as impotence, urinary incontinence, and death.

Testicular Cancer Testicular cancer occurs mostly among young men between the ages of 18 and 35, who are not normally at risk of cancer. Testicular cancer starts in the cells of the testicle. At highest risk are men with an undescended testicle (a condition that is almost always corrected in childhood to prevent this danger). To detect possibly cancerous growths, men should perform monthly testicular self-exams (TSE), as shown in Figure 10-11.

Although college- and university-age men are among those at highest risk of testicular cancer, Daley, in a study on college men's knowledge, attitudes, and beliefs about testicular cancer, found that male college students have a poor understanding of this type of cancer. Most of the participants of the study disclosed that they did not know what causes testicular cancer and were not able to describe risk factors. They did not practise testicular self-examinations, nor were they sure of how to do one.[121]

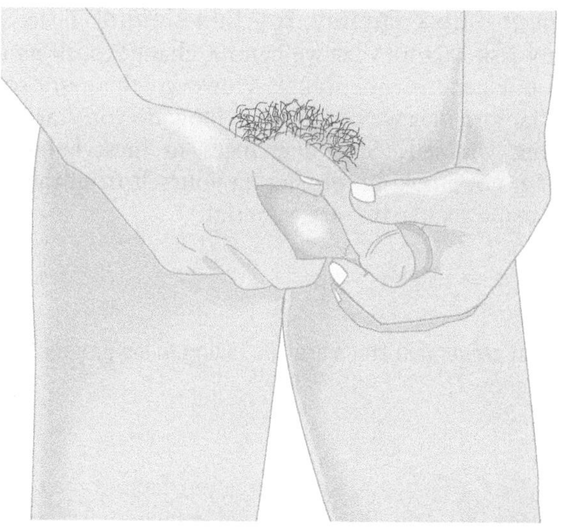

Figure 10-11 Testicular Self-Exam

The best time to examine your testicles is after a hot bath or shower, when the scrotum is most relaxed. Place your index and middle fingers under each testicle and the thumb on top, and roll the testicle between the thumb and fingers. If you feel a small, hard, usually painless lump or swelling, or anything unusual, consult a urologist.

Often the first sign of this cancer is a slight enlargement of one testicle. There also may be a change in the way it feels when touched. Sometimes men with testicular cancer report a dull ache in the lower abdomen or groin, along with a sense of heaviness or sluggishness. Lumps on the testicles also may indicate cancer.

A man who notices any abnormality should consult a physician. If a lump is indeed present, a surgical biopsy is necessary to find out if it is cancerous. If the biopsy is positive, a series of tests generally is needed to determine whether the disease has spread.

Treatment for testicular cancer generally involves surgical removal of the diseased testis, sometimes along with radiation therapy, chemotherapy, and the removal of nearby lymph nodes. The remaining testicle is capable of maintaining a man's sexual potency and fertility. Only in rare cases is removal of both testicles necessary. Testosterone injections following such surgery can maintain potency. The chance for a cure is very high if testicular cancer is spotted early.

A popular initiative on college and university campuses is the Movember Campaign where male students grow moustaches for 30 days to champion men's health issues. This event supports the Movember Foundation and raises money to fund projects focusing on prostate cancer, testicular cancer, poor mental health, and physical inactivity. Check out the Canadian Movember website at https://ca.movember.com/ and get involved.

✓ CHECK-IN

If you are a male, do you examine your testicles regularly?

Cancer—Risk Factors You Can Control There are many risk factors that we cannot change, such as age and our genetic inheritance. However, there are some risk factors that we can change. How do you start protecting yourself? Simple changes in lifestyle—smart eating, not smoking, protecting yourself from the sun, exercising regularly—are essential.

> **✓ CHECK-IN**
>
> What preventive steps are you taking to lower your risk of cancer?

Possible Carcinogens Environmental factors may cause between 80 and 90 percent of cancers. At least in theory, these cancers can be prevented by avoiding cancer-causing substances or using substances that protect against cancer-causing factors. It may not be possible to avoid all possible **carcinogens** (cancer-causing chemicals), but you can take steps to minimize your danger. Many chemicals used in industry, including nickel, chromate, asbestos, and vinyl chloride, are carcinogens. Employees and anyone living near a factory that creates smoke, dust, or gases are at risk. If your job involves their use, follow safety precautions at work. If you are concerned about possible hazards in your community, check with local environmental-protection officials.

Women and men who frequently dye their hair, particularly with permanent colouring, may be at increased risk for leukemia (cancer of blood-forming cells), non-Hodgkin's lymphoma (cancer of the lymph system), multiple myeloma (cancer of the bone marrow), and, in women, ovarian cancer.

Early Detection Cancers that can be detected by screening account for approximately half of all new cancer cases. Screening examinations, conducted regularly by a healthcare professional, can lead to early diagnosis of cancers of the breast, colon, rectum, cervix, prostate, testicles, and oral cavity and can improve the odds of successful treatment. If we all participated in regular cancer screenings, we could lower our risk of many types of cancers.

Cancer-Smart Nutrition Diets high in antioxidant-rich fruits and vegetables have long been linked with lower rates of esophageal, lung, colon, and stomach cancers.[122] It appears that antioxidants—substances that prevent the damaging effects of oxidation in cells—can block genetic damage induced by free radicals that could lead to some cancers. However, we are still waiting for conclusive evidence that any specific antioxidant, particularly in supplement form, can prevent cancer.

The mineral selenium, which promotes antioxidant activity, may protect against prostate cancer and possibly also lower the risk of cancers of the lung, colon, and esophagus. Diets rich in Vitamin C, Vitamin D, and folate also may have some specific benefits against breast cancer.

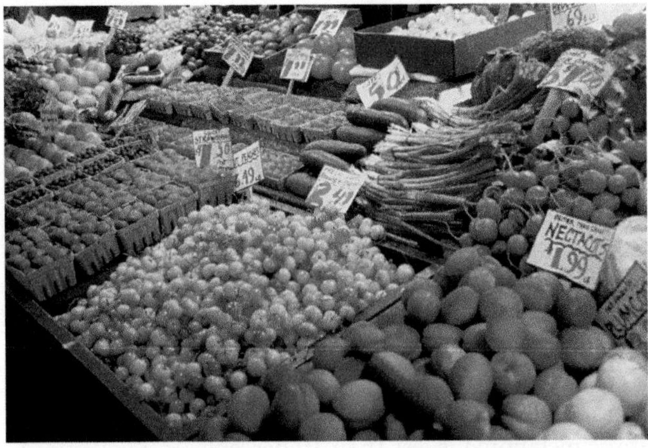

Eating seven to eight servings of vegetables and fruits a day for women aged 19–50 and 8–10 servings a day for men the same age can help reduce your cancer risk.

An awareness campaign by the Canadian Cancer Society encourages us to follow the *Eating Well with Canada's Food Guide* and to increase the number of servings of vegetables and fruits we eat per day to reduce our risks of cancer, heart disease, and stroke.[123]

Many people are not aware of the health benefits of eating a variety of fruits and vegetables as recommended by Health Canada and the Canadian Cancer Society. Lack of basic cooking skills and the ready option of fast-food restaurants are also cited as reasons why consumption of fruits and vegetables are low among many Canadian families. As we face the growing research that suggests Canada is heading toward a cancer crisis, we must figure out ways to make healthy eating realistic and manageable. As a student, you face many pressures—studying, working, tight budgets, stress, residence cafeteria food choices, or lack of cooking facilities.

The good news is that healthy eating does make a difference. Attempting to make small changes in our nutrition habits is the best place to start.

Tobacco Smoke Cigarette smoking is the single most devastating and preventable cause of cancer deaths in Canada. As has already been mentioned, cigarettes cause most cases of lung cancer. Smoking also increases the risk of cancers of the mouth, pharynx, larynx, esophagus, pancreas, and bladder. Pipes, cigars, and smokeless tobacco also increase the danger of cancers of the mouth and throat. Unfortunately, second-hand tobacco smoke can also increase the risk of cancer even among those who have never smoked. More information on the risks of smoking is presented in Chapter 12.

Physical Activity Research has shown that participating in regular physical activity throughout our lifetime can protect against some cancers. Activity during adolescence reduces the risk of premenopausal breast cancer. Long-term physical activity also lowers the risk for post-menopausal breast cancer.[124] Physical activity might reduce the risk of colon cancer by up to 20 percent. Other studies suggest a 30 percent reduction risk in endometrial cancer and a protection of the more aggressive forms of prostate cancer.[125]

Cancer—Risk Factors You Cannot Control

Age and heredity are two risk factors that we do not have control over when it comes to developing cancer. Yet, information about heredity can help individuals become more aware of their family history and cancer. Learning about your personal family risk of cancer can sometimes be the catalyst in making lifestyle changes that can lower the risks.

Age Age is a known risk for developing cancer. One example is prostate cancer. It is rarely diagnosed in men under the age of 60 years, and 22 percent of reported cases are in men over the age of 80 years.[126] As we age we can expect our risk of numerous types of cancer to rise; however, lifestyle changes and healthy living can mitigate this risk factor in many ways.

Heredity The most likely sites for inherited cancers to develop are the breast, brain, blood, muscles, bones, and adrenal glands. The telltale signs of inherited cancers include the following:

- **Cancer family syndrome.** Some families with unusually large numbers of relatives affected by cancer seem clearly cancer-prone. For instance, in Lynch syndrome (a form of colon cancer), more than 20 percent of the family members in at least two generations develop cancer of both the colon and the endometrium.
- **Early development.** Genetic forms of certain diseases strike earlier than non-inherited cancers. For example, the average age of women diagnosed with breast cancer is 62. But if breast cancer is inherited, the average age at diagnosis is 44, an 18-year difference.
- **Family history.** Anyone with a close relative (mother, father, sibling, child) with cancer has about three times the usual chance of getting the same type of cancer.
- **Multiple targets.** The same type of hereditary cancer often strikes more than once—in both breasts or both kidneys, for instance, or in two separate parts of the same organ.
- **Unusual sex pattern.** Genes may be responsible for cancers that generally do not strike a certain sex—for example, breast cancer in a man.

Women who have a first-degree (mother, sister, or daughter) family history of breast cancer have about a twofold increased risk of developing breast cancer compared with women who do not have a family history of the disease. This means that they are about twice as likely to develop breast cancer.

In hereditary cancers, such as retinoblastoma (an eye cancer that strikes young children) or certain colon cancers, a specific cancer-causing gene is passed down from generation to generation. The odds of any child with one affected parent inheriting this gene and developing the cancer are 50–50. Tracing cancers through a family tree is one simple way of checking your own risk.

DIABETES MELLITUS

Our bodies get energy by making glucose from foods we eat. In order to utilize the glucose, the body needs insulin. Insulin is a hormone that assists in controlling the level of glucose (sugar) in the blood. In individuals who have diabetes, the pancreas, which produces insulin (the hormone that regulates carbohydrate and fat metabolism) does not function as it should. About 11 million Canadians are living with diabetes mellitus or prediabetes. This number is expected to increase dramatically as the population ages.[127] Figure 10-12 illustrates the percentage of Canadians who have self-reported a diagnosis of diabetes by a health professional throughout the period 2001–2014.

There are three main types of diabetes. **Type 1 diabetes** (sometimes called *insulin-dependent diabetes*) is a disease in which the pancreas does not

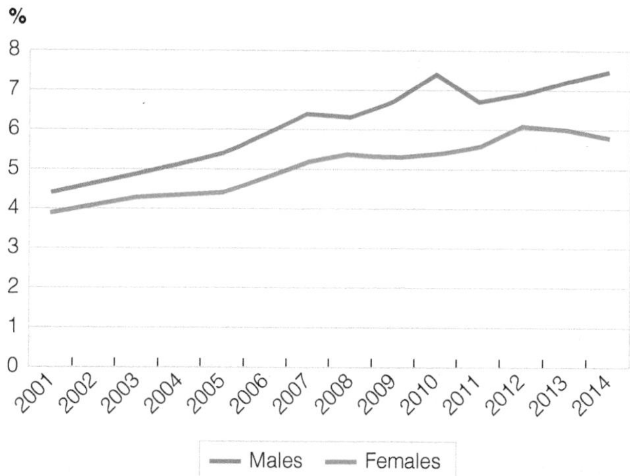

Figure 10-12 **Percentage Reporting a Diagnosis of Diabetes, by Sex, Household Population Aged 12 and Older, Canada, 2001–2014**

Source: Statistics Canada. (2015, November 27). Diabetes, 2014. Publications. 82-625-X. Chart 1. http://www.statcan.gc.ca/pub/82-625-x/2015001/article/14180-eng.htm.

produce insulin. Glucose builds up in the blood instead of being used for energy. Scientists do not know what causes type 1 diabetes. Most people are diagnosed with this type of diabetes before they are 30 years of age, with a diagnosis usually being made in children or teenagers.[128]

Type 2 diabetes is a disease in which the pancreas doesn't produce sufficient insulin to meet the body's needs or does not properly use the insulin it does make (sometimes called *non-insulin-dependent diabetes*). It is a progressive, lifelong condition. Keeping blood glucose levels in a healthy target range becomes a daily commitment.[129]

Gestational diabetes mellitus (GDM), a third type of diabetes, is a temporary condition that occurs during pregnancy. It is defined as hyperglycemia or high blood sugar with the first recognition of pregnancy.[130] It carries an increased risk of developing diabetes for both mother and child.

✓ CHECK-IN

Have you ever had your blood glucose tested?

Who Is at Risk for Developing Diabetes? Clinical practice guidelines launched by the Canadian Diabetes Association describe "at-risk" individuals as having **prediabetes** or impaired glucose intolerance (IGT), meaning that blood glucose levels are near but not quite reaching the level that defines a diabetes diagnosis. The clinical guidelines, published every five years, emphasize the importance of early identification of risk factors in the prediabetes stage in order to prevent the onset of diabetes and the serious health complications that accompany the disease.[131]

Other factors for developing diabetes include being a member of a high-risk ethnic group (Aboriginal, Hispanic, Asian, South Asian, or African descent) and being overweight—especially if you carry that weight around your middle. Between 80 and 90 percent of type 2 diabetes cases are attributable to overweight and obesity.[132]

Children are now at an increased risk for developing diabetes, too. Although type 2 diabetes was once a disease occurring almost exclusively in adults, it is now appearing in increasing rates in children.[133] This could be in part due to the fact that being overweight is now one of the most common medical conditions of childhood and many children with type 2 diabetes are overweight at diagnosis.[134] Of special concern are First Nations communities, in which type 2 diabetes is being diagnosed in children, and rates appear to be increasing rapidly.[135]

Uncontrolled glucose levels slowly damage blood vessels throughout the body, so individuals who become diabetic early in life may face challenging complications even before they reach middle age. Diabetes is the number-one cause of blindness, non-traumatic amputations, and kidney failure. Diabetes also increases the risk of heart attack or stroke by two or three times.

A lack of physical activity is a major risk factor for developing type 2 diabetes. Television watching is strongly associated with weight and obesity, a risk factor for diabetes in both children and adults. In a study by Urrutia-Rojas and Menchaca, children who reported watching television and playing video games two or more hours a day were 73 percent more likely to be at risk for developing type 2 diabetes. This environmental factor can be changed if parents, teachers, and children themselves understand the importance of choosing healthy lifestyle choices such as regular physical activity.[136]

College and university students are at risk too. In a study by Wood et al., diabetic college students had to become much more responsible for their diabetic care. Without the usual help from parents and medical professionals, there was much to learn about healthy eating, the importance of physical activity, and choosing healthy lifestyle behaviours so as not to compromise their diabetic management plans. Students not previously diagnosed with diabetes sometimes discover their condition at college or university and must become educated about the disease and how they might best manage their lifestyle.[137]

Those at highest risk include relatives of diabetics (whose risk is two and a half times that of others), males, older persons (see Figure 10-13), obese persons, and mothers of large babies (an indication of maternal prediabetes). A child of two parents with type 2 diabetes faces an 80 percent likelihood of also becoming diabetic.

The early signs of diabetes are frequent urination, excessive thirst, a craving for sweets and starches, and

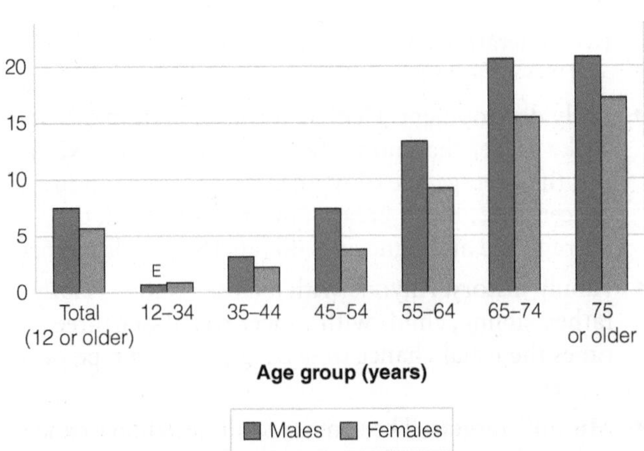

^{E} use with caution (these data have a coefficient of variation from 16.6–33.3%)

Figure 10-13 Percentage Reporting a Diagnosis of Diabetes, by Age Group and Sex, Household Population Aged 12 and Older, Canada, 2014

Source: Statistics Canada. (2015, November 27). Diabetes, 2014. Publications. 82-625-X. Chart 1. http://www.statcan.gc.ca/pub/82-625-x/2015001/article/14180-eng.htm.

weakness. Diagnosis is based on tests of the sugar level in the blood. Researchers are working to develop a test that would help identify telltale antibodies in the blood; this could indicate that pancreas cells are being destroyed years before the first signs of diabetes.

✓ CHECK-IN

Does anyone in your family have diabetes?

Dangers of Diabetes Before the development of insulin injections, diabetes was a fatal illness. Today, diabetics can have normal lifespans. However, both types of diabetes can lead to complications, including an increased risk of heart attack or stroke, kidney failure, blindness, and loss of circulation to the extremities.

Diabetic women who become pregnant face higher risks of miscarriage and babies with serious birth defects; however, precise control of blood sugar levels before conception and in early pregnancy can lower the likelihood of these problems. Women who develop gestational diabetes are more than three times as likely to develop type 2 diabetes if they have a second pregnancy; their infants may be at increased risk of cardiovascular disease later in life.

Managing this disease is also a tremendous challenge. Many people with type 2 diabetes do not have their blood sugar under control. They may also be dealing with serious health conditions such as obesity, heart disease, stroke, and kidney and eye disease.[138]

Diabetes and Ethnic Minorities Researchers now believe that the interaction of environmental factors and genes varies among different racial and ethnic groups. Of concern is the number of Aboriginal peoples living with diabetes. The prevalence of diabetes does vary among First Nations, Inuit, and Métis peoples; however, one common finding is that diabetes appears to be diagnosed at a younger age in Aboriginal peoples than non-Aboriginal peoples. Aboriginal females also experience higher rates of gestational diabetes than non-Aboriginal females. Health professionals also report that complications of diabetes are more frequently seen among Aboriginal peoples compared to non-Aboriginal peoples.

The diabetes rate differs between Aboriginal groups: First Nations people living on-reserve, 17.2 percent; those living off-reserve, 10.3 percent; and among Métis, 7.3 percent. This compares to 5 percent of non-Aboriginal peoples and 6.8 percent of all Canadians living with diabetes.[139]

Treatment There is no cure for diabetes at this time. The best treatment option is to keep blood sugar levels as stable as possible to prevent complications such as kidney damage. Home glucose monitoring allows diabetics to check their blood sugar levels as many times a day as necessary and to adjust their diet or insulin doses as appropriate.

Those with type 1 diabetes require daily doses of insulin via injections, an insulin infusion pump, or oral medication. Those with type 2 diabetes can control their disease through a well-balanced diet, exercise, and weight management. However, insulin therapy may be needed to keep blood glucose levels near normal or normal, thereby reducing the risk of damage to the eyes, nerves, and kidneys.

Medical advances hold out hope for diabetics. Laser surgery, for instance, is saving eyesight. Bypass operations are helping restore blood flow to the heart and feet. Dialysis machines and kidney and pancreas transplants save many lives. Researchers are exploring various approaches to prevention, including early low-dose insulin therapy, oral insulin to correct immune intolerance, and immunosuppressive drugs. On the horizon is the search for a true cure through transplanting insulin-producing cells from healthy pancreases.

We must also remember that we do have solid clinical evidence that it is possible to prevent one of the most common and costly chronic diseases affecting Canadians. Type 2 diabetes and its related complications can be prevented by lifestyle modifications—moderate weight loss and regular exercise—and in some people by the appropriate use of drugs.

X AND Y FILES

Sex Differences in Disease

Disease doesn't discriminate. In general, men and women are vulnerable to the same illnesses, but there are differences in the diseases that strike each sex. Women are more prone to arthritis, osteoporosis, and joint problems, while men are more likely to be felled by heart attacks and cancer.

Half of all men, compared to a third of women, develop cancer. Smoking, which for many years was much more prevalent among men, accounts for some of this difference. As more women have become smokers in the last 30 years, lung cancer rates in women have doubled.

In some cancers, estrogen may somehow protect against distant metastases. This protection may be why women have a 12 percent lower death rate from cancer of the stomach and lung than men and a 33 percent greater chance of surviving malignant melanoma.

Some diseases, such as diabetes, afflict more women than men and pose a graver threat to their health. While more men develop ulcers and hernias, women are three to four times more likely to get gallbladder disease. Irritable bowel syndrome (IBS), one of the most common digestive disorders, causes such varied symptoms in the sexes that some gastroenterologists think of it as a completely different disease in men and women. IBS affects women three times as often as men.

SELF-SURVEY

Are You at Risk of Cancer?

Answer the following questions:

1. Do you protect your skin from overexposure to the sun? ___
2. Do you abstain from smoking or using tobacco in any form? ___
3. If you're over 40 or if family members have had colon cancer, do you get routine digital rectal exams? ___
4. Do you eat a balanced diet that includes the recommended daily value for Vitamins A, B, and C? ___
5. If you're a woman, do you have regular Pap tests and pelvic exams? ___
6. If you're a man over 40, do you get regular prostate exams? ___
7. If you have burn scars or a history of chronic skin infections, do you get regular checkups? ___
8. Do you avoid smoked, salted, pickled, and high-nitrite foods? ___
9. If your job exposes you to asbestos, radiation, cadmium, or other environmental hazards, do you get regular checkups? ___
10. Do you limit your consumption of alcohol? ___
11. Do you avoid using tanning salons or home sunlamps? ___
12. If you're a woman between 40 and 49, do you have clinical breast exams by a trained healthcare professional? ___
13. Do you eat plenty of vegetables and other sources of fibre? ___
14. If you're a man, do you perform regular testicular self-exams? ___
15. Do you wear protective sunglasses in sunlight? ___
16. Do you follow a low-fat diet? ___
17. Do you know the cancer warning signs? ___

Answers to Self-Survey

If you answered no to any of the questions, your risk for developing various kinds of cancer may be increased.

Chapter Summary

1. Which statement about the heart is true?
   a. It has four chambers, which are responsible for pumping blood into the veins for circulation through the body.
   b. It pumps blood first to the lungs where it picks up oxygen and discards carbon dioxide.
   c. It beats about 10 000 times and pumps about 300 litres of blood per day.
   d. It has specialized cells that generate electrical signals to control the amount of blood that circulates through the body.

2. Which of the following is a risk factor for heart disease that cannot be controlled?
   a. male pattern baldness
   b. diabetes mellitus
   c. sedentary lifestyle
   d. blood fat cells

3. Which statement about your lipoprotein profile is true?
   a. It provides a breakdown of the different types and levels of blood fats circulating in your body.
   b. It is best obtained at a health fair where the results are uniformly accurate.
   c. It will give a total cholesterol level, which is the amount of triglycerides and LDL cholesterol levels added together.
   d. It should be evaluated after eating a full meal.

4. Which statement about hypertension is true?
   a. It is diagnosed when blood pressure is consistently less than 130/85 mm Hg.
   b. It may be treated with dietary changes, which include eating low-fat foods and avoiding sodium.
   c. It can cause fatty deposits to dissolve on the artery walls.
   d. It usually does not respond to medication, especially in severe cases.

5. Which statement about a heart attack is true?
   a. It occurs when the myocardium receives an excessive amount of blood from the coronary arteries.
   b. It is typically suffered by individuals who have irregular episodes of atherosclerosis.
   c. It can be treated successfully up to four hours after the event.
   d. It occurs when the myocardial cells are deprived of oxygen-carrying blood, causing them to die.

6. How can you protect yourself from certain types of cancer?
   a. by eating a diet rich in antioxidants
   b. by avoiding people who have had cancer
   c. by wearing sunscreen with an SPF of less than 15
   d. by using condoms during sexual intercourse

7. Which statement about skin cancer is true?
   a. Individuals with a large number of moles are at decreased risk for melanoma.
   b. The most serious type of skin cancer is squamous cell carcinoma.
   c. The safest way to get a tan and avoid skin cancer is to use tanning salons and sunlamps instead of sunbathing in direct sunlight.
   d. Individuals with a history of childhood sunburn are at increased risk for melanoma.
8. Which of the following increases a woman's risk of developing breast cancer?
   a. if she began menstruating before 12 years of age
   b. if she had her first child when in her teens or 20s
   c. if her husband's mother had breast cancer
   d. if she has fibrocystic breast disease
9. Which statement about prostate cancer is true?
   a. It occurs mostly among men between the ages of 18 and 35.
   b. It has been linked to having a vasectomy.
   c. It is the most commonly diagnosed cancer in Canadian men.
   d. Risk does not increase with age.
10. Which statement about diabetes mellitus is false?
   a. The two types of diabetes are insulin-dependent and non-insulin-dependent.
   b. The incidence of diabetes in Canada has decreased in the last decade, especially among women and children.
   c. Individuals with diabetes must measure the levels of glucose in their blood to ensure that it does not rise to unsafe levels.
   d. Untreated or uncontrolled diabetes can lead to coma and eventual death.

Answers to these questions can be found on page 284.

SELF-RESPONSIBILITY—SOCIAL RESPONSIBILITY

SELF-RESPONSIBILITY

It's not that some people have willpower and some don't. It's that some people are ready to change and others are not.

James Gordon, M.D.

As you have discovered throughout this chapter, lowering your risk of major diseases takes knowledge, commitment, time, and energy. Where are you on the continuum of Prochaska's Stages of Change model when it comes to self-care and self-responsibility? What risk factors can you change with regard to heart disease, cancer, and diabetes? How can you move forward on a healthy living plan?

SOCIAL RESPONSIBILITY

So many people spend their health gaining wealth, and then have to spend their wealth to regain their health.

A.J. Reb

Many nonprofit organizations have opportunities for volunteer work: arranging conference setup, canvassing for fundraising, participating in education fairs, and organizing fundraising events such as the CIBC Run for the Cure. Consider giving of your time for a health cause.

CRITICAL THINKING

1. Have you had a lipoprotein profile lately? Do you think it's necessary for you to obtain one? If your reading was or is borderline or high, what lifestyle changes could you make to help control your cholesterol level?
2. Do you have family members who have had cancer? Were these individuals at risk for cancer because of specific environmental factors, such as long-term exposure to tobacco smoke? If no particular cause was identified, what other factors could have triggered their diseases? Are you concerned that you might have inherited a genetic predisposition to any particular type of cancer because of your family history?
3. A friend of yours, Karen, discovered a small lump in her breast during a routine self-examination. When she mentions it, you ask if she has seen a doctor. She tells you that she hasn't had time to schedule an appointment; besides, she says she's not sure it's really the kind of lump one has to worry about. What advice would you give her?

WEB LINKS

Canadian Cancer Society

www.cancer.ca

You will find comprehensive information about different kinds of cancer: statistics, early detection, prevention, treatment options, alternative treatments, and coping strategies for families.

Canadian Diabetes Association

www.diabetes.ca

Here you will find the latest information on both type 1 and type 2 diabetes mellitus, including suggestions regarding diet and exercise. The online bookstore features meal planning guides, cookbooks, and self-care guides.

Heart and Stroke Foundation of Canada

www.heartandstroke.com

This comprehensive site features a searchable database of all major cardiovascular diseases, plus information on healthy lifestyles and current research. You can find out about your own personal risk profile by completing the Heart & Stroke Risk Assessment™. This profile will provide a free, confidential, customized action plan for healthy living.

The Lung Association of Canada

www.lung.ca

At this site you can access information and programs that are conducted at the national, provincial, and municipal levels. Current research and general information about respiratory health is abundant.

Please note that links are subject to change. If you find a broken link, use a search engine such as www.google.ca and search for the website by typing in keywords.

Key Terms

The terms listed here are used within the chapter on the page indicated. Definitions of the terms are in the Glossary at the end of the book.

angioplasty 260
aorta 256
aortic valve 257
arteriosclerosis 259
arteries 256
atherosclerosis 259
capillaries 256
carcinogens 278
cardiovascular disease (CVD) 256
cholesterol 264
chordae tendineae 258
coronary arteries 256
coronary bypass 260
coronary heart disease (CHD) 259
coronary veins 256
diabetes mellitus 265
diastole 257
diastolic blood pressure 261
gestational diabetes mellitus (GDM) 280
hypertension 261
inferior vena cava 256
infiltration 270
ischemic heart disease 259
left atrium 257
left ventricle 257
lipoproteins 264
lumpectomy 273
male pattern baldness 269
mammography 273
mastectomy 273
metabolic syndrome 265
metastasize 270
mitral valve 257
myocardial infarction (MI) 259
neoplasms 270
papillary muscles 258
plaque 259
prediabetes 280
pulmonary artery 256
pulmonary valve 257
pulmonary vein 256
right atrium 256
right ventricle 257
sinoatrial node (SA node) 256
stages or staging of cancer 271
stroke 262
superior vena cava 256
systole 257
systolic blood pressure 261
transient ischemic attack (TIA) 263
tricuspid valve 257
triglyceride 264
type 1 diabetes 279
type 2 diabetes 280
veins 256

Answers to Chapter Summary Questions

1. b; 2. a; 3. a; 4. b; 5. d; 6. a; 7. d; 8. a; 9. c; 10. b

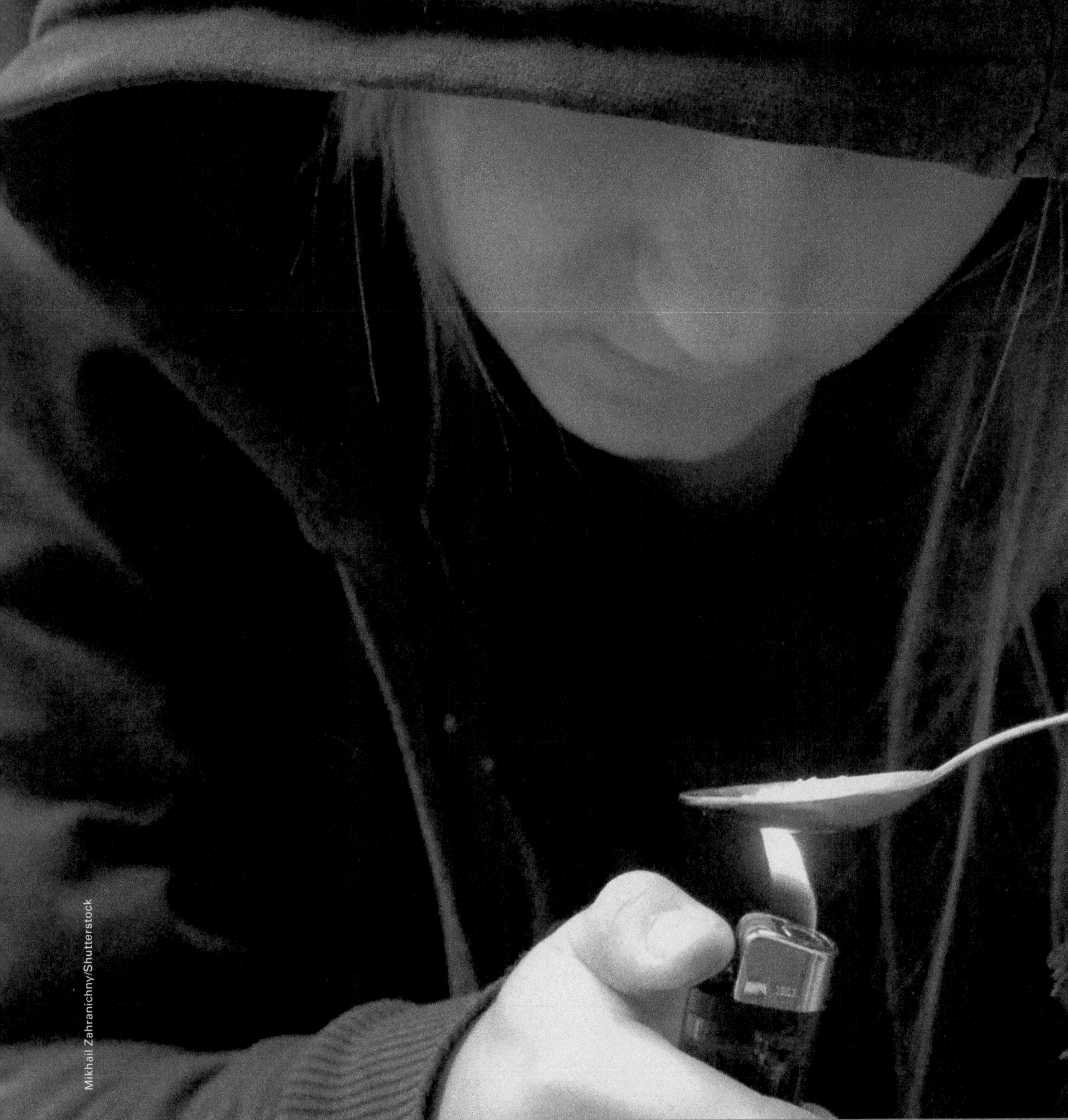

AFTER READING THIS CHAPTER, YOU WILL BE ABLE TO:

- **describe** the factors affecting individuals' responses to drugs
- **give examples** of appropriate and inappropriate use of over-the-counter and prescription medications
- **discuss** the factors affecting drug dependence
- **describe** the methods of use and the effects of common drugs of abuse
- **describe** the treatment methods available for drug dependence

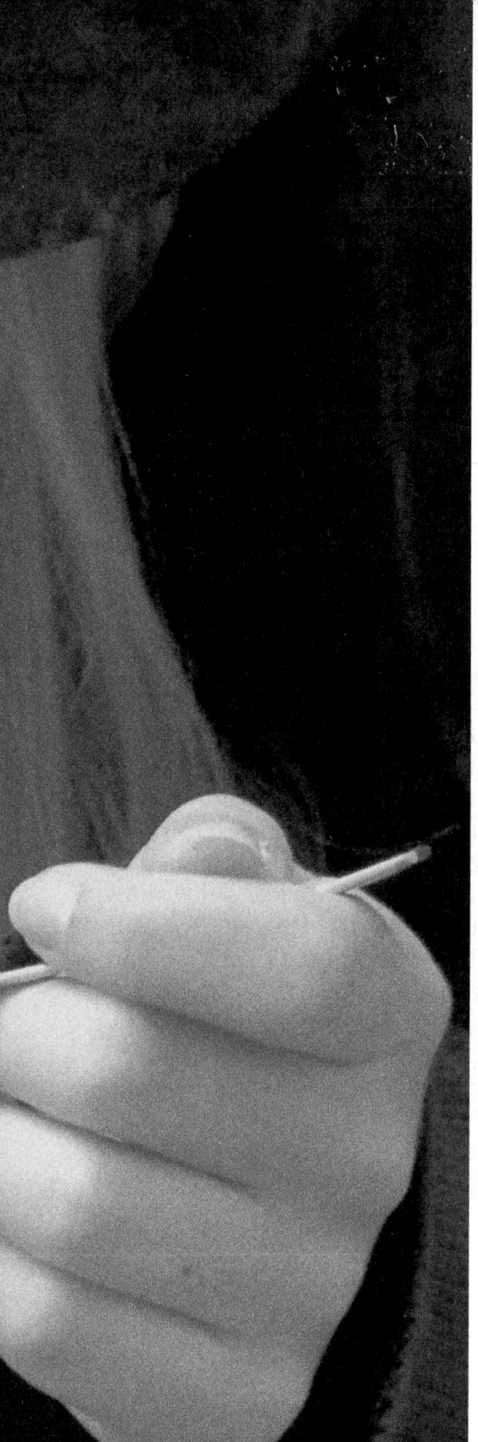

11

Drug Use, Misuse, and Abuse

People who try illegal drugs do not think they will ever lose control. Even regular users believe they are smart enough, strong enough, or lucky enough not to get caught or addicted. However, with continued use, drugs produce changes in an individual's body, mind, and behaviour. Eventually a person's need for a drug can outweigh everything else, including the values, people, and relationships he or she once held close.

Substance use, misuse, and abuse have long been important public-health concerns in Canada. The challenges of drug use and abuse are many—injection-drug use and HIV/AIDS, drug labs and grow operations, street use of prescription drugs, methamphetamine abuse, and social problems. According to findings from the *Canadian Tobacco, Alcohol and Drugs Survey (CTADS) 2013*, 11 percent of Canadians (approximately 3.1 million) reported the use of at least one of six illicit drugs—cannabis, cocaine or crack, speed, ecstasy, hallucinogens, or heroin—in the past 12 months. The rate for males was 14 percent (approximately 2.0 million) compared to females at 8 percent (about 1.0 million). The rate of drug use of one of the six illicit drugs by young adults aged 20–24 was 23 percent compared to adults over 24 at 8 percent.[1] Of added concern is that 2 percent of Canadians aged 15 years and older said they had used a psychoactive pharmaceutical drug for purposes other than as a medical prescription such as getting high.[2]

The impacts of drug addictions in college and university students range from short-term consequences, such as academic difficulties, to long-term physical and psychological problems. This chapter provides information on the nature and effects of drugs, the impact of drugs on individuals and society, and the drugs Canadians most commonly use, misuse, and abuse. It also includes a section on treating drug dependence and abuse with options for individual programs and information about how some communities in Canada are finding ways to address this important health issue.

FREQUENTLY ASKED QUESTIONS

FAQ: What should I know about buying over-the-counter drugs? p. 289

FAQ: What causes drug dependence and abuse? p. 295

FAQ: How common is drug use on campus? p. 296

UNDERSTANDING DRUGS AND THEIR EFFECTS

A **drug** is any substance that is taken to change the way you feel and function. In some circumstances, taking a drug can help the body heal or relieve physical and mental distress. In other circumstances, taking a drug can distort reality, undermine well-being, and threaten survival. No drug is completely safe; all drugs have multiple effects that vary greatly in different people at different times. Knowing how drugs affect the brain, body, and behaviour is crucial in understanding their impact and making responsible decisions about their use.

Drug misuse is the taking of a drug for a purpose or by a person other than that for which it was medically intended. Borrowing a friend's prescription for Ritalin is an example of drug misuse. It can also mean inadvertently not complying with prescription medication instructions.[3] **Drug abuse** is excessive drug use that is inconsistent with accepted medical practice.[4] Drug abuse can mean taking prescription painkillers or illicit drugs to get high.

Risks are involved with all forms of drug use. Even medications that help cure illnesses or soothe symptoms have side effects and can be misused. Some substances that millions of people use every day, such as caffeine, pose some health risks. Others—like the most commonly used drugs in our society—alcohol and tobacco—can lead to potentially life-threatening problems. With some illicit drugs, any form of use can be dangerous.

Many factors determine the effects a drug has on an individual. These include how the drug enters the body, the dosage, the drug action, and the presence of other drugs in the body—as well as the set and setting in which the drug is used.

Drugs can enter the body in a number of ways (see Figure 11-1). The most common way of taking a drug is by **oral ingestion**—swallowing a tablet, capsule, or liquid. However, drugs taken orally don't reach the bloodstream as quickly as drugs introduced into the body by other means. A drug taken orally may not have any effect for 30 minutes or more.

Drugs can enter the body through the lungs by **inhalation**. An example is smoke from marijuana—or by inhaling gases, aerosol sprays, or fumes from solvents or other compounds that evaporate quickly.

Injection is another way of administering drugs. It is often done with a syringe and can be done intravenously (directly into a vein), intramuscularly (into muscle tissue, which is richly supplied with blood vessels), or subcutaneously (beneath the skin). **Intravenous (IV) injection** gets the concentrated form of a drug into the bloodstream immediately (within seconds in most cases). Effects are felt within minutes. In emergency situations, medical personnel will use an intravenous injection as a powerful intervention. However, if illicit drugs are injected there is an elevated risk of an overdose. An **intramuscular injection** provides a slower and more consistent diffusion of the drug. It is usually administered with a hypodermic needle into the muscular tissue. This is the method used for vaccinations or for administering antibiotics. A **subcutaneous injection**, administered into the fatty layer beneath the skin, is absorbed more slowly because there is very little blood flow in this tissue. The medication is absorbed sometimes within 10 minutes or can take up to 24 hours. Medications injected this way include

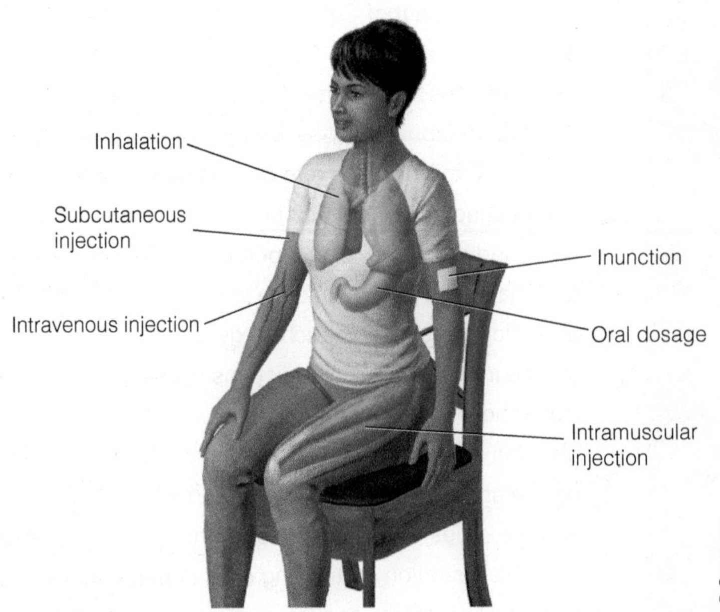

Figure 11-1 Routes of Administration of Drugs

insulin, epinephrine, some types of anesthetics, and growth hormones.

Injection can be extremely dangerous if not done in a safe manner because many diseases, including hepatitis and the human immune deficiency virus (HIV), can be transmitted by sharing contaminated needles. Injection drug users who are HIV-positive are the chief source of transmission of HIV among heterosexuals.

One other option for administering drugs is through **inunction.** Defined as anointing or applying an ointment by rubbing, inunction is also done by applying small adhesive patches containing a drug to the skin. The patches slowly release the medical ingredient transdermally. An example would be a nicotine patch.

Dosage and Toxicity The effects of any drug depend on the amount an individual takes. Increasing the dose usually intensifies the effects produced by smaller doses. Also, the kind of effect may change at different dose levels. For example, low doses of barbiturates may relieve anxiety, while higher doses can induce sleep, loss of sensation, and even coma and death.

The dosage level at which a drug becomes poisonous to the body, causing either temporary or permanent damage, is called its **toxicity.** In most cases, drugs are eventually broken down in the liver by special body chemicals called *detoxification enzymes*.

Individual Differences in Response to Drugs Each person responds differently to different drugs, depending on the set or setting. The **set** can be defined as the internal environment or *mind-set*—a person's expectations or preconceptions about using the drug. Personality, psychological attitude, and physical factors play a role. Often drugs intensify the emotional state of a person. If you're feeling depressed, a drug may make you feel more depressed. A generalized physical problem, such as having the flu, may make your body more vulnerable to the effects of a drug. Genetic differences among individuals may account for varying reactions. The enzymes in the body reduce the levels of drugs in the bloodstream; because there can be 80 variants of each enzyme, every person's body may react differently. One person may have a frighteningly bad trip on the same dosage of a drug on which another person has a positive experience.

The **setting** is the external environment that a drug user is in. The setting can include the number and type of people you are surrounded by, the level of noise and lighting, and the type of room you are in. Setting can also link to culture. Kerr, Kimber, and Rhodes found that high-risk settings can impact both the amount and frequency of drugs used.[5]

Medications Many of the medications and pharmaceutical products available in this country do relieve symptoms and help cure various illnesses. However, improper use of medications leads to hospitalizations and added healthcare costs for Canadians. Because drugs are powerful, it is important to know how to use them appropriately.

What Should I Know about Buying Over-the-Counter Drugs?

More than half a million health products are readily available without a doctor's prescription. This does not mean that they are necessarily safe or effective. Indeed, many widely used **over-the-counter (OTC) drugs**—medications that can be obtained without a prescription from a medical professional—pose unsuspected hazards.

Among the most potentially dangerous is aspirin, the "wonder drug" in practically everyone's home pharmacy. When taken by someone who has been drinking (often to prevent or relieve hangover symptoms), aspirin increases blood-alcohol concentrations. Along with other non-steroidal anti-inflammatory drugs, such as ibuprofen (brand names include Advil® and Nuprin®), aspirin can damage the lining of the stomach and lead to ulcers in those who take large daily doses for arthritis or other problems. Kidney problems have also been traced to some pain relievers, including acetaminophen (Tylenol®). Some health products that are not even considered true drugs can also cause problems. Many Canadians take food supplements, even though they have not been approved for any medical disorder.[6]

A growing number of drugs that once were available only with a doctor's prescription can now be bought over-the-counter. These include Monistat®, which combats vaginal yeast infections, and nicotine replacement patches and gum to aid smokers trying to quit. For consumers, the advantages of this greater availability include lower prices and fewer visits to the doctor. The disadvantages, however, are the risks of misdiagnosing a problem and misusing or overusing medications.

Like other drugs, OTC medications can be used improperly, often simply because of a lack of education about proper use. Among those most often misused are the following:

- **Nasal sprays.** Nasal sprays relieve congestion by shrinking blood vessels in the nose. If they are used too often or for too many days in a row, the blood *vessels widen instead of contracting*, and the surrounding tissues become swollen, causing more congestion. The result can be complete loss of smell.
- **Laxatives.** Brands that contain phenolphthalein irritate the lining of the intestines and cause muscles to contract or tighten, often making constipation worse rather than better. A high-fibre diet and more exercise are safer and more effective remedies for constipation.
- **Eye drops.** Eye drops make the blood vessels of the eye contract. With overuse (several times a day for

several weeks), the blood vessels expand, making the eye look redder than before.

- **Sleep aids.** Although over-the-counter sleeping pills are widely used, there has been little research on their use and possible risks.
- **Cough syrup.** Chugging cough syrup is a growing problem, in part because young people think of dextromethorphan (DXM), a common ingredient in cough medicine, as a "poor man's version" of the popular drug ecstasy.

Prescription Drugs Medications are a big business in this country. In 2014 total prescription sales reached 23.2 billion dollars. This is a notable increase since 2006 when Canadian prescription drug sales were 17.8 billion dollars. Sales of brand-name prescriptions reached 18 billion dollars in 2014 and generic prescriptions reached 5.2 billion dollars.[7]

Both doctors and patients make mistakes when it comes to prescription drugs. The most frequent mistakes doctors make are overdosing or underdosing, omitting information from prescriptions, ordering the wrong dosage form (a pill instead of a liquid, for example), and not recognizing a patient's allergy to a drug. College and university students, like other consumers, often take medicines without discussing them with their physician.

Figures 11-2, 11-3, and 11-4 illustrate the prevalence of self-reported prescription use of opioid pain relievers, sedatives, and stimulants among Canadians by age categories between 2008 and 2013. Overall, opioid pain reliever use in the general population (15 years and older) decreased from 21.6 percent in 2008 to 14.9 percent in 2013. Among the general population the use of prescription sedatives in 2013 was 10.4 percent, similar to use in 2008. The use of prescription stimulants has also remained steady since 2008 at about 1 percent in the general population; however, youth (age 15–24) use is higher and less stable, fluctuating between 2 and 4 percent.[8]

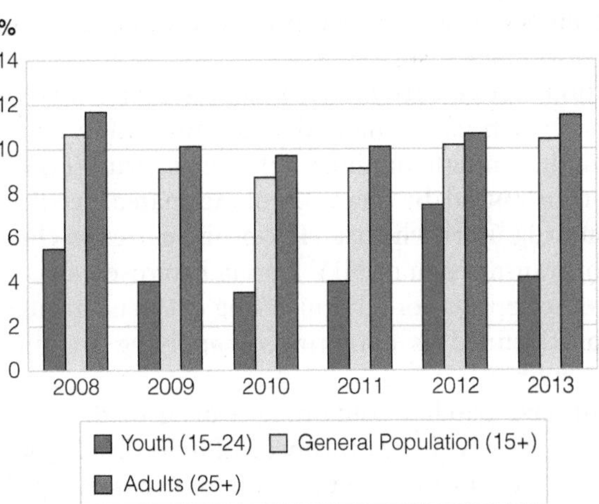

Note: Because of methodological differences between CADUMS and CTADS, comparisons of prevalence estimates between CADUMS (2008–2012) and CTADS (2013) data should be made with caution. Many of the prevalence estimates included in this summary are qualified because of high sampling variability and should be interpreted with caution.

Figure 11-3 Prevalence of Self-Reported Prescription Sedative Use among Canadians by Age Category

Source: Canadian Centre on Substance Abuse (2016). Canadian drug summary: Prescription sedatives. http://www.ccsa.ca/Resource%20Library/CCSA-Canadian-Drug-Summary-Prescription-Sedatives-2015-en.pdf (page 3, Figure 1). Reproduced with permission from the Canadian Centre on Substance Abuse.

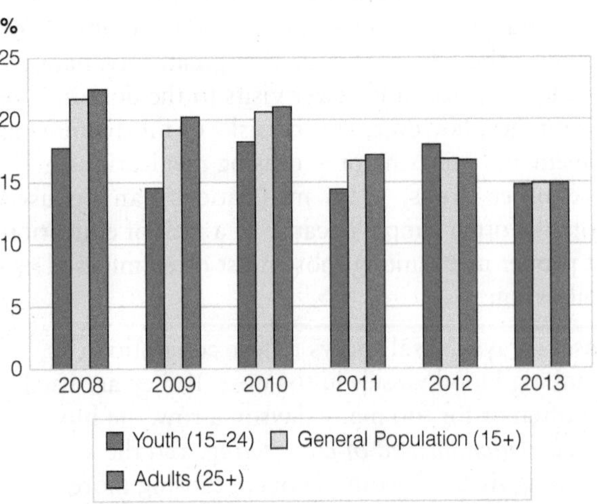

Note: Because of methodological differences between CADUMS and CTADS, comparisons of prevalence estimates between CADUMS (2008–2012) and CTADS (2013) data should be made with caution. Several of the prevalence estimates included in this summary are qualified because of high sampling variability and should be interpreted with caution.

Figure 11-2 Prevalence of Self-Reported Opioid Pain Reliever Use among Canadians by Age Category

Source: Source: Canadian Centre on Substance Abuse. Canadian drug summary: Prescription opioids. http://www.ccsa.ca/Resource%20Library/CCSA-Canadian-Drug-Summary-Prescription-Opioids-2015-en.pdf (page 3, Figure 1). Reproduced with permission from the Canadian Centre on Substance Abuse.

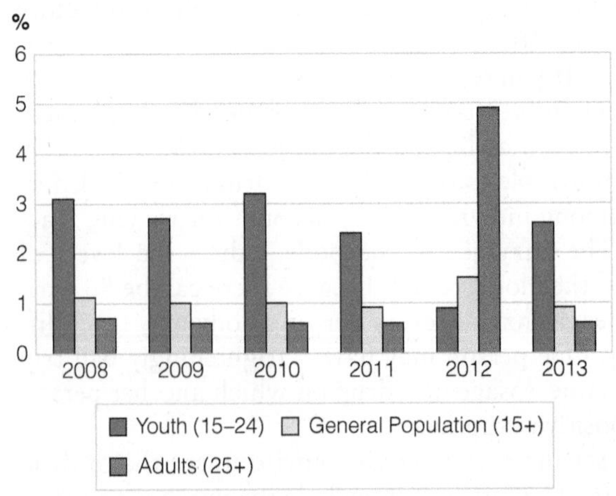

Note: Because of methodological differences between CADUMS and CTADS, comparisons of prevalence estimates between CADUMS (2008–2012) and CTADS (2013) data should be made with caution. Several of the prevalence estimates included in this summary are qualified because of high sampling variability and should be interpreted with caution.

Figure 11-4 Prevalence of Self-Reported Prescription Stimulant Use among Canadians by Age Category

Source: Canadian Centre on Substance Abuse. Canadian drug summary: Prescription stimulants. http://www.ccsa.ca/Resource%20Library/CCSA-Canadian-Drug -Summary-Prescription-Stimulants-2016-en.pdf#search=self%2Dreported%20prescription%20stimulant (page 3, Figure 1). Reproduced with permission from the Canadian Centre on Substance Abuse.

Non-adherence Many prescribed medications are not taken the way they should be; millions simply are not taken at all. Many people have trouble understanding dosage information or cannot read standard labels. In a study of 5732 Canadians, about one in ten people reported that the cost of the prescription was the reason for their non-adherence.[9] Other reasons for non-adherence include using the drug for the experience, for the feeling it causes, or to get high.

The dangers of **non-adherence** (not properly taking prescription drugs) include recurrent infections, serious medical complications, and emergency hospital treatment. The drugs most likely to be taken incorrectly are those that treat problems with no obvious symptoms (such as high blood pressure), require complex dosage schedules, treat psychiatric disorders, or have unpleasant side effects. Some people skip prescribed doses or stop taking medications because they fear that any drug can cause tolerance and eventual dependence. Others fail to let doctors know about side effects, such as stomach irritation.

✓ CHECK-IN

Have you ever taken a medication for a purpose other than the reason for which it was prescribed? If so, why?

Physical Side Effects Most medications, taken correctly, cause only minor complications. However, no drug is entirely without side effects for all individuals taking it. Serious complications that may occur include heart failure, heart attacks, seizures, kidney and liver failure, severe blood disorders, birth defects, blindness, memory problems, and allergic reactions.

Allergic reactions to drugs are common. The drugs that most often provoke allergic responses are penicillin and other antibiotics (drugs used to treat infection). Aspirin, sulpha drugs, barbiturates, anticonvulsants, insulin, and local anesthetics can also provoke allergic responses. Allergic reactions range from mild rashes or hives to anaphylaxis—a life-threatening constriction of the airways and sudden drop of blood pressure that causes rapid pulse, weakness, paleness, confusion, nausea, vomiting, unconsciousness, and collapse. This extreme response, which is rare, requires immediate treatment with an injection of epinephrine (adrenaline) to open the airways and blood vessels.

Psychological Side Effects Dozens of drugs—over-the-counter and prescription—can cause changes in the way people think, feel, and behave. Unfortunately, neither patients nor their physicians usually connect such symptoms with medications. Doctors may not even mention potential mental and emotional problems because they don't want to scare patients away from what otherwise may be a very effective treatment.

Among the medications most likely to cause psychiatric side effects are drugs for high blood pressure, heart disease, asthma, epilepsy, arthritis, Parkinson's disease, anxiety, insomnia, and depression. Some drugs—such as the powerful hormones called *corticosteroids*, used for asthma, autoimmune diseases, and cancer—can cause different psychiatric symptoms, such as mania, depression, and mood disturbances, depending on dosage and other factors.[10] Other drugs, such as ulcer medications, can cause delirium and disorientation, especially when given in high doses or to elderly patients. More subtle problems that are likely to be ignored or dismissed, such as forgetfulness or irritability, are common reactions to many drugs. The older you are, the sicker you are, and the more medications you are taking, the greater your risk of developing some psychiatric side effects. Even medications that do not usually cause problems, such as antibiotics, can cause psychiatric side effects in some individuals.

Any medication that slows down bodily systems, as many high blood pressure and cardiac drugs do, can cause depressive symptoms. Estrogen in birth control pills can cause mood changes. Many women using oral contraceptives have reported feeling depressed or moody. For many people, switching to another medication quickly lifts a drug-induced depression.

All drugs that stimulate or speed up the central nervous system can cause agitation and anxiety—including the almost 200 allergy, cold, and congestion remedies containing pseudoephedrine hydrochloride (Sudafed®). Other common culprits in inducing anxiety are caffeine and theophylline, a chemical relative of caffeine found in many medications for asthma and other respiratory problems. These drugs act like mild amphetamines in the body, making people feel hyperactive and restless.

Drug Interactions OTC and prescription drugs can interact in a variety of ways. For example, mixing some cold medications with tranquilizers can cause drowsiness and coordination problems, thus making driving dangerous. Moreover, what you eat or drink can impair or completely wipe out the effectiveness of drugs or lead to unexpected effects on the body. For instance, aspirin takes five to ten times as long to be absorbed when taken with food or shortly after a meal than when taken on an empty stomach. If tetracyclines encounter calcium in the stomach, they bind together and cancel each other out.

To avoid potentially dangerous interactions, check the label(s) for any instructions on how or when to take a medication, such as "with a meal." If the directions say that you should take a drug on an empty stomach, take it at least one hour before eating or two or three hours after eating. Do not drink a hot beverage with a medication; the temperature may interfere with the effectiveness of the drug. Do not open, crush, or dissolve tablets or capsules without checking first with your physician or pharmacist.

Whenever you take a drug, be especially careful of your intake of alcohol, which can change the rate of metabolism and the effects of many different drugs. Because it dilates the blood vessels, alcohol can add to the dizziness sometimes caused by drugs for high blood pressure, angina, or depression. Also, its irritating effects on the stomach can worsen stomach upset from aspirin, ibuprofen, and other anti-inflammatory drugs.

Caffeine Use and Misuse Caffeine, which has been drunk, chewed, and swallowed since the Stone Age, is the most widely used **psychotropic** (mind-affecting) drug in the world. Coffee has exploded into a multibillion-dollar worldwide fascination, spawning a massive global industry.[11]

Although there is no nutritional requirement for caffeine in our diet, coffee is the number-one food-service beverage choice of Canadian adults, with a total of 2.3 billion cups of coffee consumed in Canada in 2015.[12] This was a 10 percent jump from 2.1 billion in 2014. Coffee purchases at coffee shops and other venues have remained stable between 2014 and 2015. When Canadians do purchase coffee away from their home they typically order a traditional hot brewed coffee. A report by the NPD Group, Inc. states that this order constitutes 76 percent of purchased coffee servings. Speciality hot coffee purchases away from home make up 14 percent of servings and iced speciality coffees 10 percent of servings.[13] The use of in-home single-serving coffee machines has increased greatly too. There was a 13 percent growth globally in the purchase and use of the single-serve cup machines in 2015. However, there has been criticism from people concerned about the environmental issues that the use of disposable plastic coffee pods create.[14]

Canadians are also drinking more tea—about 500 million cups in 2014.[15] Worldwide tea is the greatest consumed beverage next to water.

An interesting side note is the amount of coffee beans needed to produce 453 grams (one pound) of coffee. Coffee beans are the seeds of the coffee cherry. Each coffee cherry produces two green beans. It takes approximately 2000 cherries or 4000 beans to produce 453 grams (one pound) of coffee. Each coffee bush produces, on average, about one to two pounds of coffee per year. It takes four to five years for a coffee bush to produce its first crop.[16]

Coffee contains 100–150 milligrams of caffeine per cup; tea, 40–100 milligrams; and cola, between 34 and 47 milligrams. Most medications that contain caffeine are one-third to one-half the strength of a cup of coffee. However, some, such as Excedrin®, are very high in caffeine (see Table 11-1). Health Canada recommends consuming no more than 400 milligrams of caffeine a day, which is about three 237-millilitre or 8-ounce cups of brewed coffee a day.[17] Popular 568-millilitre jumbo cups of coffee served at many coffee shops deliver this dose in a single serving. Some popular energy drinks have caffeine content that ranges from 50 milligrams to over 500 milligrams per can or bottle. While college and university students report that they use energy drinks to improve their attention span, stay awake, and increase energy for sports, many of them are not aware of the health risks that include raising heart rate and blood pressure, dehydrating our bodies, and interrupting sleep patterns.[18]

TABLE 11-1

Caffeine Counts

Substance (Typical Serving)	Caffeine (Milligrams)
Coffee (brewed), 227 ml cup	100–150
Espresso, 56 ml cup	100
Instant coffee, 227 ml cup	95
Red Bull, 250 ml can	80
Excedrin, two pills	130
No Doz, one pill	200
Coca-Cola Classic, 355 ml	34–47
Diet Coke, 355 ml	46.5
Tea, 227 ml cup	40–100
Dark chocolate, 28 ml	20
Milk chocolate, 28 ml	6
Cocoa, 142 ml	4
Decaffeinated coffee, 227 ml cup	5

The effects of caffeine vary. As a **stimulant**, it relieves drowsiness, helps in the performance of repetitive tasks, and improves the capacity for work. Some athletes feel that caffeine gives them an extra boost that allows them to go farther and longer in endurance events. Consumption of high doses of caffeine can lead to dependence, anxiety, insomnia, rapid breathing, upset stomach and bowels, and dizziness.

In a study of college men and women who normally consumed fewer than three caffeinated beverages per day, caffeine boosted anxiety but did not significantly affect performance on various low-intensity tasks, except for hand-eye coordination, which improved.[19]

Although there is no conclusive proof that caffeine causes birth defects, it does cross the placenta into the tissues of a growing fetus. Because of an increased risk of miscarriage, Health Canada has recommended that pregnant women avoid or restrict their caffeine intake. Some fertility specialists also have urged couples trying

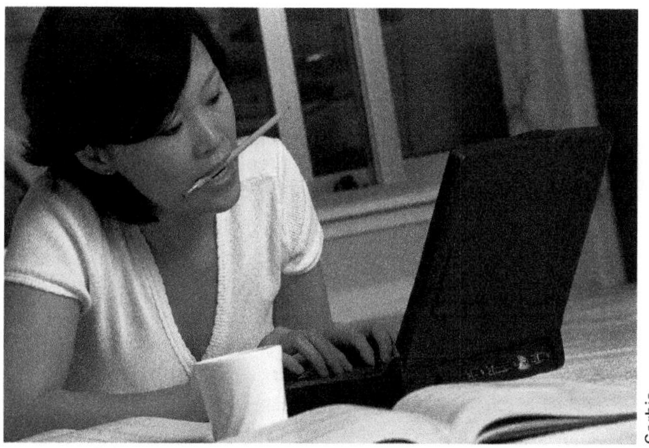

Corbis

Coffee and work often go hand in hand, but too much caffeine can lead to dependence, anxiety, and other problems.

to conceive to reduce caffeine intake to increase their chance of success. Women who are heavy caffeine users tend to have shorter menstrual cycles than non-users. A review of the literature by Pelluchi et al. suggests that coffee drinkers have a moderately high relative risk of bladder cancer compared to non–coffee drinkers.[20] However, other studies have not shown a coffee–cancer link—possibly because of the numerous compounding lifestyle factors of study participants.

✓ CHECK-IN

How much coffee do you drink each day? Are you aware of how much caffeine is in the coffee you make at home or purchase at a coffee shop?

Substance Use and Disorders People have been using **psychoactive** (mood-altering) chemicals for centuries. Citizens of ancient Mesopotamia and Egypt used opium. More than 3000 years ago, Hindus included cannabis in religious ceremonies. For centuries the Inca in South America have chewed the leaves of the coca bush. Although drugs existed in most ancient societies, their use was usually limited to small groups. Today millions of people regularly turn to drugs to pick them up, bring them down, alter perceptions, or ease psychological pain.

Both men and women are vulnerable to substance-use disorders, although they tend to have different patterns of drug use (see X & Y Files: "Men, Women, and Drugs"). The 1960s ushered in an explosive increase in drug use and in the number of drug users in our society. Marijuana use soared in the 1960s and 1970s; cocaine, in the 1980s. In 1986, crack—a cheap, smokeable form of cocaine—hit the streets, and the number of regular cocaine users zoomed. Club drugs, such as ecstasy (MDMA), methamphetamine (crystal meth), and cocaine are now the drug of choice among young people.

The word **addiction** refers to a dependence on an illegal drug or medication. It also means compulsive use of a substance, loss of control, negative consequences, and denial.[21] Mental health professionals describe drug-related problems in terms of *dependence* and *abuse*.

Dependence Individuals may develop **psychological dependence**, the emotional or mental attachment to the use of a drug, and feel a strong craving for a drug because it produces pleasurable feelings or relieves stress and anxiety. **Physical dependence** occurs when a person develops *tolerance* to the effects of a drug and needs larger and larger doses to achieve intoxication or another desired effect. Individuals who are physically dependent and have a high tolerance to a drug may take amounts many times those that would produce intoxication or an overdose in someone who was not a regular user.

Men and women with a substance-dependence disorder may use a drug to avoid or relieve withdrawal symptoms, or they may consume larger amounts of a drug or use it over a longer period than they'd originally intended. They may repeatedly try to cut down or control drug use without success; spend a great deal of time obtaining or using drugs or recovering from their effects; give up or reduce important social, occupational, or recreational activities because of their drug use; or continue to use a drug despite knowledge that the drug is likely to cause or worsen a persistent or recurring physical or psychological problem.

Specific symptoms of dependence vary with particular drugs. The degree of dependence also varies. In mild cases, a person may function normally most of the time. In severe cases, the person's entire life may revolve around obtaining, using, and recuperating from the effects of a drug.

Individuals with drug dependence become intoxicated or high on a regular basis—whether every day, every weekend, or several binges a year. They may try repeatedly to stop using a drug and yet fail, even though they realize their drug use is interfering with their health, family life, relationships, and work.

Abuse Some drug users do not develop the symptoms of tolerance and withdrawal that characterize dependence, yet they use drugs in ways that clearly have a harmful effect on them. These individuals are diagnosed as having a *psychoactive substance-abuse disorder*. They continue to use drugs despite their awareness of persistent or repeated social, occupational, psychological, or physical problems related to drug use, or they use drugs in dangerous ways or situations (before driving, for instance).

✓ CHECK-IN

Do you know anyone who has been treated for substance abuse?

X AND Y FILES

Men, Women, and Drugs

Beginning at an early age, males and females show different patterns in drug use. Among 12-year-olds who have been offered drugs, boys are more likely to have received those offers from other males or their parents. Girls are most likely to have been offered drugs by a female friend or family member. Boys are more likely to receive offers in a public setting, such as on the street or in a park, and the offers typically emphasize "benefits," such as improved status or self-image. Girls are more likely to receive a straightforward, "Do you want some?" offer or one that minimizes the risks of drug use. For girls, these offers are usually made in a private setting, such as a friend's home.

Later in life, men generally encounter more opportunities to use drugs than women, but given an opportunity to use drugs for the first time, both genders are equally likely to do so and to progress from initial use to dependence. However, men are more likely than women to use illicit drugs. According to the findings of the *Canadian Tobacco, Alcohol and Drugs Survey (CTADS) for 2013,* the overall rate of cannabis use among males was 14 percent (2.1 million) compared to females at 7.0 percent (1.0 million). With regard to the age that males and females were initiated to the use of cannabis, there was little difference, with males at 17.8 years and females at 18.1 years.[22]

The occurrence of overall use of at least one of the five most common illicit drugs excluding cannabis (cocaine or crack, speed, ecstasy, heroin, and hallucinogens including salvia) in 2013 was 2.0 percent of Canadians (458 000). About three times as many males (342 000) as females (116 000) reported using these drugs.[23]

Vulnerability to some drugs varies between men and women. Both are equally likely to become addicted to or dependent on cocaine, heroin, hallucinogens, tobacco, and inhalants. Women are more likely than men to become addicted to or dependent on sedatives and drugs designed to treat anxiety or sleeplessness, and less likely than men to abuse alcohol and marijuana.

Males and females may differ in their biological responses to drugs. Women may be more sensitive than men to the cardiovascular effects of cocaine. In studies, women and men given equal doses of cocaine experienced the same cardiovascular response, despite the fact that blood concentrations of cocaine did not rise as high in women as in men. Male and female long-term cocaine users showed similar impairment in tests of concentration, memory, and academic achievement following sustained abstinence, even though women in the study had substantially greater exposure to cocaine. Female cocaine users also were less likely than men to exhibit abnormalities of blood flow in the brain's frontal lobes. These findings suggest a sex-related mechanism that may protect women from some of the damage cocaine inflicts on the brain. However, women are more vulnerable to poor nutrition and below-average weight, depression, physical abuse, and, if pregnant, preterm labour or early delivery.

Women are nearly twice as likely as men to become infected with HIV by sharing needles with other injection-drug users and by engaging in unprotected sex.

There are also differences between men and women who seek treatment for drug abuse. Women in treatment programs are less likely than men to have graduated from high school and to be employed and are more likely than men to have other health problems, to have sought previous drug treatment, to have attempted suicide, and to have suffered sexual abuse or other physical abuse. Traditional drug-treatment programs, created for men, have proven to be less effective for women than programs that provide more comprehensive services, including child care, assertiveness training, and parenting training.

Intoxication and Withdrawal **Intoxication** refers to maladaptive behavioural, psychological, and physiologic changes that occur as a result of substance use. **Withdrawal** is the development of symptoms that cause significant psychological and physical distress when an individual reduces or stops drug use. (Intoxication and withdrawal from specific drugs are discussed later in this chapter.)

Polyabuse Most users prefer a certain type of drug but also use several others; this behaviour is called **polyabuse.** The average user who enters treatment is on five different drugs. The more drugs anyone uses, the greater the chance of side effects, complications, and possibly life-threatening interactions.

Concurrent Disorders A biennial publication of the Canadian Centre on Substance Abuse describes the term **concurrent disorder** as a situation where a person has both a mental health and a substance abuse problem.[24] This is a major health issue in Canada with reports of over 50 percent of people seeking help for addiction having a mental illness, and 15–20 percent of people who ask for help to deal with a mental illness living with an addiction.[25] Individuals with concurrent disorders require careful evaluation and appropriate treatment for the complete range of complex and chronic difficulties they face.

Many individuals with concurrent disorders have a very limited ability to cope with everyday living responsibilities. They often experience higher unemployment, social anxiety, and homelessness, and some turn to crime to deal with their addictions. Even with assistance they have frequent relapses. Following are some of the key findings of this report:[26]

- Exposure to traumatic events can increase both alcohol and drug use, which in turn can lead to more traumatic experiences, resulting in a stress–substance use cycle.
- Individuals with anxiety disorders are two to five times more likely than others to have a problem with drugs or alcohol. In 75 percent of people with both an anxiety disorder and a substance addiction, the anxiety disorder began first.

- Individuals who have difficulty with impulse control are at risk for future substance abuse. It is the single strongest predictor. Inherited genetic susceptibilities can be increased due to prenatal exposure to drugs, alcohol, and nicotine.
- Individuals dealing with mood disorders are also more likely to have a substance abuse problem. Conversely, people who use and misuse drugs and alcohol are more likely to suffer from mood disorders.
- People with psychotic disorders such as schizophrenia are almost five times more likely to have a substance use disorder (three times higher for alcohol and six times higher for illicit drugs) than those who do not. There are studies that have determined that heavy use of cannabis results in a risk for schizophrenia six times higher than in non-users.

What Causes Drug Dependence and Abuse? No one fully understands why some people develop drug dependence or abuse disorders, whereas others, who may experiment briefly with drugs, do not. Inherited body chemistry, genetic factors, and sensitivity to drugs may make some individuals more susceptible. These disorders may stem from many complex causes.

Biology of Dependence Some scientists now view drug dependence as a brain disease triggered by frequent use of drugs that change the biochemistry and anatomy of neurons and alter the way they work.[27] A major breakthrough in understanding dependence has been the discovery that certain mood-altering substances and experiences—a puff of marijuana, a slug of whiskey, a snort of cocaine, a big win at blackjack—trigger a rise in a brain chemical called *dopamine*, which is associated with feelings of satisfaction and euphoria. This brain chemical or neurotransmitter, one of the crucial messengers that link nerve cells in the brain, rises during any pleasurable experience, whether it be a loving hug or a taste of chocolate.

Addictive drugs have such a powerful impact on dopamine and its receptors (its connecting cells) that they change the pathways within the brain's pleasure centres. Various psychoactive chemicals create a craving for more of the same. According to this hypothesis, addicts do not specifically yearn for heroin, cocaine, or nicotine but for the rush of dopamine that these drugs produce. Other brain chemicals, including glutamate, GABA (gamma-aminobutyric acid), and possibly norepinephrine, may also be involved. Some individuals who are born with low levels of dopamine may be particularly susceptible to addiction.

Other Routes of Addiction Scientists believe certain individuals are at greater risk of drug dependence because of psychological factors, including difficulty controlling impulses, a lack of values that might constrain drug use (whether based in religion, family, or society), low self-esteem, feelings of powerlessness, and depression. The one psychological trait most often linked with drug use is denial. Some young people in particular are absolutely convinced that they will never lose control or suffer in any way as a result of drug use.

Many drug users have been diagnosed with at least one mental disorder, particularly depression or anxiety. Disorders that emerge in adolescence, such as bipolar disorder, may increase the risk of substance abuse. Many people with psychiatric disorders abuse drugs. Individuals may self-administer drugs to treat psychiatric symptoms; for example, they may take sedating drugs to suppress a panic attack.

Individuals who are isolated from friends and family or who live in communities where drugs are widely used have higher rates of drug abuse. Young people from lower socio-economic backgrounds are more likely to use drugs than their more affluent peers, possibly because of economic disadvantage; family instability; a lack of realistic, rewarding alternatives and role models; and increased hopelessness.

Those whose companions are substance abusers are far more likely to use drugs. Peer pressure to use drugs can be a powerful factor for adolescents and young adults. The likelihood of drug abuse is also related to family instability, parental rejection, and divorce.

When researchers followed families for a decade and a half and interviewed both children and their mothers, they found that youngsters who felt attached to their parents and showed greater responsibility and less rebelliousness were less likely to use drugs. Their attitudes and behaviours insulated them from socializing with drug-using peers, resulting in less drug use in their early and late 20s.[28] Clear rules and expectations from parents also can go a long way toward preventing or delaying alcohol and marijuana use in children, even if there is tension in the parent–child relationship.[29]

STRATEGIES FOR PREVENTION

Saying No to Drugs

If people offer you a drug, here are some ways to say no:

- Let them know you're not interested. Change the subject. If the pressure seems threatening, just walk away.
- Have something else to do: "No, I'm going to see another friend now."
- Be prepared for different types of pressure—teasing, persuasion, coercion.
- Keep it simple. "No, thanks," "No," or "No way" all get the point across.
- Choose your friends wisely. Connect with people who won't offer you drugs and who want to bring out the best in you.

Parents' own attitudes and drug-use history can also affect their children's likelihood of using drugs. In one study, parents who perceived little risk associated with marijuana use had children with similar attitudes, and the children of parents who had used marijuana were about three times more likely to try the drug than children whose parents had never used the drug.[30] In another study, parental drug attitudes and adult drug use had significant direct effects on adolescent drug use outside of the strong effects of peer influence.[31]

Drugs such as crack cocaine that produce an intense, brief high lead to dependence more quickly than slower-acting agents such as cocaine powder. Drugs that cause uncomfortable withdrawal symptoms, such as barbiturates, may lead to continued use to avoid such discomfort.

Drug use involves certain behaviours, situations, and settings that users may, in time, associate with getting high. Even after long periods of abstinence, some former drug users find that they crave drugs when they return to a site of drug use or meet people with whom they used drugs. Former cocaine users report that the sight of white powder alone can serve as a cue that triggers a craving.

Most individuals who use drugs first try them as adolescents. Teens are likely to begin experimenting with tobacco, beer, wine, or hard liquor and then smoke marijuana or sniff inhalants. Teens who smoke cigarettes are more likely to use drugs and to drink heavily than nonsmoking youths. Some then go on to try sedative-hypnotics, stimulants, and hallucinogens. A much smaller percentage of teens try the opioids. Over time, some individuals give up certain drugs, such as hallucinogens, and return to old favourites, such as alcohol and marijuana. A smaller number continues using several drugs.

The Toll of Drugs Drugs affect a person's physical, psychological, and social health. The effects of drugs can be *acute* (resulting from a single dose or series of doses) or *chronic* (resulting from long-term use). Acute effects vary with different drugs. Stimulants may trigger unpredictable rage; an overdose of heroin may lead to respiratory depression, a breathing impairment that can be fatal.

Over time, chronic drug users may feel fatigued, cough constantly, lose weight, become malnourished, and ache from head to toe. They may suffer blackouts, flashbacks, and episodes of increasingly bizarre behaviour, often triggered by escalating paranoia. Their risk of overdose rises steadily, and they must live with constant stress: the fear of getting busted for possession or of losing a job if they test positive for drugs, the worry of getting enough money for their next fix, and the dangers of associating with dealers and other users.

Reported drug use also has been linked to harm. Research has shown that one in every five Canadians who reported illicit drug use or abuse of psychoactive pharmaceuticals suffered from some harm during the past year prior to completing a survey. Males experienced some sort of harm two times higher (4 percent) than females (2 percent).[32] Within a party context, undergraduate students who drank alcohol, used marijuana, and took other illicit drugs experienced the most harm. Female students who drank alcohol and used marijuana and illicit drugs experienced more harm than the male students, even though their level of use of alcohol and drugs was less.[33]

The toll of drug use can be especially great on young people because it disrupts many critical developmental tasks of adolescence and young adulthood. Early use of drugs can lead to drug-related crime; poor achievement in high school, college, or university; and job instability. Data from the Canadian Tobacco, Alcohol and Drugs Survey (CTADS) found that both younger women and men aged 20–24 report a four times higher level of harm than those in an adult age group of 25 and older.[34]

How Common Is Drug Use on Campus? Alcohol is the number-one drug of abuse on college and university campuses. Marijuana remains the most commonly used illegal drug. Cocaine has also become a popular drug of choice. However, there is a large gap between actual drug use on campus and how prevalent students believe drug use to be. When researchers compared students' frequency of drug use with what students perceived to be the frequency of drug use by "the average student," they found that students greatly overestimate the use of a variety of drugs. Martens et al. found that while 3 percent of college students reported drinking alcohol daily, 43 percent of students perceived that a typical student consumes alcohol on a daily basis.

This research team also discovered that while 69 percent of the students indicated that they had not used marijuana within the past 30 days, 94 percent of the students surveyed believed that a typical student had done so. With regard to cocaine use, 96 percent of the college students surveyed reported they had not used cocaine in the past 30 days, whereas 60 percent of the students surveyed believed that a typical student used cocaine at least once in the past 30 days.[35]

Data from the *National College Health Assessment—NCHA II, Canadian Reference Group Executive Summary, Spring 2013*[36] shows a low prevalence of actual use of any marijuana within the last 30 days prior to the survey, at a total of 16.0 percent for both male and female undergraduate students, compared to the perceived use of 83.8 percent. Any actual use within the last 30 days of all other drugs combined (cocaine, methamphetamine, sedatives, hallucinogens, MDMA, and other illegal drugs) for both males and females was 10.7 percent, whereas the perceived use was 72.5 percent. This data was collected from 8192 undergraduate students attending one of eight Canadian postsecondary institutions.

Data from the *National College Health Assessment—NCHA II, American College Health Association, Spring 2015* also shows a low prevalence of any actual marijuana use within the last 30 days prior to the survey, at 16.9 percent for both male and female undergraduate students, compared to the perceived use of 81.9 percent. Any actual use within the last 30 days of all other drugs combined (cigars, smokeless tobacco, cocaine, methamphetamine, sedatives, hallucinogens, anabolic steroids, opiates, inhalants, MDMA, other club drugs, and other illegal drugs) for both males and females was 10.9 percent, whereas the perceived use was 76.2 percent. The American data was collected from 93 034 students from 148 postsecondary institutions.[37]

Various factors influence which students use drugs, including the following:

- **Perception of risk.** Students seem most likely to try substances they perceive as being safe or low risk. Of these, the top three are caffeine, alcohol, and tobacco; marijuana is listed fourth in terms of perceived safety.
- **Alcohol use.** Individuals often engage in more than one risk behaviour, and researchers have documented correlations among smoking, drinking, and drug use. Among college and university students, those who report binge drinking are much more likely than other students to report current or past use of marijuana, cocaine, or other illegal drugs.[38]
- **Environment.** As with alcohol use, students are influenced by their friends, their residence, the general public's attitude toward drug use, and even the Internet.

Increasingly, college and university health officials are realizing that they must change the environment to promote healthier lifestyle choices. One successful innovation is the Living, Learning, and Lifestyle residence themed communities at McMaster University. Students can choose from a number of options such as an Alcohol Free Living Community or a Healthy Active Living Community dorm.[39]

In addition to illicit drug use there is a growing concern about the increased recreational or non-medical use of over-the-counter and prescription medication among college and university students. Using medication for purposes other than what it is developed or prescribed for can result in serious medical problems.

In a study by Sharp and Rosén,[40] 8 percent of students surveyed reported personally giving away or selling their stimulant prescription medication to another student who did not have a prescription. Almost 63 percent of participants in this study reported knowing someone who had sold or given away a prescribed stimulant medication for recreational use. Almost 67 percent of students reported knowing someone who had taken prescribed stimulant medication on a recreational basis. One of the most popular stimulant prescriptions used improperly is ADD/ADHD medication, which includes methylphenidate, dextroamphetamine, and amphetamine salts. The most common reasons reported for misusing over-the-counter or prescription medication were to be able to prolong a night of partying (about 26 percent) or to be able to stay up later or focus on studying (60 percent).[41]

In the past couple of years, college and university student use of *Salvia divinorum*, a species of the mint family, has seen an increased use as a hallucinogen. The leaves of this plant can be chewed or smoked. The psychoactive compound, salvinorin A, is then released. Internet sources include a dried leaf product or oral tincture.[42] Due to the potential health risks to young people who use this substance, Health Canada added salvia to Schedule IV of the Controlled Drugs and Substances Act (CDSA) in February 2016. This means that it is now illegal to sell, export, or produce this psychedelic herb in Canada. Simple possession is not banned.[43]

There are so many good health-related reasons not to use alcohol and drugs. Another reason is the reported increase in intimate partner violence (IPV) among college and university students whose lifestyle choices include drug use. In one study of 1938 college students, cannabis users were 35 percent more likely to take part in a physical assault against their intimate partner compared to those who did not use the drug. The use of a depressant was even more alarming, with 57 percent of students more likely to assault a partner compared to those who did not use a form of depressant substance.[44]

If you are a student who has experienced partner abuse or has violated someone due to your substance abuse, counselling and assistance from resident advisors (RAs), community leaders (CLs), or medical and counselling professionals are ways you might address this very serious situation.

✓ CHECK-IN

How widespread is drug use on your campus?

Drugs and Driving Drugs affect driving ability in different ways. Impairment of driving skills is evident with cannabis, or THC (delta-9-tetrahydrocannabinol, a major psychoactive ingredient) levels of 2–5 ng/ml (using oral fluid as the test medium that is reflective of the concentration of THC in the blood). The risk of a car crash begins to increase at THC levels of 1 ng/ml. Notable impairment includes the ability to stay in the lane through curves, brake quickly, and maintain speed and a safe distance between cars. It also slows thinking and reflexes. Normal driving skills remain impaired for four to six hours after smoking a single joint. There is an elevated risk of traffic collisions among heavy cannabis users.

Amphetamines, after repeated use, impair coordination. They can also make a driver more edgy and less coordinated, and thus more likely to be involved in an accident. Hallucinogens distort judgment and reality and cause confusion and panic, thus making driving extremely dangerous. Sedatives, hypnotics, and antianxiety agents slow reaction time and interfere with hand-eye coordination and judgment. The greatest impairment is in the first hour after taking the drug. The effects depend on the particular drug.

A mixture of alcohol and drugs can affect driving ability even more. Alcohol, which affects perception, coordination, and judgment, can also increase the sedative effects of tranquilizers and barbiturates.

Here are some of the findings from the *Alcohol & Drug Use Among Drivers, British Columbia Roadside Survey 2012*, where 89 percent of drivers from 2513 vehicles (from five separate communities—Prince George, Kelowna, Saanich, Vancouver, and Abbotsford) provided breath samples and 70.4 percent provided oral fluid samples:[45]

- Of the drivers who provided breath samples, 8.3 percent had a positive blood alcohol concentration (BAC ≥ 5 mg/dL). The highest recorded BAC was 400 mg/dL. Kelowna and Prince George had the highest percentage of drivers with positive BACs (9.6 percent) and Abbotsford had the lowest (5.4 percent). There was a reduction in alcohol-positive drivers in all five communities in 2012 compared to 2010.
- Of the 1757 drivers who agreed to provide oral fluid samples, 10.1 percent tested positive for drugs. Eighty-three percent tested positive for one drug and 16.9 percent tested positive for more than one drug.
- While there were a total of 216 drugs detected in the drivers tested in 2012, cannabis use was the most frequently found substance at 43.6 percent. The minimum level found was 2 ng/ml. The highest recorded level was greater than 40 ng/ml. Data showed that in 2012, 61.5 percent of the samples were over 40 ng/ml.
- Cocaine accounted for the second-most-detected drug at 33 percent.
- The frequency of amphetamines/methamphetamines detected was 14.2 percent, opiates 8.7 percent, and benzodiazepines 0.5 percent.

If you are drinking or using drugs, understand that your driving skills are compromised. Make the decision not to drive. Be safe. Be respectful of others and yourself.

> **✓ CHECK-IN**
>
> Do you or your friends use drugs and then drive?

COMMON DRUGS OF ABUSE

The psychoactive substances most often associated with both abuse and dependence include alcohol (discussed in Chapter 12), amphetamines, cannabis (marijuana), cocaine, club drugs, hallucinogens, inhalants, opioids, phencyclidine (PCP), and sedative-hypnotic drugs. Table 11-2 groups the common drugs of abuse by their effect on the mind.

Amphetamines **Amphetamines,** stimulants that were once widely prescribed for weight control because they suppress appetite, have emerged as a global danger. They trigger the release of epinephrine (adrenaline), which stimulates the central nervous system. Amphetamines are sold under a variety of names: amphetamine (brand name Benzedrine®, street name bennies), dextroamphetamine (Dexedrine®, dex), methamphetamine (Methedrine®, meth, speed), and Desoxyn® (copilots). Related *uppers* include the prescription drugs methylphenidate (Ritalin®), pemoline (Cylert®), and phenmetrazine (Preludin®). Amphetamines are available in tablet or capsule form. Abusers might grind and sniff the capsules or make a solution and inject the drug.

Methamphetamine (MA), also known as **crystal meth,** is a white, odourless, bitter-tasting crystalline powder that readily dissolves in water or alcohol. It can be snorted, swallowed, or injected.[46] *Ice* (or crank, crystal, glass, tina, bulb baby, chore boy, hitter, pink glass, freshies, Geek, Gack, Geet, hooking up) is a smokeable form of methamphetamine. This drug is very popular among young people across Canada, and its potential to harm users is greater than ever.[47] Because of the significant health, social, and economic harm caused by this drug for young people, their families, law enforcement officers, and our environment, stiff new penalties for possession, trafficking, importation, exportation, and production of methamphetamine were announced in August 2005.

Methamphetamine was moved to Schedule 1 of the *Controlled Drugs and Substances Act* in 2009 in Canada and further revisions were made in 2010. These changes allow for the highest maximum penalties.[48] This is just one of a number of strategies (education, laws for illegal possession of chemicals for purposes of producing this drug, and rehabilitation) being taken to deal with the devastation methamphetamine is having on communities everywhere.

"Meth" is made by heating many chemical ingredients together and includes these not-so-appealing ingredients:[49]

- Red phosphorus—used to make safety matches, fireworks, and pesticides
- Hydrochloric acid—used to treat industrial waste
- Anhydrous ammonia—a source of fertilizer for farm crops

TABLE 11-2

Drug Categories and Descriptions

Type of Drug	Drug Name	Common Name	Description	How It's Used	Related Paraphernalia	Signs and Symptoms of Use
Cannabis	Marijuana	Pot, grass, reefer, weed, Colombian hash, sinsemilla, joint, blunts, Acapulco gold, Thai sticks, skunk, 420	Like dried oregano or tea leaves, from a pale green to a brown colour	Usually smoked in hand-rolled cigarettes, pipes, or thin cigars or ingested. The use of vaporizers are common now too.	Rolling papers, pipes, bongs, baggies, roach clips	Sweet burnt odour, neglect of appearance, loss of motivation, slow reactions, red eyes, memory lapses
	Hash	Hash, resin, brown, boom, chronic gangster, hemp	Substance varying from soft to very hard in consistency; light brown to black in colour	Smoked or ingested	Pipes, bong pipes, safety pins, hot knives	Loss of inhibitions, relaxation, reduction of anxiety, hilarity, fatigue, drowsiness
	Hash oil	Oil, honey oil, liquid hash	Thick liquid substance; yellow, orange-yellow, dark brown, or black in colour	Smoked	Spoons, hash pipe	Odour, red eyes, pasty mouth, slurred speech, slowed mental reactions, increased appetite
Depressants (Depress the nervous system)	Alcohol	Booze, hooch, juice, brew, alcopops (hard lemonade or fruit juices)	Clear or amber-coloured liquid; sweet, fruit-flavoured malt-based drinks	Swallowed in liquid form	Flask, bottles, cans, use of food colour to disguise it; colourful and innocent-looking labels	Impaired judgment, poor muscle coordination, lowered inhibitions
	Barbiturates Amyl®, Seconal®, Nembutal®, Butisol®, Tuinal® Phenobarbital®	Barbs, downers, yellows, yellow jackets, reds, red birds, phennies, tooies, red devils, blue devils	Variety of tablets, capsules, powder	Swallowed in pill form or injected	Syringe, needles	Drowsiness, confusion, impaired judgment, slurred speech, needle marks, staggering gait
	Tranquilizers/ Benzodiazepines Ativan®, Halcion®, Valium®, Librium®, Miltown®, Xanax®	Vs, blues, downers, candy, sleeping pills	Variety of tablets	Swallowed in pill form or injected	Syringe, pill bottles, needles	Drowsiness, faulty judgment, disorientation
	GHB (gamma hydroxybutyrate)	Georgia home boy, grievous bodily harm, liquid ecstasy, G	Clear liquid, tablet, capsule	Swallowed, dissolved in drinks	Drinks, pop cans	Can relax or sedate, drowsiness, nausea, vomiting, headache, loss of consciousness, loss of reflexes, seizures, coma, death

(Continued)

TABLE 11-2

Drug Categories and Descriptions *(Continued)*

Type of Drug	Drug Name	Common Name	Description	How It's Used	Related Paraphernalia	Signs and Symptoms of Use
Depressants (Depress the nervous system)	Rohypnol®	Roofies, roche, love drug, forget-me pill	Tablet	Dissolved in drinks, swallowed	Drinks, pop cans	Amnesia, decreased blood pressure, urinary retention, sedative effect
Opioids and Morphine Derivatives	Heroin	Brown sugar, dope, H, horse, junk, skag, skunk, smack, white horse, point	White or brown powders, tablets, capsules, liquid	Injected, smoked, snorted; may be blended with marijuana	Syringes, spoon, lighter, needles, medicine dropper	Lethargy, loss of skin colour, track marks, constricted pupils, decreased coordination
	Morphine (Roxanol, Duramorph)	M, Miss Emma, monkey, white stuff	Oral solutions, immediate and sustained-release tables and capsules, suppositories, and injectable preparations	Swallowed, injected, inhaled, smoked	Hypodermic needles, small cotton balls, spoons or bottle caps, tie-offs, razor blades, straws, pipes	Reduced gut motility, faintness, bradychardia, palpitations, flushing, dry mouth, visual distortions
	Oxycodone HCL, Percocet		White, odourless, crystalline power, or pink oval tablet, blue round tablet, peach oval tablet, yellow capsule-shaped tablet	Chewed and swallowed, crushed and snorted, crushed, dissolved in water and then injected	Spoons, needles, water	Respiratory depression, apnea, respiratory arrest, shock, light-headedness, dizziness, nausea, drowsiness, vomiting
Stimulants (Stimulate the nervous system)	Amphetamines, Biphetamine, Dexedrine	Speed, uppers, bennies, dexies, meth, crank, black beauties, white crosses, LA Turnaround, hearts, truck drivers	Variety of tablets, capsules, and crystal-like rock salt	Swallowed in pill or capsule form, smoked, or injected	Syringe, needles	Excess activity, irritability, nervousness, mood swings, needle marks, dilated pupils, talkativeness then depression
	MDMA (Methylenedioxy-methamphetamine)	Adam, clarity, Ecstasy, Eve, lover's speed, peace, STP, X, XTC, beans, disco biscuits, smarties, scoobies, peanut, dove	Tablets, imprinted logos	Usually swallowed in tablet form, or crushed and sniffed	Razor blade, straws, glass surface	Increased alertness, excitation, insomnia, loss of appetite, panic attacks, respiratory failure
	Methamphetamine, Desoxyn	Chalk, crank, crystal, fire, glass, go fast, ice, meth, speed, P	White, odourless, bitter-tasting crystalline powder, fine transparent shiny crystals, or tablets with various logos and colours	Snorted, injected, or smoked	Needles, pipes	Impaired memory and learning, hyperthermia, cardiac toxicity, renal failure, liver toxicity

TABLE 11-2

Drug Categories and Descriptions (*Continued*)

Type of Drug	Drug Name	Common Name	Description	How It's Used	Related Paraphernalia	Signs and Symptoms of Use
Stimulants (Stimulate the nervous system)	Cocaine	Coke, snow, toot, white lady, blow, bump, flake, rock	White odourless powder	Usually inhaled; can be injected, swallowed, or smoked	Razor blade, straws, glass surfaces	Restlessness, dilated pupils, oily skin, talkativeness; euphoric short-term high, followed by depression
	Tobacco/Nicotine	Smokes, butts, cigs, cancer sticks, snuff, dip, chew, plug	Dried brown organic material, bidis flavoured with mint or chocolate; moist for electronic cigarettes	Burned and inhaled as cigarettes, pipes, cigars, cigarillos; chewed or inhaled through the nose as snuff	Rolling papers, pipes, spit cups, cigar cutters, lighters, matches	Shortness of breath, respiratory illnesses; oral, lung, and other cancers
Hallucinogens (Alter perceptions of reality)	PCP (phencyclidine)	Angel dust, killer weed, supergrass, hog, peace pill, boat, Crazy Eddie, mess	White powder or tablet	Usually smoked, can be inhaled (snorted), injected, or swallowed in tablets	Tinfoil	Slurred speech, blurred vision, lack of coordination, confusion, agitation, violence, unpredictability, "bad trips"
	LSD (lysergic acid diethylamide)	Acid, cubes, blotter, boomers, microdot, yellow sunshines, purple haze, white lightning	Odourless, colourless, tasteless powder	Absorbed orally in blotter paper, liquid, or tablets	Blotter papers, tinfoil	Dilated pupils, illusions, hallucinations, disorientation, mood swings, nausea, flashbacks
	Mescaline	Mesc, buttons, cactus, caps, peyote	Capsules, tablets, tops of cactus, dried roots	Smoked, chewed, or brewed as tea	Water, pots	Anxiety, racing heart, dizziness, diarrhea, vomiting, headache
	Psilocybin	Magic mushrooms, purple passion, shrooms, mush, Fly agaric, liberties	Dry, fibrous substance of varying colours	Ingestion, eaten raw or brewed as a tea	Water, pots	Fear, paranoia; distortion of colour, sound, and objects; time sped up or slowed down
Inhalants (Substances abused by sniffing)	Solvents, aerosols	Airplane glue, gasoline, dry cleaning solution, correction fluid	Chemicals that produce mind-altering vapours	Inhaled or sniffed, often with the use of paper or plastic bags	Cleaning rags, empty spray cans, tubes of glue, baggies	Poor motor coordination; bad breath; impaired vision, memory, and thoughts; violent behaviour

(*Continued*)

TABLE 11-2

Drug Categories and Descriptions *(Continued)*

Type of Drug	Drug Name	Common Name	Description	How It's Used	Related Paraphernalia	Signs and Symptoms of Use
Inhalants (Substances abused by sniffing)	Nitrates (amyl & butyl)	Poppers, locker room, rush, snappers	Clear yellowish liquid	Inhaled or sniffed from gauze or single-dose glass vials	Cloth-covered bulb that pops when broken, small bottles	Slowed thought, headache
	Nitrous oxide	Laughing gas, whippets	Colourless gas with sweet taste and smell	Inhaled or sniffed by mask or cone	Aerosol cans such as whipped cream, small canisters	Light-headed, loss of motor control

Sources: From "A Parent's Guide for the Prevention of Alcohol, Tobacco and Other Drug Use." Copyright © 2000 Lowe Family Foundation, Inc., Revised 2001. (Lowe Family Foundation, 3339 Stuyvesant Pl. NW, Washington DC, 20015, 202-362-4883.); National Institute on Drug Abuse (NIDA Home, Drugs of Abuse/Related Topics, Commonly Abused Drugs.) Found at: www.drugabuse.gov/DrugPages/DrugsofAbuse.html; Report on the Illicit Drug Situation in Canada, 2009. Criminal Intelligence, RCMP. Found at www.rcmp-grc.gc.ca/drugs-drogues/2009/drug-drogue-2009-eng.pdf.

How Users Feel Amphetamines produce an initial intense, pleasurable rush that lasts for a few minutes. This rush is then followed by a prolonged physical and psychological high, a state of hyper-alertness and energy that can last from 4 to 12 hours. Higher doses make users feel wired: talkative, excited, restless, and irritable.

Adverse effects include confusion, rambling or incoherent speech, anxiety, mood swings, headache, and palpitations. Individuals may become paranoid; be convinced they are having profound thoughts; feel increased sexual interest; and experience unusual perceptions, such as ringing in the ears, a sensation of insects crawling on their skin, or hearing their name called. Methamphetamine produces exceptionally long-lasting toxic effects, including psychosis, violence, seizures, and cardiovascular abnormalities. Brain-imaging studies show changes in heavy users' brains that might affect learning and memory.[50]

Risks Dependence on amphetamines can develop with episodic or daily use. Users typically take amphetamines in large doses to prevent crashing. Bingeing—taking high doses over a period of several days—can lead to an extremely intense and unpleasant crash characterized by a craving for the drug, shakiness, irritability, anxiety, and depression. Two or more days are required for recuperation. Other risks include increased heart rate, dilated pupils, elevated blood pressure, perspiration or chills and nausea or vomiting, impaired breathing, chest pain, heart arrhythmia, confusion, seizures, impaired movements or muscle tone, or even coma.

Withdrawal Amphetamine withdrawal usually persists for more than 24 hours after cessation of prolonged, heavy use. Its characteristic features include fatigue, disturbing dreams, much more or less than usual sleep, increased appetite, and speeding up or slowing down of physical movements. Those who are unable to sleep despite their exhaustion often take sedative-hypnotics to help them rest and may then become dependent on them as well as amphetamines. Symptoms usually reach a peak in two to four days, although depression and irritability may persist for months. Suicide is a major risk.

Experts say that crystal meth is one of the most addictive and hardest-to-treat street drugs. Some addiction counsellors suggest that the relapse rate is 92 percent. Tragic stories are becoming public across Canada as this drug takes over the lives of young people everywhere.

Cannabis **Marijuana** (pot) and **hashish** (hash)—the most widely used illegal drugs—are derived from the cannabis plant. The major psychoactive ingredient in both is *THC (delta-9-tetrahydrocannabinol)*.[51]

THC triggers a series of reactions in the brain that ultimately lead to the high that users experience when they smoke marijuana. Heredity influences an individual's response to marijuana—research suggests that there may be a genetic basis for an individual's response to THC.

Different types of marijuana have different percentages of THC. Because of careful cultivation, the strength of today's marijuana is much greater than that used in the 1970s; the physical and mental effects are therefore greater. Usually, marijuana is smoked in a joint (hand-rolled cigarette) or pipe; it may also be eaten as an ingredient in other foods (as when baked in brownies), though with a less predictable effect. The circumstances in which marijuana is smoked, the communal aspects of its use, and the user's experience all can affect the way a marijuana-induced high feels.[52]

Some individuals use medical marijuana to deal with certain medical and health conditions. In Canada, these individuals must legally access marijuana through the Marijuana Medical Access Regulations (MMRAs). The cannabis that is provided through this program is monitored so that contamination with unknown substances is prevented. It is available in plant, pill, and oral spray form. It is approved only to relieve symptoms caused by anticancer therapy, to help AIDS patients, and for relief from symptoms of some diseases such as muscular sclerosis.[53]

In addition to concerns about the current medical use of cannabis, there is an ongoing debate in public and political circles about decriminalizing and legalizing marijuana use for Canadians. On one side of the debate are people who believe any legal use of cannabis would lead to increased drug use by Canadians. On the other side are people who believe that more control could be put in place if cannabis was legalized. At the time of revising this chapter the Government of Canada had begun work on legalizing cannabis. A federal–provincial–territorial task force was created to direct this process.[54]

✓ CHECK-IN

Do you think the federal government's commitment to decriminalizing and legalizing marijuana in Canada is a good decision? Why? Why not?

How Users Feel In low to moderate doses, marijuana typically creates a mild sense of euphoria, a sense of slowed time, a dreamy sort of self-absorption, and some impairment in thinking and communicating. Users report heightened sensations of colour, sound, and other stimuli; relaxation; and increased confidence. The sense of being *stoned* peaks within half an hour and usually lasts about three hours. Even when alterations in perception seem slight, as noted earlier, it is not safe to drive a car for as long as four to six hours after smoking marijuana.[55] Some users experience acute paranoia or anxiety, which may be accompanied by a panicky fear of losing control. They may believe that their companions are ridiculing or threatening them and experience a panic attack, a state of intense terror.

The immediate physical effects of marijuana include increased pulse rate, bloodshot eyes, dry mouth and throat, slowed reaction times, impaired motor skills, increased appetite, and diminished short-term memory (see Figure 11-5). The drug remains in the body's fat cells 50 hours or more after use, so people may experience psychoactive effects for several days after use. Drug tests may produce positive results for days or weeks after last use.

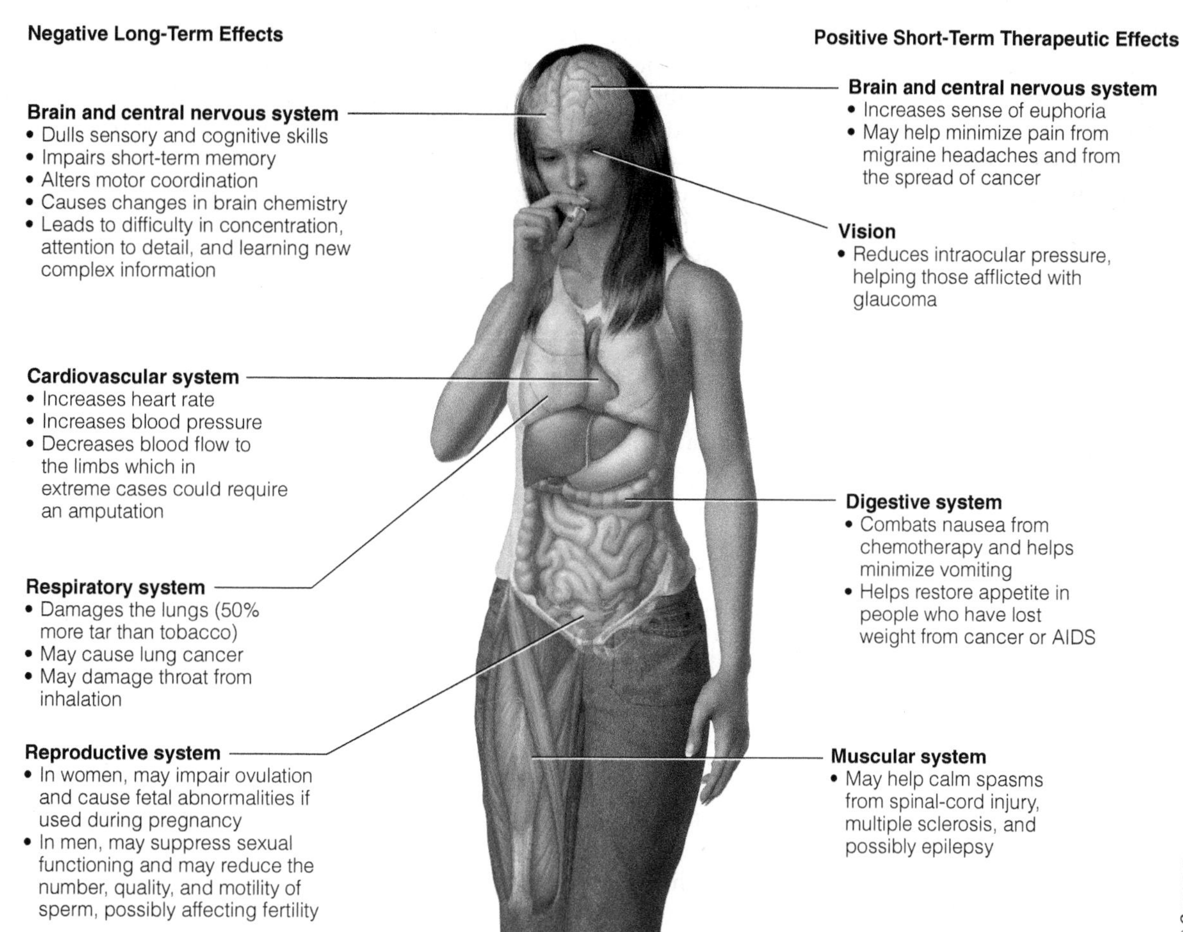

Figure 11-5 Some Effects of Marijuana on the Body

There are both negative long-term effects and positive short-term therapeutic effects of marijuana use.

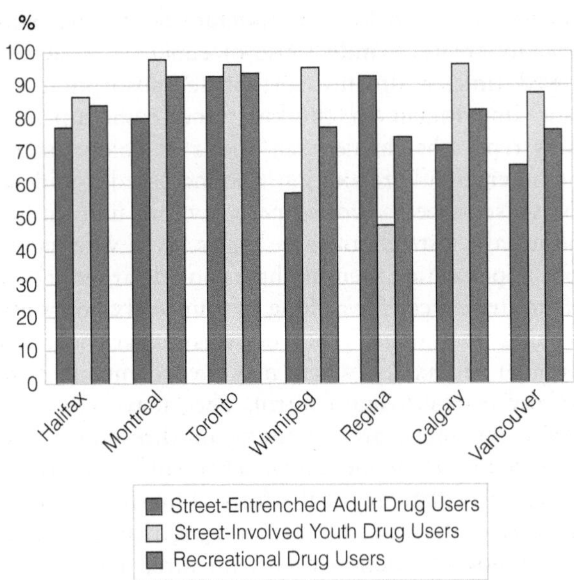

Figure 11-6 Prevalence of Past-Year Cannabis Use among High-Risk Population by City (2013)

Source: Canadian Centre on Substance Abuse (2016). Canadian drug summary: Cannabis. http://www.ccsa.ca/Resource%20Library/CCSA-Canadian-Drug-Summary-Cannabis-2015-en.pdf (page 4, Figure 2). Reproduced with permission from the Canadian Centre on Substance Abuse.

Risks Marijuana produces a range of effects in different bodily systems, such as diminished immune responses and impaired fertility in men. Other risks include damage to the brain, lungs, and heart and to babies born to mothers who use marijuana during pregnancy or while nursing. Health Canada considers three specific groups as high-risk populations. Figure 11-6 illustrates the prevalence of past-year cannabis use among these groups. Recreational drug users are considered an at-risk group. To be a recreational drug user in the Health Canada study, individuals had to have used at least one drug (excluding alcohol and tobacco) at least once in the last six months prior to their interview.

Brain THC produces changes in the brain that affect learning, memory, and the way the brain integrates sensory experiences with emotions and motivations. Short-term effects include problems with memory and learning, distorted perceptions, difficulty thinking and problem-solving, loss of coordination, increased anxiety, and panic attacks. Long-term use produces changes in the brain similar to those seen with other major drugs of abuse. As stated earlier in this chapter, there also appears to be a possible link to a greater risk of developing schizophrenia as individuals age.[56]

Lungs Regular marijuana smokers have many of the same respiratory problems as tobacco smokers, including daily cough and phlegm, chronic bronchitis, and more frequent chest colds. This could be because cannabis smoke does contain many of the same poisons and carcinogens that are in tobacco smoke. As well, THC, the active ingredient in cannabis, may make the lungs and airways more susceptible to respiratory problems. Chronic use can lead to bronchitis and Chronic Obstructive Pulmonary Disease (COPD), a progressive lung disease that damages air sacs in the lungs and narrows and blocks the airways. Some research suggests a strong link between lung cancer and smoking marijuana too. One study reported a case of small-cell lung cancer in a 22-year-old male who had smoked one marijuana joint three times a week for three years. He had not smoked cigarettes. He also had no known genetic history of cancer. Treatment resulted in a 16-month reprieve of the disease, but the cancer metastasized to the liver and para-aortic lymph nodes.[57] The authors of this study suggest that although the association between lung cancer and cannabis has not been proven to date, more studies are needed.

Heart Otherwise healthy people have suffered heart attacks shortly after smoking marijuana. However, the research about the health effects of marijuana is still confusing. A longitudinal study by Frost et al. determined that while there was no statistically significant association between marijuana use and mortality, the rate of mortality in patients who used marijuana and died from myocardial infarctions (heart attack) was 29 percent higher than patients who reported no use of marijuana.[58] In another study, the data suggested that older people who use marijuana might be at greater risk of coronary artery or cerebrovascular disease. Arayna and Williams state that we might not be recognizing the connection between marijuana and heart attacks.[59] Much more research is needed but research can be difficult due to the fact that many people who use marijuana also smoke tobacco. There are also legal issues to deal with.

Pregnancy While research on the use of marijuana during pregnancy has some conflicting results, some studies have found that pre-school–aged children born to mothers who had heavy cannabis use demonstrate shortfalls in memory, verbal and perceptual skills, and visual reasoning. In older children links to impaired abstract and visual reasoning and deficits in reading and spelling were found. Children aged 10 showed a higher level of depressive and anxious symptoms than children of non-users. Poorer scores on academic achievement at the age of 14 years have also been recorded, especially in reading tests.[60]

Withdrawal Marijuana users can develop a compulsive, often uncontrollable, craving for the drug. Stopping after long-term marijuana use can produce *marijuana withdrawal syndrome*, which is characterized by insomnia, restlessness, loss of appetite, and irritability.

Cocaine Cocaine (coke, snow, lady) is a white crystalline powder extracted from the leaves of the South American coca plant. Usually mixed with various sugars and local anesthetics such as lidocaine and procaine, cocaine powder is generally inhaled. When sniffed or snorted, cocaine anesthetizes the nerve endings in the nose and relaxes the lung's bronchial muscles.

Cocaine can be dissolved in water and injected intravenously. The drug is rapidly metabolized by the liver, so the high is relatively brief, typically lasting only about 20 minutes. This means that users will commonly inject the drug repeatedly, increasing the risk of infection and damage to their veins. Many intravenous cocaine users prefer the practice of *speedballing*, the intravenous administration of a combination of cocaine and heroin.

Cocaine alkaloid, or *freebase*, is obtained by removing the hydrochloride salt from cocaine powder. *Freebasing* is smoking the fumes of the alkaloid form of cocaine. *Crack*, pharmacologically identical to freebase, is a cheap, easy-to-use, widely available, smokeable, and potent form of cocaine named for the popping sound it makes when burned. Because it is absorbed rapidly into the bloodstream and large doses reach the brain very quickly, it is particularly dangerous. However, its low price and easy availability have made it a common drug of abuse. In a 2013 study of high-risk populations, researchers found that cocaine was the second most commonly used illicit substance after cannabis among street-entrenched and recreational adult drug users. See Figure 11-7 for prevalence of past-year cocaine use among these groups in a number of cities across Canada.[61]

How Users Feel A powerful stimulant to the central nervous system, cocaine targets several chemical sites in the brain, producing feelings of soaring well-being and boundless energy. Users feel they have enormous physical and mental ability, yet are also restless and anxious. After a brief period of euphoria, users slump into

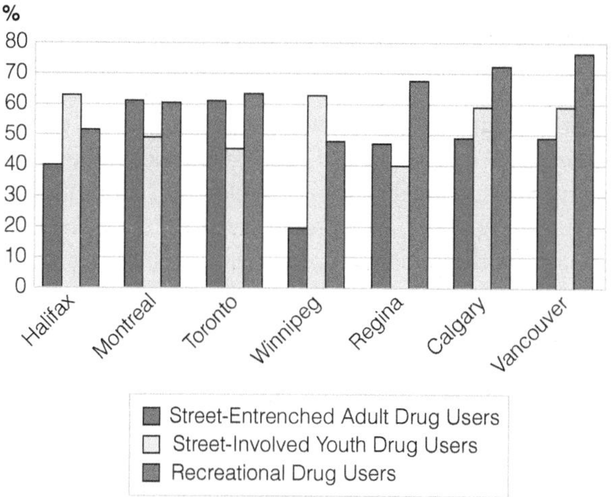

Figure 11-7 Prevalence of Self-Reported Past-Year Cocaine Use among High-Risk Population by City (2013)

Source: Canadian Centre on Substance Abuse (2016). Canadian drug summary: Cocaine. http://www.ccsa.ca/Resource%20Library/CCSA-Cocaine-Drug-Summary-2015-en.pdf (page 4, Figure 2). Reproduced with permission from the Canadian Centre on Substance Abuse.

a depression. They often go on cocaine binges, lasting from a few hours to several days, and consume large quantities of cocaine.

With crack, dependence develops quickly. As soon as crack users come down from one high, they want more crack. Whereas heroin addicts may shoot up several times a day, crack addicts need another hit within minutes. Thus, a crack habit can quickly become more expensive than heroin addiction. Police have traced many brutal crimes and murders to young crack addicts, who often are extremely paranoid and dangerous. Smoking crack doused with liquid PCP, a practice known as *space-basing*, has especially frightening effects on behaviour.

With continuing use, cocaine users experience less pleasure and more unpleasant effects. Eventually they might reach a point at which they no longer experience euphoric effects and crave the drug simply to alleviate their persistent hunger for it.

Risks Cocaine dependence is an easy habit to acquire. There are many effects on the body (see Figure 11-8). With repeated use, the brain becomes tolerant of the drug's stimulant effects, and users must take more of it to get high. Those who smoke or inject cocaine can develop dependence within weeks. Those who sniff cocaine may not become dependent on the drug for months or years.

The physical effects of acute cocaine intoxication include dilated pupils, elevated or lowered blood pressure, perspiration or chills, nausea or vomiting, speeding up or slowing down of physical activity, muscular weakness, impaired breathing, chest pain, and impaired movements or muscle tone.[62] Prolonged cocaine snorting can result in ulceration of the mucous membrane of the nose and damage to the nasal septum (the membrane between the nostrils) severe enough to cause it to collapse. Men who use cocaine regularly have problems maintaining erections and ejaculating. They also tend to have low sperm counts, less active sperm, and more abnormal sperm than non-users. Both male and female chronic cocaine users tend to lose interest in sex and have difficulty reaching orgasm.

Cocaine use can cause blood vessels in the brain to clamp shut and can trigger a stroke, bleeding in the brain, and potentially fatal brain seizures. Cocaine users can also develop psychiatric or neurological complications. Repeated or high doses of cocaine can lead to impaired judgment, hyperactivity, non-stop babbling, feelings of suspicion and paranoia, and violent behaviour.

Cocaine can damage the liver and cause lung damage in freebasers. Smoking crack causes bronchitis as well as lung damage and may promote the transmission of HIV through burned and bleeding lips. Some smokers have died of respiratory complications, such as pulmonary edema (the buildup of fluid in the lungs).

Cocaine causes the heart rate to speed up and blood pressure to rise suddenly. Its use is associated with many cardiac complications, including arrhythmia (disruption

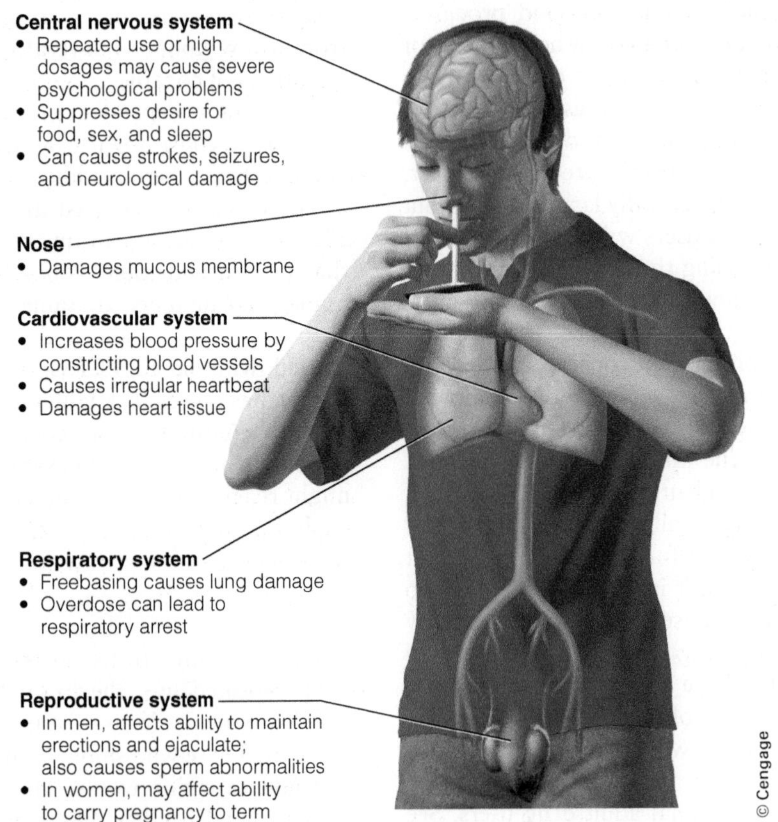

Figure 11-8 Some Effects of Cocaine on the Body

of heart rhythm), angina (chest pain), and acute myocardial infarction (heart attack). These cardiac complications can lead to sudden death.[63] The most common ways of dying from cocaine use are persistent seizures that result in respiratory collapse, cardiac arrest from arrhythmias, myocardial infarction, and intracranial hemorrhage or stroke. Cocaine-induced elevations in blood pressure can lead to kidney failure.

Cocaine users who inject the drug and share needles put themselves at risk for another potentially lethal problem: HIV infection. Other complications of injecting cocaine include skin infections, hepatitis, inflammation of the arteries, and infection of the lining of the heart.

The combination of alcohol and cocaine is particularly lethal. When people mix cocaine and alcohol, they compound the danger each drug poses. The liver combines the two agents and manufactures cocaethylene, which intensifies cocaine's euphoric effects while possibly increasing the risk of sudden death.

Cocaine is dangerous for pregnant women and their babies, causing miscarriages, developmental disorders, and life-threatening complications during birth. Infants born to cocaine and crack users can suffer withdrawal and may have major complications or permanent disabilities. Cocaine babies have higher-than-normal rates of respiratory and kidney troubles, visual problems, and developmental retardation, and they may be at greater risk of sudden infant death syndrome.

Withdrawal When addicted individuals stop using cocaine, they often become depressed. Other symptoms of cocaine withdrawal include fatigue, vivid and disturbing dreams, excessive or too little sleep, irritability, increased appetite, and physical slowing down or speeding up. This initial crash may last one to three days after cutting down or stopping the heavy use of cocaine. Some individuals become violent, paranoid, and suicidal.

Symptoms usually reach a peak in two to four days, although depression, anxiety, irritability, lack of pleasure in usual activities, and low-level cravings may continue for weeks. As memories of the crash fade, the desire for cocaine intensifies. For many weeks after stopping, individuals may feel an intense craving for the drug. Experimental medical approaches for treating cocaine dependence include antidepressant drugs, anticonvulsant drugs, and the naturally occurring amino acids tryptophan and tyrosine. Research has found that, depending on personal characteristics such as abstract reasoning ability and religious motivation, some cocaine abusers fare better with cognitive-behavioural therapy, while others do better with 12-step programs.[64]

✓ CHECK-IN

What is your impression of the dangers of crack cocaine?

Club Drugs **Club drugs** include MDMA (ecstasy), gamma hydroxy-butyrate (GHB), flunitrazepam (Rohypnol®), LSD and amphetamines, and methamphetamine (see Table 11-2). Their primary users are teens and young adults at nightclubs, bars, and raves or trance events, night-long dances often held in warehouses. They try these low-cost drugs to increase their stamina and experience a high.

Some club drugs, although illegal in Canada, are sold elsewhere in the world as legitimate drugs. Two examples are **gamma hydroxybutyrate (GHB)**, a depressant with potential benefits for people with narcolepsy, and Rohypnol®, used as a tranquilizer. GHB is usually found in liquid form. Rohypnol® comes in a small pill or white tablet form. Both are colourless, odourless, and have no taste when mixed with a drink.

Although users may think of club drugs as harmless and fun, they can produce a range of unwanted effects, sometimes even causing death. GHB can cause dizziness, nausea, vomiting, seizures, unconsciousness, coma, and memory loss. Rohypnol® causes sedation, loss of inhibitions, blackouts, and amnesia. Sexual violence is often linked with the use of these drugs.[65] When used with alcohol or other drugs, club drugs can be even more harmful because they involve the same brain mechanism.[66] Some people have been known to have extreme, even fatal, reactions the first time they use club drugs. Club drugs found in party settings are often adulterated or impure and thus even more dangerous.

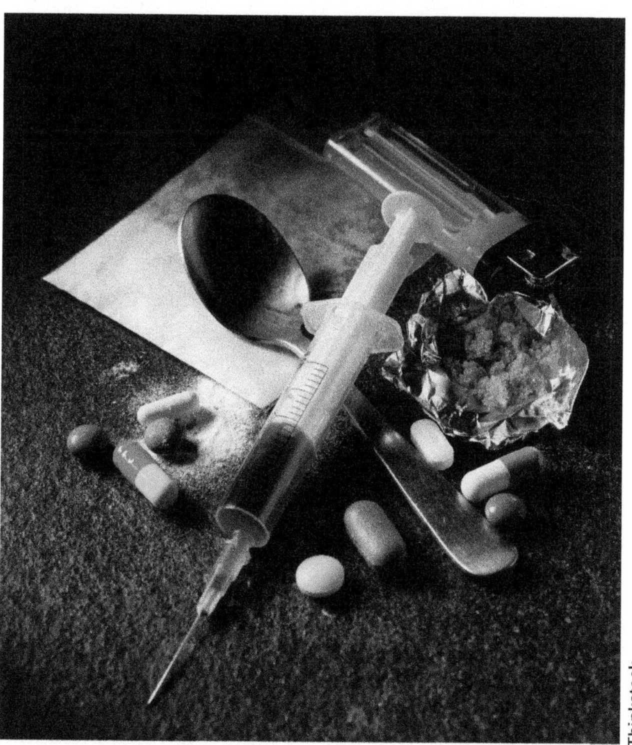

Club drugs, made in a laboratory and sold on the street, are not subject to quality controls and do not always contain what the buyer expects.

Ecstasy Ecstasy is the most common street name for methylenedioxymethamphetamine (**MDMA**), a synthetic compound with both stimulant and mildly hallucinogenic properties. Ecstasy use has been increasing substantially, particularly among young people. Although it can be smoked, inhaled (snorted), or injected, ecstasy is almost always taken as a pill or tablet. Its effects begin in 45 minutes and last for two to four hours.

Studies have shown that in addition to recreational use of ecstasy, some young adults also use this drug to cope with stress or difficult life situations, to improve their mood, and to allow them to function successfully with their friends on a daily basis.[67] Figure 11-9 shows that recreational drug users had the highest self-reported rate of use in 2013 compared to street-entrenched adult and youth drug users, with the exception of Toronto and Montreal. Recreational drug users in Vancouver, British Columbia, reported the highest rate among users in major Canadian cities.

How Users Feel MDMA belongs to a family of drugs called *enactogens*, which literally means "touching within." As a mood elevator, it produces a relaxed, euphoric state but does not produce hallucinations. Users of ecstasy often say they feel at peace with themselves and at ease and empathic with others. Like hallucinogenic drugs, MDMA can enhance sensory experience, but it rarely causes visual distortions, sudden mood changes, or psychotic reactions. Regular users may experience depression and anxiety the week after taking MDMA.

Risks Ecstasy poses risks similar to those of cocaine and amphetamines. These include psychological difficulties (confusion, depression, sleep problems, drug craving, severe anxiety, and paranoia) and physical

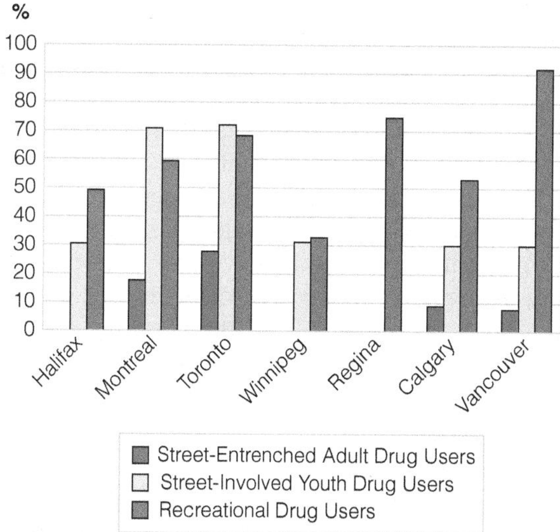

Figure 11-9 **Prevalence of Self-Reported Past-Year Ecstasy Use among High-Risk Population by City (2013)**

Source: Canadian Centre on Substance Abuse (2016). Canadian drug summary: MDMA (ecstacy, molly). http://www.ccsa.ca/Eng/topics/Monitoring-Trends/Canadian-Drug-Trends/Pages/default.aspx (page 3, Figure 2). Reproduced with permission from the Canadian Centre on Substance Abuse.

symptoms (muscle tension, involuntary teeth clenching, nausea, vomiting, dizziness, blurred vision, rapid eye movement, faintness, chills, sweating, and increases in heart rate and blood pressure, which pose a special risk for people with circulatory or heart disease).[68] When combined with extended physical exertion such as dancing, club drugs can lead to hyperthermia (severe overheating), severe dehydration, serious increases in blood pressure, strokes, and heart attacks.

Continued use of ecstasy can lead to psychological dependence because users seek to recreate the exhilarating high and avoid the plunge into unhappiness and emptiness that comes after use. Because ecstasy is *neurotoxic* (damaging to brain cells), it depletes the brain of serotonin, a messenger chemical involved with mood, sleep, and appetite, and can lead to depression, anxiety, and impaired thinking.[69]

According to some brain-imaging studies, ecstasy alters neuronal function in a brain structure called the hippocampus, which helps create short-term memory (see Figure 11-10). Regular ecstasy use has been shown to affect memory, learning, and general intelligence.[70] However, new research commissioned by the National Institute on Drug Abuse (NIDA) reports that there were no differences between cognitive ability of MDMA and ecstasy users and a control group.[71] Whether or not these findings prove to be replicable in further studies, there are still other serious health risks for individuals using ecstasy.

MDMA has been implicated in some cases of acute hepatitis, which can lead to liver failure. Another danger comes from the practice of taking Prozac®, a drug that modulates the mood-altering brain chemical serotonin, before ecstasy. This can cause jaw clenching, nausea, tremors, and, in extreme cases, potentially fatal elevations in body temperature.

Although not a sexual stimulant (if anything, MDMA has the opposite effect), ecstasy fosters strong feelings of intimacy that may lead to risky sexual behaviour. The psychological effects of ecstasy become less intriguing with repeated use, and the physical side effects become more uncomfortable.

Verhees et al. have studied the effects of ecstasy on litters of rats and suggest that there may be risks to a developing human fetus if a woman uses this drug during her pregnancy. Results so far include a greater likelihood of heart and skeletal abnormalities and long-term learning and memory impairments.[72]

✓ CHECK-IN

How aware are you or your friends of the risks of using ecstasy?

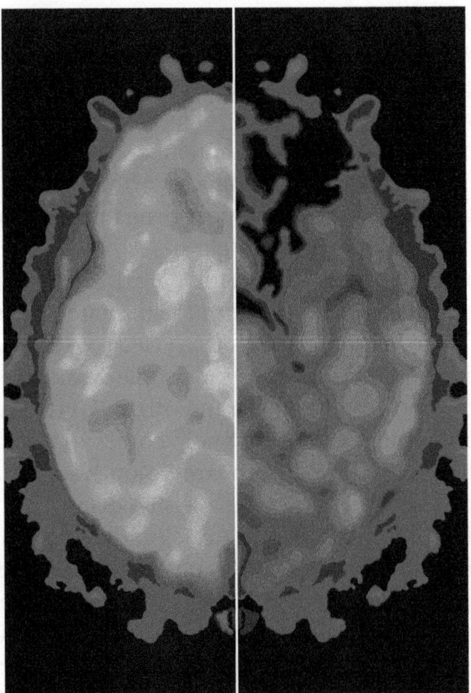

Figure 11-10 **Effects of Ecstasy on the Brain**

These brain scans show the sharp difference in human brain function for an individual who had never used drugs (left) and one who had used the club drug ecstasy many times but had not used any drugs for at least three weeks before the scan (right). In the left scan, the bright reddish colour shows active serotonin sites in the brain. Serotonin is a critical neurochemical that regulates mood, emotion, learning, memory, sleep, and pain. In the right scan, the dark sections indicate areas where serotonin is not present even after three weeks without any drugs.

Source: National Institute on Drug Abuse. Found at: www.clubdrugs.org. Courtesy of U.S. Department of Health & Human Services.

Hallucinogens The drugs known as **hallucinogens** produce vivid and unusual changes in thought, feeling, and perception. The most widely used is *LSD (lysergic acid diethylamide* or acid), which was initially developed as a tool to explore mental illness. It became popular in the 1960s and resurfaced among teenagers in the 1990s. LSD is taken orally, either blotted onto pieces of paper that are held in the mouth or chewed along with another substance, such as a sugar cube. LSD is also known as acid, back breaker, California sunshine, purple haze, and window pane.[73]

Ketamine is another hallucinogen used as an illegal drug. This drug also acts as a stimulant and a depressant. Mainly used by veterinarians as an anesthetic drug, it makes a person feel detached from their body. It is both tasteless and odourless and is sometimes put in drinks. It is classified as one of the date rape drugs. This drug goes by many names including big K, breakfast cereal, lady K, Vitamin K, and wonk. Much less commonly used is *peyote*, whose active ingredient is *mescaline*. Researchers Halpern and Sewell suggest that more education might be necessary for the general public with regard to the use of botanical drugs as they are potent intoxicants.[74]

How Users Feel LSD produces hallucinations, including bright colours and altered perceptions of reality. Effects from a single dose begin within 30–60 minutes and last 10–12 hours. During this time, there are slight increases in body temperature, heart rate, and blood pressure. Sweating, chills, and goose pimples may appear. Some users develop headache and nausea.

Mescaline produces vivid hallucinations—including brightly coloured lights, animals, and geometric designs—within 30–90 minutes of consumption. These effects may persist for 12 hours.

The effects of hallucinogens depend greatly on the dose, the individual's expectations and personality, and the setting for drug use. Many users report religious or mystical imagery and thoughts; some feel they are experiencing profound insights. Usually the user realizes that perceptual changes are caused by the hallucinogen, but some become convinced that they have lost their minds. Drugs sold as hallucinogens are frequently mixed with other drugs, such as PCP and amphetamines, combinations that can produce unexpected and frightening effects.

Risks Physical symptoms include dilated pupils, rapid heart rate, sweating, heart palpitations, blurring of vision, tremors, and poor coordination. These effects may last 8–12 hours. Hallucinogen intoxication also produces changes in emotions and mood, such as anxiety, depression, fear of losing one's mind, and impaired judgment.

LSD can trigger irrational acts. LSD users have injured or killed themselves by jumping out of windows, swimming out to sea, or throwing themselves in front of cars. Some individuals may experience *flashbacks* (re-experiencing symptoms felt while intoxicated), which include geometric hallucinations, flashes of colour, halos around objects, and other perceptual changes. Rickert et al. also determined that there is a relationship between LSD use among young women and high-risk sexual behaviours.[75]

Inhalants **Inhalants** or **deliriants** are chemicals that produce vapours with psychoactive effects. The most commonly abused inhalants are solvents, aerosols, model-airplane glue, cleaning fluids, and petroleum products such as kerosene and butane. Some anesthetics and nitrous oxide (laughing gas) are also abused. The use of inhalants is on the rise in Canada—especially among Inuit and Aboriginal peoples in isolated communities.[76]

How Users Feel Inhalants very rapidly reach the lungs, bloodstream, and other parts of the body. Intoxication often occurs within five minutes and can last more than an hour. Inhalants interfere with thinking and impulse control, so users may act in dangerous or destructive ways.

Often there are visible external signs of use: a rash around the nose and mouth; breath odours; residue on face, hands, and clothing; redness, swelling, and tearing of the eyes; and irritation of throat, lungs, and nose that leads to coughing and gagging. Nausea and headache also may occur.

Risks Regular use of inhalants leads to tolerance, so the sniffer needs more and more to attain the desired effects. Younger children who use inhalants several times a week may develop dependence. Chronic users experience a range of mental health problems, from mild impairment to severe dementia.

Although some young people believe inhalants are safe, this is far from true. Users risk the loss of motor skills, seizures, diarrhea, anxiety, and even death from a single use. Inhalation of butane from cigarette lighters displaces oxygen in the lungs, causing suffocation. Users also can suffocate while covering their heads with a plastic bag to inhale the substance or from inhaling vomit into their lungs while high. Shaw et al. found a higher rate of Hepatitis C in solvent users (81 percent) compared to non-solvent users (55 percent) in Aboriginal injection-drug users.[77]

In Canada, treatment centres have been established in a number of provinces through the Native Youth Solvent Abuse program (NYSA). Research continues about the type of treatment program that best helps youth who abuse solvents.

Opioids The **opioids** include *opium* and its derivatives (*heroin, morphine, codeine*). The opioids come from a resin taken from the seedpod of the Asian poppy. **Non-opioids**, such as *meperidine* (Demerol®), *methadone*, and *propoxyphene* (Darvon®), are chemically synthesized. A common prescribed semi-synthetic opioid is oxycondone hydrochloride (OxyContin®). Whether natural or synthetic, taken illegally or prescribed by doctors, these drugs are powerful *narcotics*, or painkillers.

Heroin (also known as horse, junk, smack, or downtown), the most widely abused opioid, is illegal in Canada. In other nations, it is used as a potent painkiller for conditions such as terminal cancer. Heroin users typically inject the drug into their veins. However, individuals who experiment with recreational drugs often prefer *skin-popping* (subcutaneous injection) rather than *mainlining* (intravenous injection); they also may snort heroin as a powder or dissolve it and inhale the vapours. Regardless of the method of administration, tolerance can develop rapidly.

Morphine, used as a painkiller and anesthetic, acts primarily on the central nervous system, eyes, and digestive tract. By producing mental clouding, drowsiness, and euphoria, it does not decrease the physical sensation of pain as much as it alters a person's awareness of the pain; in effect, he or she no longer cares about it.

Codeine, a weaker painkiller than morphine, is an ingredient in liquid products prescribed for relieving coughs and in tablet and injectable form for relieving pain. The synthetic narcotic propoxyphene (Darvon®), a somewhat less potent painkiller than codeine, is no more effective than aspirin in usual doses. It has been one of the most widely prescribed drugs for headaches, dental pain, and menstrual cramps. At higher doses, Darvon® produces a euphoric high, which may lead to misuse.

In the past decade, concern about the drug *OxyContin®* has increased. Since its introduction in 1995, it has become a popular prescription medication used to control moderate to severe pain and chronic pain related to cancer and other terminal conditions. Used to gain euphoric effects, it induces a high similar to heroin, is highly addictive, and produces side effects, such as confusion, altered mental state, vomiting, nausea, and even death.

Research on the widespread use of this drug showed that there were about 2.2 million prescriptions dispensed in 2010 for OxyContin products.[78] Among non-medical users, OxyContin also became a drug of choice for many individuals across Canada.[79] The concern about the addictive qualities of this drug and the impact it was having upon users resulted in major changes with regard to access to OxyContin. In 2012, the drug's manufacturer, Purudue Pharma, replaced OxyContin with OxyNeo, a formula that was apparently more "abuse-proof." Seven of Canada's 10 provinces removed OxyContin and OxyNeo from their provincial drug formularies, which meant that this drug would only be available by prescription in special exemption circumstances. The federal government did the same for all federal drug plans.[80] In the past few years generic oxycodone products have proven to be deadly with a reported high percentage of overdoses in Canada. In May 2015 the federal government decided to reverse an earlier decision made in 2012 to allow the generic products on the Canadian market. However, other alternative drugs such as Hydromorph Contin® have taken the place of oxycodone and medical experts have discovered these new opioids are also highly addictive and hazardous too.[81]

Fentanyl, a prescription synthetic opiate narcotic, is a drug that is used for people in severe pain. It is 50–100 times more toxic than morphine. The use of prescribed and illicit fentanyl has become a national public health concern. A recent study by Friesen, Woelk, and Bugden on the use of fentanyl painkiller patches found that half of the patients prescribed the patch were at risk for an overdose because the doctors did not follow proper prescription protocol.[82] Illicit use of fentanyl, where it is being mixed with other drugs in power, liquid, or pill form, has resulted in an escalation of overdoses and deaths nationwide.[83] Canadians are being warned about the potential risks of fentanyl overdoses. Presently, there is no quick way for a drug user to test whether or not a drug has been lace with fentanyl. Overdose symptoms include trouble breathing, walking, or talking; severe sleepiness; slow heartbeat; and shallow breathing. A person's skin may also feel cold and clammy.

How Users Feel All opioids relax the user. When injected, they can produce an immediate *rush* (high) that lasts 10–30 minutes. For two to six hours thereafter, users may feel indifferent, lethargic, and drowsy; they may slur their words and have problems paying attention, remembering, and going about their normal routine. Some people experience very unpleasant feelings, such as anxiety and fear. Other effects include a sensation of warmth or heaviness, dry mouth, facial flushing, and nausea and vomiting (particularly in first-time users).

Risks Addiction is common. Almost all regular users of opioids rapidly develop drug dependence, which can lead to lethargy, weight loss, loss of sex drive, and the continual effort to avoid withdrawal symptoms through repeated drug administration. In addition, they experience anxiety, insomnia, restlessness, and craving for the drug. Users continue taking opioids as much to avoid the discomfort of withdrawal, a classic sign of opioid addiction, as to experience pleasure.

Opioid intoxication is characterized by changes in mood and behaviour, such as initial euphoria followed by apathy or discontent and impaired judgment. Over time, users who inject opioids may develop infections of the heart lining and valves, skin abscesses, and lung congestion. Infections from unsterile solutions, syringes, and shared needles can lead to hepatitis, tetanus, liver disease, and HIV transmission. Depression is common and may be both an antecedent and a risk factor for needle-sharing.

Opioid poisoning or overdose causes shock, coma, and depressed respiration and can be fatal.[84]

Withdrawal If a regular user stops taking an opioid, withdrawal begins within 6–12 hours. The intensity of the symptoms depends on the degree of the addiction; they may grow stronger for 24–72 hours and gradually subside over a period of 7–14 days, though some symptoms, such as insomnia, may persist for several months. Irritability, nausea or vomiting, muscle aches, runny nose or eyes, dilated pupils, sweating, diarrhea, and fever are other symptoms.

The Canadian Centre for Substance Abuse (CCSA) indicates that presently the best practice for treatment includes a period of detoxification followed by behaviour-oriented therapies.

Methadone Maintenance Opioid dependence is a very difficult addiction to overcome. Studies demonstrate that only 10–30 percent of heroin users are able to maintain abstinence. Treatment for opioid dependence includes substitution therapies such as methadone, naltrexone, and buprenoprphine to help with the symptoms of withdrawal.[85]

Methadone is used in two basic ways to treat opioid dependence: as an opioid substitute for detoxification, usually with a gradual tapering of methadone over a period of 21–180 days, and as a maintenance treatment. Methadone maintenance has been criticized by some as substituting one drug for another, although research has documented several positive benefits including decreased use of illicit opioids; decreased criminal behaviour; decreased risk of contracting HIV infection; and improvements in physical health, employment, and other lifestyle factors.

Phencyclidine PCP (**phencyclidine** or Sernyl®, angel dust, peace pill, lovely, and green) is an illicit drug manufactured as a tablet, capsule, liquid, flake, spray, or crystal-like white powder that can be swallowed, smoked, sniffed, or injected. Sometimes it is sprinkled on crack, marijuana, tobacco, or parsley, and smoked. A fine-powdered form of PCP can be snorted or injected. Once, PCP was thought to have medicinal value as an anesthetic, but its side effects, including delirium and hallucinations, make it unacceptable for medical use.

How Users Feel The effects of PCP are utterly unpredictable. It may trigger violent behaviour or irreversible psychosis the first time it is used, or the twentieth time, or never. In low doses, PCP produces changes—from hallucinations or euphoria to feelings of emptiness or numbness—similar to those produced by other psychoactive drugs. Higher doses may produce a stupor that lasts several days, increased heart rate and blood pressure, flushing, sweating, dizziness, and numbness.

The behavioural changes associated with PCP intoxication include belligerence, aggressiveness, impulsiveness, unpredictability, agitation, poor judgment, and impaired functioning at work or in social situations. The physical symptoms of PCP intoxication include involuntary eye movements, increased blood pressure or heart rate, numbness or diminished responsiveness to pain, impaired coordination and speech, muscle rigidity, seizures, and a painful sensitivity to sound.[86]

Sedative-Hypnotic Drugs **Sedative-hypnotics**, also known as anxiolytic or anti-anxiety drugs, depress the central nervous system, reduce activity, and induce relaxation, drowsiness, or sleep. They include the benzodiazepines and the barbiturates.

The **benzodiazepines**—the most widely used drugs in this category—are commonly prescribed for tension, muscular strain, sleep problems, anxiety, panic attacks, anesthesia, and in the treatment of alcohol withdrawal. They include such drugs as *chlordiazepoxide* (Librium®), *diazepam* (Valium®), *oxazepam* (Serax®), *lorazepam* (Ativan®), *flurazepam* (Dalmane®), and *alprazolam* (Xanax®). They differ widely in their mechanism of action, absorption rate, and metabolism, but all produce similar intoxication and withdrawal symptoms.

Benzodiazepine sleeping pills have largely replaced the **barbiturates**, which were used medically in the past for inducing relaxation and sleep, relieving tension, and treating epileptic seizures. These drugs are usually taken by mouth in tablet, capsule, or liquid form. When used as a general anesthetic, they are administered intravenously. Barbiturates such as *pentobarbital* (Nembutal®, yellow jackets), *secobarbital* (Seconal®, reds), and *thiopental* (Pentothal®) are short-acting and rapidly absorbed into the brain. The longer-acting barbiturates, such as *amobarbital* (Amytal®, blues, downers) and *phenobarbital* (Luminal®, phennies), are usually taken orally and absorbed slowly into the bloodstream, take a while to reach the brain, and have an effect for several days.

How Users Feel Low doses of these drugs may reduce or relieve tension, but increasing doses can cause a loosening of sexual or aggressive inhibitions. Individuals using this class of drugs may experience rapid mood changes, impaired judgment, and impaired social or occupational functioning. High doses produce slurred speech, drowsiness, and stupor.

Risks All sedative-hypnotic drugs can produce physical and psychological dependence within two to four weeks. A complication specific to sedatives is cross-tolerance (cross-addiction), which occurs when users develop tolerance for one sedative or become dependent on it and develop tolerance for other sedatives as well.

McCabe[87] found that college students using prescription benzodiazepines for non-medical use had higher rates of risky lifestyle behaviours and substance abuse than students using this medication in a prescribed way. Taken in combination with alcohol, these drugs have a synergistic effect that can be dangerous or even lethal. Alcohol in combination with sedative-hypnotics leads to respiratory depression and may result in respiratory arrest and death.

Withdrawal Withdrawal from sedative-hypnotic drugs may range from relatively mild discomfort to a severe syndrome with grand mal seizures, depending on the degree of dependence. Withdrawal symptoms include malaise or weakness, sweating, rapid pulse, coarse tremors (of the hands, tongue, or eyelids), insomnia, nausea or vomiting, temporary hallucinations or illusions, physical restlessness, anxiety or irritability, and grand mal seizures. Withdrawal may begin within two to three days after stopping drug use, and symptoms may persist for many weeks. Regular users of any of these drugs should not try to quit suddenly, as they run the risk of seizures, coma, and death.

Anabolic Steroids **Anabolic steroids** are a synthetic artificial version of the male sex hormone testosterone. This hormone is responsible for the growth of bones and muscles. Steroids are controlled substances, legally available by prescription in Canada. They are sometimes used to treat specific medical conditions such as delayed puberty and loss of muscle mass in cancer and AIDS patients. Non-medical use is also common among athletes and bodybuilders to enhance physical performance. Other individuals use anabolic steroids to improve physical appearance.[88]

Berning et al., in a study of non-athlete college students, found that the reasons students used anabolic androgenic steroids were a desire to increase their physical performance, their friends were using them, and they wanted to enhance their physical appearance.[89]

How Users Feel Many young people believe that the use of steroids will help them feel more confident, that by having a well-developed body they will gain respect and admiration from their peers. Unfortunately, people who use steroids often experience negative physical and psychological side effects. Physically, users can expect to have persistent headaches, nosebleeds, and stomach aches. Severe acne and hair loss are other side effects. Psychologically, users often experience increased aggressiveness and bursts of anger, known as "roid rage."

Risks There are many serious health risks associated with the use of steroids. For males, shrunken testes and lowered sperm count, which may lead to sterility and impotence, is a risk. For females, irregular periods are common. Other risks include damage and tumour growth in the liver and kidneys, high blood pressure, and increased cholesterol levels that may lead to heart disease. Steroids can prevent bones from growing and also cause premature fusion of the long bones. This can result in stunted growth. Mood swings sometimes cause aggressive and violent behaviour. Using steroids can also be life threatening. Sharing needles to inject steroids can result in Hepatitis B and C and HIV infection.

The use of steroids is also a risk for athletes, since it is a violation of the Sport Federation and International Olympic Committee anti-doping rules. A first offence results in a two-year ban from the sport and a lifetime ban from government funding. A second offence results in a lifetime ban from the sport. Both bans result in a loss of any record or medal obtained while using steroids.[90]

Withdrawal As with many other drugs, withdrawal can be difficult. You can't stop using steroids and keep the muscle mass and weight gain. Fatigue and depression are common. As well, the effects of steroids may be permanent in both males and females.

✓ CHECK-IN

How prevalent is the use of steroids on your campus? How aware are you of the risks of using steroids?

TREATING DRUG DEPENDENCE AND ABUSE

The most difficult step for a substance user is to admit that he or she *is* in fact misusing or abusing drugs and alcohol. The second step is to determine the level of addiction. If drug and alcohol abusers are not forced to deal with their problem through some unexpected trauma, such as being fired or going bankrupt, those who care—family, friends, co-workers, doctors—may have to confront them and insist that they do something about their addiction.

Canada Drug Rehab is one online agency that provides a free referral service for substance abuse. Information on overcoming drug addiction is comprehensive. The list of addiction treatment options are as follows:[91]

- **Pre-rehabilitative care**—for individuals whose addictions are so serious that medical services are needed prior to any type of residential or community-based rehabilitation program. Services include medical detox and psychiatric support.
- **Intervention**—a meeting or forced psychiatric, medical, or physical intervention, often begun by friends and family of the user or addict in an attempt to force an individual to make a decision to change his or her lifestyle. Research has shown that intervention might be an important turning point for a user or addict.[92]
- **Medically assisted detox**—used when an individual has a physical addiction to a substance. Common drugs that create health risks in the withdrawal process are heroin, barbiturates, alcohol, and a number of prescription medications. This process is especially complicated in a polysubstance abuser. Medical doctors and health professionals are required to monitor the detox and treatment process of potentially fatal withdrawal symptoms.
- **Rapid detox**—a form of detoxification developed for users of opiate drugs such as heroin, OxyContin, or morphine. The addict is put in a chemically induced coma so they do not have to endure the physical pain that occurs during the detoxification stage. Medical administration of Naltroxin is often used in a rapid detox as it effectively purges and blocks the absorption of opiates.
- **Buprenorphine and suboxone**—new substances that are sometimes used for opiate detoxification. They are becoming a substitute for the more traditionally prescribed drug methadone, which has long been used in detoxification processes. They block the absorption of opiates and ease the individual's withdrawal symptoms.
- **In-patient rehabilitation**—usually done in a drug rehab facility. Programs range from 28 days to one year or more in length. New life skills are learned. Old behaviour patterns are deconstructed.
- **Behaviour modification**—often based on modified 12-step programs. Individuals are confronted with their lifestyle choices and behaviours. The programs are sometimes described as very rigorous and can be difficult to complete.
- **Dual diagnosis**—programs based in facilities that assist addicts who have both an addiction disorder and a mental health disorder. Programs often include both psychiatric care and a monitored prescription medication intervention.

- **Religious or spiritual guidance**—some addicts are helped through a connection to a church- or spiritual-based rehabilitation program. A moral code of ethics model is used to assist individuals to heal physically, emotionally, and spiritually and begin to serve others.
- **Post-rehabilitative care**—facility- or community-based support groups are offered for individuals who have completed detox and rehabilitation programs. Ongoing education and individual accountability are often an important part of the continued rehabilitative process.
- **Family counselling**—used during or as a follow-up to a detox or rehabilitation program to assist the family unit in dealing with addiction issues and challenges.
- **Out-patient rehabilitation**—an ongoing, sometimes optional program in which clients access counselling and medical services to prevent a relapse of addiction.

HUMAN POTENTIAL

Ashlie—The Other Side of Drug Addiction

We often hear very poignant stories about people who struggle with drug addiction. However, there is another side of drug addiction too—the stories from family members and friends. This story is about one young woman's attempt to watch, assist, and learn from her sister's drug addiction.

Ashlie's story begins when she was in Grade 5. She lived with her mother, grandmother, and older sister. The two girls were involved in numerous sporting activities. She lived in a middle-class family dealing with typical sister rivalry. A change in their relationship would occur when Ashlie's sister entered middle school, where she began skipping classes and pulling back from the family activities that had been the norm for them. Then the drug use started.

To deal with the changes that were occurring, Ashlie became even more competitive, working hard in school to "get on the straight-A wall," doing better in sports, and attempting to be the "good girl" in the family. "I couldn't do the things my sister was doing because I could see how it was hurting my mom and my grandma." Over the years regular drug use would become an issue that the entire family had to face. The focus on Ashlie's sister became all-consuming. Each day everyone had to deal with the uncertainty that comes with someone using drugs. Would Ashlie's sister come home? Would she ask for more money? Would she be angry or sad? Would she continue to use drugs, or would she recognize that her drug use was destroying lives? What could anyone do? What should everyone do?

When you speak with Ashlie, you sense that she is wise beyond her years. As a high-school student, she tried to figure things out. She was convinced that giving her sister money to buy drugs was not the answer. She didn't want the police coming to their home. She wanted someone to take action. She has learned that it is not easy to "figure things out." As her grandmother said, "What if your sister called in the night and needed picking up and we didn't go to her? What if that one time would have made a difference—that 1 percent chance that she might reach out to us? What if that one time we didn't go she didn't make it?"

Ashlie found ways to escape. Hiding her feelings, getting involved "in a million things"—she kept busy. She started to question whether or not she was happy or depressed. She felt a deep level of anger. She recalls a breakdown in Grade 12. During a visit with a counsellor, she "unloaded all this stuff." She realizes now that she is a "bundler." She knows now that "eventually the weight of the bundle gets too heavy."

And while she was doing all the right things—getting good marks in school, participating in activities, and helping her mother and grandmother—she knew she had to leave her home. She did not find the solace or support she needed on her dad's side of the family. She lived with an aunt for a time.

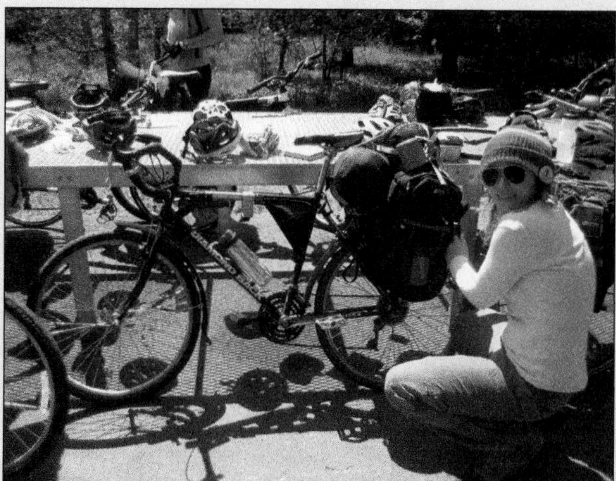

Courtesy of Ashlie

Ashlie, on a road trip through the Canadian Rocky Mountains.

A turning point for Ashlie was when she found out her sister was pregnant. She was worried for the baby. She was moved deeply—knowing that this child might have to start her life without the best chance possible. Ashlie believes that this was crossing the line—it was unethical. The pregnancy did not "save her sister." Ashlie's grandmother is now raising her niece.

Ashlie feels responsible in many ways. She senses that she will need to become a surrogate mother for her niece as her grandmother and mother age. She says she has learned that while she feels alone at times, she believes we are all unified at the same time too. "We all know so little about the people we meet. What people see from the outside is just a glance. Everyone has their story."

Her advice to others who face similar challenges is this: "Know that lifestyle choices you make do impact others. Be responsible for your own actions. Know that your life story will keep on changing. Give the rest of 'you' a chance, too. The family or relationship issues are only a fraction of who you are. You are still your own person, and you have control over what you want to achieve and who you want to be. Know, also, that challenges we face do make us stronger and wiser, and help us push past obstacles that sometimes seem impossible to deal with. Also, there is 'no perfect.' Finally, know that everyone's grass is not greener than yours—people you know and admire may be going through the same thing. I often look at other people and wish I could be that cool. It took my roommate to help me understand that I am that person to other people, too—I am cool, too, and I have a lot to offer and a lot to give."

12-Step Programs Since its founding in 1935, Alcoholics Anonymous (AA)—the oldest, largest, and most successful self-help program in the world—has spawned a worldwide movement.[93]

As many as 200 different recovery programs are based on the spiritual **12-step program** of AA. Participation in 12-step programs for drug abusers, such as Substance Anonymous, Narcotics Anonymous, and Cocaine Anonymous, is of fundamental importance in promoting and maintaining long-term abstinence.

The basic precept of 12-step programs is that members have been powerless when it comes to controlling their addictive behaviour on their own because addiction is a disease that must be managed. These programs don't recruit members. The desire to stop must come from the individual, who contacts a local AA group.

Meetings of various 12-step programs are held daily in almost every city in Canada. Some chapters, whose members often include the disabled or those in remote areas, meet via Internet chat rooms or electronic bulletin boards. Many individuals belong to several programs because they have several problems, such as alcoholism, substance abuse, and pathological gambling.

Relapse Prevention The most common clinical course for substance abuse disorders involves a pattern of multiple relapses over the course of a lifespan. When relapses do occur, they should be viewed neither as a mark of defeat nor evidence of moral weakness. While painful, they do not erase the progress that has been achieved and ultimately may strengthen self-understanding. They can serve as reminders of potential pitfalls to avoid in the future. Therapists emphasize that every lapse does not have to lead to a full-blown relapse. Users can turn to the skills acquired in treatment—calling people for support or going to meetings—to avoid a major relapse.

One key to preventing relapse is learning to avoid obvious cues and associations that can set off intense cravings. This means staying away from the people and places linked with past drug use.

Four Pillars Drug Strategy—City of Vancouver Many political groups and a variety of agencies across Canada are attempting to find ways to address substance abuse in their communities. One such example is the city of Vancouver, which adopted an approach called the Four Pillars Drug Strategy—originally begun in both Switzerland and Germany in the 1990s. The aim of this strategy was to reduce drug-related harm in Vancouver, B.C. There are four pillars of the city's drug policy:[94]

- *Harm reduction*—reducing the spread of deadly communicable diseases, preventing drug overdose deaths, increasing substance users' contact with healthcare services and drug treatment programs, and reducing consumption of drugs in the street.
- *Prevention*—using a variety of strategies to educate people about substance misuse and the negative health impacts and legal risks associated with drug use, and to encourage people to make healthy choices.
- *Treatment*—offering individuals access to services such as counselling, methadone programs, daytime and residential treatment, housing support, and medical care.
- *Enforcement*—targeting organized crime, drug dealing, drug houses, and problem businesses, and improving coordination with health services and other drug-treatment agencies.

Studies have shown that the fatal overdose rate in Vancouver's Downtown Eastside has decreased by 35 percent since the opening of InSite, a supervised injection facility. Although a review by the federal government recommended closing the site, the Supreme Court of Canada denied an appeal by the Attorney General of Canada on September 30, 2011, allowing InSite to continue operating.[95] Research on this facility and programs and services it offers has found many health benefits. They include a decrease in individuals participating in risky injection behaviour, fewer fatal drug overdoses, and a lower number of HIV infections.[96]

All Nations' Healing Hospital—Fort Qu'Appelle, Saskatchewan In June 2004, the All Nations' Healing Hospital was opened in Fort Qu'Appelle, Saskatchewan. The facility, located on First Nations' land, operates as an independent, nonprofit corporation affiliated with the Regina Qu'Appelle Regional Health Authority. Traditional First Nations values and concepts are integrated with healthcare services. In addition to medical services, community-oriented and

STRATEGIES FOR PREVENTION

Relapse-Prevention Planning

The following steps, from Terence Gorski and Merlene Miller's *Staying Sober: A Guide for Relapse Prevention*, can lower the likelihood of relapses:

- *Stabilization and self-assessment.* Get control of yourself. Find out what's going on in your head, heart, and life.
- *Education.* Learn about relapse and what to do to prevent it.
- *Warning sign identification and management.* Make a list of your personal relapse warning signs. Learn how to interrupt them before you lose control.
- *Inventory training.* Learn how to become consciously aware of warning signs as they develop.
- *Review of the recovery program.* Make sure your recovery program is able to help you manage your warning signs of relapse.
- *Involvement of significant others.* Teach them how to help you avoid relapses.

integrated mental-health therapy services are offered—with a culturally sensitive approach. These include addiction and support services in which there is a recognition of the relationship between mind, body, spirit, and community healing.[97]

Harm Reduction—Street Works, Edmonton, Alberta Another exemplary program developed and implemented to reduce the harm of drug dependence and use is the Street Works program in Edmonton, Alberta. It began in 1989 as Needleworks where eight city agencies worked together to address the issue of HIV among injection-drug users and sex trade workers. By responding to the health concerns affecting this target population, the program also addresses health concerns for the broader community.

The program is based on three principles: harm reduction, health promotion, and primary health care:[98] Health education about HIV/AIDS, hepatitis, and universal precautions is offered. Health services include nursing, health assessments, screening, and immunizations. A needle exchange and supply program, a prison program, and a referral program also support these three principles. Funding is received from research dollars, donations, and grants.

Health Canada Health Canada continues to contribute to the Drug Strategy Community Initiatives Fund and the Alcohol and Drug Treatment and Rehabilitation Program for national, regional, and community initiatives that address substance abuse in Canada.[99]

SELF-SURVEY

Do You Have a Substance-Use Disorder?

Check the statements that apply to you.

1. I use prescription medication for a longer period of time than I desire or intend.________
2. I use illicit drugs.________
3. I try, repeatedly and unsuccessfully, to cut down or control drug use.________
4. I spend a great deal of time doing whatever is necessary in order to get drugs, take them, or recover from their use.________
5. I am so high or feel so bad after drug use that I often cannot work or fulfill other responsibilities.________
6. I give up or cut back on important social, work, or recreational activities because of drug use. ________
7. I continue to use drugs even though I realize that they are causing or worsening physical or mental problems. ________
8. I use a lot more of a drug in order to achieve a "high" or desired effect or feel fewer such effects than in the past. ________
9. I use drugs in dangerous ways or situations. ________
10. I have repeated drug-related legal problems, such as arrests for possession. ________
11. I continue to use drugs, even though the drug causes or worsens social or personal problems, such as arguments with a spouse. ________
12. I develop hand tremors or other withdrawal symptoms if I cut down or stop drug use. ________
13. I take drugs to relieve or avoid withdrawal symptoms. ________

Answers to Self-Survey

The more blanks that you (or someone close to you) checks, the more reason you have to be concerned about drug use. The most difficult step for anyone with a substance-use disorder is to admit that he or she has a problem. Sometimes a drug-related crisis, such as being arrested or fired, forces individuals to acknowledge the impact of drugs. If not, those who care—family, friends, boss, or a physician—may have to confront them and insist that they do something about it. This confrontation, planned beforehand, is called an *intervention* and can be the turning point for drug users and their families.

Chapter Summary

1. Which statement about drugs is false?
   a. Toxicity is the dosage level of a prescription.
   b. Drugs can be injected into the body intravenously, intramuscularly, or subcutaneously.
   c. Drug misuse is the taking of a drug for a purpose other than that for which it was medically intended.
   d. An individual's response to a drug can be affected by the setting in which the drug is used.
2. Which strategy should you use to help ensure that an over-the-counter or prescription drug is safe and effective?
   a. Take smaller dosages than indicated in the instructions.
   b. Test your response to the drug by borrowing a similar medication from a friend.
   c. Ask your doctor or pharmacist about possible interactions with other medications.
   d. Buy all of your medications online.

3. Which drug does NOT cause withdrawal symptoms?
   a. caffeine
   b. marijuana
   c. heroin
   d. aspirin
4. Which statement about individuals with substance-use disorders is true?
   a. They are usually not physically dependent on their drug of choice.
   b. They have a compulsion to use one or more addictive substances.
   c. They require less and less of the preferred drug to achieve the desired effect.
   d. They suffer withdrawal symptoms when they use the drug regularly.
5. Which of the following drugs affects the central nervous system very similarly to amphetamine?
   a. marijuana
   b. heroin
   c. cocaine
   d. alcohol
6. Which statement about marijuana is false?
   a. People who have used marijuana may experience psychoactive effects for several days after use.
   b. Marijuana has shown some effectiveness in treating chemotherapy-related nausea.
   c. Unlike long-term use of alcohol, regular use of marijuana does not have any long-lasting health consequences.
   d. Depending on the amount of marijuana used, its effects can range from a mild sense of euphoria to extreme panic.
7. Which of the following is NOT a possible result of cocaine dependence?
   a. stroke
   b. paranoia and violent behaviour
   c. heart failure
   d. enhanced sexual performance
8. Which statement about club drugs is true?
   a. Club drugs can produce many unwanted effects, including hallucinations and paranoia.
   b. Most club drugs do not pose the same health dangers as "hard" drugs such as heroin.
   c. MDMA is the street name for ecstasy.
   d. When combined with extended physical exertion, club drugs can lead to hypothermia (lowered body temperature).
9. Which statement about the opioids is true?
   a. They are not addictive if used in a prescription form such as codeine or Demerol®.
   b. They produce an immediate but short-lasting high and a feeling of euphoria.
   c. They include morphine, which is typically used for cough suppression.
   d. They are illegal in Canada, but are allowed in other countries to help control severe pain.
10. Which statement about drug dependence treatment is false?
   a. Chemical-dependence treatment programs usually involve medications to alleviate withdrawal symptoms.
   b. Detoxification is usually the first step in a drug treatment program.
   c. Relapses are not uncommon for a person who has undergone drug treatment.
   d. The 12-step recovery program modelled after Alcoholics Anonymous has been shown to not be effective with individuals with drug dependence disorders.

Answers to these questions can be found on page 317.

SELF-RESPONSIBILITY—SOCIAL RESPONSIBILITY

SELF-RESPONSIBILITY

Courage is not the lack of fear. It is acting in spite of it.

Mark Twain

Learning to say yes to healthy lifestyle choices takes courage. If you find yourself moving toward choices that include substance abuse, reflect on the reasons why you are willing to put your body, mind, and spirit at risk. Use Prochaska's Stages of Change model to determine what preparations you can make to change this way of thinking. What would an action plan look like that would move you away from destructive lifestyle habits to habits that could enhance your well-being? What encouragement do you need to help you move into maintenance of a healthy and well life?

SOCIAL RESPONSIBILITY

The willingness to accept responsibility for one's own life is the source from which self-respect springs.

Joan Didion

Careers in social work, youth programming, addictions counselling, and government can be both rewarding and meaningful. Many agencies offer cooperative education or internship opportunities.

CRITICAL THINKING

1. Some people in Canada argue that marijuana should be a legal drug such as alcohol and tobacco. What is your opinion on this issue? Defend your position.
2. Suppose a close friend is using crystal meth. You fear that she is developing a substance-abuse disorder. What can you do to help her realize the dangers of her behaviour? What resources are available at your school or in your community to help her deal with both her drug problem and her financial needs?

WEB LINKS

Canadian Centre on Substance Abuse (CCSA)

www.ccsa.ca

You can access many reports, publications, and research articles on substance use and abuse at this site.

Canadian Centre for Ethics in Sport

www.cces.ca

If you are an athlete, coach, or educator, this site will provide you with the latest information on the Canadian anti-doping program.

United Native Friendship Centre

www.unfc.org

The goal of this agency is to assist Aboriginal peoples in addressing alcohol and drug issues. Information about education and prevention programs, treatment programs, and counselling is available at this site.

Please note that links are subject to change. If you find a broken link, use a search engine such as www.google.ca and search for the website by typing in keywords.

Key Terms

The terms listed here are used within the chapter on the page indicated. Definitions of terms are in the Glossary at the end of the book.

Answers to Chapter Summary Questions

1. a; 2. c; 3. d; 4. b; 5. c; 6. c; 7. d; 8. a; 9. b; 10. d

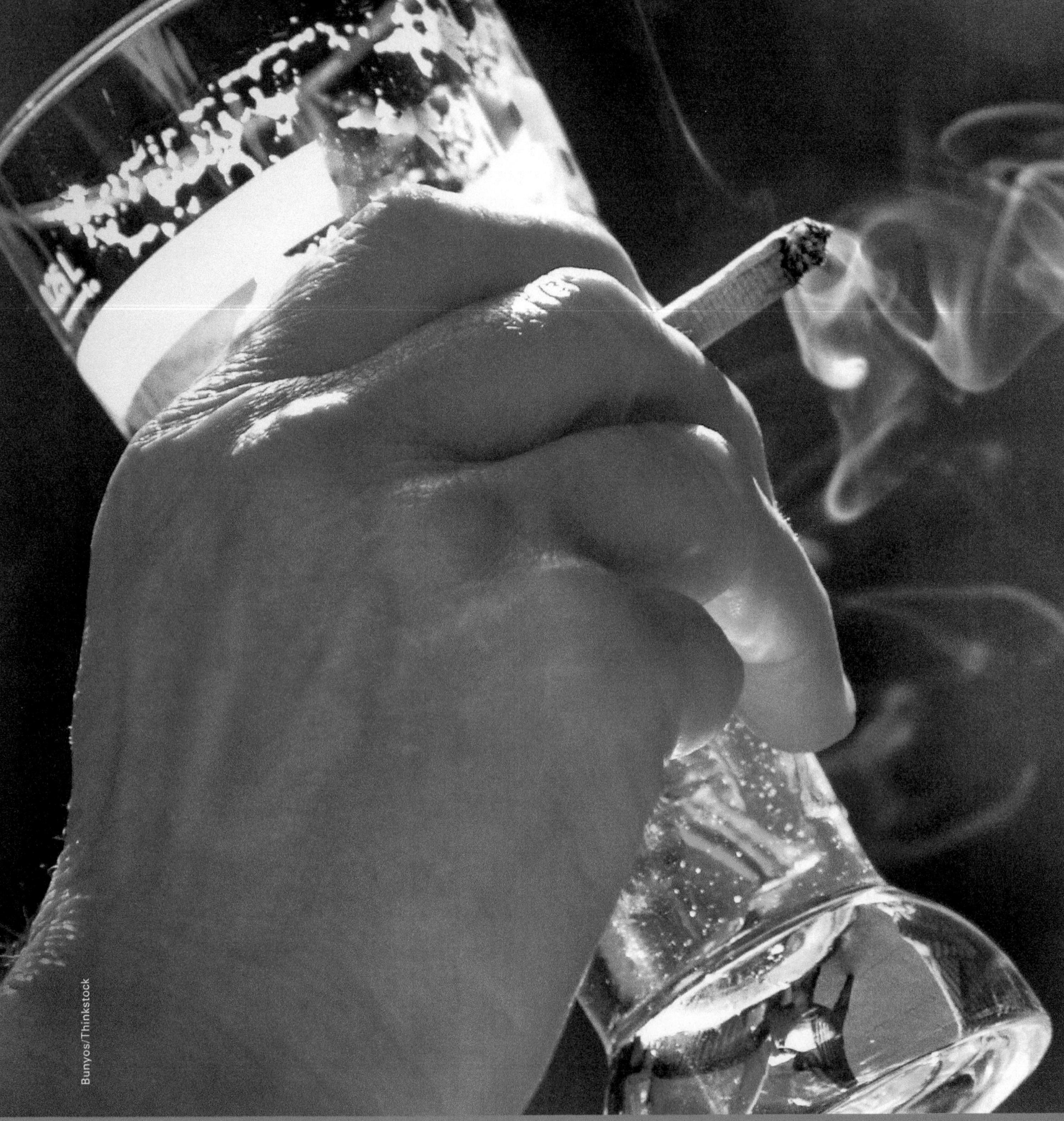

AFTER READING THIS CHAPTER, YOU WILL BE ABLE TO:

- **describe** the effects of alcohol on the body, behaviour, and brain
- **define** alcohol abuse, dependence, and alcoholism, and list their symptoms
- **list** the negative consequences to individuals and to our society from alcohol abuse
- **list** the health effects of smoking tobacco or using smokeless tobacco
- **describe** the social impact of tobacco use
- **list** the health effects of second-hand smoke

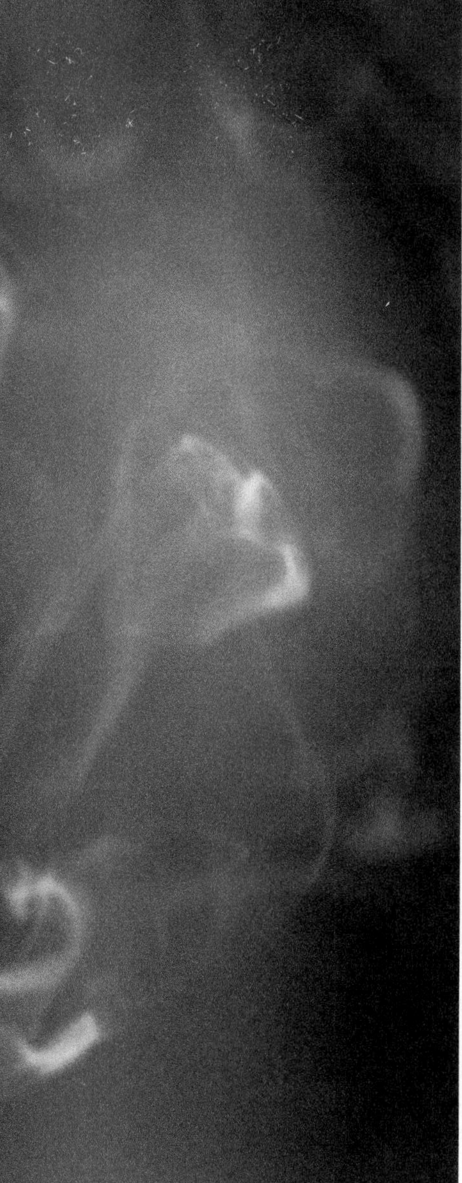

12

Alcohol and Tobacco Use, Misuse, and Abuse

Alcohol and tobacco are the most widely used mind-altering substances in the world. The use of alcohol and tobacco on college and university campuses is no exception. Although some studies reveal that many university students are making healthy choices about alcohol,[1] an increasing number engage in the dangerous practice of binge drinking.[2] In a study of 428 undergraduate students attending a Canadian university, 72 percent of the participants reported drinking at or above binge drinking thresholds on a regular basis. The study also showed that the consumption of alcohol and binge drinking among female students was higher than in earlier studies.[3]

Tobacco use continues to be a health issue among Canadians, although the overall smoking rate has declined in the past decade. Twenty-five percent of Canadians age 15 and older reported smoking in 1999. Data collected for 2013 shows that 14.6 percent of Canadians age 15 and older (about 4.2 million people) are current smokers.[4]

Although some people view smoking and drinking as recreational activities, the more individuals smoke and drink, the less likely they are to eat a nutritious diet and follow a healthy lifestyle. This chapter provides information that can help you understand, avoid, and change behaviours that could have an impact on your health, happiness, and life.

FREQUENTLY ASKED QUESTIONS

FAQ: How much alcohol can I drink and still legally drive? p. 320

FAQ: How much alcohol is too much? p. 323

FAQ: How common is drinking on college and university campuses? p. 331

FAQ: What causes alcohol dependence and abuse? p. 335

FAQ: Why do people start smoking? p. 339

FAQ: What are the risks of second-hand smoke? p. 344

ALCOHOL AND ITS EFFECTS

Pure alcohol is a colourless liquid obtained through the fermentation of a liquid containing sugar. **Ethyl alcohol**, or *ethanol*, is the type of alcohol in alcoholic beverages. Another type—methyl or wood alcohol—is a poison that should never be drunk. Any liquid containing 0.5–80 percent ethyl alcohol by volume is an alcoholic beverage. However, different drinks contain different amounts of alcohol.

One drink can be any of the following:

- One glass, 341 millilitres (12 ounces) of beer, which is 5 percent alcohol.
- One standard bottle or can, 341 millilitres (12 ounces) of beer, cider, or cooler, which is 5 percent alcohol.
- One glass, 142 millilitres (5 ounces) of table wine, such as burgundy, which is 12 percent alcohol.
- One small glass, 71 millilitres (2 1/2 ounces) of fortified wine, which is 20 percent alcohol.
- One shot, 43 millilitres (1.5 ounces) of distilled spirits (such as whiskey, vodka, or rum), which is 50 percent alcohol.

All of these drinks contain close to the same amount of alcohol. With distilled spirits (such as bourbon, scotch, vodka, gin, and rum), alcohol content is expressed in terms of **proof**, a number that is *twice* the percentage of alcohol: 100-proof bourbon is 50 percent alcohol; 80-proof gin is 40 percent alcohol.

But the words *bottle* and *glass* can be deceiving in this context. Drinking a 454-millilitre (16-ounce) bottle of malt liquor, which is 6.4 percent alcohol, is not the same as drinking a 340-millilitre (12-ounce) glass of 3.2 percent beer. Two bottles of high-alcohol wines packaged to resemble much less powerful wine coolers can lead to alcohol poisoning, especially in those who weigh less than 68 kilograms (150 pounds). This is one reason alcoholic drinks are a serious danger for young people.

We will discuss many health-related issues that link to alcohol consumption in this chapter, but we start with a common question raised by many young people about drinking and driving.

How Much Alcohol Can I Drink and Still Legally Drive? The best way to drive is to be alcohol free. Some people find that their reaction times and fine-muscle coordination are affected by very small amounts of alcohol. If you are going to drink and want to drive legally, you must determine your **blood-alcohol concentration (BAC)**. BAC is expressed in terms of the percentage of alcohol in the blood. It can be measured by a blood test, from a breathalyzer, or from urine samples. Food, kind and quantity of beverage, weight, sex, and rate of elimination determine BAC after the consumption of alcohol. A BAC of 0.05 percent indicates approximately five parts alcohol to total blood volume. Most people reach a 0.05 level after consuming one or two drinks and experience all the sensations of drinking—relaxation and euphoria—without feeling intoxicated. If they continue to drink past the 0.05 percent BAC level, they gradually lose control of speech, balance, and emotions (see Table 12-1). At a BAC of 0.2 percent, they may pass out. At a BAC of 0.3 percent, they could lapse into a coma; at 0.4 percent, they could die.

For some people, even very low blood alcohol concentrations can cause a headache, upset stomach, or dizziness. These reactions often are inborn. People who have suffered brain damage, often as a result of head trauma or encephalitis, may lose all tolerance for alcohol, either temporarily or permanently, and behave abnormally after drinking small amounts. The elderly, as well as those who are unusually fatigued or have a debilitating physical illness, may also have a low tolerance for alcohol and respond inappropriately to a small amount.

If you are planning on travelling abroad, it is wise to find out the BAC limits for driving and drinking before you land in a foreign country. The range of acceptable limits of BAC (blood alcohol concentration) and BrAC (breath alcohol concentration) varies greatly. The *International Alliance for Responsible Drinking* has developed a comprehensive document titled BAC and BrAC Limits[5] to assist travellers. When referring to the international charts it is important to note that BAC is often expressed in milligrams of ethanol per millilitre of blood (mg/ml)—for example, 0.8. In Canada we define BAC as the amount in milligrams of alcohol in 100 millilitres of blood—or 0.08.

Law-enforcement officers use BAC to determine whether a driver is legally drunk. There are two levels of government that deal with impaired driving in Canada. The federal *Criminal Code of Canada*, section 253(b), puts the BAC legal limit at 0.08. At a provincial level, there are a number of different laws, costs, court-ordered fines, and penalties. In addition to charging drivers with impaired driving, some provinces also impose administrative licence suspensions on drivers whose BAC is under 0.08. One example is the immediate roadside suspensions in British Columbia given to drivers with a BAC of 0.05–0.08. Drivers in B.C. might also have their vehicles impounded for 3–30 days.[6] Table 12-2 illustrates the roadside prohibitions of impaired driving in British Columbia. If you live in a different province check out your own provincial laws and penalties. More provinces are considering or have implemented "warning ranges" or lowering the legal limit of BAC while driving. See Table 12-3 for Blood Alcohol Concentration (BAC) Estimation Charts for Men and Women.

Impaired driving is no longer the leading criminal cause of death in Canada, but it remains a leading cause.

TABLE 12-1

Dose-Specific Effects of Alcohol Intoxication

BAC	Dose-Specific Effects of Alcohol Intoxication*
0.02–0.03	No loss of coordination, slight euphoria, and loss of shyness. Depressant effects are not apparent.
0.04–0.06	Feeling of well-being, relaxation, lower inhibitions, sensation of warmth. Euphoria. Some minor impairment of reasoning and memory, lowering of caution. Driving skills may be impaired at this level of intoxication.
0.07–0.09	Slight impairment of balance, speech, vision, reaction time, and hearing. Euphoria. Judgment and self-control are reduced and caution, reason, and memory are impaired. Driving skills are always impaired at this level of intoxication. It is illegal to operate a motor vehicle in Manitoba at this level of intoxication. (Check levels in your province.)
0.10–0.125	Significant impairment of motor coordination and loss of good judgment. Speech may be slurred; balance, vision, reaction time, and hearing will be impaired. Euphoria.
0.13–0.15	Gross-motor impairment and lack of physical control. Blurred vision and major loss of balance. Euphoria is reduced, and dysphoria (anxiety, restlessness) is beginning to appear.
0.16–0.20	Dysphoria predominates; nausea may appear.
0.25	Needs assistance in walking; total mental confusion. Dysphoria with nausea and some vomiting.
0.30	Loss of consciousness.
0.40 and up	Onset of coma, possible death due to respiratory arrest.**

***The effects of alcohol intoxication vary from person to person and are influenced by such factors as weight, age, and sex.**
****Death can occur at lower blood alcohol levels in some individuals.**

Source: Adapted from: William J. Bailey, *Drug Use in American Society*, 3rd ed., (Minneapolis: Burgess, 1933); The University of Manitoba Security Services, University of Manitoba Alcohol Education Program. Dose-Specific Effects of Alcohol Intoxication. Copyright © 2005 University of Manitoba.

TABLE 12-2

Immediate Roadside Prohibitions (IRPs) for Drivers in British Columbia—Summary Table of Consequences and Costs, Effective April 2016

"WARN" (BAC 0.05–0.08) 1st sanction	• 3-day driving prohibition • Possible 3-day vehicle impoundment • $200 monetary penalty
"WARN" (BAC 0.05–0.08) 2nd sanction (within 5 years)	• 7-day driving prohibition • Possible 7-day vehicle impoundment • $300 monetary penalty
"WARN" (BAC 0.05–0.08) 3rd sanction (within 5 years)	• 30-day driving prohibition • 30-day vehicle impoundment • $400 monetary penalty • Potential referral to remedial programs
"FAIL" (BAC over 0.08) or refuse breath test	• 90-day driving prohibition • 30-day vehicle impoundment • $500 monentary penalty • Mandatory referral to remedial programs
24-Hour Driving Prohibition & Vehicle Impoundment	• If reasonable and probable grounds that a driver's ability to operate a vehicle is affected by alcohol, drugs, or both, a police officer can issue, at roadside, a 24-hour driving prohibition notice. • Impoundment of the vehicle can be made at roadside at the police officer's discretion.

NOTE: Graduated Licensing Program drivers with any alcohol in their system continue to face GLP-specific consequences and reviews, in addition to the penalties outlined above.

Source: Reproduced with permission of the Province of British Columbia. www.ipp.gov.bc.ca

TABLE 12-3

BAC Estimation Charts[1]
Approximate Blood Alcohol Percentage, Men

Drinks	Body Weight in Kilograms (pounds in brackets)								
	45 (100)	54 (120)	64 (140)	73 (160)	82 (180)	91 (200)	100 (220)	109 (240)	
1	.04	.03	.02	.02	.02	.02	.02	.02	Impairment
2	.08	.06	.05	.05	.04	.04	.03	.03	Begins
3	.11	.09	.08	.07	.06	.06	.05	.05	
4	.15	.12	.11	.09	.08	.08	.07	.06	
5	.19	.16	.13	.12	.11	.09	.09	.08	Legally
6	.23	.19	.16	.14	.13	.11	.10	.09	Impaired
7	.26	.22	.19	.16	.15	.13	.12	.11	For
8	.30	.25	.21	.19	.17	.15	.14	.13	Driving
9	.34	.28	.24	.21	.19	.17	.15	.14	
10	.38	.31	.27	.23	.21	.19	.17	.16	

Subtract 0.01% for each 40 minutes of drinking.
One drink is 43 ml (1.5 oz) of spirits @ 40% alc/vol
or 341 ml (12 oz) of beer @ 5% alc/vol
or 142 ml (5 oz) of wine @ 12% alc/vol.
[1] BAC Estimation Chart data should not be relied upon without considering other factors and individual conditions.

Source: Smart Responsible Drinking. AGLC Smart Training Programs (ProTect Security Staff Training and ProServe Liquor Staff Training) 2004. Found at: http://protect.aglc.ca/protectuploads/document/BAC%20Estimation%20Chart_ProTect.pdf.

BAC Estimation Charts[1]
Approximate Blood Alcohol Percentage, Women

Drinks	Body Weight in Kilograms (pounds in brackets)									
	41 (90)	45 (100)	54 (120)	64 (140)	73 (160)	82 (180)	91 (200)	100 (220)	109 (240)	
1	.05	.05	.04	.03	.03	.03	.02	.02	.02	Impairment
2	.10	.09	.08	.07	.06	.05	.05	.04	.04	Begins
3	.15	.14	.11	.10	.09	.08	.07	.06	.06	
4	.20	.18	.15	.13	.11	.10	.09	.08	.08	Legally
5	.25	.23	.19	.16	.14	.13	.11	.10	.09	Impaired
6	.30	.27	.23	.19	.17	.15	.14	.12	.11	For
7	.35	.32	.27	.23	.20	.18	.16	.14	.13	Driving
8	.40	.36	.30	.26	.23	.20	.18	.17	.15	
9	.45	.41	.34	.29	.26	.23	.20	.19	.17	
10	.51	.45	.38	.32	.28	.25	.23	.21	.19	

Subtract 0.01% for each 40 minutes of drinking.
One drink is 43 ml (1.5 oz) of spirits @ 40 % alc/vol
or 341 ml (12 oz) of beer @ 5% alc/vol
or 142 ml (5 oz) of wine @ 12% alc/vol.
[1] BAC Estimation Chart data should not be relied upon without considering other factors and individual conditions.

Source: Smart Responsible Drinking. AGLC Smart Training Programs (ProTect Security Staff Training and ProServe Liquor Staff Training) 2004. Found at: http://protect.aglc.ca/protectuploads/document/BAC%20Estimation%20Chart_ProTect.pdf.

According to the Canada Safety Council, most Canadians consider drinking and driving to be unacceptable. Yet, drinking and driving is still causing tragic accidents. Because of the efforts of MADD (Mothers Against Drunk Driving) Canada,[7] SADD (Students Against Destructive Decisions), and other lobbying groups, provincial and federal governments are cracking down on drivers who drink. More detailed information on drinking and driving is included in Chapter 14, Staying Safe: Preventing Injury, Violence, and Victimization.

To keep drunk drivers off the road, many cities have set up checkpoints to stop cars and inspect drivers for intoxication. National Safe Driving Week—December 1–7—reminds Canadians of the hazards of driving under the influence of alcohol. Key campaign messages are that it is unsafe to operate any vehicle after drinking and that if you have been drinking, you should use a designated driver, call a family member or friend who has not been drinking and ask for a ride, take a cab, or stay where you are overnight.[8]

✓ **CHECK-IN**

What experience have you had with drinking and driving? Do you or your friends drink and drive? Do you offer to be a designated driver?

How Much Alcohol Is Too Much? According to Canadian guidelines for low-risk drinking, weekly alcohol intake should not exceed 15 standard drinks for males and 10 drinks for females. Males should have no more than three drinks a day, most days, and females should have no more than two drinks a day, most days.[9] Your own limit might well be less, depending on your sex, size, and weight. Some people—such as women who are pregnant or trying to conceive; individuals with problems, such as ulcers, that might be aggravated by alcohol; those taking medications such as sleeping pills or antidepressants; and those driving or operating any motorized equipment—shouldn't drink at all. See Figure 12-1 for

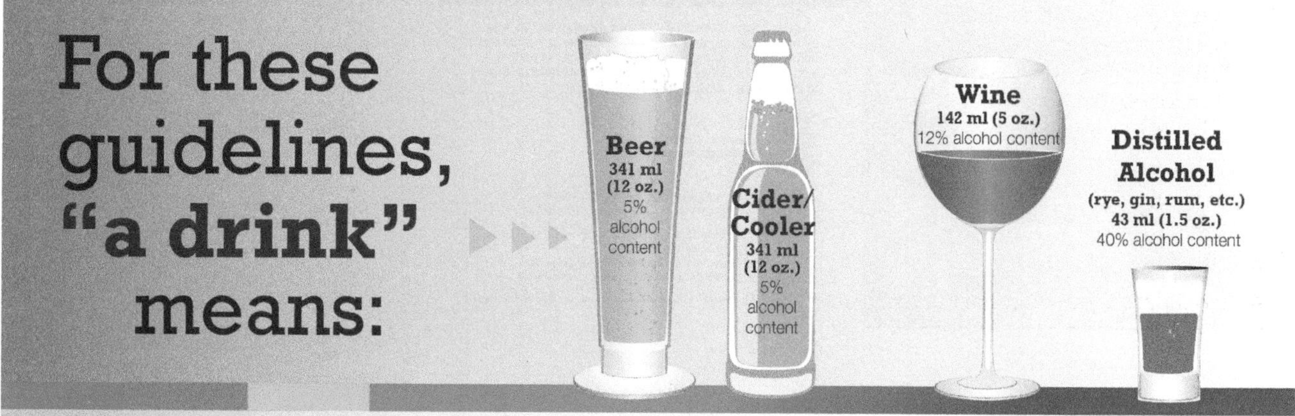

Your limits

Reduce your long-term health risks by drinking no more than:

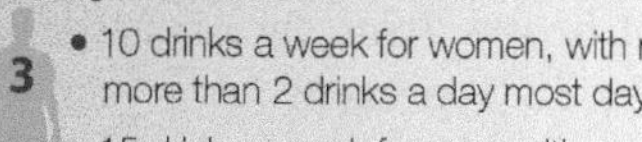

- 10 drinks a week for women, with no more than 2 drinks a day most days
- 15 drinks a week for men, with no more than 3 drinks a day most days

Plan non-drinking days every week to avoid developing a habit.

Special occasions

Reduce your risk of injury and harm by drinking no more than 3 drinks (for women) or 4 drinks (for men) on any single occasion.

Plan to drink in a safe environment. Stay within the weekly limits outlined above in ***Your limits***.

When zero's the limit

Do not drink when you are:

- driving a vehicle or using machinery and tools
- taking medicine or other drugs that interact with alcohol
- doing any kind of dangerous physical activity
- living with mental or physical health problems
- living with alcohol dependence
- pregnant or planning to be pregnant
- responsible for the safety of others
- making important decisions

Pregnant? Zero is safest

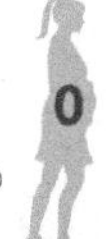

If you are pregnant or planning to become pregnant, or about to breastfeed, the safest choice is to drink no alcohol at all.

Delay your drinking

Alcohol can harm the way the body and brain develop. Teens should speak with their parents about drinking. If they choose to drink, they should do so under parental guidance; never more than 1–2 drinks at a time, and never more than 1–2 times per week. They should plan ahead, follow local alcohol laws and consider the ***Safer drinking tips*** listed in this brochure.

Youth in their late teens to age 24 years should never exceed the daily and weekly limits outlined in ***Your limits***.

(a)

Figure 12-1 Low-Risk Alcohol Drinking Guidelines (LRDG)

Source: Canadian Centre on Substance Abuse (2016). Drinking guidelines. Topics. http://www.ccsa.ca/Eng/topics/alcohol/drinking-guidelines/Pages/default.aspx; http://www.ccsa.ca/Resource%20Library/2012-Canada-Low-Risk-Alcohol-Drinking-Guidelines-Brochure-en.pdf. Reproduced with permission from the Canadian Centre on Substance Abuse.

Safer drinking tips

- Set limits for yourself and stick to them.
- Drink slowly. Have no more than 2 drinks in any 3 hours.
- For every drink of alcohol, have one non-alcoholic drink.
- Eat before and while you are drinking.
- Always consider your age, body weight and health problems that might suggest lower limits.
- While drinking may provide health benefits for certain groups of people, do not start to drink or increase your drinking for health benefits.

Low-risk drinking helps to promote a culture of moderation.

Low-risk drinking supports healthy lifestyles.

CCSA wishes to thank the partners who supported development of Canada's Low-Risk Alcohol Drinking Guidelines. For a complete list of the organizations supporting the guidelines, please visit www.ccsa.ca/Eng/topics/alcohol/drinking-guidelines/Pages/Supporters-LRDG.aspx

Visit our website to find out more!

www.ccsa.ca

Reference:

Butt, P., Beirness, D., Gliksman, L., Paradis, C., & Stockwell, T. (2011). *Alcohol and health in Canada: A summary of evidence and guidelines for low-risk drinking*. Ottawa, ON: Canadian Centre on Substance Abuse.

The Canadian Centre on Substance Abuse changes lives by bringing people and knowledge together to reduce the harm of alcohol and other drugs on society. We partner with public, private and non-governmental organizations to improve the health and safety of Canadians.

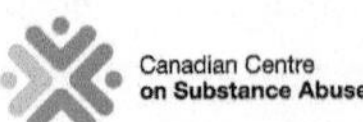

500–75 Albert Street, Ottawa, ON K1P 5E7
Tel: 613-235-4048 | Fax: 613-235-8101

Charitable #: 122328750RR0001 | ISBN 978-1-927467-55-6
Developed on behalf of the
National Alcohol Strategy Advisory Committee

Cette publication est également disponible en français.

Canada's Low-Risk Alcohol Drinking Guidelines

Drinking is a personal choice. If you choose to drink, these guidelines can help you decide when, where, why and how.

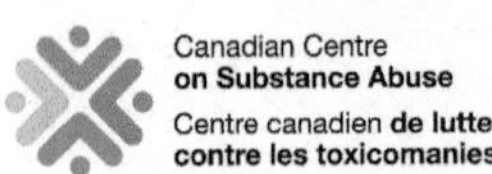

Partnership. Knowledge. Change.
Collaboration. Connaissance. Changement.

(b)

Figure 12-1 *(Continued)*

more information on Canada's Low Risk Drinking Guidelines (LRDG) developed by Canadian and international experts.

The dangers of alcohol increase along with the amount you drink. Heavy drinking[10] means having five drinks or more on one occasion for men and four or more drinks on one occasion for women at least once a month in the past year. Heavy drinking destroys the liver, weakens the heart, elevates blood pressure, damages the brain, and increases the risk of cancer. Individuals who drink heavily have a higher mortality rate than those who have two or fewer drinks a day. However, the boundary between safe and dangerous drinking isn't the same for everyone. For some people, the upper limit of safety is zero: once they start, they can't stop.

Statistics Canada reports that in 2013, 18.9 percent (5.5 million) of Canadians aged 12 and over stated that their alcohol consumption categorized them as heavy drinkers. Among males, 24.5 percent reported they were heavy drinkers. For females it was 13.4 percent. See Figure 12-2 for the percentage of heavy drinkers between 2001 and 2013.[11]

The highest rate of heavy drinking occurred among males aged 20–34, at 38.3 percent. For females, the highest rate of heavy drinking was among the 18- to 19-year-old age group.[12] See Figure 12-3 for an illustration of the percentage of heavy drinking by age group overall and Canadians aged 12–65 years and older.

✓ CHECK-IN

If you drink alcohol, when and why do you drink?

Intoxication If you drink too much, the immediate consequence is that you get drunk—or, more precisely, intoxicated. **Intoxication** is defined as an "abnormal state that is essentially a poisoning."[13,*] Alcohol intoxication, which can range from mild inebriation to loss of consciousness,

*By permission. From Merriam-Webster's Collegiate® Dictionary, 11th Edition © 2016 by Merriam-Webster, Inc. (www.Merriam-Webster.com).

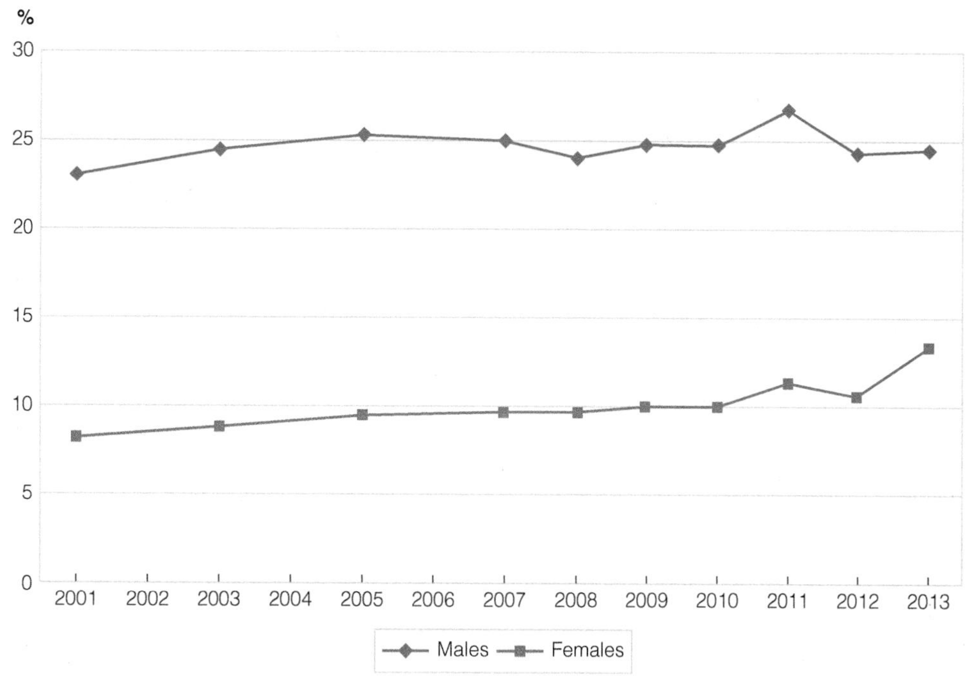

Figure 12-2 **Percentage Who Reported Heavy Drinking in the Last Year, by Sex, Household Population Aged 12 or Older, Canada, 2001–2013**

Source: Statistics Canada (2015, November 27). Heavy drinking, 2013. Health Fact Sheets. Publications. Catalogue no. 82-625-X. http://www.statcan.gc.ca/pub/82-625-x/2014001/article/14019-eng.htm.

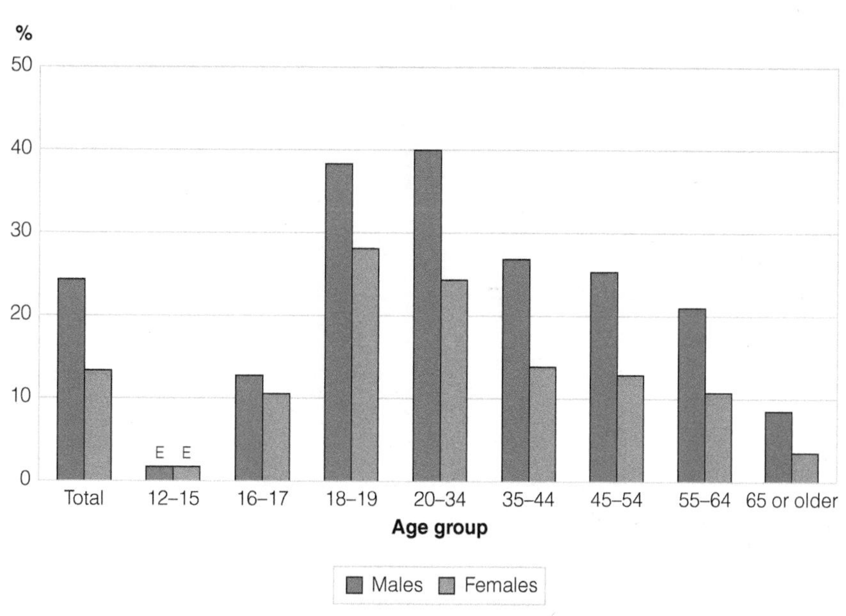

Figure 12-3 **Percentage Who Reported Heavy Drinking in the Last Year, by Age Group and Sex, Household Population Aged 12 or Older, Canada, 2013**

Source: Statistics Canada (2015, November 27). Heavy drinking, 2013. Health Fact Sheets. Publications. Catalogue no. 82-625-X. http://www.statcan.gc.ca/pub/82-625-x/2014001/article/14019-eng.htm.

is characterized by at least one of the following signs: slurred speech, poor coordination, unsteady gait, abnormal eye movements, impaired attention or memory, stupor, or coma. Medical risks of intoxication include falls, hypothermia in cold climates, and increased risk of infections because of suppressed immune function.

Time and a protective environment are the recommended treatments for alcohol intoxication. Anyone who passes out after drinking heavily should be monitored regularly to ensure that vomiting (the result of excess alcohol irritating the stomach) doesn't block the breathing airway. Always make sure that an unconscious drinker is lying on his or her side, with the head lower than the body. Intoxicated drinkers can slip into shock, a potentially life-threatening condition characterized by a weak pulse, irregular breathing, and skin-colour changes. This is an emergency, and professional medical care should be sought immediately.

✓ CHECK-IN

Do you know how best to help someone who's intoxicated? Do you know what to do if you suspect alcohol poisoning? Call 911 immediately for help.

Impact of Alcohol Unlike drugs in tablet form or food, alcohol is directly and quickly absorbed into the bloodstream through the stomach walls and upper intestine. The alcohol in a typical drink reaches the bloodstream in 15 minutes and rises to its peak concentration in about an hour. The bloodstream carries the alcohol to the liver, heart, and brain.

Alcohol is a *diuretic*, a drug that speeds up the elimination of fluid from the body. Most of the alcohol you drink can leave your body only after it has been metabolized by the liver, which converts about 95 percent of the alcohol to carbon dioxide and water. The other 5 percent is excreted unchanged, mainly through urination, respiration, and perspiration. Alcohol lowers body temperature, so you should never drink to get or stay warm.

Alcohol affects the major organ systems of the body and is a known risk factor for several cancers (see Figure 12-4). Drs. Boffetta and Hashibe reviewed numerous studies on alcohol and cancer. They report that researchers from around the world have determined that there is evidence of a high risk of cancer of the head and neck area, specifically in the anatomical sites that are in close contact on ingestion of alcohol such as the oral cavity, tongue, pharynx, larynx, and

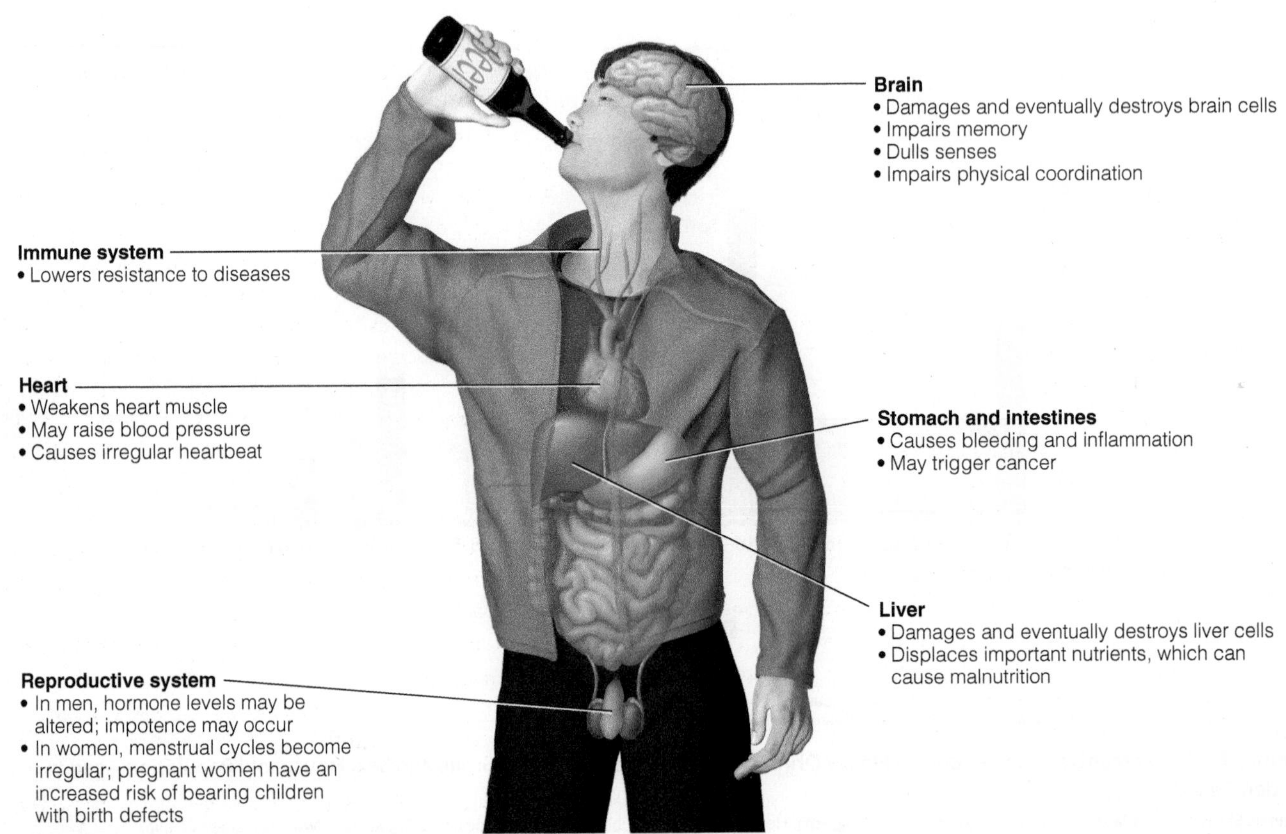

Figure 12-4 The Effects of Alcohol Abuse on the Body

Alcohol has a major effect on the brain, damaging brain cells, impairing judgment and perceptions, and often leading to accidents and altercations. Alcohol also damages the digestive system, especially the liver.

esophagus. These studies have been consistent since the mid-1950s.[14]

Studies have identified alcohol consumption as a risk factor for breast cancer, too. Boyle and Boffetta completed an extensive review of the literature on the effects of alcohol and the link to breast cancer.[15] They determined that there is a large body of evidence that shows alcohol consumption increases the risk of breast cancer. Research showed that even moderate alcohol consumption increases this risk. Further review by Boffetta and Hashibe confirmed this link and indicated that although the extent of additional risk of breast cancer due to alcohol is not very large, the high incidence of this cancer results in more women with breast cancer attributable to alcohol than for any other type of cancer.

Then there is the other side of the story—some studies suggest that light to moderate consumption of alcohol can have positive effects. Benefits include an increase of high-density lipoproteins, which lowers the risk of coronary heart disease.[16] However, it may be that light to moderate drinkers may participate in regular physical activity, make healthy food choices, and see their physicians for regular checkups, which might account for their overall health status. We must recognize that any benefits may be specific to individuals and also depend on their genetic makeup.[17] The risks of alcohol consumption can outweigh the benefits, especially for young people. Pregnant women *should not drink*, and people who do not drink should not necessarily be encouraged to start.

Digestive System Alcohol reaches the stomach first, where it is partially broken down. The remaining alcohol is absorbed easily through the stomach tissue into the bloodstream. In the stomach, alcohol triggers the secretion of acids, which irritate the stomach lining. Excessive drinking at one sitting may result in nausea; chronic drinking may result in peptic ulcers (breaks in the stomach lining) and bleeding from the stomach lining.

The alcohol in the bloodstream eventually reaches the liver. The liver, which bears the major responsibility of fat metabolism in the body, converts this alcohol to fat. After a few weeks of four or five drinks a day, liver cells start to accumulate fat. An increase of fat levels increases the risk of diabetes and cirrhosis of the liver. Alcohol also stimulates liver cells to attract white blood cells, which normally travel throughout the bloodstream engulfing harmful substances and wastes. If white blood cells begin to invade body tissue, such as the liver, they can cause irreversible damage.

Cardiovascular System Alcohol gets mixed reviews regarding its effects on the cardiovascular system. People who drink moderate amounts of alcohol have lower mortality rates after a heart attack, as well as a lower risk of heart attack, compared to abstainers and heavy drinkers. It also appears that beer, distilled spirits, and red wine might positively influence our platelets and lipids. However, Lindberg and Amsterdam remind us that the benefits might be linked to the socio-economic levels of individuals instead of the alcohol itself.[18] It is also important to remember that heart health can be improved through regular physical activity, lowering stress levels, and healthy eating.

Heavier drinking triggers the release of harmful oxygen molecules called free radicals, which can increase the risk of heart disease and stroke. Alcohol can weaken the heart muscle, causing a disorder called *cardiomyopathy*. The combined use of alcohol and other drugs, including tobacco and cocaine, greatly increases the likelihood of damage to the heart.

Immune System Chronic alcohol use can inhibit the production of both white blood cells, which fight off infections, and red blood cells, which carry oxygen to all the organs and tissues of the body. Alcohol may increase the risk of HIV infection by altering the judgment of users so that they more readily engage in activities, such as unsafe sexual practices, that put them in danger. If you drink when you have a cold or the flu, alcohol interferes with the body's ability to recover. It also increases the chance of bacterial pneumonia in flu sufferers.

Brain and Behaviour At first, when you drink, you feel "up." In low dosages, alcohol affects the regions of the brain that inhibit or control behaviour, so you might feel more relaxed. However, you also experience losses of concentration, memory, judgment, and fine motor control, and you have mood swings and emotional outbursts. Moderate and heavy drinkers show signs of impaired intelligence, slowed-down reflexes, and difficulty remembering. Research has shown that heavy drinking also depletes the brain's supplies of crucial chemicals, including dopamine, gamma amino butyric acid, upload peptides, and serotonin, that are responsible for our feelings of pleasure and well-being. At the same time, alcohol promotes the release of stress chemicals, such as corticotrophin releasing factor (CRF), that create tension and depression.

Heavy alcohol use may pose special dangers to the brains of drinkers at both ends of the age spectrum. Studies show that binge drinking or heavy episodic drinking in adolescence (15–21 years) damages the corticolimbic or frontal lobe region of the brain. This alcohol-induced brain damage leads to mood changes, a decreased level of cognitive and neurological performance, increased risk of dementia, and a susceptibility to alcoholism in later life. It also decreases the ability to regulate the normal process of anticipation and reward, resulting in impatience, lack of judgment, impulsiveness, and, at times, lack of understanding consequences for behaviours.[19] What concerns researchers is the finding that the brain damage can occur after very few and infrequent binge drinking sessions.[20]

Elderly people who drink heavily appear to have more brain shrinkage, or atrophy, than those who drink lightly or not at all. Because alcohol is a central nervous system depressant, it slows down the activity of the neurons in the brain, gradually dulling the responses of the brain and nervous system. One or two drinks act as a tranquilizer or relaxant. Additional drinks result in a progressive reduction in central nervous system activity, leading to sleep, general anesthesia, coma, and even death. Older adults misusing or abusing alcohol often suffer from long-term depression, too.[21]

Even moderate amounts of alcohol can have disturbing effects on perception and judgment, including the following:

- **Impaired perceptions.** You're less able to adjust your eyes to bright lights because glare bothers you more. Although you can still hear sounds, you can't distinguish between them or accurately determine their source.
- **Dulled smell and taste.** Alcohol itself may cause some vitamin deficiencies, and the poor eating habits of heavy drinkers result in further nutrition problems.
- **Diminished sensation.** On a freezing winter night, you may walk outside without a coat and not feel the cold.
- **Altered sense of space.** You may not realize, for instance, that you have been in one place for several hours.
- **Impaired motor skills.** Writing, typing, driving, and other tasks involving your muscles are impaired. Drinking large amounts of alcohol impairs reaction time, speed, accuracy, and consistency, as well as judgment.

Increased Risk of Harm and Dying Although most people do not have a problem with alcohol and do not suffer from harm when they drink, findings from a 2015 report on alcohol consumption in Canada confirmed that people who do use alcohol without care and attention are at an increased risk of harm—either to themselves or from drinking by others. Of the 22 million Canadians who indicated they drank alcohol, 3.1 million drank a sufficient amount to put themselves at risk for injury and harm.[22] Alcohol can increase your risk for cirrhosis of the liver and a number of cancers. It can also cause anemia, can affect cardiorespiratory health, is linked to dementia, can disrupt the sympathetic nervous system that impacts blood pressure, and can cause seizures. Misusing alcohol can also affect personal and professional lives and impact friendships, social life, financial stability, relationships, and employment opportunities, and can create legal problems. Findings from the 2015 *National College Health Assessment (NCHA)* illustrate the risk. Students who drank alcohol experienced the following in the twelve months prior to the survey:[23]

- 29.2 percent of students did something that they later regretted.
- 25.2 percent of students forgot where they were or what they did.
- 2.1 percent got in trouble with the police.
- 20.4 percent of students had unprotected sex.
- 11.7 percent of students injured themselves.
- 1.3 percent of students injured someone else.
- 2.9 percent of students seriously considered suicide.

Alcohol and driving also injures and kills. MADD Canada estimates that there are somewhere between 1250 and 1500 alcohol-impairment-related crash deaths each year, or 3.4–4.1 deaths per day.[24]

Alcohol also plays a role in homicides and suicides and is the leading cause of cirrhosis of the liver, a chronic disease that causes extensive scarring and irreversible damage. Drinkers over age 50 face the greatest danger of premature death from cirrhosis of the liver, hepatitis, and other alcohol-linked illnesses.

Mortality rates increase with the amount of alcohol consumed. The mortality rate for alcoholics is two and a half times higher than for non-alcoholics of the same age.

✓ CHECK-IN

Have you ever experienced any alcohol-related problems or harm?

Interaction with Other Drugs Alcohol can interact with other drugs—prescription and non-prescription, legal and illegal. Of the 100 most frequently prescribed drugs, more than half contain at least one ingredient that interacts adversely with alcohol. Because alcohol and other psychoactive drugs may work on the same areas of the brain, their combination can produce an effect much greater than that expected of either drug by itself. The consequences of this synergistic interaction can be fatal (see Table 12-4). Alcohol is particularly dangerous when combined with depressants and anti-anxiety medications.

Aspirin, long used to prevent or counter alcohol's effects, may actually enhance its impact by significantly lowering the body's ability to break down alcohol in the stomach, resulting in a higher BAC. This increase could make a difference in impairment for individuals driving cars or operating machinery.

If you want to drink while taking medication, be sure you read the warnings on non-prescription drug labels or prescription-drug containers; ask your doctor about possible alcohol–drug interactions; and check with your pharmacist if you have any questions about your medications, especially over-the-counter (OTC) products.

TABLE 12-4

Alcohol and Drug Reactions

Drug	Possible Effects of Interaction
Analgesics (painkillers); narcotics (codeine, Demerol®, Percodan®)	Increase in central nervous system depression, possibly leading to respiratory failure and death
Non-narcotics (Aspirin®, Tylenol®)	Irritation of stomach resulting in bleeding and increased susceptibility to liver damage
Antabuse	Nausea, vomiting, headache, high blood pressure, and erratic heartbeat
Anti-anxiety drugs (Valium®, Librium)	Increase in central nervous system depression, decreased alertness, and impaired judgment
Antidepressants	Increase in central nervous system depression; certain antidepressants in combination with red wine could cause a sudden increase in blood pressure
Antihistamines (Actifed®, Dimetapp®, and other cold medications)	Increase in drowsiness; driving more dangerous
Antibiotics	Nausea, vomiting, headache; some medications rendered less effective
Central nervous system stimulants (caffeine, Dexedrine®, Ritalin®)	Stimulant effects of these drugs may reverse depressant effect of alcohol but do not decrease its intoxicating effects
Diuretics (Diuril®, Lasix®)	Reduction in blood pressure resulting in dizziness upon rising
Sedatives (Dalmane®, Nembutal, Quaalude)	Increase in central nervous system depression, possibly leading to coma, respiratory failure, and death

Source: *Canadian addiction survey.* Health Canada 2007. Reproduced with the permission of the Minister of Health, 2013.

DRINKING IN CANADA

Approximately 22 million Canadians (15 years and older) reported that they drank alcohol in the previous year when surveyed in 2013. The highest percentage of past year drinkers was in the 30- to 34- year-old age group. Canadians in the 20- to 29-year-old age group were found to have the highest percentage of risky drinkers—individuals who drank more alcohol than the low-risk drinking guidelines recommend[25] (see Figure 12-1).

Since 2004, the rate of past-year drinking has declined with 79 percent of Canadians reporting they drank in 2004, compared to 75 percent of Canadians in 2013. Many Canadians are also choosing not to drink. Close to seven million Canadians disclose that they do not drink at all.[26]

While men drink more than women and have riskier drinking patterns, women are starting to report increased risky drinking behaviour, especially those who are 35 years and older.[27]

Why People Drink The most common reason people drink alcohol is to relax (see Figure 12-5). Because it depresses the central nervous system, alcohol can make people feel less tense. Other motivations for drinking include the celebration of important occasions, friendship, lowering inhibitions, self-medication, and role modelling. Some of our most admired celebrities appear regularly in commercials for alcohol. This can be a powerful form of advertising—an encouragement to drink.

Canadian undergraduate students report similar reasons for drinking, although social reasons appear to be their primary motivation. These include aesthetic reasons—to enjoy the taste or to enhance a meal, to celebrate, and to be sociable or polite. Other reasons are to get drunk, to feel good, to relax, and to comply with others.[28]

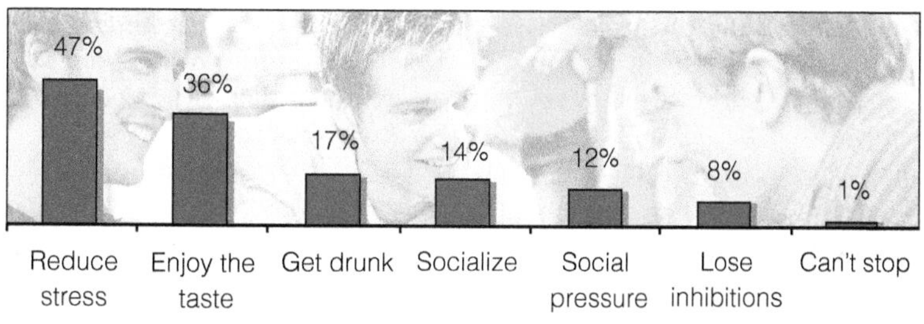

Figure 12-5 **Why Students Drink**

Source: *Wasting the Best and the Brightest: Substance Abuse at America's Colleges and Universities.* New York: The National Center on Addiction and Substance Abuse at Columbia University, March 2007.

HUMAN POTENTIAL

Duncan Campbell—From Tragedy to Triumph

You have heard it before. If you are going to drink, drink responsibly. This Human Potential story is about someone who has lived with the consequences of an accident that occurred, in part, because of drinking. It is also a story of someone who took responsibility for his actions and lived with the consequences.

When Duncan Campbell was 17 he was drinking with friends at a shallow, artificial lake in Winnipeg, Manitoba. Everyone knows you should not drink and swim. You shouldn't drink and dive either, but that is what Duncan did. The result of a dive into the shallow lake was a broken neck. In a moment's time he became a C7 quadriplegic. He cannot walk, but he does have good use of his arms, is mobile in a manual wheelchair, drives a car, and works. Duncan says that "there are definitely consequences to drinking and diving or doing anything else where alcohol would put you or others at risk. Accidents involving brain and spinal cord injuries involve alcohol almost one-third of the time. It doesn't mean that you have to completely abstain but you have to be diligent in taking precautions. If you develop a more active healthy lifestyle you probably won't have problems with drinking."

Duncan was in rehab for nine months. He had to learn how to dress himself, go to the bathroom, get into bed, and wheel his chair. He also had to figure out how to stay involved in sports. Back in 1976, there were no team sports for quadriplegics—hockey was no longer an option. Hanging out in the rehab facility's gym one day, Duncan and a group of new friends, also in rehab, started to "throw some stuff around." From that chance beginning, Duncan helped to create and develop wheelchair rugby, also known as murderball, a sport that would end up being played in 36 countries, have an annual world championship event, and become a Paralympic sport in 2000 for quadriplegics.

Duncan says that he does not consider himself to be any kind of hero; however, he does consider himself to be a strong promoter of fitness and sport. "I feel that getting involved with wheelchair sports permanently changed my life. Through volunteering with the organizational needs of wheelchair sports I changed my career choices. It allowed me to become a healthier, more active, and more independent individual. It facilitated me meeting numerous friends around the world who I will have forever." Duncan has had a lifetime of helping others. He worked for 16 years as a recreation therapist at the G.F. Strong Rehabilitation Centre in Vancouver, British Columbia, a centre that specializes in spinal cord injuries; here he helped 13- to 19-year-olds explore options that assisted them in rebuilding through rehabilitation. He was passionate about his work. "Recreation therapy is something I truly believe in with all my heart. When the kids are at a rehab centre classes and programs are scheduled for them. When they return home, many of them don't know what to do—they don't know what options they have in their community. Recreation therapy shows people all the choices they have to stay active." Duncan helped to make the G.F. Strong Rehabilitation facility become a leader in spinal-cord rehabilitation in Canada and the world. When asked about his job at that facility, Duncan says that it was the kids that were the highlight of his work. "They were amazing. They made every day a new day. I feel privileged that I had the opportunity to work at G.F. Strong and meet so many wonderful young people."

Currently Duncan works with the Canadian Wheelchair Sports Association as the national coordinator of a wheelchair sports recruitment program called Bridging the Gap, a program intended to expand wheelchair sport awareness, recruitment, development, and retention across Canada. He is also the national development director of wheelchair rugby in Canada.

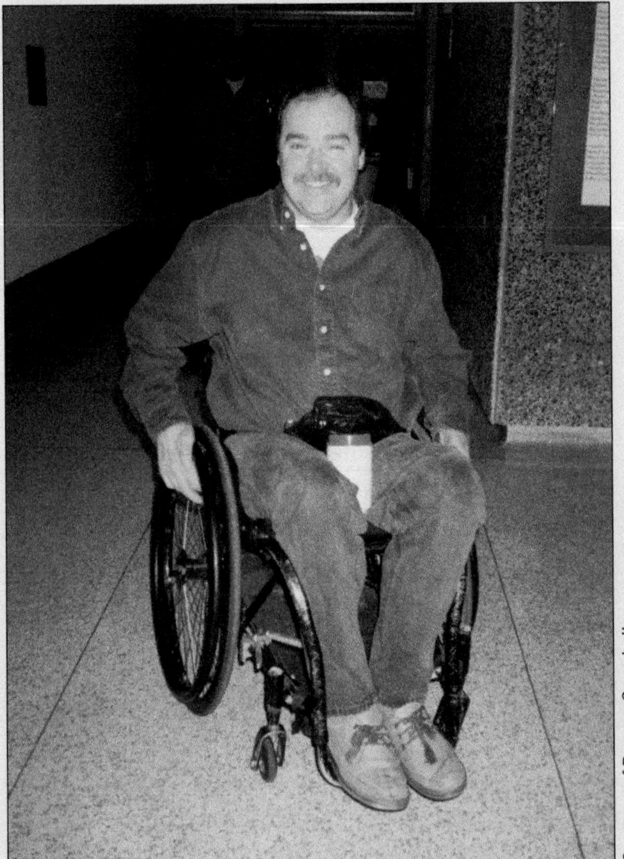
Courtesy of Duncan Campbell

Duncan Campbell, National Coordinator for Bridging the Gap.

He participates in physical activity on a regular basis himself. He often hand-cycles to work in a wheelchair designed for cycling. He plays rugby and hockey and he cross-country skis. Some of his other accomplishments include two university degrees and worldwide travel. "One very special trip involved a good friend of mine, also a quadriplegic, securing all our gear to our wheelchairs and pushing the bike routes from Amsterdam to Northern France over a six-week period."

He was inducted into the Canadian Paralympic Sports Hall of Fame as a "Builder" in 2005. He also was selected as a Paralympic torchbearer for both the 2008 Paralympics in China and the 2010 Paralympics in Whistler, British Columbia, representing the City of Vancouver, British Columbia, and the International Wheelchair Rugby Federation. He was inducted into the University of Alberta Alumni Hall of Fame in 2014.

Duncan managed the Canadian National Wheelchair Rugby Team including the Sydney Paralympics. The one constant in Duncan's life has been his passion for sport, especially wheelchair rugby. Duncan's words of wisdom for all of us: Don't drink and dive, but more importantly, no matter what life throws at you, don't dwell on the past—it can't be changed—and keep on going.

How Common Is Drinking on College and University Campuses? Drinking has long been part of the college and university experience. As can be expected, undergraduates display diverse drinking patterns. Data from the National College Health Assessment found that there was a difference between actual alcohol use and perceived use among college and university students.[29] *Actual* alcohol use for both males and females within the 30 days prior to the survey was as follows:

- *Never Used*—25.5 percent
- *Used, but not in the last 30 days*—15.0 percent
- *Used 1–9 days*—45.5 percent
- *Used 10–29 days*—12.9 percent
- *Used all 30 days*—1.1 percent
- *Actual any use within the last 30 days*—59.5 percent

Perceived use was as follows:

- *Never used*—5.3 percent
- *Used, but not in the last 30 days*—2.6 percent
- *Used 1–9 days*—37.3 percent
- *Used 10–29 days*—40.7 percent
- *Used all 30 days*—14.1 percent
- *Perceived any use within the last 30 days*—92.1 percent

The data also showed a difference between any actual use and perceived use among males and females:

- Actual any use within the last 30 days (males)—59.5 percent
- Actual any use within the last 30 days (females)—59.6 percent
- Perceived any use within the last 30 days (males)—91.1 percent
- Perceived any use within the last 30 days (females)—92.8 percent[30]

The Canadian Centre for Social Norms Research also studied the perceptions and beliefs of university students across the country to gain a greater understanding of the behaviours of students and alcohol use. This study concluded the following:[31]

- The majority of students (63 percent) drink twice per month or less.
- When students do drink, most (64 percent) consume one to four drinks at parties or bars.
- Most students overestimate both the quantity and frequency of drinking by their peers.
- Eighty percent of students believe that their peers typically drink once per week or more often.
- One-third believe that their fellow students drink at least three times per week.
- Sixty-seven percent of students believe that their peers consume five or more drinks per occasion. One-quarter believe the average consumption is seven or more drinks.
- Ninety-three percent thought they should not drink to levels that interfered with academics or other responsibilities.

To address the alcohol-use problems on college and university campuses, administrators, faculty, student services, and students are developing many innovative alcohol-reduction programs and initiatives. Lane,[32] in a study of 103 college students who were taking first-year experience courses, evaluated the benefits of a computer-assisted online program called eChug and a skills training self-management program. The students who were classified as heavy drinkers benefited from the e-Chug program. The lighter drinkers benefited more greatly from the skills training self-management program. However, there is still work to be done. Roosen and Mills,[33] in a large-scale study on 3400 first-year Canadian psychology students, found a new phenomenon—**drunkorexia**—occurring on campuses across Canada. Findings revealed that approximately 1 in 5 students intentionally cut back on food consumption prior to drinking alcohol. Both male and female students indicated they did this for two main reasons: watching calories and having the ability to get drunk faster. This research reminds us that a variety of alcohol-reduction strategies need to be available for students who are unaware of the major health risks of over-drinking and for those who are attempting to lower their alcohol consumption.

✓ CHECK-IN

How widespread is drinking on your campus?

Binge Drinking **Binge drinking**—defined as the consumption of five or more alcoholic drinks in a row by men and four or more by women—is the leading cause of preventable death among undergraduates and the most serious threat to their intellectual, physical, and psychological development.

Adlaf et al.[34] discovered that heavy or binge drinking among Canadian undergraduates is common. The groups that reported the highest rates of binge drinking were among males, students living in residence, students with low academic orientation, and those with what the researchers described as a high recreational orientation. In recent years, many students have died after consuming numerous drinks in a short period of time, while others have sustained serious injuries or caused others to be injured.

Why do students binge? Some educators view bingeing as a product of the college or university environment.[35] More students binge drink at the beginning of the school year and then cut back as the semester progresses and academic demands increase. Binge drinking also peaks following exam times, during athletic home-game weekends, and during reading break. Many new students engage in binge drinking for the first time very soon after they arrive on campus. Kubacki et al. found that opportunities for binge drinking were created by students living together in residence halls without parental supervision. Intensive consumption of alcohol was also linked to the need for students to belong to certain groups, and their desires to fit in and to follow friends.[36] Another finding was that binge drinking decreased in subsequent years for some students. Although the amount of alcohol consumption for the students did not change, the drinking pattern evolved from binge drinking to a more regular consumption of smaller amounts of alcohol at one time.[37]

Surveys consistently show that students who engage in binge drinking, particularly those who do so more than once a week, experience a far higher rate of problems than other students. Frequent binge drinkers are likely to miss classes, vandalize property, and drive after drinking.[38] Frequent binge drinkers are also more likely to experience five or more different alcohol-related problems and to use other substances, including nicotine and drugs.[39]

✓ CHECK-IN

Is binge-drinking common among your friends? Is it common on your college or university campus?

The Toll of Drinking for College and University Students A lack of awareness of the consequences of alcohol consumption seems to be common among college and university students. However, alcohol use can become problematic and even tragic. Alcohol combined with poor judgment or bad luck can lead to life-altering and sometimes life-threatening consequences.

Results from the *Canadian Campus Survey* show that university students report a number of consequences of drinking: having a hangover, regretting their actions, memory loss, missing classes, having unplanned sexual relations and unsafe sex, and drinking and driving.[40] According to the Commission on Substance Abuse at Colleges and Universities in the United States, alcohol is involved in two-thirds of college student suicides, 9 of 10 rapes, and 95 percent of violent crimes on campus.[41]

Smith et al. used a Web-based survey with 891 students at a large Midwestern university in the U.S.A. to uncover what undergraduates perceived to be the most severe alcohol-related harms and what behaviours might be put in place to prevent the harm.[42] The nine most severe harms identified were

- forced sex,
- legal trouble,
- physically injuring another person,
- unprotected sex,
- relationship damage,
- regretting something you did,
- physically injuring yourself,

X AND Y FILES

Alcohol, Tobacco, Men, and Women

In the past, far more men than women drank. Today, both genders are likely to consume alcohol. However, there are well-documented differences in how often and how much men and women drink. In general, men drink more frequently, consume a larger quantity of alcohol per drinking occasion, and report more problems related to drinking.

Women are at greater risk of organ damage from heavy alcohol use and have higher rates of liver cirrhosis. One reason is that females do not respond to long-term heavy use of alcohol with the same protective physiological mechanisms as men. Excessive drinking causes more damage to the female liver. Women drinkers also are at greater risk of heart disease, osteoporosis, and breast cancer.

In recent years, researchers have been comparing and contrasting the reasons why men and women drink. Undergraduate women and men are equally likely to drink for stress-related reasons; both perceive alcohol as a means of tension relaxation. Some psychologists theorize that men engage in *confirmatory drinking*—that is, they drink to reinforce the image of masculinity associated with alcohol consumption. Both genders may engage in *compensatory drinking*, consuming alcohol to heighten their sense of masculinity or femininity.

Male and female smokers share certain characteristics: Most start smoking as teenagers; the lower their educational level, the more likely they are to smoke. But there are gender differences in tobacco use. In the last decade, smoking rates among adult women stopped their previous decline and have risen sharply among teenage girls. Men of all ages are more likely than women to use other forms of tobacco, such as cigars and chewing tobacco.

Men smoke to decrease boredom and fatigue and to increase arousal and concentration. Women smoke to control their weight and to decrease stress, anger, and other negative feelings.

Women tend to be less successful than men in quitting smoking. Possible reasons include gender differences in the effectiveness of therapies, a greater fear of weight gain among women, the inability to take certain anti-smoking drugs while pregnant, and the menstrual cycle's effect on withdrawal symptoms. Women drop out at higher rates from traditional stop-smoking programs and are less responsive to nicotine-replacement therapies. The approaches that work best for them combine medication and behavioural treatments, including support groups.

- forgetting where you were or what you did, and
- getting involved in a fight.

When asked what behaviours could be used to prevent these harms, the students shared many ideas, with the top five listed here:

- Accept personal responsibility (32.3 percent).
- Stay with the same group of friends (13.0 percent).
- Do not party with strangers or by yourself (5.7 percent).
- Choose not to drink (4.5 percent).
- Watch out for companions (3.7 percent).[43]

Other protective behaviours that were identified include arranging for an escort, not travelling alone, acting responsibly in public, avoiding confrontations, having a friend let you know when you have had enough, and not drinking and driving. The findings have both positive and negative implications. It is noteworthy that undergraduate students have ranked personal responsibility as the number-one protective behaviour to lower the risk of harm when drinking. As the authors of this study suggest, the finding shows that undergraduate students do recognize the importance of taking personal responsibility for their actions.

However, when people partake in heavy or extreme drinking, the ability to "take care of oneself" is diminished. Self-monitoring is not an easy thing to do when you are intoxicated. Alcohol-related harm on some college and university campuses appears to be widespread. It is linked with serious physical, social, and psychological consequences. We must all continue to do more to bring awareness to the negative aspects of alcohol misuse and abuse.

Aboriginal Communities—Reaching Out and Moving Forward Alcohol abuse is a leading self-reported threat to the health and quality of life for many Aboriginal peoples. The misuse of alcohol has been traced to stresses related to acculturation, poverty, racial discrimination, and powerlessness. Certainly not all Aboriginal peoples drink, and not all who drink do so to excess. But experts in alcohol treatment are increasingly recognizing racial and ethnic differences in risk factors for drinking problems, patterns of drinking, and most effective types of treatment.

Within the First Nations and Inuit Health Department of the Government of Canada, the National Native Alcohol and Drug Abuse Program (NNADAP)[44] supports First Nations and Inuit with prevention activities such as school programs, intervention activities such as native spiritual and cultural programs, and aftercare activities such as sharing circles and support groups.

Support also comes from First Nations people themselves. The First Nations Health Authority (FNHA) in British Columbia has embarked on community-centred care, multidisciplinary health teams, Elders' gatherings, youth wellness quests, and urban on-reserve care clinics to reinforce healthy living options and healing from alcohol abuse and misuse.[45]

Women and Alcohol—Special Considerations Problems directly related to a woman's alcohol use range from the consequences of risky sexual behaviour after alcohol consumption to severe physiological problems related to fertility and pregnancy. Because women have a far smaller quantity of a protective enzyme in the stomach to break down alcohol before it is absorbed into the bloodstream, women absorb about 30 percent more alcohol into their bloodstream than men. The alcohol travels through the blood to the brain, so women become intoxicated much more quickly. Because there's more alcohol in the bloodstream to break down, the liver may also be adversely affected. In alcoholic women, the stomach seems to completely stop digesting alcohol, which may explain why women alcoholics are more likely to suffer liver damage than men.

Alcohol brings many other health dangers to women:

- Gynecologic problems. Moderate to heavy drinking may contribute to infertility, menstrual problems, sexual dysfunction, and premenstrual syndrome.
- Breast cancer. As mentioned previously, numerous studies have suggested an increased risk of breast cancer among women who drink, and many physicians feel that those at high risk for breast cancer should stop, or at least reduce, their consumption of alcohol.
- Osteoporosis. As women age, their risk of osteoporosis, a condition characterized by calcium loss and bone thinning, increases. Alcohol can block the absorption of many nutrients, including calcium, and heavy drinking may worsen the deterioration of bone tissue.
- Heart disease. Women who are very heavy drinkers are more at risk of developing irreversible heart disease than men who drink even more.

Women who abuse alcohol also face a special burden: intense social disapproval. Many become cross-addicted to prescription medicines, or they develop eating disorders or sexual dysfunctions. Also, women are more likely to blame their symptoms on depression or anxiety, whereas men attribute them directly to alcohol. As a result, women often obtain treatment later in the course of their illness, at a point when their problems are more severe.

Fetal Alcohol Spectrum Disorders Of very special concern is the combination of women, alcohol consumption, and pregnancy. According to the authors of *Fetal Alcohol Spectrum Disorder: A Guideline for Diagnosis*

STRATEGIES FOR PREVENTION

How to Prevent Drunk Driving

- Don't drink and drive.
- When going out in a group, always designate one person who won't drink at all to serve as the driver.
- Never let intoxicated friends drive home. Call a taxi, drive them yourself, or arrange for them to spend the night in a safe place.

across the Lifespan, abstinence from alcohol should be recommended to all women during pregnancy. Women who are planning to become pregnant are also encouraged to abstain.[46] Why the concern? Because there is no safe amount or no safe time to drink alcohol during pregnancy.[47] Alcohol puts the fetus at risk. When a woman drinks while pregnant, the alcohol passes through the placenta into the bloodstream of the fetus. The BAC of the fetus will be much higher than the mother's due to its small size. Alcohol is oxidized more slowly in the fetus because the liver is underdeveloped. Alcohol in the fetus's system can result in a cluster of physical and mental defects known as **fetal alcohol spectrum disorder** (FASD).

FAS or **fetal alcohol syndrome** can result in a lifetime of developmental and cognitive disabilities. The physical symptoms include small head, abnormal facial features, jitters, poor muscle tone, sleep disorders, sluggish motor development, failure to thrive, short stature, delayed speech, mental challenges, a higher risk for spinal bifida, possible congenital heart problems, hyperactivity, and multi-faceted behaviour problems. There is also a noted increase in the risk of learning disabilities such as dyslexia. Many more babies suffer from **fetal alcohol effects** (FAE): low birth weight, irritability as newborns, and possible permanent mental impairment.[48]

As pregnancies are not always planned, extra precaution needs to be made to lower the risk of becoming pregnant when drinking alcohol. FASD cannot be cured. Be aware of the risks of drinking alcohol and conceiving a child. Societal pressures to drink should be weighed carefully when it comes to drinking and pregnancy.

ALCOHOL-RELATED PROBLEMS

By the simplest definition, problem drinking is the use of alcohol in any way that creates difficulties, potential difficulties, or health risks for an individual. Like alcoholics, problem drinkers are individuals whose lives are in some way impaired by their drinking. The only difference is one of degree. Alcohol becomes a problem and a person becomes an alcoholic when the drinker can't "take it or leave it." He or she spends more and more time anticipating the next drink, planning when and where to get it, buying and hiding alcohol, and covering up secret drinking.

Alcohol abuse involves continued use of alcohol despite awareness of social, occupational, psychological, or physical problems related to drinking or drinking in dangerous ways or situations (before driving, for instance). A diagnosis of alcohol abuse is based on one or more of the following occurring at any time during a 12-month period:

- a failure to fulfill major role obligations at work, school, or home (such as missing work or school)
- the use of alcohol in situations in which it is physically hazardous (such as before driving)
- alcohol-related legal problems (such as drunk-driving convictions)
- continued alcohol use despite persistent or recurring social or interpersonal problems caused or exacerbated by alcohol (such as fighting while drunk)

Alcohol dependence is a separate disorder in which individuals develop a strong craving for alcohol because it produces pleasurable feelings or relieves stress or anxiety. Over time, they experience physiological changes that lead to *tolerance* of its effects; this means that they must consume larger and larger amounts to achieve intoxication. If they abruptly stop drinking, they suffer *withdrawal,* a state of acute physical and psychological discomfort. A diagnosis of alcohol dependence is based on three or more of the following symptoms occurring during any 12-month period:

- tolerance, as defined by either a need for markedly increased amounts of alcohol to achieve intoxication or desired effect or a markedly diminished effect with continued drinking of the same amount of alcohol as in the past
- withdrawal, including at least two of the following symptoms: sweating, rapid pulse, or other signs of autonomic hyperactivity; increased hand tremor; insomnia; nausea or vomiting; temporary hallucinations or illusions; physical agitation or restlessness; anxiety; or grand mal seizures
- drinking to avoid or relieve the symptoms of withdrawal
- consuming larger amounts of alcohol or drinking over a longer period than was intended
- persistent desire or unsuccessful efforts to cut down or control drinking
- a great deal of time spent in activities necessary to obtain alcohol, drink it, or recover from its effects
- important social, occupational, or recreational activities given up or reduced because of alcohol use
- continued alcohol use despite knowledge that alcohol is likely to cause or exacerbate a persistent or recurring physical or psychological problem

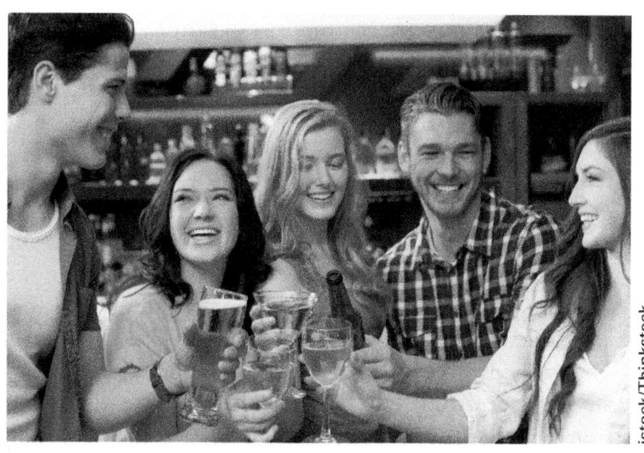

istock/Thinkstock

Alcohol dependence may spring from the perception that alcohol relieves stress and anxiety or creates a pleasant feeling. Social drinking sometimes becomes chronic drinking with college and university students.

Alcoholism is a primary, chronic disease in which genetic, psychosocial, and environmental factors influence its development and manifestations. The disease is often progressive and fatal. Its characteristics include an inability to control drinking, a preoccupation with alcohol, continued use of alcohol despite adverse consequences, and distorted thinking, most notably denial. Like other diseases, alcoholism is not simply a matter of insufficient willpower, but a complex problem that causes many symptoms, can have serious consequences, and yet can improve with treatment.

What Causes Alcohol Dependence and Abuse?

Although the exact causes of alcohol dependence and alcohol abuse are not known, certain factors—including biochemical imbalances in the brain, heredity, cultural acceptability, and stress—all seem to play a role. They include the following:

- Genetics. Scientists who are working toward mapping the genes responsible for addictive disorders have not yet been able to identify conclusively a specific gene that puts people at risk for alcoholism. However, epidemiological studies have shown evidence of heredity's role. Foroud et al. reviewed studies of twins, adoption, and families, and suggest that studies conclusively demonstrate that genetic factors are associated with the risk of becoming an alcoholic.[49] Analysis of genetic markers continues and may someday explain the genetic basis of alcoholism.
- Stress and traumatic experiences. Many people start drinking heavily as a way of coping with psychological problems. Alcohol often is linked with depressive and anxiety disorders. Men and women with these problems may start drinking in an attempt to alleviate their anxiety or depression.[50]
- Parental alcoholism. According to researchers, alcoholism is four to five times more common among the children of alcoholics, who may be influenced by the behaviour they see in their parents.[51]
- Drug abuse. Alcoholism is associated with the abuse of other psychoactive drugs, including marijuana, cocaine, heroin, amphetamines, and various anti-anxiety medications.[52] Adults under age 30 and adolescents are most likely to use alcohol plus several drugs of abuse. Middle-aged men and women are more likely to combine alcohol with benzodiazepines, such as anti-anxiety medications or sleeping pills, which may be prescribed for them by a physician.

Whatever the reason they start, some people keep drinking out of habit. Once they develop physical tolerance and dependence, they may not be able to stop drinking on their own.

Complications of Alcohol Dependence and Abuse

The previous section on the impact of alcohol demonstrated how excessive alcohol use adversely affects virtually every organ system in the body, including the digestive system, the cardiovascular system, our immune system, and our brain. Alcohol abuse can lead to major complications:

- Liver disease. Because the liver is the organ that breaks down and metabolizes alcohol, chronic heavy drinking can lead to alcoholic hepatitis (inflammation and destruction of liver cells) and, in people who continue drinking beyond this stage, cirrhosis (irreversible scarring and destruction of liver cells). The liver eventually may fail completely, resulting in coma and death.
- Cancer. Alcohol use may contribute to cancer of the liver, stomach, and colon, as well as malignant melanoma, a deadly form of skin cancer.
- Vitamin deficiencies. Alcoholism is associated with vitamin deficiencies, especially of thiamin (B_1), which may be responsible for certain diseases of the neurological, digestive, muscular, and cardiovascular systems. Lack of thiamin may result in Wernicke Korsakoff syndrome, which is characterized by disorientation, memory failure, hallucinations, and jerky eye movements and can be disabling enough to require lifelong custodial care.
- Reproductive and sexual dysfunction. Alcohol interferes with male sexual function and fertility through direct effects on testosterone and the testicles. Damage to the nerves in the penis by heavy drinking can lead to impotence. In women who drink heavily, a drop in female hormone production may cause menstrual irregularity and infertility. While drinking may increase your interest in sex, it may also impair sexual response, especially a man's ability to achieve or maintain an erection.
- Accidents and injuries. Alcohol contributes to deaths caused by car accidents, burns, falls, and choking.

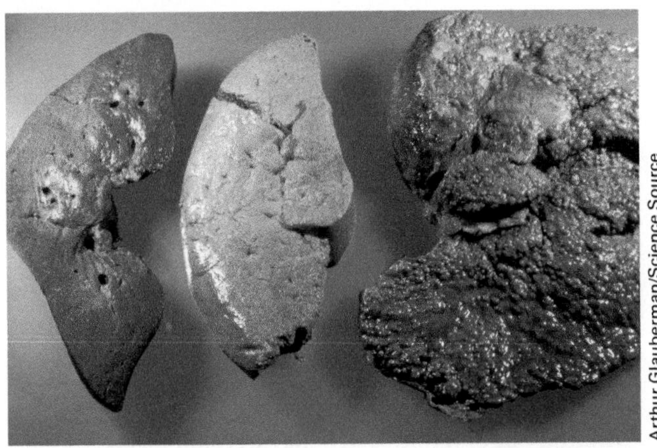
Arthur Glauberman/Science Source

Normal liver (left), fatty liver (middle), liver with cirrhosis (right).

- Higher mortality. Alcohol is a factor in suicides, too. Alcoholics who attempt suicide may have other risk factors, including major depression, poor social support, serious medical illness, and unemployment.
- Withdrawal dangers. Withdrawal can be life-threatening when accompanied by medical problems, such as grand mal seizures, pneumonia, liver failure, or gastrointestinal bleeding.

Alcoholism Treatments Today, individuals whose drinking could be hazardous to their health may choose from a variety of approaches. Treatment that works well for one person may not work for another. As research into the outcomes of alcohol treatments has grown, more attempts have been made to match individuals to approaches tailored to their needs and more likely to help them overcome their alcohol problems.

In a study of 222 men and women who had seriously abused alcohol, those who remained sober for more than a decade credited a variety of approaches, including Alcoholics Anonymous, individual psychotherapy, and other groups such as Women for Sobriety. There is no one sure path to sobriety—a wide variety of treatments may offer help and hope to those with alcohol-related problems.[53] Studies done on campus-based initiatives show that the most successful approaches include a commitment from the institution to address the issue of student drinking; the provision of funds for preventive and recovery programs; accessible community services that can provide support for students; encouraging municipal, provincial, and federal governments to take action; and involving students themselves in designing student-centred alcohol awareness and recovery programs.[54]

TOBACCO AND ITS EFFECTS

Tobacco, a herb that can be smoked or chewed, directly affects the brain. While its primary active ingredient is nicotine, tobacco smoke contains almost 400 other compounds and chemicals, including gases, liquids, particles, tar, carbon monoxide, cadmium, pyridine, nitrogen dioxide, ammonia, benzene, phenol, acrolein, hydrogen cyanide, formaldehyde, and hydrogen sulfide.

How Nicotine Works A colourless, oily compound, **nicotine** is the addictive substance of cigarettes. It is also poisonous in concentrated amounts. If you inhale while smoking, 90 percent of the nicotine in the smoke is absorbed into your body. Even if you draw smoke only into your mouth and not into your lungs, you still absorb 25–30 percent of the nicotine. Nicotine is a dangerous drug that is regulated in Canada.

Nicotine stimulates the cerebral cortex, the outer layer of the brain that controls complex behaviour and mental activity, and enhances mood and alertness. Investigators have shown that nicotine may enhance smokers' performance on some tasks but leaves other mental skills unchanged. Nicotine also acts as a sedative. How often you smoke and how you smoke determine nicotine's effect on you. If you're a regular smoker, nicotine will generally stimulate you at first, then tranquilize you. Shallow puffs tend to increase alertness because low doses of nicotine facilitate the release of the neurotransmitter *acetylcholine*, which makes the smoker feel alert. Deep drags, on the other hand, relax the smoker because high doses of nicotine block the flow of acetylcholine.

Nicotine stimulates the adrenal glands to produce adrenaline, a hormone that increases blood pressure, speeds up the heart rate by 15–20 beats a minute, and constricts blood vessels (especially in the skin). Nicotine also inhibits the formation of urine, dampens hunger, irritates the membranes in the mouth and throat, and dulls the taste buds so foods don't taste as good as they would otherwise. Nicotine is a major contributor to heart and respiratory diseases.

Tar and Carbon Monoxide As it burns, tobacco produces **tar**, a thick, sticky dark fluid made up of several hundred different chemicals—many of them poisonous, some of them *carcinogenic* (enhancing the growth of cancerous cells). As you inhale tobacco smoke, tar and other particles settle in the forks of the branch-like bronchial tubes in your lungs, where precancerous changes are apt to occur. In addition, tar and smoke damage the mucus and the cilia in the bronchial tubes, which normally remove irritating foreign materials from your lungs.

Smoke from cigarettes, cigars, and pipes also contains **carbon monoxide**, the deadly gas that comes out of the exhaust pipes of cars, in levels 400 times those considered safe in industry. Carbon monoxide interferes with the ability of the hemoglobin in the blood to carry oxygen, impairs normal functioning of the nervous system, and is at least partly responsible for the increased risk of heart attacks and strokes in smokers.

Health Effects of Cigarette Smoking Figure 12-6 shows some effects of smoking on the body. If you're a

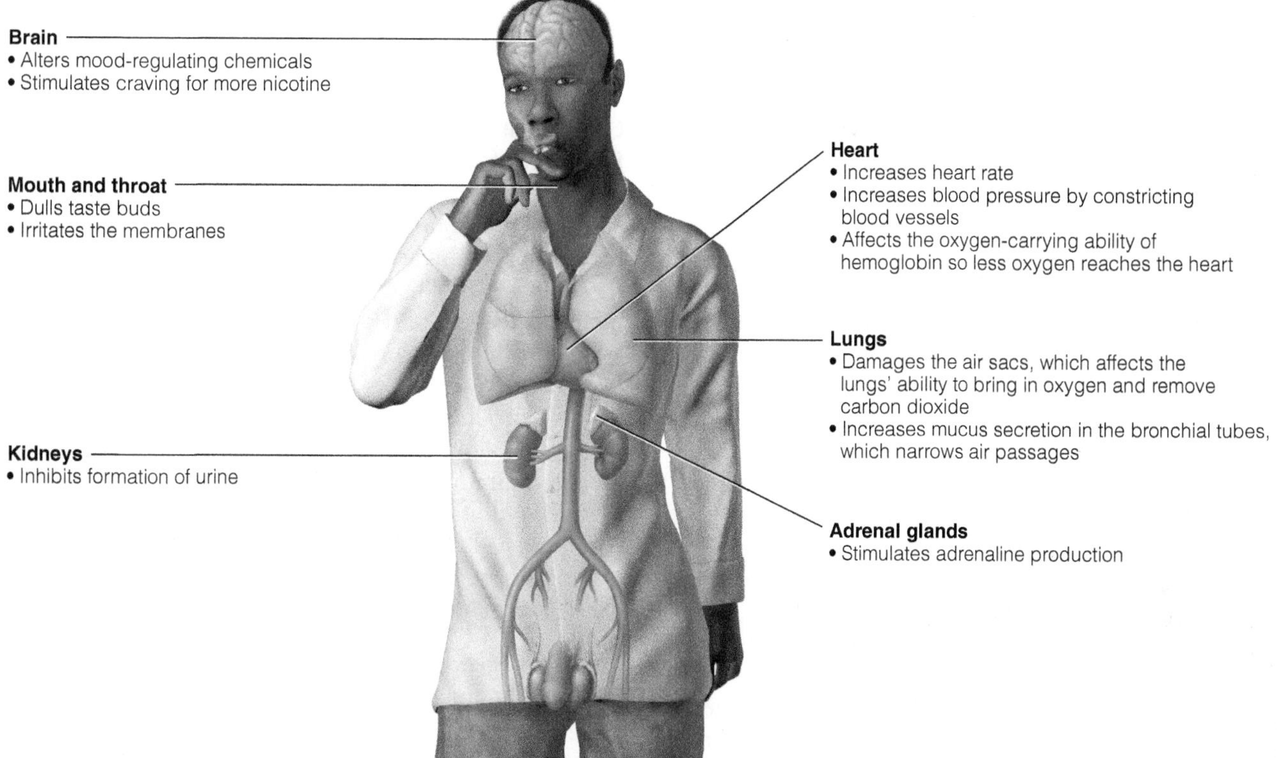

Figure 12-6 Some Effects of Smoking on the Body

smoker who inhales deeply and started smoking before the age of 15, you are trading a minute of future life for every minute you now spend smoking. On average, smokers die nearly 10 years earlier than non-smokers.[55] Smoking not only eventually kills, it also ages you: smokers get more wrinkles than non-smokers.

But the effects of smoking are far more than skin-deep. A cigarette smoker is 10 times more likely to develop lung cancer than a non-smoker and 20 times more likely to have a heart attack. Those who smoke two or more packs a day are 15–25 times more likely to die of lung cancer than non-smokers.

✓ CHECK-IN

Have you ever smoked? If so, how old were you when you tried your first cigarette?

Heart Disease and Stroke Although a great deal of publicity has been given to the link between cigarettes and lung cancer, heart attack is actually the leading cause of death for smokers. Smoking doubles the risk of heart disease, and smokers who suffer heart attacks have only a 50 percent chance of recovering. Smokers have a 70 percent higher death rate from heart disease than non-smokers, and those who smoke heavily have a 200 percent higher death rate.

Smoking is more dangerous than the two most notorious risk factors for heart disease: high blood pressure and high cholesterol. If smoking is combined with one of these, the chances of heart attack are four times greater. Women who smoke and use oral contraceptives have a 10 times higher risk of suffering heart attacks than women who do neither.

Smoking also causes a condition called *cardiomyopathy*, which weakens the heart's ability to pump blood.[56] Although researchers do not know precisely how smoking poisons the heart muscle, they speculate that either nicotine or carbon monoxide has a direct toxic effect. Other coronary diseases may be associated with smoking. *Aortic aneurysm* is a bulge in the aorta (the large artery attached to the heart) caused by a weakening of its walls.[57] *Pulmonary heart disease* is a heart disorder caused by changes in blood vessels in the lungs.

Even people who have smoked for decades can reduce their risk of heart attack if they quit smoking.[58] However, some irreversible damage to blood vessels may occur. Progression of atherosclerosis (hardening of the arteries) among former smokers continues at a faster pace than among those who never smoked.

In addition to contributing to heart attacks, cigarette smoking increases the risk of stroke two to three times in men and women, even after other risk factors are taken into account. According to one study of middle-aged men, giving up smoking leads to a considerable decrease in the risk of stroke within five years of quitting.[59] The risk for heavy smokers declines but never reverts back to that of men who never smoked.

Cancer The more people smoke, the longer they smoke, and the earlier they start smoking, the more likely they are to develop lung cancer.[60] Lung cancer is the leading cause of cancer death for both women and men in Canada.[61] Smokers of two or more packs a day have lung cancer mortality rates 15–25 times greater than non-smokers. If smokers stop smoking before cancer has started, their lung tissue tends to repair itself, even if there were already precancerous changes. Former smokers who haven't smoked for 15 or more years have lung cancer mortality rates only somewhat above those for non-smokers.

Chemicals in cigarette smoke and other environmental pollutants switch on a particular gene in the lung cells of some individuals. This gene produces an enzyme that helps manufacture powerful carcinogens, which set the stage for cancer. The gene seems more likely to be activated in some people than others, and people with this gene are at much higher risk of developing lung cancer. However, smokers without the gene still remain at risk because other chemicals and genes also may be involved in the development of lung cancer.

Smokers who are depressed are more likely to get cancer than non-depressed smokers. Although researchers don't know exactly how smoking and depression may work together to increase the risk of cancer, one possibility is that stress and depression cause biological changes that lower immunity, such as a decline in natural killer cells that fight off tumours.

Despite some advances in treating lung cancer, fewer than 10 percent survive for five years after diagnosis. This is one of the lowest survival rates of any type of cancer. If the cancer has spread from the lungs to other parts of the body, only 1 percent survive for five years after diagnosis.

Respiratory Diseases Smoking quickly impairs the respiratory system. Even some teenage smokers show signs of respiratory difficulty—breathlessness, chronic cough, excess phlegm production—when compared with non-smokers of the same age. Cigarette smokers are up to 18 times more likely than non-smokers to die of non-cancerous diseases of the lungs.

Cigarette smoking is the major cause of chronic obstructive pulmonary disease (COPD), which includes emphysema and chronic bronchitis. COPD is characterized by progressive limitation of the flow of air into and out of the lungs. In emphysema, the limitation of airflow is the result of disease changes in the lung tissue, affecting the bronchioles (the smallest air passages) and the walls of the alveoli (the tiny air sacs of the lung). Eventually, many of the air sacs are destroyed, and the lungs become much less able to bring in oxygen and remove carbon dioxide. As a result, the heart has to work harder to deliver oxygen to all organs of the body. Findings of a study done by the Canadian Lung Association showed that approximately 20 percent of smokers or ex-smokers over the age of 40 years may have COPD, but may not know it. The study also showed that 8 percent of smokers still smoke in their cars even when children are passengers. Children breathe faster than adults so their bodies are at risk for second-hand smoke because of the higher rate of absorption of pollutants in their lungs.[62] Prolonged exposure to second-hand smoke increases the risk of COPD.

In chronic bronchitis, the bronchial tubes in the lungs become inflamed, thickening the walls of the bronchi, and the production of mucus increases. The result is a narrowing of the air passages. Smoking is more dangerous than any form of air pollution, but exposure to both air pollution and cigarettes is particularly harmful. Although each may cause bronchitis, together they have a synergistic effect—that is, their combined impact exceeds the sum of their separate effects.

Other Smoking-Related Problems Smokers are more likely than non-smokers to develop gum disease, and they lose significantly more teeth. Smoking may also contribute to the loss of teeth-supporting bone, even in individuals with good oral hygiene.

Cigarette smoking is associated with stomach and duodenal ulcers; mouth, throat, and other types of cancer; and cirrhosis of the liver. Smoking may worsen the symptoms or complications of allergies, diabetes, hypertension, peptic ulcers, and disorders of the lungs or blood vessels. Some men who smoke 10 cigarettes or more a day may experience sexual impotence. Cigarette smokers also tend to miss work one-third more often than non-smokers, primarily because of respiratory illnesses. In addition, each year cigarette-ignited fires claim thousands of lives.

Cigarette smoking may also increase the likelihood of anxiety, panic attacks, and social phobias. The exact mechanism is unknown, but one theory is that nicotine may have anxiety-generating effects that act on the nervous system.[63]

✓ CHECK-IN

Have you, family members, or friends ever experienced any health-related problems or harm from smoking?

Financial Cost of Smoking Tobacco use continues to cost our Canadian healthcare system 4.4 billion dollars in direct healthcare costs and 2.2 million in acute-care hospital days per year.[64] The total cost of cigarette smoking to Canadian society includes greater work absenteeism, higher insurance premiums, increased disability payments, and the training costs to replace employees who die prematurely from smoking. In the course of a lifetime, the average smoker can expect to spend tens of thousands of dollars on cigarettes—but that's only the beginning. The potential costs for medical services that might be needed for smoking-related diseases is even higher. But the greatest toll—the pain and suffering of cancer and cardiac disease victims and their loved ones—obviously cannot be measured in dollars and cents.

The Government of Canada has invested millions of dollars since 2007 in programs and tobacco initiatives aimed at reducing tobacco use among Canadians. One example of where the federal funding is going is the Federal Tobacco Control Strategy.[65] However, there is concern that the federal government is still not doing enough to address the challenges of smoking in Canada, and there are calls for an integrated and sustainable strategy to deal with the healthcare costs attributed to this issue.

Why Do People Start Smoking? Most people are aware that an enormous health risk is associated with smoking, but many don't know exactly what that risk is or how it might affect them. The two main factors linked with the onset of a smoking habit are age and education. Other factors associated with the reasons for smoking are also discussed in the following sections.

Genetics Researchers speculate that genes may account for smoking behaviour, with environment playing an equally important role.[66] Studies have shown that identical twins, who have the same genes, are more likely to have matching smoking profiles than fraternal twins. If one identical twin is a heavy smoker, the other is also likely to be; if one smokes only occasionally, so does the other.

This suggests that some individuals do have a strong genetic predisposition toward tobacco use. However, when smoking is strongly discouraged, they do not express that genetic tendency. On the other hand, if smoking is socially acceptable, the genetic tendency to smoke emerges.

Parental Role Models Children who start smoking are 50 percent more likely than youngsters who don't smoke to have at least one smoker in their family. A mother who smokes seems a particularly strong influence on making smoking seem acceptable. Parental role modelling has a powerful influence on youth behaviour, including unhealthy habits such as smoking. Having siblings who smoke also impacts the adoption of smoking behaviour among young people. The majority of youngsters who smoke say that their parents also smoke and are aware of their own tobacco use.[67]

Adolescent Experimentation and Rebellion Young people who are trying out various behaviours may take up smoking because they're curious or because they want to defy adults. Others simply want to appear grown-up or "cool." Teenagers often misjudge the addictive power of cigarettes. Many, sure that they'll be able to quit any time they want, figure that smoking for a year or two won't hurt them. But when they try to quit, they can't. Like older smokers, most young people who smoke have tried to quit at least once.

Wolburg studied the smoking habits of college students and found that a number of them had a misguided optimism about quitting. Many of the students planned to quit smoking by the time they graduated, but very few actually succeeded and the students who were finally successful had many failed attempts.[68]

Limited Education People who have graduated from college or university are much less likely to smoke than high school graduates; those with fewer than 12 years of education are most likely to smoke.

Weight Control Smokers burn up an extra 100 calories a day—probably because nicotine increases metabolic rate. Once they start smoking, many individuals say they cannot quit because they fear they'll gain weight. Smoking can also suppress appetite. Women who stop smoking gain an average of 3.7 kilograms (8 pounds), while men put on an average of 2.7 kilograms (6 pounds). The reasons for this weight gain include nicotine's effects on metabolism as well as emotional and behavioural factors, such as the habit of frequently putting something into one's mouth. Bean et al. conducted a study on students living in a rural area who smoked. Their findings determined that current student smokers did believe that they would gain weight if they quit smoking.[69] Yet as a health risk, smoking can be a greater danger than carrying extra weight.

Weight gain can be counteracted by aerobic exercise and limiting alcohol and foods high in sugar and fat.

Aggressive Marketing Most television and radio tobacco advertising ceased in the early 1970s, and the Canadian Tobacco Act banned the promotion of tobacco company sponsorships in 2003.[70] However, tobacco companies use

STRATEGIES FOR PREVENTION

Why Not to Light Up

Before you start smoking—before you ever face the challenge of quitting—think of what you have to gain by *not* smoking:

- a significantly reduced risk of cancer of the lungs, larynx, mouth, esophagus, pancreas, and bladder
- half the risk of heart disease that smokers face
- a lower risk of stroke, chronic obstructive pulmonary disease (COPD), influenza, ulcers, and pneumonia
- a lower risk of having a low-birth-weight baby
- a longer lifespan
- potential savings of tens of thousands of dollars that you would otherwise spend on tobacco products and medical care

very sophisticated methods to continue to market their product. Full-page ad campaigns are only one way to sell cigarettes. Tobacco product placement is another—a familiar name or logo being used by or placed behind actors in movies, music videos, and television shows. Tobacco products are glamorized. Experts generally conclude that tobacco advertising attempts to reassure us that smoking is okay and not a threat to our health. A report titled *The Influence of Tobacco Powerwall Advertising on Children*[71] indicates that tobacco companies spend over 300 million dollar annually in Canada on point-of-purchase advertising, displays, and listing allowances. Canadians are also exposed to crossover marketing from the United States—especially in magazine advertising.[72]

In Canada, three companies dominate tobacco manufacturing. They are Imperial Tobacco Canada, Rothmans Inc., and JTI-Macdonald Corporation. The largest company, Imperial Tobacco, is owned by British American Tobacco in the United Kingdom—the third-largest tobacco company in the world. Outside of the United States, British American Tobacco sells the most cigarettes worldwide.[73] Even though scientists have proven that smoking is dangerous to our health and cigarette production and sales in Canada have dropped over the past two decades, cigarette companies are now focusing their marketing efforts on Third World countries where the regulations are not as stringent.

Stress In studies that have analyzed the impact of life stressors, depression, emotional support, marital status, and income, researchers have concluded that an individual with a high stress level is approximately 15 times more likely to be a smoker than a person with low stress. About half of smokers identify workplace stress as a key factor in their smoking behaviour.

Addiction According to recent research, the first symptoms of nicotine addiction can begin within a few days of starting to smoke and after just a few cigarettes, particularly in teenagers.[74] The findings, based on a study of almost 700 adolescents, challenge the conventional belief that nicotine dependence is a gradual process that takes hold after prolonged daily smoking.

SMOKING IN CANADA

Even though there has been a decline in the overall current smoking rate among Canadians who are 15 years and older (see Figure 12-7), tobacco use remains the most serious and widespread addictive behaviour in our country and the world. It is also the major cause of preventable deaths in our society. Over 27 percent of all cancer deaths in Canada can be attributed to lung cancer, the cancer that causes the most deaths.[75]

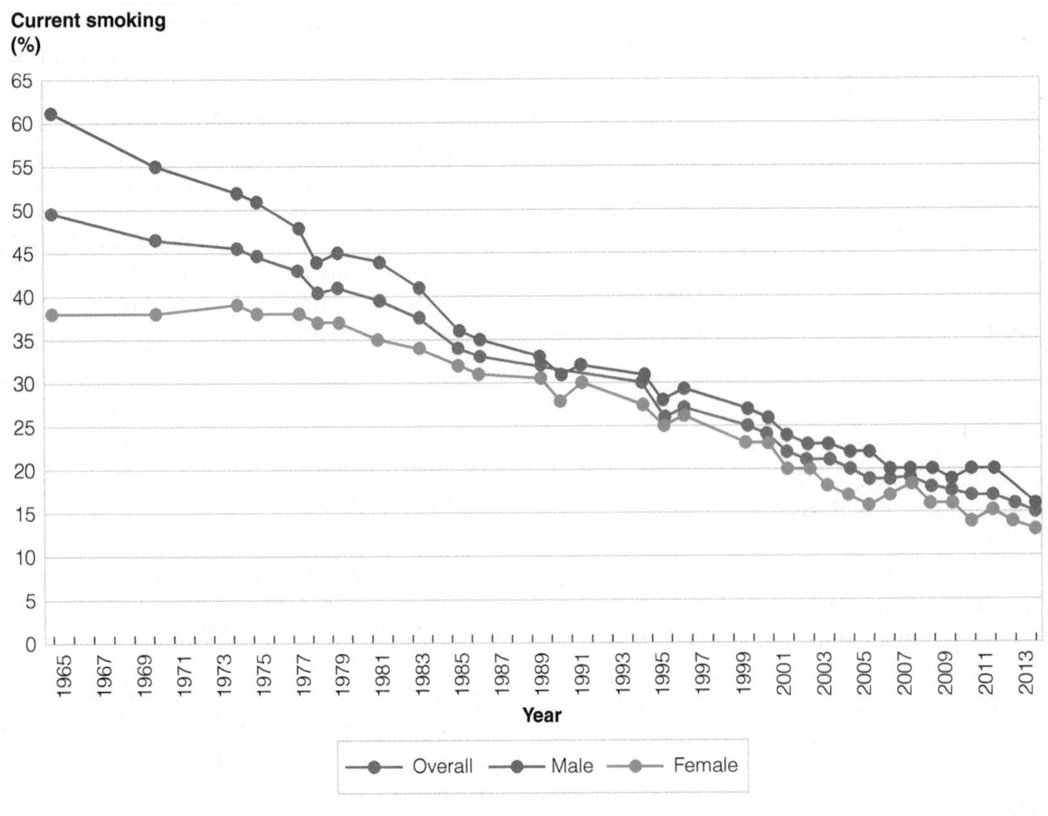

Figure 12-7 Smoking Prevalence* in Canada, Adults Aged 15+, 1965–2013

Source: Tobacco use in Canada: Patterns and trends, 2015. http://tobaccoreport.ca/2015/TobaccoUseinCanada_2015.pdf. Used with permission.

In 2013, about 4.2 million Canadians smoked.[76] About 3.1 million of Canadians smoked daily. Approximately 1.1 million Canadians reported that they were non-daily smokers. People who smoked on a daily basis smoked an average of 13.9 cigarettes per day. This was a decrease from 2012 of 15 cigarettes per day. As could be predicted, males reported smoking daily more than females, at 15.2 percent and 12.5 percent respectively. Canadians aged 25–34 had the highest prevalence of smoking at 18.5 percent followed by young people aged 20–24 at 17.9 percent.[77]

There was a notable difference of smoking rates between provinces. Three provinces—New Brunswick, Newfoundland and Labrador, and Nova Scotia—had the highest rates at almost 20 percent of people smoking. This was above the national average of 14.6 percent. British Columbia had the lowest rate of smokers at 11.4 percent.[78] See Figure 12-8 for an illustration of the prevalence of smoking in all provinces in 2013.

Tobacco Use on Campus Today's students use a broad range of tobacco products: cigarettes, cigars, pipes, smokeless tobacco, and waterpipes (hookahs). There is also a range of perceptions by students on how to define whether or not they are a smoker. Berg et al. examined how college students defined the term "smoker" and how their definition impacted their smoking behaviour and attitudes.[79] Some interesting findings emerged from this study:

- Over half of the college students surveyed who had smoked in the past 30 days did not identify themselves as a smoker.
- Smoking alone indicated that a person was a smoker, but smoking at a party did not necessarily mean you were a smoker.

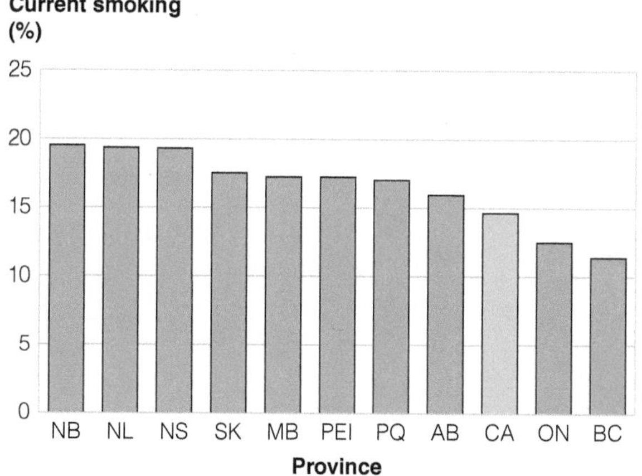

Figure 12-8 Smoking Prevalence* by Province, 2013

Source: Tobacco use in Canada: Patterns and trends, 2015 (Figure 2.1, page 22). http://tobaccoreport.ca/2015/TobaccoUseinCanada_2015.pdf. Used with permission.

- Smokers purchase cigarettes, while non-smokers borrow cigarettes.
- Smokers would have difficulty quitting, but non-smokers would be able to quit without great effort.
- Many students who smoked in the past 30 days, but defined themselves as non-smokers, did not believe that they needed to "quit."

Tobacco use is often higher among students who use alcohol[80] or marijuana, and students who use tobacco are more likely to smoke marijuana, binge drink,[81] have more sexual partners, have lower grades, rate parties as important, and spend more time socializing with friends.

Despite concern about student smoking, many colleges and universities do not offer smoking-cessation programs to students who want to quit or do not have a comprehensive smoking policy on campus. Those that do mainly refer students to campus support groups or community-based programs. Yet, first-year students who did not smoke regularly in high school and who lived in smoke-free residences were 40 percent less likely to smoke than those in unrestricted housing, according to a study of the smoking behaviour of 4495 students at 101 schools.[82] Borders et al., in another study on college campus smoking policies and students' smoking behaviours, discovered that tobacco prevention and education programs helped to reduce student smoking rates more than governing the sale and distribution of cigarettes did.[83] Fletcher and Camblin, in a study of first-year Canadian students entering a university in a city where smoke-free legislation had been put in place, found that smoking rates were lower than those found on other university campuses where no similar legislation was in place.[84]

A Canadian study on tobacco control policy among postsecondary institutions in Canada by Hammond et al.[85] illustrates the other side of the tobacco story. The researchers found that every university and half of all the colleges that they surveyed (35 academic institutions in all) had participated in some form of tobacco marketing in the past year. Among the universities surveyed, 80 percent had run a tobacco advertisement in their paper, and 18 percent had hosted a tobacco-sponsored nightclub event.

Tobacco control policies varied greatly between the institutions. Some campuses had campus-wide outdoor smoking restrictions, tobacco sales bans, and indoor smoking restrictions; other institutions had yet to introduce smoking restrictions.

Students smoke for a number of reasons, including having the option to smoke, no parental rules to follow or defiance of parental norms, fears of weight gain, inability to manage stress, denial of nicotine addiction, and drinking behaviour.[86]

Working toward campus-wide non-smoking policies and tobacco/smoke-free environments will take effort from both administration and students. Ideas that are

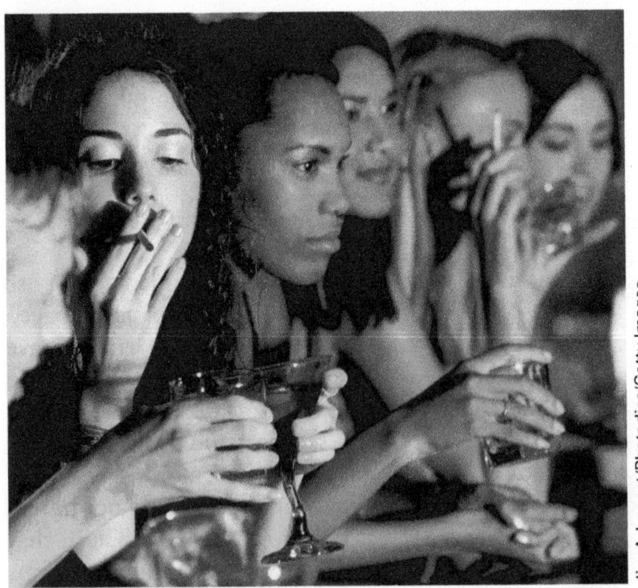
Jim Arbogast/Photodisc/Getty Images

Social smoking has negative short- and long-term health effects and can lead to dependence.

being implemented in colleges and universities across Canada include the following:

- prohibition of campus-controlled advertising, sales, or free sampling of tobacco products and of sponsorship of campus events by tobacco-promoting organizations
- prohibition of smoking in all public areas, including classrooms, auditoriums, laboratories, libraries, gymnasiums, meeting rooms, stadiums, buses, vans, private offices, and dining facilities
- prohibition of smoking in residences
- prevention and education initiatives directed against tobacco use
- programs that include practical steps to quit tobacco use
- smoke-free campuses

✓ CHECK-IN

What policies are in place with regard to smoking on your college or university campus? Are you a "smoke-free" campus?

Smoking and Aboriginal Peoples Cigarette smoking is a major cause of disease and death in all population groups; however, the smoking rates in First Nations and Inuit communities are more than double the rate in the overall population of Canada. This has resulted in a serious and growing health concern. At one time, tobacco was used in ceremonies and prayer by First Nations Peoples. It was also used as a purifying agent and had deep spiritual meanings. Tobacco was highly valued and considered to be a sacred substance. Unfortunately, cigarette smoking and the chewing of smokeless tobacco is sometimes defended on the grounds of the traditional use of tobacco. However, the teachings of many Elders suggest that there is a critical difference between traditional and non-traditional tobacco practices.

The First Nations and Inuit Health Branch is working with Aboriginal groups across Canada to develop and support culturally sensitive and effective smoking cessation programs and initiatives. An Aboriginal health strategy has been developed to include core values that respect all cultures, and encourage responsibility of community members to practise lifestyles free of tobacco misuse.[87]

Smoking and Women As reported in the Smoking in Canada section, males smoke more than females in almost all age groups. However, young women continue to start smoking and 15 percent of females aged 20–24 years smoke.[88] With the known health risks of smoking and the addictive properties of cigarettes, young females need to heed the advice from medical and educational professionals and not start smoking in the first place.

As discussed in X & Y Files: "Alcohol, Tobacco, Men, and Women," women smoke for different reasons and in different ways than men. They also suffer unique consequences.[89]

If a woman smokes, her annual risk of dying more than doubles after age 45 compared with a woman who has never smoked. Women who smoke face an increased risk of lung cancer and cancers of the pharynx and bladder. Smoking may also increase the risk of liver, colon, cervical, kidney, and pancreatic cancers. Links to other health risks include depression, stroke, bleeding in the brain, diseases of the blood vessels, and respiratory diseases such as chronic obstructive pulmonary disease.

The risk of heart attack in women who smoke 25 or more cigarettes a day is more than 500 percent greater than the risk in women who don't smoke. Even smoking just one to four cigarettes a day doubles the risk. Women who smoke low-nicotine cigarettes are four times more likely to have a first heart attack than women who don't smoke—the same risk as for those who smoke high-nicotine cigarettes.

Women who smoke also are more likely to develop osteoporosis, a bone-weakening disease. They tend to be thin, which is a risk factor for osteoporosis, and they enter menopause earlier, thus extending the period of jeopardy from estrogen loss.

Smoking directly affects women's reproductive organs and processes. Women who smoke are less fertile and experience menopause one or two years earlier than women who don't smoke. Smoking also greatly increases the possible risks associated with taking oral contraceptives. Older women who smoke are weaker, have poorer balance, and are at greater risk of physical disability than non-smokers.

Women who smoke during pregnancy increase their risk of miscarriage and pregnancy complications, including bleeding, premature delivery, and birth defects such as cleft lip or palate. Women who smoke are twice as likely to have an ectopic pregnancy (in which a fertilized egg develops in the fallopian tube rather than in the uterus) and to have babies of low birth weight as those who have never smoked. However, women who stop smoking before pregnancy reduce their risk of having a low-birth-weight baby to that of women who don't smoke. Even those who quit three or four months into the pregnancy have babies with higher birth weights than those who continue smoking throughout pregnancy.

OTHER FORMS OF TOBACCO

Cigars, pipes, and smokeless and chewing tobacco all put the user at risk of cancer of the lip, tongue, mouth, and throat, as well as other diseases and ailments.

Cigars After cigarettes, cigars are the tobacco product most widely used by college and university students. In a study by Callison, Karrh, and Zillman, who evaluated the character traits of men and women seen smoking cigars, both male and female college undergraduates judged cigar smokers, compared to cigarette smokers, as being more confident and secure. Female students also rated cigar smokers as being as appealing as non-smokers.[90]

These findings are disconcerting because cigar smoking is as dangerous as cigarette smoking even though smokers do not inhale. Cigars are known to cause cancer of the lung and the digestive tract. The risk of death related to cigars approaches that of cigarettes as the number of cigars smoked and the amount of cigar smoke inhaled increases. Cigar smoking can lead to nicotine addiction, even if the smoke is not inhaled. The nicotine in the smoke from a single cigar can vary from an amount roughly equivalent to that in a single cigarette to that in a pack or more of cigarettes.

In 2013, about 3 percent of all Canadians who were aged 15 and older reported smoking cigars (of a variety of types) within the past 30 days. About 5 percent of young people aged 15–19 and about 7 percent of young adults aged 20–24 reported smoking some type of cigar in the past 30 days when surveyed. Not all of the cigar smokers were of legal age. Five percent were under the legal age but purchased them anyway.

About 4 percent of Canadians who were 15 years and older indicated they smoked little cigars or cigarillos in the 30 days previous to the survey date. Sixty-two percent smoked the flavoured type.[91]

Pipes Many cigarette smokers switch to pipes to reduce their risk of health problems. But former cigarette smokers may continue to inhale, even though pipe smoke is more irritating to the respiratory system than cigarette smoke. People who have only smoked pipes and who do not inhale are much less likely to develop lung and heart disease than cigarette smokers. However, they are as likely as cigarette smokers to develop—and die of—cancer of the mouth, larynx, throat, and esophagus.

Waterpipes (Hookahs) In a study done by Roskin and Aveyard,[92] waterpipe (hookah) smoking appears to be on the rise on college and university campuses in Toronto, Canada, and in Birmingham, England. This type of smoking was viewed as a novel and communal activity. Students believed that since there were no apparent warnings about waterpipe smoking, it must be safer than cigarette smoking. They also believed that the mildness of the smoke, the fruit flavours, and the filtering of the smoke by the water lessened the risks of smoking in this way. The authors encourage further longitudinal studies to determine the impact of this type of smoking on the health of students.

Smith-Simone, Curbow, and Stillman also found that there was a surge of waterpipe use among the 411 American college students that they surveyed.[93] However, the results from the 2013 Canadian Tobacco, Alcohol and Drugs survey (CTADS) show a different story. While 2.8 million (10 percent) of Canadians aged 15 years and older and 694 000 (29 percent) of young adults aged 20–24 state that they have tried using a water-pipe in their lifetime, 229 000 or less than 1 percent of Canadians 15 years and older and 86 000 (4 percent) of young adults aged 20–24 confirm they used a water-pipe for smoking in the last 30 days before the survey.[94]

Smokeless Tobacco The consumption of smokeless tobacco products presents health risks too.[95] These substances include snuff, finely ground tobacco that can be sniffed or placed inside the cheek and sucked, and chewing tobacco, tobacco leaves mixed with flavouring agents such as molasses. With both, nicotine is absorbed through the mucous membranes of the nose or mouth.

Many young people who use smokeless tobacco are emulating professional baseball players who keep wads of tobacco jammed in their cheeks. These users often lack awareness of its dangers. Smokeless tobacco can cause cancer and non-cancerous oral conditions and lead to nicotine addiction and dependence. Smokeless tobacco users are more likely than non-users to become cigarette smokers. Powerful carcinogens in smokeless tobacco include nitrosamines, polycyclic aromatic hydrocarbons, and radiation-emitting polonium. Its use can lead to the development of white patches on the mucous membranes of the mouth, particularly on the site where the tobacco is placed. Most lesions of the mouth lining that result from the use of smokeless tobacco dissipate six weeks after the use of the tobacco products is stopped. However, when first found, about 5 percent of these lesions are cancerous or exhibit changes that progress to cancer within 10 years if not properly treated. Cancers of the lip, pharynx, larynx, and esophagus have all been linked to smokeless tobacco.

In recent years, there has been a decline in chewing tobacco, but an increase in the use of moist snuff, a product that is higher in nicotine and potential cancer-causing chemicals. The use of snuff increases the likelihood of oral cancer by more than four times. Other effects include bad breath, discoloured or missing teeth, cavities, gum disease, and nicotine addiction.

E-cigarettes E-cigarettes were invented in 2003. An e-cigarette is a cylindrical appliance or device that looks like a real cigarette. It is made up of a battery, a heating element, and cartridges that may come with nicotine, water, and other ingredients such as propylene glycol and vegetable glycerine, as well as candy-like flavourings. The solution in the cartridge is electronically vapourized. A smoker inhales the mist into their lungs, then exhales the residue. E-cigarettes simulate the act of smoking without exposing people's bodies to the high level of carcinogens found in tobacco smoke.

E-cigarettes and e-liquids that contain nicotine have not yet been approved for sale by Health Canada. Because they contain nicotine they are defined as a drug or drug delivery device under the national *Food and Drugs Act*, and therefore need authority through Health Canada prior to importation, marketing, and sales. However, there is a strong international market and they are available through the Internet. Nicotine-free e-cigarettes are for sale legally in Canada as long as health claims for these products in advertisements or marketing materials are not included. Provincial and municipal governments are developing further policies for their sale.[96]

People use e-cigarettes as a smoking cessation aid or to supplement their cigarette smoking. Research is starting to show that there are some potential health risks to users of e-cigarettes and that their use does not necessarily assist people in quitting smoking. Some people have complained of irritation of their throat and mouth. Others suffer from nausea. Headaches and dry cough have also been reported. Years of research has shown that exposure to nicotine is harmful, especially during pregnancy and brain development of young people. As well, there have been no long-term studies on the impact of continued inhalation of propylene glycol.[97]

There have also been reports in Canada and the United States of the cartridge containing the heating element exploding and causing major facial and head burns. These incidents have started a conversation about the need for federal regulation.[98] In Alberta, bylaws in Edmonton and Calgary now ban smoking e-cigarettes or vaping anywhere cigarettes are banned. Nova Scotia is the first province to pass legislation that includes bans on the use of e-cigarettes in indoor public spaces. Anyone under the age of 19 is prohibited from purchasing e-cigarettes. British Columbia, New Brunswick, and Quebec have also passed legislation where e-cigarettes are not allowed in public spaces or municipal offices. Ontario has banned the sale of e-cigarettes to anyone under the age of 19.[99]

The Canadian Lung Association position statement does not support e-cigarettes as a method to help people quit smoking.[100] Members of this association are concerned that users of e-cigarettes are inhaling unknown, unregulated, and potentially harmful substances. At this time there is no consistent evidence-based research that documents the risks or benefits of e-cigarettes. Some health professionals fear that e-cigarettes may actually increase nicotine addiction. There is also alarm that the use of e-cigarettes may glamorize smoking, which could lead more young people to start smoking. However, there are other health professionals who suggest electronic cigarettes are a safe alternative to tobacco cigarettes.

✓ CHECK-IN

Have you or any of your friends used e-cigarettes? Do you think they are a healthy alternative to smoking tobacco products?

Second-Hand Tobacco Smoke Maybe you don't smoke—never have, never will. That doesn't mean you don't have to worry about the dangers of smoking, especially if you live or work with people who smoke. **Second-hand cigarette smoke**, or environmental tobacco smoke, is the most hazardous form of indoor air pollution and ranks behind cigarette smoking and alcohol as the third-leading preventable cause of death.

On average, a smoker inhales what is known as **mainstream smoke** eight or nine times with each cigarette, for a total of about 24 seconds. However, the cigarette burns for about 12 minutes, and everyone in the room (including the smoker) breathes in what is known as **sidestream smoke**. Incomplete combustion from the lower temperatures of a smouldering cigarette makes sidestream smoke dirtier and chemically different from mainstream smoke. It has twice as much tar and nicotine, five times as much carbon monoxide, and 50 times as much ammonia. Because the particles in sidestream smoke are small, this mixture of irritating gases and carcinogenic tar reaches deeper into the lungs.[101]

What Are the Risks of Second-Hand Smoke? Even a little second-hand smoke is dangerous. According to the Canadian Cancer Society, exposure to second-hand smoke causes over 800 deaths in Canadian non-smokers per year.[102] Approximately 80 percent of exposure to second-hand smoke occurs in the workplace. Lobbying by non-smokers and health advocates has resulted in smoking being prohibited in federal, provincial, and municipal workplaces, on inter-provincial transit, and on airplanes.

The hospitality sector, with over one million workers, is one of the most significant areas where workplace exposure to second-hand smoke is an issue. Some workplaces such as restaurants and bars are now designated as "smoke-free." One of the main arguments put forth by groups and individuals opposed to smoke-free legislation is that businesses, especially bars and restaurants, will lose revenue. However, many studies have shown that smoke-free legislation has no long-term negative impact on restaurant, bar, hotel, and tourism receipts.[103]

Most provinces have now enacted laws and bylaws that also address the issue of second-hand smoke in public places. Table 12-5 illustrates how smoking bans in some provinces began in one city or municipality and then grew to include the entire province or territory. There is not yet a consistent level of protection but work on banning smoking in public places continues.

TABLE 12-5

Public Smoking Bans by Province and Territory

Province or Territory	Regulations
British Columbia	• August 1, 2001—Victoria, B.C., bans smoking in all public spaces and workplaces. There is no option for designated smoking rooms. • 2008—Province-wide ban on smoking in public places including restaurants, bars, bingo halls, bowling alleys, and casinos. • 2008—Restaurant and bar owners in some jurisdictions can build smoking rooms or operate open outside areas where staff can volunteer to serve. Smoking is legal on outdoor patios that are not partially or fully enclosed. Some municipalities have complete smoking bans including in parks and on beaches. 2009—No citizen can smoke in a vehicle in the presence of anyone under the age of 16.
Alberta	• January 1, 2006—*Smoke-Free Places Act* becomes effective, restricting smoking in any public place or space and workplaces, including outdoor patios. • Stronger bylaws are in effect in some municipalities such as Edmonton, Strathcona, and Calgary. • 100 percent ban on smoking in public places takes place in, for example, Peace River, Stettler, Wainwright, Drumheller, Olds, Airdrie, and Jasper. • Smoking in a car with young passengers is not banned province-wide, but is punishable by a fine in some municipalities.
Saskatchewan	• December 31, 2002—Bingo halls, bars, casinos, and restaurants are required to designate 40 percent of their space as non-smoking. • 2004—Requirements for non-smoking spaces increase to 60 percent. • January 2005—Under the *Tobacco Control Act*, all public places, including outdoor areas and veterans' clubs, become smoke-free. Fines up to 10 000 dollars for violators. • January 19, 2005—"Shower curtain law" requires store owners to keep tobacco products out of sight. • 2009—Smoking bylaw prohibits smoking in all enclosed public spaces, including restaurants, bars, private clubs, bingo halls, bowling alleys, and casinos. • Drivers who smoke while with a passenger under 16 face a fine of 220 dollars.
Manitoba	• January 2002—Illegal to smoke in any indoor location in Winnipeg where minors are present. • September 1, 2003—All public places in Winnipeg become smoke-free. • October 2004—*Non-Smokers' Health Protection Act* bans smoking in public spaces. Exceptions include group-living facilities and hotel rooms. • Further bans now include all enclosed public spaces and indoor workplaces (including work vehicles). The ban does not apply to Reserve Lands. • Drivers with passengers under 16 cannot smoke in the car.
Ontario	• August 1, 2001—City of Ottawa bans smoking in all workplaces and public spaces. No option for designated smoking rooms. • Illegal to sell tobacco products at hospitals, psychiatric facilities, nursing homes, long-term care facilities, and charitable institutions. • January 1, 2003—Northwestern (Ontario) Health Unit bans smoking in all public places and private businesses. Fines range from 5000 to 25 000 dollars. • 2004—In Toronto, all bars, pool and bingo halls, casinos, and racetracks become smoke-free. • May 31, 2006—*Smoke-Free Ontario Act* prohibits smoking at all workplaces and enclosed spaces open to the public, except for private homes and hotel rooms. • Also prohibits smoking in vehicles used for work, in reserved seating at open-air stadiums, and in underground parking areas.

(Continued)

TABLE 12-5

Public Smoking Bans by Province and Territory *(Continued)*

Province or Territory	Regulations
Ontario	• 2008—Retail displays of tobacco are banned. • 2009—Smoking in vehicles carrying any passengers under 16 is outlawed. • As of January 1, 2016, it is illegal to sell or supply electronic cigarettes and their parts to anyone under 19 years of age.
Quebec	• May 31, 2006—Quebec's *Tobacco Act* introduces a 100 percent smoke-free environment in all indoor public places. • Smoking is also banned within nine metres of any doorway leading to a health or social services institution, college, university, or child-care facility. • It also becomes illegal to sell tobacco by mail order, over the Internet, on school grounds, or in health-care, social services, or child-care facilities. • May 2008—Smoking is prohibited in all private designated smoking rooms.
New Brunswick	• October 2004—Province-wide ban on smoking in all public areas. Restaurants and bars are prohibited from having smoking sections in outdoor eating and drinking areas or glassed-in smoking areas.
Nova Scotia	• January 1, 2003—Smoking ban in effect in taxicabs, bowling alleys, schoolyards, and other public places. In bars and restaurants, smoking is restricted after 9:00 p.m. to an enclosed, separately ventilated, adult-only room. • December 1, 2006—*Nova Scotia Smoke-Free Act* implements a province-wide ban on smoking in indoor workplaces and all public spaces including outdoor bars and patios. Only exception—designated rooms in nursing homes and long-term care facilities. • Drivers cannot smoke if there are passengers younger than 19. • Prominent displays of tobacco products in stores is prohibited. • April 2008—Smoking banned in prisons. Smoking banned in vehicles carrying children. • October 2009—Halifax regional council restricts smoking in about 480 outdoor venues where children are present (parks, rinks, sports fields). • Drivers cannot smoke if they carry passengers younger than 16.
Prince Edward Island	• June 1, 2003—*PEI Smoke-Free Places Act* bans smoking in public places, but allows hospitality venues to build enclosed, separately vented smoking rooms. • September 15, 2009—Amendments to the *PEI Smoke-Free Places Act* ban designated smoking rooms in public places and smoking in vehicles carrying anyone under 19 years of age. • Smoking on outdoor patios limited to between 10:00 p.m. and 3:00 a.m. • Smoking on hospital property is banned with the exception of one hospital in Charlottetown.
Newfoundland and Labrador	• 1994—*Smoke-Free Environment Act* comes into effect. Smoking is prohibited or restricted in public places such as daycares, schools, retail stores, recreational vehicles, public transportation vehicles, hospitals, and some food premises and liquor establishments. • 2002—Amendments to the act restrict smoking on more food premises, games arcades, passenger terminals, and common areas of hotels and motels. • July 1, 2005—Further amendments are made to the act banning smoking in bars, bingo halls, private clubs, community centres, and decks and patios of licensed liquor and food outlets. • No smoking in cars with passengers younger than 16.
Yukon	• May 2008—The last of the provinces and territories to ban smoking in all public places. • Group-living facilities can have designated smoking rooms. • Drivers cannot smoke if they carry passengers younger than 18.
Northwest Territories	• March 1, 2004—Workers' Compensation Board bans smoking in all enclosed businesses and work sites. Smoking rooms are only allowed in workplaces that are private residences. • March 2006—Legislation passes enforcing the Workers' Compensation ban on smoking in workplaces. • Group homes can have designated smoking rooms.
Nunavut	• May 1, 2004—Workers' Compensation Board bans smoking in all enclosed businesses, work sites, and bars. It also bans smoking within a 3-metre radius of entrances and exits of buildings and within a 15-metre radius of schools.

Sources: FindLaw Canada. 2015. Smoking laws by province. http://findlaw.ca/learn-about-the-law/health-care/article/smoking-laws-by-province/; Statistics Canada, http://www.statcan.gc.ca/pub/82-003-x/2006008/article/smoking-tabac/t/4060721-eng.htm.

Children are also regularly exposed to second-hand smoke. They are more than 50 percent more likely to suffer damage to their lungs and have breathing problems such as asthma. They are also much more likely to be at risk of brain tumours. Much of their exposure comes from living with smoking parents or guardians. Table 12-5 also lists provinces that have passed smoking bans in personal vehicles where children are passengers.

✓ CHECK-IN

How would you describe your lifetime exposure to second-hand smoke?

POLITICS OF TOBACCO

More than four decades after government health authorities began to warn of the dangers of smoking, tobacco remains a politically hot topic. In the United States, after many years of difficult negotiations, the tobacco industry and the Attorney Generals from nearly 40 states reached a historic settlement. Major tobacco companies agreed to pay more than 200 billion dollars to settle smoking-related lawsuits filed by 46 states, to finance anti-smoking campaigns, to restrict marketing, to permit federal regulation of tobacco, and to pay fines if tobacco use by minors does not decline.[104]

Provincial governments in Canada are modelling their own lawsuits after the successful negotiations in the U.S.A. In 2005, in British Columbia, the Supreme Court of Canada cleared the way for the province to sue Imperial Tobacco, JTI-Macdonald, Rothmans, Benson and Hedges, the Canadian Tobacco Manufacturers' Council, and nine foreign firms for the cost of treating smoking-related illnesses.[105] The lawsuit is still making its way through the courts. The cigarette companies have launched countersuits, and Imperial Tobacco launched a third-party lawsuit to involve the Government of Canada.

In September 2009, the province of Ontario also began a 50-billion-dollar lawsuit against 14 tobacco companies based in Canada, the United States, and England, seeking damages for past and ongoing health-care costs that link to tobacco-related illnesses. The latest piece of the lawsuit puzzle is an approved appeal for the province of Ontario to go forward with their lawsuit now that a countersuit by Imperial Tobacco Canada, Ltd. was thrown out of court.[106]

On the positive side of politics and smoking, Canadian federal politicians are working to support the *Framework Convention on Tobacco Control (FCTC)*—the first-ever international legal public-health treaty.[107] The *FCTC* was developed as an international response to a global concern about the devastating health, social, environmental, and economic consequences of tobacco consumption and exposure to tobacco smoke. This agreement seeks to protect present and future generations from these consequences.

Closer to home, we are guided by our national Federal Tobacco Control Strategy,[108] which includes a combination of tobacco-control efforts in protection, prevention, cessation, and harm-reduction initiatives. One example is the commitment of the federal government to strengthen cigarette and cigar package labelling. The new labelling requirements will include the following features:[109]

- an increased size of health warnings and images on the front and back of the packages—up from 50 percent to 75 percent
- photographs of people severely affected by smoking-related diseases
- testimonials from smokers
- a national toll-free *Quitline* number and website address for support for quitting
- eight new full-colour warning messages inside the packages
- improved toxic emissions warnings on the sides of the packages

Non-smokers' Bills of Rights are also being developed in many communities across Canada (see Figure 12-9).

QUITTING

Most people who eventually quit on their own have already tried other methods. In recent studies, some people who tried to quit smoking reported a small improvement in withdrawal symptoms over two weeks, but then their symptoms levelled off and persisted. Others found that their symptoms intensified rather than lessened over time. For reasons scientists cannot yet explain, former smokers who start smoking again put their lungs at even greater jeopardy than smokers who never quit.

According to therapists, quitting usually isn't a one-time event but a dynamic process that may take several years and four to ten attempts. The good news is that half of individuals who ever smoked have managed to quit. Thanks to new products and programs, it may be easier now than ever before to become an ex-smoker.

Quitting on Your Own More than 90 percent of former smokers quit on their own—by throwing away all their cigarettes, by gradually cutting down, or by first switching to a less-potent brand. One characteristic of successful quitters is that they see themselves as active participants in health maintenance and take personal responsibility for their own health. Often they experiment with a variety of strategies, such as learning relaxation techniques. Exercise has proven especially effective for quitting and avoiding weight

Non-smokers' Bill of Rights

Non-smokers Help Protect the Health, Comfort, and Safety of Everyone by Insisting on the Following Rights:

The Right to Breathe Clean Air

Non-smokers have the right to breathe clean air, free from harmful and irritating tobacco smoke. This right supersedes the right to smoke when the two conflict.

The Right to Speak Out

Non-smokers have the right to express—firmly but politely—their discomfort and adverse reactions to tobacco smoke. They have the right to voice their objections when smokers light up without asking permission.

The Right to Act

Non-smokers have the right to take action through legislative means—as individuals or in groups—to prevent or discourage smokers from polluting the atmosphere and to seek the restriction of smoking in public places.

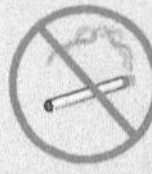

Figure 12-9 Non-smokers' Bill of Rights

gain. Making your home and car smoke-free zones also increases your likelihood of successfully quitting.

> *Health Canada has an extensive Quit Now Web-based program you can access. If you are a smoker who wants to quit, you will find information on dealing with withdrawal and an On the Road to Quitting program.*[110] *There is also an online Cost calculator*[111] *to help you put in perspective the money you spend on cigarette smoking. Learning about the financial costs of smoking sometimes help people make a commitment to quit.*

There are so many benefits to quitting—health, financial, emotional, physical, social, environmental, and more. The benefits also start quickly.[112]

- **Within 20 minutes** after smoking your last cigarette your body begins to change.
- **Twenty minutes** after quitting your heart rate drops.
- **Twelve hours** after quitting the carbon monoxide level in your blood drops to normal.
- **Two weeks to three months** after quitting your heart attack risk begins to drop. Your lung function begins to improve.
- **One to nine months** after quitting your coughing and shortness of breath decrease.
- **One year** after quitting your added risk of coronary heart disease is half that of a smoker's.
- **Five to 15 years** after quitting your stroke risk is reduced to that of a non-smoker's.
- **Ten years** after quitting your cancer death rate is about half that of a smoker's. Your risk of cancers of the mouth, throat, esophagus, bladder, kidney, and pancreas decreases.
- **Fifteen years** after quitting your risk of heart disease is back to that of a non-smoker's.

Quitting with the Help of Others Joining a support group doubles your chances of quitting for good. Instructors explain the risks of smoking, encourage individuals to think about why they smoke, and suggest ways of unlearning their smoking habit. A quitting day is often set for the third or fourth session.

Smoking cessation programs are sometimes available through student health services on many college and university campuses, as well as through public-health departments. Many businesses sponsor smoking-cessation programs for employees, available through Employee Assistance Programs (EAPs). Motivation may be even higher in these programs than in programs outside the workplace because of the social support.

Some smoking-cessation programs rely primarily on **aversion therapy**, which provides a negative experience every time a smoker has a cigarette. This may involve taking drugs that make tobacco smoke taste unpleasant, having smoke blown at you, or rapid smoking (the inhaling of smoke every six seconds until you're dizzy or nauseated).

Researchers have found that the use of cellphones and text messaging to individuals who participate in group smoking cessation programs is beneficial.[113] Daily messages of encouragement and information provided incentive for students on a college campus in their attempts to quit smoking. Health and wellness courses, trained peer facilitators, and online smoking cessation programs also proved to help students quit smoking.[114]

Nicotine-Replacement Therapy This approach uses a variety of products that supply low doses of nicotine in a way that allows smokers to taper off gradually over a period of months. There are four different nicotine-replacement therapy options available in Canada. They include gum, patches, lozenges, and an inhaler.[115] Because nicotine is a powerful, addictive substance, using nicotine replacements for a prolonged period is not advised. Pregnant women and individuals with heart disease shouldn't use them at all. Nicotine-replacement therapies don't affect the psychological dependence that makes quitting smoking so hard. That's why the key to long-term success in quitting smoking is getting support in addition to using replacement therapies.

Nicotine Gum, Lozenges, and Inhalers Nicotine gum, sold under brand names such as Nicorette®, the oldest and most widely known, can be purchased without a prescription.[116] The gum contains a nicotine resin that's gradually released as it is chewed. Absorbed through the mucous membrane of the mouth, the nicotine doesn't produce the same rush as a deeply inhaled drag on a cigarette. However, the gum maintains enough nicotine in the blood to diminish withdrawal symptoms. To use the gum, which comes in either 2 or 4 milligram doses, you bite, park it between your cheek for one minute, and then repeat the bite and park for up to 30 minutes. If you use lozenges, which are available in 1, 2, and 4 milligram doses, you suck until a strong taste is released, rest it between your cheek and gum for one minute, and then repeat for up to 30 minutes.

The NRT Inhaler delivers up to 4 milligrams of nicotine and is absorbed through the lining of the mouth and throat. Place the tapered end of the inhaler in your mouth. Inhale deeply into the back of your throat or take short puffs.

Side effects of the gum or lozenge can include mouth soreness, jaw ache, mild indigestion, sore jaws, nausea, heartburn, and stomach ache. Also, because nicotine chewing gum is heavier than regular chewing gum, it may loosen fillings or cause problems with dentures. Drinking coffee or other beverages may block absorption of the nicotine in the gum or lozenge; individuals trying to quit smoking shouldn't ingest any substance immediately before or while chewing nicotine gum. Side effects from the use of an inhaler include throat irritation, runny nose, and cough.

Between 5 and 10 percent of users transfer their dependence from cigarettes to these nicotine replacement therapies. When they stop using the products they experience withdrawal symptoms, although the symptoms tend to be milder than those prompted by quitting cigarettes.

Nicotine Patches Nicotine transdermal-delivery system products, or patches, provide nicotine, their only active ingredient, via a patch attached to the skin by an adhesive. The nicotine patch minimizes withdrawal symptoms, such as intense craving for cigarettes. Nicotine patches, now available without a prescription,[117] are replaced daily during therapy programs that run between 6 and 16 weeks. There is no evidence that continuing their use for more than eight weeks provides added benefit.

Some patches deliver nicotine for 24 hours while others for just 16 hours (during waking hours). Those most likely to benefit from nicotine-patch therapy are people who smoke more than a pack a day, are highly motivated to quit, and participate in counselling programs. When combined with counselling, the patch can be about twice as effective as a placebo, enabling 26 percent of smokers to abstain for six months.

Patch wearers who smoke or use more than one patch at a time can experience a nicotine overdose; some users have even suffered heart attacks. Occasional side effects include redness, itching, or swelling at the site of the patch application; insomnia; dry mouth; and nervousness.

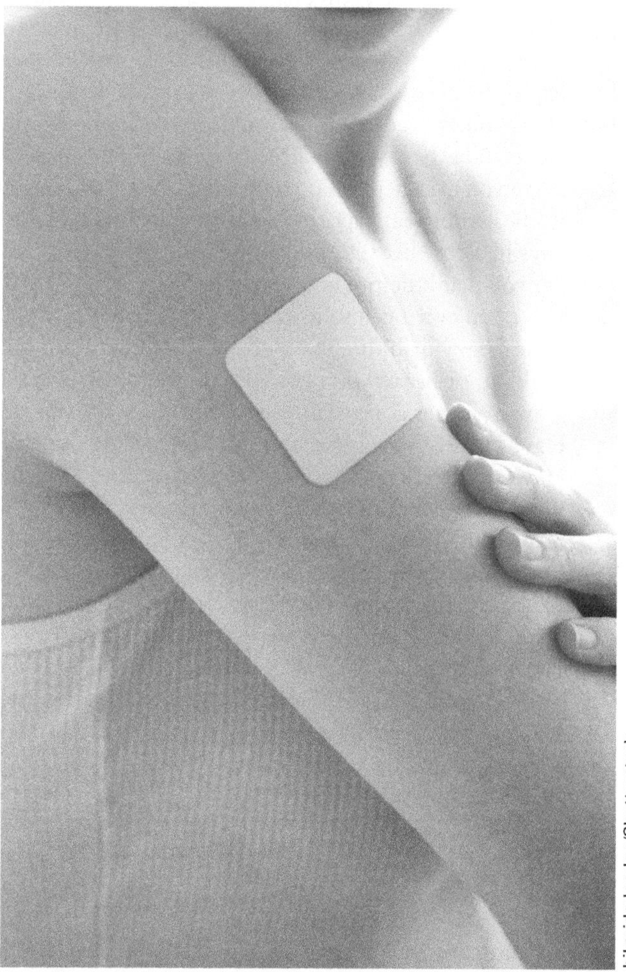

bikeriderlondon/Shutterstock

A nicotine patch releases nicotine transdermally (through the skin) in measured amounts, which are gradually decreased over time.

SELF-SURVEY

Do You Have a Drinking Problem?

This self-assessment, the Michigan Alcoholism Screening Test (MAST), is widely used to identify potential problems.

This test screens for the major psychological, sociological, and physiological consequences of alcoholism.

Answer Yes or No to the following questions, and add up the points shown in the right column for your answers.

	Yes	No	Points
1. Do you enjoy a drink now and then?	___	___	(0 for either)
2. Do you think that you're a normal drinker? (By normal, we mean that you drink less than or as much as most other people.)	___	___	(2 for no)
3. Have you ever awakened the morning after some drinking the night before and found that you couldn't remember part of the evening?	___	___	(2 for yes)
4. Does your boyfriend, girlfriend, partner, wife, husband, parent, or other near relative or friend ever worry or complain about your drinking?	___	___	(1 for yes)
5. Can you stop drinking without a struggle after one or two drinks?	___	___	(2 for no)
6. Do you ever feel guilty about your drinking?	___	___	(1 for yes)
7. Do friends or relatives think that you're a normal drinker?	___	___	(2 for no)
8. Do you ever try to limit your drinking to certain times of the day or to certain places?	___	___	(0 for either)
9. Have you ever attended a meeting of Alcoholics Anonymous?	___	___	(2 for yes)
10. Have you ever gotten into physical fights when drinking?	___	___	(1 for yes)
11. Has your drinking ever created problems for you and your boyfriend, girlfriend, partner, wife, husband, a parent, friend, or other relative?	___	___	(2 for yes)
12. Has your boyfriend, girlfriend, partner, wife, husband, parent, friend, or other family members ever gone to anyone for help about your drinking?	___	___	(2 for yes)
13. Have you ever lost friends because of your drinking?	___	___	(2 for yes)
14. Have you ever gotten into trouble at work or school because of your drinking?	___	___	(2 for yes)
15. Have you ever lost a job because of your drinking?	___	___	(2 for yes)
16. Have you ever neglected your obligations, your family, your academic studies, your team sports commitments, or your work for two or more days in a row because of drinking?	___	___	(2 for yes)
17. Do you drink before noon fairly often?	___	___	(1 for yes)
18. Have you ever been told you have liver trouble? Cirrhosis?	___	___	(2 for yes)
19. After heavy drinking, have you ever had delirium tremens (DTs) or severe shaking, or heard voices or seen things that weren't actually there?	___	___	(2 for yes*)
20. Have you ever gone to anyone for help about your drinking?	___	___	(5 for yes)
21. Have you ever been in a hospital because of your drinking?	___	___	(5 for yes)
22. Have you ever been a patient in a psychiatric hospital or on a psychiatric ward of a general hospital where drinking was part of the problem that resulted in hospitalization?	___	___	(2 for yes)
23. Have you ever been seen at a psychiatric or mental health clinic or gone to any doctor, social worker, or clergyman for help with any emotional problem where drinking was part of the problem?	___	___	(2 for yes)
24. Have you ever been arrested for drunk driving, driving while intoxicated, or driving under the influence of alcoholic beverages?	___	___	(2 for yes)
25. Have you ever been arrested or taken into custody, even for a few hours, because of drunken behaviour?	___	___	(2 for yes)
(If Yes how many times?) **	___	___	

Answers to Self-Survey

*Five points for delirium tremens
**Two points for each arrest

Scoring

In general, five or more points places you in an alcoholic category; four points suggests alcoholism; three or fewer points indicates that you're not an alcoholic.

Chapter Summary

1. Which statement about the effects of alcohol on the body systems is true?
   a. In most individuals, alcohol sharpens the responses of the brain and nervous system, enhancing sensation and perception.
   b. Alcohol speeds up the elimination of fluid from the body.
   c. French researchers have found that drinking red wine with meals may have a positive effect on the digestive system.
   d. The leading alcohol-related cause of death is liver damage.

2. Which statement about drinking on college and university campuses is true?
   a. The percentage of students who frequently binge drink has increased.
   b. The number of female students who binge drink has decreased.
   c. Because of peer pressure, students tend to drink less alcohol when they live in residences.
   d. Students who live in substance-free dormitories tend to binge drink when alcohol is available.

3. Which statement about fetal alcohol syndrome (FAS) is true?
   a. Women who plan to get pregnant can drink in moderation.
   b. Alcohol is oxidized more slowly in the fetus because the liver is underdeveloped.
   c. Drinking during pregnancy will not affect the fetus because it is protected by the placenta.
   d. It is difficult to distinguish a baby with FAS.

4. Which statement about women who have drinking problems is true?
   a. They often suffer from fetal alcohol syndrome as a result of their mother's alcohol consumption.
   b. They are less likely to have an alcoholic parent than men with drinking problems.
   c. They are at higher risk for osteoporosis than women who are not heavy drinkers.
   d. They are less likely to suffer liver damage than men.

5. Which statement about alcohol abuse and dependence is false?
   a. Alcohol dependence involves a persistent craving for and an increased tolerance to alcohol.
   b. An individual may have a genetic predisposition for developing alcoholism.
   c. Alcoholics often abuse other psychoactive drugs.
   d. Alcohol abuse and alcohol dependence are different names for the same problem.

6. Which statement about tobacco and its components is true?
   a. Nicotine settles in the lungs, eventually causing precancerous changes.
   b. Tobacco stimulates the kidneys to form urine.
   c. Carbon monoxide contained in tobacco smoke impairs oxygen transport in the body.
   d. Tar is the addictive substance in tobacco.

7. Which statement about cigarette smokers is true?
   a. They are more likely to die of lung cancer than heart disease.
   b. They usually develop lung problems after years of tobacco use.
   c. They have two to three times the risk of suffering a stroke than non-smokers.
   d. They may completely reverse the damage to their blood vessels if they quit smoking.

8. Which statement about tobacco use on college and university campuses is true?
   a. Tobacco use is most often in the form of smokeless tobacco products used by students to avoid detection.
   b. Tobacco use is more prevalent among those students who also use marijuana, binge drink, and spend more time socializing with friends.
   c. Tobacco use has decreased in the past 10 years because almost all schools have adopted a no-smoking policy on their premises.
   d. Tobacco use is considered a minor problem by most student health centre directors, since less than a third of students smoke.

9. Which statement about second-hand tobacco smoke is true?
   a. It is the smoke inhaled by a smoker.
   b. It is more hazardous than outdoor pollution as a cancer-causing agent.
   c. It is less hazardous than mainstream smoke.
   d. It is less likely to cause serious health problems in children than in adults.

10. Which statement about quitting smoking is true?
    a. Quitting smoking usually results in minor withdrawal symptoms.
    b. Quitting smoking will do little to reverse the damage to the lungs and other parts of the body.
    c. Quitting smoking can be aided by joining a support group.
    d. Quitting smoking is best done by cutting down on the number of cigarettes you smoke over a period of months.

Answers to these questions can be found on page 353.

SELF-RESPONSIBILITY—SOCIAL RESPONSIBILITY

SELF-RESPONSIBILITY

It makes absolutely no sense to put something in your mouth and set it on fire.

George Sheehan

Sometimes it is hard to let go of a lifestyle habit that has become comfortable, even though it might not be a healthy habit. If you are someone who has been thinking about making some changes with regard to alcohol consumption or tobacco use, you are already in the contemplation stage of Prochaska's Stages of Change model. Ask yourself what next steps would move you into preparation and action. What would maintenance look and feel like to you? Can you visualize yourself at the termination stage where a healthy lifestyle habit becomes the habit of choice for you? Start slowly, embrace change, and move along the continuum of the change model toward healthy living.

SOCIAL RESPONSIBILITY

We cannot live only for ourselves. A thousand fibres connect us with our fellow men.

Herman Melville

Healthy lifestyle habits make a difference not only to personal health and wellness, but also to global health and wellness. Connect with campus initiatives that support healthy living options. Educate other students about responsible alcohol consumption. Work toward a smoke-free campus.

CRITICAL THINKING

Driving home from a night out partying, 20-year-old Rick has had too much to drink. As he crosses the dividing line on the two-lane road, the driver of an oncoming car—a young mother with two young children in the backseat—swerves to avoid an accident. She hits a concrete wall and dies instantly, but her children survive. Rick has no record of drunk driving. Should he go to prison? Is he guilty of manslaughter? How would you feel if you were the victim's husband or if you were Rick's friend?

1. Have you ever been around people who have been intoxicated when you have been sober? What did you think of their behaviour? Were they fun to be around? Was the experience not particularly enjoyable, boring, or difficult in some way? Have you ever been intoxicated? How do you behave when you are drunk? Do you find the experience enjoyable? What do the people around you think of your actions when you are drunk?
2. Has smoking become unpopular among your friends or family? What social activities continue to be associated with smoking? Can you think of any situation in which smoking might be frowned upon?
3. How would you motivate someone you care about to stop smoking? What reasons would you give for them to stop? Describe your strategy.

WEB LINKS

Canadian Centre on Substance Abuse

www.ccsa.ca

At this site you can access current and comprehensive reports such as the *Canadian Addiction Survey (CAS)* and research articles on substance abuse.

QuitNow—The Lung Association

www.quitnow.ca

News, announcements, and current and historical research articles are available at this site. Information on strategies for smoke-free workplaces is also available.

Healthy Canadians—Smoking and Tobacco

http://healthycanadians.gc.ca/healthy-living-vie-saine/tobacco-tabac/index-eng.php

A national one-stop shop for information about tobacco and smoking. Here you will find smoking cessation programs, a cost calculator, and information on nicotine addiction and how to help yourself or others to quit.

Government of Ontario—Health and Wellness

www.ontario.ca/page/support-quit-smoking

This site provides some excellent information about how to quit smoking. Learn about the longer-term benefits of quitting and read tips to help you quit.

Ontario Tobacco Research Unit

www.otru.org

The Ontario Tobacco Research Unit is the research component of the Ontario Tobacco Strategy. Led by a multidisciplinary team, this unit carries out research and evaluation and explores data sources and questions about tobacco use in Canada.

Please note that links are subject to change. If you find a broken link, use a search engine such as www.google.ca and search for the website by typing in keywords.

Key Terms

The terms listed here are used within the chapter on the page indicated. Definitions of terms are in the Glossary at the end of the book.

Answers to Chapter Summary Questions

1. b; 2. a; 3. b; 4. c; 5. d; 6. c; 7. c; 8. b; 9. b; 10. c

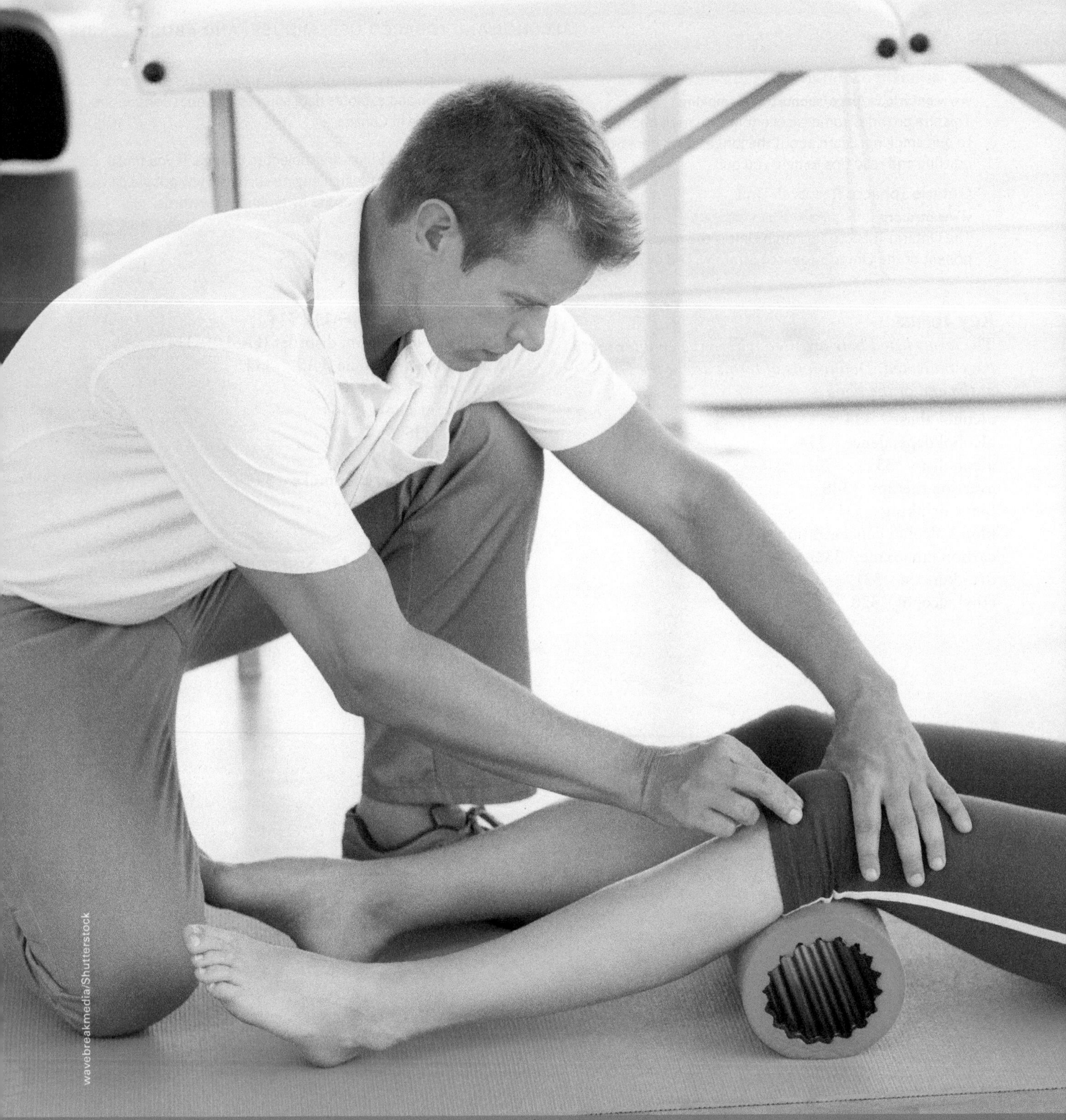

AFTER READING THIS CHAPTER, YOU WILL BE ABLE TO:

- **list** and **describe** the five principles of the *Canada Health Act*
- **describe** the difference between activity-based and bundle-payment healthcare funding
- **list** ways of evaluating online medical advice and health news
- **list** your medical rights
- **describe** the different types of complementary and alternative medicine therapies and **explain** what research has shown about their effectiveness
- **explain** what managed care is

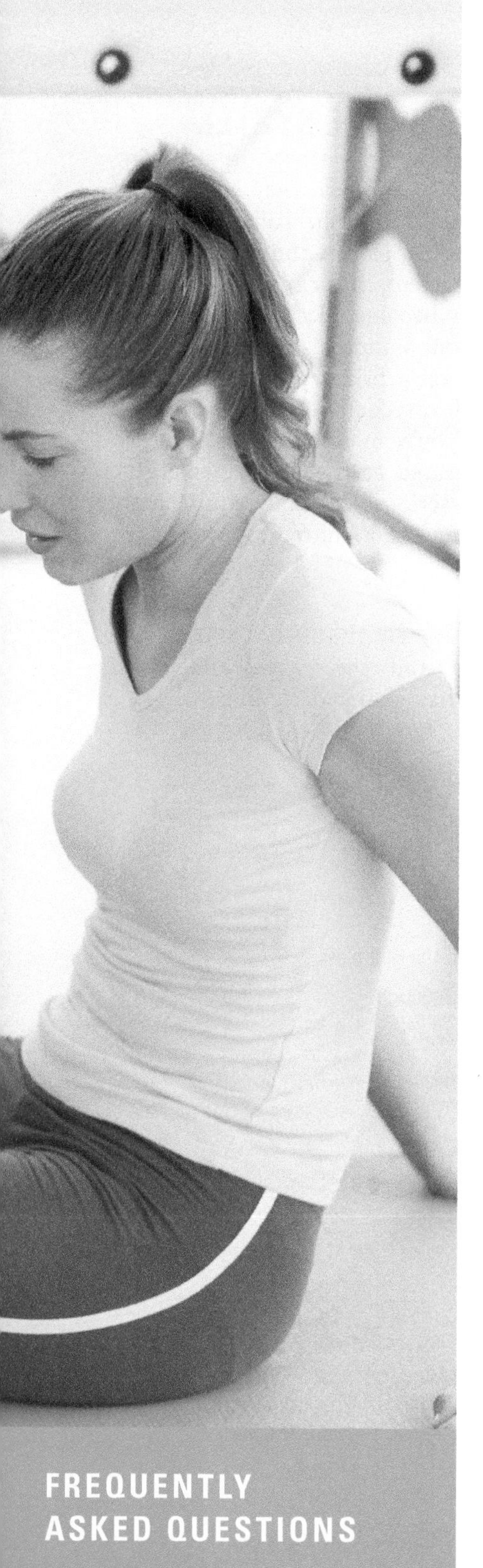

13

Traditional and Complementary Healthcare Approaches

Canadians have access to more healthcare services and health practitioners, undergo more surgery, take more prescription drugs, and spend more time in hospitals today than they have in past decades. According to the National Health Expenditure Trends, 1975–2015 report,[1] total healthcare spending in 2015 in Canada was estimated at 219.1 billion dollars (see Figure 13-1). This was an average of 6105 dollars per person. The largest expenditures in 2015 were for hospitals at 29.5 percent, followed by drugs at 15.7 percent, and physician services at 15.5 percent.[2] Spending for drug costs was estimated at 959 dollars per person, which was an increase of 0.7 percent from 2014.[3] Healthcare spending does vary across the country. Quebec and British Columbia had the lowest healthcare expenditures per capita in 2015. Newfoundland and Labrador and Alberta had the highest[4] (see Figure 13-2).

Canadians are also accessing complementary and alternative medicine (CAM), also known as complementary and alternative health care (CAHC). This term includes a broad range of healing philosophies, approaches, and therapies not traditionally taught in medical schools or provided in hospitals. Metcalfe et al. report that a large proportion of Canadians use CAM services.[5]

College and university health can be thought of as the caring intersection between health and education. As a college or university student, you are concerned with and responsible for both. This chapter will help prepare you for making informed healthcare choices. As Dr. Donald Ardell states, "All dimensions of high-level wellness are equally important, but self-responsibility seems more equal than all the rest."[6]

FREQUENTLY ASKED QUESTIONS

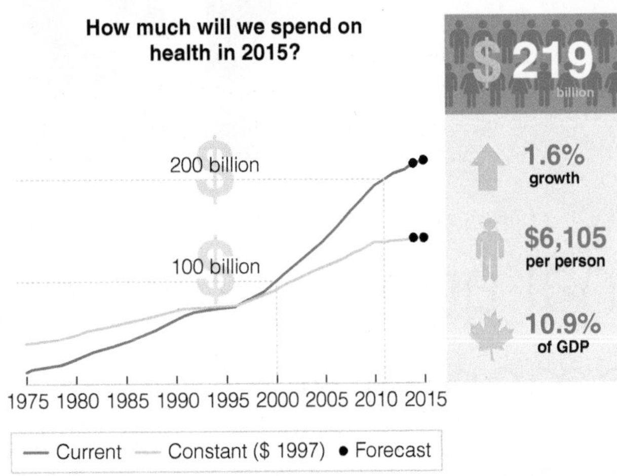

Figure 13-1 Total Healthcare Expenditure in Canada (Estimated), 2015

Source: Canadian Institute for Health Information (CIHI) National Health Expenditure Trends. Found at https://www.cihi.ca/sites/default/files/document/nhex_trends_narrative_report_2015_en.pdf (page 6)

CANADA'S HEALTHCARE SYSTEM

In the past, when people were sick, they went to their family physician and paid in cash. Today, healthcare involves many more people, places, and processes. As a college or university student, you can turn to student health services if you become ill. There, a medical doctor may evaluate your symptoms and provide basic care, or you may rely on a primary-care physician in your hometown to perform regular checkups or manage a chronic condition. If you're injured in an accident, you will most likely be treated at the nearest emergency room. If you become seriously ill and require highly specialized care, you may be admitted to a hospital to receive treatment.

A Brief History of Our Healthcare System "The practice of medicine and the range and nature of treatment options has changed significantly since

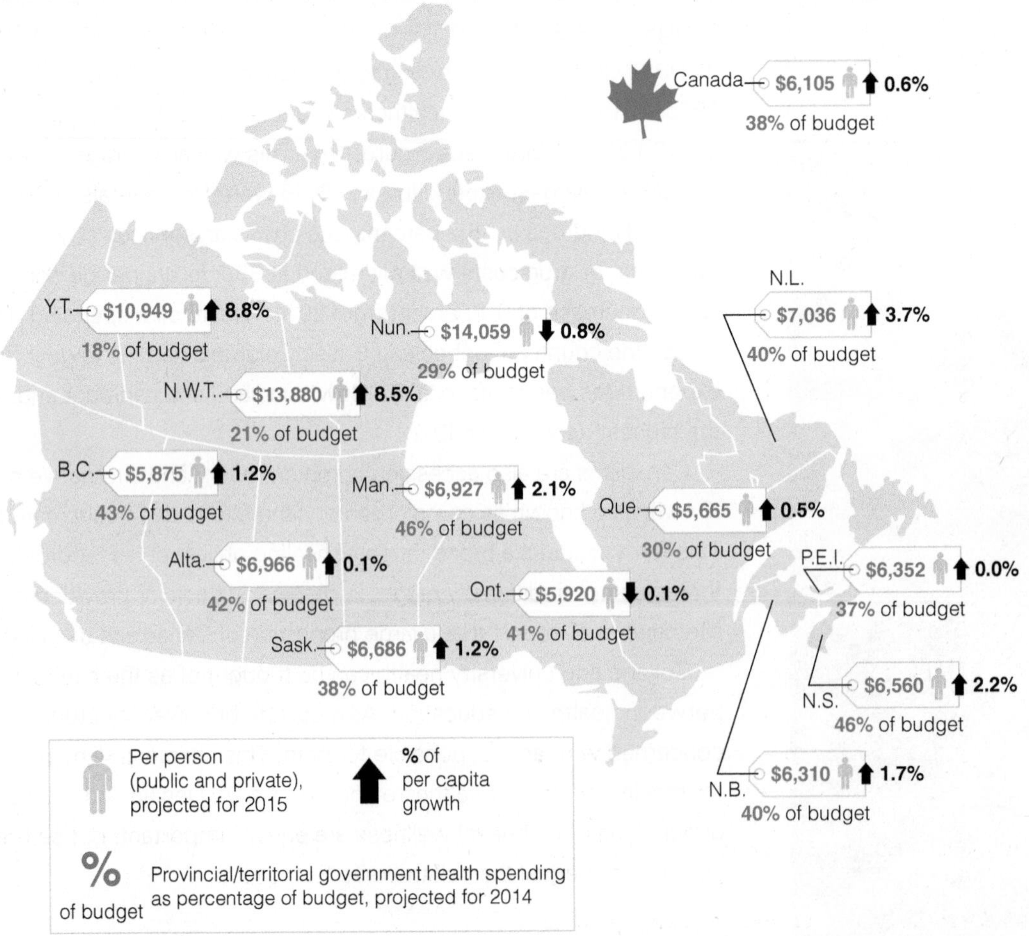

Figure 13-2 Health Expenditure in the Provinces and Territories

Source: Canadian Institute for Health Information (CIHI) National Health Expenditure Trends. Found at https://www.cihi.ca/sites/default/files/document/nhex_trends_narrative_report_2015_en.pdf (page 17)

Medicare was introduced 40 years ago," said Roy Romanow, in his *2002 Final Report of the Commission on the Future of Health Care in Canada*.[7] What you might know and understand as healthcare today did look very different in the past.

The person credited with establishing Canada's healthcare system is Tommy Douglas, the late premier of Saskatchewan. In 1948, his governing party, the Co-operative Commonwealth Federation (CCF), introduced a universal hospital insurance plan for the residents of the province. In 1957, his government introduced an insurance scheme for physician services.[8] Then, in 1964, the federal government, under the *Hospital Insurance and Diagnostic Services Act (HIDSA)*, agreed to reimburse provinces for a portion of the costs of providing insurance to their residents. By 1972, all of the provinces had joined the plan, creating a nationwide medicare program for hospital and physician services.[9]

In 1985, the *Medical Care Act* and the *HIDSA* were replaced by the *Canada Health Act (CHA)*. The act is based on five principles:[10]

1. **Public administration**—Provincial and territorial healthcare insurance plans must be administered and operated on a nonprofit basis by a public authority. It does not prohibit private facilities or providers from supplying insured health services, but no eligible provincial or territorial resident can be charged for these services.
2. **Comprehensiveness**—Provincial or territorial healthcare insurance plans must cover all insured health services that are provided by hospitals, physicians, or dental work requiring a hospital setting.
3. **Universality**—All health-insured residents are entitled to any insured health service provided in their province or territory. There can be a three-month waiting period for immigrants or Canadian citizens returning from living abroad or moving to another province.
4. **Portability**—If a Canadian resident moves from one province to another province or territory, the "home" province must continue health-insurance coverage for any waiting period required by the new province. The new province or territory then assumes responsibility for healthcare coverage. The resident is required to inform their provincial or territorial healthcare insurance plan of any move or new residency. Portability does not allow a person to search for services in other provinces, territories, or countries. It is intended only for urgent or necessary services on a temporary basis such as a vacation or business trip.
5. **Accessibility**—Reasonable access of health services has been interpreted to mean "where and as available" in the province or territory. It also is meant to ensure that any insured resident has reasonable access to insured hospital, medical, and surgical-dental services without incurring user charges or extra billing. Insured residents are not to be discriminated against on the basis of age, health status, or financial circumstances either.

These principles have become the conditions that provinces must abide by to receive federal transfer funds that support the national health-insurance plan. The 13 interlocking provincial and territorial health-insurance plans share common features and basic standards of coverage. Residence in a province or territory is the basic requirement for insured healthcare coverage. Each province determines minimum residence requirements.

We appear to be at a crossroads with regard to our medicare system. Healthcare costs are prohibitive, waiting lists are long, and there is a physician shortage in some areas of Canada. More and more people are advocating a move toward private healthcare or public–private healthcare partnerships. In April 2001, the Commission on the Future of Health Care in Canada was established. Roy J. Romanow was appointed as its commissioner. Mr. Romanow's mandate was to review medicare, engage Canadians in a national dialogue on its future, and make recommendations to enhance our health system's quality and sustainability. His assessment was that while medicare is as sustainable as Canadians want it to be, we need to take steps toward transforming it into a truly national, more comprehensive, responsive, and accountable healthcare system.[11]

What Are Federal, Provincial, and Territorial Healthcare Responsibilities? The federal government is responsible for[12]

- setting and administering national principles or standards for the healthcare system through the *Canada Health Act*;
- assisting in the financing of provincial healthcare services through fiscal transfers;
- delivering direct health services to specific groups, including veterans, Native Canadians living on reserves, military personnel, inmates of federal penitentiaries, and the Royal Canadian Mounted Police; and
- fulfilling other health-related functions, such as health protection, disease prevention, and health promotion.

The provincial and territorial governments are responsible for

- managing and delivering healthcare services;
- planning, financing, and evaluating the provision of hospital care;
- physician and allied healthcare services; and
- managing some aspects of prescription care and public health.

We are fortunate to have one of the best medical systems in the world, and support for our public healthcare system is still strong. Our current healthcare structure depends upon approximately 70 percent of funding coming from the public sector and about 30 percent from the private sector.[13] However, some provinces have implemented new funding structures to deal with high healthcare expenditures. **Activity-based funding** is one of these structures.[14] Instead of the traditional block-funding model that provides hospitals with a lump-sum budget on an annual basis, the activity-based model provides funding on a patient-focused system, where a healthcare unit or institution gets funding based on the volume and the complexity of the patients that are treated. There are advantages to this type of funding. Hospitals are allowed to keep any overage funding—the difference between the amount they were paid and the actual cost of the medical services they provided. This type of funding is also described as a visible funding method as every hospital is paid the same amount for the same type of services.

In Ontario a health-based allocation model (HBAM) for local health integration networks (LHINs) is determined by population-based factors that include age, gender, socio-economic status, rural geography, and patient flows.

The British Columbia government is distributing funds to the largest hospitals based on a patient-focused service, where dedicated funding will be available to the hospitals offering the lowest prices for surgery. Goals include reducing wait times for some common surgical procedures and decreasing the number of overnight patient stays.

Alberta Health Services introduced activity-based funding with its new Seniors Care Plan. Activity-based funding is also being used in Quebec. If hip and knee replacement operations cannot be performed at a government-funded hospital within six months, the province will pay for surgery at a private clinic affiliated with the province. Ontario, British Columbia, and Quebec are also implementing reforms to reduce the cost of generic drugs.

Bundled payments are another funding option for healthcare services. If a patient needs a set of treatments and services to recover from a specific health issue, such as a stroke, a single funding amount will be awarded to the healthcare provider.[15] Bundled payment funding is designed to cover a fixed-time recovery period. The risk to a healthcare provider with this type of funding is the possibility that overall costs might be more than the bundled payment award. The healthcare provider is expected to pay any overrun. However, if the treatment plan is less than the actual costs of the medical service, the provider keeps the difference.

Canada's Healthcare Providers According to a report from the Canadian Institute for Health Information (CIHI),[16] there was a 2.9 percent increase in the number of physicians in Canada between 2013 and 2014. The number of physicians rose to 79 000. This increase was felt in every province except Prince Edward Island, Nova Scotia, and Manitoba. Nunavut (9.1 percent), Yukon (7.5 percent), and Alberta (5.5 percent) had the largest growth in physician to population ratios.[17]

The number of doctors graduating from universities in Canada is also increasing. In 2014, 2804 students graduated as physicians from Canadian universities. This was a 5.5 percent increase in graduates from 2013. The number of physicians working in rural areas increased by almost 10 percent between 2007 and 2011. Another change is the demographic makeup: in 2014, 43.8 percent of Canada's physicians were women and 34 percent were specialists. The number of female physicians increased by 23.7 percent between 2010 and 2014, whereas male physicians increased by 9.5 percent.[18]

In 2014, more regulated nurses left the nursing profession than those who entered the profession. The reasons for this reduction included a lower number of graduates from nursing programs, nurses choosing not to renew their registration status, retirement, and nurses leaving their profession.[19]

However, there were 406 817 regulated nurses employed in the profession in 2014; registered nurses (RNs) numbered 289 239, nurse practitioners (NPs) numbered 3966, licenced practical nurses (LPNs) numbered 107 923, and registered psychiatric nurses numbered 5689.[20]

The skills needed by healthcare professionals working in Canada vary, and the scope of practice of healthcare providers is changing. A number of younger doctors are seeing fewer patients than doctors their age did 10 years ago,[21] and there has been a decrease in the number of family doctors performing surgeries, delivering babies, and providing care to patients in a hospital setting, although more are providing mental-health counselling in their practices.[22]

Canada has many universities and colleges that train physicians. If you are interested in becoming a doctor, you can find out more about medical schools in Canada by accessing *The Association of Faculties of Medicine of Canada* for careers in the medical and healthcare field.[23] To become a doctor, some universities require that you must complete three years of an undergraduate degree before applying for medical school. Other universities require that you earn an undergraduate degree before you apply for medical school. Students in their final year of studies in medicine must take examinations set by the Medical Council of Canada before they can be licensed to practise. Medical students can decide if they would like to work as a general practitioner (GP) or a specialist. A GP has general knowledge in all health and medical areas. He or she will direct patients to specialists if more care is needed.

According to the *National Physician Survey*, 79 percent of all physicians and other specialists stated that intellectual stimulation and challenge were factors leading to their career choice.[24] In one survey of medical students, Scott et al. found that the choice of family medicine as a career when entering into medical school was the best predictor of the eventual career.[25] Further specialist studies in various fields such as family medicine, internal medicine, and general surgery can be taken at a postgraduate level.

Nurses must take academic courses, too. Some university schools of nursing have accelerated programs that allow students to complete a Bachelor of Science in Nursing (BScN) in two or three years. Many community and university colleges offer nursing diploma programs. The Canadian Nurses Association (CNA) provides information about nursing schools in Canada.[26]

Nurses can work in hospital settings, care homes, schools, and community outreach programs. Nurse specialties include cardiovascular, critical care, emergency, gerontology, hospice palliative care, occupational health, and psychiatric and mental health.

Other types of medical professionals include the following:

- *Gynecologists*—who deal with the care of women during pregnancy, childbirth, and recovery. They also diagnose and treat disorders that affect the female reproductive organs.
- *Dermatologists*—who specialize in skin physiology and pathology and diagnose and treat skin diseases.
- *Family practitioners*—who help diagnose long-term health issues that are passed on through generations.
- *Orthopedic doctors*—who deal with the prevention and correction of injuries or disorders of the skeletal system and muscles, joints, and ligaments.
- *Urologists*—who specialize in the diagnosis and treatment of diseases of the urinary tract and urogenital system.
- *Pediatricians*—who specialize in the care of infants and children.
- *Endocrinologists*—who study the glands and hormones and their related disorders, such as diabetes.
- *Oncologists*—who deal with the diagnosis, treatment, and prevention of tumours.

Careers in the healthcare field also include those in allied health sectors. Dietitians, nutritionists, medical laboratory technicians, dentists, health-information educators, addiction counsellors, and pharmacists are just some examples. Working with an allied health professional may support personal healthcare. We have included information about chiropractors, kinesiologists, massage therapists, and physiotherapists in the Complementary and Alternative Medicine Programs and Services section.

> **✓ CHECK-IN**
>
> Do you have a good, ongoing relationship with a primary-care physician?

Your Medical Rights Certain rights in healthcare are recognized in Canada. Canadians have access to their own medical records and the right to have those records kept private. Privacy is becoming an issue as patients' records are now being computerized and stored in large databases. Patients also have the right to receive treatment that is provided with a reasonable degree of care.[27] As a consumer, you have basic rights to help ensure that you know about any potential dangers, receive competent diagnosis and treatment, and retain control and dignity in your interactions with healthcare professionals. You can designate someone else to make decisions about your care if and when you cannot.

Some hospitals in Canada have a patient advocate or representative. These individuals can help you communicate with physicians, make any special arrangements, and get answers to questions or complaints.

Canadians also have the right to give consent to donate an organ while alive or have organs removed in the event of an accident, injury, or illness that leaves them brain dead. However, you cannot agree to donate a body part for money or other compensation.

Your Right to Information By law, you have the right to give your informed consent for hospitalization, surgery, and other major treatments. **Informed consent** is a right, not a privilege. Use this right to its fullest. Ask questions. Seek other opinions. Make sure that your expectations are realistic and that you understand the potential risks, as well as the possible benefits, of a prospective treatment. Informed consent is also required for research studies. You have the right to know whether a procedure is experimental.

> **✓ CHECK-IN**
>
> Think back on your healthcare experiences. Were your rights as a patient respected?

BECOMING A KNOWLEDGEABLE HEALTHCARE CONSUMER

The term **health literacy** describes your ability to know how to spot health problems, how to evaluate health news, what to expect from healthcare professionals, and where to turn for health information and appropriate treatment so that you can ensure you receive the best possible healthcare—when you need it.

Self-Care Most people do treat themselves. You might have self-prescribed aspirin or acetaminophen for a headache, had some chicken soup or orange juice for a cold, or taken a weekend trip to unwind from stress. At the very least, you should know what your **vital signs** are and how they compare against normal readings. Vital signs are indicators for overall health and should be taken at rest:

- Body temperature—The average body temperature is 37° C. It is taken with a thermometer and is usually lower in the morning than later in the day. It can vary due to exercise, when drinking hot or cold fluids, and when you are fighting an infection.
- Pulse or heart rate—A resting adult heart rate should be between 60 and 80 beats per minute. Pulse checks can be taken at your radial pulse (wrist) or at the carotid pulse (neck). Use your index or middle finger to measure your pulse rate.
- Respiratory rate—The normal adult rate is 12–18 breaths per minute. Count the number of times your chest rises in one minute while breathing normally.
- Blood pressure—The average blood pressure is 120 mmHg (systolic)/80 mmHg (diastolic). A resting blood pressure of over 90 diastolic is considered mildly elevated.

Once a thermometer was the only self-testing equipment found in most Canadian homes. Now there are numerous home tests available to help consumers monitor everything from pregnancy to blood pressure. The new tests are generally as accurate as those administered by a professional. You should always follow directions precisely, and if your concerns persist, see your doctor.

How Can I Evaluate Online Health Advice? The Internet has changed the way people obtain information. Canadians have adopted the Internet and broadband technology with enthusiasm. Nearly 8 out of 10 Canadians are daily users of the Internet. Canadians spend an average of 34.6 hours per month online using personal computers. They also access the Internet through smartphones with three out of four Canadians owning a smartphone and spending 49 percent of time spent on-line using their mobile devices.[28]

Many people use the Internet to search for health or medical information. Seventy percent of Canadians state they look for online sites about specific diseases, medical issues, or health-related products. A growing group of Canadians also visit online chat rooms and support groups for medical concerns.[29] What is troubling for some medical professionals is that many Canadians who do use the Internet for medical advice say that they trust the information they have found. Research in the area of Internet medical information suggests that some websites may have incorrect or outdated information.[30]

Some doctors are embracing technology and use the Internet to support their medical practice. Findings from the 2014 *National Physician Survey* showed that 75 percent of physicians reported that they use electronic records to support their patient-care program.[31] However, some doctors are finding that it complicates the doctor–patient relationship. Research also shows that 20 percent of Canadians believe that their electronic health records are open to security risks.[32]

Behaviour of health users also differed somewhat from other users:[33]

- Health users were more likely to access the Internet daily.
- Health users spent at least five hours a week online.
- B.C. residents were the Canadians most likely to look for online health information. Residents of Ontario and Alberta were close behind.
- Half of health users reported searching for information on lifestyle, diet, nutrition and exercise, medications, and alternative therapies.

The Internet permits ease of access to cutting-edge medical knowledge and bridges the communication gap created by high-tech medicine. However, it can have serious drawbacks. Simple queries for terms such as *obesity* or *depression* often lead to irrelevant sites, relevant sites with incomplete information, or sites that are difficult for most consumers to understand.[34] Even when information is technically precise, people may not know how to interpret it properly.

The sale of Internet prescriptions has become a controversial issue in Canada and the United States.[35] The concerns are about public safety. Many physicians do not examine patients before they write prescriptions for those who are purchasing drugs online. Another concern is rooted in protecting the pharmaceutical industry's profitability. A large proportion of Internet prescription sales are to customers in the United States, with estimates of upward of 1 billion U.S. dollars in sales per year.

The Canadian Medical Protective Association (CMPA) has warned their members not to prescribe or co-sign prescriptions for Americans seeking prescription drugs, either on the Internet or in person. As well, if any licensed pharmacy offers Internet services, they must meet the standards of practice within the home province.[36] Presently there are more questions than answers in how to deal with the blend of technology and medicine. Online prescription drugs can be illegal or unapproved. Many Internet pharmacies have an "offshore" location so it is difficult to know where they are located, where they get their drugs, and how to reach them if there is a problem with a prescription.[37] You can put yourself at risk for drug interactions or harmful side effects if the drugs have dangerous additives or ingredients. You might also be at a financial risk if the prescription you ordered is never shipped, or is stopped at the Canadian border.

Other "cyberdocs" offer "virtual house calls" with board-certified physicians who engage in private chat sessions on minor illnesses and prescribe medicine. In the future, video conferencing may allow doctors to examine patients in cyberspace. However, there are no professional standards for doctors on the Internet, and experts advise caution. The doctor who treats your allergies may be a urologist or pathologist who is not up to date on new therapies or is unaware of potential side effects.

Health Canada is attempting to play a role in electronic health (e-health) issues. Health experts recognize that information and communications technology might help to overcome the challenges of delivering healthcare in Canada. Collection, management, and use of patient health information; convenient access to health education; and increased communication among healthcare providers are all positive benefits of an e-health or telehealth system. However, ethical considerations and evaluation of the effectiveness of such a system need to be addressed to protect both medical professionals and the general public. The National Association of Pharmacy Regulatory Authorities has developed standards for pharmacists offering services over the Internet.[38]

Here are some specific guidelines for evaluating online health sites:[39]

- **Check the creator.** Websites are produced by health agencies, health-support groups, school health programs, health-product advertisers, health educators, health-education organizations, and provincial and federal governments. Read site headers and footers carefully to distinguish biased commercial advertisements from unbiased sites created by scientists and health agencies.
- **Look for possible bias.** Websites may be attempting to provide healthful information to consumers, but they also may be attempting to sell a product. Many sites are merely disguised advertisements.
- **Check the date.** If you are looking for the most recent research, check the date the page was created and last updated as well as the links. Several non-working links signal that the site isn't carefully maintained.
- **Check the references.** As with other health-education materials, Web documents should provide the reader with references. Unreferenced suggestions may be unwarranted, scientifically unsound, and possibly unsafe.
- **Consider the author.** Is he or she recognized in the field of health education or otherwise qualified to publish a health-information Web document? Does the author list his or her occupation, experience, and education?

✓ CHECK-IN

Which websites have you used to find health information? Which ones do you trust? Which ones don't you trust?

Evaluating Health News Cure! Breakthrough! Medical miracle! These words make catchy headlines. Remember that although medical breakthroughs and cures do occur, most scientific progress is made one small step at a time.

Medical opinions invariably change over time, sometimes going from one extreme to another. For instance, several decades ago the treatment of choice for breast cancer was radical mastectomy—removal of the woman's breast, lymph nodes, and chest wall. Since then, much less extensive surgery (lumpectomy), coupled with chemotherapy or radiation, or both, has proven equally effective. There was also a time when individuals who had suffered heart attacks were advised to limit all physical activity. Today, a progressive exercise program is a standard component of rehabilitation.

Health researchers are struggling to find better ways of assessing what they know and need to know in order to offer more complete and balanced information to consumers. However, sometimes the only certainty is uncertainty. Try to gather as much background information and as many opinions as you can. Weigh them carefully—ideally with a trusted physician—and make the decision that seems best for you.

When reading a newspaper or magazine article, listening to a radio or television report about a medical advance, or searching the Internet, look for answers to the following questions:

- Who are the scientists involved? Are they recognized, legitimate health professionals? What are their credentials? Are they affiliated with respected medical or scientific institutions? Be wary of individuals whose degrees or affiliations are from institutions you've never heard of, and be sure that the person's educational background is in a discipline related to the area of research reported.
- Where did the scientists report their findings? The best research is published in peer-reviewed professional journals. One example is the *British Medical Journal*. Research developments also may be reported at meetings of professional societies.[40] Is the information based on personal observations? Does the report include testimonials from cured patients or satisfied customers? If the answer to either question is yes, be wary.[41]
- Does the article, report, or advertisement include words like *amazing, secret,* or *quick?* Does it claim to be something the public has never seen or been offered before? Such sensationalized language is often a tip-off to a dubious treatment.

- Is someone trying to sell you something? Manufacturers who cite studies to sell a product have been known to embellish the truth.
- Does the information defy all common sense? Be skeptical. If something sounds too good to be true, it probably is.

Evaluating Health Claims Every year thousands of Canadians search for medical miracles that never happen. Millions of dollars are spent on medical **quackery**, unproven health products and services. Those who lose only money are the lucky ones. Many people end up wasting precious time, during which their conditions worsen. Some suffer needless pain, along with crushed expectations. Far too many risk their lives on a false hope—and lose.

Watch out for marketing techniques such as *bait and switch*, where retailers advertise a product at a low price to lure you into their store, but are sold out when you arrive. Attempts are then made to persuade you to purchase a higher-quality product at a higher price. The *brand-loyalty approach* is also used to sell health products. A retailer or advertiser might try to convince you that a specific brand name means quality, but they do not tell you that in many cases the active ingredients of the product are the same as those in lower-priced products. *Product misrepresentation* is yet another approach used. If the sales pitch says that 9 out of 10 doctors endorse a certain product, be sure to ask questions: Which doctors? What are their credentials? Were they paid to endorse the product? It is also important to check out the legitimacy of health food or lifestyle stores. Where one health store might have reputable and qualified personnel, others might not.

✓ CHECK-IN

Where do you turn for health information? What sources do you consider the most reliable?

In the fitness and health industry, there is a direct emphasis on physical appearance and sales pitches that attempt to make you believe that getting or staying fit is easy—no effort is needed to lose weight, become muscular, or look great. Noted personalities are used to endorse products that they may not even use. Before and after pictures are also used to encourage you to buy the product. Computer technology is often the reason why the model looks terrific in the after picture. Multi-level marketing of nutrition supplements or health products is also a problem in Canada. Many fitness facilities hire people with no knowledge of medicine or health to sell, on commission, products such as nutrition supplements.

STRATEGIES FOR PREVENTION

Protecting Yourself against False Health Claims

- Arm yourself with up-to-date information about your condition or disease from reputable organizations, such as the Canadian Institute for Health Information (CIHI).
- Ask for a written explanation of what a treatment does and why it works, evidence supporting all claims (not just testimonials), and published reports of the studies that have been done, including specifics on numbers treated, doses, and side effects.
- Be skeptical of self-styled "holistic practitioners," treatments supported by crusading groups, and endorsements from self-proclaimed experts or authorities.
- Don't quickly part with your money. Be especially careful because provincial medical plans and employee insurance companies won't reimburse for unproven therapies.
- Don't discontinue your current treatment without your physician's approval. Many physicians encourage supportive therapies—such as relaxation exercises, meditation, or visualization—as a supplement to standard treatments.

COMPLEMENTARY AND ALTERNATIVE MEDICINE

The last decade has seen an increase in the use of a broad range of therapies sometimes called complementary, alternative, unconventional, or holistic. Alternative treatments are typically given outside the mainstream medical system. Many have not been corroborated by clinical trials.[42]

The medical research community uses the terms **complementary and alternative medicine** (CAM) or **complementary and alternative health care** (CAHC) to apply to all healthcare approaches, practices, and treatments not widely taught in medical schools and not generally used in hospitals. They include many healing philosophies, approaches, and therapies, including preventive techniques designed to delay or prevent serious health problems before they start and **holistic** methods that focus on the whole person and the physical, mental, emotional, and spiritual aspects of well-being (see Figure 13-3). Some examples are nutritional therapies, herbal and botanical therapies, physical therapies, body/energy or life-force therapies, mind–body practices, and complementary and alternative health systems such as traditional Chinese medicine, Ayurvedic medicine, First Nations healing traditions, naturopathic medicine, and environmental medicine.[43]

Fees for treatment vary from one health practice to another and from one province or territory to another. As a general rule, Canadians are expected to cover a large part of the cost of CAM services. In some provinces,

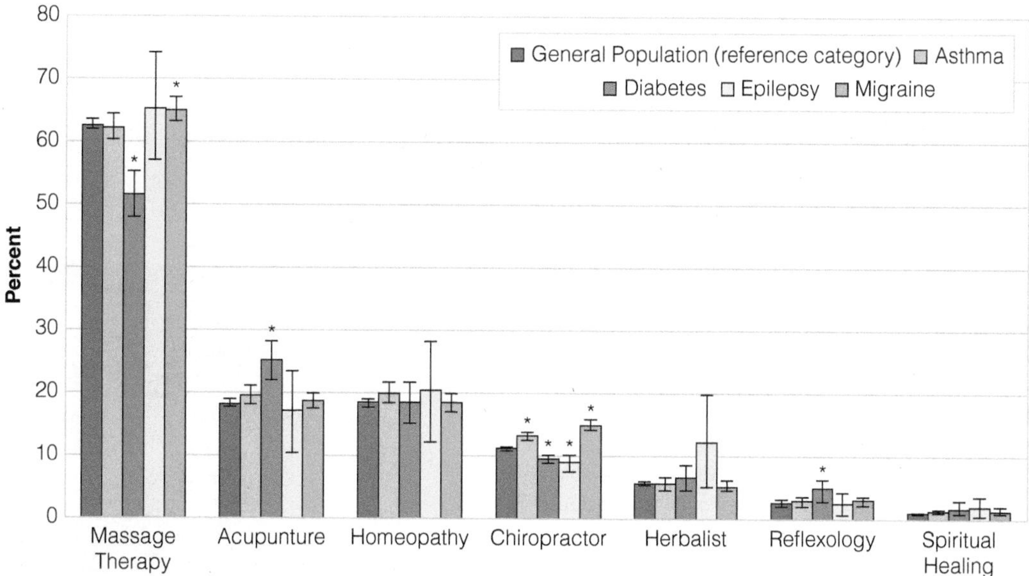

Figure 13-3 **Common Types of CAM Use**

Rates presented as a percentage of those who reported using any CAM services in the past two months.

*significantly different from the general population

Source: A. Metcalfe, J. Williams, J. McChesney, S.B. Patten, & N. Jetté, "Use of complementary and alternative medicine by those with a chronic disease and the general population—results of a national population based survey," *BMC Complementary and Alternative Medicine*, Vol. 10 (1), Pg. 58–63, 2010. Found at http://www.biomedcentral.com/1472-6882/10/58

depending on the service, individuals must pay the entire cost of the treatment.[44]

Why People Use Complementary and Alternative Therapies Many Canadians try complementary and alternative medicine for a variety of reasons. Most people who use CAM say that it fits with their values and beliefs about life and health. They may have concerns about side effects from conventional medical treatments and drug therapies, or they may have had a disappointing experience with mainstream medicine. They often believe that body, mind, and spirit are all involved in health.

Metcalfe et al. found that individuals with asthma and migraines tend to utilize alternative medicine therapies as do Canadians who have arthritis and back pain.[45] Massage therapy is the most common type of treatment used by people in Canada. Almost 63 percent of Canadians had seen a massage practitioner in the past 12 months. Acupuncture treatments were also popular at 18.3 percent followed by homeopathy treatments at 18.2 percent. Other treatments included chiropractic care, herbalists, reflexology, and spiritual healing. The team of researchers also discovered that the higher the level of education and income, the higher the possibility that a person would use alternative therapies. Women were also more likely than men to access complementary healthcare. Age made a difference too, with 25- to 44-year-olds using this type of health service the most.

Results from a survey of 33 557 U.S. adults revealed that the use of alternative medicine therapies was common. Multivitamins, vitamins, minerals, and herbal treatments were the top four choices. People who had two or more chronic health conditions used alternative medicine therapies more than those with one or no chronic condition.[46]

Littlewood and Vanable[47] found that complementary and alternative medicine is common among HIV-positive individuals and is used to prevent or alleviate HIV-related symptoms, reduce side effects of traditional treatments, and improve their quality of life.

Most Canadians who do try CAM do so as a complementary health practice. They rarely abandon all conventional healthcare. However, findings from Busse et al.'s research from a survey of patients accessing care from the Canadian College of Naturopathic Medicine showed that only 58.5 percent of Canadians who report using alternative healing methods and strategies discuss their use of alternative medicine with their family practitioners, whereas 90.9 percent discuss their traditional prescription medication with their naturopathic physician.[48]

Doctors and CAM **Integrative medicine**, which combines selected elements of both conventional and alternative medicine in a comprehensive approach to diagnosis and treatment, is gaining greater acceptance within the medical community.[49] More medical schools are teaching courses in CAM.[50] Canadian physicians who offer CAM services as part of their medical practice are expected to provide care that is within their scope of clinical training.[51]

Many doctors are calling upon their colleagues not to dismiss or embrace CAM but to consider each

HUMAN POTENTIAL

Julia Pritchard—A Young Woman's Dream of Medical School

Our Human Potential story for this chapter is about a young woman who grew up "wanting to be a doctor." Her story is one of commitment, tenacity, and belief in herself. It is also a story about a young woman who wants to make a difference.

Getting into medical school is not an easy task. In addition to excellent undergraduate marks, selection committees are looking for students who can take on leadership roles within our healthcare system. In Julia's story, we see how she put the pieces of the "application puzzle" together and gained one of the revered places at the University of British Columbia's medical school. Her story also highlights her belief that career choice is not made from one conscious decision, but a lifetime of experiences that shape the idea of how we hope our lives to be.

When asked about her teenage years, Julia talks about her life as an elite competitive gymnast. "Gymnastics taught me self-discipline and self-motivation from a young age," says Julia. In a sport that can be very demanding both physically and emotionally, Julia soon learned that success was measured by setting well-defined short- and long-term goals, time management, and organizational skills. Little did she know that she was developing essential skills that would be vital in her path toward medical school.

Participation in a Grade 10 Trek outdoor education program was another important experience for Julia. The focus on adventure, environmental education, and character development helped Julia grow from a shy, young woman to someone who took on leadership roles. As Julia reflects on her participation in this program she says, "It is clear that teamwork is essential in today's multidisciplinary nature of medicine, and as a graduate of the Trek program, I gained enough self-confidence to both lead groups and also be effective in group decision-making."

However, it was Julia's volunteer work at *Camp Goodtimes*, a summer camp for children with cancer, that helped her discover her true inspiration for medicine. "Until this point, I had the ambition to become a physician, but I couldn't pinpoint why I had made that career goal. Working so closely with these children and their families and experiencing their strength and courage, I was inspired." She also learned that you get back what you give.

Work as a volunteer support worker with the Victoria Women's Sexual Assault Centre, as a scientist at the B.C. Cancer Research Centre, and as a research assistant at the Healthy Heart Society of British Columbia have challenged Julia's scientific thinking, problem-solving, and troubleshooting skills. Julia believes that, as a physician, these skills are essential in providing a treatment plan that balances the need to cure disease with any physical, emotional, or cultural limitations of the patient. This work has also introduced Julia to the Aboriginal culture's holistic approach to healthcare and helped her gain a broader understanding of the World Health Organization's definition of health as "a state of complete physical, mental, and social well-being and not merely the absence of disease or infirmity."

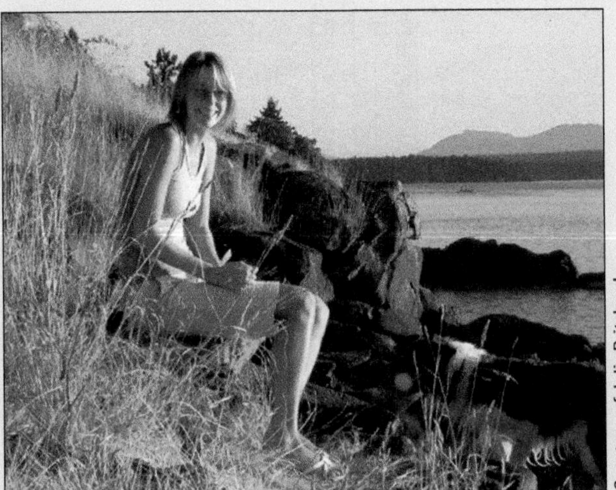

Courtesy of Julia Pritchard

Julia Pritchard enjoying a family getaway on Galiano Island with her dog Samson.

Taken together, all of these achievements and experiences have provided Julia with an excellent footprint on which to become a skilled and ethical physician. To quote from Julia's application to medical schools: "I believe I am prepared, through my academic progress; I am a participant, shown through my volunteerism and advocacy activities; and I am professional, shown by my work ethic and drive toward lifelong learning. I am ready to become a physician."

Julia has completed her medical training at the Vancouver Fraser Medical Program at UBC. Further training is now underway at the University of Calgary in the Faculty of Medicine. She knows that her early experiences helped her to get into medical school, but she also believes that they will assist her to become a self-motivated, lifelong learner who will emerge as a skilled, yet self-reflective, physician. Her next step is her residency program in internal medicine with a possible specialization in respirology. Her advice to other students who may be considering a career as a medical professional: "Set goals, work hard, ask for help when needed, and understand that we all have special gifts and skills to share with others. We can all make a difference in this world, and we can do this by trusting in our own abilities and reaching out with care and compassion."

approach thoroughly and evaluate its potential to benefit patients.[52] In a survey of physicians, most—60 percent more women than men—wanted to learn more about CAM. The most common reasons were "to dissuade patient if alternative method is unsafe and/or ineffective" and "to recommend method to patient if safe and effective." The physicians who felt "very positive" or "somewhat positive" about CAM therapies were more interested in education but no more comfortable in discussing CAM with patients.[53]

The World Health Organization is creating a Web-based classification system for "traditional" or complementary health medicine to bridge the divide between Western medicine and historical traditional medicine long practised in countries around the world. The WHO has also published the *WHO Traditional Medicine (TM)*

X AND Y FILES

Men and Women as Healthcare Consumers

The genders differ significantly in the way they use healthcare services. Women see more doctors than men, take more prescription drugs, are hospitalized more, and control the spending of three of every four healthcare dollars.

Many experts believe that the need for birth control and reproductive health services gets women into the habit of making regular visits to healthcare professionals, primarily gynecologists. There are no comparable specialists for men, who tend to visit urologists (specialists in male reproductive organs) only when they develop problems. Men also are conditioned to take a stoic, tough-it-out attitude to early symptoms of a disease.

Men feel they are not allowed to manifest illness unless it's overt, says family practitioner Martin Miner, who has conducted research on men and healthcare. One reason men die earlier than women is because of the length of time they wait to go for treatment.

Men and women also differ in the symptoms and syndromes they develop. For instance, men are more prone to back problems, muscle sprains and strains, allergies, insomnia, and digestive problems. Men develop heart disease about a decade earlier in life than women. More men develop ulcers and hernias; women are more likely to get gallbladder disease and irritable bowel syndrome. More women than men suffer from migraines. Yet women and men spend similar proportions of their lifetimes—about 81 percent—free of disability.

The genders also differ in access to health services. Women and men are about equally likely to use complementary and alternative medicine—but different types. Men outnumber women in use of chiropractic services and acupuncture, while women are more likely to try herbal medicine, mind-body remedies, folk remedies, movement and exercise techniques, and prayer or spiritual practices. Both genders turn to alternative treatments for the same reason: a desire for greater control over their health.

Strategy, 2014–2023 to advance the potential use of alternative healthcare traditions in safe and effective ways and to help countries regulate medicines and make them safer and more accessible to their populations.[54]

Fundamental to integrative care is the necessity of establishing links between traditional and complementary healthcare options and enhancing communication between patients, doctors, complementary healthcare providers, and government agencies that oversee healthcare in Canada. Consumers have been bridging this gap and appear to have been the driving force behind the current move toward integrative healthcare.[55]

Is Complementary and Alternative Medicine Safe and Effective? Safety and effectiveness have specific meanings in healthcare. Health practices are usually considered safe if the benefits outweigh the risks. By scientifically studying a practice under controlled conditions, researchers can determine whether a practice is harmful. Health practices are considered to be effective if they are helpful when used or experienced in a research study, under usual conditions.[56]

Scientifically studying the safety and effectiveness of complementary and alternative medicine is relatively new. Much of the information about CAM has been based upon opinion—anecdotal evidence and folklore, not controlled studies. The research that has been done has focused mostly on medicinal herbs, chiropractic, homeopathy, and acupuncture.[57] As studies are conducted, some alternative therapies are gaining acceptance, while others have shown little or no demonstrable benefits.[58] In 2004, IN-CAM Canada Research Network was launched to support a CAM research community. Members link with organizations and educational institutes to develop formal CAM research partnerships and initiatives. They also share their research in a biannual IN-CAM Research Symposium.[59]

Many people have criticized healthcare providers for giving alternative therapies a "free ride" by not demanding the same proof and regulation required of traditional treatments.[60] In Canada, training standards have been set by governing organizations for specific alternative health practices. Among these licensed therapies, training standards are not necessarily "standard." They do vary widely from province to province or territory. If you are interested in becoming a complementary and alternative health practitioner, it is important that you research the provincial or national agencies thoroughly to determine the qualifications and credentials of the instructors of the workshops and diploma or degree programs. For example, chiropractors must be registered or licensed, and the Council of Chiropractic Education of Canada supervises chiropractic education in Canada.

Homeopathic physicians are not regulated in Canada, except in Ontario, although members of the Canadian College of Homeopathic Medicine have been advocating for regulation and a coordinated education system since 1991.[61] Massage therapists are regulated in only four provinces in Canada: British Columbia, with the most stringent education standards in North America, requiring individuals to have three years of training prior to practising; Ontario; Newfoundland and Labrador, and New Brunswick.[62] In 2015, the government of Manitoba approved regulation of massage therapists, but it will take some time to establish a college and educational standards in this province.[63] Acupuncturists are regulated in British Columbia, Alberta, Ontario, Newfoundland, and Quebec.[64]. There is no uniform regulation system for alternative medicine in Canada.[65]

If you decide to seek complementary and alternative medicine, ask yourself the following questions:

- Is it safe? The fact that a treatment does not require hospitalization or surgery does not guarantee it is safe.

- Is it effective? Research the type of therapy you are considering. Know the risks.
- Is the practitioner qualified? Find out what licences are necessary for the practitioner to practise. What is his or her educational background?
- What has been the experience of other people who have been cared for by the practitioner you are considering?
- What are the costs? Many CAM services are not covered fully by provincial medical plans. Find out if your extended health benefits cover any of the charges.

✓ CHECK-IN

Have you used complementary healthcare approaches to support your health and wellness? If so, what type of approaches?

Natural Health Products In response to growing concerns about the regulatory environment for Natural Health Products (NHPs), a term used to describe a variety of products such as herbal medicines, homeopathic remedies, and nutritional supplements, Health Canada developed a regulatory framework that came into effect January 1, 2004. The Natural Health Products Directorate (NHPD) now oversees regulations for all NHPs sold in Canada.[66]

All NHPs sold in Canada now require pre-market assessment and authorization of their safety and effectiveness. A listing of each product's medicinal and non-medicinal ingredients must also appear on product labels. However, it is worth noting that NHPs do not have to have a nutrient facts box, so they may a high calorie count of sugar. In some cases overall caloric content is not known either. An example would be vitamin water. Although the regulations for these products are not embraced fully by all alternative healthcare practitioners and NHP manufacturers, it is hoped that they will allow for industry innovation in bringing new products to the market while ensuring that Canadians have access to NHPs that are safe, effective, and of high quality.[67]

Complementary and Alternative Medicine—Programs and Services

Aboriginal Healing Many Aboriginal healthcare providers experience and understand the gaps in the current healthcare system for Aboriginal peoples. These gaps include access and appropriateness of services. Aboriginal healing is a way of integrating health services available through our Canadian health system and using a uniquely Aboriginal perspective that incorporates the four aspects of health—spiritual, emotional, intellectual, and physical.[68] Healing circles, sweat lodges, traditional medicine, and the use of medicine wheels and healing ceremonies are some of the approaches that are being used to support the health and wellness of Aboriginal peoples.

Acupuncture An ancient Chinese form of medicine, **acupuncture** is based on the philosophy that a cycle of energy circulating through the body controls health. Pain and disease are the result of a disturbance in the energy flow, which can be corrected by inserting long, thin needles at specific points along longitudinal lines, or *meridians*, throughout the body. Each point controls a different corresponding part of the body. Once inserted, the needles are rotated gently back and forth or charged with a small electric current for a short time. Western scientists aren't sure exactly how acupuncture works, but some believe that the needles alter the functioning of the nervous system.

There are two main approaches to training in Canada within this field. Acupuncture training can be part of a degree in Traditional Chinese Medicine (TCM) or taught as a stand-alone practice. Medical acupuncture

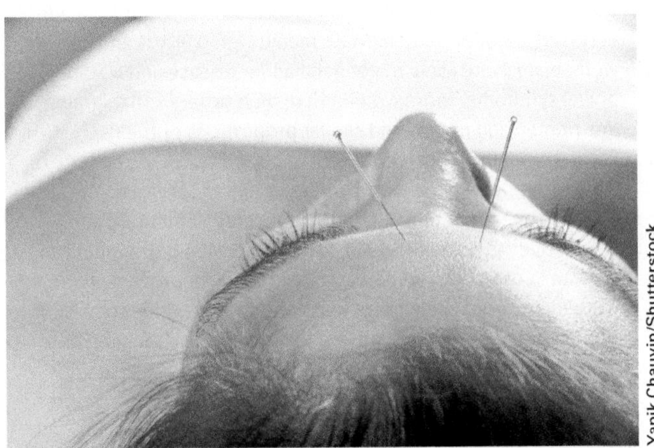

Yanik Chauvin/Shutterstock

The ancient Chinese practice of acupuncture produces healing through the insertion and manipulation of needles at specific points throughout the body.

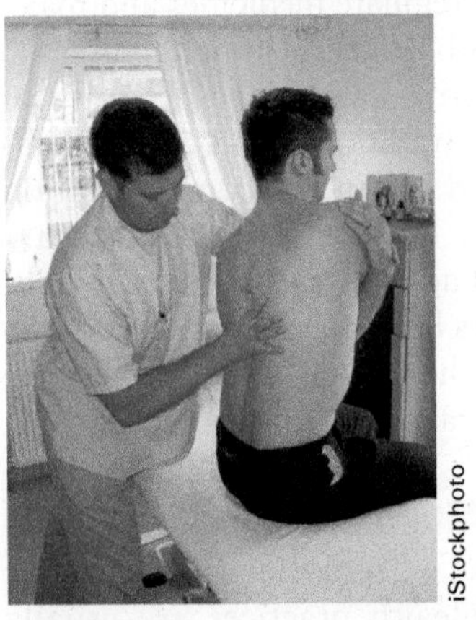

iStockphoto

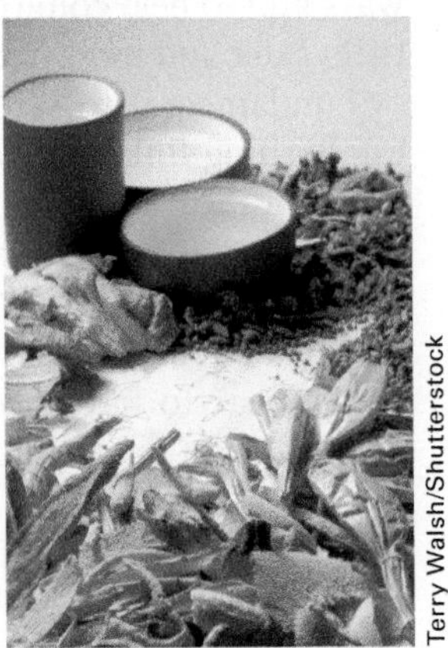

Terry Walsh/Shutterstock

A chiropractor can help relieve shoulder and back pain; herbal medicines are a popular form of alternative medicine.

training is geared toward licensed health professionals, such as doctors, physiotherapists, dentists, naturopaths, and chiropractors.[69]

An NIH consensus development panel that evaluated current research into acupuncture concluded that there is "clear evidence" that acupuncture can control nausea and vomiting in patients after surgery or while undergoing chemotherapy and relieve post-operative dental pain.[70] Ongoing studies are evaluating the efficacy of acupuncture for chronic headaches and migraines.

In *acupressure*, the therapist uses his or her finger and thumb to stimulate certain points, relieve pain, and relax muscles. **Reflexology** is based on the theory that massaging certain points on the foot or hand relieves stress or pain in corresponding parts of the body. These methods seem most effective in easing chronic pain, arthritis, and withdrawal from nicotine, alcohol, or drugs.[71]

Ayurveda **Ayurveda** is a traditional form of medical treatment in India, where it has evolved over thousands of years. Its basic premise is that illness stems from incorrect mental attitudes, diet, and posture. Practitioners use a discipline of exercise, meditation, herbal medication, and proper nutrition. In India, students enter Bachelors of Ayurvedic Medicine and Surgery programs after high-school graduation. In Canada, portions of this program of study are taught in general-interest courses and programs for health professionals through the International Institute of Ayurveda and Complementary Medicines.[72]

Biofeedback **Biofeedback** uses machines that measure temperature or skin responses and then relay this information to the subject. People can learn to control involuntary functions, such as circulation to the hands and feet, tension in the jaws, and heart rates. Biofeedback has been used to treat dozens of ailments, including asthma, epilepsy, pain, and Reynaud's disease (a condition in which the fingers become painful and white when exposed to cold). Some extended health-benefit plans now cover biofeedback treatments. Training in biofeedback therapeutic services in Canada is offered through the College of International Holistic Studies (CIHS), a registered educational institution with the federal government.[73]

Chiropractic **Chiropractic** is a treatment method based on the theory that many human diseases are caused by misalignment of the bones (subluxation). Each provincial chiropractic regulatory body has the authority to grant a licence to practise chiropractic. Registered or licensed chiropractors, or D.C.s (Doctors of Chiropractic), must complete a four- to five-year course of full-time study.[74] Research in the last 10 years has demonstrated its efficacy for acute lower-back pain. Research is also being conducted on other potential benefits, including headaches and arthritis, but findings are inconclusive at this time. Some medical professionals do not recommend using chiropractic for any condition not clearly related to disorders of the back or neck.

Herbs, Botanical Medicines, and Dietary Supplements Herbs, **botanical medicines**, and dietary supplements are the most popular form of complementary and alternative medicine in North America. Natural healthcare products are used to treat both internal and external conditions. They can be taken by mouth or applied to the body. They are sold in many different forms—raw herbs and teas, salves and creams, liquid extracts, and tablets or capsules.

Natural healthcare products are not necessarily safe just because they are from natural sources. Some may cause side effects or allergic reactions. Others may be harmful to people with certain health conditions, such as pregnancy or heart disease. They may also interact with other medications, even non-prescription drugs such as aspirin (see Table 13-1). It is important to tell your doctor about any natural health products you are taking—especially when he or she may be prescribing medications.

An example of a potentially harmful natural medication is St. John's wort, which affects the action of drugs such as the anti-clotting agent warfarin (Coumadin). When taken with dextromethorphan, an ingredient in cough syrup, St. John's wort can cause serotonin syndrome, a potentially fatal condition characterized by rapid pulse, high fever, and convulsions. Another example is the amphetamine-like herb called ***ephedra****, or Ma huang, sold as an energy booster and weight-loss aid. It can cause dangerous rises in blood pressure and speed up the heart rate. More than 800 injuries and 17 deaths have been linked to this herb.*[75]

Homeopathy **Homeopathy** is based on three fundamental principles: "like cures like," treatment must always be individualized and holistic, and less is more—the idea that increasing dilution (and lowering the dosage) can increase efficacy.[76] Doses of animal, vegetable, or mineral substances are administered as serially diluted solutions. The more diluted the solution, the stronger it is thought to be—the opposite of the way we usually think about the strength of pharmaceutical drugs. Homeopathic remedies may be given directly as drops, or the diluted solution may be sprayed onto granules or powder. Remedies taken in solid forms are held in the mouth until they dissolve—they are not to be swallowed.

Kinesiology **Kinesiology** can be described as the study of the human body in motion. Individuals working in

TABLE 13-1

Some Popular Herbal Remedies

Herb	Used For	Does It Work?	Warning
Acidophilus	Diarrhea, digestive problems, upset stomach, or yeast infections caused by use of antibiotics	Acidophilus, either in live lactobacillus acidophilus cultures in yogurt or in capsules, can restore the body's normal bacterial balance.	Refrigerate to preserve potency.
Aloe vera	Sunburn, cuts, burns, eczema, psoriasis	In studies on both humans and animals, aloe vera applied directly to the skin has been shown to speed healing and have antibacterial, anti-inflammatory, and mild anesthetic effects.	Refrigerate gel to extend its shelf life.
Chamomile	Relaxation, better sleep, stomach aches, menstrual cramps	Laboratory and animal studies indicate that chamomile's active compounds have properties that combat inflammation, bacterial infection, and spasms.	People allergic to plants in the daisy family, such as ragweed, may have an allergic reaction.
Echinacea	Colds and flu	Inconsistent findings, although some studies found that flu sufferers who used Echinacea extract recovered more quickly than others.	Use for more than eight weeks at a time may lessen its effectiveness and suppress immunity. Should not be taken by pregnant women and those with diabetes, tuberculosis, or autoimmune disorders.
Garlic	Fighting infection, preventing heart disease and cancer, stimulating the immune system	Extensive laboratory and animal studies and a review of clinical trials have shown that the active ingredient in garlic has anti-infective and anti-tumour properties and lowers cholesterol.	Check with your doctor if you take blood-thinning medication, including aspirin or ibuprofen, because garlic also is an anticoagulant.
Ginkgo biloba	Improving memory, cognition, and circulation	There is some evidence that ginkgo biloba can help stabilize mental deterioration in patients with early Alzheimer's disease or stroke-related dementia. One study found that healthy seniors who took ginkgo performed mental tasks better.	Do not take with aspirin because of the risk of excessive bleeding. Should not be used during pregnancy. Side effects include upset stomach, headache, and an allergic skin reaction.
Ginseng	Improving mental and physical energy and stamina	Small studies have shown that ginseng can help improve mental performance and respiratory function during exercise.	If used for more than two weeks, ginseng can cause nervousness and heart palpitations, especially in those with high blood pressure.
Goldenseal	Colds, allergies, upper respiratory tract infections	Little research has been done, but some laboratory and animal studies suggest that one of goldenseal's components may have some antibiotic and antihistamine effects.	Goldenseal should not be used instead of traditional antibiotics or for more than ten days at a time. Long-term use may interfere with the normal bacterial balance in the digestive system.
St. John's wort	Anxiety and depression	Older studies showing benefits had serious flaws. Recent, more rigorous research has shown that St. John's wort is not effective against major depression.	Side effects include stomach pain, bloating, constipation, nausea, fatigue, dry mouth. St. John's wort should never be taken in combination with prescription antidepressants.

this field are called kinesiologists. They provide exercise therapy, injury assessment and rehabilitation, ergonomics and workplace design, health and fitness courses and workshops, and gait analysis services using biomedical technology.

In many countries kinesiology is not yet considered a "profession," but since 2013, in Canada, kinesiologists in Alberta, British Columbia, New Brunswick, Newfoundland and Labrador, Ontario, and Quebec have had provincial kinesiology associations and can apply for a professional designation of Registered Kinesiologist or RKin. The Canadian Kinesiology Alliance[77] is working with provincial organizations to promote the professional designation of kinesiologists in all provinces. Undergraduate degrees in kinesiology are available at colleges and universities across the country. There are also many online courses available too.

Massage Therapy **Massage therapy** is a general term for a number of techniques that involve manipulation of the muscles and connective tissues. Massage is used to relieve muscle tension and stress, improve flexibility, and enhance a patient's sense of well-being. Different types of massage vary with approaches that range from the very light touches used in lymphatic drainage massage to deep tissue manipulation. Examples are Swedish massage, Ayurvedic massage, Thai massage, and Shiatsu massage.

Provincial governing bodies called "colleges" set training requirements for the profession in British Columbia, Ontario, Newfoundland and Labrador, and New Brunswick. In the other provinces and territories, massage therapy is overseen by professional associations. Members of the Canadian Massage Therapists Alliance (CMTA) are urging provincial and territorial governments to regulate the profession of massage therapy.[78]

Naturopathy **Naturopathy** or naturopathic medicine is a comprehensive, holistic health system that incorporates therapies from traditional Chinese medicine, Ayurveda, homeopathy, and Western herbalism, as well as nutritional approaches, body therapies, and other healing practices. This system also emphasizes natural remedies, such as sun, water, heat, and air, as treatments for disease. Naturopathic doctors take health histories and perform physical examinations using standard diagnostic instruments and laboratory tests. Lifestyle information is also an important part of the naturopathic practice.[79] A recent study done in Ontario exploring the experiences and perceptions of providing and receiving naturopathic care within an Aboriginal community found that the services provided at the naturopathic clinic contributed in a positive way and helped to address unmet health needs in this population. Naturopathic medicine was seen to link to Aboriginal care needs, in part, because of the traditional knowledge approaches to the body, mind, and spirit connection.[80]

Naturopathic medicine is regulated in British Columbia, Alberta, Saskatchewan, Manitoba, and Ontario. Other provinces and the territories are working toward regulation.[81] Education requirements include three years of undergraduate-level academic university courses and four years of full-time education at an accredited naturopathic training institution. Education is then followed up by provincial and national licensing examinations.[82]

Physiotherapy **Physiotherapy** is sometimes considered a complementary or alternative healthcare profession. Due to its popularity in Canada, it is now seen by some medical professionals as part of the primary healthcare system. Physiotherapists, also known as physical therapists, are educated and trained to assess, restore, and maintain physical function. They can assess the strength and endurance of muscles. They can also assess the impact of an injury or a physical disability on physical function. They provide treatment with modalities such as ultrasound and assist in program planning and exercise rehabilitation to restore movement and reduce pain.[83]

The minimum entry-level educational qualification for a physiotherapist is a master's degree from one of the 14 accredited universities offering physical therapy education programs. To practise, physiotherapists must register with the College of Physiotherapists in their home province or territory. Registered physiotherapists can use the professional designation of PT or PHT.[84] Some physiotherapists take advanced training in specific areas such as orthopedics and sports physiotherapy.

Other alternative therapies include Alexander technique, aromatherapy, reiki, therapeutic touch, and visualization.

SELF-SURVEY

Are You a Savvy Healthcare Consumer?

Circle the answer that best describes how you would act or react in the following situation. Then compare your answers to the suggested answers below.

1. You want a second opinion, but your doctor dismisses your request for other physicians' names as unnecessary. What do you do?
   a. Assume that he or she is right and you would merely be wasting time.
   b. Suspect that your physician has something to hide and immediately switch doctors.
   c. Contact your health-plan administrator and request a second opinion.
2. As soon as you enter your doctor's office, you get tongue-tied. When you try to find the words to describe what's wrong, your physician keeps interrupting. When giving advice, your doctor uses such technical language that you can't understand what it means. What do you do?
   a. Prepare better for your next appointment.
   b. Pretend that you understand what your doctor is talking about.
   c. Decide you'd be better off with someone who specializes in complementary/alternative therapies and seems less intimidating.
3. You feel like you're running on empty, tired all the time, worn to the bone. A friend suggests some herbal supplements that promise to boost energy and restore vitality. What do you do?
   a. Immediately start taking them.
   b. Say that you think herbs are for cooking.
   c. Find out as much as you can about the herbal compounds and ask your doctor if they're safe and effective.
4. Your hometown physician's office won't give you a copy of your medical records to take with you to college or university. What do you do?
   a. Hope you won't need them and head off without your records.
   b. Threaten to sue.
   c. Politely ask the office administrator to tell you the particular law or statute that bars you from your records.
5. Your doctor has been treating you for an infection for three weeks, and you don't seem to be getting any better. What do you do?
   a. Talk to your doctor, by phone or in person, and say, "This doesn't seem to be working. Is there anything else we can try?"
   b. Stop taking the antibiotic.
   c. Try a herbal remedy that your roommate recommends.
6. Your doctor suggests a cutting-edge treatment for your condition, but your health plan refuses to pay for it. What do you do?
   a. Try to get a loan to cover the costs.
   b. Settle for whatever treatment options are covered.
   c. Challenge your health plan.
7. You call for an appointment with your doctor and are told nothing is available for four months. What do you do?
   a. Take whatever time you can get whenever you can get it.
   b. Explain your condition to the nurse or receptionist, detailing any symptoms and pain you're experiencing.
   c. Give up and decide you don't need to see a doctor at all.
8. Even though you've been doing sit-ups faithfully, your waist still looks flabby. When you see an ad for waist-whittling liposuction, what do you do?
   a. Call for an appointment.
   b. Talk to a healthcare professional about a total fitness program that may help you lose excess pounds.
   c. Carefully research the risks and costs of the procedure.
9. You have a condition that you do not want anyone to know about, including your health insurer and any potential employer. What do you do?
   a. Use a false name.
   b. Give your physician a written request for confidentiality about this condition.
   c. Seek help outside the healthcare system.
10. Your doctor suggests a biopsy of a funny-looking mole that's sprouted on your nose. What would you do?
   a. Follow up with your doctor's request to have the mole biopsy.
   b. Tell your doctor that you will keep an eye on the mole and get back to him/her if you notice any changes.
   c. Hope that if you don't do anything the mole might go away.
   d. Check in with your friends to see what they suggest you do.

Answers to Self-Survey

1. c; 2. a; 3. c; 4. c; 5. a; 6. c; 7. b; 8. b and c; 9. b; 10. a

Chapter Summary

1. Which of the following statements is false?
   a. Home health tests are available for pregnancy.
   b. Vital signs include temperature, blood pressure, pulse, and cholesterol level.
   c. Health expenditures in Canada are expected to continue to rise in the next five years.
   d. Most students do not have access to health information from their college or university.

2. Which statement about health information on the Internet is true?
   a. Chat rooms are the most reliable source of accurate medical information.
   b. The Canadian Medical Protective Association (CMPA) has warned their members not to prescribe or co-sign prescriptions for Americans seeking prescription drugs via the Internet.
   c. All sponsored Internet sites are reliable sources of accurate healthcare information.
   d. The Internet is a safe and cost-effective source of prescription drugs.

3. Which of the following is NOT a right held by patients?
   a. to access their medical records
   b. to medical care that meets accepted standards of quality
   c. to donate a body part for compensation
   d. to get a second opinion from another health professional

4. What does informed consent mean?
   a. The patient has informed the doctor of his or her symptoms and has consented to treatment.
   b. The physician has informed the patient about the treatment to be given and has consented to administer the treatment.
   c. The patient has informed the doctor of his or her symptoms, and the doctor has consented to administer treatment.
   d. The physician has informed the patient about the treatment to be given, and the patient has consented to the treatment.

5. Why do people use complementary and alternative therapies?
   a. to spend less money on healthcare
   b. to take an active role in their own treatment
   c. to show their disdain for the medical establishment
   d. to take more prescription drugs

6. Which of the following is NOT an example of a complementary and alternative therapy?
   a. psychiatry
   b. acupuncture
   c. chiropractic
   d. homeopathy

7. Which herbal remedy appears to have positive health effects?
   a. Ayurveda for controlling asthma
   b. acidophilus for improving memory
   c. aloe vera for diabetes
   d. garlic for preventing infection and tumour growth

8. Which statement about complementary and alternative therapies is false?
   a. Acupuncture has been shown to control nausea in patients after surgery.
   b. Reflexologists massage points on the foot or hand to relieve stress or pain in corresponding parts of the body.
   c. People can learn to control involuntary functions through biofeedback.
   d. Naturopathy is based on the premise that "like cures like."

9. Which statement regarding healthcare in Canada is true?
   a. Medicare was designed after a private-care system.
   b. Provincial residency is not a requirement for medicare.
   c. Canadians have reasonable access to medically necessary hospital and physician services on a prepaid basis.
   d. Canadians have a fee-for-service medical system.

10. Which service is NOT provided by physiotherapists?
    a. assessing muscular strength
    b. prescribing medication
    c. assisting in exercise rehabilitation
    d. assessing the physical limitations of an injury

Answers to these questions can be found on page 373.

SELF-RESPONSIBILITY—SOCIAL RESPONSIBILITY

SELF-RESPONSIBILITY

The first wealth is health.

Ralph Waldo Emerson

Sometimes the pressures of studying and working prevent students from assessing their health and accessing healthcare. Have you been ignoring some signs and symptoms of health-related issues? If so, how can you move from contemplation to preparation to action? Taking responsibility for our own health is an important step toward living life to its fullest.

SOCIAL RESPONSIBILITY

The patient should be made to understand that he or she must take charge of his [or her] own life. Don't take your body to the doctor as if he [or she] were a repair shop.

Quentin Regestein

Taking care of yourself allows you to then take care of others when they need it. Try to think of self-care as a path to personal potential.

CRITICAL THINKING

1. Have you used any complementary or alternative approaches to healthcare? If so, were you satisfied with the results? How did your experience with the CAM practitioner compare with your most recent experience with a traditional medical practitioner?
2. Jocelyn has been experiencing a great deal of fatigue and frequent headaches for the past couple of months. She doesn't have a family doctor and doesn't want to spend the time trying to find one. So she did some research on the Internet about ways to relieve her symptoms and was considering taking a couple of herbal supplements that were touted as potential treatments. If she asked you for your advice, what would you tell her? Do you think self-care is appropriate in this situation?

WEB LINKS

Aboriginal Healing Foundation

www.ahf.ca

The site has articles, educational material, stories, and links to other agencies and organizations that promote awareness of healing issues.

Canadian Institute for Health Information (CIHI)

www.cihi.ca

This site offers current health research, quick statistics, client services, information about health standards, and an annual report titled *Health Care in Canada.*

Canadian Public Health Association—Health Literacy Resources

http://www.cpha.ca/en/programs/portals/h-l/resources.aspx

This site offers many health literacy resources including reports and research articles. There are also Web links to international resources.

IN-CAM Canada Research Network

www.incamresearch.ca/

Access this site for current CAM information and resources including links to academic complementary and alternative medicine research journals.

Please note that links are subject to change. If you find a broken link, use a search engine such as www.google.ca and search for the website by typing in keywords.

Key Terms

The terms listed here are used within the chapter on the page indicated. Definitions of the terms are in the Glossary at the end of this book.

activity-based funding 358
acupuncture 366
Ayurveda 367
biofeedback 367
botanical medicines 367
bundled payments 358
chiropractic 367
complementary and alternative health care (CAHC) 362
complementary and alternative medicine (CAM) 362
ephedra 367
health literacy 359
holistic 362
homeopathy 367
informed consent 359
integrative medicine 363
kinesiology 367
massage therapy 369
naturopathy 369
physiotherapy 369
quackery 362
reflexology 367
vital signs 360

Answers to Chapter Summary Questions

1. b; 2. b; 3. c; 4. d; 5. b; 6. a; 7. d; 8. d; 9. c; 10. b

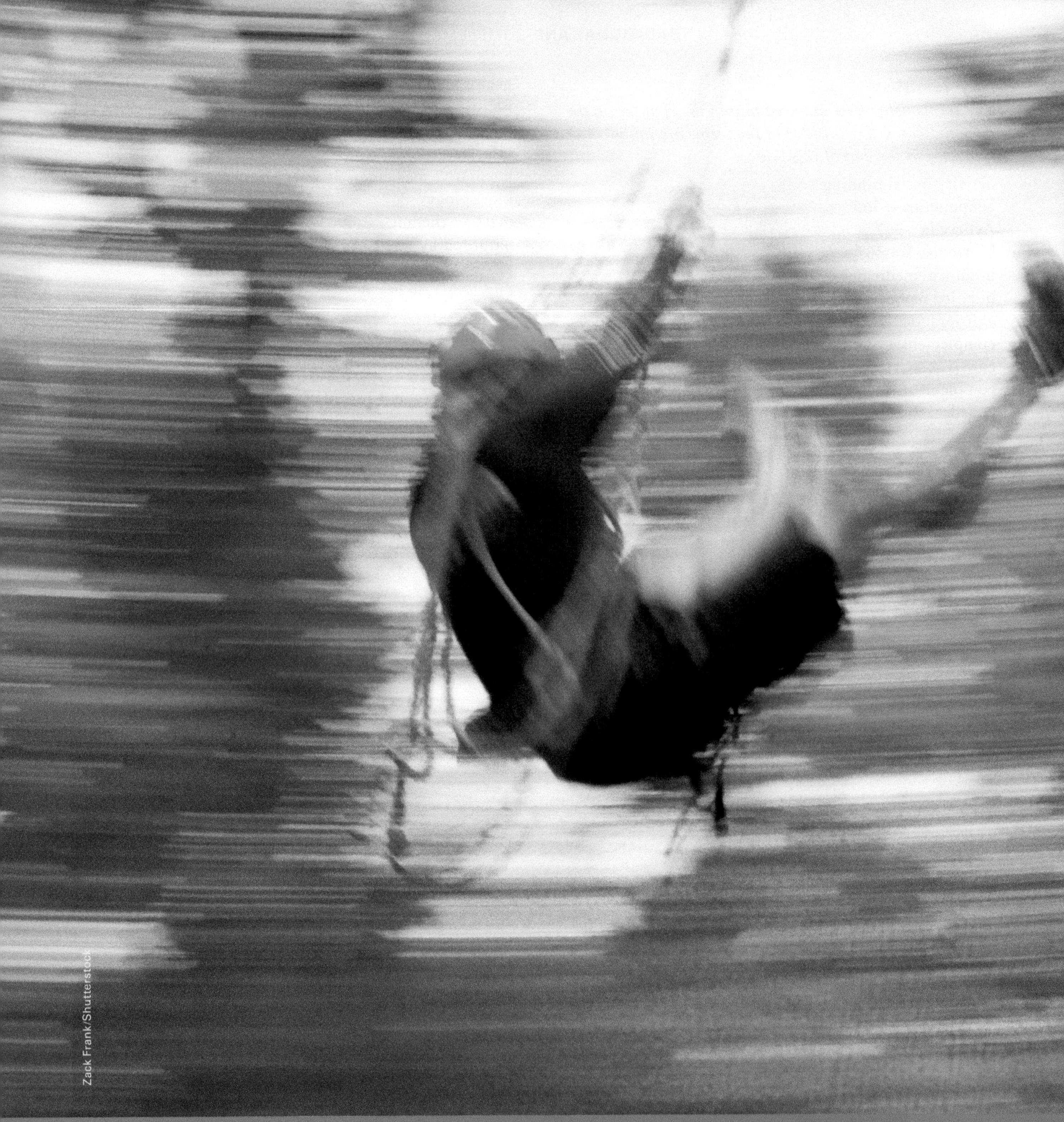
Zack Frank/Shutterstock

AFTER READING THIS CHAPTER, YOU WILL BE ABLE TO:

- **describe** ways you can prevent injury while at home
- **list** the three basic factors that support a safe work environment
- **discuss** reasons why legislation has been put in place to ban the use of cellphones while driving
- **describe** safety procedures for outdoor recreational and sport activities
- **define** sexual victimization, sexual harassment, and sexual coercion
- **describe** recommended actions for preventing rape

14

Staying Safe: Preventing Injury, Violence, and Victimization

Accidents, injuries, assaults, and crimes may seem like things that happen only to other people. But no one is immune from danger. Recognizing the threat of unintentional and intentional injury is the first step to ensuring your personal safety. You may think that the risk of something bad happening is simply a matter of chance, of being in the wrong place at the wrong time. That's not always the case. Common injuries include falls, traffic accidents, sports mishaps, and physical and sexual assaults.[1] Behaviours such as using alcohol or drugs and not buckling your seat belt also increase the risk of harm. Ultimately, you have more control over your safety than anyone or anything else in your life.

Being prepared for natural disasters such as earthquakes, floods, severe storms, and fires is also an important part of personal and community safety. Emergency services may not be readily available and it is important for all of us to be able to take care of ourselves for at least 72 hours.

This chapter is a primer in self-protection. Included are recommendations for safety at home, on campus, and at your workplace. Common-sense safety on the road is discussed. As well, information about safe participation in recreation and sport activities is presented. This chapter also explores other serious threats to personal safety in our society, such as sexual victimization and violence on college and university campuses. Living life to the fullest means taking some risks; however, we can all take steps to stay safe and prevent injuries.

FREQUENTLY ASKED QUESTIONS

FAQ: What is sexual harassment? p. 392

FAQ: How can I prevent date rape? p. 394

PERSONAL SAFETY

The concept of personal safety is a complex one. It can be defined as a freedom from fear or worry of physical and psychological harm. It has also been described as an awareness of situations, conditions, or events that are harmful or dangerous to one's well-being.[2] Men and women often view personal safety in different ways. Cultural backgrounds and personality traits also have a bearing on how we take care of ourselves. Personal safety demands[3]

- an awareness of your environment,
- an awareness of yourself,
- healthy lifestyle choices,
- the ability to assess danger,
- vigilance,
- avoidance, and
- knowing how to defend yourself.

Personal injury is the leading cause of death of children and young adults. It is also one of the major causes of short- and long-term harm and disability for Canadians of all ages. According to the 2013–2014 *Canadian Community Health Survey*, 15.8 percent of Canadians aged 12 and older experienced an injury that was serious enough to affect day-to-day routines.[4] Males were more likely to suffer an injury at 17.4 percent compared to females at 14.3 percent. Sprains were the most-reported injury with 51.5 percent of Canadians disclosing this information. Fractures and broken bones were the second-most-reported injury at 15.5 percent. The leading cause of injuries was involvement in sports at 33.5 percent. Unpaid work was the second-leading cause of injuries at 15.0 percent, followed by injuries sustained at a job or a business at 13.3 percent. (See Table 14-1 for information about types and causes of injury.)

TABLE 14-1

Most Serious Injury in the Past 12 Months, by Type and Cause of Injury, Household Population Aged 12 and Older, Canada, 2013/2014.

Most Serious Injury in the Previous 12 Months	
Type of Injury	**%**
Multiple serious injuries	1.3
Broken or fractured bones	15.5
Burn, scald, chemical burn	3.2
Dislocation	2.6
Sprain or strain	51.5
Cut, puncture, animal or human bite	9.6
Scrapes(s), bruise(s), blisters(s)	6.2
Concussion or other brain injury	3.2
Other[1]	6.9
Cause of Injury	
Sports or physical exercise	33.5
Leisure or hobby	6.7
Working at a job or business	13.3
Unpaid work[2]	15.0
Sleeping, eating, or personal care	3.4
Going up and down stairs	4.4
Driver or passenger in/on a motor vehicle[3]	5.0
Walking	12.5
Other	6.1

Note(s): Figures by cause of injury do not add up to 100% as a result of rounding.

[1]Includes poisoning, injuries to internal organs, and other.
[2]Includes household chores, outdoor yard maintenances, home renovations, or other unpaid work.
[3]Includes road and off-road motor vehicles.

Sources: Canadian Community Health Survey, 2013/2014 (Record no. 3226). Statistics Canada. (2015, June 24). Canadian community health survey: Combined data, 2013/2014, The Daily. Table 5. http://www.statcan.gc.ca/daily-quotidien/150624/dq150624b-eng.htm

SAFETY AT HOME

Injuries can and do occur in the home. Falls, the most common cause of injury, frequently happen within the home or yard. Approximately 50 percent of injuries among young people result from a fall. For older adults the proportion is even higher.[5] Falls are the leading cause of injury among seniors. They also result in hospitalization with 84 828 older adults in Canada in 2013 needing to be hospitalized from falls.[6]

Falls result from slips, where there is not enough traction between footgear and the walking surface. Common causes are wet or oily surfaces, loose carpets or rugs, and slippery or uneven walkways. Trips happen when feet strike or hit an object, causing a loss of balance. Common causes of tripping include poor lighting, clutter on the floor, broken stairs, or uneven steps and thresholds.

Poison also poses a great threat. The third most frequent type of injury that leads to hospitalization in Canada is poisoning. Studies show that medications are the most common substance in all poisonings.

Adults may be poisoned by mistakenly taking someone else's prescription drugs or taking medicines in the dark and swallowing the wrong one. Prescription medication poisoning is a major concern among older adults.[7] Children are also at risk. Those who are under six years of age make up half of all poison exposures. Nine hundred young people, 14 years and younger, are hospitalized each year from unintentional poisoning.[8] An iPhone

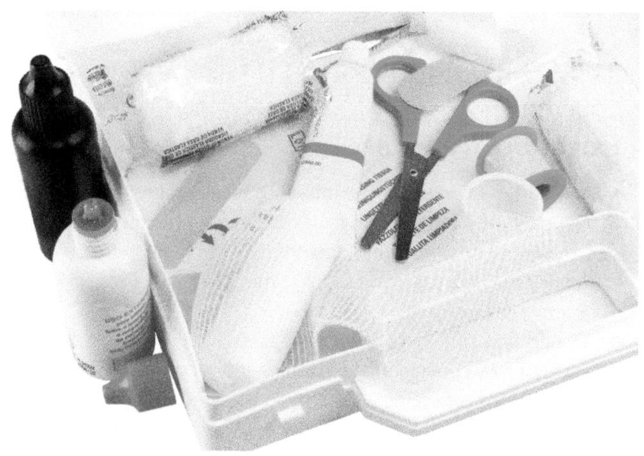
Thinkstock

Your home first-aid kit should include (at minimum) bandages, sterile gauze pads, adhesive tape, scissors, cotton, antibiotic ointment, a needle, safety pins, calamine lotion, syrup of ipecac to induce vomiting, and a thermometer.

application called MyMedRec is now available and can assist people in keeping track of necessary medications.[9]

If you have medications in your home or dorm room, make sure that they are all kept in their original containers and locked in a cabinet—out of reach of children or others who might be at risk should they take your medication. If you suspect that someone has been poisoned, call 911 and your local Poison Control Centre immediately.

Fires can cause many home injuries and result from three ingredients—fuel, a heat source, and oxygen. Paper, wood, flammable liquids such as oils, gasoline, some paints, and burning cigarettes are often the cause of fires—even in resident housing at colleges and universities. If a fire does start, you might have only two to five minutes to get out of a building alive. Whether you live in a house, an apartment, or in residence, a fire-escape plan can save time and lives. If a fire breaks out, get out as quickly as possible, but don't run. If you're on an upper floor and your escape routes are blocked, open a window (top and bottom, if possible) and wait or signal from the window for help. Never try to use an elevator in a fire. Make sure everyone is familiar with escape routes. Designate an area outside where all dorm residents, roommates, or family members should meet after escaping from a fire.

Think about purchasing an emergency first-aid kit to have in your dorm room, apartment, or house. According to the Canadian Red Cross, a first-aid kit should be readily available and stored in a dry place, and outdated contents or items should be replaced when needed.[10] First-aid kit items include

- emergency telephone numbers for EMS/911, local poison control centre, and your personal healthcare providers;
- sterile gauze pads, in small and large squares, and bandages to hold dressings in place;
- adhesive tape and adhesive bandages in assorted sizes;
- scissors, tweezers, and safety pins;
- instant ice packs;
- antiseptic wipes;
- disposable non-latex gloves, pocket mask, and face shield;
- flashlight, with extra batteries or a windup no-battery-needed flashlight; and
- emergency blanket.

For additional emergency supply kits, consider investing in extra bottled water (four litres of water per person per day—replace every six months), candles and matches or a lighter, additional flashlight and batteries, and packaged or canned food and a can opener; also have readily available personal supplies such as walking shoes, change of clothing, blankets or sleeping bags, toilet paper, extra pair of glasses, and contact information for family, friends, and medical personnel.[11] Check out your campus security division to find out more about emergency preparedness or contact your provincial or territorial emergency management organization.

SAFETY ON CAMPUS

Safety issues on campuses across Canada and the United States have become an important topic of discussion and have consequences for the health and wellness of all campus members. Administration and health and safety units have addressed safety problems by offering workshops, developing brochures and information packages, and posting ongoing Web bulletins and information to assist college and university campus communities to become more aware of ways they can prepare for emergencies and prevent unintentional and intentional injuries. Common concerns are dorm and vehicle break-ins, poor lighting, lack of proper signage and emergency telephones, fire safety issues, bullying threats, sexual violence, and food safety.[12] More information about crime on campus is presented later in this chapter.

Some effective strategies that have been put in place to build safer campus environments include Safewalk programs and campus escort services, campus security patrols, emergency planning programs such as earthquake preparedness, and law enforcement practices that help to lower sexual victimization.[13] A number of universities have set up an early warning system to be used in emergency situations. Students, staff, and faculty who provide the university with their cellphone numbers will be sent a text message should there be a crisis on the campus. The Guardly free mobile emergency phone service is offered to students at 67 Canadian universities and colleges. It is available as a free download on iPhone, BlackBerry, and Android devices.[14]

SAFETY AT THE WORKPLACE

Safe work is good for business.[15] As you begin to look for career options or change jobs, attention to the safety of the workplace environment that you are about to enter into is of utmost importance. You should also assess the safety practices of the work environment you might be in currently. There are three basic factors that support a safe work environment:[16]

- **Environmental factors**—safe physical conditions such as noise, air quality and ergonomics; reasonable work schedules; and the relationships and responsibilities of workers and employers
- **Personal resources**—employees' sense of control over their health; an opportunity to participate in the decision-making process at a workplace; support from co-workers and supervisors; access to safety training and a work environment that supports safe working policies and procedures
- **Health practices**—lifestyle choices that include physical activity, nutrition, and sleeping habits

Staying safe on the job demands that we follow safety procedures when performing tasks. Be sure to wear protective equipment when necessary, learn how to identify hazards, participate in safety training workshops and courses, and learn what to do when an accident does occur.[17]

STRATEGIES FOR PREVENTION

How to Drive Safely

- Don't drive while under the influence of alcohol or other drugs, including medications that may impair your reflexes, cause drowsiness, or affect your judgment.
- Never get into a car if you suspect the driver may be intoxicated or affected by a drug.
- Be alert and anticipate possible hazards. Don't let yourself be distracted by conversations, passenger directions, arguments, food or drink, or scenic views. If you become exhausted, pull over and rest.
- Don't get too comfortable. Alertness matters. Use the rearview mirror often. Use the turn signals when changing lanes or making a turn.
- If you are transporting small children, make sure they are in safety or booster seats or buckled up. Children under 12 years of age are not permitted in the front seat of a car that has an airbag.
- Drive more slowly if weather conditions are bad. Make sure that your car has the proper equipment, such as chains or snow tires, and that you know how to respond in case of a skid.
- Properly maintain your car, replacing windshield wipers, tires, and brakes when necessary. Keep flares and a fire extinguisher in your car for use in emergencies.
- To avoid a head-on collision, generally veer to the right—onto a shoulder, lawn, or open space. Steer your way to safety; avoid hitting the brakes hard once you leave the pavement. If you have to hit something stationary, look for a soft target.

SAFETY ON THE ROAD

Since 1970, when statistics on motor vehicle collisions were first collected, fatalities have decreased and serious injuries have declined. However, deaths and injuries resulting from traffic collisions continue to be the major transportation safety problem in Canada. In 2014, the number of motor vehicle fatalities was 1834, which was down slightly from 1923 in 2013.[18] Of great concern is the number of young driver and passenger fatalities. About 18 percent of all motor vehicle fatalities in 2014 were young drivers aged 15–24, and approximately 27 percent were passengers.[19] The societal costs of traffic collisions are enormous; economic losses are estimated to be in the billions of dollars.[20]

Responsibility for road safety is shared between our federal and provincial/territorial levels of government. The federal government, through Transport Canada, develops motor vehicle safety regulations and is responsible for the *Criminal Code of Canada.* The provincial and territorial governments have direct jurisdiction over driver and vehicle licensing. Municipalities are becoming involved in road safety too, through police services and injury prevention efforts.[21] To ensure road safety Canadians need to adopt safe driving habits.

Safe Driving The vision of Canada's Road Safety Strategy 2015 is to have the safest roads in the world. Over the next five years, the Canadian Council of Motor Transport Administrators will target drivers under the age of 25 years; medically at-risk drivers; vulnerable road users such as pedestrians, motorcyclists, cyclists, and individuals with wheelchairs and scooters; transport truck, bus, and high-risk drivers.[22]

The key causes of collisions include impaired driving, speed and aggressive driving, occupant protection, and environmental factors. Strategies that will be put in place to address these key causes will include education and training, communication, and awareness about road safety issues; enforcement for driving infractions; the gathering of important crash and victim data; introduction of improved regulation; and the use of technology such as electronic stability controls, side curtain airbags, and seat belt interlocks.[23]

Basic precautions can greatly increase your odds of reaching a destination alive, without injuring yourself or others. Vehicles equipped with seat belts, airbags, padded dashboards, safety glass windows, a steel frame, and side-impact beams all help protect against injury or death. The size and weight of a vehicle also matter.

Airbags Airbags supplement the protection provided by using seat belts. They are connected to sensors that detect sudden deceleration. When activated, the sensors send an electrical signal that ignites a chemical propellant. When ignited, the propellant produces nitrogen gas, which inflates the airbag. This process occurs in less than 1/20th of a second. Most airbags have internal tether straps that shape the fabric and limit the movement of the bag. Vents in the rear allow the bag to deflate slowly to cushion the passenger's head as it moves forward into the bag.

In low- to moderate-speed collisions, your seat belt is usually sufficient to prevent serious injury. However, in high-speed crashes, your seat belt may not be able to prevent your head (if you are the driver) from striking the steering wheel or your passenger's head from hitting the dashboard. Front airbags are designed to protect the head and upper body in frontal crashes. They are not designed to open in rear-end collisions, side impacts, or rollovers. You should adjust the vehicle's front seats as far to the rear as possible to give the airbags as much room as possible in which to inflate.[24] Side airbags are designed to prevent head and chest injuries in side crashes. When deployed, the side air bag provides a cushion between the driver or passenger and the vehicle interior such as the window glass or side door frame.[25] Although airbags have been found to save lives, Transport Canada has been receiving complaints from the public about injuries caused by airbags that inflate in low-speed collisions and about incidents in which airbags did not open when they were supposed to open. Airbags sometimes cause injuries because they must inflate very quickly with great force. Most of the injuries incurred are minor—bruises and abrasions—but some are more serious, such as broken arms. There have been some cases when the head or chest was against the module when the airbag opened and fatal injuries occurred.[26]

Children or people of small stature are vulnerable. Children under age 12 should be seated in the back of vehicles that have airbags installed. You should also never install a rear-facing infant car seat in a seat equipped with an airbag. If it were to deploy, the infant car seat would be propelled into the back of the seat.

Airbag systems of the future are already being developed. Known as "smart" airbags, some will possess two levels of activation. One will be appropriate for occupants who are using their seat belts; the other will work for an unbelted occupant. New airbag systems might also have proximity sensors that will gauge how close you are to the airbag module. They will be equipped with a warning system that will signal when someone is too close. Some vehicles already have a manual cut-off switch that allows an occupant to switch off the passenger-side airbag when an infant-restraint system is being used.[27]

✓ CHECK-IN

Have you ever had a car accident? Were airbags involved? If so, were they protective?

Alcohol and Drugs Although rates of impaired-driving incidents over the past 20 years have been falling, the percentage of fatally injured drivers who had been drinking (HBD) or were impaired with blood alcohol levels (BAC) over 80 mg (also equal to 0.08 percent and described as 0.08 BAC) in 2012 was still disturbing.[28]

Male drivers accounted for 84.4 percent of all fatally injured drivers who had been drinking and 84.3 percent of all the fatally injured drivers who were legally impaired. Male drivers who were fatally injured were more likely to have been drinking than female drivers (35.9 vs. 23.8 percent). It is troublesome to discover that most of the male and female drivers who were drinking had BACs over the legal limit at 85.6 percent for males and 86.3 percent for females.[29]

Age makes a difference too. (See Figure 14-1 for a comparison of all fatally injured drinking and legally impaired drivers). The highest percentage of drinking drivers who were fatally injured was the 26- to 35-year-old age group at 28.1 percent, followed by 20.8 percent for those aged 20–25. Almost 18 percent were between the ages of 46–55, followed closely by Canadians aged 36–45 at 16.5 percent. Only 9.5 percent of fatally injured drivers who were impaired

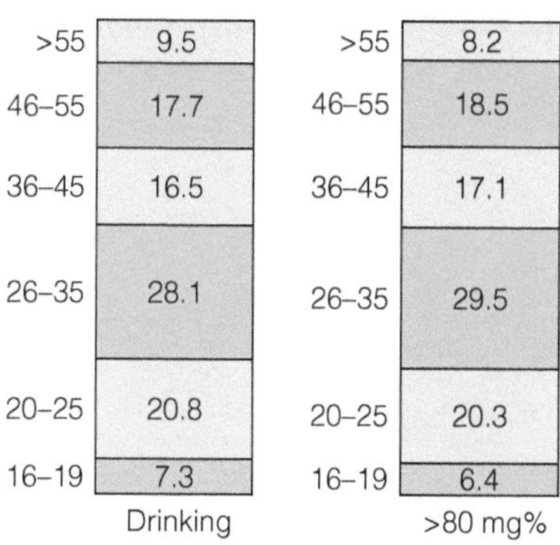

Figure 14-1 Percent of All Fatally Injured Drinking and Legally Impaired Drivers Accounted for by Each Age Group: Canada, 2012

Source: Brown, S.W., Valar, W.G.M., & Robertson, R.D. (2015, December). Alcohol and drug-crash problem in Canada. 2012 report. CCMTA Road Safety Research Report Series. Canadian Council of Motor Transport Administrators (CCMTA) (Figure 3-3, page 18). http://ccmta.ca/images/publications/pdf//2012_Alcohol_Drug_Crash_Problem_Report_ENG.pdf. Reprinted with the permission of the Canadian Council of Motor Transport Administrators.

were over 55 years of age. Young people aged 16–19 accounted for 7.3 percent of fatally injured drivers. For drivers who were fatally injured and legally impaired at the time of death (BACs over 80 mg), again, the highest percentage—29.5 percent—was between 26 and 35 years old, followed by the 20- to 25-year-old age group at 20.3 percent, the 46- to 55-year-old age group at 18.5 percent, and the 36- to 45-year-old age group at 17.1 percent. Of fatally injured drivers over the legal limit, 8.2 percent were in the 55-and-over group and 6.4 percent were 16- to 19-year-olds.[30]

According to research on impaired driving, 4.2 percent of Canadians reported that they had driven when they thought they were over the legal limit in the past 12 months in 2015. This is an increase from 3.6 percent in 2012.[31] Reports from police indicate that 50 percent of impaired driving accidents happen between 11 p.m. and 4 a.m. with the majority of these accidents occurring between 2 a.m. and 3 a.m.—just after bars close in most provinces.[32]

A study of full-time college students revealed that 20 percent of students drove after drinking some amount of alcohol, 10 percent drove after drinking five or more drinks, and 23 percent rode with a driver who was high or drunk.[33] Students who attended schools with more restrictions on underage drinking and that devoted more resources to enforcing drunk-driving laws reported less drinking and driving.[34]

A growing movement of young people—MADD Parkland, Youth in Canada[35] and Students Against Drinking and Driving[36]—are doing a lot to educate students about the consequences of drinking and driving. MADD Youth, working with Mothers Against Drunk Driving (MADD), has grown to become a dominant peer-to-peer youth education and prevention organization. Provincial agencies, such as the Insurance Corporation of British Columbia (ICBC), are also targeting high-school, college, and university students with programs such as Road Sense. A speaker's bureau and resource package support this educational program, which also includes student visits to local morgues and demonstrations and videos of vehicle crashes.[37] Other provinces have similar programs.

While it is more difficult to measure the impact of drugs and traffic accidents, tests do show that of all Canadian drivers who were fatally injured and tested for drug use in 2012, 40 percent of them were found to be positive for drugs.[38] They included prescription drugs such as Valium, over-the-counter drugs such as cold remedies, and illegal drugs such as cannabis, cocaine, and benzodiazepines.[39] There is evidence that a moderate or high dose of psychoactive drugs impairs driver performance.[40] Some studies have reported that the largest degree of impairment is observed with tasks involving attention, tracking, and psychomotor skills. Other studies show that drug use is often combined with alcohol use. The effects of alcohol in combination with another drug can be multiplicative—greater than the addition of the effects of each substance. It is more common to find younger people mixing alcohol and drugs. (See Figure 14-2, which shows the percentage of drivers who engaged in impaired-driving behaviours.)

The *Criminal Code of Canada*, Section 253a, permits police to lay a charge of impaired driving if they believe a person's ability to operate a vehicle is impaired by "alcohol or a drug." In some provinces in Canada drinking-driving laws are now becoming more stringent. While most provinces have a BAC legal limit of 80 milligrams (called 0.08), police in a number of provinces can now issue immediate roadside suspensions to a driver with a BAC of 0.05 or higher. One example is in Ontario, where police are able to issue an immediate driver's licence suspension for up to three days for a first occurrence if a driver is caught driving in the "warn-range" with a BAC from 0.05 to 0.08. A driver is also required to pay a $180 administrative monetary penalty. After a second occurrence within five years, police can

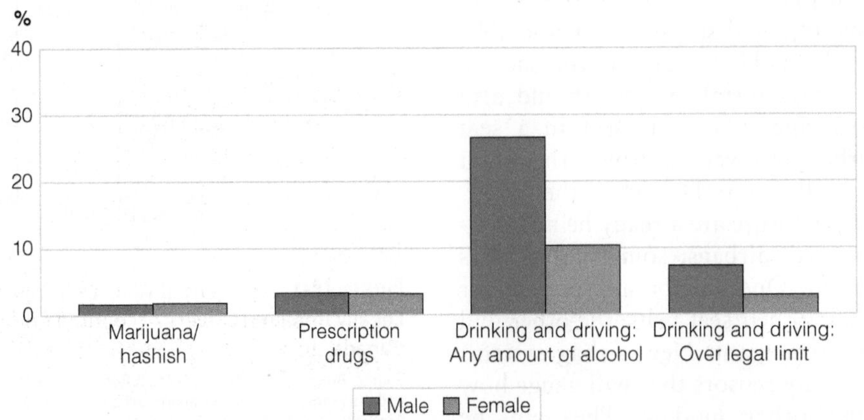

Figure 14-2 Percentage of Drivers Who Engaged in Impaired-Driving Behaviours, by Drug Classification and Gender, 2013

Source: Pashley, C.R., Robertson, R.D., & Vanlaar, W.G.M. (2013, September). The road safety monitor 2013. Drugs and driving. Traffic Injury Research Foundation. Ottawa, Ontario. Available at http://www.tirf.ca/publications/PDF_publications/2013_RSM_Drugs&Driving_6.pdf. Page 15.

suspend a driver's licence for seven days, apply the $180 administrative monetary penalty, and require the driver to attend a mandatory alcohol education program. For a third or subsequent occurrence within five years, the same suspensions, administrative fees, and mandatory education programs apply as the second occurrence with an added penalty of a six-month ignition interlock licence condition.[41]

With regard to testing for drugs and driving, presently there are no national standardized roadside tests that are available so that police officers can detect specific types and levels of drugs in a person's system. Another difficulty is the driver's use of more than one drug and the combination of drugs and alcohol, which confounds the testing protocol that is available. However, the Criminal Code of Canada (CCC) has been strengthened and does enable police officers who suspect a driver might be under the influence of drugs to submit to some physical coordination tests that are also used for alcohol testing. Police officers are now being trained as Drug Recognition Evaluators (DREs). If further examination of the driver is determined to be important then further tests can be requested, which include oral fluid, urine, or blood. These tests can determine the presence of drugs and alcohol in the body.[42]

There is a new message being sent out by the Canada Safety Council and it is "Don't drink and walk." Some people attempting to find alternatives to drinking and driving choose to walk home after a social event. Unfortunately, statistics are showing that this option might not be the best alternative. Once again, it is younger people who are most at risk.[43] Approximately 25 percent of 20- to 25-year-olds and 26- to 35-year-olds who were fatally injured while walking had BACs over 80 milligrams. Fifteen percent were young people aged 16–19 years. Close to 82 percent of all fatally injured pedestrians who had been drinking were males. Of the males who were fatally injured, 47.3 percent had been drinking. Approximately 91.5 percent of the male pedestrians had BACs over 0.08. Only 23.5 percent of fatally injured female pedestrians had been drinking; however, of this group, approximately 93.8 percent had BACs over 0.08.[44]

The healthy choice is to find a designated driver or take a cab. Being responsible can lower the risk of unintentional injury to yourself and others.

✓ CHECK-IN

Have you ever driven after you drank alcohol? Have you ever taken a ride from someone who had been drinking? If so, why?

Cellphones and Distracted Driving According to the Canadian Wireless Telecommunications Association (CWTA), there were approximately 29.3 million wireless phone subscribers as of May 2016. Mobile broadband subscribers are increasing and opting for smartphone voice/data plans. Canadians are sending more than 270 million text messages a day. Over half of the 911 calls made in Canada are from mobile phones.[45]

Mobile phones can be of great benefit if you need to call for help or report an accident. Unfortunately, cellphones have also been cited as a major contributing factor to motor vehicle accidents. The Canadian Automobile Association (CAA) reports that drivers using cellphones while driving are three to four times more likely to be in a car crash than drivers who are focused on the road. And if you text and drive you are more than 23 times more likely to have a collision than drivers who do not text and drive.[46] The reason is that text messaging takes your eyes off the road for about 4.6 seconds out of a 6-second interval. Visually this means you would be driving the full length of a football field without looking at the road while travelling 90 kilometres per hour.[47]

A meta-analysis of the effects of cellphones on driver performance found that drivers needed a 25 percent longer reaction time (RT) to respond to general driving tasks when they used either a hand-held or hands-free phone. The researchers also suggest that their laboratory study most likely underestimates the true behaviour of drivers using cellphones in their own vehicles: reaction time when using a hand-held or hands-free phone could be even longer. One other important finding was that the drivers using either type of phone do not compensate while driving by giving greater headway or reducing speed.[48]

Another study done on college students revealed some disturbing statistics. The students reported that 21 percent of the accidents or near-accidents that they had experienced involved at least one driver using a cellphone. The most frequently cited reason for the

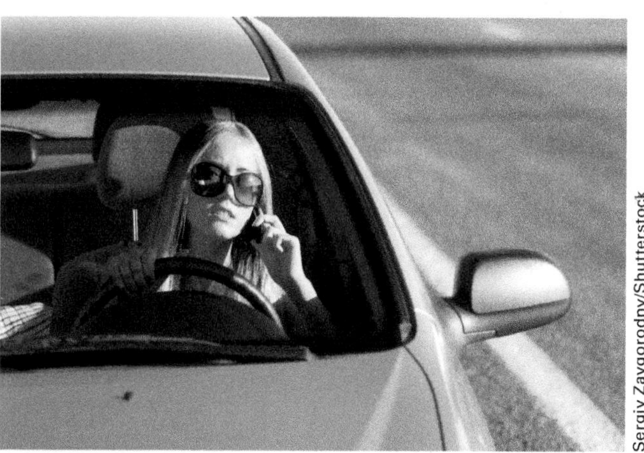

Sergiy Zavgorodny/Shutterstock

Any form of distraction, including talking on a cellphone, can put you and others at risk.

accident or near-accident was the driver's talking while driving (TWD), rather than their attempt to dial or answer. Contrary to the researchers' expectations, more students who experienced accidents were using hands-free rather than hand-held models. Female students were more likely than male students to use a cellphone while driving.[49]

With the new generation of cellphones now available, drivers are not only talking but also attempting to read emails, send text messages, and access the Internet. Due to the increasing fatalities linked to cellphone use and driving, many provinces have put legislation in place either banning or limiting use of a variety of hand-held devices. Table 14-2 shows the

TABLE 14-2

Current Legislation for Driver Distractions

Province/ Territory	Prohibitions on Hand-held Devices	Prohibitions on Hands-free Devices	Restrictions on other Distractions
British Columbia	All hand-held electronic equipment is banned. Sending or receiving text messages or email on any type of electronic device, including while stopped at a red light, is banned.	Drivers in Graduated Driver Licensing (GDL) program are not allowed to use hands-free electronic equipment.	Careless driving legislation; television sets cannot be visible to the driver.
Alberta	Holding, viewing, or manipulating a communications device or a hand-held or wireless electronic device is banned even while stopped at a red light.	None	With exceptions (e.g., GPS systems fixed to the car), electronic screens cannot be visible to the driver; reading, writing, hygiene, or any other activity that distracts a driver.
Saskatchewan	All hand-held communication equipment is banned.	Drivers in Graduated Driver Licensing (GDL) program not allowed to use hands-free communication equipment. Experienced drivers allowed to use hands-free devices, but recommended to pull over when making or receiving a call.	Careless driving legislation; electronic screens visible to the driver must be attached to the car and can only be used to aid the driver with the task of driving.
Manitoba	All hand-held electronic devices are banned. As an exception to above prohibition, a person may use a hand-operated electronic device by hand to call or send a message to a police force, fire department, or ambulance service about an emergency.	Cellphone must be configured and equipped to allow hands-free use as a telephone and used in a hands-free manner.	Imprudent driving legislation.
Ontario	All hand-held wireless communication devices are banned.	None	Careless driving legislation; with exceptions (e.g., GPS systems), electronic screens cannot be visible to the driver.
Quebec	All hand-held devices that include a telephone function are banned.	Hands-free devices that include a telephone function are permitted.	Careless driving legislation.
New Brunswick	All hand-held devices that include a telephone or text function are banned. If there is an emergency you can call 911.	None	Manual programming and adjusting of any GPS navigation system while driving is banned. Television screens, monitors, DVD players, and computer screens not permitted within the visual range of the operator of a motor vehicle.

(Continued)

TABLE 14-2

Current Legislation for Driver Distractions *(Continued)*

Province/ Territory	Prohibitions on Hand-held Devices	Prohibitions on Hands-free Devices	Restrictions on other Distractions
Nova Scotia	All hand-held cellular phones are banned; text messaging is banned on any communications device. Hand-held cellphone use only allowed in emergency situations.	None	Careless driving legislation; screens cannot be visible to the driver.
Prince Edward Island	All hand-held wireless communication devices are banned. Includes the use of GPS systems and laptops.	Can use hands-free technology activated by a single touch to a button or when safe to do so can pull over and stop vehicle to talk or email.	Careless driving legislation; operational televisions cannot be in any position within a vehicle.
Newfoundland & Labrador	All hand-held cellular phones are banned; text messaging is banned on any communications device.	None	Programming GPS when car is in motion is banned; careless driving legislation.
Yukon Territory	Hand-held devices used for talking, texting, or emailing are prohibited.	Graduated driver's license holders are not allowed to use hand-held electronic devices for talking, texting, or emailing or any hands-free devices.	Exceptions: Citizen's band (CB) and other simple push-to-talk two-way radios may be used as long as they are not used in a telephone function or transmitting or receiving email or texts.
Northwest Territories	All hand-held electronic devices including cellphones, laptops, devices for playing audio or video recordings, and handheld GPS systems are banned.	None	Careless driving legislation.
Nunavut	None at this time. Government is considering a new graduated licensing system and penalties for distracted-driving texting, or using a cellular phone while behind the wheel.		None at this time. Considering penalties for distracted driving including eating.

Sources: Based on data from Transport Canada and CAA.

current legislation for driver distractions in all provinces and territories.[50] Table 14-3 shows fines and demerits.

The Insurance Corporation of British Columbia (ICBC) provides smart driving tips with regard to cellphone use and driving:[51]

- Turn off your cellphone while driving to avoid the temptation to answer the call.
- Let voicemail do its job. Call back later when it is safe to do so.
- Have your passenger(s) answer your cellphone for you.
- If you must answer the call, pull off the road safely. Your life and the lives of people around you are more important than a telephone call.
- Use a hands-free device if you need to take a call. Keep your conversation brief. Keep your speed safe and consistent. Make sure your device is securely fastened.

✓ CHECK-IN

What is most likely to distract you while driving?

Seat Belts Reports from the Traffic Injury Research Foundation show that seat belt use has increased in Canada from 93 in 2007 to 95 percent in 2010. If Canadians would increase their seat belt use to 100 percent, thousands of lives would be saved each year. Who is the least likely to wear seat belts? Young males—aged 18–24 years. Young drivers who drive late at night and who have passengers who are under 29 years of age or have passengers who have been drinking tend not to use seat belts either. Canadians who live in urban areas are also more likely to wear seat belts compared to people living in rural areas. Data also show that "risky" drivers—those who follow too closely to vehicles in front of them, do not stop at red lights, or

TABLE 14-3

Distracted Driving Laws in Canada

Province	Fine	Demerits	Into Effect
British Columbia*	$ 543** first offense $ 888*** second offense	4	June 01, 2016
Alberta	$ 287	3	January 01, 2016
Saskatchewan	$ 280	4	June 2014
Manitoba	$ 200	5	July 2015
Ontario*	$ 490–1000	3	September 01, 2015
Quebec	$ 80–100	4	April 2015
Newfoundland and Labrador	$ 100–400	4	April 2003
Prince Edward Island	$ 500–1200	5	Summer 2015
Nova Scotia	$ 233.95 first offence	4	February 2015
	$ 348.95 second offence		
	$ 578.95 subsequent offences		
New Brunswick	$ 172.50	3	June 2011
Yukon	$ 250	3	April 2011
Northwest Territories	$ 322–644****	3	May 2016
Nunavut	-	-	Nothing at this time

*In addition to banning hand-held communication devices, British Columbia and Ontario also ban the use of hand-held electronic entertainment devices while driving.

**B.C.'s base fine is $368 plus $175 for ICBC's driver penalty point premiums.

***A second offense within 12 months has a base fine of $368 plus $520 for ICBC's driver penalty point premiums. Repeat offenders will also have their driving record subject to automatic review, which could result in a 3–12 month driving prohibition.

****The fine increases to $644 for distracted driving in school and construction zones.

Note: British Columbia and Saskatchewan prohibit GDL (Graduated Driver Licensing) drivers from using both hand-held and hands-free devices. No Canadian jurisdiction bans ALL drivers from using hands-free cellphones while driving.

Source: CAA. *Hand-Held Cell Phone Legislation in Canada*. Found at: http://distracteddriving.caa.ca/education/distracted-driving-laws-in-canada.php.

speed—are less likely to use seat belts. They are more likely to experience a car crash too. The good news is that the older people get, the more likely they are to wear their seat belts. Unfortunately drivers who drink and drive are also less likely to use their seat belts.[52]

One of the targets of Canada's Road Safety Strategy 2015 is increasing seat belt use. National collision data reveal that approximately 60 percent of all fatally injured drivers and passengers (26.2 percent of drivers and 33.2 percent of passengers) and almost 29.5 percent of those seriously injured (11.8 percent of drivers and 17.7 percent of passengers) were not wearing seat belts at the time of the collision.[53] Transport Canada is currently evaluating possible ignition interlock approaches to promote seat belt use. One idea being tested is that of requiring a time delay before unbelted drivers would be able to put their vehicle into gear.[54]

When lap-shoulder belts are used properly, they reduce the risk of fatal injury to front-seat passengers by 45 percent and the risk of moderate to critical injury by 50 percent. The risk of death or severe injury increases nearly five times for front-seat passengers when back-seat passengers are not wearing seat belts. In a collision, unbelted back-seat passengers may be thrown forward, pushing the front-seat passengers into the dashboard and the windshield.[55]

✓ CHECK-IN

Do you always buckle up your seat belt when you are driving or are a passenger in a car? If not, why not?

Safe Cycling Cycling is popular with Canadians of all ages. It is good for your heart, improves your balance and coordination, helps with weight control, and helps the environment. But there are some inherent risks in riding a bicycle. About 7500 cyclists are injured each year in Canada. Most cycling accidents occur during the afternoon rush-hour time. Intersections and areas where there are traffic signals or traffic lights are the most likely areas where cyclists are injured. Sixty-four percent of cyclist fatalities occur on city roads where the speed limit is up to 70 kilometres per hour.[56] Most injuries suffered by bicyclists are fractures, dislocations, and other non-life-threatening injuries. Head injuries are the most dangerous, accounting for an estimated two-thirds of cyclist fatalities. Even a mild head injury can have serious long-term consequences.

A Canada Safety Council survey found that although 97 percent of Canadians realize helmets prevented serious injury, over half of Canadian adults who ride bicycles don't wear helmets.[57] Topping the list of reasons: they just don't bother (14 percent), they didn't like the appearance (14 percent), they weren't "cool" (13 percent), they were uncomfortable (11 percent), and they were inconvenient or cumbersome (10 percent).

While children, by law, must wear bicycle helmets in most provinces, laws for adults are not consistent across the country. New Brunswick was the first province to mandate bicycle helmets for all ages in 1995. British Columbia was the second province in 1996. Nova Scotia followed in 1997, and Prince Edward Island is the fourth province that has an "all ages" helmet law, which passed in July 2003. Alberta, Manitoba, and Ontario now all have legislation mandating the use of helmets for anyone under 18 years of age. Saskatchewan, Quebec, Newfoundland, the Yukon, and the Northwest and Nunavut Territories do not have any helmet legislation in place at this time.[58] Having a law in place is only part of the solution. Helmets worn too far back and straps that are too loose or not clipped at all do not prevent head injuries. The Canadian Association of Emergency Physicians (CAEP) advocates for the use of helmets by everyone and disagrees with some research that suggests the use of helmets does not lower head-injury risks. Instead, the members of this association believe that they have a responsibility to encourage the enactment of legislation for all provinces in Canada with regard to mandatory helmet use.[59]

Alcohol use is another factor for cycling injuries and fatalities. A Canadian Council of Motor Transport Administrators' report found that although only 26.5 percent of fatally injured bicyclists had been drinking at the time of a collision, 84.6 percent had BACs over the legal limit.[60]

If you are going to ride a bicycle for sport or commuting, use road smarts:

- Obey the rules of the road. A bicycle is classified as a vehicle.
- Equip your bike with a horn and lights—front and back. Wear reflective gear and a CSA-approved helmet.
- Ride defensively. Anticipate the actions of other road users. Watch for car doors, debris, grates, or holes in the road.
- Fit your bike correctly. You should be able to straddle it comfortably with both feet on the ground.
- Keep it well maintained—chain clean and oiled, brakes adjusted, gears in working order, tires in good condition.

✓ CHECK-IN

Do you always wear a helmet when you are riding a bicycle?

SAFETY AND RECREATIONAL ACTIVITIES

Every year Canadians are injured during recreational activities such as hiking, skiing, snowboarding, off-roading, or boating.[61] Many of the victims suffer from head injuries requiring emergency room or hospital treatment. Environmental concerns such as heat and cold also need to be considered to keep outdoor enthusiasts safe.

Sport and Recreational Activities Canada's parks, forests, and wilderness areas are well used by hikers, campers, backpackers, climbers, canoeists, ATV riders, and others who seek adventure or just want to enjoy nature. If you are going to participate in an outdoor or sports field trip, think ahead: What conditions might you face? Find out about the area you plan to explore. Bring a good map and check the weather forecast. Tell other people about your plans—are you going surfing, skiing, or hiking in the mountains? What is your intended route and timetable? Go with others and stay with your group. Wear proper clothes, footwear, and sport-activity protection such as helmets, pads, and mouth guards. Invest in a wilderness survival kit that you can take along. Use common sense and take precautions. Manage your risks.[62]

Skiing and snowboarding are popular Canadian sports. However, the Canadian Institute for Health Information (CIHI) reports that in the 2010–2011 season there were 2329 hospital admissions for skiing and snowboarding accidents. Children younger than 10 years of age were hospitalized most often for injuries resulting from these sports. Unfortunately, in the 2010–2011 season, nearly one-third of serious head injuries occurred while skiing or snowboarding.[63]

Wearing protective equipment, including a helmet specifically designed for skiing and snowboarding, can reduce the severity and the risk of fatal injury. The Canadian Ski Council recommends wearing helmets for both sports. In 2009, the Canadian Standards Association (CSA) developed the first recreational alpine skiing and snowboard helmet standard. They updated the standard in 2014.[64] Even though this is still a voluntary standard, more manufacturers are beginning to design helmets to meet these standards. The Canadian Ski Council is working with ski operator associations to promote helmet use. Helmets are now available for rent or sale at all ski hills across Canada. Helmet use for snow sports increased from 32 in 2002–2003 to 86 percent in 2015. Among children under 14 years of age, 99.5 percent use helmets.[65]

Injuries and deaths from snowmobile accidents in North America are on the rise. These accidents lead to more serious injuries than any other sport. The problem is thrill-seekers who speed, ride after drinking—often at night, and misuse the equipment, zooming across roads, thin ice, or rough terrain. The Canadian Council of Motor Transport Administrators report that 72.7 percent of snowmobile drivers surveyed had been drinking and driving and 78.1 percent had BACs over the legal limit in 2012.[66] The Canadian Council of Snowmobile Organizations (CCSO) has published a position statement titled *Zero Alcohol—Your Smart Choice*[67] encouraging all snowmobile users to take responsibility for themselves and their passengers to drive impairment-free.

Boating is the number-one cause of drowning in Canada.[68] In Canada, 53 percent of boating deaths occur on lakes. Almost all boating victims are male (91 percent).[69] Wear a lifejacket or a personal flotation device (PFD) if you boat. A lifejacket is designed to turn the wearer's body face up. A PFD is designed to keep a conscious person's head out of water in calm conditions and assist them in rough water. PFDs offer comfort, style, and flexibility and come in a wide range of models and sizes. There are also PFDs with hypothermia protection—a valuable feature in some of our cold Canadian waters.

There are new rules for personal watercraft use. Since September 15, 2002, all operators of personal watercrafts (PWC) must have proof of competency. All operators born after April 1, 1983, must have proof of competency on board the craft. Proof of competency includes a pleasure craft operator card or proof of having taking a boating-safety course prior to April 1, 1999, or a completed rental boat safety checklist. Accredited courses and tests are available. Experienced boaters can take the test without completing the course. A new *Safe Boating Guide* is available from Transport Canada.[70]

It is also important to remember that driving a boat under the influence of alcohol or drugs is a criminal offence. If your BAC is over the legal limit of 80 milligrams you can be fined and/or go to prison. The maximum fines do vary in each province. Most fines and penalties are similar to drunk- or drug-driving infractions. Consuming alcohol on a boat is legal if the boat is anchored or secured to a dock, and has permanent cooking facilities, sleeping facilities, and a toilet.[71]

Handling Heat Two common heat-related maladies are **heat cramps** and **heat stress.** Heat cramps are caused by hard work and heavy sweating in the heat. Heat stress may occur simultaneously or afterward, as the blood vessels try to keep body temperature down. **Heat exhaustion**, a third such condition, is the result of prolonged sweating with inadequate fluid replacement (see Table 14-4). The first step in treating these conditions is to stop exercising, move to a cool place, and drink plenty of water. Don't resume work or activity until all the symptoms have disappeared; see a doctor if you're suffering from heat exhaustion.

Heat stroke is a life-threatening medical emergency caused by the breakdown of the body's mechanism for cooling itself. The treatment is to cool the body down: move to a cooler environment, sponge down with cool water, and apply ice to the back of the neck, armpits, and groin. Immersion in cold water could cause shock. Get medical help immediately.

Being safe in the sun is also important. Incidents of skin cancer in Canada have risen. According to reports from Health Canada, skin cancer is the most common diagnosed cancer in both Canada and the world.[72] The main cause of skin cancer is too much UV radiation. Dermatologists encourage all Canadians to use sunscreen. The problem of overexposure to UV rays is also an indoor issue.

A study done on 487 college students found that despite their awareness of the risks associated with ultraviolet light exposure, many students used tanning beds to get a so-called healthy tan. Thirty-seven percent of the students had used a tanning lamp or bed. Of the current users, 86 percent of

TABLE 14-4

Heat Dangers

Illness	Symptoms	Treatment
Heat cramps	Muscle twitching or cramping; muscle spasms in arms, legs, and abdomen	Stop exercising; cool off; drink water.
Heat stress	Fatigue, pale skin, blurred vision, dizziness, low blood pressure	Stop exercising; cool off; drink water.
Heat exhaustion	Excessive thirst, fatigue, lack of coordination, increased sweating, elevated body temperature	Stop exercising; cool off; drink water. See a doctor.
Heat stroke	Lack of perspiration, high body temperature (over 40.5°C [105°F]), dry skin, rapid breathing, coma, seizures, high pulse	Cool the body; sponge down with cool water; apply ice to the back of the neck, armpits, and groin. Get immediate medical help.

the females and 100 percent of the males said that they used tanning lamps because they thought they looked better when they were tanned. Of the past tanners, 64.5 percent of the females and 60.9 percent of the males also enjoyed a tanned appearance. The second most common reason for tanning for both female and male current and past tanners was to prepare for the summer. Other reasons for tanning included having more confidence, relaxation, and influence of friends, media, and celebrities. The authors of the study also noted that students used tanning beds because the service was free or available at a low cost.[73] *They suggest that education on the risks of tanning might benefit college students.*

Concerned about the health risks of tanning beds, Nova Scotia, British Columbia, and Ontario have passed legislation banning the use of tanning equipment for anyone under the age of 18.[74]

Coping with Cold The tips of the toes, fingers, ears, nose, chin, and cheeks are most vulnerable to exposure from high wind speeds and low temperatures, which can result in **frostnip.** Because frostnip is painless, you may not even be aware of it occurring. Watch for a sudden blanching or lightening of your skin. The best early treatment is warming the area by firm, steady pressure with a warm hand; blowing on it with hot breath; holding it against your body; or immersing it in warm (not hot) water. As the skin thaws, it becomes red and starts to tingle. Be careful to protect it from further damage. Don't rub the skin vigorously or with snow, since you could damage the tissue.

More severe is **frostbite,** which can be either superficial or deep. *Superficial frostbite,* the freezing of the skin and tissues just below the skin, is characterized by a waxy look and firmness of the skin, although the tissue below is soft. Initial treatment should be to slowly re-warm the area. As the area thaws, it will be numb and turn bluish or purple, and blisters may form. Cover the area with a dry, sterile dressing, and protect the skin from further exposure to cold. See a doctor for further treatment. **Deep frostbite,** the freezing of skin, muscle, and even bone, requires medical treatment. It usually involves the tissues of the hands and feet, which appear pale and feel frozen. Keep the victim dry and as warm as possible on the way to a medical facility. Cover the frostbitten area with a dry, sterile dressing.[75]

The gradual cooling of the centre of the body may occur at temperatures above, as well as below, freezing—usually in wet, windy weather. When body temperature falls below 35°C (95°F), the body is incapable of re-warming itself because of the breakdown of the internal system that regulates its temperature. This state is known as **hypothermia.** The first sign of hypothermia is severe shivering. Then the victim becomes uncoordinated, drowsy, listless, confused, and is unable to speak properly. Symptoms become more severe as body temperature continues to drop, and coma or death can result.[76]

HUMAN POTENTIAL

Ashleigh Hawes—Travel and Academics—Take a Risk

This human potential story shows that by asking for help and taking risks, it is possible to combine academic studies with adventure.

Ashleigh's love for travel began as a child as she watched her older sister travel all over the world prior to attending university. Ashleigh was inspired to do something similar. After high school she worked to save money in order to complete her goal of also seeing the world. After a few small trips, she travelled for eight months. She travelled with her sister in India, on her own in Nepal, and with friends new and old through Southeast Asia and Australia. When asked about what she learned from that first trip, she talks about the importance of understanding different cultures. She shares how travelling helped her develop personal confidence and independence, and increase trust in her own abilities to cope in challenging situations.

Upon her return she started university. The first term was challenging. While prepared for academic demands, she found it difficult to find time to prepare proper meals, exercise, and study. Living 22 kilometres out of town, she had to get up at 5:30 a.m. and catch a 6:30 bus to get to her early-morning classes. She got home so late that she did not have the energy to cook so would go to bed hungry.

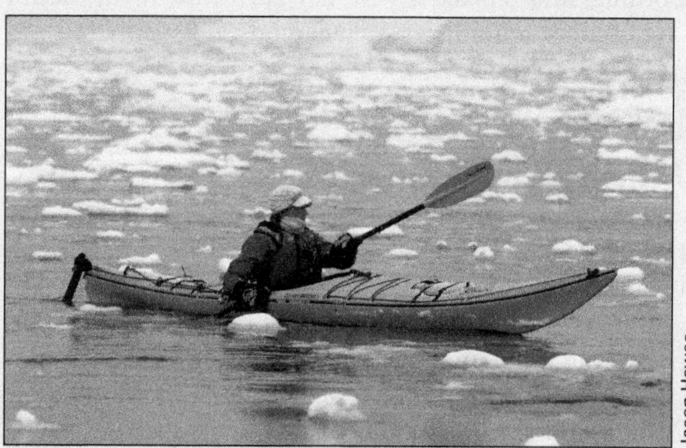
Jason Hawes

Ashleigh Hawes, a university student who balances academics and adventure, kayaking off the Antarctic Peninsula.

She also began to appreciate that she was an outdoor person who was spending most of her time indoors. She was surviving—not thriving. Additionally she dealt with a "long-distance relationship" and breakup.

With words of concern from friends and family, she realized it was time for a change. She moved closer to school and adjusted her

(Continued)

priorities for school and physical and emotional health. Then an opportunity for a trip of a lifetime came her way. Her older sister, who was working as a kayak guide in Antarctica, invited Ashleigh to visit her. She would be "on standby" for a trip scheduled during the mid-term exam period early in the New Year. Ashleigh was torn. Here was an opportunity that might never come again. Ashleigh had certain perceptions of being a student—academics were supposed to come first. How could she combine travelling and school, especially at such an important time in the semester?

In one of her first-term courses Ashleigh had learned about the importance of "asking for help" and "just saying yes." These two concepts would lead her to a conversation with one of her professors who suggested she contact her second-term professors and ask for permission to reschedule her mid-term exams. She was hesitant to do so, but emailed all of her professors. To her surprise, all of them wrote back and four out of five professors encouraged Ashleigh to go on the trip. Only one professor was unable to accommodate her request. The ability to ask for help was a lesson learned that has helped her again and again. But she now had another challenge ahead. The one course that she actually needed to support her application to a Recreation and Health Education program she hoped to apply for was the one course where she could not be accommodated. Dropping this course would mean her application to the program would have to be put on hold for one year. It was a difficult decision but she decided to take the risk and go on the trip.

When asked to describe her trip she says it was surreal. She still has difficulty explaining the sense of awe she felt when there. The uniqueness of the environment was exceptional. She got close to penguins, whales, and icebergs. She says there is nothing like it. The 100 guests on the trip ranged from teenagers to older adults. They were from all over the world and from varying cultures. Some people had saved up for a large part of their life for this trip.

She learned about respecting the environment and the power of nature. It can take just one drop of water to flip an iceberg. She learned that the animals in Antarctica have not yet become fearful of humans. They check you out and are happy to show off. She also reconnected with her brother who joined her for the trip. She was able to see her sister in her element working as a successful sea kayak guide. She was reminded about how important family connections are. Upon her return she wrote her missed exams, did well, and discovered that the self-study sessions done while on the trip had helped her keep pace with the other students.

Her advice for students wondering what they should do when surprise opportunities arise at university is to ask for advice and help and start with the thought that a trip or new experience might be possible. She learned that professors are willing to help students who are keen and responsible. She began to understand that life does not have to be put on hold just because you are a college or university student. She came to know that she had a high level of resilience and tenacity and could accomplish much more than she had given herself credit for. The most important lesson—that academics are just one part of your life. Taking time out from academic studies does not mean you will not complete a degree or fulfill your academic potential. She has now completed a Recreation and Health Education undergraduate degree, is working as a Recreation Programmer, and is excited about her life ahead. And she has only one more continent to visit!

Hypothermia requires emergency medical treatment. Try to prevent any further heat loss: Move the victim to a warm place, cover him or her with blankets, remove wet clothing, and replace it with dry garments. If the victim is conscious, administer warm liquids, not alcohol.

UNINTENTIONAL INJURY: WHY ACCIDENTS HAPPEN

Injuries can be classified as unintentional or intentional. Unintentional injuries are often linked to transportation accidents, falls, drowning, fire, burns, unintentional poisoning, and sport. They are a serious public-health concern in Canada. Unintentional injuries accounted for 26 billion dollars in total economic costs in 2010.[77] The leading cause of unintentional injury resulting in death was falls at 4071 in 2010. Fall-related injuries resulted in 128 389 000 hospitalizations and over one million emergency-room visits. Transport incidents were the second-leading cause of death with 4071 deaths. Hospitalizations numbered 28 350.[78] Many non-fatal injuries result in disabilities and physical impairments such as blindness, spinal cord injury, and brain injury. Many factors influence an individual's risk of unintentional injury, including age, alcohol and drug use (discussed in the safe driving section), stress, and thrill-seeking. The majority of unintentional injuries are not only preventable but also predictable.[79]

Age Injuries (not including adverse events in medical care) are the leading cause of death for Canadians between the ages of one and 44 and the third-leading cause of death of Canadians aged 45–64.[80] Unintentional injuries accounted for almost 70 percent of injury-related deaths among children and youth. Another group affected is seniors. The most common cause of injury among seniors is falls. University students are also at risk for injuries. Peltzer and Pengpid surveyed 19 111 (41.5 percent male and 58.5 percent female) undergraduate university students from 27 different universities in 26 low-, middle- and high-income countries (Asia, Africa, and the Americas) and discovered that 25.2 percent of students reported one or more serious injuries within the past 12 months of completing the survey. Male students had a higher rate of injuries compared to female students at 28.8–21.1 percent respectively. Health-risk behaviours, post-traumatic stress disorder (PTSD) symptoms, and lack of personal control and social support were found to be factors for both male and female students. Living in residence on campus was also associated with injuries for female students.[81]

Stress Demanding schedules have led to changes in lifestyle. More and more college and university students are attempting to balance studying and part- or full-time work. If you are stressed out or sleep-deprived, you pose a risk to yourself and to others.[82] Paying less attention to what we're doing can result in an increase in accidents. The findings of a Canada Safety Council driving survey showed that 84 percent of drivers admit to acts of aggressive driving. Passing on the right-hand side of the road, speeding, passing cars under risky conditions, and showing visible anger toward other drivers were some examples cited. Stress was the main reason given.[83] As well, over half the drivers surveyed drove while tired during the year, including one in ten who admitted to falling asleep behind the wheel. Ninety-seven percent of drivers in the 18- to 49-year-old age group admitted to multitasking (drinking coffee, putting on music, reaching for objects in the car, talking on cellphones) while driving. If you find yourself having a series of small mishaps or near-misses, do something to lower your stress level, rather than waiting for something more harmful to happen.

Thrill-Seeking To some people, activities that others might find terrifying—such as skydiving or parachute jumping—are stimulating. Thrill-seekers may have lower-than-normal levels of the brain chemicals that regulate excitement. Because the stress of potentially hazardous sports may increase the levels of these chemicals, they feel pleasantly aroused rather than scared. However, these activities can result in numerous injuries. Adventure racing is an extreme sport that is becoming popular. The world's top expedition racers run, bike, hike, and paddle for sometimes five or six days almost non-stop. Even marathoners and triathletes often push their bodies to a level that takes a significant toll. Structural damage to joints, bones, and muscles can occur. Lack of sleep, poor nutrition, and dehydration can cause the body's metabolic systems to overheat, and damage to the kidneys and heart can be the result.[84]

In some cases, taking risks can enhance personal well-being. Preparation, planning, and an understanding of inherent risks can help to prevent unintentional injuries.

✓ **CHECK-IN**

What type of emergencies, if any, have you experienced?

INTENTIONAL INJURY: LIVING IN A DANGEROUS WORLD

The World Health Organization (WHO) describes intentional injuries as interpersonal violence that can include homicide, sexual assault, neglect and abandonment, suicide, and war. Some people or groups of people are more vulnerable to intentional injuries than others. Living in unsafe environments can raise these risks.[85] Suicide and other forms of self-harm are the leading causes of all intentional injury deaths. In 2010, there were 3948 deaths as a result of suicide. There were 16 131 hospitalizations and 34 677 visits to hospital emergency departments.[86] Older adult males aged 85 years and older were most likely to die from suicide or self-harm at 26 per 100 000 followed by males aged 25–64 at 23 per 100 000. Females most likely to die from suicide or self-harm were those aged 25–64 at 88 per 100 000.[87]

Violence in Canada According to crime statistics in Canada[88] the police-reported crime rate decreased between 2013 and 2014 (see Figure 14-3). The Crime Severity Index (CSI), which measures the volume and severity of a crime, also fell by 3 percent from 2013–2014. Both the crime rate and the CSI either decreased or remained the same in almost all provinces in 2014. Data showed that Prince Edward Island had the largest drop in both crime rate (17 percent) and the CSI (20 percent). However, while the Yukon's crime rate stayed the same between 2013 and 2014, the CSI went up by 11 percent. In British Columbia the crime rate increased (3 percent) and the CSI also increased (2 percent) over the same time period.[89]

When comparing crime rates between males and females, males still account for the majority of criminal offences. It is interesting to note, though, that the rate of adult male offences has been declining over the past 20 years while the rate of adult female offences has been increasing.

Family Violence Family violence has long-lasting impacts on not only on the family unit but also our entire society and increases the risk for future alcohol and drug use, loss of jobs, performance at school, and various chronic illnesses. In 2014, common physical assault—pushing, slapping, or punching—accounted for 80 percent of family violence. Major assault, including use of a weapon that involves bodily harm, was the next most frequently reported offence. Uttering threats (11 percent) and sexual offenses (8 percent) affected nearly one in five family members.[90] Twenty-six percent of victims who reported violent crime to police were maltreated by other family members such as a spouse, parent, child, sister, brother, or other extended members of the family. The majority of victims—7 out of 10—were young girls or women. No matter what age, females are at a greater risk of family violence than men.[91]

Police-reported violence against family members has declined by 16 percent between 2009 and 2014. However, it is important to remember that family violence is often not reported.[92]

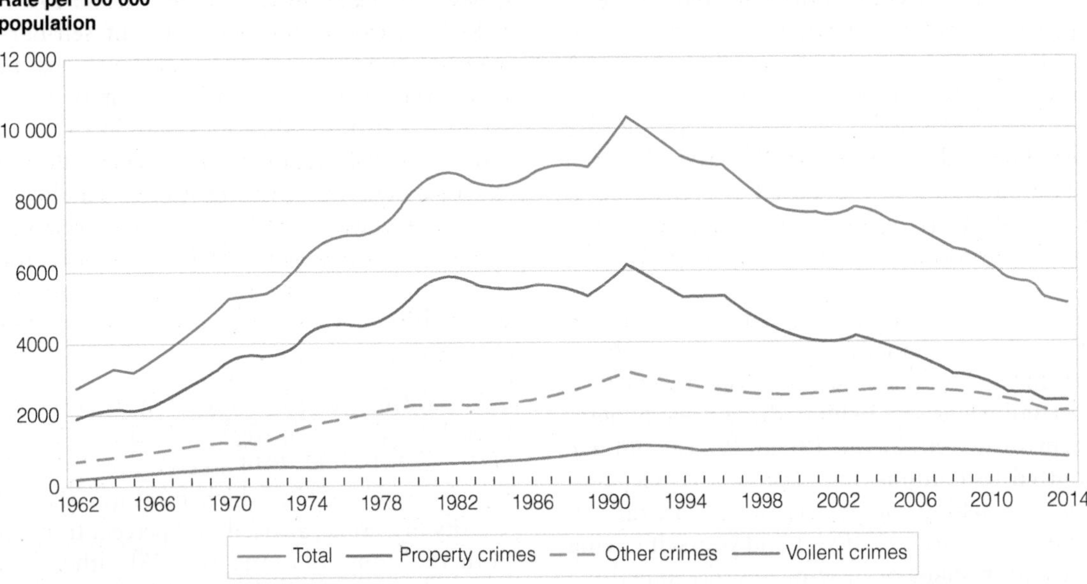

Note: Information presented in this chart represents data from the UCR Aggregate (UCR1) Survey, and permits historical comparisons back to 1962. New definition of crime categories were introduced in 2009 and are only available in the new format back to 1998. As a result, numbers in this chart will not match data released in the new UCR2 format. Specifically, the definition of violent crime has been expanded. In addition, UCR1 includes some different offences in the 'Other' crimes category. Populations are based upon July 1st estimates from Statistics Canada, Demography Division.

Figure 14-3 Police-Reported Crime Statistics in Canada, 1962–2014

Source: Boyce, J. (2015, November 30). Police-reported crime statistics in Canada, 2014, *Juristat*. Catalogue no. 85-002-x. Publications (Chart 1). http://www.statcan.gc.ca/pub/85-002-x/2015001/article/14211-eng.htm.

Crime on Campus While most college and university campuses provide a safe environment for living and studying, there are reports of increasing crime rates. Property crimes such as burglary and theft are the most common. However, students today must also cope with the dangers of alcohol, drugs, fire, and gambling.[93] Cyberbullying is also on the rise. The consequences of this type of crime range from personal embarrassment and harassment to suicide and homicide.[94]

Because of concerns about safety on college and university campuses, many academic institutions are taking tougher stands on student behaviour. Many have established codes of conduct that restrict the use of alcohol and drugs in residences, and address verbal and physical abuse, sexual harassment, racism, and homophobia issues. Some campuses have instituted policies requiring suspension or expulsion for students who violate these codes.

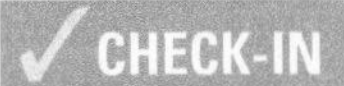

Do you feel safe on your college or university campus? Why or why not?

Public safety initiatives include safe-walk programs, campus security patrols, and emergency phones. Sexual-assault services provide counselling, crisis intervention, and educational programs. Students are urged to walk in groups and lock their doors and windows.

X AND Y FILES

Which Gender Is at Greater Risk?

Just like illness, injury doesn't discriminate against either gender. Both men and women can find themselves in harm's way—but for different reasons. Here are some gender differences in vulnerability with statistics taken from *Family Violence in Canada: A Statistical Profile 2014*.[95]

- Men are more likely to die of an occupational injury than women.
- Males are most often the victims and the perpetrators of homicides in Canada.
- Boys and men are more likely to be perpetrators of interpersonal violence, including homicide, physical assault, sexual assault, domestic abuse, and hate-related crimes. Men are more likely than women to be assaulted as an adult.
- Males are more likely to be harassed by an acquaintance. Women are more likely to be harassed by their spouse or partner.
- Females continue to be the most likely victims of police-reported spousal violence. This holds true for every province and territory across Canada.
- Female victims of spousal violence are more than twice as likely to be injured as male victims.
- Women are three times more likely to fear for their lives than men and twice as likely to be targets of more than 10 violent episodes.

Student and parent orientations often include mandatory sessions on campus safety and sexual assault.

Here's how to keep yourself safe:[96]

- Visit your campus security division to learn about safety on the campus.
- Drink responsibly. Stay away from drinking games and contests.
- Be aware of who is serving you drinks. Don't accept any drinks from strangers.
- Be especially vigilant about date-rape drugs. Don't leave your drink where someone can slip a drug into it.
- Take advantage of your campus's safe-walk services.
- Lock up your valuables. If you cycle, keep your bike locked up.
- Don't give out your dorm, apartment, or house key to anyone. Don't let strangers into your dorm or apartment.
- Take all fire alarms seriously.
- Stay away from Internet gambling sites. Avoid any type of illegal gambling.
- If you are a victim of cyberbullying, ask for help. This can include the consequences of "sexting" photographs to friends and acquaintances that end up being used as a form of cyberbullying. Find a counsellor or professor who can assist you in dealing with this problem. Do not withdraw or isolate yourself.

Most student crime is committed by students themselves. The more aware you are that crime is a possibility on campus, the better prepared you will be to prevent crime in the first place or deal with crime should it happen to you.

Hate Crimes Recent years have seen a slight reduction of violent crimes motivated by hatred. In Canada, in 2013, there were 1167 hate crimes reported by the police. This was a reduction of 17 percent from 2012.[97] Hate crimes linked to race or ethnicity represented over half of the total hate crimes. This was followed by religious hate crimes and crimes motivated by sexual orientation[98] (see Figure 14-4).

Unfortunately hate crimes related to race and ethnicity are still of great concern and equal 51 percent of police-reported hate crimes in 2013. Black populations are targeted most frequently. With regard to hate crimes that are religiously motivated, Jewish populations continue to be the most targeted. However, a new report from the National Council of Canadian Muslims indicates that hate crimes against Muslims doubled between 2012 and 2014.[99] Males tend to be the both the perpetrators and victims of hate crimes. Eighty-one percent of male victims were part of a violent incident because of hatred of sexual orientation.[100]

The most common types of hate-crime violations include mischief or vandalism, assault, uttering threats, and hate propaganda. Often violent hate crimes involve

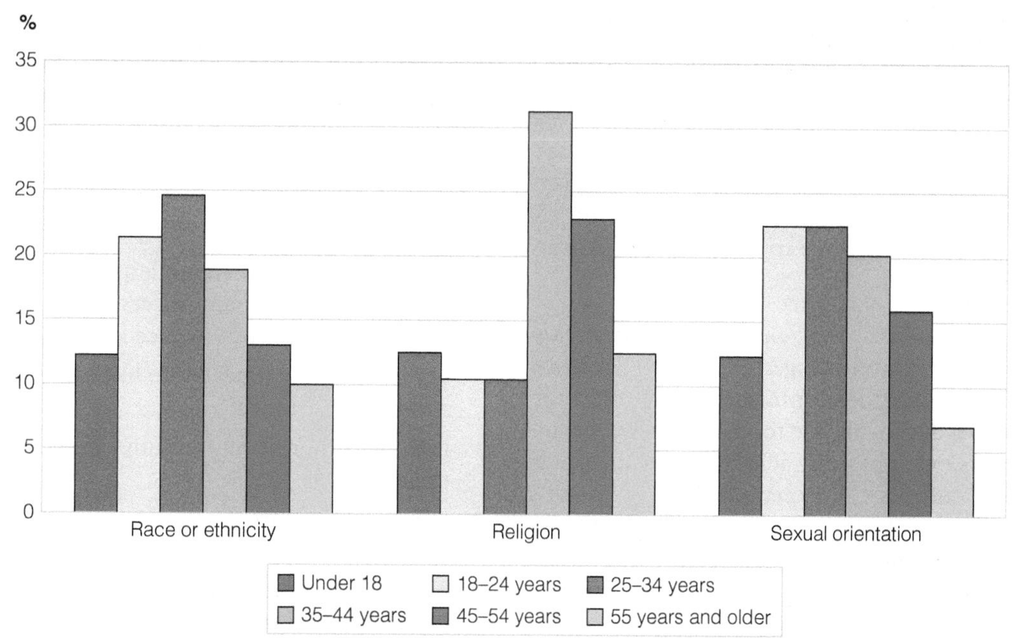

Note: Information in this chart reflects data reported by police services covering 86% of the population of Canada. It does not include municipal police services in Toronto, Calgary, Québec, and Saint John reporting to the UCR2.2 Supplemental Survey. Information on victims is limited to incidents involving violent offences. In 2013, information on 412 victims was reported in 336 violent hate crime incidents. In 16% of hate crime incidents involving victims, more than one victim was identified.

Figure 14-4 **Age Distribution of Victims in Hate Crime Incidents, by Motivation, Canada, 2013**

Source: Police-reported hate crime in Canada, 2013, Juristat, 35 (1), (Chart 5, page 12). Catalogue no. 85-002-x, ISSN 1209-6393, by Mary Allen Canadian Centre for Justice. Release date: June 9, 2015. http://www.statcan.gc.ca/access_acces/alternative_alternatif.action?l=eng&loc=/pub/85-002-x/2015001/article/14191-eng.pdf.

the threat of force. Physical force using weapons such as knives and pellet guns is common. Many injuries sustained during hate crimes are deemed to be minor, but many victims suffer major injuries—sometimes death. In almost half of all hate crimes, the perpetrator was a stranger.

Many administrators at Canadian colleges and universities are denouncing hate crime and doing more to educate faculty, staff, and students about this issue. Perry[101] surveyed 807 students from one Canadian college and one university campus to determine the type and frequency of hate crimes. Verbal assaults were common with one in 10 students reporting that they dealt with racial comments and threats. Students were also exposed to offensive online images. Other incidents included being spat upon, being pushed and shoved, sexual harassment, being chased, and receiving offensive phone calls and emails. In a healthy community differences are celebrated, not feared.

✓ CHECK-IN

What initiatives are being put in place on your campus to prevent hate crimes?

Sexual Victimization and Violence Sexual victimization refers to any situation in which a person is deprived of free choice and forced to comply with sexual acts. This is not only a woman's issue—men are also victimized. In recent years, researchers have come to view acts of sexual victimization along a continuum, ranging from street hassling, stalking, and obscene telephone calls, text, or Facebook messages, to rape, battering, and incest.

What Is Sexual Harassment? All forms of sexual harassment or unwanted sexual attention—from the display of pornographic photos to the use of sexual obscenities to a demand for sex by anyone in a position of power or authority—are illegal.

Sexual Harassment on Campus Sexual harassment can undermine a student's well-being and academic performance. Its effects include diminished ambition and self-confidence, reduced ability to concentrate, sleeplessness, depression, physical aches, and numerous other ailments. Students can experience sexual harassment from their professors, staff, or other students. To combat hostile or offensive sexual environments, many colleges and universities have set up committees to handle student complaints and to take action should sexual harassment occur. Universities also are discouraging and, in some cases, restricting consensual relationships between teachers and students, especially any dating of students and their academic professors or advisers. Although such relationships may seem consensual, in reality they may not be because of the power faculty members have to determine students' grades and futures.[102]

If you encounter sexual harassment report it to your department chair, dean, and police. Talk with counsellors, who can help you deal with the emotional issues that you might be faced with and assist you in reporting this crime. Sexual-harassment guidelines prevent any discrimination against you in terms of grades or the loss of a job if you report harassment.

Sexual Victimization of Students As our society has become more aware of issues such as sexual harassment and coercion, there has been growing recognition that both women and men need to take care to protect themselves, even on college and university campuses. According to a report about sexual assault and rape on United States college campuses, approximately 27 percent of female students reported at least some type of unwanted sexual contact since they began their academic studies. Other studies show a statistical link between sexual assault and the use of alcohol by students. College males also report victimization of sexual assault and rape.[103] A special task force—RAINN—Rape, Abuse, and Incest National Network, recommended a three-step approach to addressing this issue on college and university campuses: 1) developing bystander education; 2) encouraging community response to sexual violence; and 3) wide-ranging education across campuses to protect students from sexual assaults.[104]

In Canada, Ontario adopted legislation to protect students from sexual violence. Dr. Andrew Weaver, the Green Party leader in British Columbia, also introduced a private member's bill that will now require academic institutions in British Columbia to report sexual misconduct incidents. The Liberal government of B.C. expanded the definition of sexual violence to include non-consensual distribution of sexually explicit photos and videos.[105]

Victims of Violence reports that:[106]

- four out of five female undergraduate students surveyed at Canadian universities reported that they had been victims of violence in a dating relationship;
- women are five times more likely to be sexually assaulted than men;
- nine out of ten sexual assaults are not reported to police;
- young females are at a greater risk of date rape from boyfriends, dates, or male classmates;
- males also report being verbally pressured, threatened, or blackmailed by female dating partners to have sex;
- 99 percent of women are raped by male offenders; and
- 95 percent of men are raped by male offenders.

Lifestyle choices can also lead to sexual victimization. In a study of 314 female college students, Lawyer examined the frequency of sexual assaults after voluntary and involuntary drug or alcohol consumption. The results of his study showed that drug-related sexual assaults are more frequent than forcible assaults and are most frequently preceded by voluntary alcohol consumption.[107]

Sexual assault can take place in intimate relationships and between dating partners, friends, acquaintances, or strangers. Rapes committed by acquaintances of the victim are the most common forms of sexual assault, closely followed by sexual assaults by dates or partners of other relationships. Incidents on college and university campuses in Canada have included student frosh week events that have encouraged various forms of sexual assault, sport team members involved in rape cases and team members or coaches not reporting the incidents, and lack of support for female or male victims due to lack of sexual misconduct policy or the reluctance of administration to deal with the complaints.[108]

✓ CHECK-IN

Have you experience or observed sexual harassment on campus?

Sexual Coercion and Rape At a bar on a weekend night, a group of intoxicated young men grab a woman and squeeze her breasts as she struggles to get free. At a party, a man offers his date drugs and alcohol in the hope of lowering her resistance to sex. Although some people don't realize it, such actions are forms of **sexual coercion** (forced sexual activity), which is very common on and off college and university campuses.

Sexual coercion can take many forms, including exerting peer pressure, taking advantage of one's desire for popularity, threatening an end to a relationship, getting someone intoxicated, stimulating a partner against his or her wishes, or insinuating an obligation based on the time or money one has expended. Men may feel that they need to live up to the sexual stereotype of taking advantage of every opportunity for sex. Women are far more likely than men to encounter physical force.

Rape refers to sexual intercourse with an unconsenting partner under actual or threatened force. *Statutory rape* refers to sexual intercourse between an adult and another person under the age of 16. On May 1, 2008, the *Tackling Violent Crime Act* raised the legal age of consent in Canada, from 14 to 16 years of age, the first time this age has been raised since 1892. There is a "close-in-age exception" included in the new law, whereby 14- and 15-year-olds can have sex with someone less than five years older than themselves.[109] The law is now in line with laws in Britain, Australia, and many jurisdictions in the United States. In *acquaintance rape*, or *date rape*, the victim knows the rapist. In *stranger rape*, the rapist is an unknown assailant. Both stranger and acquaintance rapes are serious crimes that can have a devastating impact on their victims.

In Canada, one in every 17 women is raped in her lifetime. Approximately 80 percent of assaults take place in a victim's home and about one-half of all rapes occur on dates. The most likely victims are girls and young women aged 15–24 years.[110]

The motives of rapists vary. Those who attack strangers often have problems establishing intimate relationships, have poor self-esteem, feel inadequate, and may have been sexually abused as children. Some rapists report a long history of fantasizing about rape and violence, generally while masturbating. Others commit rape out of anger that they can't express toward a wife or girlfriend. The more sexually aggressive men have been, the more likely they are to see such aggression and violence as normal and to believe rape myths, such as that it's impossible to rape a woman who doesn't really want sex. Sexually violent and degrading photographs, films, books, magazines, and videos may contribute to some rapists' aggressive behaviours. Hardcore pornography depicting violent rape has been strongly associated with judging oneself capable of sexual coercion and aggression and with engaging in such acts.

Alcohol and drugs also play a major role. Many rapists drink prior to an assault, and alcohol may interfere with a victim's ability to avoid danger or resist attack.

For many years, the victims of rape were blamed for doing something to bring on the attack. Researchers have since shown that women are raped because they encounter sexually aggressive men, not because they look or act a certain way. Although no woman is immune to attack, many rape victims are children or adolescents. Women who were sexually abused or raped as children are at greater risk than others. Scientists are exploring the reasons for this greater vulnerability.

Women who successfully escape rape attempts do so by resisting verbally and physically, usually by yelling and fleeing. Women who use forceful verbal or physical resistance (screaming, hitting, kicking, biting, and running) are more likely to avoid rape than women who try pleading, crying, or offering no resistance.

✓ CHECK-IN

Have you encountered any form of sexual coercion? Do you know any victims of sexual assault? Do you know any perpetrators?

Acquaintance or Date Rape Most rapes are committed by someone who is known to the victim. Both women and men report having been forced into sexual activity by someone they know. Many college and university students are in the age group most likely to face this threat: women aged 16–25 and men under 25.

Women who describe incidents of sexual coercion that meet the legal definition of rape often don't label it as such. They may have a preconceived notion that true rape consists of a blitz-like attack by a stranger, or they may blame themselves for getting into a situation from which they couldn't escape. They may feel some genuine concern for others who would be devastated if they knew the truth (e.g., if the rapist were the brother of a good friend or the son of a neighbour).

The same factors that lead to other forms of sexual victimization can set the stage for date rape. Socialization into an aggressive role, acceptance of rape myths, and a view that force is justified in certain situations increase the likelihood of a man's committing date rape. Some men also believe that when a woman is silent or acts in a passive way that she might want to be touched or have sex.[111]

Other factors can also play a role:

- **Personality and early sexual experiences.** Certain factors may predispose individuals to sexual aggression, including first sexual experience at a very young age, earlier and more frequent than usual childhood sexual experiences (both forced and voluntary), hostility toward women, irresponsibility, lack of social consciousness, and a need for dominance over sexual partners.
- **Situational variables (what happens during the date).** Men who initiate a date, pay all expenses, and provide transportation are more likely to be sexually aggressive, perhaps because they feel they are in a power position.
- **Acceptance of sexual coercion.** Some social groups, such as athletic teams, may encourage the use of alcohol; reinforce stereotypes about masculinity; and emphasize violence, force, and competition. The group's shared values, including an acceptance of sexual coercion, may keep individuals from questioning their behaviour.
- **Drinking.** Alcohol use is one of the strongest predictors of acquaintance rape. Men who have been drinking may not react to subtle signals, may misinterpret a woman's behaviour as a come-on, and may feel more sexually aroused. At the same time, drinking may impair a woman's ability to effectively communicate her wishes and to cope with a man's aggressiveness.
- **Date-rape drugs.** Drugs such as Rohypnol (roofie, La Rocha, rope, Mexican Valium, Rib Roche, R-2), a tranquilizer used overseas, and gamma hydroxybutyrate (GHB), a depressant with potential benefits for people with narcolepsy, have been implicated in cases of acquaintance or date rape. Since both are odourless, colourless, and tasteless, victims have no way of knowing whether their drink has been tampered with. The subsequent loss of memory leaves victims with no explanation for where they've been or what has happened. Rohypnol can cause impaired motor skills and judgment, lack of inhibitions, dizziness, confusion, lethargy, very low blood pressure, coma, and death. Deaths also have been attributed to GHB overdoses.
- **Gender differences in interpreting sexual cues.** In research comparing college men and women, the men typically overestimated the woman's sexual availability and interest, seeing friendliness, revealing clothing, and attractiveness as deliberately seductive. In one study of date rape, the men reported feeling "led on," in part because their female partners seemed to be dressed more suggestively than usual.

✓ CHECK-IN

What steps do you take to prevent acquaintance rape?

How Can I Prevent Date Rape? Take note of the following points:

- Remember that it's okay to not "score" on a date. And don't assume that a sexy dress or casual flirting are an invitation to sex.
- Be aware of your partner's actions. If she/he pulls away or tries to get up, understand that a message is being sent—one you should acknowledge and respect.
- Restrict drinking, drug use, or other behaviours (such as hanging out with a group known to be sexually aggressive in certain situations) that could affect your judgment and ability to act responsibly.
- Think of the way you would want your friend to be treated by her/his date. Behave in the same manner.
- Back away from a man who pressures you into other activities you don't want to engage in on a date, such as chugging beer or drag racing with his friends.
- Be aware that some messages and behaviour may be interpreted as sexual teasing.
- Despite your clearly stated intentions, if your date behaves in a sexually coercive manner, use a strategy of escalating forcefulness—direct refusal, vehement verbal refusal.
- Avoid using alcohol or other drugs when you definitely do not wish to be sexually intimate with your date.

It has been many years since Parliament rewrote the *Criminal Code* (1999) to make it clear that voluntary consent is a prerequisite to any sexual activity. Unfortunately, old myths and stereotypes continue to surface in Canada's courtrooms and in the minds of some Canadians. *No Means No* campaigns, on many campuses across the country, continue to raise the issue of violence against women. Attitudes, behaviours, and beliefs that discourage violence at the individual, community, and societal levels must be embraced.[112]

Male Rape No one knows how common male rape is because men are less likely to report such assaults than women. Researchers estimate that the victims in about 10 percent of acquaintance rape cases are men. These hidden victims often keep silent because of embarrassment, shame, or humiliation, as well as their own feelings and fears about homosexuality and conforming to conventional gender roles.[113]

Although many people think men who rape other men are always homosexuals, most male rapists consider themselves to be heterosexual. Young boys aren't the only victims. The average age of the male rape victim is 24. Rape is a serious problem in prison, where men may experience brutal assaults by men who usually resume sexual relations with women once they are released.

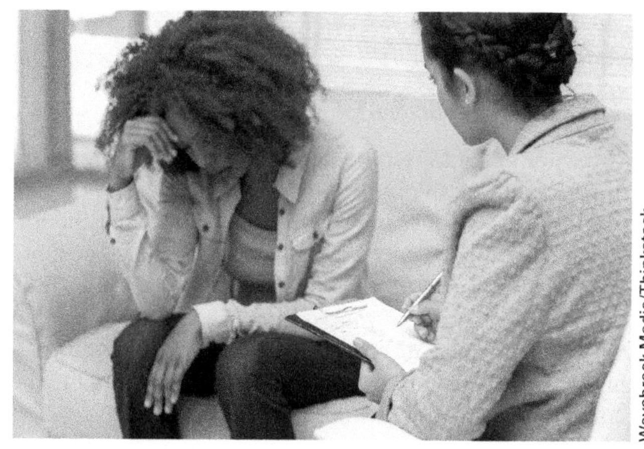

Wavebreak Media/Thinkstock

Counselling from a trained professional can help ease the trauma suffered by a rape victim.

Impact of Rape Rape-related injuries include unexplained vaginal discharge, bleeding, infections, multiple bruises, and fractured ribs. Victims of sexual violence often develop chronic symptoms, such as headaches, backaches, high blood pressure, sleep disorders, pelvic pain, and fertility problems, as well as STIs and HIV infections. But sexual violence has both a physical and a psychological impact. The psychological scars of a sexual assault take a long time to heal. Therapists have linked sexual victimization with hopelessness, low self-esteem, high levels of self-criticism, and self-defeating relationships. An estimated 30–50 percent of women develop post-traumatic stress disorder following a rape. Many do not seek counselling until a year or more after an attack, when their symptoms have become chronic or intensified.[114]

Acquaintance rape may cause fewer physical injuries but greater psychological torment. Often too ashamed to tell anyone what happened, victims may suffer alone, without skilled therapists or sympathetic friends to reassure them. Women raped by acquaintances blame themselves more, see themselves less positively, question their judgment, have greater difficulty trusting others, and have higher levels of psychological distress. Nightmares, anxiety, and flashbacks are common. The women may avoid others, become less capable of protecting themselves, and continue to be haunted by sexual violence for years. A therapist can help these victims begin the slow process of healing.

What to Do in Case of Rape If a person has been raped, she/he will have to decide whether to report the attack to the police. Even an unsuccessful rape attempt should be reported because the information provided about the attack—the assaulter's physical characteristics, voice, clothes, car, even an unusual smell—may prevent another person from being raped.

Only a small percentage of college and university students who are raped report their assault to police; many don't even tell a close friend or relative about the assault. If you are raped you should call a friend or a rape-crisis centre. A rape victim should not bathe or change her/his clothes before calling the police. Semen, hair, and material under fingernails or on apparel all may be useful in identifying the person who was the rapist.

A rape victim who chooses to go to a doctor or hospital should remember that she/he might not necessarily have to talk to police. A doctor can collect the necessary evidence, which will then be available later if the decision is made to report the rape to police. All rape victims should talk with a doctor or healthcare worker about testing and treatment for sexually transmitted infections and post-intercourse conception.

Many rape victims find it very helpful to contact a rape-crisis centre, where qualified staff members assist in dealing with the trauma. These individuals can also put victims in touch with other survivors of rape and support groups. Many colleges and universities have such programs. It is important to remember that the victim hasn't committed a crime.

Halting Sexual Violence: Prevention Efforts Sexual violence has its roots in social attitudes and beliefs that demean women and condone aggression. According to international research, much sexual violence takes place within families, marriage, and dating relationships. In many settings, rape is a culturally approved strategy to control and discipline women. In these places, laws and policies to improve women's status are critical to ending sexual coercion.

All men and women should recognize misleading rape myths and develop effective ways of communicating to avoid misinterpretation of sexual cues. Students should also know to whom they can turn to learn more about and seek help for sexual victimization: counsellors, campus police, deans of student affairs, and campus chaplains.

First Nations groups are moving forward on family-violence programs. One such program is administered by Indigenous and Northern Affairs Canada (INAC).[115]

SELF-SURVEY

How Safe Is Your School?

There are many aspects to consider when thinking about staying safe on campus or moving to a new home or new city to attend a college or university. Ask yourself the following questions. Check a "yes" or "no" answer. The more "yes" checks, the more support you have to stay safe. Take responsibility to make your own Safety Plan so you can enjoy college and university living. The focus of this self-survey is for students living on campus, but many of the safety tips are helpful to students living off campus too.

Staying Safe on Campus—In the Residence

Are there single-sex residence dorms?	❑ YES	❑ NO
Are there first-year student residence dorms?	❑ YES	❑ NO
Are there health and wellness–themed residence floors or dorms?	❑ YES	❑ NO
Is alcohol prohibited for students under the legal age for consumption?	❑ YES	❑ NO
Is illegal drug use prohibited for all students?	❑ YES	❑ NO
Does your building have door alarms?	❑ YES	❑ NO
Are students asked NOT to prop doors open?	❑ YES	❑ NO
Are the doors to the residences or dorms kept locked day and night?	❑ YES	❑ NO
Are the individual residence floors locked day and night?	❑ YES	❑ NO
Do the residence buildings have smoke alarms?	❑ YES	❑ NO
Do the residence buildings have carbon monoxide alarms?	❑ YES	❑ NO
Do the individual dorm rooms have smoke alarms?	❑ YES	❑ NO
Do you know where your fire escape exits are?	❑ YES	❑ NO
Are you aware of a fire escape plan?	❑ YES	❑ NO
Do you have a fire extinguisher in your dorm room?	❑ YES	❑ NO
Do you and your roommates know how to use a fire extinguisher?	❑ YES	❑ NO
Are there Resident Advisors, community leaders, or equivalent who oversee security of the residence, the dorms, and the students on a 24-hour basis?	❑ YES	❑ NO
Is the exterior well lit?	❑ YES	❑ NO
Are lower-floor windows secured?	❑ YES	❑ NO
Are shrubs and trees around the building windows cut back?	❑ YES	❑ NO
If you are on an upper floor, are you able to secure your windows?	❑ YES	❑ NO
Does your door include a peephole?	❑ YES	❑ NO
Is there a deadbolt on your room door?	❑ YES	❑ NO
Is your bathroom in your dorm room?	❑ YES	❑ NO
Are the bathrooms shared?	❑ YES	❑ NO
Do you have single-sex bathrooms?	❑ YES	❑ NO
Are single-sex bathrooms kept locked?	❑ YES	❑ NO
Is there safety education programming?	❑ YES	❑ NO
Are there support groups for students?	❑ YES	❑ NO

Health Services

Is a rape crisis centre accessible?	❑ YES	❑ NO
Are alcohol or drug counsellors available?	❑ YES	❑ NO
Are student AA meetings available?	❑ YES	❑ NO
Is there protocol for disciplinary probation?	❑ YES	❑ NO
Is there protocol for residence or dorm violations?	❑ YES	❑ NO
Is there protocol for off-campus citations?	❑ YES	❑ NO
Is there support for sexualized harassment or violence?	❑ YES	❑ NO
Is there support for LGBTQ-identified students, staff, and faculty?	❑ YES	❑ NO

Campus Security Services

Is there a community police force connected to the college or university campus?	❑ YES	❑ NO
Is there a campus and security service department or unit on your campus?	❑ YES	❑ NO
Do security guards patrol overnight?	❑ YES	❑ NO
Do security guards patrol during the day?		
Do security guards carry firearms?	❑ YES	❑ NO
Are there security guard bicycle patrols?	❑ YES	❑ NO
Are there surveillance cameras in the residence buildings or on the campus?	❑ YES	❑ NO
Are the emergency phones located on campus and in the residences in working condition?	❑ YES	❑ NO
Does the college or university offer programs such as Safewalk, Campus Alone, or campus escort services 24 hours/day?	❑ YES	❑ NO
Are there shuttle services available on campus for transportation between academic and recreation buildings?	❑ YES	❑ NO
Does the college or university offer emergency updates and alerts on mobile devices? These can include mobile safety apps, Twitter feeds, or voice mail notifications.	❑ YES	❑ NO

Tips for Students

Act Now—to put a safety plan in place.

1. Always lock your dorm room door and don't loan your key to anyone.
2. Be very careful about sharing personal information on social networking sites.
3. Never walk alone at night. Use the campus escort services, Safewalk, or the buddy system.

4. Share your daily class and activities schedule with close friends and family. If you are going somewhere alone, tell a friend or family member where you will be and when you are coming back.
5. Know where emergency phones are located. Program the campus security number into your cellphone. Keep your cellphone charged!
6. Don't take a drink, alcoholic or otherwise, from anyone. It may be spiked with a date-rape drug.
7. Purchase tenant insurance for personal belongings. Many students are now insured for theft or fire.

Sources: *How safe is your college?* Retrieved September 17, 2009, from http://www.thedailybeast.com/; Lucier, Kelci Lynn. *15 ways to stay safe while in college*, ©2013. http://collegelife.about.com/od/healthwellness/qt/SafetyTips.htm. All rights reserved; *How to stay safe in the dorms*. http://www.sheknows.com; Safety Services Company. (n.d.). *The complete university guide. Top tips to staying safe*. www.thecompleteuniversityguide.co.uk/preparing-to-go/staying-safe-and-secure/top-tips-to-stay-safe/; University of Victoria. (2013). *Campus and personal safety*. www.uvic.ca/future-students/undergraduate/safety/

Chapter Summary

1. You can help keep yourself safe by doing all of the following except which factor?
   a. using seat belts when driving or a passenger
   b. wearing pyjamas made of non-flammable materials
   c. removing or fixing loose carpets
   d. hiking without an emergency plan
2. Which factor affects an individual's risk of accident or injury?
   a. a first-aid kit in the car
   b. stress level
   c. amount of automobile insurance coverage
   d. knowledge of CPR
3. Which of the following is NOT a safe-driving tip?
   a. Avoid driving at night for the first year after getting a licence.
   b. Make sure your car has snow tires or chains before driving in hazardous, snowy conditions.
   c. If riding with an intoxicated driver, keep talking to him so that he doesn't fall asleep at the wheel.
   d. Don't let packages or people obstruct the rear or side windows of a car.
4. Which statement about home safety is true?
   a. Falls do not pose the greatest threat of injury in the home.
   b. The three ingredients of fire are fuel, a heat source, and oxygen.
   c. The risk of falls is lowest in the elderly.
   d. When using cleaning products, make sure that windows are tightly closed.
5. Which statement about recreational safety hazards is true?
   a. Hypothermia is a life-threatening medical emergency caused by the inability of the body to cool itself.
   b. The most common heat-related condition is heat stroke.
   c. Most drownings occur at organized facilities.
   d. Frostbite usually affects the tissues of the hands and feet.
6. Which statement about hate crimes is false?
   a. Over half of all hate crimes are motivated by race or ethnicity.
   b. Often violent hate crimes involve the threat of force.
   c. Hate-crime victims sustain only minor injuries.
   d. The most common types of hate-crime violations include mischief or vandalism, assault, uttering threats, and hate propaganda.
7. Which statement about violence on college and university campuses is false?
   a. Property crimes account for most crimes on campus.
   b. On college and university campuses, crimes are most often committed by outside community members.
   c. Students must cope with the dangers of alcohol, drugs, fire, and even gambling.
   d. Crime statistics for colleges and universities are posted on the Internet.
8. Which statement about sexual victimization is true?
   a. It includes sexual harassment, sexual coercion, and rape.
   b. It is gender-specific, affecting women who are violated emotionally or physically by men.
   c. It is rare in academic environments such as college campuses.
   d. It most commonly takes the form of physical assault and stalking.
9. Which statement about rape is true?
   a. When a person is sexually attacked by a stranger, it is referred to as rape. When a person is sexually attacked by an acquaintance, it is referred to as sexual coercion.
   b. Statutory rape is defined as sexual intercourse initiated by a woman under the age of consent.
   c. Men who rape other men usually consider themselves heterosexuals.
   d. Women who are raped flirt and dress provocatively. They are typically more willing to participate in aggressive sex than women who dress conservatively and do not flirt.
10. What should you do if you have been raped?
    a. report the attack
    b. refrain from bathing, showering, or changing your clothes
    c. not talk to any of your friends or family
    d. both a & b

Answers to these questions can be found on page 399.

SELF-RESPONSIBILITY—SOCIAL RESPONSIBILITY

SELF-RESPONSIBILITY

I want to LIVE my life. For me that means taking chances. I will not let fear stop me from doing things that I really want to do.

Ray Greenlaw

SOCIAL RESPONSIBILITY

Relationships are all there is. Everything in the universe only exists because it is in relationship to everything else. Nothing exists in isolation. We have to stop pretending we are individuals that can go it alone.

Margaret Wheatley

Taking good care in risky situations is possible if you recognize potential risks and prepare for them. There is a balance to living with purpose and living recklessly. What Stage of Change are you in when it comes to safety on the road, safety at home or work, recreational safety, and safety within your relationships? How can you stay safe—yet challenge yourself to reach your goals and visions? How do you treat others when in a relationship? Take good care of others—take good care of yourself. Respect others—respect yourself.

CRITICAL THINKING

1. Can you name two risk factors in your daily life that might increase the likelihood of accidental injury? What actions have you taken to keep yourself safe?
2. A friend of yours, Eric, frequently makes crude or derogatory comments about women. What might you say to him?
3. At one university, women raped by acquaintances or dates scrawled the names of their assailants on the walls of women's restrooms on campus. Several young men whose names appeared on the list objected, protesting that they were innocent and were being unfairly accused. Do you think it violates the rights of men? How do you feel about naming women who've been raped in news reports?

WEB LINKS

Canada Safety Council
www.safety-council.org
At this site you can find safety education information that can help you avoid injury. Information on safety legislation and links to public safety awareness campaigns are also available.

Centre for Children and Families in the Justice System
www.lfcc.on.ca/
Many comprehensive handbooks, manuals, publications, and reports, such as *Helping a Child Be a Witness in Court* (2011), are available online.

National Aboriginal Circle against Family Violence (NACAFV)
http://www.nacafv.ca/
This site provides you with information about culturally appropriate programs and services that address family violence. Publications, reports, and newsletters are available.

Parachute—Preventing Injuries Saving Lives
http://www.parachutecanada.org/concussion
This is a national, charitable organization that educates and encourages safety—focusing on motor vehicles, sports and recreation, and seniors' falls. If you want to know more about concussions this website will be of great interest.

Please note that links are subject to change. If you find a broken link, use a search engine such as www.google.ca and search for the website by typing in keywords.

Key Terms

The terms listed here are used within the chapter on the page indicated. Definitions of terms are in the Glossary at the end of the book.

deep frostbite 387
frostbite 387
frostnip 387
heat cramps 386
heat exhaustion 386
heat stress 386
heat stroke 386
hypothermia 387
rape 393
sexual coercion 393

Answers to Chapter Summary Questions

1. d; 2. b; 3. c; 4. b; 5. d; 6. c; 7. b; 8. a; 9. c; 10. d

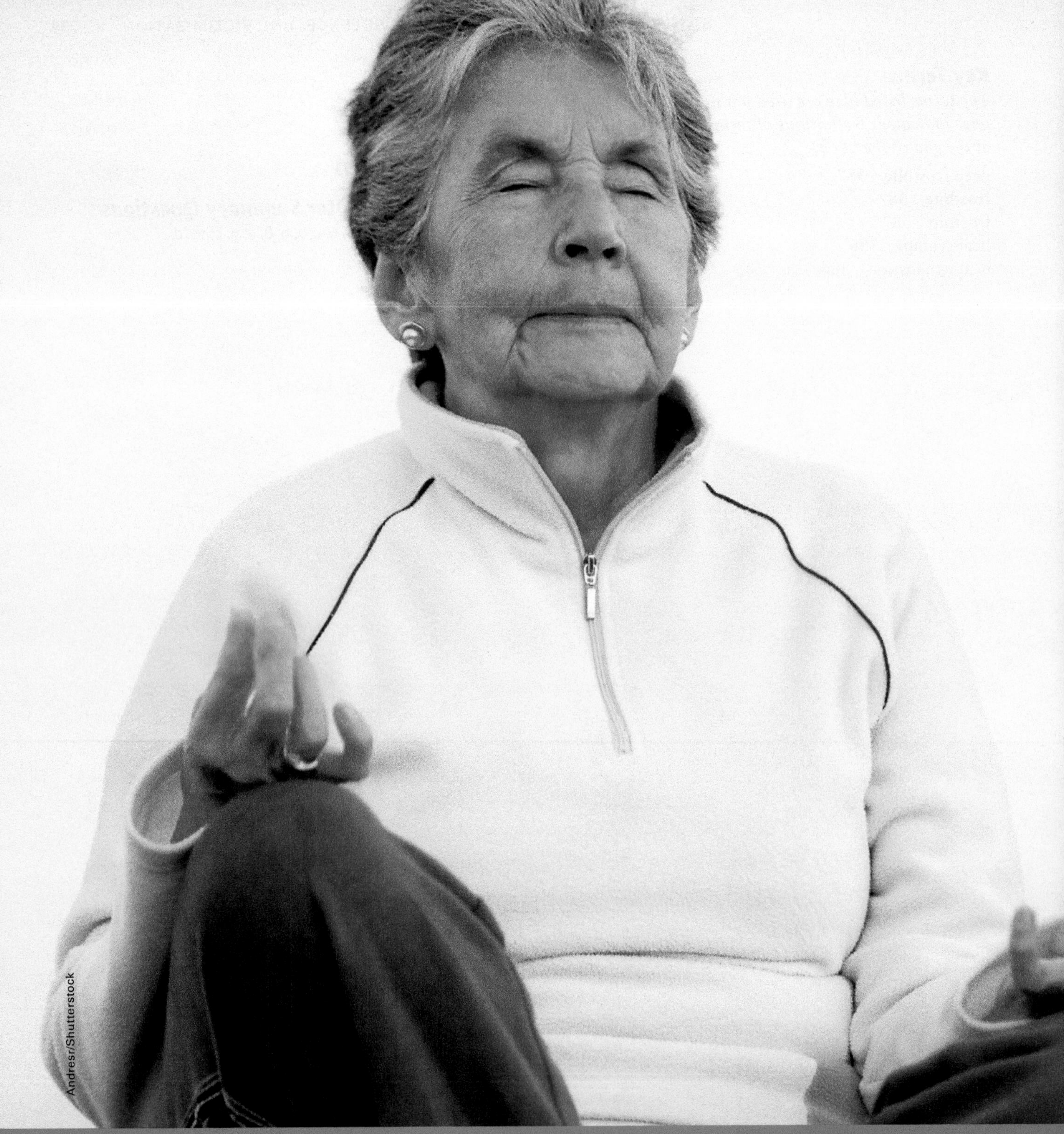
Andresr/Shutterstock

AFTER READING THIS CHAPTER, YOU WILL BE ABLE TO:

- **discuss** the various ways we define aging
- **list** the benefits that older adults can gain from physical activity
- **describe** three memory skills that diminish with age
- **explain** why many elderly people suffer from poor nutrition
- **describe** the mid-life changes in the female reproductive system
- **identify** some of the challenges of aging
- **define** death and **explain** the stages of emotional reaction experienced in facing death
- **explain** the purposes of a living will

15

Healthy Aging

Too young to worry about getting old? Think again. Whether you are in your teens, 20s, 30s, or older, you can take steps that will add healthy, active, productive years to your life.

Gerontologists,[1] health professionals who study the ways in which we adapt to **aging**,[2] define this term as the characteristic pattern of normal life changes that occur as humans grow older. Research has shown that at any age, at any stage of life, and at any level of fitness, you can do a great deal to influence the impact that the passage of time has on you. As Onedera and Stickle suggest, getting older can be a positive thing, and there are ways in which we can be active participants in the aging process.[3] More and more Canadians are extending not just their lifespan but also their *health span*—their years of health and vitality. You can do the same. Our later years can be a stage of continued personal growth, both physiologically and psychologically. There may be new opportunities to try fitness or sport pursuits and time for introspection, mentoring others, attending educational workshops or academic courses, and finishing off projects that have been on a list of things to do.

This chapter provides a preview of the changes that occur as we age and the steps you can take to age healthfully. It also explores the meaning of death, dying, and end-of-life issues. It concludes with information on advance directives and wills, and offers advice on comforting the dying and helping their survivors.

FREQUENTLY ASKED QUESTIONS

LIVING IN AN AGING SOCIETY

Older adults are now the fastest-growing age group in Canada. According to Statistics Canada, there were 5 780 900 Canadians who were 65 years of age or older in 2015.[4] This is the first time in Canadian history that the number of citizens aged 65 years and older surpassed the number of children aged 0–14 years.[5] By 2024 the estimate for older adults aged 65 years and older is expected to reach 20.1 percent of the Canadian population. While the number of people aged 65 years and older has grown in every G7 country (the seven major advanced economic countries—Canada, France, Germany, Italy, Japan, the United Kingdom, and the United States), both the United States and Canada actually have the lowest proportions of this age group at 15 percent and 16.1 percent respectively.[6] The age of Canadians does vary among the provinces and territories. Quebec, Ontario, British Columbia, and the Atlantic provinces had the highest number of adults aged 65 years and older as of July 2015. The Prairie provinces and territories reported more children aged 0–14 years old compared to people aged 65 and older.[7] Low fertility rates, an increase in life expectancy, and the effects of the baby boom are the main reasons for the aging of the Canadian population. See Figure 15-1 for a historical overview of the population of Canadians aged 0 to 14 years and 65 years and older between 1995 and 2015 and projected estimates from 2015 to 2035. See Figure 15-2 for a comparison of the proportion of the population in Canada, the provinces and territories for July 2015.[8]

Women form about 17.4 percent of the Canadian older adult population of 65 years and over. Men form about 14.7 percent.[9] This is due in part to the higher life expectancy of women, which is 84 years compared to 80 years for men.[10] Aboriginal seniors make up a relatively small proportion of Canada's Aboriginal population. However, they are living longer, and their population is growing significantly. In 2001, 39 000 Aboriginal seniors represented 4 percent of the total Aboriginal population. This percentage is expected to rise to 6.5 percent by 2017.[11] War veterans who served in World Wars I and II or the Korean conflict make up a significant segment of our senior population. In Canada, approximately one in five male seniors has served in wartime.

It is estimated that just over one in four Canadian seniors was born outside Canada. Many of them immigrated when they were children or young adults. While a number of seniors can speak one or both of Canada's official languages, there are older adults who are unable to speak either English or French. More females than males are unable to converse in either of our official languages.

Throughout your life, you will confront a variety of issues related not just to your own age but also to that of the overall aging Canadian population. These include the following:

- **Retirement costs.** Unless changes are made to decrease the demand on the Old Age Security program (OAS) and the Canada/Quebec pension plans (CPP/QPP), taxes on workers may be increased.
- **Health costs.** Some experts argue that health costs will soar because people over age 65 use more health services and require more medical care than those who are younger. However, others contend

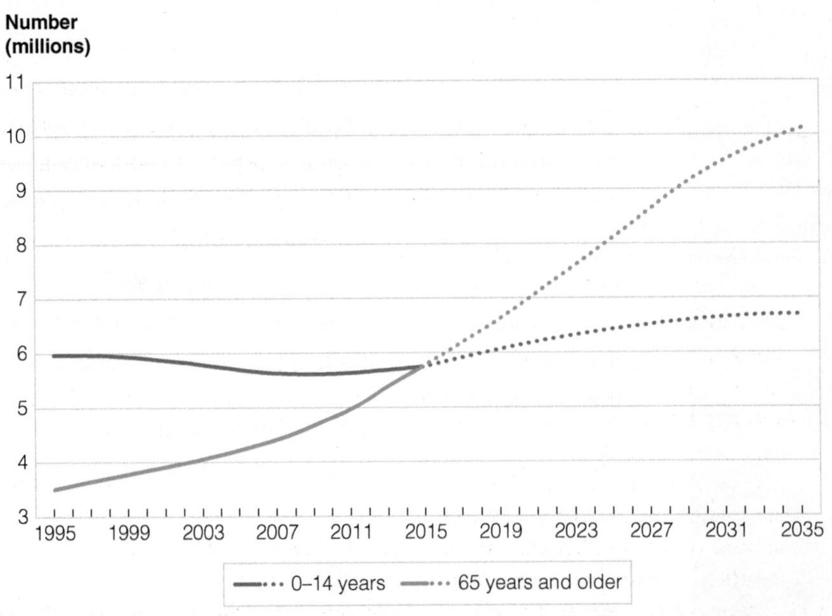

Figure 15-1 Population Aged 0 to 14 Years and 65 Years and Older, as of July 1, 1995 to 2035, Canada.
Source: Canada's population estimates: Age and sex, July 1, 2015. *The Daily*. http://www.statcan.gc.ca/daily-quotidien/150929/dq150929b-eng.htm (Chart 3).

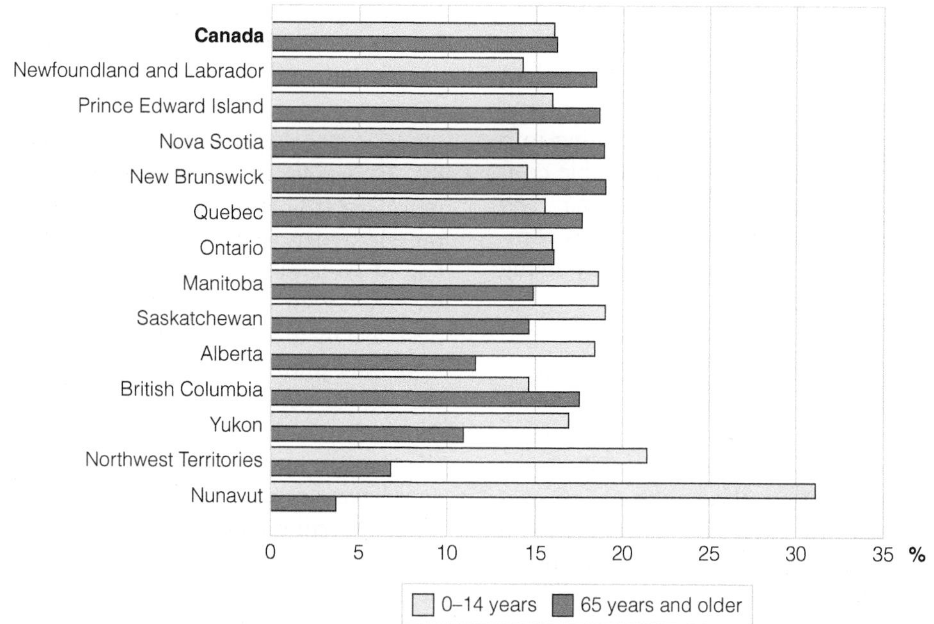

Figure 15-2 **Proportion of the Population Aged 0 to 14 Years and 65 Years and Older, July 1, 2015, Canada, Provinces and Territories**
Source: Canada's population estimates: Age and sex, July 1, 2015. *The Daily.* http://www.statcan.gc.ca/daily-quotidien/150929/dq150929b-eng.htm (Chart 4).

that nations with a large elderly population do not necessarily spend more of their national wealth on healthcare.

- **Grey-power politics.** Senior citizens go to the polls in larger numbers than younger voters. With such voting power, programs for the elderly may make up a larger share of future federal budgets.

✓ CHECK-IN

How old is the oldest person you know? Do you expect to live as long as that person? Why? Or why not?

SUCCESSFUL AGING

The life expectancy of Canadian seniors has risen substantially over the course of the last century. Canadians are not only living longer but also are staying healthy and independent longer. According to a report from the Canadian Institute for Health Research,[12] the majority of Canadians who are under the age of 85 do not report any limitations in functional capacity. Fewer seniors are smoking, and obesity rates among seniors who are 65–74 years of age have also decreased. Among the factors contributing to a longer health span are improved medical care, diet, exercise, and public-health advances.

Genes, as studies of identical twins have revealed, influence only about 30 percent of the rate and ways in which we age. "The rest is up to us," says Michael Roizen, M.D., author of *RealAge*, who notes that it's possible to become healthier, fitter, and biologically younger with time. "With relatively simple changes, someone whose chronological age is 69 can have a physiological age of 45. And the most amazing thing is that it's never too late to live younger."[13] Roizen's comment reminds us that there are a number of different ways we can define aging:

- **Chronological age**—how old we are in calendar years measured by time such as years and months[14]
- **Functional age**—a combination of chronological, physiological, and emotional ages[15]
- **Physiological age**—the normal functioning of our bodies as controlled by the interactions between physical and chemical bodily states
- **Psychological age**—an individual perception of how "old" a person feels, sometimes based on an individual's behaviour[16]
- **Social age**—determined by how well people cope with their social roles[17]

✓ CHECK-IN

How successfully do you think you will age? What do you think will help you the most? What may get in your way?

FIT FOR LIFE

At one time, medical experts thought that aging meant weakness, frailty, and declining strength. Certainly, there are physiological changes that alert us to the aging process and they will be discussed in this section; however, we do know that no one is ever too old to benefit from a regular exercise program. Rather than telling seniors to take it easy, the Active Living Coalition for Older Adults recommends engaging in a full range of physical activities, including aerobic conditioning, muscle fitness, and flexibility training.[18] As much as 50 percent of the physiological declines commonly attributed to aging are due to sedentary living and can be dramatically reversed.

Why Is Physical Activity Important as We Age? A proactive health-promoting behaviour, such as exercising, contributes to a high quality of life, even when begun late in life.[19] People who are not physically fit are more likely to die younger than those who are, even if they are physically healthy. Exercise is so effective in preserving well-being that gerontologists sometimes describe it as the closest thing to an anti-aging pill. It slows many changes associated with advancing age, such as loss of lean muscle tissue, increase in body fat, and decreased work capacity. It lowers the risk of heart disease and stroke in the elderly—and greatly improves general health.[20] Male and female runners over age 50 have much lower rates of disability and much lower healthcare expenses than less active seniors. Even less intense activities, such as gardening, dancing, and brisk walking, can delay chronic disability.[21]

Cardiovascular Fitness and Aging As we age, one of the major changes of the cardiovascular system is the decrease of elasticity of the aorta and arteries. The job of the left ventricle of the heart is to eject blood into the aorta that is then pumped to all parts of our body through the arteries. With increased stiffness of the aorta and arteries, there is an increased resistance to accepting the blood volume when the heart pumps. The result is an increase in the systolic aortic pressure, a decrease in the lower diastolic pressure, and an increase in pulse pressure.[22] Continued pressure places great wear and tear on artery walls, which in turn can lead to a stroke or a heart attack. We do know, though, that regular physical activity can lower this risk.[23]

Despite these potential benefits, 60 percent of older adults in Canada are inactive.[24] Yet as Sharatt states, it is never too late to gain significant benefits from participating in an exercise program.[25] Results from a number of studies have shown that regular physical exercise can help keep older adults functioning and mobile. The Canadian Society of Exercise Physiology has developed Physical Activity Guidelines for Older Adults, 65 years and older[26] (see Figure 15-3). Older adults are encouraged to accumulate at least 150 minutes of moderate- to vigorous-intensity aerobic physical activity per week in bouts of 10 minutes or more. Suggested activities include brisk walking, biking, swimming, and cross-country skiing.

Skeletal Muscle Fitness and Aging Skeletal muscles cover 40–50 percent of the human body. As we age, skeletal muscles get both smaller and weaker.[27] This change in muscle structure is called **sarcopenia**—the degenerative loss of skeletal muscle mass and strength.[28] By the time we are about 70 years of age, muscle strength can decrease by about 30–40 percent. We maintain muscle fibre bulk until we are about 40–50 years of age, but by the age of 80, loss of muscle fibre bulk can be up to 30 percent.[29] Fat tissue replaces the muscle fibre and there is often an increase in fibrosis. Muscle weakness can have an impact on the overall health of older adults. Getting in and out of chairs, going up and down stairs, lifting items, walking, and functioning on a daily basis can become difficult.[30]

The Canadian Physical Activity Guidelines for Older Adults, 65 years and older, suggest that muscle- and bone-strengthening activities using major muscle groups be done at least two days a week (see Figure 15-3). Stronger muscles help to prevent falls and enhance balance. Strength or resistance training does not stop the process of sarcopenia but helps to maintain and, in some cases, even build muscle mass and strength at any age. Ploutzt-Snyder, Druger, and Manini's study reconfirms that strength exercise is an effective way to improve strength of older adults. A progressive program that increases the intensity of the exercise is important for optimal benefits.[31]

Bone Health and Aging Bones are an important organ of our body. They are made up of bone tissue known as osseous tissue (the major structural and supportive connective tissue of the body), bone marrow, blood vessels, and nerves. They not only produce red and white blood cells but also support our body, help us move, and protect other organs. They are both lightweight and hard and come in a variety of shapes and sizes. It is the osseous tissue (the mineralized connective tissue) that gives bones their rigidity and also their honeycomb-like three-dimensional internal structure.

In our younger years, bones grow stronger because bone mineral accumulates and lays down more bone tissue. When we fully mature, the bone mineral accumulation and loss of bone mineral are about equal. However, as we move into our middle and adult years, bone mineral loss surpasses the bone mineral growth. The results include a deterioration of our bone tissue, bones becoming fragile, brittle, and porous, and the onset for many older adults of a condition called **osteoporosis**.

Canadian Physical Activity Guidelines

FOR OLDER ADULTS - 65 YEARS & OLDER

Guidelines

To achieve health benefits, and improve functional abilities, adults aged 65 years and older should accumulate at least 150 minutes of moderate- to vigorous-intensity aerobic physical activity per week, in bouts of 10 minutes or more.

It is also beneficial to add muscle and bone strengthening activities using major muscle groups, at least 2 days per week.

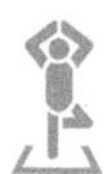

Those with poor mobility should perform physical activities to enhance balance and prevent falls.

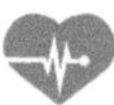

More physical activity provides greater health benefits.

Let's Talk Intensity!

Moderate-intensity physical activities will cause older adults to sweat a little and to breathe harder. Activities like:

- Brisk walking
- Bicycling

Vigorous-intensity physical activities will cause older adults to sweat and be 'out of breath'. Activities like:

- Cross-country skiing
- Swimming

Being active for at least **150 minutes** per week can help reduce the risk of:

- Chronic disease (such as high blood pressure and heart disease) and,
- Premature death

And also help to:

- Maintain functional independence
- Maintain mobility
- Improve fitness
- Improve or maintain body weight
- Maintain bone health and,
- Maintain mental health and feel better

Pick a time. Pick a place. Make a plan and move more!

☑ Join a community urban poling or mall walking group.
☑ Go for a brisk walk around the block after lunch.
☑ Take a dance class in the afternoon.
☑ Train for and participate in a run or walk for charity!
☑ Take up a favourite sport again.
☑ Be active with the family! Plan to have "active reunions".
☑ Go for a nature hike on the weekend.
☑ Take the dog for a walk after dinner.

Now is the time. Walk, run, or wheel, and embrace life.

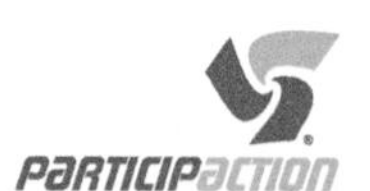

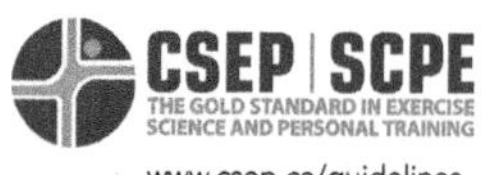

PARTICIPACTION

CSEP | SCPE
THE GOLD STANDARD IN EXERCISE SCIENCE AND PERSONAL TRAINING
www.csep.ca/guidelines

Figure 15-3 Canadian Physical Activity Guidelines for Older Adults, 65 Years and Older

Source: Canadian Physical Activity Guidelines, © 2011, 2012. Used with permission from the Canadian Society for Exercise Physiology, www.csep.ca/guidelines.

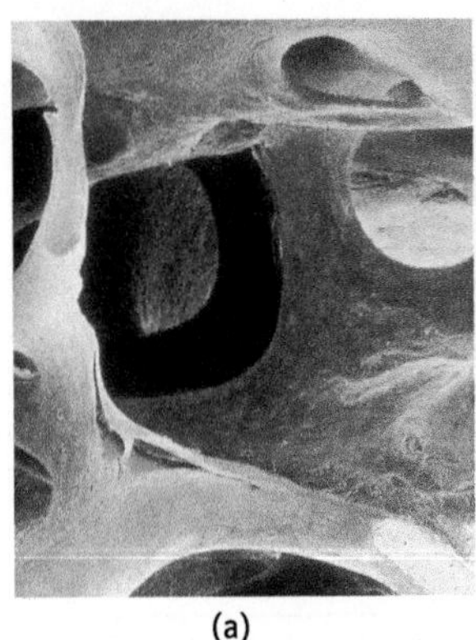

(a)

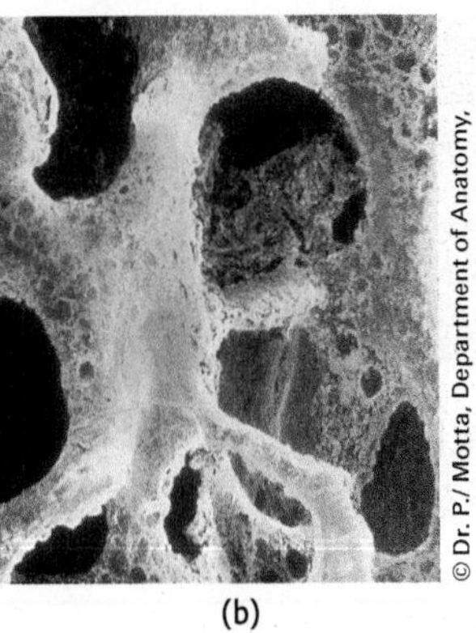

(b)

Figure 15-4 The Effect of Osteoporosis on Bone Density

(a) Normal bone tissue.

(b) After the onset of osteoporosis, bones lose density and become hollow and brittle.

If someone has osteoporosis the loss in bone density can become so severe that a bone will break after even slight trauma or injury (see Figure 15-4). Women have smaller skeletons and are more vulnerable than men; in extreme cases, their spines may become so fragile that just bending causes severe pain.

The Osteoporosis Society of Canada states that two million Canadians suffer from osteoporosis and that one in three women and one in five men will suffer from an osteoporosis fracture sometime in their lifetime. The cost of treating this disease and the fractures it caused was estimated to be $2.3 billion in Canada in 2010.[32]

Various factors can increase a woman's risk of developing osteoporosis, including family history (a mother, grandmother, or sister with osteoporosis, fractures, height loss, or humped shoulders); petite body structure; Caucasian or Asian background; menopause before age 40; the rate of postmenopausal bone loss; smoking; heavy alcohol consumption; loss of ovarian function through chemotherapy, radiation, or hysterectomy; low calcium intake; and a sedentary lifestyle.

In the past, doctors often prescribed hormone replacement therapy to protect aging bones; this is no longer the recommended practice. Alternatives include raloxifene (Evista®), bisphosphonates (Didrocal®, Fosamax®, and Actonel®) that slow the breakdown of bone and may even increase bone density, and calcitonin, a naturally occurring hormone that increases bone mass in the spine. Other possible therapies are sodium fluoride, parathyroid hormone (PTH), and some forms of Vitamin D.[33]

Osteoporosis doesn't begin in old age. In fact, the best time for preventive action is early in life. Increased calcium intake and Vitamin D are important. So is regular physical activity, especially in the first three decades of life. When we are physically active we increase the load or force on our bones. The bones then respond by forming new bone and remodelling old bone to become stronger. Bones in our legs, back, and wrists must be stimulated by physical activity so that their structure and strength can be maintained. Starting a regular physical activity program at a young age helps to build peak bone mass. Staying active throughout mid- and older life helps to maintain the bone mass. Physical activity not only improves the strength of the bone but also helps to reduce the risk of falls because of increased muscle strength and endurance, which helps balance and coordination issues and can sometimes reduce joint pain and help people with osteoporosis to function better on a daily basis.

Older adults who have not exercised regularly throughout their lifetime and have osteoporosis are still encouraged to participate in regular physical activity, although the exercise session would have to be adapted so as not to increase the risk of injury. There are many specialized physical activity programs offered for older adults in community recreation and fitness centres across Canada. One such program is called Osteofit,[34] developed with assistance from specialists from the B.C. Women's Osteoporosis Program.

Flexibility and Aging As we age, physiological changes can result in a decrease in our musculoskeletal flexibility level. As our connective tissue becomes stiffer and we lose muscle function, a decreased range of motion (ROM) can lead to incorrect body alignment and tight muscles. These changes can result in the risk of accidents such as falling.[35]

Incorporating stretching exercises into daily life at any age can help. However, stretching is especially important as we age. Other activities that improve flexibility are Tai Chi,[36] yoga, and chair stretching. Research does show that, just like aerobic conditioning and muscle strength and endurance training for older adults, a regular stretching routine can maintain or increase flexibility levels of older adults.[37]

✓ CHECK-IN

Are you active enough to keep your body as strong and fit as possible?

Nutrition Issues for Older Adults Many elderly people who live independently do not get adequate amounts of one or more essential nutrients. Among the nutrients often lacking in older adults are folate, Vitamin D, calcium, Vitamin E, magnesium, Vitamins B^6 and B^{12}, Vitamin C, and zinc. The reasons are many: limited income, difficulty getting to stores, chronic illness, medications that interfere with the metabolism of nutrients, problems chewing or digesting, poor appetite, inactivity, illness, depression, and lack of sunshine in some parts of Canada.

STRATEGIES FOR PREVENTION

Lowering Your Risk of Osteoporosis

Regardless of your age and gender, you can prevent future bone problems by taking some protective steps now. The most important guidelines are as follows:

- Get adequate calcium. Aim for 1200 milligrams a day.
- Exercise regularly. Both aerobic exercise and weight training can help preserve bone density.
- Drink alcohol only moderately. More than two or three alcoholic beverages a day interferes with intestinal calcium absorption.
- Don't smoke. Smokers tend to be thin (a risk factor for osteoporosis) and enter menopause earlier, thus extending the period of jeopardy from estrogen loss.
- Let the sunshine in (but don't forget your sunscreen). Vitamin D, a vitamin produced in the skin in reaction to sunlight, boosts calcium absorption.

Dietitians urge the elderly, as they do all Canadians, to concentrate on eating healthful foods; many also recommend daily nutritional supplements, which may provide the added benefit of improving cognitive function in healthy people over 65. In a study of 86 older people living independently who took either a supplement or a placebo, those taking the supplement showed significant improvements in short-term memory, problem-solving ability, abstract thinking, and attention.[38]

In Canada, many seniors are widowed. Among widowed seniors, eating disorders are considered to be one of the most troubling problems related to bereavement. A disruption of normal patterns of eating, meal skipping, less dietary variety, and reduced home food preparation often result in poor health.[39]

Does Body Composition Change with Age? Both weight and body-fat percentage typically increase in adulthood. Starting in their 20s, many men and women put on an average of 0.45 kilograms (1 pound) of weight a year. By age 65, they have gained about 18 kilograms (40 pounds). Because activity levels decline with age, the average individual also loses 0.22 kilograms (0.5 pounds) of lean body mass a year. The result is a change in body composition over time: a 9-kilogram (20-pound) loss of lean tissue and an 18-kilogram (40-pound) gain in body fat.

Body composition can affect how well older adults function.[40] Researchers have documented that physical activity—both aerobic workouts and resistance exercise—can increase and maintain lean body tissue.

✓ CHECK-IN

What effects do you think your weight and body mass index may have on the way you age?

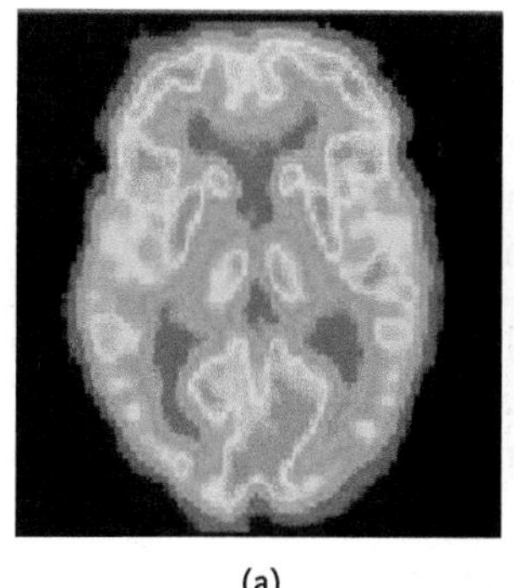

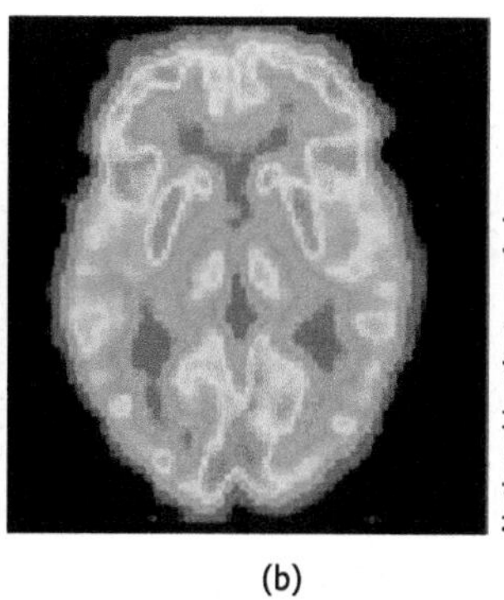

National Institute on Aging

(a) (b)

(a) PET scan of a 20-year-old brain (b) PET scan of an 80-year-old brain

In these PET scans, the red and yellow show greater neuron activity in the young adult. The brain of the older person shows less activity and more dark areas, indicating that the fluid-filled ventricles have grown larger. Recent research shows, however, that older brains do repair themselves.

THE AGING BRAIN

Scientists used to think that the aging brain, once worn out, could never be fixed. Now they know that the brain can and does repair itself. The photographs of the PET scans compare the difference between a 20-year-old brain and an 80-year-old brain. When neurons (brain cells) die, the surrounding cells develop "fingers" to fill the gaps and establish new connections, or synapses, between surviving neurons. Although self-repair occurs more quickly in young brains, the process continues in older brains. Even individuals suffering from Alzheimer's disease, the most devastating form of senility, have enough healthy cells in the diseased brain to re-grow synapses.[41] Scientists hope to develop drugs that someday may help the brain repair itself.

Mental ability does not decline along with physical vigour. Researchers have been able to reverse the supposedly normal intellectual declines of 60- to 80-year-olds by tutoring them in problem solving. Reaction time, intellectual speed and efficiency, nonverbal intelligence, and maximum work rate for short periods may diminish by age 75. However, understanding, vocabulary, ability to remember key information, and verbal intelligence remain about the same.

Thinking Young The healthiest seniors are actively engaged in life, resilient, optimistic, productive, and socially involved, observes John Rowe, M.D., of the MacArthur Foundation Research Network on Successful Aging.[42] While seniors are not immune to life's slings and arrows, successful "agers" bounce back after a setback and have a can-do attitude about the challenges they face. They also tend to be lifelong learners who may take up entirely new hobbies late in life—pursuits that stimulate production of more connections between neurons and that may slow aging within the brain.

Just as with muscles, the best advice for keeping your brain healthy as you age is "use it or lose it." Some memory loss among healthy older people is normal, but this is reversible with training in simple methods, such as word associations, that improve recall.

Memory Some memory skills, particularly the ability to retrieve names and quickly process information, inevitably diminish over time. What normal changes should you expect? Here is a preview:

- **Recalling information takes longer.** As individuals reach their mid- to late 60s, the brain slows down, but usually by just a matter of milliseconds. As long as they're not rushed, older adults eventually adapt and perform just as well as younger ones.
- **Distractions become more disruptive.** Many college and university students can study and listen to music at the same time. Thirty-something moms can soothe the baby, field questions about homework, and put together a dinner all at once. But as individuals pass age 50, they find it much more difficult to divide their attention or to remember details of a story after having switched their attention to something else.
- **"Accessing" names gets harder.** The ability to remember names, especially those you don't use frequently, diminishes by as much as 50 percent between ages 25 and 65. Preventive strategies can help, such as repeating a person's name when introduced, writing down the name as soon as possible, and making obvious associations with the name.
- **Learning new information is harder.** The quality of memory doesn't change, just the speed at which we receive, absorb, and react to information. Strategies like taking notes or outlining material become critical for older students, especially when learning new skills. However, adding to existing knowledge remains as easy as ever.
- **Wisdom matters.** In any memory test involving knowledge of the world, vocabulary, or judgment, older people outperform their younger counterparts.

Dementia and Alzheimer's Disease Dementia[43] is a syndrome that describes a group of disorders that includes a number of symptoms such as loss of memory, judgment, and reasoning, and changes in mood and behaviour. It can be caused by more than 50 different disorders, but 50–70 percent of dementia cases are caused by Alzheimer's disease, and 20–30 percent are caused by vascular disease.

Alzheimer's disease[44] is the most common form of dementia. In 2016, the government of Canada reported that there were 395 000 Canadians, 40 years and over, living with Alzheimer's and other forms of dementia. That number is predicted to rise and the estimated number of Canadians who will suffer from Alzheimer's and dementia is 674 000 in 2031.[45]

Alzheimer's involves a gradual onset and progressive deterioration of brain cells and mental capacity. At first, the symptoms resemble ordinary memory lapses. Eventually, people with Alzheimer's lose their ability to learn and remember anything new, the names of their family and friends, and their way around. People with Alzheimer's often begin avoiding social contact, become upset at otherwise trivial events, and end up having trouble dressing or feeding themselves because they are unable to remember how to function. Once their brains lose the capacity to regulate elementary body functions, people with Alzheimer's die of malnutrition, dehydration, infection, or heart failure. The average interval between early symptoms and death is 7–10 years, although it can last between 2 and 20 years.

Women are more likely to develop Alzheimer's than men. By age 85, as many as 28–30 percent of women suffer from Alzheimer's, and women with this form of dementia perform significantly worse than men in various visual, spatial, and memory tests.

Even though medical science cannot restore a brain that is in the process of being destroyed by an organic brain disease such as Alzheimer's, medications can control difficult behavioural symptoms and enhance or partially restore cognitive ability. It is important to help individuals with Alzheimer's to stay socially active and maintain relationships.[46] Often physicians find other medical or psychiatric problems, such as depression, in these patients; recognizing and treating these conditions can have a dramatic impact.

✓ CHECK-IN

How do you exercise your brain to keep it healthy? Have any of your close relatives developed cognitive impairment or Alzheimer's?

MOVING THROUGH MID-LIFE

Although men don't experience the dramatic mid-life hormonal changes that women do, their primary sex hormone, testosterone, gradually declines by 30–40 percent between ages 48 and 70. This change, sometimes called *andropause*, may cause decreased muscle mass, greater body fat, loss of bone density, flagging energy, lowered fertility, and impaired virility. Some researchers are experimenting with testosterone supplements, but their safety and efficacy are not yet known.

The major changes that occur during a woman's middle years are more evident than those in men. Women enter into **perimenopause**, the period from a woman's first irregular cycles to menopause, the end of menstruation.

Perimenopause The average onset for perimenopause is 45 years, but it can start anytime between the

HUMAN POTENTIAL

Dr. Martin Collis—A Lifelong Educator

Our human potential story for this chapter celebrates the work and achievements of Dr. Martin Collis, someone who has spent a lifetime inspiring others to adopt healthy lifestyles. He was a past university professor of mine and continues to be a mentor, colleague, and friend.

Dr. Martin Collis grew up in England during World War II, and his early years were spent in various locations as he was evacuated to escape the London bombing. After the war he got a scholarship to an English public school where his passion for soccer—not the popular school sport of rugby—and his offbeat sense of humour presented many challenges. He left school at 16 and worked for two years before serving in the military. During his military service his love of sports grew. He then decided to go university to qualify to teach physical education and English. He also made plans to coach sports. One of his guiding principles as an educator was to find a way to inspire and encourage children to reach their potential. He did not want to teach how he had been taught.

As a teacher in England, he built his school swim team into the premier club in South London. With his coaching success and deepening interest in exercise physiology, Martin set out to further his education. He moved to California, U.S.A., and completed a Ph.D. at Stanford University. He also began coaching at the Santa Clara Swim Club where he worked with world- class swimmers. This was the leading swim team, with Mark Spitz among its many Olympians. It was here Martin met Claudia Kolb, a young, dedicated swimmer who struggled through her first years of training to eventually become a two-time Olympic gold medalist. Martin was so inspired by her commitment as an athlete and her improbable success that he wrote a song titled *Claudia*, a song that is still used to motivate young athletes today.

From Stanford Dr. Collis joined the School of Physical Education at the University of Victoria where he conducted research and taught for 30 years. His first major research project with two UVic colleagues was a study designed to measure the effect of cold-water immersion on human hypothermia. This research led to the rewriting of the science of cold-water survival. It was embraced by the Red Cross, U.S. and Canadian Coast Guards, and water safety groups throughout the world. The research scientist team developed re-warming techniques that are now standard among first responders. When analyzing their own research data, they discovered every physiology textbook used in science courses was incorrect in saying that shivering was driven by core temperature alone. They patented a survival jacket, the UVic Thermofloat, which is still sold today.

The other main area of research Dr. Collis was associated with was physical activity and health. This work also saved lives, although in a less dramatic way. In order to facilitate the use of the Canada Home Fitness Test, Dr. Collis and colleagues created a simple screening test named PAR-Q (Physical Activity Readiness Questionnaire), which is still used throughout the world. He wrote the first North American book on workplace wellness titled *Employee Fitness* and followed that with a behaviour modification lifestyle book, *The Phacts of Life*, which was translated into multiple languages.

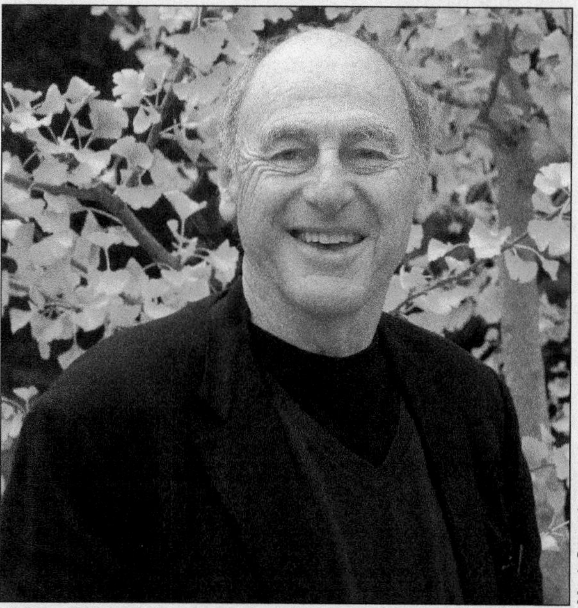
Mark Cacovic

Dr. Martin Collis, lifelong educator, motivational speaker, songwriter, and healthy living advocate.

He also encouraged and taught thousands of UVic students over the years, motivating them to "move a little more often" and make healthy lifestyle choices. His courses, such as Human Wellness and Active Health, were always oversubscribed. He had students begging to be moved from the long waiting lists into the classes, and when they did get registered, they were willing to sit in the aisles just to hear his zany lectures and the results from his latest song-writing efforts.

Dr. Collis became a major proponent of walking and walking programs and cooperated with the Taiwan manufacturer Bestek to create inexpensive but accurate pedometers. He has supervised walking programs in schools, workplaces, and recreation centres. His book *Walking, Weight and Wellness* offered a definitive guide to pedometers and current information on the role of exercise in weight loss and weight control. He is an internationally renowned health and wellness speaker who has criss-crossed the globe sharing his passion of active health for every age level. His distinctive talks are always humorous and often feature songs he has written and recorded.

At 81 years of age, Dr. Collis is still speaking, still practising what he's always preached, still coaching soccer, and preparing for his next 20 years on the planet. The music and sport that served him so well as a boy still serves him today. He has been influenced by many, but perhaps none more than Dr. Kenneth Cooper, who gave us the word *aerobics*, and Bob Dylan, who has been in his head for more than 50 years. He takes pleasure from the achievements of his former students and stays in touch with many of them. Currently he is writing a book titled *Hungry for Health*.

ages of 39 and 51. The average time frame for perimenopause is about five years, but this stage has a range of two to eight years.[47] During this time, the egg cells, or oocytes, in a woman's ovaries start to *senesce* or die off at a faster rate. Eventually, the number of egg cells drops to a tiny fraction of the estimated two million packed into her ovaries at birth. Trying to coax some of the remaining oocytes to ripen, the pituitary gland churns out extra follicle-stimulating hormone (FSH). This surge is the earliest harbinger of menopause, occurring 6–10 years before a woman's final periods. Eventually the other menstrual messenger, luteinizing hormone (LH), also increases, but at a slower rate.

These hormonal shifts can trigger an array of symptoms. The most common are night sweats (a *subdromal hot flash*, in medical terms), which can be just intense enough to disrupt sleep. About 10–20 percent of perimenopausal women also experience daytime hot flashes, a symptom that becomes more prevalent with the more drastic and enduring hormonal changes of menopause itself.

Menopause **Menopause**, defined as the complete cessation of menstrual periods for 12 consecutive months, generally arrives at age 51 or 52. About 10–15 percent of women breeze through this transition with only trivial symptoms. Another 10–15 percent are virtually disabled. The majority fall somewhere in between. Women who undergo surgical or medical menopause (the result of removal of their ovaries or chemotherapy) often experience abrupt symptoms, including flushing, sweating, sleeplessness, early morning awakenings, involuntary urination, changes in libido, mood swings, perception of memory loss, and changes in cognitive function.

Dwindling levels of estrogen subtly affect many aspects of a woman's health, from her mouth (where dryness, unusual tastes, burning, and gum problems can develop) to her skin (which may become drier, itchier, and overly sensitive to touch). The drop in estrogen levels also may cause hot flashes (bursts of perspiration that last from a few seconds to 15 minutes), which often happen at night, disturbing sleep and causing fatigue. With less estrogen to block them, a woman's androgens, or male hormones, may have a greater impact, causing acne, hair loss, and, according to some anecdotal reports, surges in sexual appetite. Other women, however, report a drop in sexual desire.

At the same time, a woman's clitoris, vulva, and vaginal lining begin to shrivel, sometimes resulting in pain or bleeding during intercourse. Since the thinner genital tissues are less effective in keeping out bacteria and other pathogens, urinary tract infections may become more common. Some women develop breast or ovarian cysts, which usually go away on their own. Eventually, a woman's ovaries don't respond at all to her pituitary hormones. After the last ovulatory cycle, progesterone is no longer secreted, and estrogen levels decrease rapidly.

Women experiencing menopause face risks of various diseases, including heart disease, stroke, and breast cancer.[48,49] Because estrogen or progestin may play a role in these risks, for many years **hormone replacement therapy (HRT)** was routinely prescribed to ease short-term symptoms of menopause, such as hot flashes, improve a woman's quality of life, and reduce long-term health risks.[50] However, recent research has challenged this practice.[51]

In 1991, the U.S. National Institutes of Health (NIH) launched a major study called the Women's Health Initiative (WHI). This was a set of studies involving healthy post-menopausal women that was carried out in 40 U.S. centres. The study included a clinical trial to evaluate the risks and benefits of two types of HRT (estrogen and progestin), which were administered in pill form. The researchers were looking for how this type of treatment affected women's health. In July 2002, after an average of 5.2 years of follow-up with the participants, the NIH prematurely ended the combined HRT component of this trial. It was found that there were more risks than benefits among the women using the combined HRT compared to the women in the placebo group. Specifically, the researchers found that there were more cases of coronary heart disease, strokes, blood clots, invasive breast cancer, and dementia. Although the actual numbers of cases in the test group of participants appeared to be low, they were very significant given that millions of women were taking combined HRT.[52]

The NIH made a decision to stop a second study in 2004 where women who had hysterectomies were taking estrogen only. It was found that estrogen alone appeared to increase the risk of stroke and blood clots, although it did decrease the risk of breast cancer compared to women who were given a placebo.

The HRT story continues. At the First Global Summit on Menopausal-Related issues, held in Zurich in March 2008, a report that had been released to the World Congress on Menopause was discussed. Experts attending the summit now suggest that HRT is safe for women entering menopause who are healthy. The researchers concluded that the women in the Women's Health Initiative study had a larger number of people with higher risk factors than normal and that the average age of the study participants was 10 years older than the age at which most women begin taking HRT. The conclusions shared at this summit suggest that HRT does not increase the risk of chronic heart disease in healthy women who are between the ages of 50–59, that the slightly increased risk of breast cancer is minimal compared to other risk factors, that HRT does not impair mental processes in healthy women in this age group, and that it might delay cognitive dysfunction as well. The experts' recommendation is that women consult with their doctor in order to decide if HRT is an appropriate plan of action for menopause.[53]

In Canada, the Society of Obstetricians and Gynecologists of Canada advises that combined HRT continue to be used to treat moderate to severe menopausal symptoms, but that the lowest effective dosage be used for short-term use. The society also asked doctors not to prescribe HRT to prevent heart disease or dementia.[54]

Because of the findings, many other medical groups have revised their guidelines for HRT. The North American Menopause Society recommends against the use of HRT for preventing heart disease in both healthy women and those who already have heart problems. Although this society considers HRT an acceptable treatment for menopausal symptoms, they advise caution regarding its prolonged use.

There are alternatives, both in terms of medication and lifestyle changes, to HRT. Testosterone creams, used in the vagina, can help with dryness and irritation. Many postmenopausal women relieve symptoms and lower their risk of future health problems by exercising—which can lower the risk of heart disease—and strengthening bones by eating calcium-rich foods and supplements.

Some women have reported relief from hot flashes, fatigue, depression, and other menopausal symptoms with vitamins and herbal therapies. Some of these herbs have undergone clinical trials. For the safest use of herbs, consult your doctor or a qualified alternative practitioner, such as a naturopathic doctor or traditional Chinese medicine practitioner. Purchase herbs that have been standardized—look for a Drug Information Number (DIN) or General Public (GP) number, which shows that Health Canada has reviewed and approved the product's information, labelling, and instructions for use.

✓ CHECK-IN

If you are a woman, do you know the age your mother entered perimenopause or went through menopause? Have you ever talked to her about her experience?

CHALLENGES OF AGING

No matter how well we eat, exercise, and take care of ourselves, common life problems, such as depression, driving risks, and substance misuse and abuse can become more challenging as we age. Living well in later life requires that we learn to adapt to our changing bodies and minds. It is helpful to be flexible and open to new ways of managing day-to-day activities so that we can shield ourselves from a sense of hopelessness that sometimes accompanies the aging process. The more we can learn about the aging process, the more options we can put in place for others and ourselves so that we can contribute to society and find ways to live a full and active life.

Depression Depression is a serious problem among the elderly. In the over-65 age group, at least one million seniors are living with a mental illness.[55] As many as 15–20 percent of seniors suffer mild to severe depression, ranging from 5 to 10 percent of seniors living in the community and 30–50 percent of seniors in long-term care facilities.[56] Depression can be hard to recognize, especially among older adults. It is often confused with aging itself. As well, many seniors hold negative attitudes about depression. This stops some of them from seeking help. It is estimated that seniors are among the most undertreated populations for mental health, with depression in more than one-third of people aged 65 or over going undetected.[57]

Older people face many challenges, including declining health, social isolation, and physical limitations. Deteriorating health can change a planned, happy retirement into one that includes fear, confusion, and chronic pain. Caring for loved ones also takes a toll. Between 20 and 50 percent of older adults who care for family members with dementia suffer from depression. This can lead to elder abuse, a growing problem in Canada. Psychological, emotional, or physical abuse includes shouting and bullying, insults, name calling, threats of violence, isolation, and physical harm.[58] Losing a loved one affects mental well-being, too. About one-third of Canadian seniors are coping with the loss of their life partners, as well as the gradual loss of their friends and relatives. Wade and Pevalin,[59] in a study on marital transitions and mental health, found that those who experience the loss of a spouse go through an adjustment phase prior to and after the death. There were significantly higher proportions of people with poor mental health during this time compared to people who remain married.

However, depressed older adults are as likely to benefit from medication as younger individuals. More than 70 percent of the depressed elderly improve dramatically with treatment. There is a downside to the medical approach to treatment though. According to reports from the National Advisory Council on Aging, up to 50 percent of all prescriptions are not taken correctly, and up to 20 percent of all hospital admissions are due to adverse reactions to medications or not following prescription-drug instructions.[60] Some of the widely prescribed medications for seniors are known to be addictive and cause side effects. Benzodiazepine medications, which include Ativan®, Valium®, Serax®, and Xanax®, commonly prescribed for treating acute anxiety and insomnia, are meant only for short-term use. In many cases, use of these drugs becomes prolonged and side effects from their use include increased fatigue, impaired performance, and decreased ability to learn new things.

Since loneliness and loss are often important contributing factors to depression, psychiatrists often combine counselling, such as psychotherapy, with medication. Maintaining positive relationships with family and friends, seeking opportunities to express feelings, pursuing activities that are enjoyable, and participating in regular physical activity can also help. Motle et al. examined the effects of a walking and low-intensity resistance and flexibility training program on depressive symptoms among older adults over a five-year period. After the six-month intervention, depressive symptom scores decreased immediately. The reduction in depressive symptom scores was also sustained for 12–60 months after the initial intervention. Both the walking and the resistance and flexibility programs were successful in reducing the depressive symptoms.[61]

Driving Risks In 2014 there were 4 112 205 Canadians aged 65 and older categorized as licensed drivers.[62] While age alone is not an indicator of impairment, age-related changes can affect driving ability. Over the years, road fatalities have dropped significantly in most age groups; however, this is not the case for people aged 70 or older. Reports indicate that these drivers have a higher accident rate per kilometre than any other age group except for young male drivers.[63] The most common contributing factors in accidents involving older drivers include pulling out from the side of the road or changing lanes without looking, careless backing up, inaccurate turning, failure to yield the right of way, and difficulty reading traffic signs. Unlike younger drivers, older drivers' accidents seldom involve high speeds. Rather, problem driving in older adults involves visual, cognitive, and motor skills, which may decline with aging.

Medications are a factor when driving—especially for older adults. Drugs that combat anxiety and insomnia can make a person drowsy. Antihistamines can affect concentration. Combining over-the-counter and prescription drugs can be very dangerous. Table 15-1 shows some of the potential side effects medications can have.

TABLE 15-1

Medication Effects for the Older Driver

Medical Condition	Type of Medication	Potential Effects
Anxiety	Sedatives	Drowsiness, staggering, blurred vision
Arthritis and rheumatism	Analgesics (pain relievers)	Drowsiness, inability to concentrate, ringing in ears
Common cold	Antihistamines, antitussives (cough suppressants)	Drowsiness, blurred vision, dizziness
Fatigue	Stimulants	Overexcitability, false sense of alertness, dizziness
Heart arrhythmia	Anti-arrhythmics	Blurred vision, dizziness
Hypertension	Anti-hypertensives (blood pressure drugs)	Drowsiness, blurred vision, dizziness

Source: *Drugs and the Older Driver. Information.* Found at www.safetycouncil.org/info/seniors/medicati.htm. ©2005 2011 Canada Safety Council.

Is It Ever Too Late to Quit Smoking? Despite the well-documented benefits of quitting, 10.8 percent of Canadians aged 55 years and older still smoke occasionally or on a daily basis. This is the second lowest rate of smokers in Canada, next to the 15- to 19-year-old age group at 10.7 percent. There has been very little change in the smoking prevalence of the 55-year-old and older age group in the past 10 years. However, adults 55 years and older who do smoke have the highest rate of average daily cigarettes per day at 15.2.[64] The smoking rate of Aboriginal seniors is higher; 24 percent of those aged 65 or older not living on a reserve smoke on a daily basis. Of the seniors who are currently smokers, almost half of them started smoking by the age of 16. Older adult smokers tend to be heavy smokers and do not intend to quit. They are also less likely to accept the health risks that are associated with smoking. The mortality rate among current older adult smokers is twice that of people who have never smoked.

Cigarette smoking is the principle cause of **chronic obstructive pulmonary disease (COPD)**, a lung disorder that causes airways to become partially obstructed. The two main forms of this disease are chronic bronchitis, an inflammation of the airways in the lungs, and emphysema, which damages and destroys lung tissue.[65] COPD often affects people over 60. The treatments include bronchodilators, inhaled steroids, antibiotics, vaccines, and supplemental oxygen.[66]

The sooner a smoker stops using tobacco, the greater the health benefits. While risks of smoking persist into old age, so do the benefits of quitting smoking—at any age.[67] A person who smokes more than 20 cigarettes a day and quits at age 65 increases life expectancy by two or three years. When older people stop tobacco use, their circulation and lung function increase, they suffer less cardiovascular illness, and their quality of life improves.[68]

Substance Misuse and Abuse Misuse and abuse of prescription and over-the-counter medications occur frequently among the elderly. This may be in part because the great majority of seniors use prescription or over-the-counter medication. Many seniors tend to have more than one health problem and receive multiple prescriptions. Sometimes they combine prescription drugs with over-the-counter products or with natural remedies. The drugs may interact and cause a confusing array of symptoms and reactions.

The most commonly misused drugs are sleeping pills, tranquilizers, pain medications, and laxatives. Sometimes a person innocently uses more than the prescribed dose or simultaneously takes several prescriptions of the same drug. Some older people are aware of their overreliance on drugs but don't like how they feel when they don't take the pills.

Problems remembering, concentrating, and thinking are the most common psychological side effects of drugs in the elderly. As we age, our bodies take longer to metabolize drugs, so medications like sleeping pills build up in the body. In some provinces, education programs such as *MedsCheck* are offered by pharmacists. Funded by the Government of Ontario, these seminars cover a variety of important topics with regard to medication use.[69] Almost 50 percent of all prescription medication taken by older adults is not used appropriately. This can reduce the effectiveness of the medication or can be dangerous. There is concern, also, about the increased number of prescriptions for anxiety and insomnia. The top five Beers list drugs (an internationally recognized list of medications identified as potentially inappropriate for seniors) were hormone replacement drugs; amitriptyline; digoxin, a treatment for heart conditions; oxybutynin, a treatment for incontinence; and temazepam, a treatment for sleep disorders.[70]

In some older adults, alcohol can make mental confusion and memory problems worse. Community surveys suggest people older than 65 consume less alcohol and have fewer alcohol-related problems than younger drinkers; however, current research has found increasing prevalence of alcoholism among older adults. In addition to the direct risks of alcohol, older individuals face related dangers when they drink, including falls, fractures, accidents, medication interactions, depression, and cognitive changes.[71]

SEXUALITY AND AGING

Health and sexuality interact in various ways as we age. A study based on 3005 participants found that older adults between 57 and 85 remain sexually active. Fifty-eight percent of sexually active respondents in the youngest age group—between 57 and 64—reported engaging in oral sex within the past 12 months, as did 31 percent in the oldest age group. Fifty-four percent of sexually active participants in the study between the ages of 75 and 85 reported having sex once a week or more.

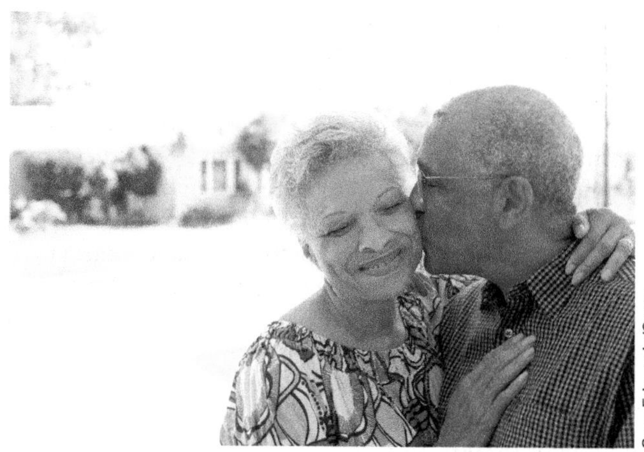

Sam Edwards/Getty

For older couples, sexual desire and pleasure can be enhanced by years of intimacy and affection.

The study also showed that when sexual activity declined, it had more to do with poor physical health than lack of desire.[72] The most commonly reported reason for sexual inactivity among individuals with a partner was the male partner's physical health. Women who had diabetes were less likely to be sexually active than women who did not, and men with this disease often suffered erectile difficulties. Dr. Lindau, one of the researchers of this study, suggests that doctors should be aware of the connection between sexual activity and health because older adult men and women might stop taking prescribed medication for other health issues if it negatively affects their sex life. According to the research findings, only 38 percent of men and 22 percent of women had discussed sex with their doctors since the age of 50.[73]

In another study by Ginsberg et al., most of the older adult participants surveyed wanted to maintain a sexual relationship and wanted more sexual experiences than were available to them. The main barrier for lack of sexual activity was lack of a partner.[74]

Aging does cause some changes in sexual response. Women produce less vaginal lubrication. An older man needs more time to achieve an erection or orgasm and to attain another erection after ejaculating. Both men and women experience fewer contractions during orgasm. However, none of these changes reduces sexual pleasure or desire.

ARE OLDER CANADIAN ADULTS USING DIGITAL TECHNOLOGY?

The use of digital technology has changed the way we communicate with family, friends, workmates, and strangers. It has also changed the way we gather information, shop, and work. Canada's older adults have embraced technology and are the fastest-growing group of users of the Internet. In 2000, only 5 percent of seniors 75 years and older were online. Now 27 percent of seniors are using the Internet. Eighty-eight percent go online at least once a day. Seven in 10 older adults think that technology is helping them live in their own home for a longer period of time and makes it easier to manage on a day-to-day basis. Email has become a popular way for this group to stay in contact with others. The *Report on Tech-Savvy Seniors* indicates that Canadian seniors are using digital technology in other ways to keep socially active. Fifty-three percent use networking sites such as Facebook, and one in five older adults uses Skype or Facetime to contact their family or friends.[75]

Sums et al., in another study on Internet use with 222 Australians over 55 years of age, determined that 90 percent of the older adult participants used the Internet at least four hours per week. Twenty-nine percent reported using it more than 16 hours per week. Ninety-seven percent had used the Internet for more than one year, and 44 percent had used the Internet for over seven years.

The primary reasons for use were communication, seeking information, entertainment, commercial purposes, and finding new people. The primary purpose for using the Internet was as a method of communication. The authors found that overall, the more hours spent using the Internet, the higher degree of social loneliness. However, they also discovered that when the participants used the Internet specifically as a communication tool there was a lower level of social loneliness. When the older adults used the Internet to find new people there was an increase in the level of reported emotional loneliness.[76] Heo et al. also studied Internet usage among older adults.[77] The findings of this study indicate that older adults who acknowledge the importance of the Internet tend to be satisfied using it as a leisure activity. Psychological benefits of using the Internet included enhanced self-confidence and a sense of accomplishment. A 2015 poll by the .CA Community Investment Program in conjunction with Ipsos Reid indicated that 86 percent of Canadians thought that better access to the Internet and training on how to become competent in using it would help older adults stay connected to their families and their communities. This included 90 percent of Canadians over 55 years of age who responded to the survey.[78]

✓ CHECK-IN

Do the older adults in your life use the Internet to stay connected? Do you think there are benefits to using the Internet to keep in touch with older family members?

DEATH AND DYING

In our society, death is not a part of everyday life as it once was. Facing death can be difficult. The process of dying can stir up emotions, increase stress levels, and make us evaluate our lives. According to mortality data from Statistics Canada, women can expect to live longer than men. (See X and Y Files: "Why Do Women Live Longer Than Men?") The three main causes of death for Canadian seniors are circulatory diseases (such as cerebrovascular and ischemic heart disease), cancers (lung, colon, breast, and prostate), and respiratory diseases (chronic obstructive pulmonary disease, influenza, and pneumonia).[79]

Defining Death The definition of death has become more complex. Because machines can now keep people alive who, in the past, would have died, there are now a number of different ways to define death:

- **Functional death**—the end of all vital functions, such as heartbeat and respiration.
- **Cellular death**—the gradual death of body cells after the heart stops beating. If placed in a tissue culture or, as is the case with various organs, transplanted to another body, some cells can remain alive indefinitely.
- **Cardiac death**—the moment when the heart stops beating.
- **Brain death**—the end of all brain activity, indicated by an absence of electrical activity (confirmed by an electroencephalogram, or EEG) and a lack of reflexes. The destruction of a person's brain means that his or her personality no longer exists; the lower brain centres controlling respiration and circulation no longer function.
- **Spiritual death**—the moment when the soul, as defined by many religions, leaves the body.

Denying Death Most of us don't quite believe that we're going to die. A reasonable amount of denial helps us focus on the day-to-day realities of living. However, excessive denial can be life-threatening. One important factor in denial is the nature of the threat. When the threat is not immediate it can be difficult to think that current lifestyle choices can impact a person's life later. One example is cigarette smoking; it can be difficult to believe that cigarette smoking might cause your death 20 or 30 years down the road. Elisabeth Kübler-Ross, a psychiatrist who extensively studied the process of dying, described the downside of denying death in *Death: The Final Stage of Growth.*

> *It is the denial of death that is partially responsible for people living empty, purposeless lives; for when you live as if you'll live forever, it becomes too easy*

to postpone the things you know that you must do. You live your life in preparation for tomorrow or in the remembrance of yesterday—and meanwhile, each today is lost. In contrast, when you fully understand that each day you awaken could be the last you have, you take the time that day to grow, to become more of who you really are, to reach out to other human beings.[80]

Emotional Responses to Dying Elisabeth Kübler-Ross identified five typical stages of reaction that a person goes through when facing death (see Figure 15-5).

1. *Denial ("No, not me").* At first knowledge that death is coming, a terminally ill patient rejects the news. The denial overcomes the initial shock and allows the person to begin to gather together his or her resources. Denial, at this point, is a healthy defence mechanism. It can become distressful, however, if it's reinforced by the relatives and friends of the dying patient.
2. *Anger ("Why me?").* In the second stage, the dying person begins to feel resentment and rage regarding imminent death. The anger may be directed at God or at the patient's family and caregivers, who can do little but try to endure any expressions of anger, provide comfort, and help the patient on to the next stage.
3. *Bargaining ("Yes, me, but . . . .").* In this stage, a patient may try to bargain, usually with God, for a way to reverse, or at least postpone, dying. The patient may promise, in exchange for recovery, to do good works or to see family members more often. Alternatively, the patient may say, "Let me live long enough to see my grandchild born" or "to see the spring again."
4. *Depression ("Yes, it's me").* In the fourth stage, the patient gradually realizes the full consequences of his or her condition. This may begin as grieving for health that has been lost and then become anticipatory grieving for the loss that is to come of friends, loved ones, and life itself. This stage is perhaps the most difficult: The dying person should not be left alone during this period. Neither should loved ones try to cheer up the patient, who must be allowed to grieve.
5. *Acceptance ("Yes, me, and I'm ready").* In this last stage, the person has accepted the reality of death: The moment looms as neither frightening nor painful, neither sad nor happy—only inevitable. The person who waits for the end of life may ask to see fewer visitors, separate from other people, or perhaps turn to just one person for support.

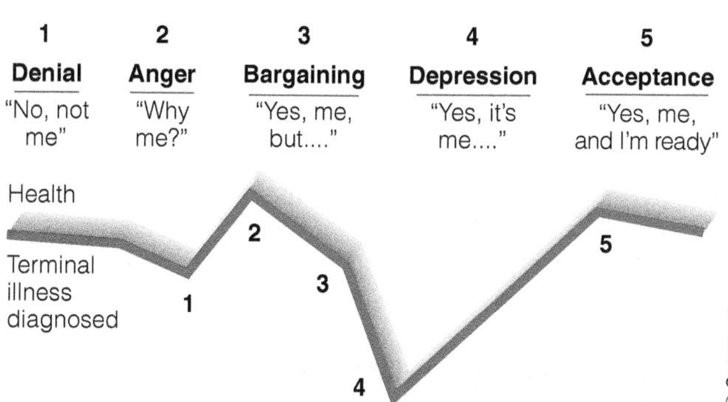

Figure 15-5 Kübler-Ross's Five Stages of Adjustment to Death

Several stages may occur at the same time, and some may happen out of sequence. Each stage may take days or only hours or minutes. Throughout, denial may come back to assert itself unexpectedly, and hope for a medical breakthrough or a miraculous recovery is forever present.

Some experts dispute Kübler-Ross's basic five-stage theory as too simplistic and argue that not all people go through such well-defined stages in the dying process.

X AND Y FILES

Why Do Women Live Longer Than Men?

The gap between men and women in terms of longevity has been shrinking since 1990; however, women still outlive men. The sex difference in mortality rates emerges from the moment of conception. Baby girls are less likely to die in the womb or after delivery than baby boys. Once past age 30, women consistently outnumber and outlive men.

Why do men die sooner? The female edge may begin at conception with the extra X chromosome, which provides a backup for defects on the X gene and a double dose of the genetic factors that regulate the immune system. In addition, the female hormone estrogen bolsters immunity and protects heart, bone, brain, and blood vessels.

In some cancers, estrogen may somehow protect against distant metastases. In contrast, testosterone may dampen the immune response in males—possibly to prevent attacks on sperm cells that might otherwise be mistaken as alien invaders. When the testes are removed from mice and guinea pigs, their immune systems become more active. In men, lessened immunity may lower resistance to cancer as well as infectious disease. Half of all men—compared with a third of women—develop cancer. Smoking, which for a long time was much more prevalent among men, accounts for some of this difference.

Testosterone also has been implicated in men's risk of heart disease and stroke. Originally designed to equip men with an instantaneous burst of power—essential for survival in Stone Age times—this potent male hormone may surge so intensely that it wreaks havoc throughout the cardiovascular system.

Males also die more often as a result of intentional and unintentional injury. Overall, men are three times more likely than women to die in accidents, mainly in cars and on the job. Men also are four times more likely to die violently.

The way a person faces death is often a mirror of the way he or she has faced other major stresses in life: those who have had the most trouble adjusting to other crises will have the most trouble adjusting to the news of their impending death.

An individual's will to live can postpone death for a while. The prospect of an upcoming birthday can delay death in women but hasten it in men. The will to live typically fluctuates in terminal patients, varying along with depression, anxiety, shortness of breath, and a sense of well-being.[81]

Preparing for Death Throughout this book we have stressed the ways in which you can determine how well and how long you live. You can also make decisions about the end of your life, particularly its impact on other people. To clarify your thinking on this difficult subject, ask yourself the following questions:

- Would I prefer to receive or refuse any specific treatments if I were unconscious or incapable of voicing my opinion?
- Would I like my bodily systems to be kept functioning by extraordinary life-sustaining measures, even though my natural systems had failed? If I could not survive without mechanical assistance, would I want to be kept alive or resuscitated if my heart were to stop?
- Would I like the province to decide how to distribute my property, or would I rather name the recipients of my estate?
- Would I like to decide how to handle my funeral arrangements?

You can assure that your wishes are heeded by several means, including advance directives, living wills, and holographic wills.

What Are Advance Directives? **Advance directives** are used to specify the kind of medical treatment individuals want in case of a medical crisis. These documents indicate a person's preferences. Hospitals and other institutions often make decisions on an individual's behalf, particularly if family members are not available or if they disagree. Advance directives also help physicians, who often do not feel comfortable making these kinds of decisions about life-extending treatments for their terminally ill patients.[82]

A *health-care proxy* is an advance directive that gives someone else the power to make decisions on your behalf. People typically name a relative or close friend as their agent. You need to let family, friends, and your primary physician know about the type of care you would or wouldn't want to receive in various circumstances, such as an accident that results in an irreversible coma.

You can also sign an advance directive specifying that you want to be allowed to die naturally—a **do-not-resuscitate (DNR)** directive indicates that you do not want to be resuscitated in case your heart stops beating.

What Is a Living Will? A **living will** isn't just for people who don't want to be kept alive by artificial means. Individuals can also use these advance directives to indicate that they want all possible medical treatments and technology used to prolong their lives. Some provinces recognize living wills as legally binding, and a growing number of healthcare professionals and facilities offer patients help in drafting living wills. Give copies to anyone who might have input in decisions on your behalf. You should also give copies to your physician.

Wills Perhaps you think that only wealthy or older people need to write wills. However, if you're married, have children, or own property, you should prepare a will. There are three types of wills: formal, notarial, and holographic. A formal will is a typed document, prepared by a lawyer or a notary, and signed by you in front of at least two witnesses who cannot be a beneficiary or your spouse. A notarial will is similar to the formal will but only used in Quebec. It is prepared by a notary and signed before the notary and a witness. A **holographic will** is prepared in your handwriting and signed by you, with no witness necessary. Experts advise against this type of will because it is often subject to misinterpretation and challenge, and it is not recognized in all provinces. It is important that you specify who you wish to raise your children and who should have your property. If you die *intestate* (without a will), the province will make these decisions for you. Even a modest estate can be tied up in court for a long period of time, depriving family members of money when they need it most.

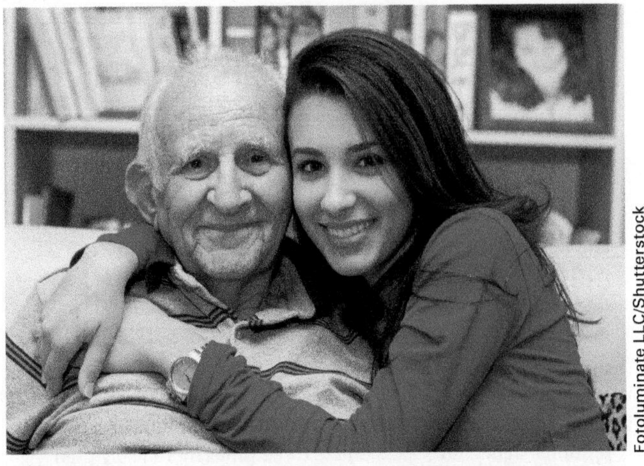

Fotoluminate LLC/Shutterstock

Communication and caring from family members can make the later years in life more meaningful and assist in the preparation of end-of-life planning.

✓ CHECK-IN

Has your family discussed each member's preferences in case of a medical crisis? Have you thought through and communicated your own preferences?

Suicide Suicide among the elderly is a danger that often goes unnoticed. Elderly men are at a far greater risk of attempting suicide than women, with almost five times as many senior men committing suicide. Of all groups in Canada, men over the age of 65 have the highest rate of completed suicides. Men over 70 are also hospitalized at higher rates than women for attempted suicide.[83]

One of the main factors leading to suicide is illness, especially terminal illness. A great deal of debate centres on quality of life, yet there is no reliable or consistent way to measure this. Patients who are dying may feel they have some quality of life, even when others do not recognize it, or their evaluations of the quality of their lives may fluctuate. Dying patients who say their lives are not worth living may be suffering from depression; hopelessness is one of its characteristic symptoms.[84]

"Rational" Suicide An elderly widow suffering from advanced cancer takes a lethal overdose of sleeping pills. A woman in her 50s, diagnosed with Alzheimer's disease, asks a doctor to help her end her life. Are these suicides "rational" because these individuals used logical reasoning in deciding to end their lives?

The question is intensely controversial. Advocates of the right to self-deliverance argue that individuals in great pain or faced with the prospect of a debilitating, hopeless battle against an incurable disease can and should be able to decide to end their lives. As legislatures and the legal system tackle the thorny issue of an individual's right to die, there are health professionals who worry that suicidal wishes, even in those with fatal diseases, often stem from undiagnosed depression.

A number of studies have indicated that most patients with painful, progressive, or terminal illnesses do not want to kill themselves. The percentage of those who report thinking about suicide ranges from 5 to 20 percent, and most of these have major depression. Many mental-health professionals argue that what makes patients with severe illnesses suicidal is depression, not their physical condition.[85]

Because depression may indeed warp the ability to make a rational decision about suicide, mental-health professionals urge physicians and family members to make sure individuals with chronic or fatal illnesses are evaluated for depression and treated with medication, psychotherapy, or both.

On April 16, 2016, the federal ministers of health and justice tabled legislation for doctor-assisted death. This bill takes into consideration ways to protect vulnerable Canadians and was designed for adults who are mentally competent and have a serious and incurable illness, disease, or disability. The bill limits access to people who are dealing with intolerable suffering or whose death is reasonably foreseeable. The bill also makes clear that doctors and nurse practitioners who provide assistance for dying will not face criminal charges. The legislation was drafted to meet a Supreme Court of Canada ruling that indicated the ban on physician-assisted dying in Canada violated Canadians' Charter rights.

There are some contentious issues. Mature minors (people under the age of 18) and individuals suffering from mental illness would not be able to access assistance to die. The bill also prevents people suffering with degenerative disorders from organizing advance consent.[86] The bill to legalize and regulate doctor assisted dying passed in Parliament on June 17, 2016.[87]

Grief The death of a loved one may be the single most upsetting and feared event in a person's life. Losing a parent in childhood can have a lasting impact. A study that followed 100 orphans found that as young adults they suffered significantly higher depressive symptoms.[88] When both parents die, individuals may feel like orphaned children. They mourn not just for the father and mother who are gone, but also for their lost role of being someone's child.

The death of a family member produces a wide range of reactions, including anxiety, guilt, anger, and financial concern. Many may see the death of an old person as less tragic than the death of a child or young person. A sudden death can be more of a shock than one following a long illness. A suicide can be particularly devastating. The death of a child can be even more traumatic.

Grieving may continue for many years. Eventually, parents may be able to resolve their grief and accept the death as "God's will" or as "something that happens." Others deal with their grief by keeping busy or by substituting other problems or situations to take their minds off their loss. Yet many parents who lose a child continue to grieve for many years. Although the pain of their loss diminishes with time, they view it as part of themselves and describe an emptiness inside—even though most have rich, meaningful, and happy daily lives.

The loss of a mate can also have a profound impact, although men's and women's responses to the death may depend on how their spouses died. Men whose wives die suddenly face a greater risk of dying themselves than those whose wives die after a long illness. Women whose husbands die after a long illness face greater risk of dying than other widows. The reason may be that men whose wives were chronically ill learned how to cope with the loss of their nurturers, while women who spend a long time caring for an ill husband may be at greater risk because of the combined burdens of caregiving and loss of financial support.

Bereavement is not a rare occurrence on college and university campuses, but it is largely an ignored problem. Counsellors have called upon universities to help students who have lost a loved one through initiatives such as training students to provide peer support and raising consciousness about bereavement.[89]

Grief's Effect on Health Men and women who lose partners, parents, or children endure so much stress that they are at increased risk of serious physical and mental illness and even of premature death. Studies of the health effects of grief have found the following:

- Grief produces changes in the respiratory, hormonal, and central nervous systems and may affect functions of the heart, blood, and immune systems.
- Grieving adults may experience mood swings between sadness and anger, guilt and anxiety. They may feel physically sick, lose their appetite, sleep poorly, or fear that they're going crazy because they "see" the deceased person in different places.
- Friendships and remarriage offer the greatest protection against health problems.
- Some widows may have increased rates of depression, suicide, and death from cirrhosis of the liver. The greatest risk factors are poor previous mental and physical health and a lack of social support.
- Grieving parents, partners, and adult children are at increased risk of serious physical and mental illness, suicide, and premature death.

✓ CHECK-IN

If you have suffered the loss of a loved one, how did you experience grief?

Methods of Mourning Grief is a psychological necessity, not self-indulgence. Psychotherapists refer to grief as work, and it is—slow, tedious, and painful. Yet only by working through grief—dealing with feelings of anger and despair, and adjusting emotionally and intellectually to the loss—can bereaved individuals make their way back to the living world of hope and love.

Some widows and widowers move through the grieving process without experiencing extreme distress. Others stop somewhere in the midst of normal grieving and continue to pine for the deceased, become overly reliant on others, or show signs of denial, avoidance, or anxiety.

How Can You Help Survivors of a Loss? Although we grieve for the dead, the living are the ones who need our help. Bereavement is such an intense state that survivors may be too numb or too stunned to ask for help. Family and friends must take the initiative and spend time with those who are mourning the loss of a loved one, even if that means sitting together silently. Offer empathy and support, and let the grieving person know with verbal and nonverbal expressions that you care and wish to help. Simply being there is enough to let your friend know you care.

Giving help over the first few days is important, but grieving people continue to need support for many months. The first anniversary of a death or the first holiday spent alone can be particularly difficult.

Most bereaved people don't need professional psychological counselling. In most instances, sharing their feelings with friends is all that's needed. However, you should urge a friend or relative to seek help if he or she shows no sign of grieving or exhibits as much distress a year after the loss as during the first months. Therapy and medication can be enormously helpful—and potentially life-saving.

SELF-SURVEY

What Is Your Aging IQ?

Answer True or False

T F 1. Everyone becomes "senile" sooner or later, if he or she lives long enough.

T F 2. Canadian families have by and large abandoned their older members.

T F 3. Depression is a serious problem for older people.

T F 4. The numbers of older people are growing.

T F 5. The vast majority of older people are self-sufficient.

T F 6. Mental confusion is an inevitable, incurable consequence of old age.

T F 7. Intelligence declines with age.

T F 8. Sexual urges and activity normally cease around ages 55–60.

T F 9. If a person has been smoking for 30 or 40 years, it does no good to quit.

T F 10. Older people should stop exercising and rest.

T F 11. As you grow older, you need more vitamins and minerals to stay healthy.

T F 12. Only children need to be concerned about calcium for strong bones and teeth.

T F 13. Extremes of heat and cold can be particularly dangerous to old people.

T F 14. Many older people are hurt in accidents that could have been prevented.

T F 15. More men than women survive to old age.

T F 16. The most common causes of death for older adults aged 65 years and older are circulatory diseases, a variety of cancers, and respiratory diseases.

T F 17. Older people on average take more medications than younger people.

T F 18. Snake-oil salesmen are as common today as they were on the frontier.

T F 19. Personality changes with age, just like hair colour and skin texture.

T F 20. Sight declines with age.

Answers to Self-Survey

Scoring

1. False. Even among those who live to be 80 or older, only 20–25 percent develop Alzheimer's disease or some other incurable form of brain disease. "Senility" is a meaningless term that should be discarded.
2. False. The Canadian family is still the number-one caretaker of older Canadians. Many older people live close to their children and see them often; many live with their spouses.
3. True. Depression, loss of self-esteem, loneliness, and anxiety can become more common as older people face retirement, along with the deaths of relatives and friends, and other such crises—often at the same time. Fortunately, depression is treatable.
4. True. By the year 2036, the number of Canadian older adults is predicted to be between 9.9 and 10.9 million.
5. True. Only a small percentage of the older population live in nursing homes. The rest live independently or with relatives or caregivers.
6. False. Mental confusion and serious forgetfulness in old age can be caused by Alzheimer's disease or other conditions that cause incurable damage to the brain, but some 100 other problems can cause the same symptoms. A minor head injury, a high fever, poor nutrition, adverse drug reactions, and depression can all be treated and the confusion will be cured.
7. False. Intelligence per se does not decline without reason. Most people maintain their intellect or improve as they grow older.
8. False. Most older people can lead an active, satisfying sex life.
9. False. Stopping smoking at any age not only reduces the risk of cancer and heart disease but also leads to healthier lungs.
10. False. Many older people enjoy—and benefit from—exercises such as walking, swimming, and bicycle riding. Exercise at any age can help strengthen the heart and lungs, and lower blood pressure. See your physician before beginning a new exercise program.
11. False. Although certain requirements, such as that for "sunshine" Vitamin D, may increase slightly with age, older people need the same amounts of most vitamins and minerals as younger people. Older people in particular should eat nutritious food and cut down on sweets, salty snack foods, high-calorie drinks, and alcohol.
12. False. Older people require fewer calories, but adequate intake of calcium for strong bones can become more important as you grow older. This is particularly true for women, whose risk of osteoporosis increases after menopause. Milk and cheese are rich in calcium as are cooked dried beans, collards, and broccoli. Some people need calcium supplements as well.
13. True. The body's thermostat tends to function less efficiently with age, and the older person's body may be less able to adapt to heat or cold.
14. True. Falls are the most common cause of injuries among the elderly. Good safety habits, including proper lighting, non-skid carpets, and keeping living areas free of obstacles, can help prevent serious accidents.
15. False. Women tend to live 5–10 percent longer than men.
16. True. Circulatory diseases include cerebrovascular and ischemic heart disease; cancers include lung, colon, breast, and prostate; and respiratory diseases include chronic obstructive pulmonary disease, influenza, and pneumonia.
17. True. Data from the *Chief Public Health Officer's Report on the State of Public Health in Canada 2010* shows that 76 percent of Canadian older adults living in private residences reported using at least one medication (prescription and/or over the counter) in the past two days and 13 percent had used five or more different medications. Among older adults living in institutions, 97 percent used one medication and 53 percent used five or more medications in the past two days.
18. True. Medical quackery is a multibillion-dollar business. People of all ages are commonly duped into "quick cures" for aging, arthritis, and cancer.
19. False. Personality doesn't change with age. Therefore, all old people can't be described as rigid and cantankerous. You are what you are for as long as you live. But you can change what you do to help yourself to good health.
20. False. Although changes in vision become more common with age, any change in vision, regardless of age, is related to a specific disease. If you are having problems with your vision, see your doctor.

Source: National Institute on Aging; Chief Public Health Officer's Report on the State of Public Health in Canada 2010.

Chapter Summary

1. Factors that contribute to a long life and successful aging include all of the following *except*
   a. healthy weight
   b. moderate smoking
   c. regular exercise
   d. social involvement
2. Which statement about physically fit people over age 60 is true?
   a. They have a lower risk of dying from chronic heart disease.
   b. They can regain the fitness level of a 25-year-old.
   c. They show no difference in levels of anxiety and depression.
   d. They increase their body-fat percentages due to age.
3. Which statement about the aging brain is false?
   a. When brain cells die, surrounding cells can fill the gaps to maintain cognitive function.
   b. Remembering names and recalling information may take longer.
   c. "Use it or lose it."
   d. Mental ability declines with age.
4. Which statement about aging is false?
   a. People over age 70 who take vitamin supplements showed improvement in short-term memory and problem-solving ability.
   b. Fitness and frequency of sexual activity are linked.
   c. Hormone replacement therapy reduces the risk of heart disease in menopausal women.
   d. Seniors who take up new hobbies late in life may slow aging within the brain.
5. Which statement about age-related problems is correct?
   a. Osteoporosis affects only women.
   b. Alzheimer's disease is a form of dementia.
   c. Depression is no more prevalent in the older population.
   d. Drug interactions do not occur in the elderly.
6. When should concern change to intervention?
   a. Uncle Charlie is 85 and continues to drive himself to the grocery store and to the senior centre during the daytime.
   b. Nana takes pills at breakfast, lunch, and dinner, but sometimes mixes them up.
   c. Mom's hot flashes have become a family joke.
   d. Your older brother can never remember where he put his car keys.
7. According to Elisabeth Kübler-Ross, which of the following is NOT one of the emotional stages an individual facing death goes through?
   a. bargaining
   b. acceptance
   c. denial
   d. repression
8. Which statement about the longevity gap between men and women is true?
   a. It is due to deficiencies in the Y chromosome.
   b. It results from the presence of a mutant gene.
   c. It may be due to the X chromosome and its hormonal influences on the immune system.
   d. It is a result of a gene responsible for maintaining the immune system.
9. What is the purpose of an advance directive?
   a. It indicates who should have your property in the event that you die.
   b. It might authorize which individuals may not participate in your healthcare if you are unable to care for yourself.
   c. It can specify your desires related to the use of medical treatments and technology to prolong your life.
   d. It should specify which physician you designate to be your healthcare proxy.
10. How can you best help a friend who is bereaved?
    a. by encouraging him to have a few drinks to forget his pain
    b. by simply spending time with her
    c. by avoiding talking about his loss because it is awkward
    d. by reminding her about all she still has in her life

Answers to these questions can be found on page 421.

SELF-RESPONSIBILITY—SOCIAL RESPONSIBILITY

SELF-RESPONSIBILITY

Our care should not be to have lived long as to have lived enough.
Seneca

Presently, you may be in the pre-contemplation or contemplation stage of preparing for older adulthood. That is the case for many college and university students, but preparation can begin at any time. Choices you make today will affect you as you age. Visualize yourself as an older adult. What activities do you hope to be doing?

SOCIAL RESPONSIBILITY

What we have done for ourselves alone dies with us; what we have done for others and the world remains and is immortal.
Albert Pike

How can lifestyle choices you make now support your vision of older adulthood? Many older adults living in assisted living or care homes would welcome a visit from a college or university student. Consider volunteering once or on a regular basis.

CRITICAL THINKING

1. How are your parents or other mentors staying fit and alert as they age? Do you think you might use similar strategies?
2. Have your living parents and grandparents written advanced directives or living wills? Have you discussed with them their preferences regarding treatment in the event of a medical crisis? If you haven't had this discussion with your family, how can you begin the process of helping your parents or grandparents communicate their wishes?
3. Many people are chronically unconscious, kept alive by artificial respirators and feeding tubes. If you were in an accident that left you in a vegetative state, would you want doctors to do everything possible to fight for your life, or would you want to have the right to decide when to end your life?

WEB LINKS

Active Living Coalition for Older Adults

www.alcoa.ca

This agency is a partnership of organizations and individuals who are interested in the field of aging. Reports, fact sheets, and information on how older adults can maintain their well-being and independence through healthy living are available at this site.

National Seniors Council

www.seniorscouncil.gc.ca/en/home.shtml

Reporting to a variety of federal government agencies, the National Seniors Council advises on quality of life and health and well-being issues of seniors. You can find reports and research at this site.

Osteoporosis Canada

www.osteoporosis.ca

Free publications, educational programs, medically accurate information for people dealing with osteoporosis and healthcare workers, and current up-to-date research are available at this site.

Please note that links are subject to change. If you find a broken link, use a search engine such as www.google.ca and search for the website by typing in keywords.

Key Terms

The terms listed here are used within the chapter on the page indicated. Definitions of the terms are in the Glossary at the end of the book.

advance directives 416
aging 401
Alzheimer's disease 408
brain death 414
cardiac death 414
cellular death 414
chronic obstructive pulmonary disease (COPD) 412
chronological age 403
dementia 408
do-not-resuscitate (DNR) 416
functional age 403
functional death 414
gerontologist 401
holographic will 416
hormone replacement therapy (HRT) 410
living will 416
menopause 410
osteoporosis 404
perimenopause 408
physiological age 403
psychological age 403
sarcopenia 404
social age 403
spiritual death 414

Answers to Chapter Summary Questions

1. b; 2. a; 3. d; 4. c; 5. b; 6. b; 7. d; 8. c; 9. c; 10. b

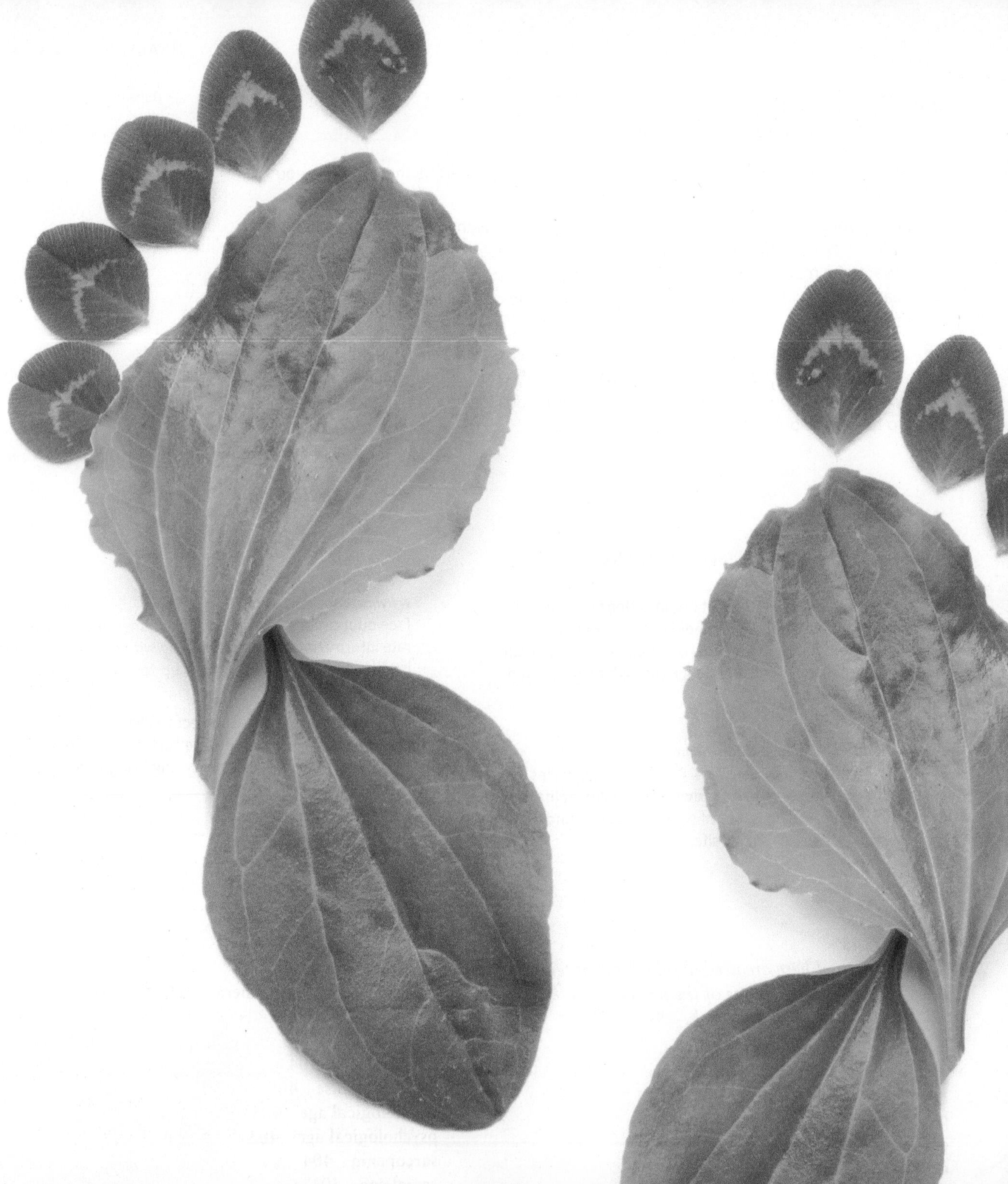

Konstanttin/Shutterstock

AFTER READING THIS CHAPTER, YOU WILL BE ABLE TO:

- **define** important environmental terms
- **describe** a number of national, provincial, and college and university campus environmental initiatives
- **list** the major types of indoor and outdoor pollution
- **list** the ecological determinants of health
- **list** and **describe** actions that individuals can take to protect the environment

16

Working Toward a Healthy Environment

Ours is a planet in peril. A report of the Intergovernmental Panel on Climate Change documents increasing dangers to the planet Earth and its inhabitants. Sea levels are rising. Forests are being destroyed. Droughts in Asia and Africa have become more frequent and more intense. At the same time, record flooding is impacting communities worldwide. Millions of people are dying every year from the effects of climate change.[1] Environmental concerns may seem so enormous that nothing any individual can do will have an effect. This is not the case. All of us, as citizens of the world, can help find solutions to the challenges confronting our planet. The first step is realizing that we have a personal responsibility for safeguarding the health of our environment and, thereby, our own well-being. We cannot be "well" in an "unwell" world.

This chapter will help you become more environmentally aware. It explores the complex interrelationships between our world and our well-being and what is being done to support environmental sustainability. There is also an introduction to some environmental experts who encourage all of us to stand up, take notice, and put an action plan into place with regard to current environmental issues. We discuss major threats to the environment, including atmospheric changes of the ecological determinants of health—air, water, and noise pollution; chemical risks; and radiation—and provide specific guidance on what you can do about them. We have also included a special section on the greening of college and university campuses.

FREQUENTLY ASKED QUESTIONS

FAQ: What is global warming? p. 425

FAQ: What can we do to protect the planet? p. 427

FAQ: What health risks are caused by pesticides? p. 438

ENVIRONMENTAL AWARENESS

Planet Earth—once taken for granted as a ball of rock and water that has existed for our use for all time—now is seen as a single, fragile **ecosystem** (a community of organisms that share a physical and chemical environment). An ecosystem approach recognizes the interrelationships between land, air, water, wildlife, human beings, and activities.[2] Our environment is a closed ecosystem, powered by the sun. The materials needed for the survival of our planet must be recycled over and over again. We have to take responsibility for our environment and embrace these interrelationships because there is no other option. This responsibility includes being more aware of the environmental costs of technological advances. While technology continues to raise the standard of living in industrialized countries, it often does so at a great environmental cost.

The dangers of technological developments became evident in the post–World War II era when we had to deal with toxic radioactive wastes because of atomic-weapons technology, the devastation of nature due to the indiscriminate use of pesticides and herbicides, and the heavy pollution of our air and water with petroleum by-products. We began to realize that we were changing our world as we knew it. We also heard from Aboriginal people and a group of distinguished scientists, philosophers, and citizens, whose writings and research have called on us to pay attention to our environment.

Over the past two decades there has been an international effort to support a more environmentally sustainable global future. One of the ways we can find out about these efforts is to access the **Environmental Performance Index (EPI)**, a joint initiative between researchers at Yale University and Columbia University. This biennial report shares important data on how 180 countries—members of the Organisation for Economic Co-operation and Development (OECD)—are attempting to protect their ecosystems and human health. The focus on these two aspects links directly to the Sustainable Development Goals (SDGs) of the United Nations.[3] Measurements are made in nine specific areas: climate and energy, biodiversity and habitat, fisheries, forests, agriculture, water resources, health impacts, air quality, and water sanitation. In the 2016 report, Finland was awarded a first-place ranking at a 90.68 rating score. Iceland, Sweden, and Denmark followed with second-, third-, and fourth-place rankings, respectively. Canada was ranked 25th with a score of 85.06 followed by the U.S.A. at 26th place with a score of 84.72.[4]

Globally, there has been improvement in developing infrastructure that targets clean drinking water and proper sewage treatment. As a result, the number of people who lack access to clean water has been cut in half. Unfortunately, there still needs to be improvements in this area. Twenty-three percent of countries do not have wastewater treatment. The report also revealed that air pollution has actually gotten worse. Half the world's population—3.5 billion people—live in countries that have hazardous levels of air pollution. With regard to habitat protection, 2.52 million square kilometres of tree canopy were lost in 2014.

In Canada, the not-for-profit organization Extended Producer Responsibility (EPR) Canada releases a report card on how well producers in each province manage the environmental impact of their products. The EPR Canada team members attempt to determine to what level the producers are taking responsibility for the consumer goods they sell.[5] The 2015 report awarded British Columbia an overall A grade. The lowest rating provincially was Alberta whose grade went down from D in 2013 to an F in 2015.[6]

CLIMATE CHANGE

Climate change is any long-term significant change in the "average weather" that a region experiences. The change includes variations within the Earth's atmosphere: the temperature and humidity of the air, the rainfall, the strength of the winds and clouds, the variations in solar radiation, the Earth's orbit, and greenhouse gas concentrations.[7] Climate change is happening on a global scale and the impacts are very real. Whereas research in this area had been focused on possible energy shortages around the world, current research is now showing this is not the main immediate problem. Instead, as Hodgson states, "There is a distinct possibility of large, unexpected, and irreversible changes that quite rapidly [could] have catastrophic consequences."[8] And these catastrophic changes seem to be directly linked to the amount of greenhouse gases in our atmosphere.

Life on earth as we know it is possible because of the solar radiation of the sun and the Earth's atmosphere. Solar radiation passes through the Earth's atmosphere, which is made up of **greenhouse gases (GHGs)**. The primary greenhouse gases are carbon dioxide (CO_2), methane (CH_4), nitrous oxide (NO_2), Ozone (O_3), and water vapour. This layer of insulation is what makes our planet livable.[9] CO_2 is the most important gas in this insulation layer. It acts like glass in a greenhouse, allowing a small amount of solar radiation through the Earth's atmosphere and trapping it so the heat generated warms the Earth. The rest of the solar radiation is bounced back into space. This process is a natural phenomenon known as the **greenhouse effect**. Without greenhouse gases the average temperature of the Earth's surface would be 18° C.[10] You might wonder why there is such an enormous concern about CO_2 emissions and the link to climate change if CO_2 is such an important gas. Wouldn't more be better? Not so, say the scientists.

Carbon is stored in plants, soil, the ocean, and our own bodies. It is released into our atmosphere by both natural causes, such as volcanic activity, and man-made causes, such as burning fossil fuels like coal, oil, and gas, and deforestation. There have been times over the Earth's history when the natural balance of CO_2 levels and dust emissions was disrupted. However, it has not been until recently that human activities have introduced **climate forcings**—physical factors that force a net increase (positive forcing) or a net decrease (negative forcing) of heat in the climate system as a whole—where the magnitude of change has occurred so quickly in such a negative way.[11] Today's atmosphere contains 32 percent more carbon dioxide than it did at the beginning of the industrial era.[12] Research from the Suzuki Foundation suggests that we have released so much carbon dioxide and other greenhouse gases such as methane and nitrous oxide into our atmosphere that we are now covered by a thick, heat-trapping blanket.[13] You can think of it as a defective thermostat. We are overheating. This is known as the **enhanced greenhouse effect.**[14] While there are a small number of climate-change deniers, there is a consensus among climate-change scientists that the main culprit of greenhouse gas emissions is CO_2 produced from the burning of fossil fuels and the foremost reason for global warming. Figure 16-1 shows changes in greenhouse gas emissions by province for the years 1990, 2005, and 2014.

In 2014, the greenhouse gas emissions in Canada were 732 megatonnes (Mt) of carbon dioxide equivalent (CO_2eq).[15] The primary sources of GHG are transportation, oil and gas production, distribution of fossil fuels (Canada's tar sands are the fastest-growing source of global warming pollution), and mining.

✓ CHECK-IN

What do you see as the greatest environmental threat?

What Is Global Warming? **Global warming** is an important measure of climate change. It can be defined as a sustained increase in the average temperature of the Earth's atmosphere that causes changes in the global climate. According to the National Aeronautics and Space Administration (NASA), the global average temperature rose by almost 0.83°C (1.5°F) over the last century. The average global temperature in 2015 was the warmest on record, rising by 0.13°C (0.23°F) from 2014 (see Figure 16-2). Most of the global warming has occurred in the last 35 years. Fifteen of the 16 warmest years on record have occurred since 2001.[16] Scientists are projecting additional warming of 1–6.4°C (2–11.5°F) over the next century if man-made greenhouse gas emissions continue at current rates.[17] Some scientists argue that the mean surface temperatures of the last 100 years are not unusual, but the extremely rapid warming in the last 15 years cannot be explained by natural forces alone.[18] Figure 16-3 shows some man-made factors.

The Impact of Global Warming No one can forecast exactly what the effects of a continuing temperature rise will be, but some experts have predicted severe drought and a rise in ocean levels of 0.6 metres (2 feet) to 6 metres (20 feet)—conditions that will affect everyone on Earth. A warmer world is expected to produce more severe flooding in some places and more severe droughts in others, jeopardizing natural resources and the safety

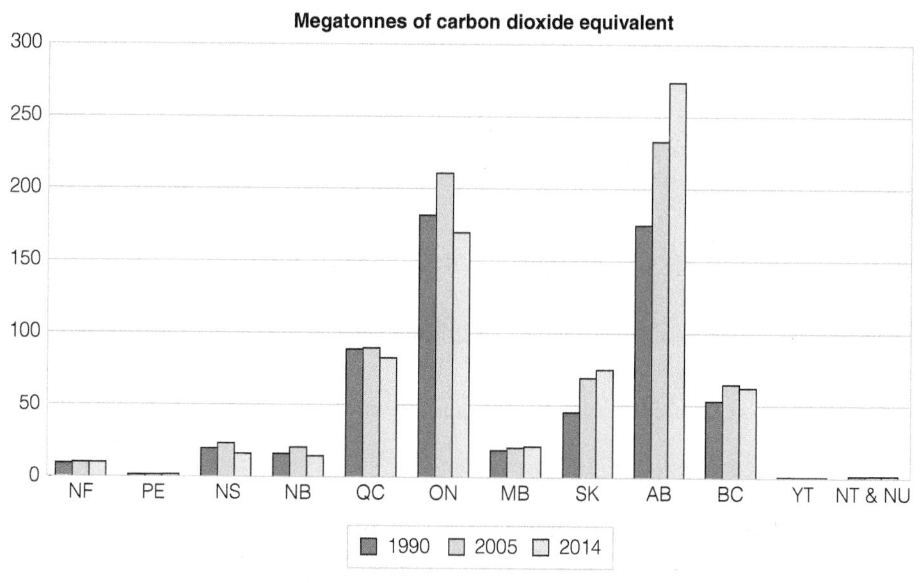

Figure 16-1 Greenhouse Gas Emissions by Province and Territory, Canada, 1990, 2005, and 2014

Source: ©Her Majesty The Queen in Right of Canada, Environment and Climate Change Canada, 2016. Available at https://www.ec.gc.ca/indicateurs-indicators/default.asp?lang=en&n=18F3BB9C-1.

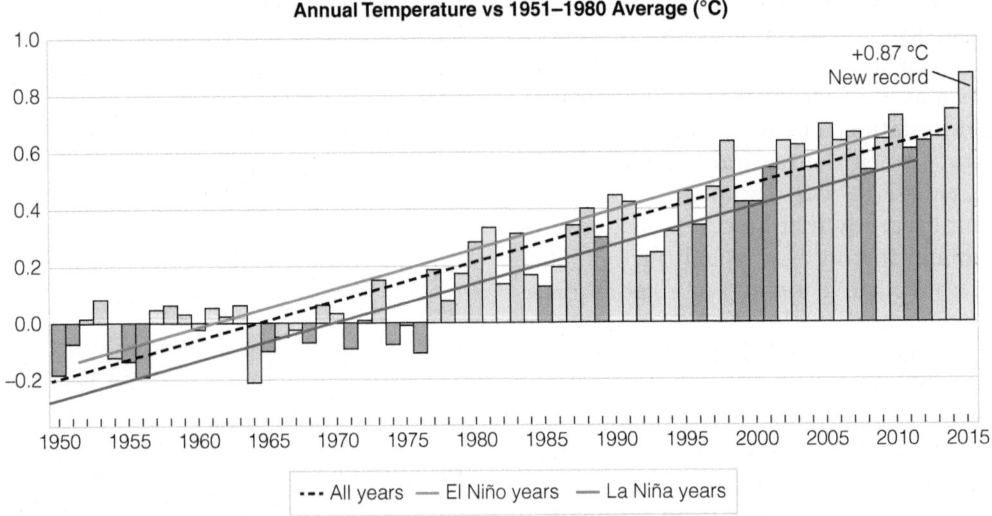

Figure 16-2 **Graph of Temperature Trends in Relation to El Niño and La Niña Events**

Red bars represent global temperature anomalies in El Niño years, with the red line showing the trend. Blue bars depict La Niña years, and the blue line shows that trend. Neutral years are shown in gray, and the dashed black line shows the overall temperature trend since 1950.

Source: NASA/GSFC/Earth Observatory; fig. upd. 2016-01-25. "NASA, NOAA Analyses Reveal Record-Shattering Global Warm Temperatures in 2015," http://www.giss.nasa.gov/research/news/20160120/

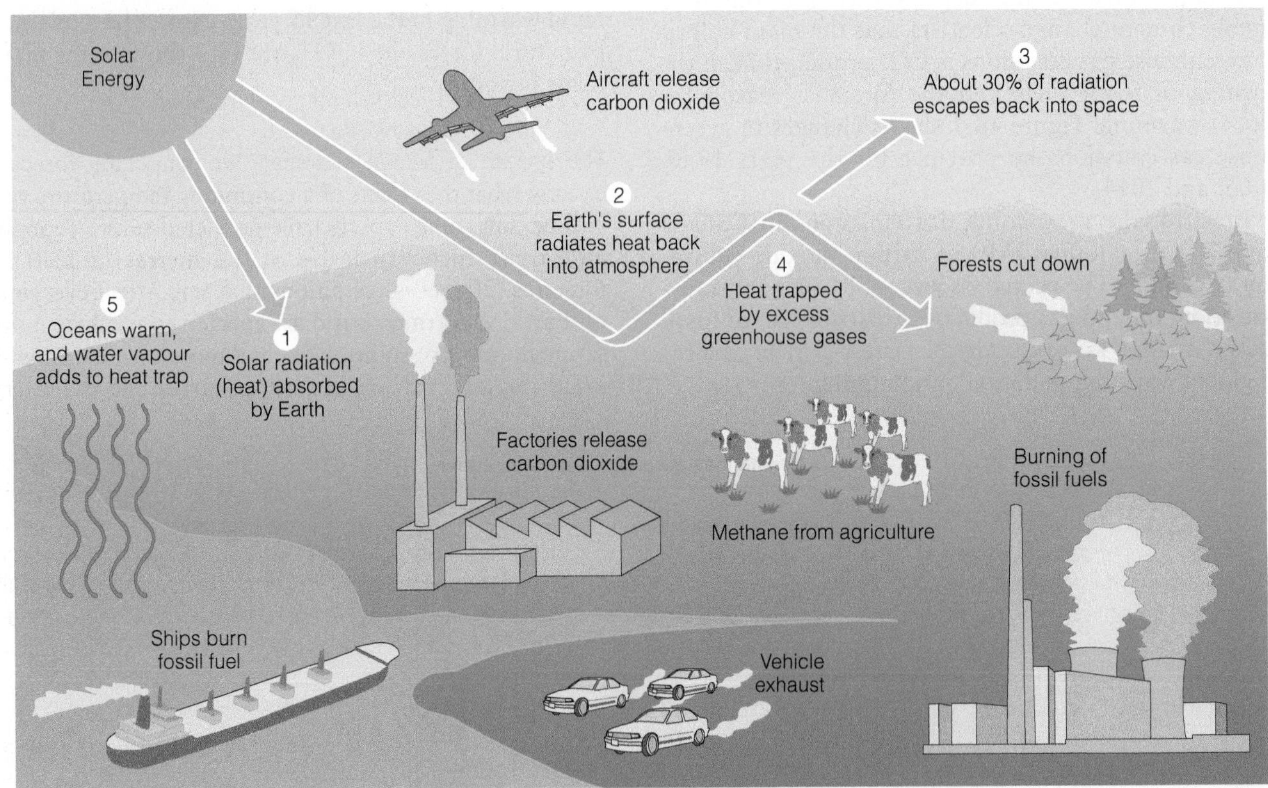

Figure 16-3 **Why the World Is Heating Up**

Source: Atlas of Canada, 2008. Natural Resources Canada, 2008. Reproduced with the permission of Natural Resources Canada, 2016.

of our water supply. Warmer weather—a consequence of changes in atmospheric gases and climate—worsens urban-industrial air pollution and, if the air also is moist, increases concentrations of allergenic pollens and fungal spores.

Extreme weather events have already become a reality around the globe. Hurricanes are becoming more intense. This could be linked to the increase in ocean temperature. As the water warms up, the hurricane draws more strength from the heat in the ocean surface waters.[19] Heat waves have become more frequent.[20] In Europe, in both 2003 and 2010, historic heat waves caused thousands of deaths and destroyed wheat crops. That resulted in rising food prices around the globe too.

These are truly problems without borders—climate change is also now a reality in Canada. In just the past decade we have witnessed

- Indigenous peoples living in the Artic suffering from sea-ice loss. Polar bears and caribou suffer because of disrupted feeding options. It has been suggested that the region might have an ice-free summer by 2040.[21]
- salmon stocks in British Columbia migrating further north as water temperature rises.[22]
- Alberta's epic flooding[23] and fires.[24]

The buildup of carbon dioxide and other greenhouse gases in the atmosphere could result in the greatest climate change in human history. A combination of factors, including the burning of fossil fuels and deforestation, is causing the atmosphere to retain heat. Scientists estimate that the world will become hotter within 100 years—the hottest it's been in two million years.

WHAT CAN WE DO TO PROTECT THE PLANET?

The choices we make and the actions we take can improve the health of our Earth. Being environmentally aware and putting plans into action do not mean that we have to sacrifice every comfort or spend great amounts of money. However, on international, national, and provincial scales and through individual commitment there is plenty of room for improvement.

International Initiatives

Kyoto Protocol In 1997, in Kyoto, Japan, an international treaty called the Kyoto Protocol was negotiated by a number of nations. In 2001, 165 countries signed onto the treaty. Kyoto committed some 40 industrialized nations to limit carbon emissions or reduce them to levels below those of 1990. On February 16, 2005, the Kyoto Protocol officially came into force—a historic milestone, according to environmental experts.[25] It was the first binding international agreement that set targets to reduce greenhouse gas emissions that cause climate change. There were 141 countries that ratified it, including every major industrialized country except the United States, Australia, and Monaco. Monaco ratified the accord in February 2006.

This treaty required countries to move to more responsible ways of producing and using energy. Under Kyoto, the target to reduce greenhouse gas emissions, between 2008 and 2012, was different for each country. Developing countries such as India and China did not have to commit to reducing their greenhouse gas emissions in the first phase. This was because their per capita emissions were much lower than those of developed countries.[26]

Although Canada was a signatory to the United Nations Framework Convention on Climate Change (UNFCCC) and legally required to meet its Kyoto targets by 2012, in October 2006, the Canadian government at the time opted to introduce Canada's *Clean Air Act* and subsequent eco-ACTION plan as an alternative plan. Then in December 2011, the federal government, at the Durban Climate Summit in South Africa, indicated that Canada would pull out of the Kyoto agreement after the first phase expired in 2012.

The Canadian plan to meet our country's targets includes mandatory cutbacks in emissions for large factories and power plants; updated standards for more energy-efficient buildings, homes, vehicles, and appliances; financial incentives for smaller businesses to cut emissions; and tax breaks or financial support for public transit and alternative fuels. There are concerns from industry lobby groups that environmental initiatives will cost Canada jobs and hurt our economy. There are also experts who suggest that they will create more jobs in alternative energy activities and produce net cost savings for Canadian consumers through energy savings and a chance to market new processes and technologies in a global market.

Bali Action Plan The Bali Climate Convention in 2007 was another important gathering of international delegates where work toward a global sustainability plan continued. The outcome of this convention laid a road map for a post-Kyoto protocol agreement for developed countries. Discussions about how to persist in the reduction of GHG emissions, how to best assist developing countries to adapt to climate change, and how to fund and use technology to shift to low carbon development worldwide were the topics of the day. A working group on long-term cooperative action (LTCA) was assembled and a working group on the Kyoto Protocol (KP) was tasked with negotiations aimed at commitments for new deep emission reductions for developed countries.[27]

Copenhagen Accord In 2009, the United Nations Climate Change Conference, commonly known as the Copenhagen Summit, was held in Copenhagen, Denmark. This was the 15th Conference of the Parties (COP15) under the United Nations Framework Convention on Climate Change. It brought together 125 heads of state, government representatives from 191 countries, and over 40 000 delegates of scientists, activists, and industrialists, the largest group of individuals interested in global environmental issues ever assembled.[28]

The goal of this international meeting was to finalize the Bali Action Plan and prepare for the expiry of the

Kyoto Protocol in 2012. While the Copenhagen Accord did not meet primary expectations that a legally binding treaty would be signed, it did result in a treaty that was not legally binding. However, it is also important to note that the Accord was not unanimously passed.[29]

Successes included the following:

- An aim of keeping global warming below 2°C and a review of the Accord by 2015.[30]
- Financing of a 100-billion-dollar-per-year Copenhagen Green Climate Fund with a fast-start funding of 10 billion dollars per year between 2010 and 2012 to assist the poorest nations adapt to climate change.[31]

Rio+20 The United Nations Conference on Sustainable Development, known as Rio+20, was held in June 2012 in Rio de Janeiro, Brazil. Member states began a process to develop a set of Sustainable Development Goals (SDGs). They also adopted guidelines on green economy policies. They also formulated an agreement to strengthen the United Nations Environment Program (UNEP) and establish a political forum for sustainable development. Another achievement was the adoption of a 10-year framework of programs that would focus on sustainable consumption and production patterns. Most notable was the attention of the world on this conference and the reminder that climate change needs continued partnership to advance sustainable development.[32]

The Paris Agreement On December 12, 2015, a new international environmental treaty, the Paris Agreement, was signed by delegates at the 21st session of the United Nations Framework Convention on Climate Change (UNFCCC).[33] The long-term goal is an agreement to keep the rise in global warming to below 2.0°C and strive to keep it within 1.5°C. The Canadian government is supporting the goal of 1.5°C.[34] Other commitments include an expectation that all countries will do their best to reach nationally determined contributions (NDCs): review and commit to new NDCs every five years; call on developed nations to provide funds to enable developing nations to reduce climate change; publish greenhouse gas reduction targets; and move toward carbon neutrality by 2050.

While enforcing the key points of the agreement has not been mandated, a mechanism will be developed to promote compliance among all countries. The Canadian government has a challenge of balancing the economy and environmental needs as the commitment to lower greenhouse gas emissions will impact many sectors such as transportation, energy, fisheries, and farming.

Carbon Offsets and Cap and Trade To solve the global environmental issues we all have to take into account our environmental footprint. Calculating our personal and organizational carbon emissions is a good first step.

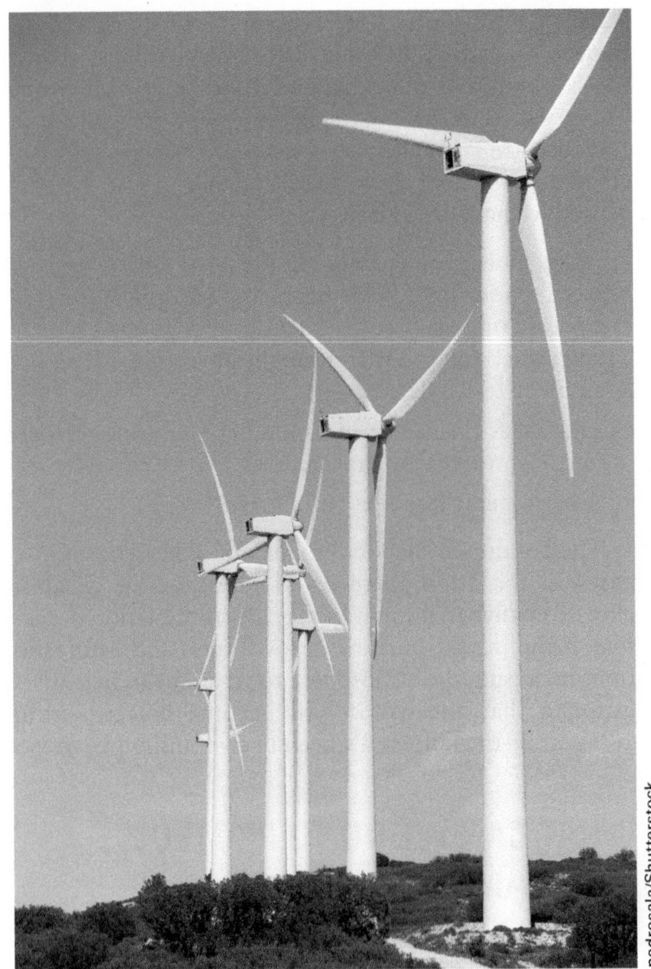

pedrosala/Shutterstock

Renewable fuel sources, such as wind turbines, can provide more environmentally friendly alternative sources of energy. However, individual choices and behaviours also have an impact on the state of our world.

Carbon offsets, defined as a credit for greenhouse gas reductions, have been promoted as one way to achieve carbon neutrality. There are two ways to look at the use of carbon offsets. First of all, businesses that are selling energy-efficient products can sell carbon offsets. One example would be a solar company that could realize a credit by selling carbon offsets to individuals or companies that are either not able to eliminate their own emissions or are in the process of making a transition to using non-polluting energy.

Individuals who want to compensate for their own GHG emissions, such as taking an airplane fight, can purchase carbon offsets as a way of supporting global sustainability. This assists the airline company with research and development of sustainable company policies. The expectation of carbon offsets is that your purchase results in a net benefit for our climate.[35]

Cap and trade is a tested and proven system for reducing pollution. The system requires that an organization, region, province, or country sets responsible

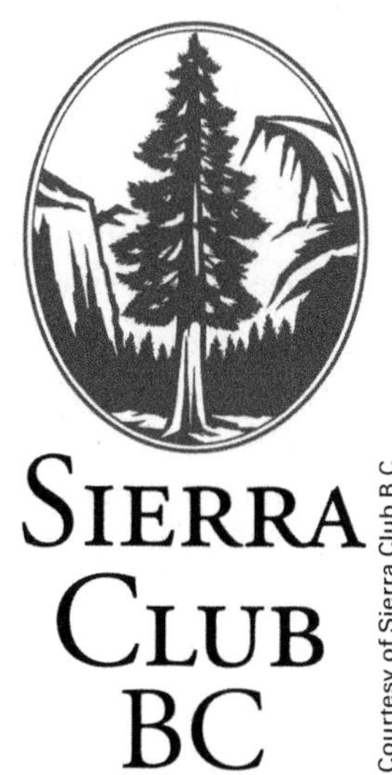

Courtesy of Sierra Club B.C

The Sierra Club BC works to protect and preserve British Columbia's natural wilderness and wildlife. Check for local, provincial, or national groups or agencies you can work with.

limits on GHG emissions and attempts to lower the emissions over time. The *cap* is the legal limit of the GHG emissions that can be emitted each year. The *trade* is a legal agreement between companies where they may swap among themselves the permission or permits to emit greenhouse gases.[36]

✓ CHECK-IN

What is your carbon footprint? Can you use carbon offsets or a cap and trade system to lower yours?

A Call to Action—Environmental Advocacy International and national governmental agencies certainly have a role to play with regard to global environmental issues. However, it takes small groups and individual action to make a difference too. We present only a few environmental advocates. Be sure to take note of organizations and individuals on your own campus or in your own community that are making a difference. Become a "change agent" yourself.

Indigenous Environmental Network The Indigenous Environmental Network (IEN) is a circle of Indigenous peoples who came together because of environmental concerns such as clear-cutting, herbicides, dams, and oil and gas exploration.[37]

The mission of IEN is to protect and restore the harmony of all life through traditional values, following the path of the ancestors. IEN is committed to connecting Indigenous peoples to the wider national and international community. While the headquarters for the IEN is in the United States, Canadian concerns are also being addressed.

There have been many changes in Canada because of the actions of the members of the IEN. Some examples include opposition to nuclear waste dumping in Saskatchewan adjacent to or on Native reserves; support for Bear Watch efforts to stop trophy hunting and poaching of black bears and grizzly bears for body parts; stopping destructive logging practices in many provinces; and efforts to stop low-level military flights to protect traditional lands. Current attempts are being made to bring attention to the Alberta tar sands project and the oil and natural gas pipelines being built across Alberta and British Columbia.

Sierra Club BC Since 1969 the Sierra Club BC[38] has been working to protect and preserve British Columbia's natural wilderness and wildlife. Members of the club want to ensure that B.C. is a global leader when tackling climate change. From an award-winning Environmental Education program, reaching 10 000 schoolchildren across the province each year, to monitoring provincial forestry and mining policy, to tracking provincial commitments to reduce greenhouse gas emissions, members of this organization are making a difference.[39]

Rachel Carson Rachel Carson, the author of one of the 20th century's most important books, *Silent Spring* (1962),[40] alerted us to the consequences of attempting to control nature with the use of poisonous chemicals to kill insects. The 40th anniversary edition of her book was published in 2002.

Sometimes called the "mother of the environmental movement,"[41] Carson challenged the practices of agricultural scientists and the U.S. government and called for new policies to protect human health and our environment.[42] Although she was attacked by individuals in the chemical industry and accused of being an alarmist, her research and writing helped to awaken public concern. This resulted in a government report that called for more research into the potential health hazards of pesticide use and urged care in the use of chemicals in homes and in industry.

Al Gore Al Gore, former vice-president of the United States, is an environmental activist and author who believes that the climate-change issue is one of the most important moral issues of our time. In 1992, he wrote a bestseller titled *Earth in the Balance: Ecology and the Human Spirit*[43] in which he explained the dire consequences of global warming.

In 2006, Gore wrote *An Inconvenient Truth: The Planetary Emergency of Global Warming and What We Can Do about It.*[44] This book struck a chord with a worldwide audience. It was followed by the production of one of the top documentaries in history and won an Academy Award for Documentary Feature.

In 2007, Gore was awarded a Nobel Peace Prize, shared with the Intergovernmental Panel on Climate

Change and given for efforts to build up and disseminate greater knowledge about human-made climate change. In his latest book, *The Future. Six Drivers of Global Change,*[45] Gore encourages all of us to be proactive when it comes to the climate-change crisis—even when the changes may be "inconvenient."

Ian McTaggart Cowan Known as the "father of Canadian ecology," Dr. Ian McTaggart Cowan was a wildlife biologist and naturalist.[46] He passed away in 2010 at the age of 99, but was still writing into his 90s and published his last major writing project, the final volume of *Birds of British Columbia*, at the age of 91.

During his 35-year tenure as a professor at the University of British Columbia (UBC), he founded the first university-based wildlife department in Canada. He was committed to educating students, colleagues, other scientists, and politicians about conservation of endangered species, the dangers of pesticides, and climate change. Celebrated for his work in the national parks system, his efforts became the foundation for wildlife environmental education in Canada.

He also pioneered nature television in the 1950s with shows such as *Fur and Feathers*, *The Web of Life*, and *The Living Sea*, which changed the way North Americans understood the important interconnection between the natural world and human actions. He helped produce 110 television documentaries and many teaching films.

He was widely honoured throughout his lifetime and won numerous awards such as the Order of British Columbia. He worked on behalf of many boards and public service agencies always advancing the application of scientific methods to wildlife management. A biography of Dr. McTaggart Cowan's life—*The Real Thing: The Natural History of Ian McTaggart Cowan*—was published in 2015.[47]

David Suzuki Dr. David Suzuki is an internationally renowned Canadian scientist, academic, broadcaster, writer, and founder of the David Suzuki Foundation. The mission of his foundation, started in 1990, is to protect the diversity of nature and the quality of life, now and for the future. The vision is that within a generation, Canadians will act on the understanding that we are all interconnected and interdependent with nature.[48]

Considered to be one of North America's leading environmentalists, Suzuki continues to encourage individual action to change the world. If you are concerned about the environment and want to make a difference, there are things you can do:[49]

1. **Queen of green.** Try to use eco-friendly cleaning products and cosmetics.
2. **Take action.** Your voice matters. Add your voice to environmental issues. Contact your politicians.
3. **Eat for healthy oceans.** Choose environmentally friendly seafood. Check out the Sea-Choice guide, www.seachoice.org/.
4. **Recycle your electronics.** Join the Think Recycle cost-free environmental fundraising program to keep your electronics out of the landfill.
5. **Green your workplace.** Commute to work if you can. Turn off lights and computers when you are not using them. Use double-sided printers.
6. **Reduce your carbon footprint.** Reduce your energy consumption. Travel in a sustainable way. Be mindful of what you purchase.
7. **Food and our planet.** Compost your food waste. Try a hundred-mile lunch.
8. **Connect youth with nature.** Download David Suzuki's *Connecting with Nature* educational guide.
9. **Be a citizen scientist.** You can join in on a SciStarter program and be connected to scientists and community leaders who are contributing to scientific research.
10. **Try the 30 × 30 nature challenge.** Add a daily dose of nature to your routine. Commit to getting outside 30 minutes a day for 30 days in a row.

If you are a student, it might be difficult to put into practice all of these suggestions. Just start with one, and then work up to 10. Linking up with community groups might be one way to start your own lifestyle changes.

Andrew Weaver We are fortunate to have in our midst yet another Canadian who is also calling for action, Dr. Andrew Weaver, a world-class climatologist, a University of Victoria professor, and the first-ever elected British Columbia Green Party MLA (Member of the Legislative Assembly) for Oak Bay–Gordon Head.[50] Alongside other colleagues, Dr. Weaver has developed an Earth systems climate model that is now used by scientists around the world. He has also been a lead author on the second, third, fourth, and fifth Intergovernmental Panel on Climate Change's (IPPC) scientific assessments.

He is a prolific writer of peer-reviewed scientific papers and two books on the environment. He is highly respected by his colleagues and his students. He has won many academic and research awards such as a Guggenheim fellowship in 2008, the Royal Society of Canada Miroslaw Romanowski Medal, and the A.G. Huntsman Award for Excellence in Marine Science in 2011. In 2008 he was appointed to the Order of British Columbia. In 2012 he was awarded the Queen's Diamond Jubilee Medal and the University of Victoria Community Leadership Award.

Dr. Weaver has now turned to politics because he believes that British Columbia needs an independent, evidence-based viewpoint in the legislature. He believes that his experience as a scientist, policy advisor, and community member will help him continue to make significant contributions both nationally and internationally.

THE GREENING OF COLLEGE AND UNIVERSITY CAMPUSES

There is a new movement at colleges and universities—campus environmental sustainability. From hiring sustainability coordinators, building LEED (Leadership and Energy in Environmental Design)[51] buildings, switching energy sources, and providing subsidized access to public transit, to educating the campus population, environmental advocacy is evident from administration, faculty, staff, and students who are attempting to "green" their campuses. Some students are basing their decisions on what institute to attend on how sustainable an institution is.[52]

Other students are forming environmental organizations. Common Energy[53] is one example. This nonprofit organization began at the University of Victoria in November 2006. Founded by a group of students, Common Energy became a network of students, staff, faculty, and community partners that focused on moving the university "beyond climate-neutral"—where it would do more to solve the problems of climate change than to cause them. A Common Energy group has now been established at the University of British Columbia, too.

To become more educated about climate-change issues, find out what environmental initiatives are in place on your campus or in your community. Volunteer, become an advocate, and make a difference. Table 16-1

TABLE 16-1

Calling All Campuses—Environmental Initiatives

Examples of Green and Sustainability Initiatives in a Sample of Canadian Universities and University Colleges

University	Who's Who, What's What	Web Link
Alberta		
University of Alberta	Office of Sustainability Student Sustainability Summit	http://sustainability.ualberta.ca/en.aspx
University of Calgary	UCalgary Sustainability	https://www.ucalgary.ca/sustainability/
University of Lethbridge	Sustainability	http://www.uleth.ca/sustainability/
British Columbia		
Royal Roads University	Sustainability at Royal Roads University	http://www.royalroads.ca/about/sustainability
Simon Fraser University	Sustainability	https://www.sfu.ca/sustainability.html
University of British Columbia	Common Energy	https://commonenergyubc.com/
University of Northern British Columbia	Canada's Green University	http://www.unbc.ca/green
University of Victoria	Campus Planning and Sustainability	http://www.uvic.ca/sustainability/
Vancouver Island University	Sustainability Starts with You	https://www2.viu.ca/sustainability/
Manitoba		
University of Manitoba	Students for Sustainability	http://www.thegrowingvillage.org/home-1.html
University of Winnipeg	Campus Sustainability Office	http://uwinnipeg.ca/sustainability/
New Brunswick		
Mount Allison University	Environmental Activism	https://www.mta.ca/Community/Academics/Faculty_of_Social_Sciences/Geography_and_Environment/Environmental_activism/Environmental_activism/
University of New Brunswick–Fredericton	Sustainability—Facilities Management	http://www.unb.ca/fredericton/fm/sustainability/
Newfoundland		
Memorial University	Sustainability at Memorial	http://www.mun.ca/sustain/
Nova Scotia		
Acadia University	Campus Sustainability	http://sustainability.acadiau.ca/campus-sustainability.html
Dalhousie University	Office of Sustainability	http://www.dal.ca/dept/sustainability.html

(Continued)

TABLE 16-1

Calling All Campuses—Environmental Initiatives *(Continued)*

University	Who's Who, What's What	Web Link
Ontario		
Brock University	Sustainability at Brock	https://brocku.ca/sustainabilityatbrock
Carleton University	Sustainability Strategic Plan	http://carleton.ca/fmp/energy-and-sustainability/sustainability-strategic-plan/
Queen's University	Queen's Green Campus	http://www.queensu.ca/about/greencampus
Ryerson University	Campus Facilities and Sustainability	http://www.ryerson.ca/campusfacilities/departments/sustainability/
University of Ottawa	Office of Campus Sustainability	https://sustainable.uottawa.ca/
University of Toronto	Sustainability Office	http://www.fs.utoronto.ca/SustainabilityOffice/
University of Waterloo	Sustainability	https://uwaterloo.ca/sustainability/
York University	Sustainability@yorku	http://sustainability.info.yorku.ca/
Prince Edward Island		
University of PEI	Sustainability and Energy Management	http://www.upei.ca/facilities/sustainability
Quebec		
Concordia University	Sustainable Concordia	http://sustainableconcordia.ca/
McGill University	Sustainability	https://www.mcgill.ca/sustainability/home
Saskatchewan		
University of Regina	Facilities Management—Sustainability Around Campus	http://www.uregina.ca/fm/campus-sustainability/
University of Saskatchewan	Office of Sustainability	http://sustainability.usask.ca/

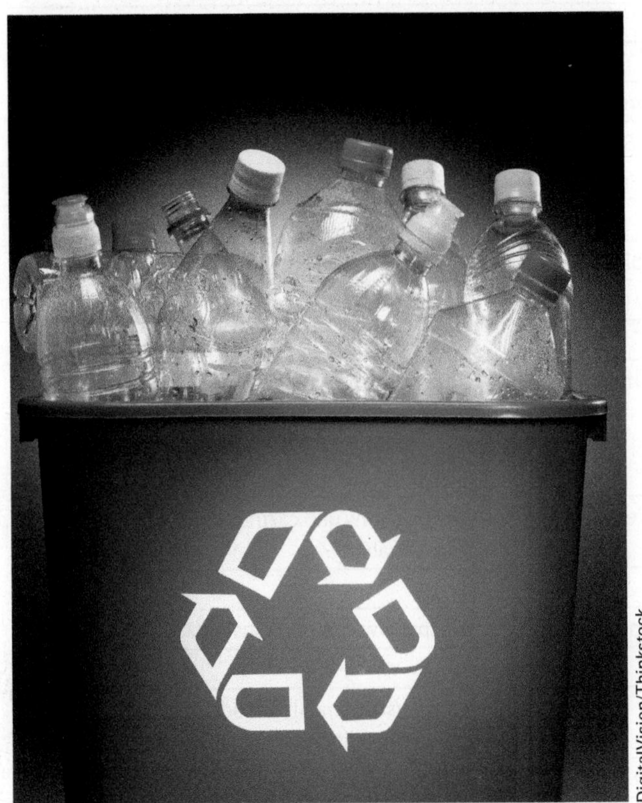

DigitalVision/Thinkstock

Recycling is an easy way to help save energy and conserve resources.

will provide you with some ideas of green and sustainability initiatives in a sample of Canadian universities across Canada such as the sustainable residence program at Mount Allison's Cuthbertson House.

✓ CHECK-IN

What type of environmental initiatives are being developed and put in place on your campus? Is there a student environmental club or group you could join?

The 4 Rs—Reduce, Reuse, Recycle, Recover Colleges and universities are also promoting the 4 Rs—Reduce, Reuse, Recycle, and Recover. Initiatives are being organized in student dorms, in common areas, and in educational and recreational buildings. Students can also compete for national environmental awards.

One basic environmental action is to **reduce**: buy products packaged in recycled materials or purchase products that have little or no packaging. Packaging makes up about half our garbage by volume, one-third by weight. Consider how you are going to dispose of a product and the packaging materials before purchasing it. How to start? Bring reusable bags when you have purchases to make. Some municipalities are moving toward banning single-use plastic bags entirely.

What you cannot reduce, try to **reuse**. When possible, repair items instead of purchasing new ones. Use jars, tins, and plastic containers to store household and food items. If you cannot reuse, **recycle**, at home, at work, and at school. Recycling—collecting, reprocessing, marketing, and using materials once considered trash—has become a necessity for several reasons: we've run out of space for all the garbage we produce; waste sites are often health and safety hazards; recycling is cheaper than landfill storage or incineration (a major source of air pollution); and recycling helps save energy and natural resources.

Some communities and college and university campuses provide regular blue box pickup of recyclables. Most programs pick up bottles, cans, and newspapers—either separated or mixed together. Other communities have drop-off centres where consumers can leave recyclables. Some recycling centres, including grocery stores, will buy back aluminum cans, plastic bottles, and tetra packs. Soft plastic recycling is another option on many campuses across Canada, as are composting facilities.

Finally, you might **recover**. One example is the refurbishing of old computers, called E-Recycle, which are then donated to schools and community groups.[54] Parts can also be salvaged. Hazardous computer parts are then disposed of safely. "Tech trash" buried in landfills is creating a new hazard because trace amounts of potentially hazardous agents, such as lead and mercury, can leak into the ground and water.

Four Laws of Ecology Every so often we need a gentle reminder about our personal responsibility for global sustainability. Some students have found the use of Barry Commoner's Four Laws of Ecology helpful. They are outlined in his book, *The Closing Circle: Nature, Man, and Technology*.[55] Although written over three decades ago, this book seems all the more relevant today.

1. *Everything Is Connected to Everything Else.* Our environment is a closed ecosystem, powered by the sun. The materials needed for the survival of this planet must be recycled over and over again. Natural ecosystems are so complex that many of us do not see or understand the entire range of connections. We must begin to understand the impact our personal and collective lives have on such a system. Ask yourself how your lifestyle choices affect our environment.
2. *Everything Must Go Somewhere.* There is no "away" to throw things. In nature, there is no concept of waste—elements excreted by one organism serve as nourishment for another. Human beings have created "industrialization," where items are designed to be disposable—thrown "away." Ask yourself the following: What did you throw away today? Where will it go? What impact will it have on the ecosystem? Presently our garbage is accumulating and will be polluting landfill sites for centuries to come.
3. *Nature Knows Best.* In nature, for every organic compound produced by a living thing, there is an enzyme somewhere in the ecosystem that is capable of breaking it down. This is essential to the harmony of the ecosystem. Unfortunately, technology has been responsible for the creation of substances that cannot be broken down. In some cases, these non-biodegradable products have created problems in diverse ecosystems. What products or services do you use that do not support sustainable living? How can you change your consumption or use of these products?
4. *There Is No Such Thing as a Free Lunch.* For every technological gain there is an ecological price tag. Sometimes, this price tag can be delayed for a time; however, we eventually pay the price. Air, water, and land pollution, which have poisoned the food we grow and eat, are examples of costs we have incurred for modern living. Unfortunately, when clean-up costs become monumental, environmental initiatives are often stalled. What are you doing to clean up after yourself?

The following online calculators can help you determine your own **ecological footprint**. Try them out.

- **Global Footprint Network calculator**[56]—estimates the amount of land and ocean required to sustain your personal consumption patterns on an annual basis. http://www.footprintnetwork.org/en/index.php/GFN/page/calculators/
- **Environmental Paper Network**[57]—estimates the environmental impacts of different types of paper choices. www.edf.org/papercalculator
- **Canadian Automobile Association**[58]—Driving Costs Calculator. Calculate your weekly, monthly, and annual commuting costs. http://caa.ca/car_costs/
- **Lifestyle Carbon Calculator**[59]—Use the LiveSmart BC Lifestyle Carbon Calculator to estimate your yearly greenhouse gas (GHG) emissions. http://www.livesmartbc.ca/homes/h_calc.html

✓ CHECK-IN

Have you determined your ecological footprint?

THE ENVIRONMENT AND OUR HEALTH

The Ecological Determinants of Health In Chapter 1, the social determinants of health were introduced and a discussion presented as to how the determinants were connected to overall human health and wellness. The

Canadian Public Health Association (CPHA) has published an important document that reminds us that ecological determinants of health are also inextricably linked to our overall well-being too.[60] Ecological determinants at the most essential level include oxygen, water, and food. The current state of our ecosystem is in peril, according to many climate scientists, who suggest that our human actions are impacting all three ecological determinants in negative ways. The following sections will address some of the environmental concerns on our ecology.

Environment and Physical Health We cannot separate our health from our environment. No individual is immune to the effects of changes in the environment. Information from the Office of Disease Prevention and Health Promotion (ODPHP) indicates that close to 25 percent of all deaths and diseases globally can be linked to environmental factors.[61] These factors include exposure to harmful elements in air, water, soil, and food that have been found to cause respiratory and cardiovascular diseases as well as various cancers. Improving indoor and outdoor air quality, water, sanitation, and hygiene could greatly reduce child mortality in the world's lowest-income countries.[62] We must address our carbon footprint; we are depleting the ozone layer and destroying many plant and animal species.[63]

Environment and Psychosocial Health Changes in our environment are also impacting our psychosocial health. Research shows that a strong relationship to a location or place is essential to human health. Human beings need a sense of belonging and familiarity. They build relationships in communities that they call home. The sense of attachment increases with the length of time we live in a certain place.[64] Shifting climates can complicate and destabilize that sense of attachment.

Elevated sea levels, drought, flooding, and extreme weather events can result in people being displaced from their homes and businesses, deaths of family and friends, economic hardships, and feelings of uncertainty, restlessness, mistrust, and concern about the future. No one can be prepared for all the consequences of climate change and global warming, but a focus on our psychosocial health will be important as we attempt to adapt to environmental changes.

THE IMPACT OF POLLUTION

Any change in the air, water, or soil that could reduce its ability to support life is a form of **pollution**. Natural events, such as smoke from fires triggered by lightning, can cause pollution. The effects of pollution depend on the concentration (amount per unit of air, water, or soil) of the **pollutant**, how long it remains in the environment, and its chemical nature. An *acute effect* is a severe, immediate reaction, usually after a single, large exposure. For example, pesticide poisoning can cause nausea and dizziness, even death. A *chronic effect* may take years to develop or may be a recurrent or continuous reaction, usually after repeated exposures. The development of cancer after repeated exposure to a pollutant such as asbestos is an example of a chronic effect.

Environmental agents that trigger changes, or **mutations**, in the genetic material (the DNA) of living cells are called **mutagens**. The changes that result can lead to the development of cancer. Many mutagens are carcinogens. Furthermore, the effects of a mutagen on an egg or a sperm cell can be passed on to future generations. Mutagens that can cross the placenta of a pregnant woman and cause a spontaneous abortion or birth defects in the fetus are called **teratogens**.

Among the health problems that have been linked with pollution are the following:

- headaches and dizziness
- eye irritation and impaired vision
- nasal discharge
- cough, shortness of breath, and sore throat
- constricted airways
- constriction of blood vessels and increased risk of heart disease
- chest pains and aggravation of the symptoms of colds, pneumonia, bronchial asthma, emphysema, chronic bronchitis, lung cancer, and other respiratory problems
- birth defects and reproductive problems
- nausea, vomiting, and stomach cancer

Human beings are exposed to pollution through a number of pathways (see Table 16-2). Toxic substances can enter our body through our lungs, our digestive system, and through skin contact. The combined interaction of two or more hazards can produce an effect greater than that of either one alone. Pollutants can affect an organ or organ system directly or indirectly.

TABLE 16-2

Pathways of Human Exposure to Pollution Sources

Examples of Pollution Sources	Environmental Elements	Route of Exposure
Carbon monoxide (CO)	Air	Inhalation Dermal contact
Pesticides	Soil	Ingestion Dermal contact Inhalation
Nitrates	Water	Ingestion Dermal contact
E. coli	Food	Ingestion

CLEARING THE AIR

Air pollution of any sort can cause numerous ill effects. As pollutants destroy the hair-like cilia that remove irritants from the lungs, individuals may suffer chronic bronchitis, characterized by excessive mucus flow and continuous coughing. Air pollution can be as harmful to breathing capacity as smoking. Residents of polluted cities are exposed to some of the same toxic gases, such as nitrogen oxide and **carbon monoxide**, found in cigarettes. Emphysema may develop or worsen as pollutants constrict the bronchial tubes and destroy the air sacs in the lungs, making breathing more difficult. Deaths caused by air pollution exceed those from motor vehicle accidents.

In addition to respiratory diseases, air pollution also contributes to heart disease, cancer, and weakened immunity. For the elderly and people with asthma or heart disease, polluted air can be life threatening. Even healthy individuals can be affected, particularly if they exercise outdoors during high-pollution periods. Carbon monoxide has been shown to impair joggers' exercise performance. Check out the Air Quality Health Index (AQHI) from Environment Canada to learn more about air quality and your risks from air pollution.[65]

Smog A combination of smoke and fog, **smog** is made up of chemical vapours from auto exhaust, industrial and commercial pollutants (volatile organic compounds, carbon monoxide, nitrogen oxides, sulphur oxides, particulates), and ozone. The most obvious sources of these pollutants are motor vehicles, industrial factories, electric utility plants, and wood-burning stoves. These chemicals react with sunlight, especially during high-pressure systems and periods of low wind speeds, to form smog.

✓ CHECK-IN

What is the air quality like where you live and work?

Sulphur dioxide smog (grey-air smog) is produced by burning oil of high sulphur content. Some larger Canadian cities are now dealing with grey-air smog. Like cigarette smoke, grey-air smog affects the cilia in the respiratory passages; the lungs are unable to expel particulates, such as soot, ash, and dust, which remain and irritate the tissues. This condition is hazardous to people with chronic respiratory problems.[66]

Photochemical smog (brown-air smog) is also found in large traffic centres. This type of smog results principally from nitric oxide in car exhaust reacting with oxygen in the air and forming nitrogen dioxide, which produces a brownish haze and, when exposed to sunlight, other pollutants.

STRATEGIES FOR CHANGE

Doing Your Part for Cleaner Air

- Drive a car that gets high gas mileage and produces low emissions. Keep your speed at or below the speed limit.
- Keep your tires inflated and your engine tuned. Seventy percent of cars and light trucks in Canada have at least one tire that is overinflated or underinflated. Maintaining the correct tire pressure could reduce your GHGs by at least one-eighth of a tonne each year. Recycle old batteries and tires. (Most stores that sell new ones will take back old ones.)
- Turn off your engine if you're going to be stopped for more than a minute. If you avoid idling for just three minutes each day of the year, CO_2 emissions could be reduced by 1.4 million tonnes annually. We could save 630 million litres of fuel— equivalent to taking 320 000 cars off the road for an entire year.[67]
- Collect all fluids that you drain from your car (e.g., motor oil, antifreeze) and recycle or properly dispose of them.

One of these, **ozone**, the most widespread pollutant, can impair the body's immune system and cause long-term lung damage. (Ozone in the upper atmosphere protects us by repelling harmful ultraviolet radiation from the sun, but ozone in the lower atmosphere is a harmful component of air pollution.) Automobiles also produce carbon monoxide, a colourless and odourless gas that diminishes the ability of red blood cells to carry oxygen. The resulting oxygen deficiency can affect breathing, hearing, and vision.

Indoor Pollutants Because people in industrialized nations spend more than 90 percent of their time inside buildings, the quality of the air they breathe can have an even greater impact on their well-being than outdoor pollution. The most hazardous form of indoor air pollution is cigarette smoke—we discussed this in Chapter 12. Table 16-3 lists some other common indoor pollutants and describes the potential health risks. Living green walls are now being used in office buildings and homes not only to beautify rooms but also to improve air quality. Adding living green wall or indoor plants can lower levels of nitrogen dioxide and particulate matter as well as toxins that leech from our indoor environment.

One other indoor pollutant viewed as an environmental risk is **mould**. One of the oldest and most widespread substances on Earth, mould is a type of fungus that decomposes organic matter and provides plants with nutrients. It has emerged as a major health concern because of its growth in buildings and homes. Common moulds include *Aspergillus, Penicillium,* and *Stachybotrys,* a slimy, dark-green mould that has been blamed for infant deaths and various illnesses, from

Alzheimer's disease to cancer, in adults that breathe its spores. Faulty ventilation systems and airtight buildings have been implicated as contributing to the increased mould problem.

Experts agree that mould may trigger or worsen a number of health problems, including dizziness, breathing problems, nausea, and asthma attacks. However, mould usually is harmful only to allergic or sensitive individuals.

THE QUALITY OF OUR DRINKING WATER

In Chapter 9, there was a discussion of water quality in Canada, so we will not look at this issue further here. For further information, you may want to access the Canadian Drinking Water Quality Guidelines, developed by Health Canada, which have made Canadians more aware of the importance of safe drinking water. These guidelines have been established for all public and private drinking-water supplies.[68]

We will, however, mention the environmental impact of bottled water. Any water sold in sealed containers is considered to be bottled water. It can be spring water, mineral water, or water from a variety of water sources that might have been treated to make it fit for human consumption.[69] The popularity of bottled water has risen in part because some people think bottled water is safer than tap water. Although bottled water is usually disinfected to remove harmful organisms, many studies have shown that bacteria are found in most bottled waters.[70] Other studies have shown that the levels of bacteria increase quickly to maximum levels after six weeks at room temperature. Since ultraviolet light destroys harmful organisms, this regrowth of harmless flora is not seen as a health hazard. Refrigeration is recommended after you open your bottled water, however.

TABLE 16-3

Common Indoor Pollutants

Indoor Pollutant	Description	Health Risks
Formaldehyde	Comes from the materials buildings are made of and the appliances inside them. Examples include carpet backing, furniture, foam insulation, plywood, and particle board.	Can cause nausea, dizziness, headaches, heart palpitations, stinging eyes, burning lungs; shown to cause cancer in animals.
Asbestos	Mineral used for building insulation. Consumer products containing asbestos are now banned under the *Hazardous Products Act*.[71]	Linked to lung and gastrointestinal cancer among asbestos workers and families.
Lead	In many homes painted with lead-based paint (prior to 1960). Also in air and water. New regulations have been set for lead content in paint and surface coating material and children's jewellery.[72] The lead content limit has been reduced from 5000 mg/kg to 600 mg/kg.	High risk to fetuses and children under seven years of age. In children, lead can kill brain cells and cause poor concentration, reduced short-term memory, slower reaction time, and learning disabilities. In adults, exposure to low levels can cause headaches, high blood pressure, irritability, tremors, and insomnia. Exposure to high levels can cause anemia, stomach pain, vomiting, diarrhea, and constipation. Long-term exposure can impair fertility, damage kidneys and the central nervous system, and result in stillbirth or miscarriage.
Mercury	A metal found in paint, enamels, varnishes, and lacquers. A new mercury content limit of 10 mg/g for all surface materials has been set by Health Canada.[73]	Health effects on children can include a decrease in intelligence, delay in walking and talking, lack of coordination, blindness, and seizures.
Carbon monoxide (CO) and nitrogen dioxide (NO_2)	CO is a tasteless, odourless, colourless, and non-irritating gas produced by the incomplete combustion of fuel in space heaters, furnaces, water heaters, and engines. NO_2 gas comes from natural gas or propane stoves. Canada's National Ambient Air Quality Objectives (NAAQOs) prescribe targets for air quality.[74]	CO can be deadly. Reduces the delivery of oxygen to the blood. Effects include headaches, nausea, vomiting, fatigue, and dizziness. NO_2 can lead to respiratory illness.

In Canada, bottled water is defined as a food product so it is controlled under the *Food and Drugs Act* and *Food and Drug Regulations.* Under this act Health Canada is responsible for establishing safety and nutritional standards and quality of food sold. The standards are enforced by the Canadian Food Inspection Agency (CFIA). This agency is also in charge of the labelling requirements. However, although nutrition labelling has become mandatory on most pre-packaged products, there are some bottled water products that are exempt from these regulations.[75]

How does bottled water link to environmental concerns? In a number of communities in Canada where large bottled-water manufacturing plants are located, citizens are concerned about the large quantities of water being removed from local water sources. Bottlers are not required to pay for the water that they take. Environmental assessments of the impact that this industry has on our local ecosystems are not being done in most cases.[76]

Another concern is the fact that plastic water bottles are environmentally unfriendly. Reports suggest that on a global scale, approximately 2.7 million tonnes of plastic are used to produce plastic water bottles each year. The production and distribution of the bottles burns fossil fuels and results in the release of thousands of tonnes of harmful emissions.[77]

Many of these water bottles—9 out of 10—end up in the garbage instead of being recycled. It is estimated that it takes 700 years before they start to decompose and up to 1000 years to fully decompose. In the United States, supplying Americans with water bottles for one year consumes more than 1.5 million barrels of oil, which is enough to fuel 100 000 cars for a year, or generate electricity for more than 250 00 homes.[78] This is just one more example of the cause-and-effect relationship between nature and our technological society.

In Canada, there is a gathering revolt, too. Students at colleges and universities across Canada are encouraging "bottled-water-free zones" and supporting the purchase of reusable coffee mugs and water bottles. The University of Winnipeg was the first university in Canada to ban the sale of plastic water bottles. At Queen's University plastic water bottles are no longer available through vending machines, retail outlets on campus, or any catered events.[79]

✓ **CHECK-IN**

Do you use a refillable water bottle when you are on campus?

Fluoride In Canada, most of us are exposed to fluorides on a daily basis—through trace amounts found in our food and the fluoride added to drinking water supplies to prevent tooth decay. Fluorides are chemical compounds that have been shown to protect tooth enamel against the acids that cause tooth decay. About 45 percent of Canadians receive fluoridated water.[80]

The risks of using fluoride appear to be very small; however, if children under the age of six ingest high levels of fluorides during the period of tooth formation, they can develop a condition known as dental fluorosis, which causes white or brown stains to appear on the teeth. It does not affect the function of the teeth, just the appearance. Health Canada has set labelling requirements for dental products such as toothpaste that contain fluoride since many young children tend to swallow these products.[81]

Health Canada also reports that high levels of fluorides consumed for very long periods of time may lead to skeletal fluorsis, a condition in which bones increase in density and become more brittle. In severe cases bones can become deformed and fracture. In mild cases, an individual may experience stiff joints.[82]

Health professionals advise consumers to use only small amounts of fluoridated toothpaste, rinse thoroughly after brushing, and use fluoride supplements only when the home water supply is known to be deficient.

Chlorine Chlorine is a disinfectant added to our drinking water to reduce or eliminate microorganisms such as bacteria and viruses. Chlorine is the most commonly used drinking-water disinfectant. Current research suggests that the health risks of drinking water treated with chlorine are much less than the risks from trihalomethanes (THMs), a common by-product of chlorine when it reacts with organic matter present in water supplies.[83] However, many Canadians are becoming concerned about chlorinated water supplies and a number of cities are now using ozone to disinfect their water. Ozonation does not produce THMs. When ozone is used as the main disinfectant, small amounts of chlorine must still be used, since ozone breaks down quickly.

CHEMICAL RISKS

Pesticides are toxic. When pesticides are used in or around your home, safe handling and proper application procedures must be followed. Before purchasing or using pesticide products, check out possible alternatives that might be available to you. Insecticidal soaps, boric acid, and pyrethrum have low toxicity to humans and can be effective.

Purchase only domestic-class products bearing a PCP registration number. Commercial or industrial class products are intended for use only by licensed applicators. People and pets should leave the area you are treating.

You should wear protective clothing such as rubber gloves, long-sleeved shirts, coveralls, and goggles. Do not use a pesticide indoors that is intended for outdoor use. Don't smoke, drink, or eat while applying pesticides. After use, make sure you wash your face and hands with soapy water. Clean your clothing before reusing it. Wash this clothing separately from your other clothing items.

What Health Risks Are Caused by Pesticides?

Although some research suggests that pest-control products can be used without posing a significant risk to our health or our environment, other studies indicate that exposure to pesticides may pose a risk to pregnant women and their fetuses. Exposure to toxic chemicals causes about 3 percent of developmental defects.[84] Other studies have shown a link to chronic diseases related to past exposure to toxic substances, including lung cancer, bladder cancer, leukemia, lymphoma, chronic bronchitis, and disorders of the nervous system. **Endocrine disruptors**, chemicals that act on or interfere with human hormones, particularly estrogen, may pose a different threat. Scientists are investigating their impact on fertility, falling sperm counts, and cancers of the reproductive organs.

Chlorinated hydrocarbons include several high-risk substances—such as DDT, kepone, and chlordane—that may cause cancer, birth defects, neurological disorders, and damage to wildlife and the environment. They are extremely resistant to breakdown.[85]

DDT, a synthetic chlorinated insecticide, kills insects by attacking biochemical processes in their nervous systems. Although it was seen as a technological triumph of the 1940s and was used widely until the 1960s, DDT proved to be a persistent pesticide, a toxin that remains in the environment for as long as 15 years before degrading. When sprayed to kill insect pests, it also killed the natural predators of that pest. The peak year for use in the United States was 1959, when nearly 80 million pounds were applied. From then, usage declined steadily to about 13 million pounds in 1971, most of it applied to cotton.

DDT has also been found in humans and appears to be a risk factor for breast cancer in women. Because of the work of Rachel Carson and others, DDT use was restricted in 1969 and banned in the United States in 1972.[86] However, it is still manufactured in the United States and sold in developing nations. It now contaminates products such as coffee, tea, and bananas, which are then sold back to consumers in Canada and the United States.

Organic phosphates, including chemicals such as malathion, break down more rapidly than the chlorinated hydrocarbons. Most are highly toxic, causing cramps, confusion, diarrhea, vomiting, headaches, and breathing difficulties. Higher levels in the blood can lead to convulsions, paralysis, coma, and death.

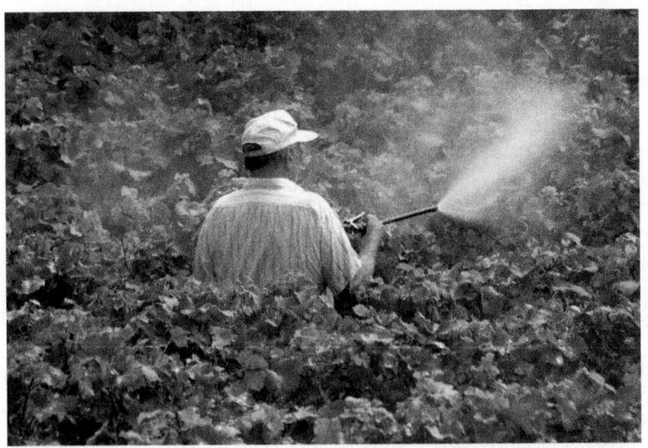

Alistair Scott/Shutterstock

Pesticides protect crops from harmful insects, plants, and fungi, but may endanger human health.

✓ CHECK-IN

Do you or your family use pesticides to control weeds in your yard or garden? Were you aware of the risks of using pesticides before reading this chapter?

Chemical Weapons Terrorist threats and weapons of war have included the use of chemical weapons. The impact of chemical weapons has contaminated soil, air, and water quality around the world. The impact of chemical weapons continues to be a major health issue.[87] Bio-terror agents include poison gases, herbicides, and other types of chemical substances that can kill, maim, or temporarily incapacitate. Chemical agents can be dispersed as liquids, vapours, gases, and aerosols that attack nerves, blood, skin, or lungs. In contrast to biological weapons, chemical weapons can kill rapidly, often within hours or minutes, and sometimes with just a small drop. Possible protection against chemical weapons includes gas masks, shelters, and sealed suits and vehicles. Treatment and antidotes can sometimes help after exposure. If contaminated, you need to flush your eyes and skin immediately for at least five to ten minutes while awaiting emergency help.

Some common chemical agents include ricin, which, when inhaled, causes weakness, fever, chest tightness, and potentially fatal fluid buildup in the lungs; sarin, a nerve gas that can cause death within minutes by paralyzing the muscles used for breathing; and VX, which kills within minutes by blocking the transmission of nerve impulses along the central nervous system, causing convulsions, respiratory paralysis, and death.

Cosmetic Chemicals When you shampoo your hair, wash your hands with soap, apply makeup, or use

HUMAN POTENTIAL

Naomi Devine—Working for Climate Change

Our Human Potential story for this chapter is about Naomi Devine, a young woman who is facing the challenge of climate change with perseverance and commitment.

Climate change is the defining issue of my generation. I often refer to myself as a child of the "David Suzuki generation." I became aware of environmental damage being done to the natural world as a young girl. My favourite place to play was in a park. Having a natural affinity to water I wanted to play in the small river that ran through it. Unfortunately, I was too young to understand how the three letters, "PCBs," were ruining my daily adventure. All I remember is that it made me upset that I could not play in an area I loved so much.

Watching so many places that were important to me become victim to pollution, development, and destruction, I began searching for solutions to insurmountable challenges. I began to realize that we need to be climate-neutral in my lifetime. Mountains are difficult to climb, but many of us find the resolve within ourselves to do what needs to be done. Climate change is our collective mountain challenge.

I enrolled at university to complete a degree in environmental studies and political science. I also became the Director of the University of Victoria's Sustainability Project and started the Victoria, British Columbia's Chapter of the B.C. Sustainable Energy Association (BCSEA). I wanted to fully immerse myself in the work on how we handle the design of our energy system. Climate change is a very large symptom of poor energy design.

In 2006, I was chosen to be a member of the Canadian Youth Delegation to the United Nations Framework Convention on Climate Change Conference in Nairobi, Kenya. As a delegate to this conference I wanted to see how our federal government would negotiate on our behalf in the international climate talks. What I found shocked and embarrassed me—Canada was de facto pulling out of the Kyoto Accord. I promised myself then that I would try to find a way to hold politicians and organizations accountable for their actions (or non-action) on the climate file.

When I returned to UVic, a group of friends and I founded an organization called Common Energy. We created a bold goal—to have UVic move "beyond climate-neutral." The organization became a network of over 100 students, staff, faculty, and community members. We researched, wrote, and published a report on institutional action on climate change that was the first of its kind in Canada. The success of Common Energy grew and expanded to the University of British Columbia. That club is now the largest student-run university sustainability organization housed on campuses in the country.

I was then honoured to be asked to sit on British Columbia's Climate Action Team. My job, along with 29 well-respected scientists, economists, and business and non-governmental organization leaders, was to provide expert advice to the premier on how B.C. could meet its newly legislated greenhouse gas emissions targets. British Columbia was the first jurisdiction in North America to legislate hard targets on GHG emission reductions—33 percent below 2007 levels by 2020.

I then began work in the University of Victoria's Sustainability Office. I set out to help create the university's first sustainability policy and five-year action plan. From there, I spent three remarkable years in Whistler, B.C., where I was the Sustainability Coordinator for the Resort Municipality—up to and including the 2010 Winter Olympics and Paralympic Games. As a lead team member I helped to develop a carbon neutral operations plan and create a climate action innovation fund for the municipality using carbon tax funds to lower municipal emissions—part of Whistler's 2020 community sustainability plan.

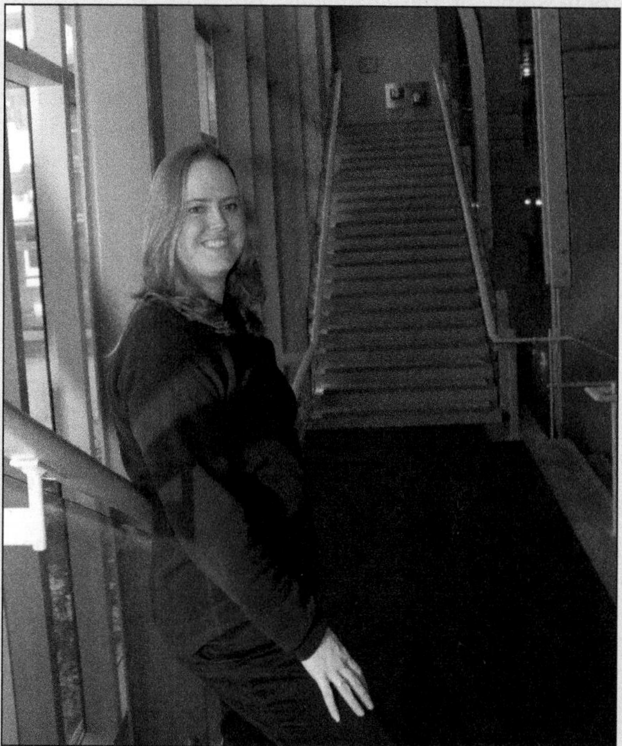
Courtesy of Naomi Devine

Naomi Devine, Co-founder of Common Energy, and a passionate advocate for solving the climate crisis.

At this stage the 20th anniversary of the Rio Conference in 1992 was approaching. With my love of adventure I decided to bike, bus, and boat to Rio. After riding thousands of kilometres on a solo journey looking for answers, I wish I could report that the Rio+20 Conference was a true success. In my opinion, it was not, but I did not despair. I did what I always do—searched for the next solutions-based opportunity—and found a marvelous one.

Renowned Canadian climate scientist Dr. Andrew Weaver decided to run for B.C. politics. I was asked to be his Communications Director and strategist. I jumped at the chance. I know that one of the most powerful levers for change is running for public office. On May 14, 2013, Dr. Weaver made history. He was elected as the first provincial Green Party Member of the Legislative Assembly (MLA) in Canada.

It is important here to note that I have never had all the answers; I am not particularly special. I have just known that we need to commit and to act. This instinct has led me on some incredible journeys. For my next adventure I want to help ensure that all Canadians have meaningful, formative outdoor experiences. I am starting an organization that will do just that. I want to work with a group of unstoppable people who are willing to do what it takes to ensure a climate-friendly future now, and for future generations. Together we will meet the challenge of climbing our generation's mountain, and solving the climate crisis.

shaving cream, do you stop to think about the ingredients that are in the products you are using? Some of you might, but many of us have not taken time to learn about some of the chemicals found in personal-care items. As a report titled *What's Inside? That Counts. A Survey of Toxic Ingredients in Our Cosmetics*[88] says, the picture is not pretty. Research in the United States determined that 10 500 industrial chemicals are used as cosmetic ingredients. Some of these ingredients are known carcinogens, pesticides, endocrine disruptors, and plasticizers.

This report also found that almost 80 percent of cosmetic and personal-care products in Canada contained at least one of twelve chemicals—the "dirty dozen"—linked to health and environmental concerns. Over half of all the products checked contained more than one of the dirty dozen ingredients. Another finding was that there are loopholes in the national *Cosmetic Regulations*[89] that allow for an incomplete ingredient list on many personal-care products.

Next time you go shopping for your personal-care products, check the labels for the dirty dozen chemicals.[90]

- **BHA and BHT**—used in moisturizers and makeup as a preservative. May cause cancer as it is a suspected endocrine disruptor. These chemicals are also harmful to fish and wildlife.
- **Coal tar dyes**—p-Phenylenediamine and colours listed as CI followed by a five-digit number—often found in hair dyes. These coal tar dyes have been linked to cancer and may also be contaminated with heavy metal that is toxic to our brain.
- **DEA-related ingredients**—found in many creamy and foaming products such as moisturizers and shampoos. May cause cancer. Harmful to fish and wildlife.
- **Dibutyl phthalate**—this product is used in some nail-care products such as nail polish. It is a plasticizer and a suspected endocrine disrupter and reproductive toxicant.
- **Formaldehyde-releasing preservatives**—used in many different cosmetic products. Look for DMDM hydantoin, diazolidinyl urea, imidazolidinyl urea, methenamine, and quarterium-15. This preservative causes cancer.
- **Parabens**—used as a preservative. May interfere with male reproductive functions.
- **Parfum (a.k.a. fragrance)**—can be a mixture of numerous fragrance ingredients. Sometimes even found in products marketed as "unscented." Can trigger allergies and asthma. Has been linked to some cancers.
- **PEG compounds**—can be contaminated with 1, 4-dioxane, which may cause cancer. Found in many cosmetic creams.
- **Petrolatum**—Marketed as helping hair "shine" and also used in some lip balms, lipsticks, and moisturizers as a moisture barrier. It is a petroleum product, which may cause cancer.
- **Siloxanes**—used in a variety of cosmetics and marketed as a way to smooth, soften, and moisturize skin. A possible endocrine disrupter and reproductive toxicant (cyclotetrasiloxane).
- **Sodium laureth sulphate**—found in foaming cosmetics such as shampoos, cleansers, and bubble baths. Can be contaminated with 1,4-dioxane, which may cause cancer.
- **Triclosan**—found in some toothpastes, cleansers, antiperspirants, and antibacterial cosmetics. May contribute to antibiotic resistance in bacteria.

Where do you start with regard to the use of products that claim to make us more beautiful or handsome? Begin by restricting your use of products that have the dirty dozen chemicals listed in the ingredient list. Ask questions of the sales representatives or companies selling these products. Look for and use alternative products when available. Don't use anti-bacterial household or personal-care products. Stand up and make your voice known to your local politicians. Support and strengthen North America's most respected **EcoLogo** certification program. Founded in 1988 by the Government of Canada, EcoLogo is now a respected environmental standard and certification mark program in North America. Products and services that bear this logo must meet stringent standards of environmental leadership. This organization is now represented by UL, a long-standing company that focuses on global safety science.[91]

You can also reduce your use of cosmetics that include **microplastics—**particles made of small (less than 5 millimetres), synthetic, solid plastic material that is non-degradable and water insoluble and used in many cosmetic and personal-care products. We are polluting our oceans because so many products such as make-up, moisturizers, shampoo and soap, deodorant, toothpaste, shaving cream, and sunscreen contain microplastics, which are going down our drains. The microplastics in these products are not collected in sewage treatment plants because they pass through any current filter system presently in use today.[92]

Research shows that microplastics can persist for centuries. Microplastics, sometimes called microbeads, are now in our food chain and are having a negative impact on marine life and, in turn, human life.[93]

✓ CHECK-IN

Do you know what ingredients are in your personal-care products?

INVISIBLE HAZARDS

Among the unseen hazards to health are various forms of *radiation*, energy radiated in the form of waves or particles.

Electromagnetic Fields and Radiation Electricity plays a central role in our society today. We use it to light our homes, prepare our food, run our computers, and operate numerous household appliances such as televisions, radios, and **video display terminals (VDTs)**. Any electrically charged conductor generates two kinds of invisible fields: electric and magnetic. Together they're called **electromagnetic fields (EMFs)**. Every time you use electrical appliances such as a microwave oven, you are exposed to EMFs or **microwaves.** For years, these fields were considered harmless. However, studies have revealed some health risks.

Laboratory research on animals has shown that alternating current, which changes strength and direction 60 times a second (and electrifies most of North America) emits EMFs that may interfere with the normal functioning of human cell membranes, which have their own electromagnetic fields. The result may be mood disorders, changes in circadian rhythms (our inner sense of time), miscarriage, developmental problems, or cancer. Researchers have documented an increase in breast-cancer deaths in women who worked as electrical engineers, as electricians, or in other high-exposure jobs, and a link between EMF exposure and an increased risk of leukemia and possibly brain cancer.[94]

Scientists at Health Canada are aware of these studies, but they have determined that the evidence is not strong enough to conclude that EMFs definitely cause cancer and suggest that more studies are needed.[95] See Table 16-4 for a description of some common invisible dangers.

There is a new concern among scientists and it has to do with cellphone use. Cellphone radiation falls between FM radio and microwaves on the electromagnetic spectrum and is able to penetrate deeper into the brain. Some scientists have found an elevated risk of tumours in cellphone users compared with people who rarely or never use cellphones. The risk was highest among those who had used cellphones for 10 years or more.[96] In the spring of 2011, both the World Health Organization (WHO) and Health Canada concluded that current available evidence did not show that cellphone use caused health risks.[97]

If you are concerned about your own cellphone use, some researchers suggest that you use the text message or speakerphone option so you can keep the phone as far away from your ear (and brain) as possible.

✓ CHECK-IN

How much time do you spend talking on your cellphone each day?

TABLE 16-4

Invisible Dangers

Invisible Dangers	Possible Health Risks
Video Display Terminals—computer monitors	VDTs have been blamed for increases in reproductive problems, miscarriages, low birth weights, and cataracts, yet research by Health Canada has shown that leakage is well below present standards for safe occupational exposure.[98]
Microwaves—extremely high-frequency electromagnetic waves; a form of radiofrequency electromagnetic energy	According to Health Canada, if the door on a microwave oven has a proper seal and there is no buildup of food or dirt around the seal, then there is no evidence that the microwave radiation emitted from the oven will pose a health risk.[99] There are concerns that the chemicals in plastic wrap or containers that are used in microwaves can cause cancer in mice. Consumers should also be cautious about plastic-encased heat receptors included in convenience food.
Cellular Phones—The World Health Organization (WHO) reports that there are 6.9 billion subscriptions for cellular phones.[100] In some parts of the world, mobile phones, or cellphones, are the most reliable or the only phones available.	Researchers have documented changes in biological tissue exposed to radiofrequency (RF) electromagnetic energy generated by cellphones.[101] Concern has grown about possible links to slow-growing tumours and brain cancer. The World Health Organization (WHO) has indicated that radiofrequency electromagnetic fields may possibly be carcinogenic to humans based on an increased risk for glioma, a malignant type of brain cancer associated with wireless phone use.[102] However, the National Cancer Institute suggests that the findings in many studies are inconsistent. Some research indicates that there is an association between cellphone use and the risk for brain cancer, while other studies report no association.[103]

OTHER ENVIRONMENTAL ISSUES

Irradiated Foods The use of radiation on food, from either radioactive substances or devices that produce X-rays, is known as **irradiation.** It doesn't make the food radioactive; its primary benefit is to prolong the food's useful life. Irradiation can kill microorganisms that might grow in food; the sterilized food can then be stored for years in sealed containers at room temperature without spoiling.

Nutritional studies have shown no significant decreases in the quality of the foods, but high-dose treatments may cause vitamin losses similar to those that occur during canning. It's also possible that the ionizing effect of radiation creates new compounds in foods that may be mutagenic or carcinogenic.

Irradiated foods are believed to be safe to eat. In Canada, several federal agencies are involved in regulating aspects of the food-irradiation process, two of which include the Health Products and Food Branch of Health Canada and the Canadian Food Inspection Agency (CFIA).[104]

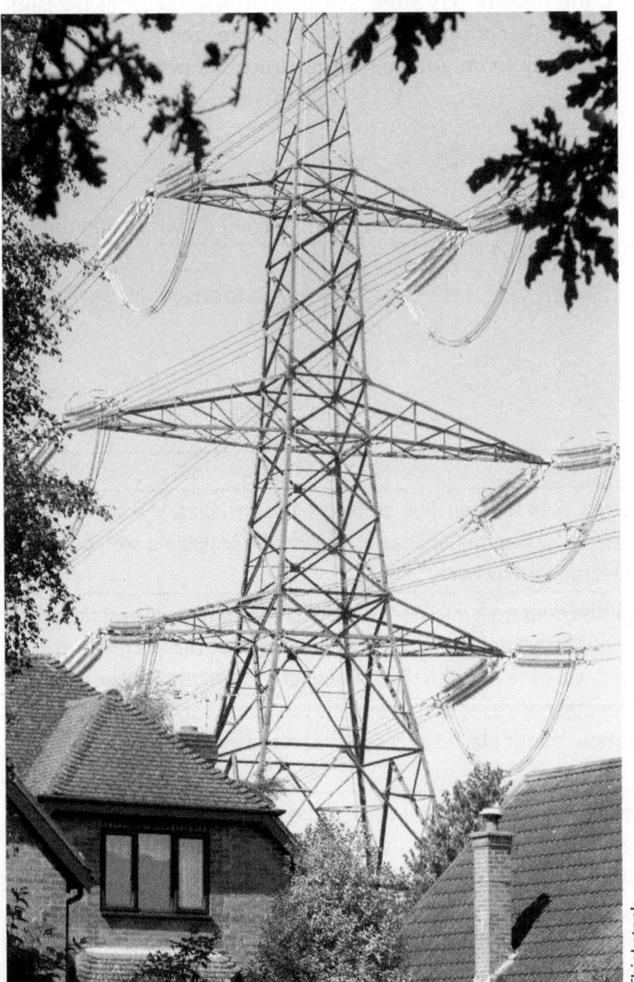
Thinkstock

Although laboratory studies on animals indicate that EMFs affect human cell membranes, research on humans has found only a weak connection between EMFs and disease.

Multiple Chemical Sensitivity The proliferation of chemicals in modern society has led to an entirely new disease, **multiple chemical sensitivity (MCS)**, also called environmentally triggered illness, universal allergy, or chemical AIDS. There is no agreed-upon definition for the condition, no medical test that can diagnose it, and no proven treatment. Symptoms can include chest pain, depression, difficulty remembering, dizziness, fatigue, headache, inability to concentrate, nausea, and aches and pains in muscles and joints. Medical professionals have become convinced that MCS is a real and serious health problem that requires investigation.[105]

NOISE POLLUTION

Data from a Canadian study on the prevalence of hearing loss of Canadians aged 20–79 showed that 19.2 percent had significant hearing loss in at least one ear and 35.4 percent had high-frequency hearing loss. The study also showed that men were more likely to have hearing loss than women.[106] In a study of college students and their MP3 listening habits, researchers found that while the majority of students listened for less than two hours daily at safe volume levels, more than one-third of the participants experienced soreness in their ears after a listening session. As well, about one-third of the students reported occasionally playing their MP3 players at maximum volume levels.[107]

Loudness, or the intensity of a sound, is measured in **decibels (dB)**. A whisper is 20 decibels; a conversation in a living room is about 50 decibels. On this scale, 50 is not two and one-half times louder than 20, but 1000 times louder: each 10-decibel rise in the scale represents a tenfold increase in the intensity of the sound. Very loud but short bursts of sounds (such as gunshots and fireworks) and quieter but longer-lasting sounds (such as power tools) can induce hearing loss.

Sounds under 70 decibels don't seem harmful. However, prolonged exposure to any sound over 85 decibels (the equivalent of a power mower or food blender) or brief exposure to louder sounds can harm hearing. The noise level at rock concerts can reach 110–140 decibels, about as loud as an air-raid siren. Portable CD players and personal listening devices such as iPods can generate potentially harmful sound levels of up to 115 decibels. Statistics Canada reports that 51 percent of Canadians, 3–79 years of age, indicated that they used earbuds or headphones when listening to

Decibels	Example	Zone
0	The softest sound a typical ear can hear	Safe
10 dB	Just audible	
20 dB	Watch ticking; leaves rustling	
30 dB	Soft whisper at 16 feet	
40 dB	Quiet office; suburban street (no traffic)	
50 dB	Interior of typical urban home; rushing stream	1000 times louder than 20 dB
60 dB	Normal conversation; busy office	
70 dB	Vacuum cleaner at 10 feet; hair dryer	
80 dB	Alarm clock at 2 feet; loud music; average daily traffic	1000 times louder than 50 dB
90 dB*	Motorcycle at 25 feet; jet 4 miles after takeoff	Risk of injury
100 dB*	Video arcade; loud factory; subway train	
110 dB*	Car horn at 3 feet; symphony orchestra; chainsaw	1000 times louder than 80 dB
120 dB	Jackhammer at 3 feet; boom box; nearby thunderclap	Injury
130 dB	Rock concert; jet engine at 100 feet	
140 dB	Jet engine nearby; amplified car stereo; firearms	1000 times louder than 110 dB

Figure 16-4 Loud and Louder

The human ear perceives a 10-decibel increase as a doubling of loudness. Thus, the 100 decibels of a subway train sound much more than twice as loud as the 50 decibels of a rushing stream.

*Note: The maximum exposure allowed on the job by federal law in hours per day is 90 decibels for eight hours, 100 decibels for 2 hours, or 110 decibels for half an hour.

music, movies, or other types of audio files within the last 12 months. Of the 51 percent, one-third said they listened at volume levels that were at or above three quarters of the maximum volume.[108] Cars with extremely loud music systems can produce an ear-splitting 145 decibels—louder than a jet engine or thunderclap (see Figure 16-4).

Most hearing loss occurs on the job. The people at highest risk are firefighters, police, military personnel, construction and factory workers, musicians, farmers, and truck drivers. Other sources of danger include live or recorded high-volume music, recreational vehicles, airplanes, lawn-care equipment, woodworking tools, some appliances, and chainsaws. Even low-level office noise can undermine well-being and increase health risks.

Noise-induced hearing loss is 100 percent preventable; it is also, unfortunately, irreversible. Hearing aids are the only treatment, but they do not correct the problem. They just amplify sound to compensate for hearing loss. Noise can also harm more than our ears: High-volume sound has been linked to high blood pressure and other stress-related problems that can lead to heart disease, insomnia, anxiety, headaches, colitis, and ulcers. Noise frays the nerves; people tend to be more anxious, irritable, and angry when their ears are constantly barraged with sound.

✓ CHECK-IN

How aware are you of the decibel levels of sounds that you hear on a daily basis?

SELF-SURVEY

Are You Doing Your Part for the Planet?

You may think that there is little you can do, as an individual, to save Earth. But every day acts can add up and make a difference in helping or harming the planet on which we live.

	Almost Never	Sometimes	Always
1. Do you walk, cycle, carpool, or use public transportation as much as possible to get around?	___	___	___
2. Do you recycle?	___	___	___
3. Do you reuse plastic and paper bags?	___	___	___
4. Do you try to conserve water by not running the tap as you shampoo or brush your teeth?	___	___	___
5. Do you use products made of recycled materials?	___	___	___
6. Do you drive a car that gets good fuel mileage and has up-to-date emission control equipment?	___	___	___
7. Do you turn off lights, televisions, and appliances when you're not using them?	___	___	___
8. Do you avoid buying products that are elaborately packaged?	___	___	___
9. Do you use glass jars and waxed paper rather than plastic wrap for storing food?	___	___	___
10. Do you take brief showers rather than baths?	___	___	___
11. Do you use cloth towels and napkins rather than paper products?	___	___	___
12. When listening to music, do you keep the volume low?	___	___	___
13. Do you try to avoid any potential carcinogens, such as asbestos, mercury, or benzene?	___	___	___
14. Are you careful to dispose of hazardous materials (such as automobile oil or antifreeze) at appropriate sites?	___	___	___
15. Do you follow environmental issues in your community and write your provincial or federal representatives to support "green" legislation?	___	___	___

Answers to Self-Survey

Count the number of items you've checked in each column. If you've circled 10 or more in the "always" column, you're definitely helping to make a difference. If you've mainly circled "sometimes," you're moving in the right direction, but you need to be more consistent and more conscientious. If you've circled 10 or more in the "never" column, carefully read this chapter to find out what you can do.

Chapter Summary

1. Which of the following is a threat to the environment?
   a. an open ecosystem
   b. depletion of the oxygen layer
   c. ecological processes
   d. global warming
2. What are mutagens?
   a. They are caused by birth defects.
   b. They are considered a chronic effect of a pollutant.
   c. They are agents that trigger changes in the DNA of living cells.
   d. They are caused by repeated exposure to soil.
3. Which statement about global warming is true?
   a. Global warming is not an environmental issue in our society.
   b. Global warming may result in severe drought and a rise in ocean levels.
   c. Increasing tree cover and agricultural lands will contribute to global warming.
   d. Increasing carbon dioxide production will slow the progress of global warming.
4. How can climate change be defined?
   a. aircraft release of carbon dioxide
   b. the Kyoto Accord
   c. any long-term significant change in the "average weather" that a given region experiences
   d. using plastic storage containers and plastic wrap to save trees from being cut down
5. Which statement about air pollution is false?
   a. Late-model automobiles emit much less pollution per kilometre than cars that were new in 1970.
   b. The two types of smog include sulphur dioxide smog, produced by burning oil of high sulphur content, and photochemical smog resulting from chemical reactions from car exhaust.
   c. Ozone in the upper atmosphere does not protect us from harmful ultraviolet radiation from the sun.
   d. Air pollution can cause the same types of respiratory health problems as smoking.
6. Which common indoor pollutant is linked to lung and gastrointestinal cancer?
   a. lead
   b. mercury
   c. asbestos
   d. carbon monoxide
7. How can you protect your hearing?
   a. by avoiding prolonged exposure to sounds under 70 decibels
   b. by exposing yourself to 100 decibels of noise for only 8 hours per day
   c. by limiting noise exposure to levels between 85 and 140 decibels
   d. by listening to very loud sounds in short bursts
8. Which statement about drinking water safety is true?
   a. Drinking water safety has been significantly increased in communities that add chlorine to the water.
   b. Fluoride is the most commonly used drinking-water disinfectant.
   c. Bottled water is completely free of chemical contaminants.
   d. Well water is safe.
9. Which statement about electromagnetic fields is true?
   a. There is no evidence that indicates a link between electromagnetic fields around power lines and cancer.
   b. The electromagnetic fields emitted by electric blankets are probably less dangerous than those from hair dryers.
   c. The amount of radiation from video display terminals exceeds present standards for safe occupational exposure.
   d. Electrical engineers and electricians who have high exposure to EMFs may be at greater risk for developing leukemia.
10. Which statement about radiation usage is false?
    a. Chemicals in plastic wrap may leak into foods heated in microwave ovens.
    b. There is no evidence that radiofrequency signals from cellphones cause brain cancer.
    c. Irradiation can be used to kill microorganisms in food.
    d. Irradiation can delay the ripening of fruits.

Answers to these questions can be found on page 447.

SELF-RESPONSIBILITY—SOCIAL RESPONSIBILITY

SELF-RESPONSIBILITY

Environmental problems affect the water we drink, the air we breathe, and the food we eat. You can start solving the world's problems in your own backyard.

David Suzuki

SOCIAL RESPONSIBILITY

After observing the planet for eight days from space, I have a deeper interest and respect for the forces that shape our world. Each particle of soil, each plant and animal is special. I also marvel at the creativity and ingenuity of our own species, but at the same time, I wonder why we all cannot see that we create our future each day, and that our local actions affect the global community, today as well as for generations to come.

Roberta Bondar

Refer to Prochaska's Stages of Change model and ask yourself where you are on the continuum? Are you in the pre-contemplation stage—not really aware of the impact you are having on the environment? Are you contemplating making some changes in how you live to lighten your environmental footprint? What could you do today that would make a difference?

CRITICAL THINKING

1. How do you contribute to environmental pollution? How might you change your habits to protect the environment?
2. An excerpt from a recent newspaper article states: "Children living near a local refinery suffer from a high rate of asthma and allergies, and an environmental group says the plant may be to blame." The refinery has met all the local air-quality standards, employs hundreds in the community, and pays taxes, which support police, fire, and social services. If you were a city council member, how would you balance health and environmental concerns with the need for industry in your community?
3. In one poll, people given a choice between a high standard of living (but with hazardous air and water pollution and the depletion of natural resources) and a lower standard of living (but with clean air and drinking water) would prefer clean air and drinking water and a lower standard of living. What about you? Do you think most people are willing to change their lifestyles to preserve the environment?

WEB LINKS

Chris Turner

http://www.speakers.ca/speakers/chris-turner-2/

Chris Turner, one of Canada's leading writers and speakers, has published two books linked to environmental sustainability. *The Geography of Hope: A Tour of the World We Need* shares stories of his globetrotting adventure where he discovered individuals and communities making a difference. His *The Leap: How to Survive and Thrive in the Sustainable Economy*, is another "must read."

The David Suzuki Foundation

www.davidsuzuki.org

Find information on climate change, forests and wild lands, oceans and fishing, and sustainability. Access numerous current environmental reports.

Earth Day Network

www.earthday.org/

Access this site and click on Your Ecological Footprint and fill out a quiz that estimates how much productive land and water you need to support what you use and what you discard. You can compare your ecological footprint to other people around the world.

Environment and Climate Change Canada

https://www.ec.gc.ca/

This site helps connect Canadians to exchange information and share knowledge for environmental decision-making.

Global Footprint Network

http://www.footprintnetwork.org/en/index.php/GFN/

Global Footprint Network serves as the steward of the National Footprint Accounts, the calculation system that measures the ecological resource use and resource capacity of nations over time.

Please note that links are subject to change. If you find a broken link, use a search engine such as www.google.ca and search for the website by typing in keywords.

Key Terms

The terms listed here are used within the chapter on the page indicated. Definitions of terms are in the Glossary at the end of the book.

Answers to Chapter Summary Questions

1. d; 2. c; 3. b; 4. c; 5. c; 6. c; 7. c; 8. a; 9. d; 10. b

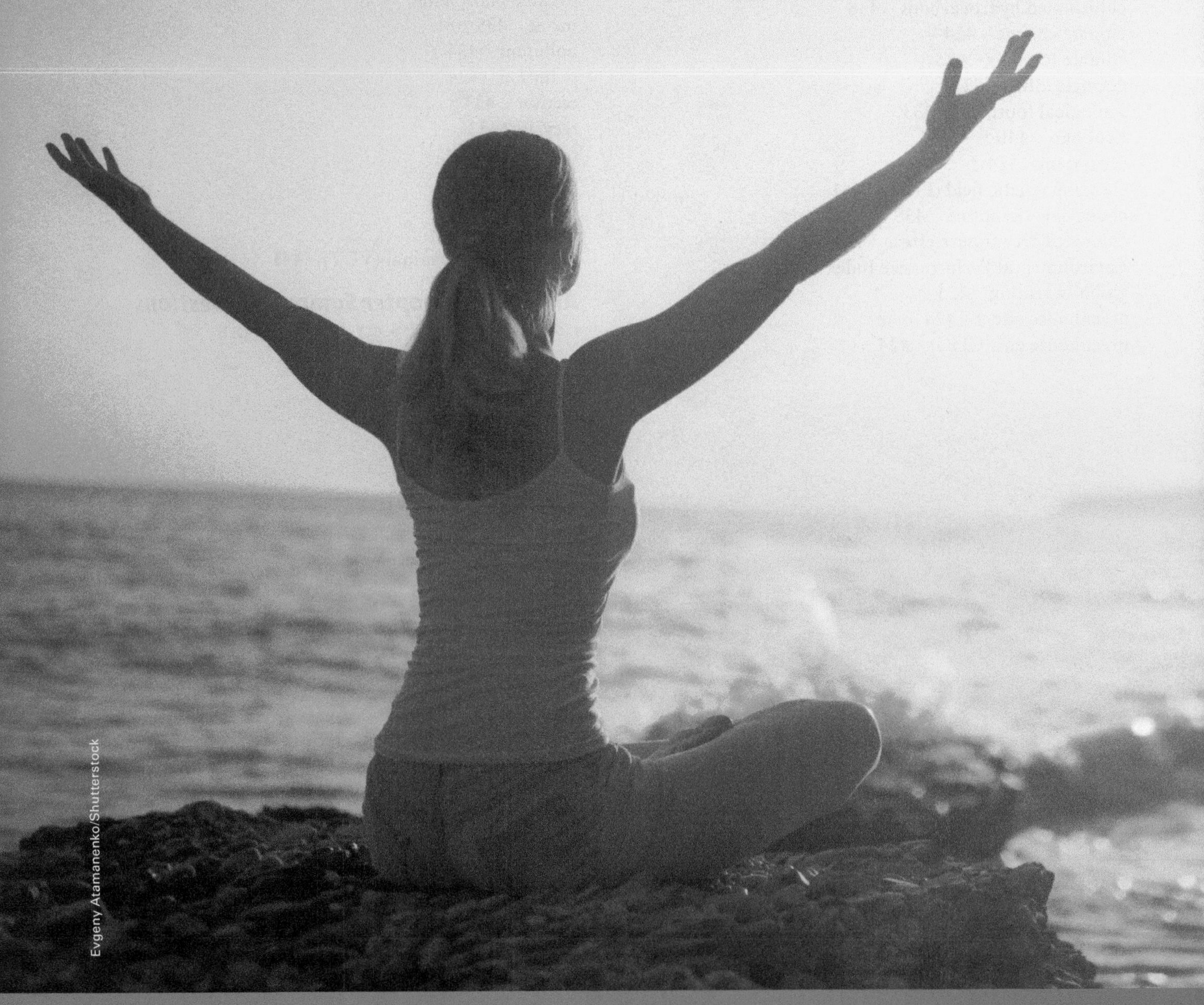
Evgeny Atamanenko/Shutterstock

AFTER READING THIS CHAPTER, YOU WILL BE ABLE TO:

- **discuss** different definitions of spirituality
- **discuss** why spirituality is important
- **list** and **describe** some of the major religions of the world
- **describe** ways in which spirituality can enhance your health, wellness, and personal potential

17

The Spirit of Health and Wellness

Spirituality can be a challenging topic to discuss. However, it is an important topic, and, as Riyad Ahmed Shahjahan says, spirituality "cannot be left on the margins" and should be part of our discussions in academic institutions.[1] Current research shows that an interest in the spiritual dimension of health and wellness is growing among college and university students.[2,3]

Spirituality means different things to different people. For some, spirituality is a discovery of our self—about finding out about our unique abilities so that we can serve humanity and leave legacies. A quest for spirituality can add a richness and depth to our lives. Spirituality can also equate with moral well-being. For others, spirituality is an organized faith or formal religion based on an association with an all-powerful being or God. It is confined to a set of doctrines or experiences that guide a "way of living."

This chapter presents various definitions of spirituality. It attempts to connect the spiritual dimension of wellness to other dimensions of wellness within your life. It examines the body, mind, and spiritual bond. We celebrate First Nations spirituality. There are discussions about the relationship between nature and spirituality and about spirituality on college and university campuses. As well, information about the ever-growing field of research that links spirituality and religion to overall health is introduced.

The chapter concludes with a brief description of the major religions of the world and Canada.

FREQUENTLY ASKED QUESTIONS

WHAT IS SPIRITUALITY?

Spirituality can be defined as having a sense of self and a set of values that link to meaning and purpose in life and a connection to others.[4] Dr. John Travis suggests that spirituality is a connection with everything in creation—an animating force, the principle of unification, shared consciousness.[5] Erriker and Erriker might agree, since they view spirituality as belonging in society.[6] The understanding of spirituality is also built upon the idea that there is a higher intelligence, a fundamental or creative power—a universal energy or source. Many words such as God, Spirit, Higher Power, the Light, Higher Self, Cosmic Intelligence, or Christ Consciousness have been used to describe this source. Scherurs supports this way of thinking—that spirituality is a personal relationship with a transcendent Being.[7] Other definitions include

- a movement toward living an authentic life, embracing a more authentic self[8]
- a search for the sacred or divine through any life experience or route[9]
- a growth process that leads to the realization of the ultimate purpose and meaning of life[10]
- a belief in unseen powers in all natural phenomena and that all things are dependent on one another[11]
- the development of a deep appreciation for the depth and expanse of life and natural forces that exist in the universe[12]

As you can see by the many definitions of spirituality, it is difficult to consistently and clearly define the term. When a common definition seems to be out of reach, it makes it difficult to measure the relationship among spirituality, religion, and health,[13] and the validity of research in this area is sometimes called into question. Estanek[14] suggests that it might even be unwise to try to agree on one definition of spirituality and that we try instead to recognize the complexity of the term. However, Ingersoll and Bauer discovered that although it is a challenge to define the term, many researchers do agree on common elements within the dimension of spiritual wellness. These elements include hope, meaning, purpose in life, connectedness, honesty, compassion, forgiveness, rituals, recognition of what is held to be sacred, and transcendent beliefs and experiences that might include a sense of a higher power.[15]

A short discussion of **spiritual intelligence** and the powerful connection to discovering our inner wisdom in our personal lives was included in Chapter 2, Psychosocial Health. Maheshwari suggests that spiritual intelligence is of utmost importance in our professional lives too.[16] She proposes that spiritual intelligence can guide us in ethical decision making, assist us in turbulent times, help us value our work, and embrace our occupational responsibilities. She advocates for an acknowledgment of spiritual intelligence within a workplace as a way of promoting tolerance of others and celebrating differences. Spiritual intelligence can help us find work that is meaningful and purposeful. The term **religion** often refers to a definition somewhat different from spirituality. Sometimes described as a specific system of beliefs about a deity or deities, often involving rituals, a code of ethics, and a philosophy of life, it usually represents a special doctrine or group of people.[17] A separate section on religion is presented later in the chapter.

Whether or not you believe that spirituality is about finding personal meaning or you follow the teachings of a formal religion, spirituality is about feeling more complete and fulfilled as a human being. To embrace the "spirit" part of our being, we must be open to the idea that while a healthy and well life can include getting a good education, a decent career, and making money, it can also mean making a difference and connecting with our inner self, nature, or a higher being. As described in Chapter 1, spiritually well individuals learn how to experience love, joy, peace, and fulfillment.

✓ CHECK-IN

How do you define spirituality? How would you describe your spiritual intelligence level?

Integration of Body, Mind, and Spirit We often talk about health and wellness as a connection of our body, mind, and spirit. In many college and university health, wellness, and physical activity courses, there is a strong emphasis on the body and mind. We seem to tiptoe around the spirit connection. Yet, academic writing and research about this connection was evident in the early 1900s, in the writings of Starbuck[18] about the psychology of religion, and James,[19] who wrote a series of lectures titled *The Varieties of Religious Experience.* Between the 1920s and 1960s, a number of psychologists began to understand this connection, too. Jung[20] wrote about the role of spirituality and psychological health. Viktor Frankl developed a counselling approach he called Logotherapy where the search for meaning in one's life is identified as the primary motivational force in human beings.[21] Seeman et al. suggest that in the past few decades "there has been a resurgence of interest" in investigating the potential impact that religion and spirituality might have on health outcomes.[22] Norman Cousins's books *Anatomy of An Illness*[23] and *Head First: The Biology of Hope and the Healing Power of the Human Spirit*,[24] which both emphasize spiritual factors in a recovery process from a serious illness, are two examples.

Dr. Pat Fosarelli suggests that the key to discovering our own spirituality is to understand that our body,

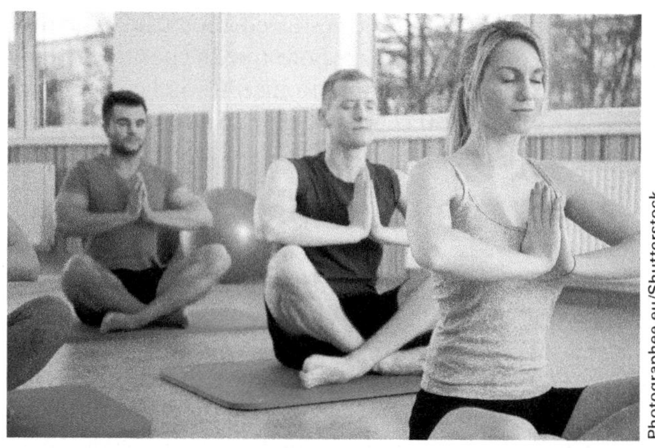

Photographee.eu/Shutterstock

Practising yoga harmonizes the body, mind, and spirit.

mind, and spirit are interconnected to our health and wellness. She also suggests that by sharing our human experiences we enhance our spirituality.[25] On college and university campuses across Canada and the United States, recreation departments have experienced a major increase in the registration of students in mind, body, and spirit classes such as yoga. Often taken, at first, for the physical benefits, many students are also discovering the spiritual benefits of yoga. As Richard Freeman, a long-time yoga practitioner and teacher, says, with regular yoga practice we become more mindful of what is important; we get insights and awakenings. He describes hatha yoga as a moving together of prana—life force or breath—and *chita*—our mind.[26] When you take positive steps to brighten your spirit, strengthen your body, or improve your mind, you can expect gains in your total well-being.

Aboriginal Spirituality In a chapter on spirituality we would be remiss if we did not honour Aboriginal spirituality. Aboriginal peoples across Canada have various spiritual beliefs, sacred items, and ceremonies. Spiritual traditions are customarily passed down orally.[27] There are differences among Aboriginal groups, but there is a common belief that the Great Spirit created the Earth and its people. There is also a central understanding that the Earth is the Mother of all life and people; plants and animals have spirits that must be respected, honoured, and cared for. Humans are the guardians of the Earth. Other widespread beliefs are that prayers of thanks should be made to the Creator each day for all living things; there is great value placed on families and extended families; respect must be shown to all people; and individuals should control their own behaviour in consideration of the community they live in.[28] Special rituals include healing circles, sweat-lodge ceremonies, and powwows. There is a growing interest from academics on the benefits of First Nations spirituality as it links to health. Wagemakers, Schiff, and Moore[29] studied the impact of a sweat-lodge ceremony on dimensions of well-being. They found that an increase in spiritual and emotional well-being of the participants who took part in the ceremony was directly attributable to the ceremony.

First Nations' spiritual life is a connectedness of all natural things. A description of this connectedness is told in *The Story of the Sacred Tree*.[30] First, the Creator planted a Sacred Tree under which the people could gather. Under this tree people would find "healing, power, wisdom, and security."[31] The roots spread into Mother Earth, and the branches reached upward to Father Sky. The fruits of the tree were the good things that the Creator gave to the people—"teachings that show the path to love, compassion, generosity, patience, wisdom, justice, courage, respect, humility, and many other wonderful gifts."[32]

Figure 17-1 shows the Four Great Meanings of the Sacred Tree. Placed within the ancient symbol of the Medicine Wheel, the four great meanings are protection, nourishment, growth, and wholeness. The following brief description does not tell the whole story. For those of you who are encouraged to read this book, it is available from the Four Worlds International Institute at www.4worlds.org.

- *Protection*—The Sacred Tree is symbolic of a gathering place for different tribes and peoples of the world. It provides a place of protection, peace, contemplation, and centring. It "gives rise to a vision, not of what we are, but of what we can become."[33]
- *Nourishment*—The Sacred Tree is symbolic of the nourishment we need to live and sustain growth. Eating the fruit of the tree represents the interaction of the human, physical, and spiritual aspects of our lives. The leaves, which fall to the ground, represent the passing of the generations and the spiritual teachings that are left behind. The wisdom of the past nourishes the present and the future.[34]

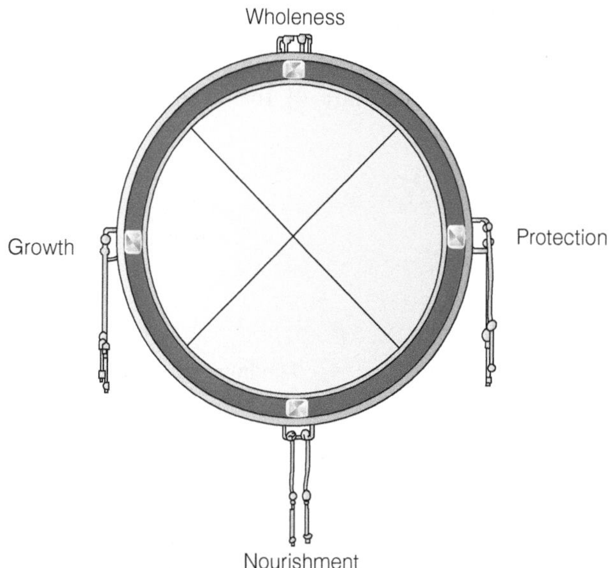

Figure 17-1 **The Sacred Tree**

Source: Worlds International Institute for human and community development. Lethbridge, Alberta. Www.4worlds.org.

- *Growth*—The Sacred Tree is symbolic of pursuing life experiences and respecting our inner spiritual growth. This includes growing in the qualities of the four directions—physically, mentally, emotionally, and spiritually. It also represents the cycles of time and life, the changing seasons, and our lifelong relationship to creation.[35]
- *Wholeness*—The Sacred Tree is symbolic of the Great Spirit as the centre pole of creation. It is here we can balance and begin to understand ourselves as human beings. The roots, which are unseen, represent the invisible aspects of our being, while the parts of the Sacred Tree that are above ground are the visible aspects of ourselves. Understanding and balancing of all of our parts provide the nurturing environment for further growth and wholeness.[36]

The First Nations authors of this book conclude with the thought that gaining an understanding of the Sacred Tree is an eternal journey. By reflecting and acting upon the teachings of the Sacred Tree, we can bring a renewal to the life of humanity.[37]

The Métis of Canada have varied religious and spiritual traditions. Some have formal Catholic or Protestant rituals such as attending church services, getting married in a church, or being buried in a church cemetery. Some honour the Patron Saint of Métis People, St. Joseph of Nazareth. Other Métis report that they lean toward New Age spirituality. There are also Métis who follow Aboriginal spiritual traditions and participate in sweat-lodge or Long House ceremonies. They may also follow a medicine wheel and use sacred pipes for certain celebrations.[38]

The Inuit believe that all living things and objects have a spirit and they must be respected. This belief system is defined as animism. Community members receive assistance in celebrating these spirits through Shamans, or Angakoqs—the central religious figure in traditional Inuit Culture. The role of the Shaman is to bless hunting expeditions and take care of the health needs of the community. This role is bestowed on male or female members, or individuals are born into the position. Many Inuit also follow traditional Roman Catholic, Anglican, or other Evangelical church doctrine and rituals.[39]

SPIRITUAL DIMENSIONS

You may wonder, as you read this chapter, how you might "fit" spirituality into your life as you are attempting to stay physically active, eat in a healthy way, keep up with your school work, and have a social life, too. Do you really need to embrace spirituality to be well? Just like physical activity and nutrition programs change over time, or the demands of school work ebb and flow, so does the spiritual dimension of your life. People working in the spiritual health and wellness area suggest that when we are ready to learn more about and embrace spirituality, we will find the time. Their suggestion is be open to the concept of spirituality and find comfortable ways to support your spiritual dimension.

How Do I Begin Learning about My Spiritual Dimension? How do you gain a greater understanding of your own spirituality? You can start by asking yourself these questions:

- What is my understanding of spirituality?
- What am I passionate about? What personal and professional experiences make me feel healthy and well?
- What kind of person am I? What kind of person do I want to be?

Just as you prepare to begin a fitness program or organize your work space to study for an exam, you can prepare for your spiritual journey by starting somewhere, taking small steps, and pondering the four domains of the spiritual dimension: interconnectedness; mindfulness; meaning, purpose and potential; and transcendence (See Figure 17-2).

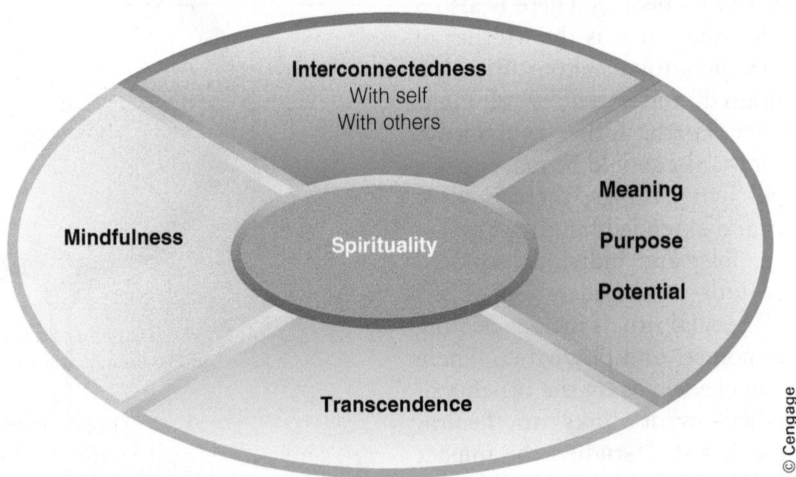

Figure 17-2 Spiritual Dimensions

✓ CHECK-IN

How would you describe your spiritual self?

Interconnectedness **Interconnectedness** can be defined as having a sense of unity, and being connected reciprocally. In a spiritual sense it has been defined as a worldview that sees a *oneness in all things*.[40] With technological advances the term "interconnectedness" has taken on a new meaning in global political, social, and ecological terms. Never before have we been so interconnected. Some examples of worldwide interconnectedness projects in Canada include meditation sessions for world peace,[41] sacred walks, and prayer circles.[42]

Interconnectedness can be understood by two distinct domains, *connectedness to self* and *connectedness to others*. Though described differently, these domains work in concert with each other.

Connectedness to Oneself Many people are very busy with day-to-day tasks or dealing with problems that come their way and don't feel the need to spend time reflecting about spirituality or connecting with their inner selves. Yet there is a growing body of research that tells us that setting aside some time to question who we are and what we want to accomplish can bring richness to our life and be healthy for us.[43]

Sometimes a focus on the spiritual wellness dimension by college and university students is neglected. Developing a personal adult identity when you are at college or university is difficult enough. Developing your spiritual self can be even more difficult, some might say even risky. Spirituality might seem to be a lofty goal, one that is difficult to achieve. You might also have feelings of anxiety about the concept of spirituality or God or are beginning to question the doctrine of a familiar religion. Yet it is the questioning and the searching that helps us discover our spiritual selves. There is no "one way" to become a spiritual person.

Listen to your intuition or hunches. Begin to notice which situations or events test your abilities and challenge your way of thinking. As you engage in reflective practice, you may start to notice that there are times you feel uncertain and experience chaos within. At other times you might experience sensations of peacefulness, a clear mind, and a feeling of centredness.

Connectedness to Others As spiritual growth takes place, some people come to believe that all human beings are connected to one another. This oneness is what some people call God. Others call it universal energy. When you come to this understanding of connectedness, you are presented with alternatives to the way you plan and live your life. You begin to believe that one person can make a difference and that person might be you.

✓ CHECK-IN

What does interconnectedness mean to you?

HUMAN POTENTIAL

Erin Pearce: See Them Run—A Story of Courage and Conviction

Sometimes we are fortunate to be inspired by individuals who seem to have found their calling, who live life with meaning and purpose. In this final human potential story, you will meet a young woman named Erin Pearce who is one of those remarkable individuals. Coupled with her strong faith and her passion for social justice issues, and known for her ability to make seemingly ludicrous ideas become a reality, Erin's life motto is this: "Life is not a journey to the grave with the intention of arriving safe and pretty, but rather arriving, skidding in broadside, thoroughly out of breath, and proclaiming loudly, 'WOW! What a ride!'"

In 2005 Erin, who was just 19 at the time, found herself frustrated with the seemingly futile direction of her competitive triathlon career. Inspired by a local newspaper article written about disabled children living in an orphanage in Maralal, Kenya, Erin decided to try to find purpose for her life by developing a summer integration sports program for these children. Raising funds to allow her to travel to Africa was just the first step in what would be a poignant time of personal transformation. Working for three months in the rural orphanage in the Samburu district with abandoned disabled kids would instill a spiritual passion within her that is still driving her today.

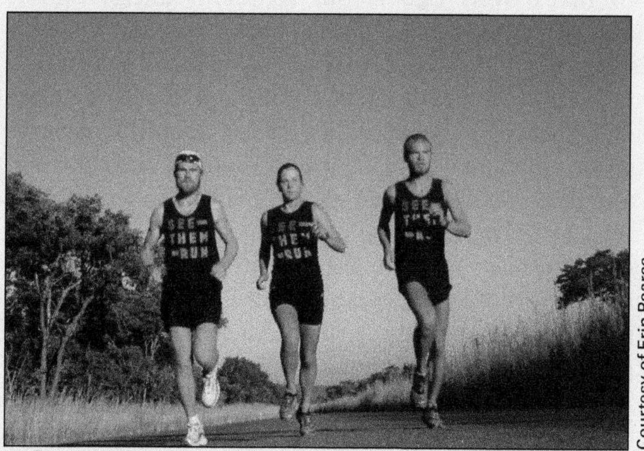

Patrick Donker, Erin Pearce, and Reuben Jentink running across Africa for their See-Them-Run fundraiser.

(Continued)

The work at the orphanage was very challenging, yet when asked about the young people she met, Erin speaks with passion and love. She tells of a girl named Nasusui. "I met Nasusui in Kenya at the orphanage and discovered that she had been burned alive, starved, and abused due to a birth defect. From ages 8–11 she was kept in solitary confinement where she was sexually abused by a family friend. No one in the village aided her because she was disabled. It wasn't until a humanitarian aid worker intervened that she was brought to safety to the orphanage I was working at.

I remember Nasusui telling me her story as a 12-year-old. The injustice brought tears to my eyes and, grabbing my hand, she asked, 'Erin, why are you crying?' I told her I was sorry. In her broken English she said, in a quiet, confident voice, 'I am blessed, Erin, because God has brought me here.'"

Erin, like Nasusui, believes that everything in life happens for a reason: "I think God's definition of success and failure is very different than our human terms. We, as humans, are so entrenched in a society that values material worth, self-promotion, and ease that we have lost the sense that there is a spiritual world woven into our daily existence. And if we could acknowledge and have faith in the divine pattern and design, we would find that God in fact weaves life's circumstances in awe-inspiring ways and shapes us into remarkable people. That doesn't mean it's always easy, but it is always worth it."

Erin has learned to have faith in what she calls "the divine agenda." Through integrating spiritual values into her own daily existence, Erin lives to help others. She devotes her life to spiritual issues and is determined to advocate for human dignity across the globe. In 2006, Erin began a project called the "100-Item Challenge" in which she lived with only one hundred things. Trying to link the gap between Western consumption and Third World poverty, Erin challenges people to redefine the word "need." Erin's presentations to groups of college and university students are life-changing. One student's comments illustrate Erin's impact. "I was truly touched by today's presentation. It was amazing to see the dedication and selflessness that Erin has. What she is doing deserves the utmost respect from all of us. To give your time, self, and money so readily to help others is not something we see every day, especially in young people. Erin has inspired me to step out of my routine everyday life, to help out those in both my community and global society."

In 2008, Erin made another commitment to the children of Africa. She decided to raise money for African education and run across the African continent. Completing a gruelling 4200 kilometres on foot across Namibia, Zambia, and Tanzania, Erin, along with friends Reuben Jentink and Patrick Donker, and supported by her sister and brother-in-law, Anna van Wiltenburg and Drew Beiderwieden, as well as an African guide, David Passon, ran five to six marathons a week for four months to raise awareness and make a difference for African children.

Erin has completed a master's degree in Social Work in International and Community Development and is currently is living in Vancouver, British Columbia, working with refugee and immigrant populations. She continues to write, speak, and reflect on her experiences as she follows her passions and convictions.

"Spirituality has taught me to love myself. And once you love yourself it is really easy to love other people. It's easy to take risks for other people when you believe you're not in control of the end result. Sometimes you don't end up where you anticipated, but you always end up a better person."

Some psychologists refer to connectedness as our **conscience.** When you listen to your conscience, you see yourself as someone who is part of a bigger world and know that what you do has an impact on others. When we don't hear or listen to our conscience our ego takes over. **Ego** is our self-centredness. Ego is important, of course. Taking care of yourself is a necessary part of taking care of others. We have said many times throughout this textbook that if you are not healthy and well, it is difficult to fulfill dreams and visions. However, when ego becomes the centre of your life, selfishness and materialism can become the focus of living. Ego without conscience allows us to behave in ways that are not healthy and well. It allows us to believe that we can abuse our bodies, our souls, and the world at large without consequences. Ego can keep us from discovering our human potential.

There are many examples of people making a difference by connecting with one another. All of the Human Potential stories included in this textbook are examples of individuals attempting to reach out to others. Take a moment to think about people you know in your own community, in your province, or in Canada who are making a difference by connecting with others. How do these individuals inspire you? If you are already reaching out, how can you begin to share with others how these experiences are meaningful to you? Can you prepare a presentation for a student group? Can you organize a workshop on spirituality and community connection?

Collective problems must be solved by us—collectively. The spiritual dimension can be a vehicle for making our contributions to the world. You can think of it as re-purposing your skills. When people get together to do good work, hope is renewed, and visions move to action. In a study investigating relational spirituality, Faver found that social caregiving renewed and refreshed people. The sense of relatedness to their work

STRATEGIES FOR CHANGE

Your Spiritual Journey

- Redefine success—include living well and doing what you like to do as part of that success.
- Work on becoming a better person. Judge less, love more, practise forgiveness, demonstrate kindness, and honour others.
- Look at the world around you with optimism.
- Spend time each day alone in receptive silence.
- Believe the best about you.

or cause became a source of energy and vitality. Some participants in her study said the consistent presence of supportive co-workers, friends, and fellow parishioners was a powerful sustaining life force.[44]

Mindfulness Kabatt-Zinn[45] has described **mindfulness** as a process of bringing attention to a moment-by-moment experience. He introduced Mindfulness-Based Stress Reduction (MBSR) as a treatment program for chronic pain management.[46] In the Buddhist tradition, mindfulness plays an important role in understanding personal suffering,[47] and in contemporary counselling and psychology it is being used to help clients deal with life stress and emotional issues.[48]

Mindfulness is considered a form of mental training, similar in ways to meditation but with a focus or emphasis on taking notice of whatever thoughts come to mind, without judgment or making plans for action.[49] To practise mindfulness we are encouraged to sit in an upright position, concentrate on our breath, and observe our thoughts and feelings in what has been described as a state of self-observation. Mindfulness helps us respond to situations in a reflective way versus a reactive way. Mindfulness practice can then be used throughout our day, calming us d]own in stressful situations or helping us become more aware of the "here-and-now."

In a study on 135 first-year Canadian university students living in residence, researchers found significant positive relationships between mindfulness and rational coping. The study also revealed that students low in mindfulness tend to experience a higher degree of perceived stress points.[50]

✓ CHECK-IN

Would mindfulness training and practice help you on your spiritual journey?

Meaning, Purpose, and Potential Meaning, purpose, and potential are connected just like the body, mind, and spirit. **Meaning** can be defined as significant quality or an implication of a hidden or special significance.[51] **Purpose** is something set up as an object or end to be attained,[52] and **potential** expresses possibility.[53] Searching for meaning or special significance makes us more aware of worthy purposes in our lives. A worthy purpose might be living in a healthy and well way and helping others to do the same. It may be completing your education or educating others. The purpose may be small or grand. Having purpose helps us grow and learn about our own human potential so that we might express our own possibility.

For many people, finding meaning, discovering purpose, and realizing potential begins when they integrate the spiritual dimension of health and wellness into daily living. Spirituality, whether based on religious or secular beliefs, allows us to move back and forth from self-reflection to serving others. It moves us beyond thinking about spirituality only as an intellectual exercise to something that guides our intentions. It opens us up to possibilities—to see the world as a place that we can be engaged in, not fearful about. It can support our health and well-being. It is a dimension that connects us to each other and all things.

Transcendence In many articles and books about spirituality, the term "transcendence" appears. **Transcendence** can be defined as extending notably beyond ordinary limits. It has also been described as being in harmony with what we do not necessarily understand—what seems distant from us, but what seems mysteriously linked to us.[54]

At some time or another, most of us have experienced moments of transcendence. These moments are different, memorable times when you experience joy, togetherness, and great satisfaction. These moments leave us changed, sometimes for a brief time and sometimes forever. Roberta Bondar, the first Canadian female astronaut to travel in space, had these words to say upon her return to earth from her space flight aboard the space shuttle *Discovery:*

> *I feel the joy inside my entire body as I gently right myself in preparation for the last dive down through the access port between the mid-deck and flight deck. . . . The image of the bright blue atmosphere as a rainbow between the black universe and the sliding sheets of Earth's landscape stays with me as I complete my tasks. It seems to promise a pot of gold at its end, the likes of which I have never known. I promise myself that I will have adventure, love, and fun each day of my life. I will always think of Earth as never before, cherishing the sense of awe that this flight has inspired within me. I cannot imagine what new dimensions of thought will surround my life's work, because of this moment in time.*[55]

These moments open us up to possibilities. They help us create new options. They show us glimpses of the connection to all things. Participants in Faver's study reported having the feeling that at certain times they were in exactly the right place and doing what they were uniquely suited to do. One participant suggested that there is a moment in which we wake up and know that what we are doing is making a difference.[56] Understanding just what it is that we are meant to do—even for a time—can support the emotional and mental dimensions of health and wellness in that moment of transcendence.

✓ CHECK-IN

Have you had moments of transcendence in your life? What meaning do those moments hold for you?

SPIRITUALITY AND HEALTH

Spirituality is also important in the healthcare field. There is evidence that suggests there is a relationship between spirituality, religious involvement, and better health outcomes. Of course, that does not mean if you are a spiritual or religious person, you will not get sick or that illness is due to a lack of faith or spiritual connection.

It does appear, however, that there is an impact on human health for individuals who belong to religious communities or congregations, attend religious services, or report they have strong spiritual beliefs. Rosmarin, Wachholz, and Ai reviewed the spirituality and health research and discovered similar results in numerous studies that showed prayer, belief in God, and living in a spiritual or religious way had positive physical effects on HIV and the immune system, heart disease, post-surgery recovery, and pain management. There was also evidence that people who identify as religious or spiritual tend to utilize healthcare resources and embrace the concept of self-care.[57]

Seeman, Dubin, and Seeman also reviewed scientific studies that measured the physiological benefits of Judeo-Christian religious practices on blood pressure and immune function.[58] The team found that some studies suffered from methodological problems, but overall, there was reasonable evidence to support that greater religious involvement appeared to lower blood pressure and the prevalence of hypertension. They encourage the development of stronger research methodology for future studies, but suggest that scientific research has the potential to provide us with important insights into the spirituality, religiosity, and health connection.

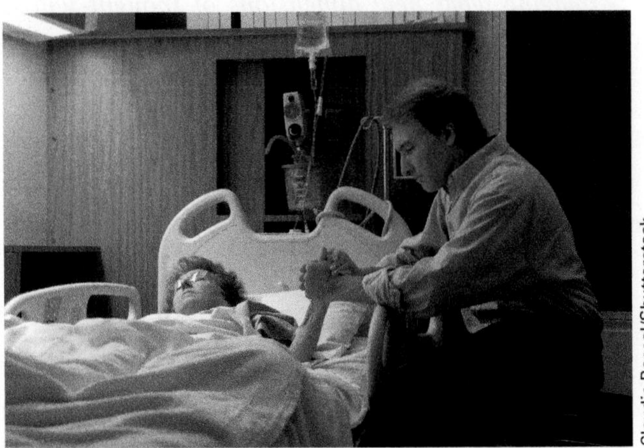

Claudio Rossol/Shutterstock

Personal connection and spiritual support have been found to positively impact patients.

Cancer patients have reported that their religious or spiritual beliefs helped them cope with the disease and improve their quality of life. Koenig found that within the 20 most methodologically rigorous studies, in a review of the literature, 60 percent of the studies found a positive association between being religious or spiritual and a lower risk of cancer or better outcomes for individuals who got cancer. None of the studies reported higher risks or worse outcomes.[59] Jim et al. conducted a meta-analysis that evaluated over 32 000 cancer patients. This team determined that a large body of research literature does show that religion and spirituality is an important factor for cancer patients and is positively linked with better physical health as reported by patients. Based on their findings, they suggest that spiritually based assistance and support for cancer patients might have the potential to enhance quality of life.[60]

Faith is important for some individuals suffering from emotional turmoil, recovering from mental illness, or dealing with post-traumatic stress disorder (PTSD). Religious and spiritual rituals such as has having conversations with God or placing trust in a higher power were just some of the ways people coped with mental distress.[61] Religious and spiritual people are also guided by a sense of meaning, social support, focus on interconnectedness, a decrease in negative self-talk, and the ability to cope when health issues are presented.[62]

Research about spirituality and the health of college and university students is also showing that students who report themselves as being healthy appear to be linking a spiritual dimension to their definition of individual health and wellness, that there appears to be a positive relationship between increased participation in physical activity and self-reported levels of spirituality, and students who report a higher level of life satisfaction with a self-reported level of spirituality might be integrating a spiritual dimension with an emotional dimension of health.[63] Balbeuna, Baetz, and Bowen[64] studied the relationship between religious attendance, spirituality, and major depression over a 14-year follow-up period. They concluded that attending religious services at least once a month had a protective effect against major depression. Their data showed there was a 22 percent lower risk of depression.

As our understanding of the complex relationships between health and healing grows, we might all begin to learn about supporting a healing process that integrates medicine, spirituality, and religion.

✓ CHECK-IN

Do you think that religion and spirituality can impact the health of an individual in a positive way?

SPIRITUALITY AND NATURE

Humans are one part of the natural world. The forces of nature are another. A growing body of literature connecting climate change and spirituality is helping us to understand our place in the natural world. As Baker and Morrison[65] suggest, spiritually motivated environmentalism can help us understand and take responsibility for our human impact on nature.

Many people are also discovering that an attachment to the land and nature contributes to their health and wellness. For centuries, throughout the world, plants have contributed to healing.[66] Plants have also been used in spiritual ceremonies, sometimes for health purposes. There are healing traditions where certain animals are perceived to have qualities that can assist humans through times of crisis. There is even research that suggests we can recover from stress more effectively if we visit a natural setting instead of staying in an urban area.[67]

In Chapter 16, Working Toward a Healthy Environment, we discussed a number of serious environmental issues that are changing the landscape of our country—of our world. Many of those issues are "people-made." If nature can heal, and the scientific evidence seems to support this concept, we must heed the cries from environmentalists, scientists, teachers, and Canadians across the country that "something must be done." Perhaps what is missing in our environmental planning processes is the spiritual dimension. This quotation from David Suzuki seems all the more meaningful when you think about your own spiritual connection to nature:

> *The way we see the world shapes the way we treat it. If a mountain is a deity, not a pile of ore; if a river is one of the veins of the land, not potential irrigation water; if a forest is a sacred grove, not timber; if other species are our biological kin, not resources; or if the planet is our mother, not an opportunity—then we will treat each one with greater respect. That is the challenge, to look at the world from a different perspective.*[68]

How do we educate ourselves and others about the importance of nature and the human spirit? We can start by rephrasing our questions about nature. Herb Hammond and Stephanie Judy, ecosystem consultants, suggest, in the following examples, that people who are sensitive to nature's spirit ask questions differently.[69]

Not, "How can we cover our tracks?" But, "How can we leave no tracks?"

Not, "How much can we take?" But, "What must we leave?"

Not, "How can we improve on nature?" But, "How can we plan with nature?"

With a sense of spiritual connection to nature, we move from managing our environment to caring for our environment. When we care for our environment, it is easier to care for ourselves and each other and stay well.

SPIRITUALITY ON CAMPUS

There has been a move in some academic institutions to integrate body, mind, and spiritual wellness into campus life. This has been done in a number of ways—through student services, counselling, and integration of spirituality curriculum to educate students about holistic living in an attempt to foster healthy campus communities.[70,71] A review of literature about spirituality and religion on campuses resulted in numerous studies. Here we present the findings of just a few.

Sorrentino set out to discover what religiously involved college students wanted with regard to religion and spirituality on campus. There were many interesting findings reported from this study:[72]

- Religious students had a commitment to a set of beliefs, regulations, symbols, and rites and wanted these particularities to be respected.
- Religious students' religion was an important element when thinking about the place of family.
- Three principles guided their thinking—*respect* for other's religious tradition; *authenticity,* where students could be true to their own beliefs and practices; and *meaning,* where planned multi-faith events were valuable for educational benefits and cultural expression and could serve to deepen relationships with other students of different faiths.*

In a study about spirituality, young women in transition from their professional education programs to their careers reported that spirituality helped them deal with their life transition, that their spiritual activities were mostly private and included individual prayer, meditation, and spending time in nature, and that the benefits of these activities were an increased level of self-awareness and encouragement.[73]

In another study on the spiritual perspectives of nursing students, a majority of the participants, 72 percent, indicated that they mentioned spiritual matters to others on a weekly basis, two-thirds of the students reported engaging in private prayer or meditation on a daily basis, and 74 percent felt that spirituality was important because it provided them with guidance in decision making.[74]

---

*P.V. Sorrentino, "What do college students want? A student-centered approach to multifaith involvement," *Journal of Ecumenical Studies,* 45(1), 79–98, 2010.

While many college and university students might not be attending formal religious services, they are searching for spiritual well-being. According to an American survey, which reflects responses from 3680 undergraduates attending 46 colleges, 77 percent of respondents said they prayed, 78 percent said they discussed religion or spirituality with their friends, and 73 percent said their spiritual or religious beliefs have helped them develop their identities.[75] Another study, which examined the association between spirituality and perceived wellness among college students, found that life purpose, optimism, and a sense of coherence were positively linked to overall health and wellness.[76]

Kuh and Gonyea analyzed data to determine how students who participated in spiritual activities spent their time on campus compared to students who did not. They learned that students who engage in spirituality-enhancing practices appear to participate more in a variety of campus activities and that students who view the campus culture or climate outside of class time as supportive of their social and non-academic needs report a deepened sense of spirituality.[77]

While education about spirituality has been traditionally found in departments of psychology, human and social development, medicine, nursing, social work, and religious or First Nations studies,[78] spirituality curriculum is now being offered in departments of kinesiology, physical education, and recreation and health education, sometimes included in health and wellness courses. This is a positive shift as more studies are beginning to show a relationship between spirituality, health beliefs, and health behaviours in college and university students. One example is research conducted by Nagel and Sgoutas-Emch, which found that younger, healthier individuals with higher spirituality scores are more active.[79]

Due in part to the findings of studies such as these, there has been an increase in the use of spiritual health models in a variety of other courses at colleges and universities such as nursing, biology, and environmental science.[80,81,82] In addition to courses and religious and spiritual campus initiatives, a new, first-of-its-kind Religion in Canada Institute (RCI) has been established at Trinity Western University. Researchers, faculty, and students associated with RCI are engaging in religious research and scholarly networking in Canada. Topics of investigation include religion and ethnicity, culture and conflict, spirituality and health, religion and globalization, and faith-based social services, to name just a few.[83]

✓ CHECK-IN

Do you participate in any religious or spiritual programs or events on your campus?

RELIGION

What Are the Major Classical World Religions?

There are many different religions of the world. Major classical world religions number 12: Baha'i, Buddhism, Christianity, Confucianism, Hinduism, Islam, Jainism, Judaism, Shinto, Sikhism, Taoism, and Zoroastrianism.[84] Alternative religions include Humanists, Unitarians, and New Age, while others find faith in cosmology and ecology.[85] First Nations spirituality might also be considered by some to be a religion and, by others, a way of life.

One thing that becomes clear when you begin to study and compare world religions or practices is that they share some universal human values and seek to create a more just and sustainable world society. Learning more about religious practices can help to increase tolerance toward others. This is an important aspect of the spiritual wellness dimension. Many of the world's religions encourage health and wellness. As you read through the following descriptions, ask yourself these questions:

- What role does religion play in the social health of the elderly? (Social dimension)
- How do the doctrines of some of these religions encourage reflection and commitment to one's life work? (Occupational dimension)
- Do the religious doctrines encourage followers to experience love, joy, peace, and fulfillment? (Spiritual dimension)
- What role does diet play in the lives of the followers of these religions? Which religions emphasize physical activity? (Physical dimension)
- Which religions encourage lifelong learning? (Intellectual dimension)
- How might prayer and meditation influence stress levels and mental and emotional health? (Emotional dimension)

Religion in Canada Canada is a religiously diverse country. An extensive public opinion poll carried out by the Angus Reid Institute in 2015[86] revealed that

- 39 percent of Canadians portrayed themselves as spiritual but not religious;
- 24 percent described themselves as spiritual and religious;
- 10 percent disclosed that they were religious but not spiritual and;
- 27 percent said they were neither religious nor spiritual (see Figure 17-3).

According to the data gathered, Canadians tend to identify themselves as spiritual almost twice as often as they identify as being religious. Canadians who believe

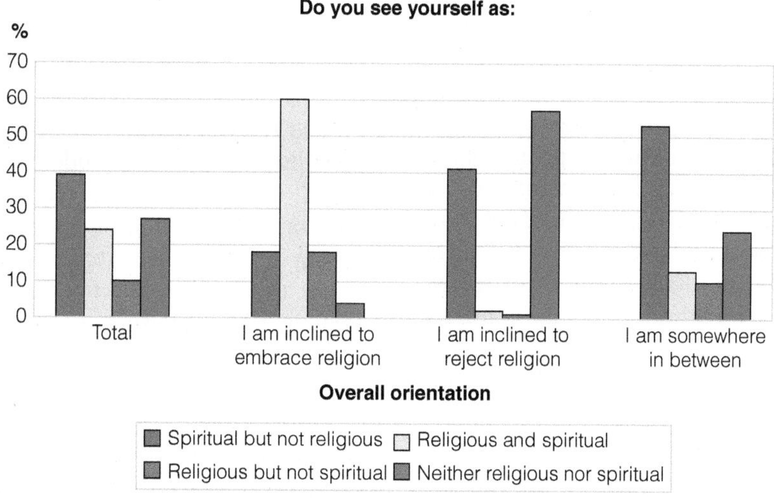

Figure 17-3 Canadians Self-Identity as Spiritual or Religious

Source: Angus Reid Institute. (2015, March 16) "Religion and faith in Canada today: strong belief, ambivalence and rejection define our views." Available at http://angusreid.org/wp-content/uploads/2016/01/2015.03.25_Faith.pdf.

that they are, to a certain degree, both spiritual and religious do attend some religious services and join in on some religious practices. They also hold on to specific traditional religious beliefs, however do not define themselves as being devout. Older adults 55 years and up lean toward embracing religion compared to younger Canadians who tend to be more indecisive about their religious beliefs. Of the women surveyed, 48 percent expressed ambivalence instead of outright rejection of religion or spirituality, compared to 40 percent of the men.

For those individuals who state that they do embrace religion, 56 percent, or more than half of the Canadians in this category, report that they attend religious services at least once a month. Eighty-six percent say that they pray in a private manner on a regular basis. Fifty-two percent declare that they read the Bible or other sacred religious texts at least once a month.

Seventy-nine percent of Canadians (eight out of ten individuals surveyed) who state they embrace religion believe they gain strength from their faith. Almost 70 percent declare that they feel God's presence on a regular basis. Figure 17-4 illustrates the percentage of Canadians who report their congregations are growing, declining, or staying the same.

> **✓ CHECK-IN**
>
> Where would you locate yourself with regard to embracing religion and spirituality?

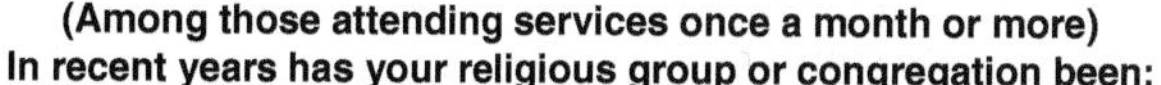

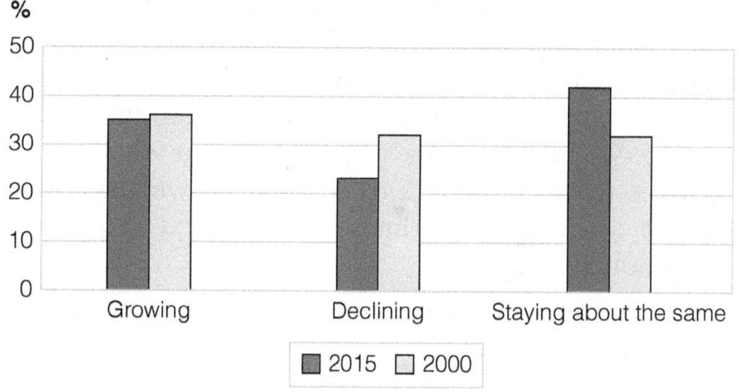

Figure 17-4 Perceived Percentage of Canadians Attending Services Once a Month or More—by Religious Group or Congregation

Source: Angus Reid Institute. (2015, March 16) "Religion and faith in Canada today: strong belief, ambivalence and rejection define our views." Available at http://angusreid.org/wp-content/uploads/2016/01/2015.03.25_Faith.pdf.

In this next section, brief descriptions of the main classical religions in Canada are presented. A description of one alternative religion is also included. Information has been drawn from various books and websites, but the information is by no means a detailed account.

The Baha'i World Faith The **Baha'i** faith was founded in Iran during the mid-19th century by Siyyid 'Ali-Muhammed. Baha'is believe that there is a single God who sends prophets into the world through whom the word of God is revealed. One of Siyyid 'Ali-Muhammed's followers, Mirza Husayn-'Ali-i-Nuri, was one of those prophets and assumed the title Baha'u'llah or "Glory of God" during the 1800s. He taught about world peace, democracy, civil rights, acceptance of scientific discoveries, and equal rights for women. These ideas were decades ahead of their time. The moral code expects virtues such as truthfulness and courtesy. Consumption of alcohol and drug abuse is forbidden. Some Muslims look upon the Baha'i faith as a breakaway sect of Islam.[87]

Buddhism **Buddhism** is the fourth-largest religion in the world. It was founded in Northern India by the first known Buddha, Siddhartha Gautama, a prince of the Sakya clan. In 535 BCE, he attained enlightenment and became Buddha the Awakened One. Buddhism encourages a connection with both the natural world and the spiritual world. It has evolved into two main forms. Thervada Buddhism, sometimes called Southern Buddhism, is largely found in Thailand, Burma, Cambodia, and Laos. The philosophy, meditation, and ethics of Thervada are based on the Pali texts that were written by Buddhists in India and Sri Lanka. Mahayana Buddhism, sometimes called Northern Buddhism, is largely found in China, Japan, Korea, Tibet, and Mongolia and is based on Sanskrit texts.[88]

Tibetan Buddhism, sometimes believed to be separate from Thervada and Mahayana, is led by the Dalai Lama, a Tibetan monk who promotes non-violence, compassion, religious harmony, world peace, and universal responsibility.[89]

The Buddha taught that we are responsible for our own happiness and suffering. What we experience is dependent on our previous actions. Good moral actions lead to happy states, and bad actions lead to future suffering. We cannot escape responsibility for what we do. This is the process of *Karma*—reaping what we sow, which can happen in this life or the next. There are four noble truths:

1. Dukkha: suffering exists.
2. Samudaya: there is a cause for suffering.
3. Niordha: there is an end to suffering.
4. Magga: to end suffering follow the eightfold path. The factors of the eightfold path are Right Understanding, Right Thought, Right Speech, Right Action, Right Livelihood, Right Effort, Right Mindfulness, and Right Concentration.

Christianity There are multiple meanings of the term **Christianity.** It can mean any person or group who believes themselves to be Christian. It can mean someone whose life has been transformed by the grace of God, anyone who has repented their sins, or anyone who has been "born again."[90] What is common is the belief that Yeshua of Nazareth, a Jewish preacher, commonly referred to as Jesus Christ, was the Son of God. He was born of the Virgin Mary, he was crucified for his beliefs and teachings, his body was resurrected after his death, and he later ascended into Heaven.

After his death, a Jewish Christian movement was formed. Other Christian movements such as Pauline Christianity and Gnostic Christianity were directed to specific groups of people. Further splits in different versions of the Christian movement resulted in Roman Catholic, Eastern Orthodox, and Protestant Reformation. There are more than 1500 different Christian faith groups in North America promoting different and sometimes conflicting beliefs about Christianity.[91]

The Ten Commandments guide Christians as they live their lives. They are intended as a universal set of rules for all people to follow. They include believing in one God only; not taking the name of God in vain; remembering to keep the Sabbath day holy; honouring our father and mother; and not killing, committing adultery, stealing, bearing false witness against neighbours, or coveting neighbours' goods. There are Protestant, Catholic, and Hebrew variations of the Ten Commandments.[92]

Christians believe that there is life after death, but the various Christian groups do not necessarily agree on the way souls are saved. All Christians believe that those who repent their sins before God will be saved and will go to Heaven. Belief in hell and purgatory, a place believed by Roman Catholics to be where there is a process of cleansing before most souls go to heaven, varies among the many Christian groups.

Confucianism Founded by K'ung Fu Tzu, **Confucianism** is an ethical system to which certain rituals at specific times during one's lifetime are practised. K'ung Fu Tzu was born in 551 BCE in the state of Lu, which is the modern-day Shantung province in China. His teachings deal with individual morality and ethics. In some areas in Asia, the social and moral ethics of Confucius are blended with Taoism and Buddhism.[93] There are approximately six million Confucians in the world. Most live in China and other parts of Asia. Approximately 26 000 live in North America.

Confucian ethical teachings include Li (ritual, propriety, etiquette), Hsiao (love within the family), Yi (righteousness), Xin (honesty and trustworthiness), Jen (benevolence, humaneness toward others—the highest Confucian virtue), and Chung (loyalty).[94] Four life passages at which the Confucian rituals are performed are birth, reaching maturity, marriage, and death.

Hinduism **Hinduism**, the world's third-largest religion after Christianity and Islam, does not have a single founder or central religious organization. It consists of thousands of different religious groups that have evolved in India since 1500 BCE[95] and is considered the world's oldest religion. There are about 120 500 Hindus in Canada.[96] Hindus recognize a single deity while honouring other Gods and Goddesses as manifestations or aspects of that supreme God. Most Hindus follow one of two major divisions with Hinduism. They are Vaishnavaism, which regards Vishnu (Krishna, The Preserver) as the ultimate deity, and Shivaism, which regards Shiva, the Destroyer, as the deity.[97]

Hindus follow the aims of Hinduism. These are Dharma (righteousness in religious life), Artha (success in economic life), Kama (gratification of the senses), and Moksa (liberation from samsara, the continuing cycle of birth, life, death, and rebirth for many lifetimes). Karma determines how you live your next life. People who live with pure acts, thoughts, and deeds can be reborn at a higher level, eventually achieving enlightenment. Hinduism is highly tolerant of other religions.

Islam Religious historians credit the founding of **Islam** to Muhammad the Prophet in 622 CE. They also suggest that the angel Jibril (or Gabriel) read the first revelation to Muhammad. However, most Muslims, followers of Islam, believe that Islam did exist before Muhammad was born, that the origins of Islam date back to the creation of the world, and that Muhammad was the last of a series of prophets.[98] Islam is the youngest of the world's largest religions, which include Christianity, Hinduism, and Buddhism. About 21 percent of all people on Earth follow Islam. If current trends continue, Islam will become the most popular world religion sometime in the mid-21st century, moving past Christianity.[99]

Muhammad the Prophet met considerable opposition to his teachings but did become the most powerful leader in Arabia, where Islam became firmly established. The two main texts Muslims consult are the *Qur'an,* or the words of God, and the *Hadith,* collections of the sayings of Muhammad.[100] The six fundamental beliefs of Islam are a single, indivisible God (Allah is often used to refer to God and is the Arabic word for God); the angels; the divine scriptures; the Messengers of God, which include Adam, Noah, Abraham, Moses, David, Jesus, and Muhammad the Prophet; the Day of Judgment; and the supremacy of God's will.

Muslims have duties to perform. They must recite the shahada (the creed: There is no God but God and Muhammad is his Prophet). They must perform the salat (prayer) five times a day if possible. They must donate regularly to charity, or zakat. They must fast during the lunar month of Ramadan, the month it is believed that Muhammad received the first revelation of the Qur'an from God, and, if able, they must make a pilgrimage to Mecca.[101]

Other practices include Jihad—the attainment of a noble goal. Jihad is probably the most misunderstood religious word in existence. From a Western perspective, it is often used to imply a holy war or a call to fight against non-Muslims in defence of Islam. Most Muslims believe it to be a personal, internal struggle with one's self. Muslims are also expected to explain Islam to followers of different faiths but do not have to recruit. This is left up to Allah. As well, suicide is forbidden. Only Allah is allowed to take a life.[102]

Jainism or Jain Dharma The roots of **Jainism** begin in ancient East India. Jainism contains a number of elements that are similar to Hinduism and Buddhism. Jainists believe that the universe, which has no beginning or end, exists as a series of layers. These layers consist of the Supreme Abode where Siddha, the liberated souls, live; the Upper World, or 30 heavens, where celestial beings live; the Middle World, which is the Earth and the rest of the universe; the Netherworld, the seven hells; the Nigoda, where the lowest forms of life live; the Universe Space, or layers of cloud that surround the upper world; and the Space Beyond, a place without soul, matter, time, or motion.[103]

Those following Jainism are expected to follow the five principles of living: Ahimsa—non-violence in all parts of a person (mental, verbal, and physical); Satya—speaking the truth; Asteya—not stealing from another; Brahma-charya or soul conduct—remaining sexually monogamous to one's spouse; and Aparigraha—detaching from people, places, and material things.[104]

Judaism **Judaism** originated with a divine covenant between the God of the ancient Israelites and the prophet Abraham. (The term "G–d" is used in some textbooks to respect the Jewish prohibition against spelling the name or title of the deity in full.) The next leader of the Israelites, Moses, led his people out of captivity in Egypt and received the Law from God. Another prophet, Joshua, later led the Israelites into "the promised land," where the Israelite kingdom was established with King Saul. The second king, David, established Jerusalem as the religious and political centre. The third king, Solomon, built the first Jewish temple. Divisions of the kingdom occurred after the death of Solomon. In 70 CE, the temple was destroyed, and the Jewish Christians were scattered throughout the world. In the 1930s, Adolph Hitler, leader of the Germany's National Socialist Party (Nazi Party), attempted to exterminate all of the Jews in Europe. About six million Jews were killed.

The creation of the state of Israel occurred in 1948. There are currently about 18 million Jews throughout the world.

Jews believe in one creator who is to be worshipped as the absolute ruler of the universe. He monitors people's activities and rewards good deeds and punishes evil. Jews believe in the inherent goodness of the world and its inhabitants as creations of God. They follow the *Tanakh,* which is composed of three groups of books, including the *Torah.* They also follow the *Talmud,* which contains stories, laws, medical knowledge, and debates about moral choices.[105] Jewish practices include observation of the Sabbath as a day of rest; strict discipline, according to the Law; regular attendance by Jewish males at Synagogue; and celebration of annual festivals that include Passover, Rosh Hashanah, Sukkoth, Hanukkah, Purim, and Shavout.[106]

Shinto **Shinto** is an ancient Japanese religion, closely connected to nature. This religion recognizes the existence of Kami, or nature deities. The first two, Izanagi and Izanami, gave birth to the Japanese Islands, and their children became the deities of the various Japanese clans. All Kami sustain and protect the people. Shintoists generally follow the code of Confucianism. Shinto also shares Buddhist beliefs. Within Shinto, Buddha is viewed as a Kami.[107]

The Four Affirmations in Shinto are tradition and the family, love of nature, physical cleanliness, and Matsuri—the worship and honour given to the Kami and ancestral spirits. Shinto practices include the recognition of many sacred places such as mountains and springs; respect for animals as the messengers of the Gods; shrine ceremonies, which include cleansing, prayers, and dances that are offered to the Kami; and seasonal celebrations held at spring planting, fall harvest, and special anniversaries of the history of a shrine or local patron spirit. Many followers are also involved in the "offer a meal movement," where they give up a meal once per month and then donate the money they saved to their religious organization for international relief.[108]

Sikhism The Sikh faith was founded by Shri Guru nanak Dev Ji in what is now known as Pakistan. **Sikhism** is sometimes believed to be a part of the Hindu religious tradition. Many Sikhs disagree and believe that their religion is a direct revelation from God. Sikh means "learner." The goal of Sikhs is to build a close, loving relationship to God. Sikhs believe in a single God with many names. They believe in samsara (the repetitive cycle of birth, life, and death), Karma (good and bad deeds), and reincarnation (the belief in a rebirth following death).[109]

They do not believe in the caste system as Hindus do. Sikhs believe that everyone has equal status. Many Sikhs follow living gurus. Their practices include prayers, which are repeated many times each day; worship; attendance in temples or shrines; and strict clothing practices.

Taoism The founder of Taoism, Lao-Tse, was a contemporary of Confucius in China. **Taoism** started as a combination of psychology and philosophy, but it became a religion in 440 CE. Tao, sometimes translated as "path," is a force that flows through all life. If you are a believer, your goal is to become one with the Tao.[110] Taoism currently has about 20 million followers in the world, with most living in Taiwan. Taoism has also provided an alternative to Confucian tradition in China. The two traditions coexist within the country.

Taoists do not pray to God. They seek answers to life's problems through meditation and observation. There is commitment to health and vitality. Development of virtue is important. Taoists search for compassion, moderation, and humility.[111] The Yin Yang symbol represents the balance of opposites in the universe. Many Taoists participate in Tai Chi, an exercise and movement technique that balances energy flow.

Unitarianism While **Unitarianism** is not included in the list of classical religions of Canada, it is considered an open-minded and alternative religion that has an individualistic approach, which supports a wide range of beliefs. It is important to discuss Unitarianism in this chapter because of its inclusivity of all society members. It grew out of the Protestant Reformation of the 16th century, starting in Poland and Transylvania in the 1560s. There are about 800 000 Unitarians worldwide.[112] In 1961, the Universalist Church of America (founded in 1793) and the American Unitarian Association (founded in 1825) merged to form the Unitarian Universalist Association in North America. In Canada, the Canadian Unitarian Council represents Unitarian congregations.

Unitarians are encouraged to search for meaning in life in a responsible way. At the heart of Unitarianism is the understanding that there are no set standards of beliefs; therefore people of all different faiths are welcomed. While there is a belief in one God, Unitarians have rejected the concept of the Trinity. A core belief is that God is present in every individual and in all parts of our natural world. They also believe that human nature is one of hope. They do not see humanity as fallen and full of sin. There is a strong conviction that religion should make a difference in the world, so social justice is another one of the important core values. The Unitarians were the first church in Britain to accept women as ministers, and they also support equal rights for gays and lesbians.[113]

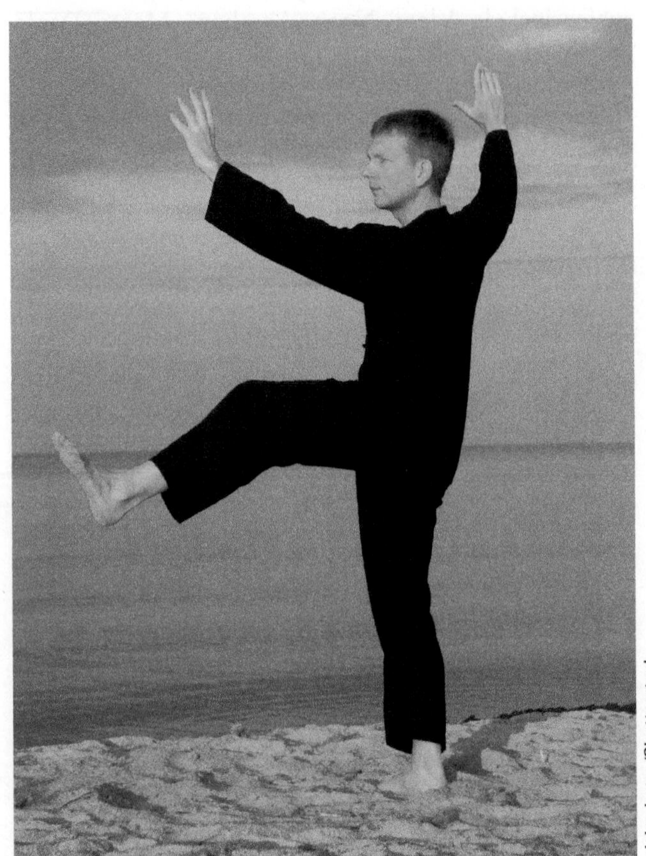

riekephotos/Shutterstock

Practising Tai Chi balances energy flow.

The debate about whether or not spirituality and religion are similar or different will most likely continue for years to come. However, we can begin to move from this debate to a thoughtful reflection on how spirituality and religion can support our personal and global health and well-being.

AN INVITATION TO HEALTH AND WELLNESS

This textbook began with an overview of health and wellness models and ended with a chapter on spirituality. In between you were presented with information on psychological and emotional health, physical activity and nutrition, and sexuality and reproductive choices. You also discovered more about major diseases and drug, alcohol, and tobacco use. There was a chapter on Canada's healthcare system, an encouragement to stay safe and protect yourself from injury, and a hint that a lifetime of health prepares us for growing older. Then there was a gentle reminder that personal wellness depends on global wellness.

You are encouraged to continue learning more about health and wellness and how lifestyle choices affect your personal potential. You are invited to continue to "live well."

SELF-SURVEY

Spiritual Self-Assessment

The purpose of this activity is to help you in identifying a sense of your spirituality. There are no "right" or "wrong" answers. It is provided to guide you as you think through what brings you a sense of meaning, purpose, and potential.

1. What are the most important relationships in your life?
   - ☐ My family of origin (parents, siblings, etc.)
   - ☐ A significant other or spouse
   - ☐ Children
   - ☐ Friends
   - ☐ God or a Higher Power
   - ☐ People I work with
   - ☐ Other ______________
2. Who or what helps you find meaning and a sense of purpose?
   - ☐ Family relationships
   - ☐ Friendships
   - ☐ Work
   - ☐ Relationships with the earth / environment
   - ☐ God / Higher Power
   - ☐ Other ______________
3. What helps you cope in difficult times?
   - ☐ Support of family / friends
   - ☐ Belief in the basic goodness of life
   - ☐ Faith in God / Higher Power
   - ☐ Music / poetry / literature
   - ☐ Prayer or meditation
   - ☐ Other ______________
4. How do you take care of yourself?
   - ☐ Time alone
   - ☐ Talking with others
   - ☐ Physical exercise, diet
   - ☐ Prayer, meditation, or other ritual
   - ☐ Nothing
   - ☐ Other ______________
5. Do you believe in God / a Higher Power?
   - ☐ Yes
   - ☐ Somewhat
   - ☐ No
6. If yes, how would you describe God / your Higher Power?
   - ☐ Angry
   - ☐ In control of all events
   - ☐ Judging
   - ☐ All-knowing
   - ☐ Kind
   - ☐ Able to do anything
   - ☐ Loving
   - ☐ Other ______________
7. If no, what are your beliefs about life?
   - ☐ Random events
   - ☐ Meaning comes from ______________
   - ☐ Hopelessness
   - ☐ Other ______________
8. Are there any spiritual practices that are important to you?
   - ☐ Attending religious services
   - ☐ Prayer
   - ☐ Reading Scripture
   - ☐ Meditation
   - ☐ Rituals
   - ☐ Yoga
   - ☐ Other ______________

There are many ways to embrace the spiritual dimension in your life. Your answers to this self-survey can help you discover your present spiritual state. Your answers can also guide you to expanding and deepening your understanding of the link between spirituality and healthy living.

Source: Chaplains On Hand. "Spiritual self-assessment." Tools & Checklists. Other Resources. http://chaplainsonhand.org/cms/resources/tools-checklists/23-spiritual-self-assessment.html.

Chapter Summary

1. What is spirituality?
   a. a formal religion
   b. a concept available only to those who attend church services
   c. a New Age term
   d. having a sense of self and a set of values that link to meaning and purpose in life and a connection to others
2. What is religion?
   a. a connection with the spirit only
   b. a specific system of belief about deity, often involving rituals and a philosophy of life
   c. something to be fearful of
   d. the only way to salvation
3. What does a holistic way of living involve?
   a. following a strict set of religious practices
   b. studying the major religions of the world
   c. a connection among body, mind, and spirit
   d. becoming physically fit
4. What have studies found is associated with a religious or spiritual connection?
   a. less cardiovascular disease, lower blood pressure, and less hypertension
   b. good jobs
   c. a perception of less control over our lives
   d. a guarantee that we will not get sick
5. What is transcendence?
   a. a major religion of the world
   b. part of many religious services around the world
   c. a spiritual practice in Christianity
   d. a moment or moments of joyful experience, togetherness, and great satisfaction
6. Which statement about First Nations peoples' traditional spiritual life is true?
   a. It is based on belief in a short-term journey.
   b. It is only available to First Nations peoples.
   c. It is a type of religion that honours the Kami.
   d. It is based on belief in a connection of all natural things.
7. Whom do followers of Islam pray to?
   a. Allah
   b. Buddha
   c. Jesus
   d. the Dalai Lama
8. Which statement about Shinto is true?
   a. Its practices include reciting the shahada.
   b. It began in ancient East India.
   c. It is an ancient Japanese religion.
   d. It is part of the Hindu religious tradition.
9. Which statement describes the results of a national survey of university undergraduate students?
   a. Most students reported that they did not discuss religion or spirituality.
   b. Seventy-eight percent of students said they discussed religion or spirituality with their friends.
   c. Forty-six percent of students said that they had no spiritual or religious beliefs.
   d. Most students did not think spirituality or religion belonged in an academic institution.
10. What is conscience?
    a. the same as ego
    b. self-centredness
    c. connectedness
    d. Shivaism

Answers to these questions can be found on page 465.

SELF-RESPONSIBILITY—SOCIAL RESPONSIBILITY

SELF-RESPONSIBILITY

Every one of us has a special place in the Life Pattern. There is guidance which comes from within to all who will listen.

Peace Pilgrim

A spiritual journey can take a lifetime. You can prepare for this journey by learning more about the spiritual dimension. Action might mean participating in a yoga class or attending a church service. Maintenance will demand from you the ability to face challenges that come your way. The spiritual journey is never easy. Human traits such as impatience, judgment, and irritability make their way into our daily lives. Yet, as we come to realize that challenges are seeds of opportunity, we become more spiritually confident and trust that things will work out.

SOCIAL RESPONSIBILITY

Service is the rent that you pay for room on this earth.

Shirley Chisholm

When we gain confidence and trust in ourselves, it becomes easier to reach out to others. When you are feeling down, try doing something for another person. Make healthy lifestyle choices so you can realize your potential.

CRITICAL THINKING

1. How do you support the spiritual dimension of your life? What actions do you take to learn more about your personal values? How might you change your lifestyle habits to become more in tune with your spiritual self?
2. How do you serve others? What type of activities do you participate in that "make a difference" or "leave legacies"?
3. What do you know about the major religions in the world? What religious doctrines or philosophies do you find meaningful? Why? How does religion link to spirituality as you define it?

WEB LINKS

Four Worlds International Institute for Human and Community Development

www.4worlds.org
This website is a family of people and organizations who are attempting to create solutions to difficult problems faced by First Nations communities across Canada and around the world.

Roberta Bondar

www.robertabondar.com/
Roberta Bondar calls herself a passionate Earthling. Visit this site to learn more about her work as a scientist and marvel at the messages of hope and the connection of nature and the human spirit.

Volunteer Abroad

www.volunteerbasecamp.com/
Volunteer Abroad, an organization owned by the Canadian Federation of Students, is a nonprofit student organization that connects motivated students with non-profit organizations, communities, and government agencies that need help around the world.

Please note that links are subject to change. If you find a broken link, use a search engine such as www.google.ca and search for the website by typing in keywords.

Key Terms

The terms listed here are used within the chapter on the page indicated. Definitions of terms are in the Glossary at the end of the book.

Baha'i 459
Buddhism 460
Christianity 460
Confucianism 460
conscience 454
ego 454
Hinduism 460
interconnectedness 453
Islam 461
Jainism 461
Judaism 461
meaning 455
mindfulness 455
potential 455
purpose 455
religion 450
Shinto 461
Sikhism 462
spiritual intelligence 450
spirituality 450
Taoism 462
transcendence 455
Unitarianism 462

Answers to Chapter Summary Questions

1. d; 2. b; 3. c; 4. a; 5. d; 6. d; 7. a; 8. c; 9. b; 10. c

Glossary

abscess A localized accumulation of pus and disintegrating tissue. (p. 229)

abstinence Voluntary refrainment from sexual activities that include vaginal, anal, and oral intercourse. (p. 194)

acquired immune deficiency syndrome (AIDS) The final stages of human immunodeficiency virus (HIV) infection, characterized by a variety of severe illnesses and decreased levels of certain immune cells. (pp. 244, 248)

action Modifying behaviour according to a plan. A commitment of time and energy is required. (p. 20)

activity-based funding A funding structure that provides a patient-focused system, where a healthcare unit or institution gets funding based on volume and the complexity of the patients that are treated. (p. 358)

acupuncture An ancient Chinese form of medicine, based on the philosophy that a cycle of energy circulating through the body controls health. The energy flow can be corrected by needles along the meridians throughout the body. (p. 366)

acute injury Physical injury, such as a sprain, bruise, or pulled muscle, that results from sudden trauma, such as a fall or collision. (p. 99)

adaptive response The body's attempt to reestablish homeostasis or stability. (p. 58)

addiction A behavioural pattern characterized by compulsion, loss of control, and continued repetition of a behaviour or activity in spite of adverse consequences. (p. 293)

additive Substance added to food to lengthen storage time, change taste in a way the manufacturer thinks is better, alter colour, or otherwise modify it to make it more appealing. (p. 129)

adrenocorticotrophic hormone (ACTH) A hormone that is released by the pituitary gland, which in turn triggers the adrenal glands to release cortisol, a hormone that helps to release nutrients the body has stored as energy. (p. 60)

advance directive Document that specifies an individual's preferences regarding treatment in a medical crisis. (p. 416)

aerobic exercise Physical activity in which sufficient or excess oxygen is continually supplied to the body. (p. 87)

agility The ability to change your body position and direction quickly and efficiently; important in many sports such as basketball, racquetball, and tennis. Agility tests include running forward and backward, then performing crossover steps. (p. 81)

aging The characteristic pattern of normal life changes that occur as humans grow older. (p. 401)

alcohol abuse Continued use of alcohol despite awareness of social, occupational, psychological, or physical problems related to its use, or use of alcohol in dangerous ways or situations, such as before driving. (p. 334)

alcohol dependence Development of a strong craving for alcohol due to the pleasurable feelings or relief of stress and anxiety produced by drinking. (p. 334)

alcoholism A chronic, progressive, potentially fatal disease characterized by an inability to control drinking, a preoccupation with alcohol, continued use of alcohol despite adverse consequences, and distorted thinking, most notably denial. (p. 335)

altruism Acts of helping or giving to others without thought of self-benefit. (p. 39)

Alzheimer's disease A progressive deterioration of intellectual powers due to physiological changes within the brain; symptoms include diminishing ability to concentrate, disorientation, depression, apathy, and paranoia. (p. 408)

amenorrhea The absence or suppression of menstruation. (p. 183)

amino acid Organic compound containing nitrogen, carbon, hydrogen, and oxygen; the essential building block of proteins. (p. 107)

amnion The innermost membrane of the sac enclosing the embryo or fetus. (p. 212)

amphetamine A stimulant that triggers the release of epinephrine, which stimulates the central nervous system; users experience a state of hyper-alertness and high energy, followed by a crash as the drug wears off. (p. 298)

anabolic steroid A synthetic artificial version of the male sex hormone testosterone. (p. 311)

anaerobic exercise Physical activity in which the body develops an oxygen deficit. (p. 87)

androgynous Refers to people who identify as neither male nor female. (p. 173)

anemia A condition marked by a deficiency of red blood cells or of hemoglobin in the blood. (p. 120)

angioplasty Surgical repair of an obstructed artery by passing a balloon catheter through the blood vessel to the area of obstruction and then inflating the catheter to compress the plaque against the vessel wall. (p. 260)

anorexia athletica A condition similar to anorexia nervosa where individuals have body image issues and over-exercise to gain a sense of control and power over their bodies. (p. 153)

anorexia nervosa A psychological disorder in which refusal to eat and/or an extreme loss of appetite leads to malnutrition, severe weight loss, and possibly death. (p. 152)

antibiotic Substance produced by microorganisms or synthetic agents that is toxic to other types of microorganisms; in diluted solutions, used to treat infectious diseases. (p. 223)

antidepressant A drug used primarily to treat symptoms of depression. (p. 46)

antioxidant Substance that prevents the damaging effects of oxidation in cells. (p. 121)

antiviral drug A substance that decreases the severity and duration of a viral infection if taken prior to or soon after onset of the infection. (p. 223)

anxiety A feeling of apprehension and dread, with or without a known cause; may range from mild to severe and may be accompanied by physical symptoms. (p. 42)

anxiety disorder Psychological disorder involving episodes of apprehension, tension, or uneasiness, stemming from the anticipation of danger and sometimes accompanied by physical symptoms; causes significant distress and impairment to an individual. (p. 43)

aorta The main artery of the body, arising from the left ventricle of the heart. (p. 256)

aortic valve One of the four valves in the heart, located at the point of exit of the left ventricle where the aorta begins. This valve lets the blood that is collected in the left ventricle move into the aorta and then prevents backflow of the blood back into the heart once it is in the aorta. (p. 257)

appetite A desire for food, stimulated by anticipated hunger, physiological changes within the brain and body, the availability of food, and other environmental and psychological factors. (p. 138)

arteriosclerosis Any of a number of chronic diseases characterized by degeneration of the arteries and hardening and thickening of arterial walls. (p. 259)

artery Any blood vessel that carries blood away from the heart. An exception is the specialized pulmonary arteries, which carry deoxygenated blood to the lungs where the blood is oxygenated. (p. 256)

artificial insemination The introduction of viable sperm into the vagina by artificial means for the purpose of inducing conception. (p. 216)

artificial reproductive technology (ART) New approaches to assisting people who deal with infertility that include microsurgery to open destroyed or blocked egg and sperm ducts, new hormone preparations to induce ovulation, and balloon tuboplasty to open blocked fallopian tubes. (p. 216)

assertive Behaving in a non-hostile, confident manner to make your needs and desires clear to others. (p. 39)

atherosclerosis A form of arteriosclerosis in which fatty substances (plaque) are deposited on the inner walls of arteries. (p. 259)

attention deficit disorder (ADD) A term often used interchangeably with attention deficit/hyperactivity disorder (ADHD). (p. 44)

attention deficit/hyperactivity disorder (ADHD) A spectrum of difficulties in controlling motion and sustaining attention, including hyperactivity, impulsivity, and distractibility. (p. 44)

attitude a feeling or way of thinking that affects a person's behaviour. (p. 17)

autoimmune disorder A disease caused by an immune response against antigens in the tissues of one's own body. (p. 232)

autonomic nervous system (ANS) A part of the central nervous system that starts in a region of the brain called the cerebral cortex and regulates our bodily functions such as our heart rate, respiratory system, and glands. (p. 59)

autonomy The ability to govern ourselves; being independent; independence from familial and societal influences. (p. 39)

aversion therapy A treatment that attempts to help a person overcome a dependence or bad habit by making the person feel disgusted or repulsed by that habit. (p. 348)

avian influenza A contagious infection that also comes from a virus that infects many kinds of birds and other animals. (p. 233)

Ayurveda A traditional Indian medical treatment involving meditation, exercise, herbal medication, and nutrition. (p. 367)

bacterial vaginosis (BV) A vaginal infection caused by overgrowth or depletion of various microorganisms living in the vagina, resulting in a malodourous white or grey vaginal discharge. (p. 237)

bacterium (plural, bacteria) One-celled microscopic organism; the most plentiful pathogen. (p. 223)

Baha'i A faith founded in Iran during the mid-19th century by Siyyid 'Ali-Muhammed. Baha'is believe that there is a single God who sends prophets into the world through which the word of God is revealed. (p. 459)

balance The body's ability to maintain proper equilibrium, which is necessary in day-to-day life as well as certain sports such as gymnastics and skiing. (p. 81)

ballistic stretching A type of stretching, sometimes called dynamic stretching, that is characterized by rapid bouncing movements, such as a series of up-and-down bobs. (p. 97)

barbiturate Anti-anxiety drug that depresses the central nervous system, reduces activity, and induces relaxation, drowsiness, or sleep; often prescribed to relieve tension, treat epileptic seizures, or as a general anesthetic. (p. 311)

barrier contraceptive Birth-control device that blocks the meeting of egg and sperm by physical barriers (such as condoms, diaphragms, or cervical caps), or by chemical barriers (such as spermicide), or both. (p. 200)

basal body temperature The body temperature upon waking, before any activity. (p. 205)

basal metabolic rate (BMR) The number of calories required to sustain the body at rest. (pp. 107, 142)

behaviour therapy Psychotherapy that emphasizes application of the principles of learning to substitute desirable responses and behaviour patterns for undesirable ones. (p. 43)

belief A state or habit of mind in which trust or confidence is placed in some person or thing (p. 18)

benzodiazepine Anti-anxiety drug that depresses the central nervous system, reduces activity, and induces relaxation, drowsiness, or sleep; often prescribed to relieve tension, muscular strain, sleep problems, anxiety, or panic attacks; also used as an anesthetic and in the treatment of alcohol withdrawal. (p. 311)

binge drinking For a man, having five or more alcoholic drinks at a single sitting; for a woman, having four drinks or more at a single sitting. (p. 331)

binge eating disorder (BED) The rapid consumption of an abnormally large amount of food in a relatively short time. (p. 153)

biofeedback An alternative healthcare technique that uses machines to measure temperature or skin responses and internal physiological activities. Information is then shared with the subjects so that they can learn to control involuntary functions such as circulation, tension, and heart rates. (pp. 69, 367)

bioterror agents The use of infectious agents such as anthrax, smallpox, botulism, and tularemia as weapons of terrorism and war. (p. 236)

bipolar disorder Severe depression alternating with periods of manic activity and elation. (p. 47)

bisexual Sexually oriented toward both men and women. (p. 174)

blood-alcohol concentration (BAC) The amount of alcohol in the blood, expressed as a percentage. (p. 320)

body composition The relative amounts of fat and lean tissue (bone, muscle, organs, water) in the body. (p. 81)

body mass index (BMI) A mathematical formula that correlates height and weight with body fat; a better predictor of disease than weight alone. (p. 139)

botanical medicine An ancient form of medical treatment using substances derived from trees, flowers, ferns, seaweeds, and lichens to treat disease. (p. 367)

botulism Possibly fatal food poisoning, caused by a type of bacterium that produces a toxin in the absence of air; found in improperly canned food. (p. 129)

brain death The end of all brain activity, indicated by an absence of electrical activity and a lack of reflexes. (p. 414)

breech birth A birth in which the infant's buttocks or feet pass through the birth canal first. (p. 215)

BSE (bovine spongiform encephalopathy) Known also as mad cow disease, this is a disease that affects the central nervous system of animals, especially cows. A human form of BSE, variant Creutzfeldt-Jakob disease, has been linked to eating beef products coming from animals infected with BSE. (p. 225)

Buddhism The fourth-largest religion in the world; founded in Northern India by the first known Buddha, Siddhartha Gautama. Buddhism encourages a connection with both the natural world and the spiritual world. (p. 460)

bulimia nervosa Episodic binge eating, often followed by forced vomiting or laxative abuse, and accompanied by a persistent preoccupation with body shape and weight. (p. 153)

bundled payments A single funding amount that pays for the care needed to restore a patient to optimal health after a specific health issue such as a stroke. (p. 358)

Caesarean delivery The surgical procedure in which an infant is delivered through an incision made in the abdominal wall and uterus. (p. 215)

calcium The most abundant mineral in the body used to build strong bone tissue throughout life; plays a vital role in blood clotting and muscle and nerve functioning. (p. 119)

calorie The amount of energy required to raise the temperature of one gram of water by one degree Celsius. In everyday usage related to the energy content of foods and the energy expended in activities, a calorie is actually the equivalent of 1000 such calories, or a kilocalorie. (p. 106)

candidiasis An infection of the yeast Candida albicans, commonly occurring in the vagina, vulva, penis, or mouth, and causing burning, itching, and a whitish discharge. (p. 237)

cap and trade A tested and proven system for reducing pollution that requires an organization, region, province, or country to set responsible limits on greenhouse gas emissions and attempts to lower emissions over time. (p. 428)

capillary A minute blood vessel that connects an artery to a vein. (p. 256)

carbohydrate Organic compound, such as starch, sugar, and glycogen, that is composed of carbon, hydrogen, and oxygen; source of bodily energy. (p. 107) carbon monoxide A colourless, odourless gas produced by the burning of gasoline or tobacco; displaces oxygen in the hemoglobin molecules of red blood cells. (pp. 336, 435)

carbon offsets A credit for greenhouse gas reductions; promoted as one way to achieve carbon neutrality. (p. 428)

carcinogen A substance that produces cancerous cells or enhances their development and growth. (p. 278)

cardiac death The moment when the hearts stop beating. (p. 414)

cardiorespiratory fitness The ability of the heart and blood vessels to efficiently circulate blood through the body. (p. 80)

cardiovascular disease (CVD) Any disease that affects the structure and function of the heart and cardiovascular system. (p. 256)

celibacy Abstention from sexual activity; can be partial or complete, permanent or temporary. (p. 175)

cell-mediated immunity The portion of the immune response that protects against parasites, fungi, cancer cells, and foreign tissue, primarily by means of T cells, or lymphocytes. (p. 228)

cellular death The gradual death of body cells after the heart stops beating. (p. 414)

cervical cap A thimble-sized rubber or plastic cap that is inserted into the vagina to fit over the cervix and prevent the passage of sperm into the uterus during sexual intercourse; used with a spermicidal foam or jelly, it serves as both a chemical and a physical barrier to sperm. (p. 200)

cervix The narrow, lower end of the uterus that opens into the vagina. (p. 181)

chain of infection Sometimes described as a series of infection events, the six links in the chain of infection are infectious agents, reservoirs, portals of exit, modes of transmission, portals of entry, and a susceptible host. All the chains much be connected for an infection to develop. (p. 222)

chancroid A soft, painful sore or localized infection usually acquired through sexual contact. (p. 244)

chiropractic A method of treating disease, primarily through manipulating the bones and joints to restore normal nerve function. (p. 367)

chlamydia A sexually transmitted infection caused by the bacterium *Chlamydia trachomatis*; often asymptomatic in women but sometimes characterized by urinary pain; if undetected and untreated may result in pelvic inflammatory disease (PID). (p. 241)

chlorinated hydrocarbon Highly toxic pesticide, such as DDT and chlordane, that is extremely resistant to breakdown; may cause cancer, birth defects, neurological disorders, and damage to wildlife and the environment. (p. 438)

cholesterol An organic substance found in animal fats; linked to cardiovascular disease, particularly atherosclerosis. (pp. 109, 263)

chordae tendineae Cord-like tendons that connect the papillary muscles to the tricuspid valve and the mitral valve in the heart. (p. 258)

Christianity A religion derived from Jesus Christ. Christians are individuals who believe their life has been transformed by the grace of God, or who have repented their sins or been born again. (p. 460)

chronic obstructive pulmonary disease (COPD) A lung disorder that causes airways to become partially obstructed. (p. 412)

chronological age How old we are in calendar years measured by time such as years and months. (p. 403)

circumcision The surgical removal of the foreskin of the penis. (p. 184)

climate change Any long-term significant change in the "average weather" that a given region experiences; variations within the Earth's atmosphere including such processes as variations in solar radiation, the Earth's orbit, and greenhouse gas concentrations. (p. 424)

climate forcings Physical factors, introduced by human activities, that force a net increase (positive forcing) or a net decrease (negative forcing) of heat in the climate system as a whole. (p. 425)

clitoris A small erectile structure on the female, corresponding to the penis on the male. (p. 181)

club drug Illegally manufactured psychoactive drug (including ecstasy, Special K, and Rohypnol) that has dangerous physical and psychological effects; often used at all-night rave or trance events. (p. 307)

cocaine A white crystalline powder extracted from the leaves of the coca plant that stimulates the central nervous system and produces a brief period of euphoria followed by depression. (p. 304)

cognitive-behavioural therapy (CBT) A technique used to identify an individual's beliefs and attitudes, recognize negative thought patterns, and educate in alternative ways of thinking. (p. 51)

cognitive-transactional model of stress and coping A non-biological stress theory, developed by Lazarus and Folkman, that looks at the relationship between demands and the power to deal with them without unreasonable or destructive costs. (p. 59)

cohabitation Two people living together as a couple, without official ties such as marriage. (p. 170)

coitus interruptus The removal of the penis from the vagina before ejaculation. (p. 194)

colpotomy Surgical sterilization by cutting or blocking the fallopian tubes through an incision made in the wall of the vagina. (p. 207)

complementary and alternative health care (CAHC) Another name for complementary and alternative medicine (CAM). (p. 362)

complementary and alternative medicine (CAM) All healthcare approaches, practices, and treatments not widely taught in medical schools and not generally used in hospitals. Examples include nutritional, herbal, and botanical therapies, body/energy or life force therapies, and mind–body practices. (p. 362)

complementary protein A pairing of two or more foods that together make up a complete protein with sufficient levels of all essential amino acids. (p. 107)

complete protein Protein that contains all the amino acids needed by the body for growth and maintenance. (p. 107)

complex carbohydrate Starches, including cereals, fruits, and vegetables. They have more than 10 units of sugar. (p. 108)

complicated grief An intense and extended period of grief that is often linked to the loss or death of a family member, friend, acquaintance, or partner relationship. Key characteristics include a sense of disbelief, anger, bitterness, recurrent intrusive thoughts, and intense yearning. (p. 63)

compulsive overeaters Individuals who eat compulsively, often as a source of comfort against feelings of inner emptiness, low self-esteem, or fear of abandonment. (p. 154)

concentric phase Decreasing the angle between two bones or contracting the muscle constitutes the concentric phase of an isotonic contraction. (p. 94)

conception The merging of a sperm and an ovum. (p. 192)

concurrent disorder A situation where an individual has both a mental health and a substance abuse problem. (p. 294)

condom A latex sheath worn over the penis during sexual acts to prevent conception and/or the transmission of disease; some condoms contain a spermicidal lubricant. (p. 200)

Confucianism An ethical system in which certain rituals at specific times during one's lifetime are practised. Teachings deal with individual morality and ethics. (p. 460)

conscience Our connectedness; our sense of moral goodness. (p. 454)

constant-dose combination pill An oral contraceptive that releases synthetic estrogen and progestin at constant levels throughout the menstrual cycle. (p. 195)

contemplation Awareness that there is a problem behaviour and the consideration of changing it within the next six months. (p. 20)

contraception The prevention of conception; birth control. (p. 192)

contraceptive patch A method of birth control consisting of a four-square centimetre patch that sticks to the skin and continuously releases estrogen and progestin into the bloodstream. (p. 197)

coordination The integration of the nervous and muscular systems, which allows for harmonious body movements. It is an important skill in sports that demand throwing, catching, and hitting. (p. 81)

core strength The ability of the body to support the spine and keep the body stable and balanced. (p. 95)

coronary artery Blood from the coronary arteries supply all parts of the heart muscle. Two major coronary arteries branch off from the aorta. (p. 256)

coronary bypass A procedure that helps restore blood flow to the heart muscle. A healthy piece of artery from a patient's leg, chest, arm, or abdomen is grafted onto a coronary artery to detour blood around the blocked area. (p. 260)

coronary heart disease (CHD) Problems with coronary arteries, which provide blood circulation to the heart. (p. 258)

coronary vein Veins that are located in the coronary sinus and collect blood from the heart muscle. They deliver deoxygenated blood to the right atrium. (p. 256)

corpus luteum A yellowish mass of tissue that is formed immediately after ovulation from the remaining cells of the follicle; it secretes estrogen and progesterone for the remainder of the menstrual cycle. (p. 181)

cortisol A hormone that is released from the adrenal glands and helps to release nutrients the body has stored for energy. (p. 60)

Cowper's gland Either of two small glands that discharge into the male urethra. (p. 184)

crucifer A plant, such as broccoli, cabbage, and cauliflower, that contains large amounts of fibre, proteins, and indoles. (p. 115)

crystal meth Also known as methamphetamine (MA). A white, odourless, bitter-tasting crystalline powder that readily dissolves in water or alcohol. It can be snorted, swallowed, or injected. Ice (or crank, crystal, glass, or tina) is a smokable form of methamphetamine. (p. 298)

culture The set of shared attitudes, values, goals, and practices of a group that are internalized by an individual within the group. (p. 34)

cunnilingus Sexual stimulation of a woman's genitals by means of oral manipulation. (p. 177)

cystitis Inflammation of the urinary bladder. (p. 237)

decibel (dB) A unit for measuring the intensity of sounds. (p. 442)

deep frostbite The freezing of skin, muscle, and bone that requires medical treatment. It usually involves the tissues of the hands and feet, which appear pale and feel frozen. (p. 387)

defence mechanism A psychological process that alleviates anxiety and eliminates mental conflict; includes denial, displacement, projection, rationalization, reaction formation, and repression. (p. 68)

deliriant Chemical, such as solvent, aerosol, glue, cleaning fluid, petroleum product, and some anesthetics, that produces vapours with psychoactive effects when inhaled. (p. 309)

dementia Deterioration of mental capability. (p. 408)

Depo-Provera® A hormonal birth control injection that contains a progestin, a synthetic version of the natural hormone progesterone; provides three months of contraceptive protection. (p. 197)

depression In general, feelings of unhappiness and despair; as a mental illness, also characterized by an inability to function normally. (p. 42)

depressive disorder A psychological disorder involving pervasive and sustained depression. (p. 46)

diabetes mellitus A disease in which the inadequate production of insulin or resistance to insulin leads to failure of the body tissues to break down carbohydrates at a normal rate. (p. 265)

diaphragm A bowl-like rubber cup with a flexible rim that is inserted into the vagina to cover the cervix and prevent the passage of sperm into the uterus during sexual intercourse; used with a spermicidal foam or jelly, it serves as both a chemical and a physical barrier to sperm. (p. 199)

diastole The period between contractions in the cardiac cycle, during which the heart relaxes and dilates as it fills with blood. (p. 257)

diastolic blood pressure The minimum arterial pressure when the heart is in a period of relaxation and dilation. (p. 261)

dietary fibre The nondigestible form of carbohydrates found in plant foods, such as leaves, stems, skins, seeds, and hulls. (p. 108)

dietary reference intake (DRI) A set of values for the dietary nutrient intake of healthy people (estimated average requirements, recommended dietary allowances, adequate intakes, and tolerable upper intake levels); used for planning and assessing diets. (p. 121)

dilation and evacuation (D&E) A medical procedure in which the contents of the uterus are removed through the use of instruments. (p. 208)

disaccharides Compounds that contain two sugar units linked by a chemical bond that must be broken down into simple sugars before they can be used by the body. Examples include sucrose, lactose, maltose, and table sugar. (p. 107)

distress A negative stress that may result in illness. (p. 58)

do-not-resuscitate (DNR) An advance directive expressing an individual's preference that resuscitation efforts not be made during a medical crisis. (p. 416)

drug Any substance, other than food, that affects bodily functions and structures when taken into the body. (p. 288)

drug abuse The excessive use of a drug in a manner inconsistent with accepted medical practice. (p. 288)

drug misuse The use of a drug for a purpose (or person) other than that for which it was medically intended. (p. 288)

drunkorexia A phenomenon on college and university campuses where students intentionally limit their food intake prior to drinking alcohol. (p. 331)

duration The amount of time of your workout. (p. 86)

dynamic stretching Controlled movements that gradually increase your reach and speed of movement; improves dynamic flexibility and takes you to the limits of your range of motion. (p. 97)

dysfunctional Abnormal or impaired functioning of a social group or partnership that does not promote healthy communication, honesty, or intimacy. (p. 169)

dysmenorrhea Painful menstruation. (p. 183)

eating disorder A bizarre, often dangerous pattern of food consumption, including anorexia nervosa and bulimia nervosa. (p. 151)

eccentric phase Increasing the angle between two bones or lengthening the muscle constitutes the eccentric phase of an isotonic contraction. (p. 94)

ecological footprint The measure of the human demand on the Earth's ecosystems. (p. 433)

EcoLogo™ The most respected environmental standard and certification mark program in North America. Products and services that bear this logo must meet stringent standards of environmental leadership. (p. 440)

ecosystem A community of organisms sharing a physical and chemical environment and interacting with each other. (p. 424)

ecstasy (MDMA) A synthetic compound, also known as methylenedioxymethamphetamine, that is similar in structure to methamphetamine and has both stimulant and hallucinogenic effects. (p. 307)

ectopic pregnancy A pregnancy in which the fertilized egg has implanted itself outside the uterine cavity, usually in the fallopian tube. (p. 212)

ego Our self and self-centredness. (p. 454)

ejaculatory duct The canal connecting the seminal vesicles and vas deferens. (p. 184)

electromagnetic field (EMF) The invisible electric and magnetic field generated by an electrically charged conductor. (p. 441)

embryo An organism in its early stage of development; in humans, the embryonic period lasts from the second to the eighth week of pregnancy. (p. 212)

emergency contraception (EC) Types of oral contraceptive pills, usually taken within 72 hours after intercourse, that can prevent pregnancy. (p. 205)

emotional abuse Any behaviour that uses fear, humiliation, or verbal assaults to control another human being. Examples include berating, belittling, and criticism. (p. 169)

emotional health The ability to express and acknowledge one's feelings and moods and exhibit adaptability and compassion for others. (p. 32)

emotional intelligence The ability to recognize and manage our own emotions and recognize, understand, and influence the emotions of others. (p. 33)

enabling factors Factors that make it possible or easier for people or populations to change their behaviours; include individual physical capabilities and mental capacities, resources, living conditions, societal support, and accessible facilities, programs, and services as well as developing skills in addition to predisposing existing skills. (p. 16)

endocrine disruptor Synthetic chemical that interferes with the way hormones work in humans and wildlife. (p. 438)

endometrium The mucous membrane lining the uterus. (p. 181)

endorphin Mood-elevating, pain-killing chemical produced by the brain. (p. 82)

enhanced greenhouse effect The release of so much carbon dioxide and other greenhouse gases into our atmosphere that we are covered by a thick, heat-trapping blanket that is causing our earth to overheat. (p. 425)

Environmental Performance Index (EPI) A biennial report that evaluates how the Organisation for Economic Co-operation and Development (OECD) member countries protect ecosystems and human health. (p. 424)

ephedra Also known as ma huang. A herbal product that comes from an evergreen plant. It has been used in the past to help people with respiratory illnesses. More recently it has been used in weight-loss programs. The use of ephedra is restricted in Canada because of its association with serious medical problems. (p. 367)

epidemiology The study of how often diseases occur in different groups of people and why. (p. 7)

epididymis That portion of the male duct system in which sperm mature. (p. 184)

epidural block An injection of anesthetic into the membrane surrounding the spinal cord to numb the lower body during labour and childbirth. (p. 214)

epinephrine A hormone also known as adrenaline that is released from the adrenal glands and initiates an increase in blood flow. (p. 59)

erectile dysfunction A common sexual arousal disorder where men have difficulty maintaining a penile erection long enough for sexual intercourse. (p. 179)

erogenous zones Areas of the human body that respond to kissing and touching; include both non-genital and genital areas. (p. 175)

Escherichia coli (E. coli) A bacteria found in undercooked or inadequately washed food that can cause a life-threatening infection. Symptoms include mild to severe diarrhea and hemolytic uremic syndrome, in which red blood cells are destroyed and the kidneys fail. (p. 224)

essential nutrient Nutrient that the body cannot manufacture for itself and must obtain from food: water, carbohydrates, fats, vitamins, and minerals. (p. 106)

estimated energy requirement (EER) The dietary energy intake that is predicted to maintain energy balance in a healthy adult of a defined age, sex, weight, height, and level of physical activity consistent with good health. (pp. 107, 142)

estrogen The female sex hormone that stimulates female secondary sex characteristics. (p. 181)

ethyl alcohol The intoxicating agent in alcoholic beverages; also called ethanol. (p. 320)

eustress A positive stress, which stimulates a person to function properly. (p. 58)

exercise Physical activity that you plan, structure, and repeat for the purpose of conditioning your body to improve health and maintain fitness. (p. 80)

exercise metabolic rate The 10 percent of energy expenditure (90 percent is attributed to resting metabolic rate—RMR) we use, which comes from all types of daily physical activities such as walking, climbing, and moving. (p. 143)

exergaming The playing of video games that require rigorous physical exercise and are intended as a workout. (p. 93)

extreme dieters Individuals who become preoccupied with what they eat and weigh and go beyond cutting back on calories or increasing physical activity. (p. 154)

failure rate The number of pregnancies that occur per year for every 100 women using a particular method of birth control. (p. 193)

fallopian tube Either of two channels that transports ova from the ovaries to the uterus; the usual site of fertilization. (p. 181)

fats An important nutrient, sometimes called lipids, that provides nine calories per gram of energy and aids in fat-soluble vitamin absorption, regulates body temperature, and plays an important role in growth and development. (p. 109)

feelings Bodily or emotional responses that help us realize we are experiencing some type of emotion that can come and go within minutes. (p. 37)

fellatio Sexual stimulation of a man's genitals by means of oral manipulation. (p. 177)

fertilization The fusion of the sperm and egg nuclei. (p. 192)

fetal alcohol effect (FAE) Milder form of fetal alcohol syndrome, including low birth weight, irritability as newborns, and permanent mental impairment; caused by the mother's alcohol consumption during pregnancy. (p. 334)

fetal alcohol spectrum disorder (FASD) A continuum of permanent birth defects that are caused by alcohol consumption by a pregnant woman. (p. 334)

fetal alcohol syndrome (FAS) A cluster of physical and mental defects in the newborn, including low birth weight, smaller-than-normal head circumference, intrauterine growth retardation, and permanent mental impairment; caused by the mother's alcohol consumption during pregnancy. (p. 334)

fetus The human organism developing in the uterus from the ninth week until birth. (p. 212)

fibre A major form of complex carbohydrates found in foods that come from plants (fruits and vegetables); made up of dietary fibre and functional fibre. (p. 107)

FITT A formula that describes the frequency, intensity, type, and length of time of physical activity. (p. 86)

flexibility The range of motion allowed by one's joints; determined by the length of muscles, tendons, and ligaments attached to the joints. (p. 81)

food toxicologist Specialist who detects toxins in food and treats the conditions toxins produce. (p. 128)

force The influence that causes movement of a body, often described as pushing or pulling. (p. 81)

friends with benefits (FWB) Relationships between friends who have sex, with no commitment for romance; benefits include trust and comfort. (p. 163)

frostbite The freezing or partial freezing of skin and tissue just below the skin, or even muscle and bone; more severe than frostnip. (p. 387)

frostnip Sudden blanching or lightening of the skin on hands, feet, and face, resulting from exposure to high wind speeds and low temperatures. (p. 387)

functional age A combination of chronological, physiological, and emotional ages. (p. 403)

functional death The end of all vital functions, such as heartbeat and respiration. (p. 414)

functional fibre Isolated, non-digestible carbohydrates with beneficial effects in humans. (p. 108)

functional fitness The performance of daily activities as well as exercises that mimic job tasks or everyday movements; can improve an individual's balance, coordination, strength, and endurance. (p. 81)

fungi Organisms that reproduce by means of spores. (p. 223)

gamma globulin The antibody-containing portion of the blood fluid (plasma). (p. 228)

gamma hydroxybutyrate (GHB) A brain messenger chemical (also known as blue nitro or the date-rape drug) that stimulates the release of the human growth hormone; commonly abused for its high and its alleged ability to trim fat and build muscles. (p. 307)

gender A term based on a sense of femininity or masculinity as defined by the society in which we live. (p. 173)

gender expression The external appearance, dress, mannerisms, and behaviour through which individuals present their gender identity, or the gender they would like to appear as. (p. 173)

gender identity A person's self-identified sense of being male, female, neither, or both. (p. 173)

gender roles Socially determined behavioural rules and standards assigned to men and women in our society. Examples include the primary role for women of caring for their family and home, and the role of the head of the household for men. (p. 173)

general adaptation syndrome (GAS) The sequenced physiological response to a stressful situation; consists of three stages: alarm, resistance, and exhaustion. (p. 58)

generalized anxiety disorder (GAD) An anxiety disorder characterized as chronic distress. (p. 43)

genetically engineered organisms (GE) Organisms that are modified through the use of new technology, where genes are either transferred into or removed from the organism. (p. 128)

genetically modified organism (GMO) A plant, animal, or bacteria that has had their genetic material altered through traditional breeding techniques where an organism is mutated and desired traits are then selected and bred together. Sometimes this term is used interchangeably with genetically engineered organisms (GE). (p. 128)

gerontologist Health professional who studies the ways in which we adapt to aging. (p. 401)

gestational diabetes mellitus (GMD) A temporary condition that occurs during pregnancy—hyperglycemia or high blood sugar. It carries an increased risk of developing diabetes for both mother and child. (p. 280)

globalization The increased transnational movement of capital, goods, people, and political systems and a rapid turnover of ideas and images through new communication technologies. (p. 13)

global warming A sustained increase in the average temperature of the Earth's atmosphere that causes changes in the global climate. (p. 425)

glucose The body's basic fuel provided by carbohydrates. (p. 107)

glycemic index (GI) A measure of how much a carbohydrate-containing food is likely to raise your blood sugar. (p. 108)

glycogen Carbohydrates (monosaccharides) that are metabolized and stored in the liver and muscles to be converted to metabolically usable energy or fuel during exercise. (p. 107)

gonads The male testes and female ovaries where the production of sex hormones takes place. (p. 173)

gonorrhea A sexually transmitted infection caused by the bacterium *Neisseria gonorrhoeae;* male symptoms include discharge from the penis; women are generally asymptomatic. (p. 241)

greenhouse effect A natural phenomenon where CO_2, an important gas in the insulation layer covering the planet, acts like a greenhouse and allows a small amount of solar radiation through the Earth's atmosphere, trapping it so heat generates warmth for the earth. (p. 424)

greenhouse gas (GHG) Earth's atmosphere is made up of greenhouse gases, including carbon dioxide (CO_2), methane (CH_4), nitrous oxide (NO_2), ozone (O_3), and water vapour. (p. 424)

guided imagery An approach to stress control, self-healing, or the motivation of life changes by means of visualizing oneself in the state of calmness, wellness, or change. (p. 69)

hallucinogen A drug that causes hallucinations. (p. 308)

happiness A state of well-being and contentment or a pleasurable or satisfying experience. (p. 37)

hashish A concentrated form of cannabis containing the psychoactive ingredient TCH; causes a sense of euphoria when inhaled or eaten. (p. 302)

health A state of complete well-being, including physical, psychological, spiritual, social, intellectual, and environmental components. (p. 5)

health belief model (HBM) Developed in the 1950s by social psychologists Hochbaum, Rosenstock, and Kegels, and updated in the 1980s, the model helps to explain and predict health behaviours. (p. 17)

health literacy The ability to access, understand, evaluate, and communicate health information to support healthy living. (p. 359)

health promotion An educational and informational process in which people are helped to change attitudes and behaviours in an effort to improve their health. (p. 5)

healthy environment The creation of conditions and surroundings conducive to health. (p. 5)

heat cramp Painful muscle spasm caused by vigorous exercise and heavy sweating in the heat. (p. 386)

heat exhaustion Faintness, rapid heartbeat, low blood pressure, an ashen appearance, cold and clammy skin, and nausea, resulting from prolonged sweating with inadequate fluid replacement. (p. 386)

heat stress Physical response to prolonged exposure to high temperature; occurs simultaneously with or after heat cramps. (p. 386)

heat stroke A medical emergency consisting of a fever of at least 40.5°C (105°F), hot, dry skin, rapid heartbeat, rapid and shallow breathing, and elevated or lowered blood pressure, caused by the breakdown of the body's cooling mechanism. (p. 386)

helminth A parasitic roundworm or flatworm. (p. 224)

hepatitis An inflammation and/or infection of the liver caused by a virus; often accompanied by jaundice. (p. 235)

herpes simplex virus (HSV) A condition caused by one of the herpes viruses and characterized by lesions of the skin or mucous membranes; herpes virus type 2 is sexually transmitted and causes genital blisters or sores. (p. 242)

heterosexual Primary sexual orientation toward members of the opposite sex. (p. 174)

Hinduism The world's third-largest religion after Christianity and Islam. Hindus recognize a single deity while honouring other Gods and Goddesses as manifestations or aspects of that supreme God. (p. 460)

HITT (high intensity interval training) Exercise training sessions that consist of up to 10 minutes of intense exercise within a 30-minute training session that includes a warm-up, interval training, recovery periods, and a cool-down. HITT training programs often mix aerobic exercise, calisthenics, and weight lifting. Equipment such as jump ropes, rowing machines, resistance bands, gymnastics rings, plyometric boxes, and kettlebells are used to increase intensity of the workouts. (p. 93)

holism An emphasis on the interconnectedness between an individual and his or her mind, body, and spirit. (p. 4)

holistic An approach to medicine that takes into account body, mind, emotion, and spirit. (p. 362)

holographic will A will entirely in the handwriting of its author. (p. 416)

homelessness Not having a home; includes absolute homelessness, being at risk for homelessness, and hidden homelessness. (p. 42)

homeopathy A system of medical practice that treats a disease by administering dosages of substances that would produce symptoms in healthy people similar to those of the disease. (p. 367)

homeostasis The body's natural state of balance or stability. (p. 58)

homophobia The irrational fear and hatred of someone who is a homosexual. Reactions range from subtle demeaning comments to gay bashing. (p. 174)

homosexual Primary sexual orientation toward members of the same sex. (p. 174)

hooking up Sexual activity with a casual partner who may be a friend or a stranger; a term used to describe a variety of sexual interactions, including kissing, fondling, oral sex, and sexual intercourse. (p. 164)

hormone replacement therapy (HRT) The use of supplemental hormones during and after menopause. (p. 410)

human immunodeficiency virus (HIV) A type of virus that causes a spectrum of health problems, ranging from a symptomless infection to the development of life-threatening diseases because of impaired immunity. (pp. 244, 246)

human papillomavirus (HPV) A pathogen that causes genital warts and increases the risk of cervical cancer. (pp. 243)

humoral immunity A portion of the immune response that provides lifelong protection against bacterial or viral infections, such as mumps, by means of antibodies whose production is triggered by the release of antigens upon first exposure to the infectious agent. (p. 227)

hunger The physiological drive to consume food. (p. 137)

hygiene Healthy; a science of the establishment and maintenance of health; conditions or practices conducive to health. (p. 4)

hyperplasia A point in time when the number of fat cells increases in our bodies; usually only occurs during infancy and puberty, but new research shows it may also happen when a person consumes more calories than they burn on a regular basis over time. (p. 138)

hypertension High blood pressure occurring when the blood exerts excessive pressure against the arterial walls. (p. 261)

hypertrophy (a) The process of a muscle getting larger by adapting to an increase in the tension on it through strength and conditioning exercises. (p. 86) (b) A process whereby the fat cells increase in size; can happen any time in life if calories taken in are greater than caloric expenditure, or calories going out. (p. 138)

hypothalamus A section of the brain that acts as our control centre and reacts to stress hormones that have been released by the sympathetic nervous system. (p. 59)

hypothermia An abnormally low body temperature; if not treated appropriately, coma or death could result. (p. 387)

hysterectomy The surgical removal of the uterus. (p. 207)

hysterotomy A procedure in which the uterus is surgically opened and the fetus inside it removed. (p. 208)

immunity Protection from infectious diseases. (p. 226)

immunization A process that helps your body fight off diseases caused by certain viruses and bacteria by exposing your body to vaccines. (p. 230)

implantation The embedding of the fertilized ovum in the uterine lining. (p. 192)

incomplete protein Protein that lacks one or more of the amino acids essential for protein synthesis. (p. 107)

incubation period The time between a pathogen's entrance into the body and the first symptom. (p. 226)

indole Naturally occurring chemical found in foods such as winter squash, carrots, and crucifers; may help lower cancer risk. (p. 115)

infectious agent The type of microbe that can cause infection—viruses, bacteria, fungi, protozoa, and helminths (parasitic worms). (p. 222)

inferior vena cava A major vein that brings deoxygenated blood from the lower body to the heart. (p. 256)

infertility The inability to conceive a child. (p. 216)

infidelity Any form of emotional or sexual intimacy with a person other than a primary dating or marriage partner. (p. 165)

infiltration A gradual penetration or invasion. (p. 270)

inflammation A localized response by the body to tissue injury, characterized by swelling and the dilation of the blood vessels. (p. 229)

influenza Illness caused by one of the highly contagious influenza viruses; symptoms include stuffy nose, headache, body aches, fever, and cough. (p. 232)

informed consent Permission (to undergo or receive a medical procedure or treatment) given voluntarily, with full knowledge and understanding of the procedure or treatment and its possible consequences. (p. 359)

inhalant Substance that produces vapours having psychoactive effects when inhaled. (p. 309)

inhalation A route of administration in which drugs enter the body through the lungs. Examples include inhaling gases, aerosol sprays, or fumes from solvents. (p. 288)

injection A method of administering drugs into the body. Can be done intravenously (directly into a vein), intramuscularly (into muscle tissue), or subcutaneously (beneath the skin). (p. 288)

integrative medicine An approach that combines traditional medicine with alternative and/or complementary therapies. (p. 363)

interconnectedness Operating as a unit, or a state of being connected reciprocally; can be understood by two distinct domains, connectedness to self and connectedness to others. (p. 453)

interpersonal therapy (IPT) A technique used to develop communication skills and relationships. (p. 51)

intersex Refers to people who were born with both male and female anatomy, or ambiguous genitalia. (p. 173)

intimacy A state of closeness between two people, characterized by the desire and ability to share one's innermost thoughts and feelings with each other, both verbally and nonverbally. (p. 167)

intoxication Maladaptive behavioural, psychological, and physiologic changes that occur as a result of substance abuse. (pp. 294, 324)

intramuscular injection A slower and consistent method of administering drugs, usually by way of hypodermic needle into the muscular tissue. (p. 288)

intrauterine device (IUD) A device inserted into the uterus through the cervix to prevent pregnancy by interfering with implantation. (p. 198)

intravenous (IV) injection A method of administration that gets a concentrated form of a drug into the bloodstream within seconds. Effects are felt within minutes. (p. 288)

inunction An option for administering drugs by anointing or applying an ointment by rubbing or by applying adhesive patches containing a drug to the skin. (p. 289)

iron An essential mineral necessary for the transport of oxygen via hemoglobin in red blood cells and for oxidation by cells. (p. 120)

irradiation Exposure to or treatment by some form of radiation. (pp. 128, 442)

ischemic heart disease Another name for coronary heart disease (CHD) or coronary artery disease (CAD). An acute or chronic cardiac disability resulting from insufficient supply of oxygenated blood to the heart. (p. 259)

Islam The youngest of the world's largest religions. The two main texts that Muslims consult are the Qur'an and the Hadith. Practices include jihad, the attainment of a noble goal. (p. 461)

isokinetic Having the same force; exercise with specialized equipment that provides resistance equal to the force applied by the user throughout the entire range of motion. (p. 94)

isometric Of the same length; exercise in which muscles increase their tension without shortening in length, such as when pushing an immovable object. (p. 94)

isotonic Having the same tension or tone; exercise requiring the repetition of an action that creates tension, such as weightlifting or calisthenics. (p. 94)

Jainism A religion that is based on the belief that the universe, which has no beginning or end, exists as a series of layers. Those following Jainism are expected to follow the five principles of living. (p. 461)

Judaism A religion developed among the ancient Hebrews and characterized by belief in one transcendent God who has revealed himself to the prophet Abraham. (p. 461) kinesiology The study of the human body in motion. Those working in the field are called kinesiologists. Services include exercise therapy, injury assessment and rehabilitation, ergonomics and workplace design, health and fitness courses and workshops, and gait analysis services using biomedical technology. (p. 367)

labia majora The fleshy outer folds that border the female genital area. (p. 181)

labia minora The fleshy inner folds that border the female genital area. (p. 181)

labour The process leading up to birth: effacement and dilation of the cervix; the movement of the baby into and through the birth canal, accompanied by strong contractions; and contraction of the uterus and expulsion of the placenta after the birth. (p. 214)

lacto-ovo-pesco-vegetarian Person who eats dairy products, eggs, poultry, and fish (but not red meat). (p. 127)

lacto-ovo-vegetarian Person who eats eggs, dairy products, and fruits and vegetables (but not meat, poultry, or fish). (p. 127)

lacto-vegetarian Person who eats dairy products as well as fruits and vegetables (but not meat, poultry, eggs, or fish). (p. 127)

Lamaze method A method of childbirth preparation taught to expectant parents to help the woman cope with the discomfort of labour; combines breathing and psychological techniques. (p. 214)

laparoscopy A surgical sterilization procedure in which the fallopian tubes are observed with a laparoscope inserted through a small incision and then cut or blocked. (p. 207)

laparotomy A surgical sterilization procedure in which the fallopian tubes are cut or blocked through an incision made in the abdomen. (p. 206)

learned helplessness The act of giving up trying as a result of consistent failure to be rewarded in life. (p. 36)

left atrium One of the upper chambers of the heart that accepts oxygenated blood from the lungs, transported through the pulmonary vein. (p. 257)

left ventricle One of the chambers of the heart that collects oxygenated blood from the left atrium. (p. 257)

lipoprotein Compound in blood that is made up of proteins and fat; a high-density lipoprotein (HDL) picks up excess cholesterol in the blood; a low-density lipoprotein (LDL) carries more cholesterol and deposits it on the walls of arteries. (p. 264)

listeria An illness caused by the bacterium *Listeria monocytogenes* that is acquired by eating contaminated food; the organism can spread to the bloodstream and central nervous system. (p. 225)

living will A written statement providing instructions for the use of life-sustaining procedures in the event of terminal illness or injury. (p. 416)

locus of control An individual's belief about the source of power and influence over his or her life; *internal influence* (from within themselves) rather than *external influence* (from others). (pp. 20, 39)

lumpectomy The surgical removal of a breast tumour and its surrounding tissue. (p. 273)

lymph node Small tissue mass in which some immune cells are stored. (p. 229)

macronutrient Nutrient required by the human body in the greatest amount, including water, carbohydrates, proteins, and fats. (p. 106)

mainstream smoke The smoke inhaled directly by smoking a cigarette. (p. 344)

maintenance Continued work at changing behaviour. The change may take six months to a lifetime. Some lapses may be temporary. (p. 20)

major depression Sadness that does not end. (p. 46)

male pattern baldness The loss of hair at the vertex, or top, of the head. (p. 269)

mammography A diagnostic X-ray exam used to detect breast cancer. (p. 273)

marijuana The drug derived from the cannabis plant; contains the psychoactive ingredient THC, which causes a mild sense of euphoria when inhaled or eaten. (p. 302)

massage therapy A therapeutic method of using the hands to rub, stroke, or knead the body to produce positive effects on an individual's health and well-being. (p. 369)

mastectomy The surgical removal of an entire breast. (p. 273)

masturbation Self-stimulation of the genitals, often resulting in orgasm. (p. 176)

meaning Significant quality or an implication of a hidden or special significance. (p. 455)

medical abortion Method of ending a pregnancy within nine weeks of conception using hormonal medications that cause expulsion of the fertilized egg. (p. 208)

meditation The use of quiet sitting, breathing techniques, and/or chanting to relax, improve concentration, and become attuned to one's inner self. (p. 69)

meningitis An extremely serious, potentially fatal illness in which the bacterium *Neisseria meningitis* attacks the membranes around the brain and spinal cord. (p. 234)

menopause The complete cessation of ovulation and menstruation for 12 consecutive months. (p. 410)

menstruation Discharge of blood from the vagina as a result of the shedding of the uterine lining at the end of the menstrual cycle. (p. 181)

mental health State of emotional and psychological well-being in which an individual is able to use his or her cognitive and emotional capabilities, function in society, and meet the ordinary demands of everyday life. (p. 32)

mental illness Behavioural or psychological syndrome associated with distress or a significantly increased risk of suffering pain, disability, loss of freedom, or death. (p. 42)

metabolic syndrome A cluster of symptoms that increases the risk of heart disease and diabetes. (p. 265)

metastasize To spread to other parts of the body via the bloodstream or the lymphatic system. (p. 270)

methicillin-resistant *S. aureus* (MRSA) A superbug that fights off traditional antibiotics and can become a major health threat. (p. 236)

micronutrient Vitamin or mineral needed by the body in very small amounts. (p. 106)

microplastics Particles that are made of small (less than 5 mm), synthetic, solid plastic material and are non-degradable and water insoluable and used in many goods including cosmetic and personal-care products. (p. 440)

microwave Extremely high-frequency electromagnetic wave that increases the rate at which molecules vibrate, thereby generating heat. (p. 441)

Middle East respiratory syndrome coronavirus (MERS-CoV) Similar to SARS virus, the symptoms include fever, cough, and shortness of breath. Current research points toward contact with live camels or camel meat or milk. (p. 234)

mindfulness A method of stress reduction that involves experiencing the physical and mental sensations of the present moment. (pp. 69, 455)

mineral Naturally occurring inorganic substance; small amounts of some minerals are essential in metabolism and nutrition. (p. 119)

minilaparotomy A surgical sterilization procedure in which the fallopian tubes are cut or sealed by electrical coagulation through a small incision just above the pubic hairline. (p. 206)

minipill An oral contraceptive containing a small amount of progestin and no estrogen; prevents contraception by making the mucus in the cervix so thick that sperm cannot enter the uterus. (p. 195)

miscarriage A pregnancy that terminates before the 20th week of gestation; also called spontaneous abortion. (p. 212)

mitral valve A heart valve that separates the left atrium from the left ventricle. (p. 257)

modelling Observing other people and emulating their behaviours, successes, or positive lifestyle choices. (p. 19)

modes of transmission A microorganism needs a mode of transmission to move from a reservoir to a host. The five ways a pathogen can be transmitted are direct contact, indirect contact, droplet contact, airborne transmission, and common vehicle transmission. (p. 226) monogamy Exclusive sexual (physical), emotional, or social relationship, only with committed partners. (p. 170)

mononucleosis An infectious viral disease characterized by an excess of white blood cells, fever, fatigue, bodily discomfort, a sore throat, and kidney and liver complications. (p. 235)

monophasic pill *See* constant-dose combination pill. (p. 195)

monosaccharides Simple sugars, sometimes known as simple carbohydrates, such as glucose, fructose, and galactose, which consist of one simple sugar unit. (p. 107)

mons pubis The rounded, fleshy area over the junction of the female pubic bones. (p. 180)

mood A conscious state of mind; a sustained emotional state that colours one's view of the world for hours or days. (p. 37)

morbidity The disease rates in one period of time or in one place. (p. 5)

mortality The number of deaths in one period of time or in one place. (p. 5)

mould A type of fungus that decomposes organic matter and provides plants with nutrients; now considered an environmental risk because of its growth in buildings and homes. Mould may trigger or worsen health problems. (p. 435)

multiphasic pill An oral contraceptive that releases different levels of estrogen and progestin to mimic the hormonal fluctuations of the natural menstrual cycle. (p. 195)

multiple chemical sensitivity (MCS) A sensitivity to low-level chemical exposure from ordinary substances, such as perfumes and tobacco smoke, that results in physiological responses such as chest pain, depression, dizziness, fatigue, and nausea; also known as environmentally triggered illness. (p. 442)

muscle dysmorphia A condition sometimes described as bigorexia—the opposite of anorexia—where men engage in excessive strength-training sessions because they have an obsessive desire to appear more muscular and lean (p. 153)

muscular endurance The ability to perform repeated muscular effort, measured by counting how many times a person can lift, push, or press a given weight. (p. 81, 94)

muscular fitness The amount of strength and level of endurance in the body's muscles. (p. 81)

muscular strength The force within muscles, measured by the absolute maximum weight that a person can lift, push, or press in one effort. (p. 81, 94)

mutagen An agent that causes alterations in the genetic material of living cells. (p. 434)

mutation A change in the genetic material of a cell or cells that is brought about by radiation, chemicals, or natural causes. (p. 434)

mutual aid The actions people take to help each other cope. (p. 5)

myocardial infarction (MI) A condition characterized by the dying of tissue areas in the myocardium, caused by interruption of the blood supply to those areas; the medical name for a heart attack. (p. 259)

naturopathy An alternative system of treatment of disease that emphasizes the use of natural remedies such as sun, water, heat, and air. Therapies may include dietary changes, steam baths, and exercise. (p. 369)

neoplasm Any tumour, whether benign or malignant. (p. 270)

nicotine The addictive substance in tobacco; one of the most toxic of all poisons. (p. 336)

non-adherence Not properly taking prescription drugs the way they should be taken. (p. 291)

non-exercise activity thermogenesis (NEAT) Unplanned daily activities, such as fidgeting and pacing, that burn calories. (p. 147)

nongonococcal urethritis (NGU) Inflammation of the urethra caused by organisms other than the gonococcus bacterium. (p. 242)

non-opioid Chemically synthesized drug that has sleep-inducing and pain-relieving properties similar to those of opium and its derivatives. (p. 309)

norm Unwritten rule regarding behaviour and conduct expected or accepted by a group. (p. 19)

nutrition The science devoted to the study of dietary needs and the effects of food on organisms. (p. 105)

NuvaRing® A contraceptive vaginal ring that releases a low dose of estrogen and progestin into the surrounding tissue. (p. 197)

obesity The excessive accumulation of fat in the body; a condition of having a body mass index (BMI) of 30 or above. (p. 140)

obsessive-compulsive disorder (OCD) An anxiety disorder characterized by obsessions and/or compulsions that impair one's ability to function and form relationships. (p. 44)

one repetition maximum (1RM) A way of measuring muscular strength by establishing how much weight a person can lift one time. (p. 94)

open relationship A relationship in which partners agree to sexual involvement with others outside of their primary relationship. (p. 170)

opioid Drug that has sleep-inducing and pain-relieving properties; includes opium (and its derivatives) and non-opioid, synthetic drugs. (p. 309)

optimistic Hoping or believing that good things will happen in the future. (p. 37)

oral contraceptive Preparation of synthetic hormones that inhibits ovulation; also referred to as birth control pills or simply the pill. (p. 195)

oral ingestion The most common way of taking a drug. Examples include swallowing a tablet, capsule, or liquid. (p. 288)

organic Term designating food produced with, or production based on the use of, fertilizer originating from plants or animals without the use of pesticides or chemically formulated fertilizers. (p. 128)

organic phosphate Toxic pesticide that may cause cancer, birth defects, neurological disorders, and damage to wildlife and the environment. (p. 438)

osteoporosis A condition common in older people in which the bones become increasingly soft and porous, making them susceptible to injury. (pp. 82, 404)

outercourse Sexual activities such as kissing, hugging, sensual touching, and mutual masturbation. (p. 195)

ovary The paired female sex organ that produces egg cells, estrogen, and progesterone. (p. 181)

overloading Method of physical training in which the number of repetitions or the amount of resistance is gradually increased to work the muscle to temporary fatigue. (p. 94)

overload principle Providing a greater stress or demand on the body than it is normally accustomed to handling. (p. 84)

over-the-counter (OTC) drug Medication that can be obtained without a prescription from a medical professional (i.e., over the counter at a retail outlet). (p. 289)

overtrain Working muscles too intensely or too frequently; results can include persistent muscle soreness, injuries, unintended weight loss, nervousness, and an inability to relax. (p. 99)

overuse injury Physical injury to joints or muscles, such as a strain, fracture, and tendonitis, which results from overdoing a repetitive activity. (p. 99)

overweight A condition of having a body mass index (BMI) between 25.0 and 29.9. (p. 140)

ovulation The release of a mature ovum from an ovary approximately 14 days prior to the onset of menstruation. (p. 181)

ovulation method A method of birth control based on the observation of changes in the consistency of the mucus in the vagina to predict ovulation. (p. 205)

ovum (plural, ova) The female egg cell. (p. 181)

ozone A colourless, unstable toxic gas that is formed from oxygen by electrical discharges or ultraviolet light. It can impair the body's immune system and cause long-term lung damage. (p. 435)

panacea To heal; a remedy for all difficulties; a cure-all. (p. 4)

pandemic flu Any virulent human flu that causes a global outbreak, or pandemic, of serious illness. (p. 234)

panic attack A short episode characterized by physical sensations of light-headedness, dizziness, hyperventilation, and numbness of extremities, accompanied by an inexplicable terror, usually of a physical disaster such as death. (p. 43)

panic disorder An anxiety disorder in which the apprehension or experience of recurring panic attacks is so intense that normal functioning is impaired. (p. 44)

papillary muscles Important anatomical structures of the heart that attach to the lower portion of the interior walls of the ventricles. (p. 258)

parasympathetic nervous system (PNS) One of two branches of the autonomic nervous system (ANS) that slows down other systems that are stimulated by the stress response. The main job of the PNS is to restore homeostasis. (p. 60)

pathogen A microorganism that produces disease. (p. 222)

PCP (phencyclidine) A synthetic psychoactive substance that produces effects similar to other psychoactive drugs when swallowed, smoked, sniffed, or injected, but may also trigger unpredictable behavioural changes. (p. 311)

pelvic inflammatory disease (PID) An inflammation of the internal female genital tract, characterized by abdominal pain, fever, and tenderness of the cervix. (p. 241)

penis The male organ of sex and urination. (p. 183)

perimenopause The period from a woman's first irregular cycles to her last menstruation. (p. 408)

perinatology The medical specialty concerned with the diagnosis and treatment of pregnant women with high-risk conditions and their fetuses. (p. 212)

perineum The area between the anus and vagina in the female and between the anus and scrotum in the male. (p. 181)

phobia An anxiety disorder marked by an inordinate fear of an object, a class of objects, or a situation, resulting in extreme avoidance behaviours. (p. 43)

physical activity All leisure and non-leisure body movement produced by the skeletal muscles and resulting in an increase in energy expenditure. (p. 78)

physical conditioning The gradual building up of the body to enhance cardiorespiratory or aerobic fitness, muscular strength, muscular endurance, and flexibility; healthy body composition. (p. 81)

physical dependence The physiological attachment to, and need for, a drug. (p. 293)

physical fitness The ability to respond to routine physical demands, with enough reserve energy to cope with a sudden challenge. (p. 80)

physiological age The normal functioning of our bodies as controlled by the interactions between physical and chemical bodily states. (p. 403)

physiotherapy Sometimes known as physical therapy, this healthcare treatment is used to assess, restore, and maintain physical function. (p. 369)

phytochemical Chemical that exists naturally in plants and has disease-fighting properties. (p. 121)

pituitary gland A gland that releases hormones called gonadotrophins, which stimulate the testes and ovaries to increase production of the female and male sex hormones. (p. 173)

placenta An organ that develops after implantation and to which the embryo attaches, via the umbilical cord, for nourishment and waste removal. (p. 212)

plaque Deposits of fat, fibrin, cholesterol, calcium, and other cell parts on the lining of the arteries. (pp. 109, 259)

plyometrics Specialized, high-intensity training exercises that develop athletic performance skills. (p. 81)

PNF (proprioceptive neuromuscular facilitation) stretching A type of stretching exercise that uses a person's own body, a partner, gravity, or a weight that serves as an external force or resistance to help joints move through their range of motion. PNF stretching can be either passive or active. (p. 96)

pollutant A substance or agent in the environment, usually the by-product of human industry or activity, that is injurious to human, animal, or plant life. (p. 434)

pollution The presence of pollutants in the environment. (p. 434)

polyabuse The misuse or abuse of more than one drug. (p. 294)

polyamory An open relationship between partners in which there is an acceptance of having intimate relationships with more than one person at a time, with both the knowledge and consent of everyone involved. (p. 170)

polysaccharides Complex carbohydrates that have more than 10 units of sugar that must be broken down in the body to be used. Examples are starches and glycogen. (p. 107)

population health A way of thinking about the social and economic forces that shape health. It builds upon public health and health promotion, but goes beyond our more traditional understanding of the causes of health and illness. (p. 6)

portal of entry The place where an infectious agent enters a reservoir. It can include excretions, secretions, wounds, respiratory and gastrointestinal tracts, and mucous membranes such as eyes, nose, and mouth. (p. 227)

portal of exit The place where an infectious agent leaves a reservoir. It can include excretions, secretions, wounds, respiratory and gastrointestinal tracts, and mucous membranes such as eyes, nose, and mouth. (p. 227)

positive visualization Creating a mental picture of a goal or a behaviour change and visualizing yourself making that change. (p. 19)

post-traumatic stress disorder (PTSD) The repeated reliving of a trauma through nightmares or recollection. (pp. 44, 62)

potential Expressing possibility. (p. 455)

power The ability to produce maximum force in the shortest time, through speed and force. (p. 81)

preconception care Healthcare to prepare for pregnancy. (p. 212)

precontemplation A stage in which you are not even aware that you have a problem and in which you have no intention to change. Others around you might be aware you have a problem. (p. 20)

prediabetes A condition where blood glucose (blood sugar) levels are higher than normal but not high enough to be called diabetes. (p. 280)

predisposing factors Factors that encourage or inhibit us from changing such as knowledge, attitudes, beliefs, values, self-efficacy, behavioural intentions, and existing skills. (p. 16)

premature ejaculation An orgasm disorder in males where ejaculation occurs very quickly after the penis is inserted into the vagina. (p. 180)

premature labour Labour that occurs after the 20th week but before the 37th week of pregnancy. (p. 214)

premenstrual dysphoric disorder (PMDD) A disorder, not related to PMS, that occurs in an estimated 3–5 percent of all menstruating women and is characterized by regular symptoms of psychological depression during the last week of a woman's menstrual cycle. (pp. 48, 181)

premenstrual syndrome (PMS) A disorder that causes bodily discomfort and emotional distress for up to two weeks, from ovulation until the onset of menstruation. (pp. 48, 181)

preorgasmic A condition where women have a difficult time achieving an orgasm. Causes can include fatigue, stress, depression, alcohol, lifestyle choices, and physical issues. (p. 180)

preparation Intent to change a problem behaviour within the next month. (p. 20)

prevention Information and support offered to help healthy people identify their health risks, reduce stressors, prevent potential medical problems, and enhance their well-being. (p. 22)

prion (proteinaceous infectious particle) Infectious self-reproducing protein structure. (p. 225)

progesterone The female sex hormone that stimulates the uterus, preparing it for the arrival of a fertilized egg. (p. 181)

progestin-only pill *See* minipill. (p. 195)

progressive overloading Gradually increasing physical challenges once the body adapts to the stress placed upon it to produce maximum benefits. (p. 86)

progressive relaxation A method of reducing muscle tension by contracting, then relaxing certain areas of the body. (p. 68)

pro-life A term that refers to the opposition to abortion and support for fetal rights. (p. 209)

proof The alcoholic strength of a distilled spirit, expressed as twice the percentage of alcohol present. (p. 320)

prostate gland A structure surrounding the male urethra that produces a secretion that helps liquefy the semen from the testes. (p. 184)

protection Measures that an individual can take when participating in risky behaviour to prevent injury or unwanted risks. (p. 22)

protein A substance that is basically a compound of amino acids; one of the essential nutrients. (p. 107)

protozoa Microscopic animals made up of one cell or a group of similar cells; their enzymes and toxins can harm or destroy healthy cells. (p. 223)

psychiatric drug Medication that regulates a person's mental, emotional, and physical functions to facilitate normal functioning. (p. 51)

psychiatrist Licensed medical doctor with additional training in psychotherapy, psychopharmacology, and treatment of mental disorders. (p. 50)

psychoactive Mood-altering effect of chemicals. (p. 293)

psychoanalyst Can be either a psychiatrist or psychologist who has taken special training in psychoanalysis. They assist clients in overcoming past traumas. (p. 51)

psychodynamic psychotherapy Interpreting behaviours in terms of early experiences and unconscious influences. (p. 51)

psychological age An individual perception of how "old" a person feels, sometimes based on an individual's behaviour. (p. 403)

psychological dependence The emotional or mental attachment to the use of a drug. (p. 293)

psychologist Mental-health professional who has completed a doctoral or graduate program in psychology and is trained in a variety of psychotherapeutic techniques, but who is not medically trained and does not prescribe medications. (p. 51)

psychoneuroimmunology (PNI) A special science that focuses on the relationship between our brain's response to stress and our immune system. (pp. 51, 59)

psychoprophylaxis *See* Lamaze method. (p. 214)

psychosocial health A complex interaction of processes or factors that are both psychological and social in nature and encompass our emotional, mental, social, and spiritual states. (p. 32)

psychotherapy Treatment designed to produce a response by psychological rather than physical means, such as suggestion, persuasion, reassurance, and support. (p. 51)

psychotropic Mind-affecting drugs. (p. 292)

puberty The period during which adolescents reach sexual maturity and become capable of reproduction. (p. 173)

pulmonary artery The artery that transports deoxygenated blood from the right ventricle to the lungs. (p. 256)

pulmonary valve A valve, located in the heart, that separates the right ventricle from the pulmonary artery; it opens to allow deoxygenated blood to flow through the pulmonary artery toward the lungs and closes as the ventricles relax to prevent backflow of blood into the heart. (p. 257)

pulmonary vein The vein that carries oxygenated blood from the lungs to the left atrium. (p. 256)

purpose Something set up as an object or end to be attained. (p. 455)

pyelonephritis Inflammation of the kidney. (p. 237)

quackery Medical fakery; unproven practices claiming to cure diseases or solve health problems. (p. 362)

rape Sexual penetration of a female or a male by means of intimidation, force, or fraud. (p. 393)

rating of perceived exertion (RPE) A self-assessment scale, developed by Dr. Gunnar Borg, that rates symptoms of exertion, such as breathlessness and fatigue. (p. 89)

rational-emotive therapy (RET) Form of therapy developed by Ellis that focuses on changing irrational beliefs and faulty interpretations, which result in negative emotions and severe anxiety. (p. 20)

recover Refurbishing old items such as computers; salvaging parts. (p. 433)

recovery principle The time it takes the body to recover from a weight-training session. For maximal gains in training, allow 48 hours but no more than 96 hours between training sessions. (p. 86)

recycle The reprocessing of used manufactured materials to reduce consumption of raw materials. (p. 433)

reduce Buying products packaged in recycled materials or purchasing products that have less packaging. (p. 432)

reflexology A treatment based on the theory that massaging certain points on the foot or hand relieves stress or pain in corresponding parts of the body. (p. 367)

reinforcement Reward or punishment for a behaviour that will increase or decrease one's likelihood of repeating the behaviour. (p. 20)

reinforcing factors Factors that reinforce behaviour change. They include praise from family and friends, rewards from others, or encouragement and recognition for meeting goals. They also include healthy community policies such as smoke-free facilities and on-site workplace health and wellness programs. (p. 17)

religion A specific system of belief about deity, often involving rituals, a code of ethics, and a philosophy of life, usually representing a special doctrine or group of people. (p. 450)

repetition (rep) The single performance of an exercise such as lifting 20 kilograms one time. (p. 94)

reservoir A place where any infectious agent can live, grow, and multiply. A reservoir can be an animal or insect, a person, food, or water. (p. 224)

resilient Tending to recover from or adjust easily to misfortune or change. (p. 37).

resting heart rate (RHR) The number of heartbeats per minute during inactivity. (p. 87)

resting metabolic rate (RMR) The largest component of our daily energy budget (approximately 90 percent). It includes our basal metabolic rate and any extra energy we expend through the day in sedentary activities such as sitting, standing, and food digestion. (p. 142)

retarded ejaculation The inability to ejaculate once a man has an erect penis. (p. 180)

reuse Repairing items instead of purchasing new ones; finding new uses for old items. (p. 433)

reversibility principle The physical benefits of exercise are lost through disuse or inactivity. (p. 86)

rhythm method A birth-control method in which sexual intercourse is avoided during those days of the menstrual cycle in which fertilization is most likely to occur. (p. 205)

right atrium A chamber of the heart that receives deoxygenated blood from the superior vena cava and inferior vena cava. (p. 256)

right ventricle A chamber of the heart that collects deoxygenated blood received from the right atrium, which is then transported through the pulmonary artery toward the lung. (p. 257)

rubella An infectious disease that may cause birth defects if contracted by a pregnant woman; also called German measles. (p. 212)

sarcopenia The degenerative loss of skeletal muscle mass and strength. (p. 404)

satiety A feeling of fullness after eating. (p. 138)

saturated fat A chemical term indicating that a fat molecule contains as many hydrogen atoms as its carbon skeleton can hold. These fats are normally solid at room temperature. (p. 109)

schizophrenia A general term for a group of mental disorders with characteristic psychotic symptoms, such as delusions, hallucinations, and disordered thought patterns during the active phase of the illness, and for a duration of at least six months. (p. 48)

scrotum The external sac or pouch that holds the testes. (p. 183)

seasonal affective disorder (SAD) Extended and severe bouts of malaise, low energy, problems with sleep and appetite; people with this disorder have difficulty functioning at home and at work during the fall and winter seasons. (p. 48)

secondary sex characteristics Features that distinguish the two sexes of a species, but that do not have a direct reproductive function. Female characteristics include the development of breasts, menarche, widening of the hips, and growth of pubic and underarm hair. Male characteristics include voice changes, the growth of facial and body hair, and the continued growth of the penis and testes. (p. 173)

second-hand cigarette smoke The most hazardous form of indoor air pollution, ranked behind cigarette smoking and alcohol as the third-leading preventable cause of death. (p. 344)

sedative hypnotic A drug that depresses the central nervous system, reduces activity, and induces relaxation and sleep; includes the benzodiazepines and the barbiturates. (p. 311)

selective serotonin reuptake inhibitor (SSRI) A class of compounds used as antidepressants in the treatment of depression, anxiety disorders, and some personality disorders. (p. 47)

self-actualization A state of wellness and fulfillment that can be achieved once certain human needs are satisfied; living and realizing one's full potential. (p. 35)

self-care The decisions and actions individuals take in the interest of their own health. (p. 5)

self-efficacy Belief in one's ability to accomplish a goal or change a behaviour. (p. 39)

self-esteem Confidence and satisfaction in oneself. (p. 36)

self-instructional methods The practice of positive self-talk to help an individual cope better with stressful situations. (p. 20)

self-talk Repetition of positive messages about one's self-worth to learn more optimistic patterns of thought, feeling, and behaviour. (p. 20)

semen The viscous whitish fluid that is the complete male ejaculate; a combination of sperm and secretions from the prostate gland, seminal vesicles, and other glands. (p. 184)

seminal vesicle Gland in the male reproductive system that produces the major portion of the fluid of semen. (p. 184)

serial monogamy A committed monogamous relationship entered into until the relationship ends and another monogamous relationship begins. (p. 170)

set (a) The number of repetitions of the same movement, such as a set of 20 push-ups. (p. 94) (b) The internal environment or mind-set, such as a person's expectations or preconceptions about using a drug. (p. 289)

setting An external environment that a drug user is in. Can include the number and type of people in the setting, the level of noise and lighting, and the type of room an individual is in. (p. 289)

severe acute respiratory syndrome (SARS) A respiratory illness caused by a previously unknown type of coronavirus. Normally, coronaviruses cause mild to moderate upper respiratory symptoms, such as the common cold. Scientists are still searching for answers about this illness. (p. 234)

sexual coercion Sexual activity forced upon a person by the exertion of psychological pressure by another person. (p. 393)

sexual dysfunction A broad term for a number of physical, psychological, or emotional problems that can interfere with healthy sexual functioning. (p. 179)

sexual fantasies Sexually arousing thoughts or dreams in which individuals fantasize about sexual experiences; also known as a form of autoerotic sexual behaviour. (p. 177)

sexual identity Sexual identity based on biology begins at the moment of conception. Female ova (eggs) carry two X chromosomes. The male sperm carry one X and one Y chromosome. If a sperm cell containing an X chromosome fertilizes an egg, the resulting one-celled organism becomes known as a zygote and will be XX, or female. If the sperm cell contains a Y chromosome, then the resulting zygote will be XY, or male. Sexual identity can also be defined from a personal self-identification perspective, and be based on how someone determines whom they are sexually attracted to. (p. 173)

sexual intercourse There are four basic types: 1) manual intercourse, when the sex organs of one partner are in contact with the hand or hands of the other partner; 2) oral intercourse, when the sex organs of one partner are in contact with the mouth of another partner; 3) genital intercourse, when the sex organs of one partner are in contact with the sex organs of the other partner; and 4) anal intercourse, when the sexual organs are in contact with the anus of the other partner. (p. 175)

sexual orientation A socially constructed pattern of emotional, romantic, or sexual fantasies, desires, behaviours, and attraction to others. Sexual orientation can include an attraction to women, men, multiple genders, neither gender, or another gender. (p. 174)

sexually transmitted infection (STI) Any of a number of infections that are acquired through sexual contact. (p. 237)

shaping Building desired behaviour in small steps and rewarding positive behaviour changes over time. (p. 19)

Shinto An ancient Japanese religion, closely connected to nature. This religion recognizes the existence of Kami, or nature deities. (p. 461)

sidestream smoke The smoke emitted by a burning cigarette and breathed by everyone in a closed room, including the smoker; contains more tar and nicotine than mainstream smoke. (p. 344)

Sikhism A monotheistic religion of India; the goal of Sikhs is to build a close, loving relationship to God. Sikhs believe in a single God, with many names. (p. 462)

simple carbohydrate Sugar; like all carbohydrates, it provides the body with glucose; consists of one simple sugar unit. (p. 107)

sinoatrial node (SA node) An impulse-generating tissue that causes the cardiac muscle tissue of the atrium to contract. (p. 256)

smog A greyish or brownish haze caused by the presence of smoke and/or chemical pollutants in the air. (p. 435)

social age Determined by how well individuals cope with their social roles. (p. 403)

social bonds The degree to which people are integrated into and attached to their families, communities, and society. (p. 33)

social determinant of health (SDOH) An aspect that is very important to health and wellness status, such as income inequality, job security, working conditions, housing and food security, education and care in early life, and social exclusion of individuals and groups. (p. 12)

social health The ability to interact with the people around us as well as our capability to function as a contributing member of society while helping others to do the same. (p. 33)

social isolation A feeling of unconnectedness with others caused and reinforced by infrequency of social contacts. (p. 41)

social phobia A severe form of social anxiety marked by extreme fears and avoidance of social situations. (p. 41)

social responsibility A principle or ethical theory that suggests governments, corporations, organizations, and individuals have a responsibility to contribute to the welfare of society. (p. 39)

social support The care and security that family, friends, colleagues, and professionals provide to us. (p. 33)

sodium A mineral that helps to maintain proper fluid balance, regulate blood pressure, transmit muscle impulses, and relax muscles. (p. 120)

specificity principle Each part of the body adapts to a particular type and amount of stress placed upon it. (p. 86) speed The ability to propel the body or part of a body rapidly from one point to another. (p. 81)

sperm The male reproductive cell produced by the testes and transported outside the body through ejaculation. (p. 184)

spermatogenesis The process by which sperm cells are produced. (p. 192)

spinal block An injection of anesthetic directly into the spinal cord to numb the lower body during labour and childbirth. (p. 214)

spiritual death The moment when the soul, as defined by many religions, leaves the body. (p. 414)

spiritual health The ability to identify one's basic purpose in life and to achieve one's full potential; the sense of connectedness to a greater power. (p. 33)

spiritual intelligence The capacity to sense, understand, and tap into the highest parts of ourselves and the world around us; also described at times as intuition. (p. 34, 450)

spirituality Having a sense of self and a set of values that link to meaning and purpose in life and a connection to others. (p. 450)

sport A form of leisure-time physical activity that is planned, structured, and competitive. (p. 81)

stages or staging of cancer The extent or the seriousness of the cancer. Each type of cancer has specific factors that determine stages. Can be labelled TNM (tumour, node, metastasis) and stage 0–4. (p. 271)

static stretching A safe and effective gradual stretch held for a short time (10–60 seconds). (p. 96)

sterilization A surgical procedure to end a person's reproductive capability. (p. 205)

stigma A severe social disapproval; also a situation where people are discriminated against, subjected to violence and abuse, and not allowed to participate fully in society. (p. 42)

stimulant An agent, such as a drug, that temporarily relieves drowsiness, helps in the performance of repetitive tasks, and improves capacity for work. (p. 292)

stress A physical, chemical, or emotional factor that causes bodily or mental tension and may be a factor in disease causation; an internal state of arousal; or the physical state of the body in response to various demands. (p. 58)

stressor Specific or non-specific agents or situations that cause the stress response in a body. (p. 58)

stretch receptors Sensory receptors found within the belly of a muscle that detect changes in the length of the muscle. (p. 96)

stroke A cerebrovascular event in which the blood supply to a portion of the brain is blocked. (p. 262)

subcutaneous injection A method of administering a drug by an injection into the fatty layer beneath the skin. The drug is absorbed more slowly because there is very little blood flow in the fatty tissue. (p. 288)

suction curettage A procedure in which the contents of the uterus are removed by means of suction and scraping. (p. 208)

suicide Taking one's own life; a leading cause of death, usually the result of a tragic consequence of emotional and psychological problems. (p. 49)

superior vena cava A major vein that brings deoxygenated blood from the head and upper body to the heart. (p. 256)

surgical abortion Surgical removal of the contents of the uterus usually performed within 12–14 weeks from the last normal menstrual period in the first trimester of the pregnancy. (p. 208)

susceptible host Someone whose health condition and level of exposure to an infectious agent or pathogen allows transmission of that agent or pathogen. Factors to consider with regard to being a susceptible host include age and current or underlying medical conditions. (p. 226)

sympathetic nervous system (SNS) One branch of the autonomic nervous system that initiates the release of stress hormones, which increase our heart rate and respiratory rate. (p. 59)

syphilis A sexually transmitted infection caused by the bacterium *Treponema pallidum;* characterized by early sores, a latent period, and a final period of life-threatening symptoms including brain damage and heart failure. (p. 242)

systemic disease A pathologic condition that spreads throughout the body. (p. 229)

systole The contraction phase of the cardiac cycle. (p. 257)

systolic blood pressure The maximum arterial pressure when the heart contracts. (p. 261)

Taoism Sometimes translated as "path," Taoism is a force that flows through all life. If you are a believer, your goal is to become one with the Tao. (p. 462)

tar A thick, sticky, dark fluid produced by the burning of tobacco; made up of several hundred different chemicals, many of them poisonous, some of them carcinogenic. (p. 336)

target heart rate The heart rate at which one derives maximum cardiovascular benefit from aerobic exercise; 55–90 percent of the maximum heart rate. (p. 89)

technostress A modern disease that consists of a feeling of anxiety or mental pressure resulting from a struggle to embrace computer technology or stress from overexposure to computer technology. (p. 66)

tension The primary load a muscle experiences when you exercise; the resistance applied against the muscle or group of muscles you are trying to strengthen. Examples include using your own body weight as the tension or resistance or using weight-training equipment. (p. 86)

teratogen Any agent that causes spontaneous abortion or defects or malformations in a fetus. (p. 434)

termination The last stage of the Stages of Change model where after two to five years, a person's behaviour becomes so deeply engrained they cannot imagine abandoning the change they have made. (p. 20)

testis (plural, testes, testicles) The paired male sex organ that produces sperm and testosterone. (p. 183)

testosterone The male sex hormone that stimulates male secondary sex characteristics. (p. 183)

total fibre The sum of both dietary fibre and functional fibre equals the total fibre in food. (p. 108)

toxicity The dosage level at which a drug becomes poisonous to the body, causing either temporary or permanent damage. (p. 289)

toxic shock syndrome (TSS) A rare, potentially deadly bacterial infection that primarily strikes menstruating women under the age of 30 who use tampons. (p. 183)

transcendence Extending notably beyond ordinary limits. (p. 455)

trans fatty acid Fat formed when liquid vegetable oils are processed to make table spreads or cooking fats, and also found in dairy and beef products; considered to be an especially dangerous dietary fat. (p. 110)

transgender/trans person/trans folk An umbrella term for people whose gender identity or gender expression differs from the sex they were assigned at birth. The term is not indicative of sexual orientation, hormonal makeup, or physical anatomy. (p. 174)

transient ischemic attack (TIA) A mini-stroke caused by a temporary interruption of blood flow to the brain. (p. 263)

trichomoniasis An infection of the protozoan *Trichomonas vaginalis;* females experience vaginal burning, itching, and discharge, but male carriers may be asymptomatic. (p. 237)

tricuspid valve A heart valve that separates the right atrium from the right ventricle, which opens and allows deoxygenated blood collected in the right atrium to flow into the right ventricle. (p. 257)

triglyceride Fat that flows through the blood after meals and is linked to increased risk of coronary artery disease. (p. 264)

tubal ligation The suturing or tying shut of the fallopian tubes to prevent pregnancy. (p. 206)

tubal occlusion The blocking of the fallopian tubes to prevent pregnancy. (p. 206)

12-step program Self-help group program based on the principles of Alcoholics Anonymous. (p. 314)

two-spirited In First Nations culture, a term used to describe gay and lesbian individuals.

The designation of this term suggests that these individuals are special and are to be respected and honoured. (p. 175)

type 1 diabetes A disease in which the pancreas does not produce insulin. Glucose builds up in the blood instead of being used for energy. (p. 279)

type 2 diabetes A disease in which the pancreas does not produce sufficient insulin to meet the body's needs or does not properly use the insulin it does make. It is a progressive, lifelong condition. (p. 280)

Unitarianism An open-minded and alternative religion where followers are encouraged to search for meaning in life in a responsible way. All people of different faiths are welcomed. There is a belief in God, but not in the concept of the Trinity. (p. 462)

unsaturated fat A fat molecule that contains fewer hydrogen atoms than its carbon skeleton can hold. These fats are normally liquid at room temperature. (p. 109)

urethra The canal through which urine from the bladder leaves the body; in the male, it also serves as the channel for seminal fluid. (p. 184)

urethral opening The outer opening of the thin tube that carries urine from the bladder. (p. 181)

urethritis Infection of the urethra. (p. 237)

uterus The female organ that houses the developing fetus until birth. (p. 181)

vagina The canal leading from the exterior opening in the female genital area to the uterus. (p. 181)

vaginal spermicide A substance that kills or neutralizes sperm, inserted into the vagina as a foam, cream, jelly, or suppository. (p. 202)

value The criteria by which one makes choices about one's thoughts, actions, goals, and ideals. (p. 36)

variant sexual behaviour Includes non-conforming, deviant, or divergent sexual behaviour, sometimes defined as unconventional sexual behaviour; can be deemed illegal in various provinces and territories. (p. 177)

vas deferens Two tubes that carry sperm from the epididymis into the urethra. (p. 184)

vasectomy A surgical sterilization procedure in which each vas deferens is cut and tied shut to stop the passage of sperm to the urethra for ejaculation. (p. 206)

vector-borne transmission The transference of a disease from an insect or an animal to a human. (p. 226)

vegan Person who eats only plant foods. (p. 126)

vein Any blood vessel that carries blood from the capillaries toward the heart. Veins often have valves at various intervals to prevent reflux of blood. An exception is the specialized pulmonary vein that carries oxygenated blood from the lungs to the left atrium. (p. 256)

video display terminal (VDT) A screen or monitor that emits electromagnetic fields from all sides; these fields may lead to increased reproductive problems, miscarriages, low birth weights, and cataracts. (p. 441)

virus Submicroscopic infectious agent; the most primitive form of life. (p. 222)

visualization An approach to stress control, self-healing, or motivating life changes by means of guided imagery. (p. 69)

vital sign Measurement of physiological functioning: temperature, blood pressure, pulse rate, and respiration rate. (p. 360)

vitamin Organic substance that is needed in very small amounts by the body and that carries out a variety of functions in metabolism and nutrition. (p. 116)

VO2 max The maximum amount of oxygen that an individual is able to use during intense or "maximal" exercise. It is measured as millilitres of oxygen used in one minute per kilogram of body weight. (p. 81)

waist circumference (WC) Used along with body mass index as a practical indicator of risk that is associated with excess abdominal fat. (p. 140)

waist-to-hip ratio (WHR) The proportion of waist circumference to hip circumference; an indicator of cardiovascular disease risk. (p. 141)

weight discrimination Policies that require individuals who are overweight to develop and pay for weight-loss plans if they are unable to meet specific weight-loss goals. (p. 148)

wellness A deliberate lifestyle choice characterized by personal responsibility and optimal enhancement of physical, mental, and spiritual health. (p. 8)

withdrawal Development of symptoms that cause significant psychological and physical distress when an individual reduces or stops drug use. (p. 294)

zygote A fertilized egg. (p. 192)

References

Chapter 1

1. Leadbetter, R. (2000, January 31). Aesculapius. In *Encyclopedia Mythica.* www.pantheon.org/articles/a/asclepius.html
2. Panacea. In *Merriam Webster Dictionary.* (2015). Available at www.merriam-webster.com/dictionary/panacea
3. Hygiene. In *Merriam Webster Dictionary.* (2015). www.merriam-webster.com/dictionary/hygiene?show=0&t =1301967525
4. Hill, D. M. (2009). Traditional medicine and restoration of wellness strategies. *Journal of Aboriginal Health,* 5(1), 26–42.
5. Kulchyski, P., McCaskill, D., & Newhouse, D. (Eds.). (1999). Introduction. *In the words of elders: Aboriginal cultures in transition* (xi–xxv). Toronto: University of Toronto Press.
6. Ibid., p. xvi.
7. First Nations Health Authority. (2016). *First Nations perspectives on health and wellness.* Wellness. Tips, Guides and Resources. Wellness and the First Nations Health Authority. www.fnha.ca/wellness/wellness-and-the-first-nations-health-authority/first-nations-perspective-on-wellness
8. World Health Organization Interim Commission. (1947). *Chronicle of the world health organization,* 1(1–2), 2. apps.who.int/iris/bitstream/10665/85582/1/Official_record3_eng.pdf
9. Preamble to the Constitution of the World Health Organization as adopted by the International Health Conference, New York, June 19–22, 1946; signed on July 22, 1946 by the representatives of 61 States (Official Records of the World Health Organization, no. 2, p. 100) and entered into force on April 7, 1948. www.who.int/about/definition/en/print.html
10. Lalonde, M. (1974). *A new perspective on the health of Canadians.* Ottawa: Government of Canada. www.phac-aspc.gc.ca/ph-sp/pdf/perspect-eng.pdf
11. The Ottawa Charter for Health Promotion. (1986). *World Health Organization, Health and Welfare Canada, and Canadian Public Health Association.* www.phac-aspc.gc.ca/ph-sp/docs/charter-chartre/pdf/charter.pdf
12. Epp, J. (1986). *Achieving health for all: A framework for health promotion.* Ottawa: Minister of Supply and Services Canada. www.hc-sc.gc.ca/hcs-sss/pubs/system-regime/1986-frame-plan-promotion/index-eng.php
13. Rosenstock, I. M. (1982). The health belief model and nutrition education. *Canadian Journal of Dietetic Practice and Research,* 43(3), 184–192.
14. Green, L. W., & Kreuter, M. S. (1999). *Health promotion and planning: An educational and ecological approach* (3rd ed.). Mountain View, CA: Mayfield Publishing.
15. The quality of life model (n.d.). Quality of Life Research Unit, University of Toronto. sites.utoronto.ca/qol/qol_model.htm
16. Canadian Institute for Health Information. (CIHI). (2016). *Population health and health care.* Population Health. www.cihi.ca/en/factors-influencing-health/population-health/population-health-and-health-care
17. Public Health Agency of Canada. (2016, February 05). Home. publichealth.gc.ca
18. Canadian Institutes of Health Research. (CIHR). (2016, February 05). Home. www.cihr-irsc.gc.ca/e/193.html
19. Health Canada. (2016, February 04). First Nations and Inuit Health Branch. www.hc-sc.gc.ca/fniah-spnia/index-eng.php
20. ParticipACTION Canada. (2013). Home. www.participaction.com/splash/
21. Physical and Health Education Canada (PHE Canada). (2016). www.phecanada.ca/
22. McGill University. (2016). *Epidemiology, biostatistics, and occupational health.* www.mcgill.ca/epi-biostat-occh/academic-programs/grad/epidemiology
23. Dunn, H. (1961). *High-level wellness. A collection of twenty-nine short talks on different aspects of high-level wellness for man and society.* Arlington, VA: R. W. Beatty.
24. Travis, J. W., & Ryan, R. S. (2004). *The wellness workbook* (3rd ed.) (xiv–xv). Berkeley, CA: Celestial Arts.
25. National Wellness Institute. (n.d.). *Sample Testwell assessments.* Resources. Testwell. http://www.nationalwellness.org/
26. National Wellness Institute. (n.d.). *The six dimensions of wellness.* www.nationalwellness.org/?page=Six_Dimensions
27. Hale, C. J., Hannum, J. W., & Espelage, D. L. (2005). Social support and physical health: The importance of belonging. *Journal of American College Health,* 53(6), 276–284.
28. Abbott, R. A., & Baun, W. B. (2015). The multi-dimensions of wellness: The vital role of terms and meanings. *American Journal of Health Promotion,* 29(5), TAHP8–10.
29. Kazanjian, V. (2013). Spiritual practices on college and university campuses: Understanding the concepts—broadening the context. *Journal of College and Character,* 14(2), 97–104. DOI: 10.1515/jcc-2013-0014
30. Reyman, L. S., Fialkowski, G. M., & Stewart-Sicking, J. A. (2015). Exploratory study of spirituality and psychosocial growth in college students. *Journal of College Counseling.* 18(2), 103–115.
31. Nelms, L., Hutchins, E., Hutchins, D., & Pursley, R. (2007). Spirituality and the health of college students. *Journal of Religion and Health,* 46(2), 249–265.
32. Clark, W. (2000, Winter). *Patterns of religious attendance.* Canadian Social Trends. Statistics Canada. Catalogue no. 11-008.
33. Jim, H. S., et al. (2015). Religion, spirituality, and physical health in cancer patients: A meta-analysis. *Cancer,* 121(21), 3760–3768. DOI: 10.1002/cncr.29353
34. Nichols, L. M., & Hunt, B. (2011). The significance of spirituality for individuals with chronic illness: Implications for mental health counseling practice. *Journal of Mental Health Counseling,* 33(1), 51–67.
35. Melton, B., Hansen, A., & Gross, J. (2010). Trends in physical activity interest in the college and university setting. *College Student Journal,* 44(3), 785–790.
36. National Wellness Institute. (n.d.). The six dimensions of wellness. www.nationalwellness.org/?page=Six_Dimensions
37. Ibid.
38. Conley, C. S., Travers, L. V., & Bryant, F. B. (2013). Promoting psychosocial adjustment and stress management in first-year college students: The benefits of engagement in a psychosocial wellness seminar. *Journal of American College Health,* 61(2), 75–86.
39. University of Guelph. (2016). Seven dimensions of health. Student Services. https://wellness.uoguelph.ca/education/about/dimensions-wellness

40. Ministry of Industry. (2015, September). *Annual demographic estimates: Canada, provinces and territories.* Statistics Canada. Demography Division. (p. 18). Catalogue no. 91-215-X. www.statcan.gc.ca/pub/91-215-x/91-215-x2015000-eng.pdf

41. Ministry of Industry. (2015, September). Annual demographic estimates: Canada, provinces and territories. Statistics Canada. Demography Division. (p. 16). Catalogue no. 91-215-X. www.statcan.gc.ca/pub/91-215-x/91-215-x2015000-eng.pdf

42. Statistics Canada. (2012, May 31). Deaths 2009. *The Daily.* www.statcan.gc.ca/daily-quotidien/120531/t120531e002-eng.htm

43. World Health Organization. (WHO). (2016). *Statistics.* Countries. Canada. www.who.int/countries/can/en/

44. Raphael, D. (2012). Educating the Canadian public about the social determinants of health: The time for local public health action is now! *Global Health Promotion,* 19(3), 54–59.

45. World Health Organization Commission on Social Determinants of Health (2008). Closing the gap in a generation—health equity through action on the social determinants of health. http://whqlibdoc.who.int/publications/2008/9789241563703_eng.pdf

46. Public Health Agency of Canada. (2011, October 21). *What determines health?* Population Health. Health Promotion. http://www.phac-aspc.gc.ca/ph-sp/determinants/index-eng.php

47. Mikkonen, J., & Raphael, D. (2010). *Social determinants of health: The Canadian facts.* Toronto: York University School of Health Policy and Management. www.thecanadianfacts.org/

48. Statistics Canada. (2015, June 03). Study: Changes in wealth across the income distribution, 1999–2012. *The Daily.* www.statcan.gc.ca/daily-quotidien/150603/dq150603b-eng.htm

49. Raphael, D. (2011). Poverty in childhood and adverse health outcomes in adulthood. *Maturitas,* 69(1), 22–26.

50. Asada, Y., Whipp, A., Kindig, D., Billard, B., & Rudolph, B. (2014). Inequalities in multiple health outcomes by education, sex, and race in 93 US counties: Why we should measure the all. *International Journal for Equity in Health,* 13(1), 2–8. DOI: 10.1186/1475-9276-13-47

51. Korpal, D., & Wong A. (2015). Education and the health of the First Nations people of Canada. *Alter-Native: An International Journal of Indigenous People,* 11(2), 132-146.

52. Trading Economics. (2016). *Canada unemployment rate 1966–2016.* Indicators. www.tradingeconomics.com/canada/unemployment-rate

53. Jackson, A., & Robinson, D. (2002). *Falling behind: The state of working Canada, 2000.* Canadian Centre for Policy Alternatives.

54. Mikkonen, J., & Raphael, D. (2010). *Social determinants of health: The Canadian facts.* Toronto: York University School of Health Policy and Management. www.thecanadianfacts.org/

55. Ibid.

56. Statistics Canada. (2015, November 27). *Food insecurity in Canada.* Publications. Health at a Glance. www.statcan.gc.ca/pub/82-624-x/2015001/article/14138-eng.htm

57. Bryant, T. (2009). Housing and health: More than bricks and mortar. In D. Raphael (Ed.), *Social determinants of health: Canadian Perspectives* (pp. 235–248; 2nd ed.). Toronto: Canadian Scholars' Press.

58. Canada Without Poverty. (2016). *Poverty. Just the Facts.* www.cwp-csp.ca/poverty/just-the-facts/

59. Mikkonen, J., & Raphael, D. (2010). *Social determinants of health: The Canadian facts.* Toronto: York University School of Health Policy and Management.www.thecanadianfacts.org/

60. Public Health Agency of Canada. (2011, October 21). *What determines health?* Population Health. Health Promotion. www.phac-aspc.gc.ca/ph-sp/determinants/index-eng.php

61. Service Canada. Employment Insurance. (2011, February 07). www.servicecanada.gc.ca/eng/sc/ei/index.shtml

62. Statistics Canada. (2016, January 21). Employment insurance, November 2015. *The Daily.* www.statcan.gc.ca/daily-quotidien/160121/dq160121a-eng.htm

63. Mikkonen, J., & Raphael, D. (2010). *Social determinants of health: The Canadian facts.* Toronto: York University School of Health Policy and Management. www.thecanadianfacts.org/

64. Korpal, D., & Wong A. (2015). Education and the health of the First Nations people of Canada. *Alter-Native: An International Journal of Indigenous People,* 11(2), 132–146.

65. Public Health Agency of Canada. (2013, January 25). *What makes Canadians healthy or unhealthy?* Health Promotion. www.phac-aspc.gc.ca/ph-sp/determinants/determinants-eng.php

66. Lasser, K., Himmelstein, D. U., & Woolhandler, S. (2006). Access to care, health status, and health disparities in the United States and Canada: Results of a cross-national population-based survey. *American Journal of Public Health,* 96(7), 1200–1307.

67. Jackson, A. (2009). *Work and labour in Canada: Critical issues.* (2nd ed.). Toronto: Canada Scholars' Press.

68. *A healthy, productive Canada: A determinant of health approach.* (2009, June). The standing senate committee on social affairs, science and technology final report of the subcommittee on population health. The Honourable Wilbert Joseph Keon, chair; The Honourable Lucie Pépin, deputy chair. www.parl.gc.ca/40/2/parlbus/commbus/senate/com-e/popu-e/rep-e/rephealth1jun09-e.pdf

69. Universities Canada. (2015, August 06). *Back to school 2015. Quick facts.*

70. Universities Canada. (2014, December 09). *Internationalization at Canadian universities. Quick Facts.* http://www.univcan.ca/universities/facts-and-stats/internationalization-at-canadian-universities-quick-facts/.

71. Davis, J., McCrae, B. P., Frank, J., Dochnahl, A., Pickering, T., Harrison, B., Zakrzewski, M., & Wilson, K. (2000). Identifying male college students' perceived health needs, barriers to seeking help, and recommendations to help men adopt healthier lifestyles. *Journal of American College Health,* 48(6), 259–267.

72. Keeling, R. (2001, September). Is college dangerous? *Journal of American College Health,* 50(2), 53–56.

73. Adlaf, E. M., Gliksman, L., Demers, A., & Newton-Taylor, B. (2001, September). The prevalence of elevated psychological distress among Canadian undergraduates: Findings from the 1998 Canadian Campus Survey. *Journal of American College Health,* 50(2), 67–72.

74. Bartlett, T. (2002, February 01). Freshman pay, mentally and physically, as they adjust to life in college. *Chronicle of Higher Education,* 48(21), A35–A38.

75. Porter, C. M. (2016). Revisiting precede-proceed: A leading model for ecological and ethical health promotion. Health Education Journal, 75(6), 753–764.

76. Janz, N. K., & Becker, M. H. (1984). The health belief model: A decade later. *Health Education Quarterly,* 11(1), 1–47.

77. Attitude. In *Merriam-Webster* Dictionary (2015). www.merriam-webster.com/dictionary/attitude

78. Belief. In *Merriam-Webster Dictionary.* (2015). www.merriam-webster.com/dictionary/belief

79. Jordan, D. J. (2007). Direct leadership techniques. In *Leadership in leisure services. Making a difference* (pp. 258–259; 2nd ed.). State College, PA: Venture Publishing, Inc.

80. Prochaska, J., Norcross, J., & DiClimente, C. (1994). *Changing for good: The revolutionary program that explains the six*

stages of change and teaches you how to free yourself from bad habits. New York: William Morrow and Company, Inc.

81. Bandura, A. (1977). Self-efficacy: Toward a unifying theory of behavioral change. *Psychological Review*, 84(2), 191–215.
82. Ellis, A. (1991). The revised ABC's of rational-emotive therapy (RET). *Journal of Rational-Emotive & Cognitive Behavior Therapy*, 9(3), 139–172.
83. Meichenbaum, D., & Cameron, R. (1974). The clinical potential of modifying what clients say to themselves. *Psychotherapy: Theory, Research and Practice*, 11(2), 103–117.
84. Seligman, Martin. Personal interview.
85. Hettler, W. (1984). Wellness: Encouraging a lifetime pursuit of excellence. *Health Values: Achieving High Level Wellness*, 8(4), 13–17.

Chapter 2

1. Morton, S., Mergler, A., & Boman, P. (2014). Managing the transition: The role of optimism and self-efficacy for first-year Australian university students. *Australian Journal of Guidance and Counselling*, 24(1), 90–108.
2. Carr, S., Colthurst, K., Coyle, M., & Elliot, D. (2013). Attachment dimensions as predictors of mental health and psychosocial well-being in the transition to university. *European Journal of Psychological Education*, 28(2), 157–172.
3. Satcher, D. (2000). Executive summary: A report of the surgeon general on mental health. *Public Health Reports*, 115(1), 89–101.
4. Adams, G. R., Berzonsky, M. D., & Keating, L. (2006). Psychosocial resources in first-year university students: The role of identity processes and social relationships. *Journal of Youth and Adolescence*, 35(1), 81–91.
5. Mental Health America (MHA). (n.d.). *10 tools to live your life well. Ways to live your life well.* http://www.mentalhealthamerica.net/live-your-life-well
6. Brown-Fraser, S., Forrester, I., Rowe, R., Richardson, A., & Spence, A. N. (2015). Development of a community organic vegetable garden in Baltimore, Maryland: A student service-learning approach to community engagement. *Journal of Hunger and Environmental Nutrition*, 10(3), 409–436. DOI: 10.1080/19320248.2014.962778
7. Morton, S., Mergler, A., & Boman, P. (2014). Managing the transition: The role of optimism and self-efficacy for first-year Australian university students. *Australian Journal of Guidance and Counselling*, 24(1), 90–108.
8. Hill, P. L., Burrow, A. L., & Bronk, K. C. (2016). An examination of purpose, commitment and positive affect as predictors of grit. *Journal of Happiness Studies*, 17(1), 257–269. DOI 10.1007/s10902-014-9593-5
9. Hales, D. (2016). *An invitation to health: Live it now!* Boston, MA: Cengage Learning (p. 22).
10. Satcher, D. (2000). Executive summary: A report of the surgeon general on mental health. *Public Health Reports*, 115(1), 89–101.
11. Hales, D. (2016). *An invitation to health: Live it now!* Boston, MA: Cengage Learning (p. 22).
12. Lazarus, R. S. (1991). Cognition and motivation in emotion. *American Psychologist*, 46(4), 352–367.
13. Simon Fraser University. (n.d.). *Emotional wellness.* Student Services. Health and Counseling Services. www.sfu.ca/students/health/resources/wellness/emotional.html
14. Hales, D. (2016). *An invitation to health: Live it now!* Boston, MA: Cengage Learning (p. 24).
15. Blank, R. Registered psychologist. Personal interview. www.bardonet.ca/
16. Goleman, D. (1997). *Emotional intelligence.* New York: Bantam Books.
17. Cazan, A., & Năstasă, E. (2015). Emotional intelligence, satisfaction with life and burnout among university students. The 6th International Conference Edu World 2014 "Education Facing Contemporary World Issues," November 7th–9th, 2014. *Procedia Social and Behavioral Sciences*, 180, 1574–1578.
18. Hales, D. (2016). *An invitation to health: Live it now!* Boston, MA: Cengage Learning (p. 76).
19. Cooke, B. D., Rossman, M. M., McCubbon, H. I., & Patterson, J. M. (1988). Examining the definition and assessment of social support: A resource for individuals and families. *National Council on Family Relations*, 37(2), 211–216.
20. Jackson, E. S., Tucker, C. M., & Herman, K. C. (2007). Health value, perceived social support, and health self-efficacy as factors in a health-promoting lifestyle. *Journal of American College Health*, 56(1), 69–74.
21. Brown, S. L., Ness, R. M., Vinokur, A. D., & Smith, D. M. (2003). Providing social support may be more beneficial than receiving it: Results from a prospective study of mortality. *Psychological Science*, 14(4), 320–327.
22. Chriss, J. J. (2007). The functions of the social bond. *The Sociological Quarterly*, 48(4), 689–712.
23. Hirchi, T. (1969). *Causes of delinquency.* Berkeley: University of California Press.
24. Wiatrowski, M., & Anderson, K. L. (1987). The dimensionality of the social bond. *Journal of Quantitative Criminology*, 3(1), 65–81.
25. Hales, D. (2016). *An invitation to health: Live it now!* (9th ed.). Boston, MA: Cengage Learning (p. 27).
26. Holst, W. (2004). "Native spirituality" gets new respect [Book review]. *National Catholic Reporter*, 41(7), 20–21.
27. Bastien, B. (2003). The cultural practice of participatory transpersonal visions: An indigenous perspective. *Revision*, 26(2), 41–48.
28. Hales, D. (2016). *An invitation to health: Live it now!* (9th ed.). Boston, MA: Cengage Learning (p. 23).
29. Miller, H. A. (2002). Traditional medicines and spirituality focus of gathering (Health). *Wind Speaker*, 20(4), 26.
30. Sorrentino, P. V. (2010). What do college students want? A student-centered approach to multifaith involvement. *Journal of Ecumenical Studies*, 45(1), 79–97.
31. Maheshwari, N. (2015). Spiritual intelligence: Occupational commitment. *SCMS Journal of Indian Management*, 12(2), 29–38, (p. 28).
32. Naparstek, B. (1997). *Your sixth sense. Unlocking the power of your potential.* San Francisco: Harper San Francisco, a Division of HarperCollins.
33. Maslow, A. H. (1943). A theory of human motivation. *Psychological Review*, 50(4), 370–396.
34. Hales, D. (2016). *An invitation to health: Live it now!* (9th ed.). Boston, MA: Cengage Learning (p. 24).
35. Koltko-Rivera, M. E. (2006). Rediscovering the later version of Maslow's hierarchy of needs: Self-transcendence and opportunities for theory, research, and unification. *Review of General Psychology*, 10(4), 302–317.
36. Erikson, E. H. (1963). *Childhood and society* (2nd ed.). New York: Norton.
37. Adams, G. R., Berzonsky, M. D., & Keating, L. (2006). Psychosocial resources in first-year university students: The role of identity processes and social relationships. *Journal of Youth and Adolescence*, 35(1), 81–91.

38. Hales, D. (2016). *An invitation to health: Live it now!* (9th ed.). Boston, MA: Cengage Learning (p. 28).

39. Rokeach, M. (1960). *The open and closed mind.* New York: Basic Books.

40. Hales, D. (2016). *An invitation to health: Live it now!* (9th ed.). Boston, MA: Cengage Learning (p. 24).

41. Tayfur, O. (2012). The antecedents and consequences of learned helplessness in work life. *Information Management and Business Review,* 4(7), 417–427.

42. Seligman, M. (1990). *Learned optimism.* New York: Knopf.

43. Hales, D. (2016). *An invitation to health: Live it now!* (9th ed.). Boston, MA: Cengage Learning (p. 26).

44. Hales, D. (2016). *An invitation to health: Live it now!* (9th ed.). Boston, MA: Cengage Learning (p. 70).

45. Eisenbarth, C. A. (2011). Does optimism moderate the negative impact of stress? *Research Quarterly for Exercise and Sport,* 82(1), A63, Supplement.

46. Lench, H. C. (2011). Personality and health outcomes: Making positive expectations a reality. *Journal of Happiness Studies,* 12(3), 493–507.

47. Hertel, J. (2003). College student generational status: Similarities, differences, and factors in college adjustment. *The Psychological Record,* 52(1), 3-18.

48. Robins, R., & Beer, J. (2001). Positive illusions about the self: Short-term benefits and long-term costs. *Journal of Personality & Social Psychology,* 80(2), 340–352.

49. Goldie, P. (2002). Emotions, feelings and intentionality. *Phenomenology and the Cognitive Sciences,* 1(3), 235–254.

50. Hales, D. (2016). *An invitation to health: Live it now!* (9th ed.). Boston, MA: Cengage Learning (p. 26).

51. Persistent bad mood leads to poor health. (2002, June 3). *Health & Medicine Week,* p. 4.

52. Howerton, A., & Van Gundy, K. (2009). Sex differences in coping styles and implications for depressed moods. *International Journal of Stress Management,* 16(4), 333–350.

53. Larsen, Randy, psychologist. Personal interview.

54. Lyubomirsky, S. (2008). *The how of happiness: A scientific approach to getting the life you want.* New York: Penguin Press.

55. Lyubormirsky, S. Personal interview.

56. Cousins, N. (1989). *Head first: The biology of hope and the healing power of the human spirit.* New York: Dutton.

57. Wei, B., Kilpatrick, M., Naquin, M., & Cole, D. (2006). Psychological perceptions to walking, water aerobics and yoga in college students. *American Journal of Health Studies,* 21(3/4), 142–147.

58. Bray, S. R., & Born, H. A. (2004). Transition to university and vigorous physical activity: Implications for health and psychological well-being. *Journal of American College Health,* 52(4), 181–189.

59. Canadian Sleep Society. (2016). *Engaging patients in sleep disorders research. Final report.* Position Papers, Guidelines & Reports. https://css-scs.ca/files/resources/publications/2015_CSS_CSCN_Report_PE_workshop.pdf

60. Law, D. (2007). Exhaustion in university students and the effect of coursework involvement. *Journal of American College Health,* 55(4), 239–245.

61. Galambos, N. L., & Dalton, A. L. (2009). Losing sleep over it: Daily variation in sleep quantity and quality in Canadian students' first semester of university. *Journal of Research on Adolescence,* 19(4), 741–761.

62. Trockel, M. Y., Barnes, M. D., & Egget, D. L. (2000). Health-related variables and academic performance among first-year college students: Implications for sleep and other behaviors. *Journal of American College Health,* 49(3), 125–131.

63. Owens, J., Adolescent Sleep Working Group, & Committee on Adolescence. (2014). Insufficient sleep in adolescents and young adults: An update on causes and consequences. Technical Report. *Pediatrics,* 34(3), e921–e932. DOI:10.1542/peds.2014-1696

64. Bandura, A. (2001). Social cognitive theory: An agentic perspective. *Annual Review Psychology,* 52, 1–26. www.annualreviews.org/doi/pdf/10.1146/annurev.psych.52.1.1

65. Bandura, A. (1994). Self-efficacy: Toward a unifying theory of behavioral change. *Psychological Review,* 84(2), 191–215. citeseerx.ist.psu.edu/viewdoc/download?doi=10.1.1.315.4567&rep=rep1&type=pdf

66. Skaalvik, E. M., & Skaalvik, S. (2014). Teacher self-efficacy and perceived autonomy: Relations with teacher engagement, job satisfaction, and emotional exhaustion. *Psychological Reports,* 114(1), 68–77.

67. Marra, J., & Wilcox, S. (2015). Self-efficacy and social support mediate the relationship between internal health locus of control and health behaviors in college students. *American Journal of Health Education,* 46(3), 122–131.

68. Hales, D. (2016). *An invitation to health: Live it now!* (9th ed.). Boston, MA: Cengage Learning (p. 78).

69. Covey, S. R. (1989). *The seven habits of highly effective people: Restoring the character ethic.* New York: Simon & Schuster.

70. Hales, D. (2016). *An invitation to health: Live it now!* (9th ed.). Boston, MA: Cengage Learning (p. 81).

71. Orlitzky, M., Siegel, D. S., & Waldman, D. A. (2011). Strategic corporate social responsibility and environmental sustainability. *Business & Society,* 50(1), 6–27.

72. Turcotte, M. (2015, November 30). *Volunteering and charitable giving in Canada.* Statistics Canada. Publications. www.statcan.gc.ca/pub/89-652-x/89-652-x2015001-eng.htm

73. Sinha, M. (2015, June 18). *Volunteering in Canada, 2004 to 2013.* Spotlight on Canadians: Results from the General Social Survey. Statistics Canada. www.statcan.gc.ca/pub/89-652-x/89-652-x2015003-eng.htm

74. Jones, S. R., & Hill. K. E. (2003). Understanding patterns of commitment: Student motivation for community service. *Journal of Higher Education,* 74(5), 516–524.

75. Ottenritter, N. W. (2004). Service learning, social justice, and campus health. (Viewpoint). *Journal of American College Health,* 52(4), 189–191.

76. Gallant, K., Smale, B., & Arai, S. (2010). Civic engagement through mandatory community service: Implications of serious leisure. *Journal of Leisure Research,* 42(2), 181–201.

77. Business students practice philanthropy. (2005, May/June). BizEd, 4(4), 6–8.

78. Government of Canada. (2015, August 08). *An implementation guide for Canadian Business.* Corporate Social Responsibility. Innovation, Science, and Economic Development. www.ic.gc.ca/eic/site/csr-rse.nsf/eng/h_rs00599.html

79. Hurst, M. (2012, May 17). *Employer support of volunteering.* Canadian Social Trends. Statistics Canada. www.statcan.gc.ca/pub/11-008-x/2012001/article/11670-eng.pdf Catalogue no. 11-008-X (p. 68).

80. Turcotte, M. (2008, November 21). *Time spent with family in a typical workday, 1986–2005.* Canadian Social Trends, Statistics Canada. Catalogue no. 11-008. www.statcan.gc.ca/pub/11-008-x/2006007/9574-eng.htm

81. Olds J., & Schwartz, R. S. (2000 April). What is the psychiatric significance of loneliness? *Harvard Mental Health Letter,* 16(10):8.

82. Clark, W. (2002, Autumn). *Time alone*. Canadian Social Trends, Statistics Canada. Catalogue no. 11-008.

83. Dittman, K. L., & Andrews, U. (2004). A study of the relationship between loneliness and Internet use among university students. *Dissertation Abstracts International: Section B: The Sciences & Engineering*, 64(7–B), 3518.

84. Odaci, H., & Kalkan, M. (2009). Problematic internet use, loneliness and dating anxiety among young adult university students. *Computers and Education*, 55(3), 1091–1097.

85. Celik, C. B., & Odaci, H. (2013). The relationship between problematic internet use and interpersonal cognitive distortions and life satisfaction in university students. *Children and Youth Services Review*, 35(3), 505–508.

86. Kim, J. H., Lau, C. H. L., Cheuk, K., Kan, P., Hui, H. L. C., & Griffiths, S. M. (2009). Brief report: Predictors of heavy internet use and associations with health promoting and health risk behaviors among Hong Kong university students. *Journal of Adolescence*, 33(1), 215–220.

87. Odaci, H. (2011). Academic self-efficacy and academic procrastination as predictors of problematic internet use in university students. *Computers and Education*, 57(1), 1109–1113.

88. Cramer, K., & Neyedley, K. (1998). Sex differences in loneliness: The role of masculinity and femininity. *Sex Roles: A Journal of Research*, 38(7), 645–653.

89. Mounts, N. S., Valentiner, D. P., Anderson, K. L., & Boswell, M. K. (2006). Shyness, sociability, and parental support for the college transition: Relation to adolescents' adjustment. *Journal of Youth and Adolescence*, 35(1), 71–80.

90. Nelson, L. J., Padilla-Walker, L. M., Badger, S., McNamara Barry, C., Carroll, J. S., & Madsen, S. D. (2008). Associations between shyness and internalizing behaviors, externalizing behaviors, and relationships during emerging adulthood. *Journal of Youth and Adolescence*, 37(5), 605–615.

91. Stein, M., et al. (2000). Social phobia symptoms, subtypes, and severity. *Archives of General Psychiatry*, 57(11), 1046–1052.

92. Government of Canada. (2006). *The human face of mental health and mental illness in Canada 2006*. www.phac-aspc.gc.ca/publicat/human-humain06/index-eng.php

93. World Health Organization (WHO). (2012, October). *mhGAP Newsletter*. Mental Health Gap Action Program. www.who.int/mental_health/mhGAP_nl_December_2012.pdf

94. Funk, M., Drew, N., Freeman, M., Edwige, F., & World Health Organization (WHO). (2010). *Mental health and development: Targeting people with mental health conditions as a vulnerable group*. Mental Health and Poverty Project. www.who.int/mental_health/policy/mhtargeting/en/

95. Government of Canada. (2006). *The human face of mental illness in Canada 2006*. www.phac-aspc.gc.ca/publicat/human-humain06/index-eng.php

96. Health Canada Editorial Board Mental Illnesses in Canada. (2002). *A report on mental illness in Canada*. Public Health Canada. Catalogue no. 0-662-32817-5. www.phac-aspc.gc.ca/publicat/miic-mmac/pdf/men_ill_e.pdf (p. 16).

97. Smetanin, P., Stiff, D., Briante, C., Adair, C. E., Ahmad, S., & Khan, M. (2011). *The life and economic impact of major mental illnesses in Canada, 2011 to 2041* (p. 89). RiskAnalytica, on behalf of the Mental Health Commission of Canada 2011. http://stg.mentalhealthcommission.ca/English/system/files/private/document/MHCC_Report_Base_Case_FINAL_ENG_0.pdf

98. Mental Health Commission of Canada. (2013). *Making the case for investing in mental health in Canada*. http://www.mentalhealthcommission.ca/sites/default/files/2016-06/Investing_in_Mental_Health_FINAL_Version_ENG.pdf

99. Ibid.

100. Mounting evidence indicates heart disease link. (2002, July 21). *Medical Letter on the CDC & FDA*, p. 14.

101. Niranjan, A., Corujo, B. S., Ziegelstein, R. C., & Nwulia, E. (2012). Depression and heart disease in US adults. *General Hospital Psychiatry*, 34(3), 254–261.

102. Parmet, S. (2002). Depression and heart disease. *Journal of the American Medical Association*, 288(6), 701–710.

103. Depression and heart disease. (2001). *Harvard Heart Letter*, 11(8).

104. Andrews, G. (2001). Should depression be managed as a chronic disease? *British Medical Journal*, 322(7283), 419–421.

105. Health Canada Editorial Board Mental Illnesses in Canada. (2002). *A report on mental illness in Canada*. Public Health Canada. Catalogue no. 0-662-32817-5. www.phac-aspc.gc.ca/publicat/miic-mmac/pdf/men_ill_e.pdf

106. Smetanin, P., Stiff, D., Briante, C., Adair, C. E., Ahmad, S., & Khan, M. (2011). *The life and economic impact of major mental illnesses in Canada: 2011 to 2041* (p. 8). RiskAnalytica, on behalf of the Mental Health Commission of Canada 2011. http://www.mentalhealthcommission.ca/sites/default/files/MHCC_Report_Base_Case_FINAL_ENG_0_0.pdf

107. Corrado, R. R., & Cohen, I. M. (2003). *Mental health profiles for a sample of British Columbia's Aboriginal survivors of the Canadian residential school system*. Publications. Research Series. Aboriginal Healing Foundation. www.ahf.ca/downloads/mental-health.pdf

108. Canadian Institute for Health Information. (2007). *Improving the health of Canadians: Mental health and homelessness*. Ottawa: CIHI. https://secure.cihi.ca/free_products/mental_health_report_aug22_2007_e.pdf

109. McClure, A. (2010). The other meal plan. *University Business*, 13(9), 14.

110. Funk, M., Drew, N., Freeman, M., Edwige, F., & World Health Organization (WHO). (2010). *Mental health and development: Targeting people with mental health conditions as a vulnerable group*. Mental Health and Poverty Project. www.who.int/mental_health/policy/mhtargeting/en/

111. Government of Canada. (2015, June 03). *Fast facts from the 2014 survey on living with chronic diseases in Canada*. Mood and Anxiety Disorders in Canada. healthycanadians.gc.ca/publications/diseases-conditions-maladies-affections/mental-mood-anxiety-anxieux-humeur/index-eng.php

112. What you should know about generalized anxiety disorders. (2000). *American Family Physician*, 62(7).

113. Phobias and panic disorder. (2015). *Canadian Mental Health Association*. www.cmha.ca/mental_health/phobias-and-panic-disorders/

114. Panic disorder. (2013). *Canadian Mental Health Association. British Columbia Division*. www.cmha.bc.ca/get-informed/mental-health-information/panic-disorder

115. Somers, J., & Queree, M. (2007, March). *Cognitive behavioural therapy*. Core information document. Centre for Applied Research in Mental Health and Addictions. (CARMHA).Faculty of Health Sciences Simon Fraser University. www.health.gov.bc.ca/library/publications/year/2007/MHA_CognitiveBehaviouralTherapy.pdf

116. Schnyder, U., et al. (2000). Incidence and prediction of posttraumatic stress disorder symptoms in severely injured accident victims. *American Journal of Psychiatry*, 158(4), 594–599.

117. Naparstek, B. (2004). *Invisible heroes: Survivors of trauma and how they heal.* New York: Bantam Books.

118. Fenske, J. N., & Schewenk, T. L. (2009). Obsessive-compulsive disorder: diagnosis and management. *American Family Physician* 80(3), 239–245.

119. American Psychiatric Association. (2014). *Diagnostic and Statistical Manual of Mental Disorders* (DSM-5). www.appi.org/products/dsm-manual-of-mental-disorders

120. Weyandt, L. L., & DuPaul, G. (2006). ADHD in college students. *Journal of Attention Disorders*, 10(1), 9–19.

121. Onninka, A. M. H., Zwiersb, M. P., Hoogmana, M., Mostertb J., Kana, C. C., Buitelaarb, J., & Frankea, B. (2014). Brain alterations in adult ADHD: Effects of gender, treatment and comorbid depression. *European Neuropsychopharmacology*, 24(3), 397–409.

122. Ursano, A. (2008). Disorders usually first diagnosed in infancy, childhood, or adolescence. In R. Hales, S. Yudofsky, & G. Gabbard (Eds.), *The American Psychiatric Publishing Textbook of Psychiatry* (pp. 505–608; 5th ed.). Washington, DC: American Psychiatric Publishing.

123. Wilmshurst, L., Peele, M., & Wilmshurst, L. (2011). Resilience and well-being in college students with and without a diagnosis of ADHD. *Journal of Attention Disorders,* 15(1), 11–17.

124. Health Canada Editorial Board Mental Illnesses in Canada. (2002). *A report on mental illness in Canada.* Public Health Canada. Catalogue no. 0-662-32817-5. www.phac-aspc.gc.ca/publicat/miic-mmac/pdf/men_ill_e.pdf

125. Pullen, L., Modrcin-McCarthy, M. A., & Graf, E. V. (2000). Adolescent depression: Important facts that matter. *Journal of Child and Adolescent Psychiatric Nursing*, 13(2), 69–75.

126. Mood Disorders Society of Canada. (2009, November; 3rd ed.). *Quick Facts: Mental illness and addiction in Canada.* www.mooddisorderscanada.ca/page/quick-facts

127. American College Health Association. *American College Health Association—National College Health Assessment II: Reference Group Executive Summary Fall 2012.* Hanover, MD: American College Health Association, 2013. (p. 14). http://www.acha-ncha.org/docs/acha-ncha-ii_referencegroup_executivesummary_fall2012.pdf

128. Eriksson, S., & Gard, G. (2011). Systematic review: Physical exercise and depression. *Physical Therapy Reviews*, 16(4), 261–268.

129. Babyak, M., Blumenthal, J. A., Herman, S., Khatri, P., Doraiswamy, M., Moore, K., Craighead, W. E., Baldewicz, T., & Krishnan, R. (2000). Exercise treatment for major depression: Maintenance of therapeutic benefit at 10 months. *Psychosomatic Medicine*, 62(5), 633–638.

130. LeTourneau, M. (2001, May–June). Pump up to cheer up. *Psychology Today*, 27.

131. Vastag, B. (2002). Decade of work shows depression is physical. *Journal of the American Medical Association*, 287(14), 1787–1788.

132. Government of Canada. (2015, June 03). *Fast facts from the 2014 survey on living with chronic diseases in Canada.* Mood and Anxiety Disorders in Canada. healthycanadians.gc.ca/publications/diseases-conditions-maladies-affections/mental-mood-anxiety-anxieux-humeur/index-eng.php

133. Straton, J., & Cronholm, P. (2002). Are paroxetine, fluoxetine, and sertraline equally effective for depression? *Journal of Family Practice*, 51(3), 285.

134. Hales, R. E., & Hales, D. (2001). *The mind-mood pill book.* New York: Bantam.

135. Currie, J. (2005). The marketization of depression: The prescribing of SSRI antidepressants to women. *Women and Health Protection.* http://www.whp-apsf.ca/pdf/SSRIs.pdf

136. Andrews, P. W., Thomson, J. A., Amstadter, A., & Neale, M. C. (2012, April 24). Primum non nocere: An evolutionary analysis of whether antidepressants do more harm than good. *Frontiers in Psychology*, 3(117), 1–19. http://journal.frontiersin.org/article/10.3389/fpsyg.2012.00117/full

137. Dunn, A., Trivedi, M., Kampers, J., Clark, C., & Chambliss, H. (2005). Exercise treatment for depression efficacy and dose response. *American Journal of Preventative Medicine*, 28(11), 1–8.

138. Rehorst, C. D., & Trivedi, M. H. (2013). Evidence-based recommendations for the prescription of exercise for major depressive disorder. *Journal of Psychiatric Practice*, 19(3), 204–212.

139. Health Canada Editorial Board Mental Illnesses in Canada. (2002). *A report on mental illness in Canada.* Public Health Canada. Catalogue no. 0-662-32817-5. www.phac-aspc.gc.ca/publicat/miic-mmac/pdf/men_ill_e.pdf

140. Ibid.

141. American Psychiatric Association (2014). Diagnostic and Statistical Manual of Mental Disorders (DSM-5). www.appi.org/products/dsm-manual-of-mental-disorders

142. UBC Mood Disorders Centre. (n.d.). Seasonal affective disorder. *Faculty of Medicine.* sad.psychiatry.ubc.ca/

143. Canadian Mental Health Association. (CMHA). North and West Vancouver Branch. British Columbia Division. (2013). *Seasonal affective disorder.* Get Informed. http://northwestvancouver.cmha.bc.ca/get-informed/mental-health-information/sad

144. Ibid.

145. American Psychiatric Association (2014). *Diagnostic and Statistical Manual of Mental Disorders* (DSM-5). www.appi.org/products/dsm-manual-of-mental-disorders

146. Health Canada Editorial Board Mental Illnesses in Canada. (2002). A report on mental illness in Canada. *Public Health Canada.* Catalogue no. 0-662-32817-5. www.phac-aspc.gc.ca/publicat/miic-mmac/pdf/men_ill_e.pdf

147. De Jong, M. A., & Mather, J. (2009). Undergraduate students' perceptions of schizophrenia. *International Journal of Mental Health and Addiction*, 7(3), 458–467.

148. Canadian Mental Health Association. (2015). Schizophrenia. *Mental Health.* www.cmha.ca/mental_health/facts-about-schizophrenia/

149. Kelley, M. E., Wan, C. R., Broussard, B., Crisafio, A., Cristofaro, S., Johnson, S., Reed, T. A., et al. (2016). Marijuana use in the immediate 5-year premorbid period is associated with increased risk of onset of schizophrenia and related psychotic disorders. *Schizophrenia Research,* 171(1–3), 62–67. DOI: 10.1016/j.schres.2016.01.015

150. World Health Organization (WHO). (2014). *Preventing suicide: A global imperative.* apps.who.int/iris/bitstream/10665/131056/8/9789241564878_eng.pdf?ua=1&ua=1

151. Canadian Association for Suicide Prevention (CASP). (n.d.). *Suicide in Canada. What is suicide?* Understanding. suicideprevention.ca/understanding/what-is-suicide/

152. Centre for Suicide Prevention. (2013). Aboriginal Resource Toolkit. suicideinfo.ca/LinkClick.aspx?fileticket=MVIyGo2V4YY%3D&tabid=516

153. Walling, A. (2000). Which patients are at greatest risk of committing suicide? *American Family Physician*, 61(8), 2487.

154. Health Canada Editorial Board Mental Illnesses in Canada. (2002). *A report on mental illness in Canada.* Public Health Canada. Catalogue no. 0-662-32817-5. www.phac-aspc.gc.ca/publicat/miic-mmac/pdf/men_ill_e.pdf

155. Canadian Mental Health Association. (2004). Your education—Your future. A guide to college and university for students with psychiatric disabilities. www.cmha.ca/youreducation/introduction.html

156. Davidson, J. (2002). Effect of hypericum perforatum (St. John's wort) in major depressive disorder: A randomized controlled trial. *Journal of the American Medical Association,* 287(14), 1807. www.healthlinkbc.ca/healthtopics/content.asp?hwid=hw260538spec

157. Health Link BC. (2015, May 22). *St. John's wort.* Health Topics A–Z. www.healthlinkbc.ca/healthtopics/content.asp?hwid=hw260538spec

Chapter 3

1. Stress. (2015). *Merriam-Webster Online Dictionary.* www.merriam-webster.com/dictionary/Stress
2. Selye, H. (1974). *Stress without distress.* New York: Lippincott.
3. Ibid.
4. Lazarus, R. S., & Folkman, S. (1984). *Stress, appraisal, and coping.* New York: Springer.
5. Lazarus, R. S. (1990). Theory-based stress measurement. *Psychological Inquiry,* 1(1), 3.
6. Folkman, S., & Lazarus, R. S. (1988). Coping as a mediator of emotion. *Journal of Personality and Social Psychology,* 54(3), 466–475.
7. Senior, K. (2001). Should stress carry a health warning? *Lancet,* 357, 126.
8. Widmaier, E. P., Raff, H., & Strang, K. T. (2006). *Vander's human physiology: The mechanisms of body function.* Boston, MA: McGraw Hill.
9. Ibid.
10. Ibid.
11. Maté, G. (2003). *When the body says no. The cost of hidden stress.* Toronto: Alfred A. Knopf Canada, a division of Random House of Canada.
12. Lazarus, R. S., & DeLongis, A. (1983). Psychological stress and coping in aging. *American Psychologist,* 38, 245–254.
13. Hamer, M., Molloy, G. J., & Stamatakis, E. (2008). Psychological distress as a risk factor of cardiovascular events: Pathophysiological and behavioral mechanisms. *Journal of the American College of Cardiology,* 52(25), 2156–2162.
14. Friedman, M., Thoresen, C. E., Gill, J. J., Ulmer, D., Powell, L. H., Price V. A., Brown, B., Thompson, L., Rabin, D. D., Breall, W. S., Bourg, E., Levy, R., & Dixon, T. (1986). Alteration of type A behavior and its effect on cardiac recurrences in post myocardial infarction patients: Summary results of the Recurrent Coronary Prevention Project. *American Heart Journal,* 112, 653–665.
15. Yusuf, S., Hawken, S., Ounpuu, S., Dans, T., Avezum, A., Lanas, F., McQueen, M., Budaj, A., Pais, P., Varigos, J., & Lisheng, L. (2004). Effect of potentially modifiable risk factors associated with myocardial infarction in 52 countries (the INTERHEART study): Case-control study. *Lancet,* 364, 937–952.
16. Daubenmier, J., Kristeller, J., Hecht, F. M., Maniger, N., Kuwata, M., Jhaveri, K., Lustig, R. H., Kemeny, M., Karan, L., & Epel, E. (2011, October 02). Mindfulness intervention for stress eating to reduce cortisol and abdominal fat among overweight and obese women: An exploratory randomized controlled study. *Journal of Obesity,* Article ID 651936. http://dx.doi.org/10.1155/2011/651936
17. Perticone, F., Ceravolo, R., Candigliota, M., Ventura, G., Iacopino, S., Sinopolo, F., & Mattioli, P. L. (2001). Obesity and body fat distribution induce endothelial dysfunction by oxidative stress. *Diabetes,* 50, 159–165.
18. Epel, E. S., McEwen, B., Seeman, T., Matthews, K., Catellazzo, G., Brownell, K. D., Bell, J., & Ickovics, J. R. (2000). Stress and body shape: Stress-induced cortisol secretion is consistently greater among women with central fat. *Psychosomatic Medicine,* 62, 623–632.
19. Thoits, P. A. (2010). Stress and health: Major findings and policy implications. *Journal of Health and Social Behavior,* 51(1), S41–S53.
20. Naperstek, B. (2006). *Invisible heroes. Survivors of trauma and how they heal.* New York: Bantam Dell, a division of Random House.
21. Klainberg, M., Ewing, B., & Ryan, M. (2010). Reducing stress on a college campus. *Journal of the New York Nursing Association,* 41(2), 4–7.
22. Enns, M. W., Cox, B. J., Sareen, J., & Freeman, P. (2001). Adaptive and maladaptive perfectionism in medical students: A longitudinal investigation. *Medical Education,* 35, 1034–1042.
23. Hameideh, S. H. (2011). Stressors and reactions to stressors among university students. *International Journal of Social Psychiatry,* 57(1), 69–80.
24. Stoliker, B., & Lafrenier, K. D. (2015). The influence of perceived stress, loneliness, and learning burnout on university students' educational experience. *College Student Journal,* 49(1), 146–160.
25. Isaak, C. A., Campeau, M., Katz, L. Y., Enns, M. W., Elias, B., & Sareen, J. (2010). Community-based suicide prevention research in remote on-reserve First Nations communities. *International Journal of Mental Health and Addiction,* 8(2), 258–270.
26. Deckro, G., et al. (2002). The evaluation of a mind/body intervention to reduce psychological distress and perceived stress in college students. *Journal of American College Health,* 50(6), 281–287.
27. Brougham, R. R., Zail, C. M., Mendoza, C. M., & Miller, J. R. (2009). Stress, sex differences, and coping strategies among college students. *Current Psychology,* 28(2), 85–97. DOI: 10.1007/s12144-009-9047-0
28. Anderson Darling, C., McWey, L. M., Howard, S. N., & Olmstead, S. B. (2007). College student stress: The influence of interpersonal relationships on sense of coherence. *Stress and Health,* 23(40), 215–229.
29. How women handle stress: Is there a difference? (2001). *Harvard Mental Health Letter,* 17(10), 7.
30. Verona, E., Reed II, A., Curtin, J. J., & Pole, M. (2007). Gender differences in emotional and overt/covert aggressive responses to stress. *Aggressive Behavior,* 33(3), 261–271.
31. Higgins, C. A., Duxbury, L. E., & Lyons, S. T. (2010). Coping with overload and stress: Men and women in dual-earner families. *Journal of Marriage and Family,* 72(4), 847–859.
32. Oman, D., Shapiro, S. L., Thoresen, C. E., Plante, T. G., & Flinders, T. (2008). Meditation lowers stress and supports forgiveness among college students: A randomized controlled trial. (Report). *Journal of American College Health, 56(5), 569–579.*
33. Welcome to the HUB. *Brock University.* (2010). www.brocku.ca/health-services/the-hub

34. Live Well Learn Well. Health and Wellness. University of British Columbia. (n.d.). students.ubc.ca/livewell
35. Cuyler, G. Byline. (2009, November 15). Coping at college: Overwhelmed students can get help on local campuses. *Reading Eagle.*
36. Bowling Green State University. Byline. (2002, May 20). Breakup of romance prompts search for spiritual healing, study of college student finds. *Ascribe Higher Education News Service.*
37. Shear, K., Fran, E., Houck, P. R., & Reynolds, C. F. (2005). Treatment of complicated grief. A randomized controlled trial. *Journal of the American Medical Association (JAMA)*, 293(21), 2601–2608.
38. Field, T., Diego, M., Pelaez, M., Deeds, O., & Delgado, J. (2009). Breakup stress in university students. *Adolescence*, 44(176), 705–728.
39. Bowling Green State University. Byline. (2002, May 20). Breakup of romance prompts search for spiritual healing, study of college student finds. *Ascribe Higher Education News Service.*
40. Burley, G., & Awad, A. (2015). *The impact of student debt.* Canadian Federation of Students. cfs-fcee.ca/wp-content/uploads/sites/2/2015/03/Report-Impact-of-Student-Debt-2015-Final.pdf
41. Ibid.
42. Statistics Canada. (2014, November 14). Graduating in Canada: Profile, labour market outcomes and student debt of the class of 2009/2010, 2013. *The Daily.* www.statcan.gc.ca/daily-quotidien/141114/dq141114b-eng.htm
43. Evans, C., Gbadamosib, G., & Richardson, M. (2014). Flexibility, compromise and opportunity: Students' perceptions of balancing part-time work with a full-time business degree. *The International Journal of Management Education*, 12(2), 80–90. DOI: 10.1016/j.ijme.2014.02.001
44. Palmer, L., Bliss, D. L., Goetz, J. W., & Moorman, D. (2010). Improving financial awareness among college students: Assessment of a financial management program. *College Student Journal*, 44(3), 659–677.
45. Statistics Canada. (2014, November 14). Graduating in Canada: Profile, labour market outcomes and student debt of the class of 2009/2010, 2013. *The Daily.* www.statcan.gc.ca/daily-quotidien/141114/dq141114b-eng.htm
46. Ipsos-Reid and Kumon Math and Reading Centre. (2005, April 12). *Canadian university students on study habits and exam-related stress.* Available by subscription at www.ipsos-na.com/news-polls/pressrelease.aspx?id=2626
47. Ibid.
48. Steinhardt, M., & Dolbier, M. S. (2008). Evaluations of a resilience intervention to enhance coping strategies and protective factors and decrease symptomatology. *Journal of American College Health*, 54(4), 445–463.
49. Ipsos-Reid and Kumon Math and Reading Centre. (2005, April 12). *Canadian university students on study habits and exam-related stress.* Available by subscription at www.ipsos-na.com/news-polls/pressrelease.aspx?id=2626
50. Jewell, L. M., & Morrison, M. A. (2010). "But there's a million jokes about everybody...": Prevalence of, and reasons for, directing negative behaviors toward gay men on a Canadian university campus. *Journal of Interpersonal Violence*, 25(11), 2094–2112.
51. Swank, E., & Raiz, L. (2007). Explaining comfort with homosexuality among social work students: The impact of demographic, contextual, and attitudinal factors. *Journal of Social Work Education*, 43(2), 257–280.
52. Currie, C. L., Wild, T. C., Schopflocher, D. P., Laing, L., & Veugelers, P. (2012). Racial discrimination experienced by Aboriginal university students in Canada. *Canadian Journal of Psychiatry*, 57(10), 617–625.
53. Walsh, B. (2010). The spill's psychic toll. *Time*, 176(6), 32–34.
54. Lübken, U., & Mauch, C. (2011). Uncertain environments: Natural hazards, risk and insurance in historical perspective. *Environment and History*, 17(1), 1–12.
55. Miller, M., & Heldring, M. (2004). Mental health and primary care in a time of terrorism: Psychological impact of terrorist attacks. *Families, Systems & Health*, 22(1), 7–30.
56. De Zulueta, C. F. (2007). Mass violence and mental health: Attachment and trauma. *International Review of Psychiatry*, 19(3), 221–233.
57. Duffy, M., Gillespe, K., & Clark, D. (2007). Post-traumatic stress disorder in the context of terrorism and other civic conflict in Northern Ireland: Randomised controlled trial. *BMJ: British Medical Journal*, 334(7604), 1147–1150.
58. Brod, C. (1984). *Technostress: The human cost of the computer revolution.* Reading, MA: Addison Wesley.
59. Kim, J. H., Lau, C. H., Cheuk, K. K., Kan, P., Hui, H. L. C., & Griffiths, S. M. (2010). Brief reports: Predictors of heavy internet use and associations with health-promoting and health risk behaviors among Hong Kong university students. *Journal of Adolescence*, 33(1), 215–220.
60. Padilla-Walker, L. M., Nelson, L. J., Carroll, J. S., & Jensen, A. C. (2010). More than just a game: Video game and Internet use during emerging adulthood. *Journal of Youth Adolescence*, 39(2), 103–113.
61. Ibid.
62. Muise, A., Christofides, E., & Desmarais, S. (2009). More information than you ever wanted: Does Facebook bring out the green-eyed monster of jealousy? *CyberPsychology & Behavior*, 12(4), 441–444.
63. Griffiths, M., & Barnes, A. (2008). Internet gambling: An online empirical study among student gamblers. *International Journal of Mental Health and Addiction*, 6(2), 194–204.
64. Petry, N. M., & Gonzalez-Ibanez, A. (2015). Internet gambling in problem gambling college students. *Journal of Gambling Studies*, 31(2), 397–408.
65. Canadian Mental Health Association. (2015). *Mental illness in the workplace.* Mental Health. www.cmha.ca/mental_health/mental-illness-in-the-workplace/
66. *How to work safely and stay healthy.* (2016, September 14). Occupational Health and Safety. Government of Alberta. https://work.alberta.ca/occupational-health-safety/resources-how-to-work-safely.html
67. Burns, J. L., Lee, R. M., & Brown, L. J. (2011). The effect of meditation on self-reported measures of stress, anxiety, depression, and perfectionism in a college population. *Journal of College Student Psychotherapy*, 25(2), 132–144.
68. Counselling and Development Centre, York University. (nd) lss.info.yorku.ca/resources/university-time-management/
69. Zarick, L. M., & Stonebraker, R. (2009). I'll do it tomorrow. *College Teaching*, 57(4), 211–215.

Chapter 4

1. Tremblay, A., & Chiasson, L. (2002). Physical fitness in young college men and women. *Canadian Journal of Applied Physiology*, 27, 563–574.

2. Canadian Society for Exercise Physiology. (2012). *Canadian physical activity guidelines. Canadian sedentary behaviour guidelines.* www.csep.ca/cmfiles/guidelines/csep_guidelines _handbook.pdf

3. Morris, J. N., & Heady, J. A. (1953). Mortality in relation to the physical activity of work: A preliminary note on experience in middle age. *British Journal of Industrial Medicine*, 10(4), 245–254.

4. Paffenbarger, R. S., & Hale, W. E. (1975). Work activity and coronary heart mortality. *New England Journal of Medicine*, 292(11), 545–550.

5. Berkman, L. F., & Breslow, L. (1983). *Health and ways of living: The Alameda County study.* New York: Oxford University Press.

6. Lewis S. F., & Hennekens, C. H. (2016). Regular physical activity: Forgotten benefits. Commentary. *American Journal of Medicine,* 129(2), 137–138.

7. Warburton, D. E. R., Nichol, C. W., & Bredin, S. S. D. (2006). Health benefits of physical activity: The evidence. *Canadian Medical Association Journal (CMAJ)*, 174(6), 801–809.

8. Public Health Agency of Canada. (2013, November 18). *Healthy living.* Health Promotion. www.phac-aspc.gc.ca/hp-ps/hl-mvs/index-eng.php

9. Janssen, I. (2012). Health care costs of physical inactivity in Canadian adults. *Applied Physiology, Nutrition, and Metabolism*, 37(4), 803–806.

10. Bounajm, F., Dinh, T., & Theriault L. (2015, February). *Moving ahead: The economic impact of reducing physical inactivity and sedentary behaviour.* Research Update. Alberta Centre for Active Living. www.centre4activeliving.ca/media/filer_public/5b/2f/5b2f73fb-cc21-46de-836d-dd49b5357ea0/2015-feb-sedentary.pdf

11. Canadian Society for Exercise Physiology. (2012). *Canadian physical activity guidelines. Canadian sedentary behaviour guidelines.* www.csep.ca/cmfiles/guidelines/csep_guidelines _handbook.pdf

12. Canadian Society for Exercise Physiology (CSEP). (2011). *Canadian physical activity guidelines for adults 18–64 years.* www.csep.ca/CMFiles/Guidelines/CSEP_PAGuidelines _0-65plus_en.pdf

13. Canadian Society for Exercise Physiology. (2012). *Canadian physical activity guidelines. Canadian sedentary behaviour guidelines.* www.csep.ca/cmfiles/guidelines/csep_guidelines _handbook.pdf

14. Statistics Canada. (2015, November 27). *Directly measured physical activity of adults, 2012 and 2013.* Health Fact Sheets. Publications. Catalogue no. 82-625-X. www.statcan.gc.ca/pub/82-625-x/2015001/article/14135-eng.htm

15. Hales, D. (2016). *An invitation to health. Live it now!* (9th ed.). Boston: Cengage Learning (p. 161).

16. Hales, D. (2016). *An invitation to health. Live it now!* (9th ed.). Boston: Cengage Learning (p. 161).

17. Liebenson, C. (2006). Functional fitness training: The functional reach. *Journal of Bodywork and Movement Therapies*, 10(2), 159–162.

18. Exercise is Medicine Canada (EMIC). (2016). *American College of Sports Medicine.* exerciseismedicine.org/canada/

19. Exercise is Medicine on Campus. (EMIC). (2016). *American College of Sports Medicine.* exerciseismedicine.org/canada/support_page.php?p=140

20. Osteoporosis Canada. (2016). *Osteoporosis facts and figures.* Osteoporosis and You. www.osteoporosis.ca/osteoporosis-and -you/osteoporosis-facts-and-statistics/

21. Yonclas, P., et al. (2002). Osteoporosis: How much exercise is enough for bone health? *Consultant,* 42(7), 829–834.

22. Rebar, A. L., Stanton, R., Geard, D., Short, C., Duncan, M. J., & Vandelanotte, C. (2015). A meta-meta analysis of the effect of physical activity on depression and anxiety in non-clinical adult populations. *Health Psychology Review*, 9(3), 366–378. DOI: 10.1080/17437199.2015.1022901

23. Dinas, P. C., Koutedakis, Y., & Flouris, A. D. (2011). Effects of exercise and physical activity on depression. *Irish Journal of Medical Science*, 180(2), 319–325.

24. Exercise as psychotherapy. (2000). *Harvard Mental Health Letter*, 17(3).

25. Babyak, M., Blumenthal, J. A., Herman, S., Khatric, P., Doraiswamy, M., Moore, K., Craighead, W. E., Baldewicz, T. T., & Ranga, K. K. (2000). Exercise treatment for major depression: Maintenance of therapeutic benefit at 10 months. *Psychosomatic Medicine*, 62(5), 633–638.

26. Burns, J. M. (2008). Cardiorespiratory fitness and brain atrophy in early Alzheimer disease. *Neurology*, 71(1), 210–216.

27. Hoffman, M. D., & Hoffman, D. R. (2008). Exercisers achieve greater acute exercise-induced mood enhancement than nonexercisers. *Archives of Physical Medicine and Rehabilitation*, 89(2), 358–363.

28. Rendi, M., Szabo, T., Szabo, A., Velenczei, A., & Kovacs, A. (2008). Acute psychological benefits of aerobic exercise: A field study into the effects of exercise characteristics. *Psychology, Health, and Medicine*, 13(2), 180–184.

29. Radak, Z., Chung, H. Y., Koltai, E., Taylor, A. W., & Goto, S. (2008). Exercise, oxidative stress and homesis. *Ageing Research Reviews,* 7(1), 34–42.

30. Neiman, D. C., Henson, D. A., Austin, M. D., & Brown, V. A. (2005). The immune response to a 30-minute walk. *Medicine and Science in Sports Exercise*, 37(1), 57–62.

31. Neiman, D. C. (2003). Current perspective on exercise immunology. *Current Sports Medicine Reports*, 2(5), 232–239.

32. Statistics Canada. (2015, December 10). *Leading causes of death, total population, by age group and sex*, Canada. CANSIM Database. www5.statcan.gc.ca/cansim/a26?lang=eng&id=1020561&p2=46

33. Sattelmair, J., Pertman, J., Ding E. L., Kohl III H. W., Haskell, W., & Lee, I-Min. (2011). Dose response between physical activity and risk of coronary heart disease. A meta-analysis. *Circulation*, 124(7), 789–795.

34. Health Topics. (2016). *Physical activity.* World Health Organization (WHO). www.who.int/topics/physical _activity/en/

35. Stessman J., & Jacobs J. M. (2014). Diabetes mellitus physical activity, and longevity between the ages of 70 and 90. *Journal of the American Geriatrics Society*, 62(7), 1329–1334.

36. Lin, Y. P., Huang, Y. H., Wu, J. S., Chang C. J., &Yang, Y. C. (2011). Non-leisure time physical activity is an independent predictor of longevity for a Taiwanese elderly population: An eight-year follow-up study. *BMC Public Health*, 11(1), 428–436. DOI: 10.1186/1471-2458-11-428

37. Gangaway, J. M. K. (2010). The need for exercise and the benefits of aquatics. *Topics in Geriatric Rehabilitation*, 26(2), 82–92.

38. Gremeauxa, V., Gaydaa, M., Leperse, R., Sosnera, P., Juneaua, M., & Nigama, A. (2012). Exercise and longevity. *Maturitas*, 73(4), 312–317.

39. Wright, H. (2007). Getting physically active may increase your chances of surviving cancer. *Environmental Nutrition*, 30(3), 1–4.

40. Grimmett, C. (2011). Exercise and cancer survivorship. *Journal of Hospital Medicine*, 72(4), 196–199.

41. Ahn, K. Y., et al. (2013). The effects of inpatient exercise therapy on the length of hospital stay in stages I-III colon cancer patients: Randomized controlled trial. *International Journal of Colorectal Disease*, 28(2), 185–194.

42. Wolin, K. Y., Yan, Y., Colditz, G. A., & Lee, I-M. (2009). Physical activity and colon cancer prevention: A meta-analysis. *British Journal of Cancer*, 100(4), 611–616.

43. Bernstein, L. (2009). Exercise and breast cancer prevention. *Current Oncology Reports*, 11(6), 490–496.

44. Canadian Diabetes Association. (2016). *Types of Diabetes*. About Diabetes. www.diabetes.ca/about-diabetes/types-of-diabetes

45. Government of Canada. (2015, December 17). *Type 2 Diabetes*. Diseases. Diseases and Conditions. healthycanadians.gc.ca/diseases-conditions-maladies-affections/disease-maladie/diabete-eng.php

46. Public Health Agency of Canada. (2012, July 04). *Diabetes in Canada: Facts and figures from a public health perspective*. Publications and Statistics. www.phac-aspc.gc.ca/cd-mc/publications/diabetes-diabete/facts-figures-faits-chiffres-2011/index-eng.php

47. American College of Sports Medicine and the American Diabetes Association: Joint Position Statement. (2010, December). Exercise and type 2 diabetes. *Medicine & Science in Sports & Exercise*, 42(12), 2282–2303.

48. OECD. (2015). *How does Canada compare?* Health at a glance, 2015. www.oecd.org/canada/Health-at-a-Glance-2015-Key-Findings-CANADA.pdf

49. Vella, C., & Kravitz, L. (2004, November/December). Exercise after-burn—A research update: What effect do intensity, mode, duration and other factors have on calorie burning after exercise? *Idea Fitness Journal*, 5, 42–46.

50. Gieck, D. J., & Olsen, S. (2007). Holistic wellness as a means to developing a lifestyle approach to health behavior among college students. *Journal of American College Health*, 56(1), 29–35.

51. Statistics Canada. (2015, November 27). *Physical activity during leisure time 2013*. Publications. www.statcan.gc.ca/pub/82-625-x/2014001/article/14024-eng.htm

52. Statistics Canada. (2015, November 27). *Directly measured physical activity of adults, 2012 and 2013*. Publications. www.statcan.gc.ca/pub/82-625-x/2015001/article/14135-eng.htm

53. Greaney, M. L., Less, F. D., White, A. A., Dayton, S. F., Riebe, D., Blissmer, B., Shoff, S., Walsh, J., & Greend, G. W. (2009). College students' barriers and enablers for healthful weight management: A qualitative study. *Journal of Nutrition Education and Behavior*, 41(4), 281–286.

54. Blair, S., Kohl, H. W. III, & Gordon, N. F. (1992). Physical activity and health: A lifestyle approach. *Medicine, Exercise, Nutrition, and Health*, 1, 54–57.

55. Ruby, M. B., Dunn, E. W., Perrino, A., Gillis, R., & Viel, S. (2011). The invisible benefits of exercise. *Health Psychology*, 30(1), 67–74.

56. Ramadan, J., & Barac-Nieto, M. (2001). Low-frequency physical activity insufficient for aerobic conditioning is associated with lower body fat than sedentary conditions. *Nutrition*, 17, 225–229.

57. Lee, I-Min., Rexrode, K. M., Cook, N. R., Manson, J. E., & Buring, J. E. (2001). Physical activity and coronary heart disease in women: Is "no pain, no gain" passé? *Journal of the American Medical Association*, 285(11), 1147–1454.

58. Chisholm, M. D., Collis, M. L., Kulak, L. L., Davenport, W., Gruber, N., & Steward, G. W. (1978). *PAR-Q* validation report: The evaluation of a self-administered pre-exercise screening questionnaire for adults*. British Columbia Ministry of Health and Welfare, Canada.

59. Canadian Society for Exercise Physiology (CSEP). (2016). *PAR-Q forms*. www.csep.ca/view.asp?ccid=517

60. Ibid.

61. Dobas, P. (2016, February). *Heart rate training 101. Fundamentals of heart rate training*. Obstacle Course Training. obstaclecourse.training/fundamentals-of-heart-rate-training/

62. Burke, E. (2002). Heart rate ABCs. *Better Nutrition*, 64(8), 48.

63. *Heart rate calculator*. www.ottawarun.com/heartrate.htm

64. Ibid.

65. Eston, R. (2012). Use of ratings of perceived exertion in sports. *International Journal of Sports Physiology and Performance*, 7(2), 175–182.

66. Crockford J. (2014, January 09). *Five reasons why you shouldn't skip your cooldown*. Family Health. American Council on Exercise (ACE). www.acefitness.org/acefit/healthy-living-article/59/3683/five-reasons-you-shouldn-t-skip-your-cool/

67. Statistics Canada. (2015, November 27). *Physical activity during leisure time 2013*. Publications. www.statcan.gc.ca/pub/82-625-x/2014001/article/14024-eng.htm

68. Lee, I-Min., Rexrode, K. M., Cook, N. R., Manson, J. E., & Buring, J. E. (2001). Physical activity and coronary heart disease in women: Is "no pain, no gain" passé? *Journal of the American Medical Association*, 285(11), 1147–1454.

69. Heart lines: Walking and gardening beneficial for heart disease patients. (2001). *Harvard Heart Letter*, 11(8).

70. Physical Activity Resource Centre (PARC). (2013). *Walk this way. Resource Guide*.parc.ophea.net/sites/parc.ophea.net/files/pdfs/WTW/WTW-User-s-Guide-English.pdf

71. Tseng I. J., Yuan R. Y., & Jeng, C. (2015). Treadmill training improves forward and backward gait in early Parkinson disease. *American Journal of Physical Medicine & Rehabilitation*, 94(10), 811–819.

72. Hatano, Y. (1993). Use of pedometers for promoting daily walking exercise. *Journal of the International Council for Health, Physical Education and Recreation*, 29(4), 4–8.

73. Croteau, K. A. (2004). A preliminary study on the impact of a pedometer-based intervention on daily steps. *Health Promotion*, 18(3), 217–220.

74. Tudor-Locke, C. E., & Myers, A. M. (2001). Methodological considerations for researchers and practitioners using pedometers to measure physical (ambulatory) activity. *Research Quarterly for Exercise and Sport*, 72(1), 1–12.

75. Tudor-Locke, C. (2008). Keynote—The art of increasing walking: The first step program. *Medicine & Science in Sports & Exercise*, 40(5), (Supplement 1), 38.

76. Bexelius, C., Löf, M., Sandin, S., Trolle Lagerros, T., Forsum, E., & Litton, J. E. (2010). Measures of physical activity using cell phones: Validation using criterion methods. *Journal of Medical Internet Research*, 12(1), e2. Open access article. www.ncbi.nlm.nih.gov/pmc/articles/PMC2821583/

77. About health. (2016). *Walking route planners and apps*. walking.about.com/od/trails/a/routeplanner.htm

78. Exergaming. In *The Free Dictionary*. (2013–2016). www.dictionary.com/browse/exergaming

79. Kraft, J. A., Russell, W. D., Bowman, T. A., Selsor III, C. W., & Foster, G. D. (2011). Heart rate and perceived exertion during self-selected intensities for exergaming compared to traditional exercise in college-age participants. *Journal of Strength and Conditioning Research*, 25(6), 1736–1742.

80. Wu, P. T., Wu, W. L., & Chu, I. H. (2015). Energy expenditure and intensity in healthy young adults during Exergaming. *American Journal of Health Behavior*, 39(4), 556–561.

81. Gillen, J. B., & Gibala, J. J., (2014). Is high-intensity interval training a time-efficient exercise strategy to improve health and fitness? *Applied Physiology and Nutrition Metabolism*, 39(3), 409–412.

82. Webb, O. J., Griffin, C., & Chambers, J. (2012). A multi-component stair climbing promotional campaign targeting caloric expenditure for worksites; A quasi-experimental study testing effects on behavior, attitude and intention. *BMC Public Health*, 12(1), 423–433.

83. Magyari, P. (2010). Resistance training intensity. Research and rationale. Health and Fitness Feature. *ACSM's Certified News*, 20(2), 3–4.

84. Ibid.

85. Streeter, C. C., Whitfield, T. H., Owen, L., Rein, T., Karri, S., Yakhkind, A., Perlmutter, R., Prescot, A., Renshaw, P. F., Ciraulo, D. A., & Jensen, J. E. (2010). Effects of yoga versus walking on mood, anxiety, and brain GABA levels: A randomized controlled MRS study. *The Journal of Alternative and Complementary Medicine*, 16(11), 1145–1152.

86. Melton, B., Hansen, A., & Gross, J. (2010). Trends in physical activity interest in the college and university setting. *College Student Journal*, 44(3), 785–790.

87. Ainsworth, B. E., Martin, M., Macera, C. A., Hootman, J. M., Blair, S. N., & Addy, C. L. (2002). Epidemiology of musculoskeletal injuries among sedentary and physically active adults. *Medicine & Science in Sports & Exercise*, 34(5), 838–844.

88. Cheung, S. S. (2010). Interconnections between thermal perception and exercise capacity in the heat. *Scandinavian Journal of Medicine & Science in Sports*, 20(Supplement 3), 53–59.

89. Flouris, A. D., & Cheung, S. S. (2010). Thermometry and calorimetry assessment of sweat response during exercise in the heat. *European Journal of Applied Physiology*, 108(5), 905–911.

Chapter 5

1. Health Canada. (2012, March 15). *Do Canadian adults meet their nutrient requirements through food intake alone?* Food and Nutrition. Catalogue no. H164-112/3-2012E-PDF. www.hc-sc.gc.ca/fn-an/surveill/nutrition/commun/art-nutr-adult-eng.php

2. Dieticians of Canada. (2014, November 27). *Guidelines for drinking fluids to stay hydrated.* Water. Nutrition A-Z. www.dietitians.ca/getattachment/becace49-3bad-4754-ac94-f31c3f04fed0/FACTSHEET-Guidelines-staying-hydrated.pdf.aspx

3. Dieticians of Canada. (2016). *Scientific basis of eaTracker.* www.eatracker.ca/background.aspx

4. Health Canada. (2014, March 20). *Estimated energy requirements.* Food Guide Basics. Food and Nutrition. www.hc-sc.gc.ca/fn-an/food-guide-aliment/basics-base/1_1_1-eng.php

5. Health Link BC. (2015). *Quick nutrition check for protein.* Healthy Eating. www.healthlinkbc.ca/healthyeating/protein.html

6. Health Link BC. (2015). *Counting carbohydrate grams or servings.* Health Topics. A–Z. www.healthlinkbc.ca/healthtopics/content.asp?hwid=tj8060

7. Canadian Sugar Institute. (2016). *Canadian sugar consumption.* Nutrition Information Service. www.sugar.ca/Nutrition-Information-Service/Health-professionals/Sugar-Consumption.aspx

8. Heart and Stroke Foundation. (2015). *Sugar and your health.* Healthy Living Features. www.heartandstroke.com/site/apps/nlnet/content2.aspx?c=ikIQLcMWJtE&b=4016859&ct=14183373

9. Health Canada. (2013, September 27). *Whole grains—get the facts.* Food and Nutrition. www.hc-sc.gc.ca/fn-an/nutrition/whole-grain-entiers-eng.php

10. Health Canada. (2011, November 11). *Eating well with Canada's food guide—A resource for educators and communicators.* Food and Nutrition. Reports and Publications. www.hc-sc.gc.ca/fn-an/pubs/res-educat/res-educat-eng.php

11. Crowe, T. C. (2005). Safety of low-carbohydrate diets. *Obesity Reviews*, 6(3), 235–245.

12. Hill, M. (2003). Dietary fibre and colon cancer: Where do we go from here? *The Proceedings of the Nutrition Society*, 62(1), 63–65.

13. Dieticians of Canada. (2012, October 04). *Healthy eating guidelines for increasing your fibre intake.* Fibre. Nutrition Resources. http://www.dietitians.ca/Downloads/Factsheets/Guidelines-for-Increasing-Fibre-Intake.aspx

14. Ibid.

15. Dietitians of Canada. (2016). *The glycemic index.* Diet and Nutrition. www.diabetes.ca/diabetes-and-you/healthy-living-resources/diet-nutrition/the-glycemic-index

16. Heart and Stroke Foundation. (2015, November). *Dietary fats, oils and cholesterol.* Healthy eating. Healthy Living. www.heartandstroke.com/site/c.ikIQLcMWJtE/b.3484237/k.D734/Healthy_living__Dietary_fats_oils_and__cholesterol.htm

17. Berkley University of California. (2014, November 14). *Is coconut oil a miracle food?* Berkley Wellness. www.berkeleywellness.com/healthy-eating/diet-weight-loss/food/nutrition/article/coconut-oil-all-its-cracked-be

18. Heart and Stroke Foundation. (2015, November). *Dietary fats, oils and cholesterol.* Healthy Eating. Healthy Living. www.heartandstroke.com/site/c.ikIQLcMWJtE/b.3484237/k.D734/Healthy_living__Dietary_fats_oils_and__cholesterol.htm

19. Siri-Tarino, P. W., Sun, Q., Hu, F. B., & Krauss, M. (2010). Meta-analysis of prospective cohort studies evaluating the association of saturated fat with cardiovascular disease. *American Journal of Clinical Nutrition*, 91(3), 535–546.

20. America Heart Association. (2010, October 29). *Monounsaturated fats.* Fats 101. Healthy Eating. Healthy Living. www.heart.org/HEARTORG/HealthyLiving/HealthyEating/Nutrition/Monounsaturated-Fats_UCM_301460_Article.jsp#.VvNpc032bIU

21. American Heart Association. (2015, October 07). *Polyunsaturated fats.* Healthy Eating. Healthy Living. www.heart.org/HEARTORG/HealthyLiving/HealthyEating/Nutrition/Polyunsaturated-Fats_UCM_301461_Article.jsp#.VvNqBU32bIU

22. American Heart Association. (2015, October 07). Trans fats. Healthy Eating. Healthy Living. www.heart.org/HEARTORG/HealthyLiving/HealthyEating/Nutrition/Trans-Fats_UCM_301120_Article.jsp#.VvNqmk32bIU

23. Health Canada. (2012, March 15). *Do Canadian adults meet their nutrient requirements through food intake alone?* Food

and Nutrition. Catalogue no. H164-112/3-2012E-PDF. www.hc-sc.gc.ca/fn-an/surveill/nutrition/commun/art-nutr-adult-eng.php

24. Health Canada. (2011, September 01). *Eating well with Canada's food guide.* Food and Nutrition. http://www.hc-sc.gc.ca/fn-an/food-guide-aliment/index-eng.php

25. Health Canada. (2007, February 05). *Canada's food guides from 1942 to 1992.* Food and Nutrition. Background on the Food Guide. www.hc-sc.gc.ca/fn-an/food-guide-aliment/context/fg_history-histoire_ga-eng.php

26. Abramovitch, S. L., Reddigan, J. I., Hamade, M. J., Jamik, V. K., Rowan, C. P., & Kuk, J. L. (2012). Underestimating a serving size may lead to increased food consumption when using *Canada's Food Guide. Applied Physiology Nutrition and Metabolism*, 37(5), 923–930.

27. Health Canada. (2011, August 24). *My food guide servings tracker.* Food and Nutrition. www.hc-sc.gc.ca/fn-an/food-guide-aliment/track-suivi/index-eng.php

28. Dietitians of Canada. (1997–2013). eaTracker. www.eatracker.ca/

29. Ware, M. (2014, January 09). *Top ten high protein vegetables.* Protein. Diet and Nutrition. www.livestrong.com/article/543186-top-ten-high-protein-vegetables/

30. Health Canada. (2015, May, 01). *Natural and non-prescription health products.* Drug and Health Products. www.hc-sc.gc.ca/dhp-mps/prodnatur/index-eng.php

31. Canadian Cancer Society. (2016). *Sunlight and vitamin D.* Sunlight and UVR Exposure. Cancer 101. www.cancer.ca/en/cancer-information/cancer-101/what-is-a-risk-factor/sun-and-uvr-exposure/sunlight-and-vitamin-d/?region=bc

32. Osteoporosis Canada. (2016). Calcium: An important nutrient that builds stronger bones. Osteoporosis and You. www.osteoporosis.ca/osteoporosis-and-you/nutrition/calcium-requirements/

33. Health Canada. (2012, June 08). *Sodium in Canada.* Nutrition and Healthy Eating. Food and Nutrition. http://www.hc-sc.gc.ca/fn-an/nutrition/sodium/index-eng.php

34. Dieticians of Canada. (2014, February 28). *Food sources of iron.* Minerals. Nutrition A–Z. www.dietitians.ca/Your-Health/Nutrition-A-Z/Minerals/Food-Sources-of-Iron.aspx

35. National Institutes of Health. (2016, February 11). *Vitamin E.* Fact sheet for professionals. Health Professional. Health Information. https://ods.od.nih.gov/factsheets/VitaminE-HealthProfessional/

36. Health Canada. (2013, April 23). *Dietary reference intakes.* Food and Nutrition. Nutrition and Healthy Eating. www.hc-sc.gc.ca/fn-an/nutrition/reference/index-eng.php

37. Health Canada. (2011, November 29). *A consumer's guide to the DRIs (dietary reference intakes).* Food and Nutrition. Nutrition and Healthy Eating. www.hc-sc.gc.ca/fn-an/nutrition/reference/cons_info-guide_cons-eng.php

38. Health Canada. (2015, June 12). *Nutrition labelling.* Food and Nutrition. www.hc-sc.gc.ca/fn-an/label-etiquet/nutrition/index-eng.php

39. Ibid.

40. Government of Canada. (2015, August 11). *Proposed food label changes to the nutrition facts table.* Consultations. Health. healthycanadians.gc.ca/health-system-systeme-sante/consultations/food-label-etiquette-des-aliments/nutrition-facts-valeur-nutritive-eng.php#s1

41. Health Canada. (2015, June 12). *Nutrition labelling.* Food and Nutrition. www.hc-sc.gc.ca/fn-an/label-etiquet/nutrition/index-eng.php

42. Smith, S. C., Taylor, J. G., & Stephen, A. M. (2000). Use of food labels and beliefs about diet-disease relationships among university students. *Public Health Nutrition*, 3(2), 175–182.

43. Food and Agriculture Organization of the United Nations. (2016). *Food-based dietary guidelines—Brazil.* Regions. Food-based Dietary Guidelines. www.fao.org/nutrition/education/food-dietary-guidelines/regions/brazil/en/

44. Ge, K. Y., Jia, J. B., & Lui, H. (2007). Food-based dietary guidelines in China: Practices and problems. *Annals of Nutrition & Metabolism*, 51, 26–31.

45. Health Canada. (2010, March 04). *Eating well with Canada's Food Guide—First Nations, Inuit and Metis.* Food and Nutrition. www.hc-sc.gc.ca/fn-an/pubs/fnim-pnim/index-eng.php

46. Receveur, O., Boulay, M., & Kuhnlein, H. V. (1997). Decreasing traditional food use affects diet quality for adult Dene/Metis in 16 communities of the Canadian Northwest Territories. *Journal of Nutrition, American Society for Nutritional Sciences*, 127, 2179–2186.

47. Bellisle, F. (2005). Nutrition and health in France: Dissecting a paradox. *Journal of the American Dietetic Association*, 105(12), 1870–1873.

48. United States Department of Agriculture (USDA). Centre for Nutrition Policy and Promotion. (2012). *Getting started with MyPlate.* Choose MyPlate.gov. www.choosemyplate.gov/content/getting-started-myplate

49. Smith, A., & MacKinnon, J. B. (2007). *The 100 mile diet. A tale of local eating.* Toronto: Random House Canada, Ltd.

50. Meal Exchange. (2006). Home. mealexchange.com/

51. Pippus, A. (2015, June 01). *Almost 12 million Canadians now vegetarian or trying to eat less meat!* Vancouver Humane Society. www.vancouverhumanesociety.bc.ca/almost-12-million-canadians-now-vegetarian-or-trying-to-eat-less-meat/

52. Dietitians of Canada. (2014, November 27). *Healthy eating guidelines for lacto-ovo-vegetarians.* Eating Guidelines for Lacto-Ovo-Vegetarians. Vegetarian Diets. www.dietitians.ca/Your-Health/Nutrition-A-Z/Vegetarian-Diets/Eating-Guidelines-for-Lacto-Ovo-Vegetarians.aspx

53. Dietitians of Canada. (2014, November 27). *Healthy eating guidelines for vegans.* Eating Guidelines for Vegans. Vegetarian Diets. www.dietitians.ca/Nutrition-Resources-A-Z/Factsheets/Vegetarian/Eating-Guidelines-for-Vegans.aspx

54. McEvoya, C. T., Temple, N., & Woodside, J. V. (2012). *Vegetarian diets, low-meat diets and health: A review.* Public Health Nutrition, 15(12), 2287–2294.

55. Euromonitor International. (2015, October). *Fast food in Canada.* Country Report, Consumer Food Service. www.euromonitor.com/fast-food-in-canada/report

56. Sturgeon, J. (2015, June 20). In Canada, new breed of fast-food chains are eating McDonald's lunch. *Global News.* global-news.ca/news/2061932/in-canada-new-breed-of-fast-food-chains-are-eating-mcdonalds-lunch/

57. Garcia, K. (2012). *Mobile fast food marketing: How Qsrs and fast casuals are getting quicker and faster.* eMarketerTM

58. Spurlock, M. (2005). *Don't eat this book: Fast food and the supersizing of America.* New York: G. P. Putnam's Sons.

59. Lum, L. (2007, April 19). Accommodating picky palates: While there remains disagreement over the prevalence of the "Freshman 15," college health and dining officials are trying to help students wade through many convoluted nutritional choices. *Diverse Issues in Higher Education*, 24(5), 13–16.

60. Adams, T. B. (2008). The association of multiple risk factors with fruit and vegetable intake among a nationwide sample of college students. *Journal of American College Health*, 56(4), 55–60.

61. Canadian Food and Inspection Agency. (2014, March 22). *Food irradiation.* Fact sheets. Information for Consumers. www.inspection.gc.ca/food/information-for-consumers/fact-sheets/irradiation/eng/1332358607968/1332358680017

62. Health Canada. (2012, December 12). *The regulation of genetically modified food.* Science and Research. Biotechnology. www.hc-sc.gc.ca/sr-sr/pubs/biotech/reg_gen_mod-eng.php

63. Okanagan Specialty Fruits. (2016). *Arctic apples.* The Perfect Fruit Just Got Even Better. www.arcticapples.com/

64. David Suzuki Foundation. (2014). *Understanding GMO. What you can do.* www.davidsuzuki.org/what-you-can-do/queen-of-green/faqs/food/understanding-gmo/?gclid=COj79IDJ38sCFYpufgodC7gMqg

65. Eat Right Ontario. (2016). *Understanding genetically modified food.* Resources. Food technology/Biotechnology/Novel Foods. www.eatrightontario.ca/en/Articles/Food-technology/Biotechnology/Novel-foods/Understanding-Genetically-Modified-Foods.aspx

66. Health Canada. (2016, January 21). *Food additives and processing aids.* Food and Nutrition. Food Safety. www.hc-sc.gc.ca/fn-an/securit/addit/index-eng.php

Chapter 6

1. World Health Organization (WHO). (2015, January). *Obesity and overweight.* Fact Sheet. Media Centre. www.who.int/mediacentre/factsheets/fs311/en

2. Statistics Canada. (2015, November 27). *Overweight and obese adults (self-reported), 2014.* Health Fact Sheets. Publications. Catalogue no. 82-625-X. www.statcan.gc.ca/pub/82-625-x/2015001/article/14185-eng.htm

3. Ibid.

4. Ibid.

5. Heart and Stroke Foundation. (2013). *2013 report on the health of Canadians.* www.heartandstroke.com/atf/cf/%7B99452D8B-E7F1-4BD6-A57D-B136CE6C95BF%7D/Report-on-Cnd-Health--D17.pdf

6. World Health Organization (WHO). (2015, January). *Obesity and overweight.* Fact Sheet. Media Centre. www.who.int/mediacentre/factsheets/fs311/en/

7. Gotay, C. C., Katzmarzyk, P. T., Janssen, I., Dawson, M. Y., Aminoltejari, K., & Bartley, N. L. (2013). Updating the Canadian obesity maps: An epidemic in progress. *Canadian Journal of Public Health,* 104(1), e64–e68. journal.cpha.ca/index.php/cjph/article/view/3513

8. Watson, S. M., Woodside, J. V., Hunter, S. J., Appleton, K. M., Young, I. S., & McKinley, M. C. (2012). Association between sleep, eating behaviours, cardiovascular risk factors and emotional states in an overweight sample. *The Proceedings of the Nutrition Society,* 71(OCE2), E114.

9. Doyle, S. (2015, November 10). Mapping calorie consumption by country. *National Geographic Magazine.* http://www.canadiangeographic.ca/article/mapping-calorie-consumption-country

10. Phelan, S. (2010). Obesity in the American population: Calories, cost, and culture. *American Journal of Obstetrics and Gynecology,* 203(6), 522–524.

11. Stender, S., Dyerberg, J., & Astrup, A. (2007). Fast food: Unfriendly and unhealthy. *International Journal of Obesity,* 31(6), 887–890.

12. Sweeny, M. M. (2011). Initiating and strengthening college and university instructional physical activity programs: The development of physical activity programs in higher education has been hindered by a number of myths. *The Journal of Physical Education, Recreation and Dance,* 82(4), 17–21.

13. Choquette, A. C., Lemieux, S., Tremblay, A., Drapeau, V., Bouchard, C., Vohle, M. C., & Pérusse, L. (2012, February 01). GAD2 gene sequence variations are associated with eating behaviors and weight gain in women from the Quebec family study. *Physiology and Behavior,* 105(3), 772–776.

14. Frayling, T. M., Timpson, N. J., Weedon, M. N., Zeggini, E., Freathy, R. M., Lindgren, C. M., et al. (2007). A common variant in the FTO gene is associated with body mass index and predisposes to childhood and adult obesity. *Science,* 316(5826), 889–894.

15. Faroogi, S., Rau, H., Whitehead, J., & O'Rahilly, S. (1998). Ob gene mutations and human obesity. *Proceedings of the Nutrition Society,* 57(3), 471–475.

16. Barabási, A. L. (2007). Network medicine—from obesity to the "diseasesome." *New England Journal of Medicine,* 357(4), 404–407.

17. Health Canada. (2012, February 23). Body mass index (BMI) nomogram. *Food and Nutrition.* Archived June 24, 2013. www.hc-sc.gc.ca/fn-an/nutrition/weights-poids/guide-ld-adult/bmi_chart_java-graph_imc_java-eng.php

18. Dieticians of Canada. (2016). BMI Weight Analyzer. www.eatracker.ca/bmi.aspx

19. Government of British Columbia. (2015, February 20). *Interactive tool: What is your child's BMI*? Health Topics A–Z. www.healthlinkbc.ca/healthtopics/content.asp?hwid=tf6820

20. Heart and Stroke Foundation. (2015, May). *Healthy waists. Healthy weights.* Health Information. www.heartandstroke.on.ca/site/c.pvI3IeNWJwE/b.3581989/k.368/Healthy_Living_Healthy_weight_and_waist.htm

21. Price, G. M., Uauy, R., Breeze, E., Bulpitt, C. J., & Fletcher, A. E. (2006). Weight, shape, mortality risk in older persons: Elevated waist-hip ratio, not high body mass index, is associated with a greater risk of death. *American Journal of Clinical Nutrition,* 84(2), 449–460.

22. Lear, S. A., James, P. T., Ko, G. T., & Kumanyika, S. (2010). Appropriateness of waist circumference and waist-to-hip ratio cutoffs for different ethnic groups. *European Journal of Clinical Nutrition,* 64(1), 42–61.

23. Canadian Society for Exercise Physiology (CEP). (2006). *Certified personal trainer's examiner's manual.* Ottawa, ON.

24. D'Alonzo, K. T., Aluf, A., Vincent, L., & Cooper, K. (2009). A comparison of field methods to assess body composition in a diverse group of sedentary women. *Biological Research for Nursing,* 10(3), 2742–2783.

25. Anderson, D. E. (2007). Reliability of air displacement plethysmography. *Journal of Strength and Conditioning Research,* 21(1), 169–172.

26. Speakman, J. R., & Selman, C. (2003). Physical activity and resting metabolic rate. *Proceedings of the Nutrition Society,* 62(3), 621–634.

27. Weibel, E. R. (2005). Exercise-induced maximal metabolic rate scales with muscle aerobic capacity. *Journal of Experimental Biology,* 208(9), 1635–1644.

28. MedicineNet.com. (2005, February 01). Calories burned during fitness activities. www.medicinenet.com/script/main/art.asp?articlekey=10289

29. Hazell, T. J. Hamilton, C. D., Olver, T. D., & Lemon, P. W. R. (2014). Running spring interval training induces fat loss in women. *Applied Physiology, Nutrition, and Metabolism,* 39(8), 944–950.

30. Shiraev, T., & Barclay, G. (2012). Evidence based exercise: Clinical benefits of high intensity interval training. *The Australian Family Physician*, 41(12), 960–962.

31. Saydah, S., Bullard, K. M., Imperatore, G., Geiss, L., & Gregg, E. (2013). Cardiometabolic risk factors among US adolescents and young adults and risk of early mortality. *Pediatrics*, 131(3), e679–e686.

32. Tobias, D., An, P., & Hu, F. B. (2014). BMI and mortality among adults with incident type 2 diabetes. *New England Journal of Medicine*, 370(14), 1361–1364.

33. Borrell, L. N., & Samuel, L. (2014). Body mass index categories and mortality risk in US adults: The effect of overweight and obesity on advancing death. *American Journal of Public Health*, 104(3), 512–519.

34. Richards, S. (2011). Weight management through the development of a healthy lifestyle. *Primary Health Care*, 21(2), 22–24.

35. MedlinePlus. (2016, March 02). *Gastric bypass surgery.* Health Topics. www.nlm.nih.gov/medlineplus/ency/article/007199.htm

36. Christian, J. G., Tsai, A. G., & Bessesen, D. H. (2010). Interpreting weight losses from lifestyle modification trials: Using categorical data. *International Journal of Obesity*, 34(1), 207–209.

37. Dietitians of Canada. (2016). *Find a dietician.* Search for a Dietician. www.dietitians.ca/Your-Health/Find-A-Dietitian/Find-a-Dietitian.aspx

38. Schlundt, David. Personal interview.

39. Dietitians of Canada. (1997–2013). eaTracker. www.eatracker.ca/

40. Kuiper, H. (2003). The scientific basis for risk assessment and regulation of genetically modified foods. *Trends in Food Science & Technology*, 14(5), 277–293.

41. Centre for Science in the Public Interest. (2000, June 22). *Health Canada rejects olestra as a food additive.* For the Record. www.cspinet.org/canada/olestra.html

42. Halton, T. L., Liu, S., Hu, F. B., & Manson, J. E. (2008). Low-carbohydrate-diet score and risk of Type 2 diabetes in women. *American Journal of Clinical Nutrition*, 87(2), 339–346.

43. Johnstone, A. M. (2012). Safety and efficacy of high-protein diets for weight loss. *Proceedings of the Nutrition Society*, 71(2), 339–349.

44. Siri-Tarino, P. W., Sun, Q., Hu, F. B., & Krauss, M. (2010). Meta-analysis of prospective cohort studies evaluating the association of saturated fat with cardiovascular disease. *American Journal of Clinical Nutrition*, 91(3), 535–546.

45. Hall, K., Bemis, T., Brychta, R., Chen, K. Y., Courville, A., Crayner, E. M., et al. (2015). Calorie for calorie, dietary fat restriction results in more body fat loss than carbohydrate restriction in people with obesity, *Cell Metabolism*, 22(3), 427–436.

46. Blanck, H. M., Serdula, M. K., Gillespie, C., Galuska, D. A., Sharpe, P. A., Conway, J. M., et al. (2007). Use of nonprescription dietary supplements for weight loss is common among Americans. *Journal of the American Dietetic Association*, 107(3), 441–447.

47. Levine, J. A. (2005). Interindividual variation in posture allocation: Possible role in human obesity. *Science*, 307(5709), 584–586.

48. Katzmarzyk, P. (2010). Physical activity, sedentary behaviour, and health: Paradigm paralysis or paradigm shift? *Diabetes*, 59(11), 2717–2725, 2723.

49. Ruff, R. R., & Zhen, C. (2014). Estimating the effects of a calorie-based sugar-sweetened beverage tax on weight and obesity in New York city adults using dynamic loss models. *Annals of Epidemiology*, 25(5), 350–357.

50. Adamy, J. (2011, April 01). Arizona proposes a Medicaid fat fee. *The Wall Street Journal.* www.wsj.com/articles/SB10001424052748704530204576235151262336300

51. Puhl, R. M., & Heuer, C. A. (2010). Obesity stigma: Important considerations for public health, *American Journal of Public Health*, 100(6), 1019–1028.

52. Heuer, C. A., McClure, K. J., & Puhl, R. M. (2011). Obesity stigma in online news: A visual content analysis. *Journal of Health Communication*, 16(9), 976–987.

53. Mavromaras, K. (2008). Policy forum: A multidisciplinary view of obesity. Economics and obesity. *The Australian Economic Review*, 41(1), 78–94.

54. Diller, P. A., & Griff, S. (2011). Regulating food retail for obesity prevention: How far can cities go? *Journal of Law, Medicine & Ethics*, 39 (Supplement), 89–93.

55. Wilcox, D., Kennedy-Hagan, K., Rhones, K., Wilkinson, R., & Painter, J. (2008). The effects of social pressure on the eating habits of college students in a restaurant environment. *Journal of the American Dietetic Association*, 108(9), A40.

56. Jung, M. E., Bray, S. R., & Ginis, K. A. (2008). Behavior change and the freshman 15: Tracking physical activity and dietary patterns in first-year university women (Report). *Journal of American College Health*, 56(5), 523–530.

57. Vella-Zarb, R. A., & Elgar, F. J. (2010). Predicting the "freshman 15": Environmental and psychological predictors of weight gain in first-year university students. *Health Education Journal*, 69(3), 321–332.

58. Jackson, R. A., Berry, T. R., & Kennedy, M. D. (2009). The relationship between lifestyle and campus eating behaviors in male and female university students. *College Student Journal*, 43(3), 860–872.

59. Yonashiro, C., Concepcion, R. Y., & Jackson, B. H. (2011). Influence of Hawaiian culture on dietary behaviors of college students. *Research Quarterly for Exercise and Sport*, 82(1), 69–71.

60. York University. (2013, April 24). *Health education and promotion at York.* healthed.scld.yorku.ca/

61. University of Saskatchewan. (2013, May 24). *Eating well on campus.* Stay Healthy, Health and Counselling. students.usask.ca/health/stay-healthy.php

62. Cohen, J. S. (2008, September 07). Friendly to planet, rude to diners: In one of the quirkiest attempts to go green, colleges are removing trays from cafeterias. *Chicago Tribune.* articles.chicagotribune.com/2008-09-07/news/0809070207_1_tray-cafeteria-food-service-provider

63. Queen's University. (n.d.). *Queen's university services.* dining.queensu.ca/todays-menus/

64. University of British Columbia. (n.d.). *Nutrition and food.* Live Well to Learn Well. students.ubc.ca/livewell/topics/nutrition-and-food

65. Lum, L. (2007). Accommodating picky palates: While there remains disagreement over the prevalence of the "Freshman 15," college health and dining officials are trying to help students wade through many convoluted nutritional choices. *Diverse Issues In Higher Education*, 24(5), 13–16.

66. University of Guelph. (2016, March 29).Eating on campus. *Office of the Registrarial Services on Campus.* https://admission.uoguelph.ca/eating

67. Lipka, S. (2011). On campus and online, students lose weight for credit. *Education Digest*, 76(5), 22–24.

68. McCaffree, J. (2001). Eating disorders: All in the family? *Journal of the American Dietetic Association*, 101(6), 622.

69. Wagener, A. M., & Much, K. (2010). Eating disorders as coping mechanisms. *Journal of College Student Psychotherapy*, 24(3), 203–212.

70. Mitka, M. (2001). Magazine ideals wrong. *The Journal of the American Medical Association*, 286(4), 409.

71. Tiggeman, M. (2001). The impact of adolescent girls' life concerns and leisure activities on body dissatisfaction, disordered eating, and self-esteem. *Journal of Genetic Psychology*, 162(2), 133–142.

72. Cohane, G., & Pope, H. (2001). Body image in boys: A review of the literature. *International Journal of Eating Disorders*, 29(4), 373–379.

73. Berry, T., & Lauzon, L. (2004). A content analysis of fitness magazines. *Avante*, 9(1), 25–33.

74. Kubo, C., & Shih, M. Y. (2005). Body shape preference and body satisfaction of Taiwanese and Japanese female college students. *Psychiatry Research*, 133(2–3), 263–271.

75. Treasure, J. (2008). Eating disorders. *Medicine*, 36(8), 430–435.

76. Prouty, A., Protinsky, H. O., & Canady, D. (2002). College women: Eating behaviors and help-seeking preferences. *Adolescence*, 37(146), 353–363.

77. O'Dea, J., & Abraham, S. (2002). Eating and exercise disorders in young college men. *Journal of American College Health*, 50(4), 273–278.

78. Cooley, E., & Toray, T. (2001). Disordered eating in college freshman women: A prospective study. *Journal of American College Health*, 49(5), 229–235.

79. Nasser, M. (2009). Eating disorders across cultures. *Psychiatry*, 8(9), 347–350.

80. Reel, J. J., Petrie, T. A., Greenleaf, C., & Carter, J. (2009). Female collegiate athletes: Prevalence of eating disorders and disordered eating behaviors. *Journal of American College Health*, 57(5), 489–496.

81. Reel, J. J., Petrie, T. A., Greenleaf, C., & Carter, J. (2008). Prevalence of 3 eating disorders and disordered eating among male collegiate athletes. *Psychology of Men and Masculinity*, 9(4), 267–277.

82. Galli, N., Reel, J., Petrie, T., Greenleaf, C., & Carter, J. (2011). Preliminary development of the weight pressures in sport scale for male athletes. *Journal of Sport Behavior*, 34(1), 47–68.

83. BC Division, Centre for Addictions Research of BC. (2015). *Eating disorders*. Fact sheets. Here to Help BC. hereto-help .bc.ca/publications/factsheets/eating-disorders

84. Ibid.

85. Serdar, K., Mazzeo, S. E., Kelly, N., Shivy, V. A., & Wingfield, N. (2011). College students' perceptions of individuals with anorexia and bulimia nervosa. *International Journal of Eating Disorders*, 44(4), 369–375.

86. National Eating Disorder Information Centre (NEDIC). (2012). *Anorexia athletica*. (Compulsive exercising). Definitions. Know the Facts. nedic.ca/know-facts/definitions

87. Serdar, K., Mazzeo, S. E., Kelly, N., Shivy, V. A., & Wingfield, N. (2011). College students' perceptions of individuals with anorexia and bulimia nervosa. *International Journal of Eating Disorders*, 44(4), 369–375.

88. Robinson, A. (2013). Integrative response therapy for binge eating disorder. *Cognitive and Behavioral Practice*, 20(1), 93–105.

89. Dymek-Valentine, M., Hamer, R. M., Bulik, C. M., Woolson, S. L., Reba-Harrelson, L., & Shapiro, J. R. (2007). Feasibility and acceptability of CD-ROM cognitive-behavioral treatment for binge-eating disorder. *European Eating Disorders Review*, 15(3), 175–184.

90. Masson, P. C., Russell-Mayhew, S., & von Ranson, K. M. (2010). How does overeaters anonymous help its members? A qualitative analysis. *European Eating Disorders Review: The Journal of the Eating Disorders Association*, 18(1), 33–42.

Chapter 7

1. Keen, C. (2010, July 07). Partner's self-revelation affects men and women differently in romance. *Ascribe Higher Education News Service*.

2. Jordan, D. J. (2007). *Leadership in leisure services: Making a difference* (2nd ed.). State College, PA: Venture Publishing, Inc.

3. Maple, Marilyn. Personal interview.

4. Ibid.

5. Gullette, D. L., & Lyons, M. A. (2006). Sensation seeking, self-esteem, and unprotected sex in college students. *Journal of the Association of Nurses in AIDS Care*, 17(5), 23–31.

6. Khanchandani, L., & Durham, T. W. (2009). Jealousy during dating among female college students. *College Student Journal*, 43(4), 1272–1278.

7. Bisson, M. A., & Levine, T. R. (2009). Negotiating a friends with benefits relationship. Behavioral Science, *Archives of Sexual Behavior*, 38(1), 66–73.

8. Bogle, K. A. (2008). *Hooking up: Sex, dating, and relationships on campus*. New York: New York University Press.

9. Gute, G., & Eshbaugh, E. M. (2008). Personality as a predictor of hooking up among college students. *Journal of Community Health Nursing*, 25(1), 25–43.

10. Holman, A., & Sillars, A., (2012). Talk about "Hooking Up": The influence of college student social networks on nonrelationship sex. *Health Communication*, 27(2), 2005–2216.

11. Kooyman, L., Pierce, G., & Zavadil, A. (2011). Hooking up and identity development of female college students. *Adultspan*, 10(1), 4–13.

12. Grello, C., Welsh, D., & Harper, M. (2006). No strings attached: The nature of casual sex in college students. *Journal of Sex Research*, 43(3), 255–267.

13. Paul, E. L., & Hayes, K. A. (2002). The casualties of "casual" sex: A qualitative exploration of the phenomenology of college students' hookups. *Journal of Social and Personal Relationships*, 19(5), 639–661.

14. Owen, J., & Fincham, F. D. (2011). Young adults' emotional reactions after hooking up encounters. *Behavioral Science. Archives of Sexual Behavior*, 40(2), 321–330.

15. Downing-Matibag, T. M., & Geisinger, B. (2009). Hooking up and sexual risk taking and college students: A health belief model perspective. *Qualitative Health Research*, 19(9), 1196–1209.

16. American College Health Association. (2009). American college health association—National college health assessment spring 2008 reference group data report (abridged). *Journal of American College Health*, 57(5), 477–488.

17. Bogle, K. A. (2008). *Hooking up sex, dating, and relationships on campus*. New York: New York University Press.

18. Gottlieb, S. L., Newman, L. M., Amin, A., Temmerman, M., & Broutet, N. (2013). Sexually transmitted infections and women's sexual and reproductive health. *International Journal of Gynecology & Obstetrics*, 123(3), 183–184.

19. Wentland, J. J., & Reissing, E. D. (2011). Taking casual sex not too casually: Exploring definitions of casual sexual relationships. *The Canadian Journal of Human Sexuality*, 20(3), 75–91.

20. Lawson, H. M., & Leck, K. (2006). Dynamics of internet dating. *Social Science Computer Review*, 24(2), 189–208.

21. Schleicher, S. S., & Gilbert, L. A. (2005). Heterosexual dating discourses among college students: Is there still a double standard? *Journal of College Psychotherapy*, 19(3), 7–23.

22. Bartoli, A. M., & Clark, M. D. (2006). The dating game: Similarities and differences in dating scripts among college students. *Sexuality & Culture*, 10(4), 54–80.

23. Knox, D., Zusman, M. E., Daniels, V., & Brantley, A. (2002). Absence makes the heart grow fonder? Long distance dating relationships among college students. *College Student Journal*, 36(3), 364–367.

24. McAnulty, R. D., & Brineman, J. M. (2007). Infidelity in dating relationships. *Annual Review of Sex Research*, 18(18), 94–114.

25. Harris, C. R. (2002). Sexual and romantic jealousy in heterosexual and homosexual adults. *Psychological Science*, 13(1), 7–12.

26. Murraya, C. E., & Kardatzke, K. N. (2007). Dating violence among college students: Key issues for college counselors. *Journal of College Counseling*, 10(1), 79–89.

27. Fisher, H. (2007). The laws of chemistry: Whom you are most attracted to reflects the biology of your brain as much as the heat of your heart. It may not have to do with us—it's all about the kids (Cover story). *Psychology Today*, 40(3), 76–81.

28. Johnson, S. (2008). *Hold me tight. Seven conversations for a lifetime of love.* New York: Little, Brown and Company, p. 15.

29. Ibid., p. 15.

30. Tennov, D. (1981). *Love and limerence: The experience of being in love.* New York: Stein and Day.

31. Ibid.

32. Sommers, J., & Vodanovich, S. (2000). Vengeance scores among college students: Examining the role of jealousy and forgiveness. *Education*, 121(1), 114–120.

33. Chapman, G. (2010). *The 5 love languages. The secret to love that lasts.* Chicago: Northfield Publishing, (p.15).

34. Ibid.

35. Love, P., & Stosny, S. (2007). *How to improve your marriage without talking about it. Finding love beyond words.* New York: Broadway Books.

36. Spring, J. A. (2004). *How can I forgive you? The courage to forgive, the freedom not to.* New York: Perennial Currents, Harper Collins Publishers.

37. Yager, J. (2009). *When friendship hurts. How to deal with friends who betray, abandon or wound you.* New York: Simon & Schuster Inc. Fireside Books.

38. Miller, L. (2007). Physical abuse in college dating relationships. *Research Quarterly for Exercise and Sport*, 78(1), A–33.

39. Anderson, E. (2010). "At least with cheating there is an attempt at monogamy": Cheating and monogamism among undergraduate heterosexual men. *Journal of Social and Personal Relationships*, 27(7), 851–872.

40. Ibid.

41. Common Law Separation Canada.com. (2012, March 26). *Common law separation Canada FAQs.* www.common-law-separation-canada.com/common-law-separation-Canada.htm; www.common-law-separation-canada.com/index.php?s=FAQs

42. Common Law Separation Canada.com. (2003–2013). *Differences.* www.common-law-separation-canada.com/differences.htm

43. Canadian Bar Association. (2014, November). *Marriage agreements and cohabitation agreements.* For the Public. www.cbabc.org/For-the-Public/Dial-A-Law/Scripts/Family-Law/162

44. Common Law Separation Canada.com. (2003–2013). *Differences.* Canada's leading resource for unmarried couples who are separating. www.common-law-separation-canada.com/

45. Grant, T. (2012, September 06). Statistics Canada to stop tracking marriage and divorce rates. *The Globe and Mail.* www.theglobeandmail.com/news/national/statistics-canada-to-stop-tracking-marriage-and-divorce-rates/article4192704/

46. Countrymeters. (2016, April 01). *Canada population.* countrymeters.info/en/Canada

47. Statistics Canada. (2015, November 02). Population by marital status and sex. *The Daily.* www.statcan.gc.ca/tables-tableaux/sum-som/l01/cst01/famil01-eng.htm

48. Sternberg, Robert. Personal interview.

49. Harder, L. (2011). After the nuclear age? Some contemporary developments in families and family law in Canada. *Vanier Institute of the Family.* vanierinstitute.ca/wp-content/uploads/2015/12/CFT_2011-10-00_EN.pdf

50. Carman, T. (2016, February 04). Large refugee families hard to house in B. C. Officials discuss sending newcomers to rural parts of B. C. *The Vancouver Sun.* www.vancouversun.com/large+refugee+families+hard+house/11696101/story.html?_lsa=5b37-d903

51. Statistics Canada. (2015, December 22). *Living arrangement of young adults aged 20 to 29.* Census in Brief. Catalogue no. 98-312-X-2011003. www12.statcan.gc.ca/census-recensement/2011/as-sa/98-312-x/98-312-x2011003_3-eng.cfm

52. Statistics Canada. (2008, October 14). *2006 Census information on same-sex common-law and married couples.* Census. 2006 Census: Reference Material. Archived Content. www12.statcan.ca/census-recensement/2006/ref/info/same_sex-meme_sexe-eng.cfm

53. Statistics Canada. (2012, September 19). 2011 Census of population: Families, households, marital status, structural type of dwelling, collectives. *The Daily.* Archived Content. www.statcan.gc.ca/daily-quotidien/120919/dq120919a-eng.htm

54. Hurley, M. D. (2005, February 02). *Bill C-38: The civil marriage act.* Parliament of Canada. www.lop.parl.gc.ca/About/Parliament/LegislativeSummaries/bills_ls.asp?ls=c38&Parl=38&Ses=1

55. DeSilver, D. (2013, June 26). *Supreme court's ruling comes as majority now supports same-sex marriage.* Fact Tank. Publications. Pew Research Centre. www.pewresearch.org/fact-tank/2013/06/26/supreme-courts-doma-ruling-comes-as-majority-now-supports-same-sex-marriage/

56. Bosse, J., & Chiodo, L. (2016). It is complicated: Gender and sexual orientation identity in LGBTQ youth. *Journal of Clinical Nursing*, 25(23–24), 3665–3675.

57. Aleshire, M.E. (2016). Sexual orientation, gender identity, and gender expression: What are they? *The Journal for Nurse Practitioners*, 12(7), e329–e330.

58. Bosse, J., & Chiodo, L. (2016). It is complicated: Gender and sexual orientation identity in LGBTQ youth. *Journal of Clinical Nursing*, 25(23–24), 3665–3675.

59. Reddy-Best, K.L., & Pedersen, E.L. (2014). The relationship of gender expression, sexual identity, distress, appearance, and clothing choices for queer women. *International Journal of Fashion Design, Technology and Education*, 8(1), 54–65.

60. Thomas, D. (2014, April 23). *The Census and the evolution of gender roles in early 20th century Canada.* Publications. Statistics Canada. Archived Content. www.statcan.gc.ca/pub/11-008-x/2010001/article/11125-eng.htm

61. Intersex. In *Dictionary.com* (2016). www.dictionary.com/browse/intersex

62. Levitt, H. M., & Ippolito, M. R. (2014). Being transgender: The experience of transgender identity development. *Journal of Homosexuality*, 61(12), 1727–1758.

63. Moser, C. (2016). Defining sexual orientation. *Archives of Sexual Behaviour*, 45(3), 505–508.

64. Carver, P.R., Egan, S.K., & Perry, D.G. (2004). Children who question their heterosexuality. *Developmental Psychology*, 40(1), 43-53.

65. Jackson, S. (2006). Gender, sexuality and heterosexuality. *Feminist Theory*, 7(1), 105–121.

66. *Kinsey's heterosexual-homosexual rating scale.* (1996–2016). The Kinsey Institute. www.kinseyinstitute.org/research/ak-hhscale.html

67. Guth, L.J., Lopez, D.F., Rojas, J., Clements, K.D., & Tyler, J.M. (2010). Experiential versus rational training: A comparison of student attitudes toward homosexuality. *Journal of Homosexuality*, 48(2), 83–102.

68. Jannini, E. A., Blanchard, R., Camperior-Ciani, A., & Bancroft, J. (2010). Male homosexuality: Nature or culture? *The Journal of Sexual Medicine*, 7(10), 3245–3253.

69. Guth, L.J., Lopez, D.F., Rojas, J., Clements, K.D., & Tyler, J.M. (2010). Experiential versus rational training: A comparison of student attitudes toward homosexuality. *Journal of Homosexuality*, 48(2), 83–102.

70. Bos, H. M. W., van Balen, F., & van den Boom, D. C. (2007). Child adjustment and parenting in planned lesbian-parent families. *American Journal of Orthopsychiatry*, 77(1), 38–48.

71. 2 Spirits.com. (2015). *2 spirited people of the 1st Nations.* Information guide. www.2spirits.com/PDFolder/2SpiritInfoGuide05.pdf

72. Elia, J.P. (2014). Bisexuality in Education: Exploring the experiences, resourcing, and representations of bisexual students, bisexual parents, and educators in educational systems – a discussion. *Journal of Bisexuality*, 14(1), 146-150.

73. Kaestle, C. E., & Allen, K. R. (2011). The role of masturbation in healthy sexual development: Perceptions of young adults. *Archives of Sexual Behavior*, 40(5), 983–994.

74. Toews, M. L., & Yazedjian, A. (2012). College students' knowledge, attitudes, and behaviors regarding sex and contraceptives. *Journal of Family and Consumer Sciences*, 104(3), 16–23.

75. American College Health Association. (2013). American college health association—national college health assessment II. *Canadian consortium reference group executive summary Spring 2013.* Hanover, MD: American College Health Association. www.cacuss.ca/_Library/documents/NCHA-II_WEB_SPRING_2013_CANADIAN_REFERENCE_GROUP_DATA_REPORT.pdf

76. Schwartz, D. (2013, June 22). We're happy with our sex lives. *CBC News.* www.cbc.ca/news/health/we-re-happy-with-our-sex-lives-canadian-university-students-say-1.1376119

77. Lam, C. B. (2013). Risky sexual behaviors in emerging adults: Longitudinal changes and within-person variations. *Archives of Sexual Behavior*, 42(4), 523–532.

78. Novik, M. G., Howard, D. E., & Boekeloo, B. O. (2011). Drinking motivations and experiences of unwanted sexual advances among undergraduate students. *Journal of Interpersonal Violence*, 26(1), 34–49.

79. Scott-Sheldon, L. A. J., Carey, M. P., & Carey, K. B. (2010). Alcohol and risky sexual behavior among heavy drinking college students. *Aids and Behavior*, 14(4), 845–853.

80. Johnson, N. L., & Johnson, D. M. (2013). Factors influencing the relationship between sexual trauma and risky behavior in college students. *Journal of Interpersonal Violence*, 28(11), 2315–2331.

81. Devdas, N. R., & Rubin, L. J. (2007). Rape myth acceptance among first- and second-generation south Asian American women. *Sex Roles*, 56(9), 701–705.

82. Whitty, M. T., & Quigley, L. L. (2008). Emotional and sexual infidelity offline and in cyberspace. *Journal of Marital and Family Therapy*, 34(4), 461–468.

83. Millner, V. S. (2008). Internet infidelity: A case of intimacy with detachment. *The Family Journal: Counseling Therapy for Couples and Families*, 16(1), 78–92.

84. Groothof, H. A. K. (2009). Sex differences in jealousy: The case of internet infidelity. *Journal of Social and Personal Relationships*, 26(8), 1119–1129.

85. Whitty, M. (2008). Liberating or debilitating? An examination of romantic relationships, sexual relationships and friendships on the Net. *Computers in Human Behavior*, 24, 1837–1850.

86. Liamputtong, P. (2008). Online dating and mating: The use of the internet to meet sexual partners. *Qualitative Health Research*, 18(2), 268–279.

87. McCown, J. A., Fischer, D., Page, R., & Homant, M. (2001). Internet relationships: People who meet people. *Cyber Psychology & Behaviour*, 4(5), 593–596.

88. Toomey, K., & Rothenberg, R. (2000). Sex and cyberspace—Virtual networks leading to high-risk sex. *Journal of the American Medical Association*, 284, 484–487.

89. Winkelman , S. B., Smith, K., Brinkley, J., & Knox, D. (2014). Sexting on the college campus. *Journal of Human Sexuality*, 17(1), 1.

90. Humphreys, T., & Herold, E. (2007). Sexual consent in heterosexual relationships: Development of a new measure. *Sex Roles*, 57(3), 305–317.

91. Beres, M. A., Herold, E., & Maitland, S. B. (2004). Sexual consent behaviors in same-sex relationships. *Archives of Sexual Behavior*, 33(5), 475–486.

92. Dimmock, P., et al. (2000). Efficacy of selective serotonin-reuptake inhibitors in premenstrual syndrome: A systematic review. *Lancet*, 356(9236), 1131-1136.

93. Harder, B. (2005). Preventing PMS. *Science News*, 167(25), 387–388.

94. Medhurst, R. (2010). Homeopathy for PMS. *Journal of the Australian Traditional-Medicine Society*, 16(1), 17–18.

95. Biggs, W. S. (2011). Premenstrual syndrome and premenstrual dysphoric disorder. *American Family Physician*, 84(8), 918–924.

96. Ravindran, L. N., Woods, A. A., Steiner, M., & Ravindran, A. V. (2007). Symptom-onset dosing with citalopram in the treatment of premenstrual dysphoric disorder (PMDD): A case series. *Archives of Women's Mental Health*, 10(3), 125–127.

97. Hochwalt, A. E. (2010). Clinical safety assessment of an ultra absorbency menstrual tampon. *Journal of Women's Health*, 19(2), 273–278.

98. Sorokan, S. T., Finlay, J. C., & Jefferies, A. L. (2015). Newborn male circumcision. *Canadian Paediatric Society*, 20(6), 311–315.

99. Ingraham, C. (2015, May 26). Americans truly are exceptional—at least when it comes to circumcision. *The Washington Post.* www.washingtonpost.com/news/wonk/wp/2015/05/26/americans-truly-are-exceptional-at-least-when-it-comes-to-circumcision/

100. SexualityandU.ca (2013, March). *Male circumcision: Recent research on its potential health benefits.* Research. Sex Information and Education Council of Canada (SIECCAN). sexualityandu.ca/uploads/files/CTR_MaleCircumcision_MAR2013-ENG.pdf

101. Ibid.

Chapter 8

1. Peipert, J. F., Madden, T., Allsworth, J. E., & Secura, G. (2012). Preventing unintended pregnancies by providing no-cost contraception. *Obstetrics & Gynecology*, 120(6), 1291–1297.

2. Miller, L. M. (2011). College student knowledge and attitudes toward emergency contraception. *Contraception*, 83(1), 68–73.

3. Huber Brunner, L. R., & Ersek, J. L. (2009). Contraceptive use among sexually active university students. *Journal of Women's Health*, 18(7), 1063–1070.

4. Moore, E. W., & Smith, W. E. (2012). What college students do not know: Where are the gaps in sexual health knowledge? *Journal of American College Health*, 60(6), 436–442.

5. Oswalt, S. B., Cameron, K. A., & Koob, J. J. (2005). Sexual regret in college students. *Archives of Sexual Behavior*, 34(6), 663–669.

6. Halifax Sexual Health Centre. (n.d.). *Spermicide.* www.hshc.ca/?q=content/spermicide

7. SexualityandU.ca (2012). *Emergency contraception (morning after pill).* Birth Control. www.sexualityandu.ca/birth-control/emergency-contraception-morning-after-pill

8. Holland, K. J., & French, S. E. (2012). Condom negotiation strategy use and effectiveness among college students. *Journal of Sex Research*, 45(5), 443–453.

9. Riley, N. S. (2005). Happy—and chaste—on the college campus. *Chronicle of Higher Education*, 51(44), 12–13.

10. Sprecher, S., & Treger, S. (2015). Virgin college students' reasons for and reactions to their abstinence from sex: Results from a 23-year study at a Midwestern U. S. university. *Journal of Sex Research*, 52(8), 936–948.

11. SexualityandU.ca (2012). *Hormonal methods.* Birth Control. www.sexualityandu.ca/birth-control/hormonal-methods

12. Planned Parenthood Federation of America. (2013). *The birth control pill: A history.* https://www.plannedparenthood.org/files/1213/9611/6329/pillhistory.pdf

13. Goldin, C., & Katz, L. (2002). The power of the pill: Oral contraceptives and women's career and marriage decisions. *Journal of Political Economy*, 110(4), 730–770.

14. Bassuk, S. S., & Manson, J. E., (2015). Oral contraceptives and menopausal hormone therapy: Relative and attributable risks of cardiovascular disease, cancer, and other health outcomes. *Annals of Epidemiology*, 25(3), 193–200.

15. Rott, H. (2012). Thrombotic risks of oral contraceptives. *Current Opinion in Obstetrics & Gynecology*, 24(4), 235–240.

16. Davidson, N., & Helzsouer, K. (2002). Good news about oral contraceptives. *New England Journal of Medicine*, 346(26), 2078–2079.

17. Marchbanks, P., McDonald, J. A., Wilson, H. G., Folger, S. G., Mandel, M. G., Daling, J. R., Bernstein, L., et al. (2002). Oral contraceptives and the risk of breast cancer. *New England Journal of Medicine*, 346(26), 2025–2026.

18. Marchbanks, P. A., Curtisa, K. M., Mandela, M. G., Wilson, H. G., Jenga, G., Folgera, S. G., et al. (2012). Oral contraceptive formulation and risk of breast cancer. *Contraception*, 85(4), 342–350.

19. Beaber, E. F., Malone, K. E., Tang, M. C., Barlow, W. E., Porter, P. L., Daling, J. R., et al. (2014). Oral contraceptives and breast cancer risk overall and by molecular subtype among young women. *Cancer Epidemiology, Biomarkers & Prevention* (A publication of the American Association for Cancer Research, cosponsored by the American Society of Preventive), 23(5), 755–764.

20. Archer, D. F. (2006). Menstrual-cycle-related symptoms: A review of the rationale for continuous use of oral contraceptives. *Contraception*, 74(5), 359–366.

21. SexualityandU.ca. (2012). *Oral contraceptive.* Hormonal Methods. Birth Control. www.sexualityandu.ca/birth-control/hormonal-methods

22. Ibid.

23. Ibid.

24. Westhoff, C., Jones, K., Robilotto, C., Heartwell, S., Edwards, S., Zieman, M., & Cushman, L. (2009). Smoking and oral contraceptive continuation. *Contraception*, 79(5), 375–378.

25. Chadwick, K. D., Burkman, R. T., Tornesi, B. M., & Mahadevan, B. (2011). Fifty years of "the pill": Risk reduction and discovery of benefits. *Toxicological Sciences*, 125(1), 2–9.

26. Walsemann, K. M., & Perez, A. D. (2006). Anxiety's relationship to inconsistent use of oral contraceptives. *Health Education and Behavior*, 33(2), 197–214.

27. National Health Service. (NHS). (2014, November 06). *What is the male pill?* Contraception Guide. Health A-Z. www.nhs.uk/Conditions/contraception-guide/Pages/male-pill.aspx

28. SexualityandU.ca. (2012). *Vaginal contraceptive ring (NuvaRing®).* Birth Control. Health Care Professionals. www.sexualityandu.ca/health-care-professionals/contraceptive-methods/vaginal-contraceptive-ring

29. Sexualityandu.ca. (2012). *Contraceptive patch.* Hormonal Methods. Birth Control. www.sexualityandu.ca/birth-control/hormonal-methods

30. Mayo Clinic. (1998–2016). *Overview. Birth control patch.* Patient Care and Health Information. www.mayoclinic.org/tests-procedures/birth-control-patch/home/ovc-20167246

31. O'Connell, K., & Burkman, R. T. (2007). The transdermal contraceptive patch: An updated review of the literature. *Clinical Obstetrics and Gynecology*, 50(4), 918–926.

32. Shulman, L. P. (2011). The state of hormonal contraception today: Benefits and risks of hormonal contraceptives: Combined estrogen and progestin contraceptives. *American Journal of Obstetrics and Gynecology*, 205(4), Supplement, S9–S13.

33. Phelps, J. Y., & Kelver, M. A. (2009). Confronting the legal risks of prescribing the contraceptive patch with ongoing litigation. *Obstetrics and Gynecology*, 113(3), 712–716.

34. Edelman, A. (2008, May). Blood clots and the patch. *OB/Gyn Clinic Alert*, 25(1), 1–8.

35. Sexualityandu.ca. (2012). *Injection (Depo-Provera®).* Hormonal Methods. Birth Control. www.sexualityandu.ca/birth-control/hormonal-methods

36. Health Canada. (2005, June 30). *Public advisory: Endorsed important safety information on DEPO-PROVERA (medroxyprogesterone acetate).* Recalls and Alerts. Archived

Content. Revised (2013, March 15). healthycanadians.gc.ca/recall-alert-rappel-avis/hc-sc/2005/14159a-eng.php

37. Options for Sexual Health. (2016, March). *Intrauterine devices (IUD)*. Birth Control Options. Birth Control and Pregnancy. www.optionsforsexualhealth.org/birth-control-pregnancy/birth-control-options/iuds

38. Ibid.

39. Ibid.

40. Paladine, H. L., Blenning, C. E., Judkins, D. Z., & Mittal, S. (2006). Clinical inquiries: What are contraindications to IUDs? *The Journal of Family Practice*, 55(8), 726–729.

41. Hirozawa, A. (2001). A first pregnancy may be difficult to achieve after long-term use of an IUD. *Family Planning Perspectives*, 33(4), 181–182.

42. Hollander, D. (2002). IUD ifs, ands and buts. *Family Planning Perspectives*, 34(2), 60.

43. Options for Sexual Health. (2009, March). *Diaphragm*. Barrier Methods. Birth Control Options. www.optionsforsexualhealth.org/birth-control-pregnancy/birth-control-options/barrier-methods/diaphragm

44. HealthLink BC. (2015, May 22). *Treatment overview*. Barrier Methods of Birth Control. Health Topics A–Z. www.healthlinkbc.ca/healthtopics/content.asp?hwid=hw138685

45. MyHealth. Alberta.ca (2015, May 22). *Diaphragm for birth control*. Health A–Z. Health Information and Tools. my-health.alberta.ca/Health/Pages/conditions.aspx?hwid=tw9508

46. Options for Sexual Health. (2009, March). *Diaphragm*. Barrier Methods. Birth Control Options. www.optionsforsexualhealth.org/birth-control-pregnancy/birth-control-options/barrier-methods

47. Yranski, P. A., & Gamache, M. E. (2008). New options for barrier contraception. *Journal of Obstetric, Gynecologic, & Neonatal Nursing*, 27(3), 384–389.

48. FemCapCanada.ca (2016). *What is the FemCap?* FemCap Details. www.femcapcanada.ca/femcap-details/

49. Options for Sexual Health. (2009, March). *(External) male condoms*. Birth Control Options. Birth Control & Pregnancy. www.optionsforsexualhealth.org/birth-control-pregnancy/birth-control-options/barrier-methods/condom-male

50. Ibid.

51. Tolani, A., & Yen, S. (2010). College students' perceptions and use of withdrawal, condoms, and emergency contraception. *Journal of Adolescent Health*, 46(2, S1), S55–S56.

52. Ford, K., Woosung, S., & Lepkowski, J. (2001). Characteristics of adolescents' sexual partners and their association with use of condoms and other contraceptive methods. *Family Planning Perspectives*, 33(3), 100–105.

53. Options for Sexual Health. (2009, March). *Internal (female condom)*. Barrier Methods. Birth Control Options. www.optionsforsexualhealth.org/birth-control-pregnancy/birth-control-options/barrier-methods/condom-female

54. Ibid.

55. Options for Sexual Health. (2016). *Spermicides*. Barrier Methods. Birth Control Options. www.optionsforsexualhealth.org/birth-control-pregnancy/birth-control-options/barrier-methods/spermicides

56. SexualityandU.ca (2012). *What is a contraceptive sponge and how does it work?* Frequently Asked Questions. www.sexualityandu.ca/health-care-professionals/contraceptive-methods/sponge

57. Options for Sexual Health. (2009, March). *Fertility awareness method (FAM)*. Birth Control Options. www.optionsforsexualhealth.org/birth-control-pregnancy/birth-control-options/natural-methods/fam

58. Government of Canada. (2014, March 26). *Emergency contraceptive pills to carry warnings for reduced effectiveness in women over a certain body weight*. Healthy Canadians. healthycanadians.gc.ca/recall-alert-rappel-avis/hc-sc/2014/38701a-eng.php

59. HealthLink BC. (2014, November). *Emergency contraception (EC)*. HealthLinkBC Files. www.healthlinkbc.ca/healthfiles/hfile91b.stm

60. Government of Canada. (2014, March 26). *Emergency contraceptive pills to carry warnings for reduced effectiveness in women over a certain body weight*. Healthy Canadians. healthycanadians.gc.ca/recall-alert-rappel-avis/hc-sc/2014/38701a-eng.php

61. Options for Sexual Health. (2009, March). *Sterilization*. Birth Control Options. Birth Control & Pregnancy. www.optionsforsexualhealth.org/birth-control-pregnancy/birth-control-options/barrier-methods/sterilization

62. Abortion Rights Coalition of Canada. (2016, March 11). *Statistics: Abortion in Canada*. www.arcc-cdac.ca/backrounders/statistics-abortion-in-canada.pdf

63. Peritz, I. (2016, April 01). In PEI, the right to choose: No longer 'the shame of being shipped off the island'. *The Globe and Mail*. www.theglobeandmail.com/news/national/prince-edward-island-to-end-its-34-year-ban-on-abortions/article29504348/

64. Options for Sexual Health. (2009, March). *Medical abortion*. Abortion. Birth Control & Pregnancy. www.optionsforsexualhealth.org/birth-control-pregnancy/pregnancy/medical-abortion

65. Options for Sexual Health. (2009, March). *Surgical abortion*. Abortion. Birth Control & Pregnancy. www.optionsforsexualhealth.org/birth-control-pregnancy/pregnancy/surgical-abortion

66. Major, B., Appelbaum, M., Beckman, L., Dutton, M. A., Russo, N. F., & West, C. (2009). Abortion and mental health. Evaluating the evidence. *American Psychologist*, 64(9), 863–890.

67. Curley, M., & Johnston, C. (2013). The characteristics and severity of psychological distress after abortion among university students. *The Journal of Behavioral Health Services & Research*, 40(3), 279–293.

68. Greene Foster, D., Gould, H., & Kimport, K. (2012). How women anticipate coping after an abortion. *Contraception*, 86(1), 84–90.

69. CBC News Canada. (2009, January 13). (Updated 2013, May 30). *Abortion rights: Significant moments in Canadian history*. www.cbc.ca/news/canada/abortion-rights-significant-moments-in-canadian-history-1.787212

70. Life Canada. (2012). *Our mission and vision*. Introduction and Mission. Who We Are. www.lifecanada.org/who-we-are/mission

71. Youth Protecting Youth. (n.d.). *About us*. youthprotectingyouth.com/about/

72. National Campus Life Network. (2016). *About*. www.ncln.ca/about/

73. Pearse, A. (2016, April 08). Personal interview.

74. Statistics Canada. (2015, September 29). *Births, estimates, by province and territory*. Births and Deaths. www.statcan.gc.ca/tables-tableaux/sum-som/l01/cst01/demo04a-eng.htm

75. Statistics Canada. (2016, February 10). Births 2012. *The Daily*. www.statcan.gc.ca/daily-quotidien/160210/dq160210b-eng.htm

76. Calleja-Agius, J., Jauniaux, E., & Muttukrishna, S. (2012). Inflammatory cytokines in maternal circulation and placenta of

chromosomally abnormal first trimester miscarriages. *Clinical and Developmental Immunology*, Article ID 175041.

77. Sater, M. S., Finan, R. R., Mustafa, F. E., Al-Khateeb, G. M., & Almawi, W. Y. (2011). Anti-annexin V lgM and IgG autoantibodies and the risk of idiopathic recurrent spontaneous miscarriage. *Journal of Reproductive Immunology*, 89(1), 78–83.
78. Government of Canada. (2013, February 04). *Fertility.* Healthy Pregnancy. healthycanadians.gc.ca/healthy-living-vie-saine/pregnancy-grossesse/fertility-fertilite/fert-eng.php
79. Government of Canada. (2013, February 05). Fertility treatment options. *Fertility.* Healthy Pregnancy. healthycanadians.gc.ca/healthy-living-vie-saine/pregnancy-grossesse/fertility-fertilite/treatment-traitement-eng.php
80. Levine, A. D. (2011). The oversight and practice of oocyte donation in the United States, United Kingdom and Canada. *HEC Forum*, 23(1), 15–30.
81. Canadian Fertility and Andrology Society. (2014, September 12). *Human assisted reproduction 2014: Live birth rates for Canada.* Media Releases. Public Affairs and News. www.cfas.ca/index.php?option=com_content&view=article&id=1363%3Ahuman-assisted-reproduction-2014-live-birth-rates-for-canada&catid=1012%3Acartr&Itemid=130
82. Norris, S., & Tiedemann, M. (2015, April 09). *Legal status at the federal level of assisted human reproduction in Canada. Background paper.* Current Publications. Law, Justice and Rights. Library of Parliament. Publication No. 2011-82-E. Ottawa, Canada. www.lop.parl.gc.ca/content/lop/ResearchPublications/2011-82-e.htm

Chapter 9

1. Chain of Infection. In *Medical Dictionary. The Free Dictionary.* (2016). medical-dictionary.thefreedictionary.com/Chain+of+Infection
2. Virus. In *Medical Dictionary. The Free Dictionary.* (2016). medical-dictionary.thefreedictionary.com/Virus+(biology)
3. International Speciality Supply. (2014). *Viruses, food safety and sprouts.* Sprout Net. www.sproutnet.com/Viruses
4. Microbe World. (2006). *Virus or bacterium?* Meet the Microbes. http://www.microbeworld.org/what-is-a-microbe/virus-or-bacterium
5. Microbe World. (2006). *Bacteria.* Meet the Microbes. http://www.microbeworld.org/types-of-microbes/bacteria
6. American Society for Microbiology (ASM). (2007, February). Basic research on bacteria. The essential frontier. *Report on the American Society for Microbiology and National Institutes of Health Workshop on Basic Bacterial Research.* www.asm.org/ccLibraryFiles/FILENAME/000000002932/NIHASM BacteriaReport.pdf
7. Microbe World. (2006). *Fungi.* Types of Microbes. Meet the Microbes. http://www.microbeworld.org/types-of-microbes/fungi
8. Ibid.
9. World Health Organization (WHO). (2015, December 09). *Fact sheet: Malaria report 2015.* www.who.int/malaria/media/world-malaria-report-2015/en/
10. Public Health Agency of Canada. (2015, June 01). *Public health reminder: West Nile virus.* West Nile Virus. www.phac-aspc.gc.ca/phn-asp/2015/wnv-vno-eng.php
11. Government of Canada. (2016, January 05). *Surveillance of West Nile virus.* West Nile Virus. Diseases. healthycanadians.gc.ca/diseases-conditions-maladies-affections/disease-maladie/west-nile-nil-occidental/surveillance-eng.php
12. Government of Canada. (2016, February 10). *West Nile virus.* Diseases. Diseases and Conditions. healthycanadians.gc.ca/diseases-conditions-maladies-affections/disease-maladie/west-nile-nil-occidental/index-eng.php
13. Government of Canada. (2016, January 05). *Surveillance of West Nile virus.* West Nile Virus. Diseases. healthycanadians.gc.ca/diseases-conditions-maladies-affections/disease-maladie/west-nile-nil-occidental/surveillance-eng.php
14. Government of Canada. (2016, January 16). *Rapid risk assessment: The risk of Zika virus to Canadians.* Diseases. Diseases and Conditions. www.healthycanadians.gc.ca/publications/diseases-conditions-maladies-affections/risks-zika-virus-risques/index-eng.php?id=publication_rapid_risk
15. Government of Canada. (2016, April 04). *Causes of Zika virus.* Diseases. Diseases and Conditions. healthycanadians.gc.ca/diseases-conditions-maladies-affections/disease-maladie/zika-virus/causes-eng.php?id=causes
16. Government of Canada. (2016, April 04). *Symptoms of Zika virus.* Diseases. Diseases and Conditions. healthycanadians.gc.ca/diseases-conditions-maladies-affections/disease-maladie/zika-virus/symptoms-symptomes-eng.php?id=symptoms
17. Government of Canada. (2016, April 04). *Risks of Zika virus.* Diseases. Diseases and Conditions. healthycanadians.gc.ca/diseases-conditions-maladies-affections/disease-maladie/zika-virus/risks-risques-eng.php?id=risks
18. Public Health Agency of Canada. (2015, October 20). *E. coli. Fact sheet.* Food Safety. www.phac-aspc.gc.ca/fs-sa/fs-fi/ecoli-eng.php
19. European Food Safety Authority. (2011). Shiga toxin-producing E. coli (STEC) O104:H4 2011 outbreaks in Europe: Taking stock. *EFSA Journal*, 9(10), 2390–2422. www.efsa.europa.eu/en/efsajournal/pub/2390
20. Public Health Agency of Canada. (2015, May 26). *Salmonella.* Fact Sheet. Food Safety. www.phac-aspc.gc.ca/fs-sa/fs-fi/salmonella-eng.php
21. Public Health Agency of Canada. (2016, March 04). Public health notice—outbreak of salmonella infections under investigation. *Public Health Notices.* www.phac-aspc.gc.ca/phn-asp/2015/salmonella-infantis-eng.php
22. Government of Canada. (2013, April 05). *Botulism (Clostridium botulinum).* Food Poisoning. Food and Nutrition. healthycanadians.gc.ca/eating-nutrition/risks-recalls-rappels-risques/poisoning-intoxication/poisoning-intoxication/botulism-botulisme-eng.php
23. Government of Canada. (2013, January 08). *Infant botulism.* Food Safety for Vulnerable Populations. www.healthycanadians.gc.ca/eating-nutrition/healthy-eating-saine-alimentation/safety-salubrite/vulnerable-populations/infant-botulism-botulisme-eng.php
24. Government of Canada. (2013, March 11). *Trichinellosis—Fact sheet.* Reportable. Diseases. Canadian Food and Inspection Agency. www.inspection.gc.ca/animals/terrestrial-animals/diseases/reportable/trichinellosis/fact-sheet/eng/1330023015817/1330023110684
25. Government of Canada. (2016, February 10). *Listeria and listeriosis.* Food Poisoning. Food Poisoning and Other Risks. healthycanadians.gc.ca/eating-nutrition/risks-recalls-rappels-risques/poisoning-intoxication/poisoning-intoxication/listeriosis-listeria-listeriose-eng.php
26. Alberta.ca. (2015, April 27). *Bovine spongiform encephalopathy (BSE) fact sheet.* Agriculture and Forestry. www1.agric.gov.ab.ca/$department/deptdocs.nsf/all/cpv8104
27. Costandi, M. (2013, February 14). Proteins behind mad-cow disease also help brain to develop. Nature. *International*

Weekly Journal of Science. www.nature.com/news/proteins-behind-mad-cow-disease-also-help-brain-to-develop-1.12428

28. World Health Organization. (WHO). (2016). *Results of round I of the WHO international scheme to evaluate household water treatment technologies.* Water, Sanitation, Hygiene and Health Unit Department of Public Health, Environmental and Social Determinants of Health World Health Organization. apps.who.int/iris/bitstream/10665/204284/1/9789241509947_eng.pdf?ua=1
29. Government of Canada. (2012, February 16). *Frequently asked questions.* Environment and Climate Change Canada. www.ec.gc.ca/eau-water/default.asp?lang=En&n=1C100657-1#ws46B1DCCC
30. Health Canada. (2015, June 05). *Guidelines for Canadian drinking water quality— summary table.* Environmental and Workplace Health. www.hc-sc.gc.ca/ewh-semt/pubs/water-eau/sum_guide-res_recom/index-eng.php
31. Livernois, J. (2001). *The Walkerton inquiry. Commissioned paper 14. The economic costs of the Walkerton water crisis.* Ministry of Attorney General. www.uoguelph.ca/~live/Livernois_14%20Final%20Report.pdf
32. O'Connor, D. R. (Hon.). (2002, January 18). *Part one: A summary report of the Walkerton inquiry: The events of May 2000 and related issues.* Ontario Ministry of the Attorney General. Toronto: Publications Ontario. http://www.archives.gov.on.ca/en/e_records/walkerton/
33. Lui, E. (2015, March). *On notice for a drinking water crisis in Canada.* Council of Canadians. canadians.org/sites/default/files/publications/report-drinking-water-0315_0.pdf
34. Health Canada. (2016, March 03). *Drinking water advisories in First Nations communities.* First Nations and Inuit Health. www.hc-sc.gc.ca/fniah-spnia/promotion/public-publique/water-dwa-eau-aqep-eng.php
35. Vector-born transmission. In *The Free Dictionary.* (2016). www.thefreedictionary.com/vector-borne+transmission
36. Scholthof, K. B. G. (2007). The disease triangle: Pathogens, the environment and society. *Nature Reviews Microbiology*, 5(2), 152–156.
37. Canadian Centre for Occupational Health and Safety. (CCOHS). (2016, April 11). *Hand washing: Reducing the risk of common infections.* Diseases, Disorders and Injuries. OHS Answers Fact Sheets. www.ccohs.ca/oshanswers/diseases/washing_hands.html
38. Immunize Canada. (2016, April 11). *What is immunization?* Learn about Immunization. immunize.ca/en/learn/what-is-immunization.aspx
39. Shen, A. K., Fields, R., & McQuestion, M. (2014). The future of routine immunizations in the developing world: Challenges and opportunities. *Global Health: The Science and Practice*, 2(4), 381–394.
40. World Health Organziation. (WHO). (2016). *Immunization.* Health Topics. www.who.int/topics/immunization/en/
41. Public Health Agency of Canada. (2015, May 20). *Canadian immunization guide.* Immunizations and Vaccines. www.phac-aspc.gc.ca/publicat/cig-gci/index-eng.php
42. Government of Canada. (2016, March 09). *Provincial and territorial immunization information.* Immunizations and Vaccines. healthycanadians.gc.ca/healthy-living-vie-saine/immunization-immunisation/children-enfants/schedule-calendrier-eng.php
43. Naus, M., Puddicombe, D., Murti, M., Fung, C., et al. (2015, July 02). Outbreak of measles in an unvaccinated population, British Columbia, 2014. Canadian Communicable Disease Report CCDR. Volume 41-7. Infectious Diseases. Public Health Agency of Canada. www.phac-aspc.gc.ca/publicat/ccdr-rmtc/15vol41/dr-rm41-07/ar-02-eng.php
44. Public Health Agency of Canada. (2015, January 19). *Mumps vaccine.* Part 4 Active Vaccines. Canadian immunization guide. Immunizations and Vaccines. www.phac-aspc.gc.ca/publicat/cig-gci/p04-mump-orei-eng.php
45. Public Health Agency of Canada. (2015, December 02). *Vaccine safety.* Immunizations and Vaccines. www.phac-aspc.gc.ca/im/safety-securite-eng.php
46. Ibid.
47. Tierra, M. (2008). An effective alternative to antibiotics. *Journal of Herbal Pharmacotherapy*, 7(2), 79–89.
48. Eby III, G. A. (2009). Zinc lozenges as cure for the common cold—A review and hypothesis. *Medical Hypotheses*, 74(3), 482–492.
49. Worall, G. (2007, November). Acute sore throat. *Canadian Family Physician.* www.ncbi.nlm.nih.gov/pmc/articles/PMC2231494/
50. Public Health Agency of Canada. (2016, April 11). *Public health reminder: Seasonal flu.* Public Health Notices. www.phac-aspc.gc.ca/phn-asp/2015/flu-grippe-1027-eng.php
51. Public Health Agency of Canada. (2015, October 16). *Prevention of flu (influenza).* Diseases. Diseases and Conditions. healthycanadians.gc.ca/diseases-conditions-maladies-affections/disease-maladie/flu-grippe/prevention-eng.php
52. Nyhan, B., Reifler, J., & Richey, S. (2012). The role of social networks in influenza vaccine attitudes and intentions among college students in the southeastern United States. *Journal of Adolescent Health*, 51(3), 302–304.
53. Centers for Disease Control and Prevention. (2015, August 07). *Live, intranasal influenza VIS.* Vaccine Information Statements. www.cdc.gov/vaccines/hcp/vis/vis-statements/flulive.html
54. Public Health Agency of Canada. (2016, March 08). *Statement on seasonal influenza vaccine for 2015–2016.* An Advisory Committee Statement (ACS)—National Advisory Committee on Immunization (NACI). www.phac-aspc.gc.ca/naci-ccni/flu-2015-grippe-eng.php#v2
55. Mutsch, M., Weigong, Z., Rhodes, P., Bopp, M., Chen, R., Linder, T., Spyr, C., & Steffen, R. (2004). Use of inactivated intranasal influenza vaccine and the risk of Bell's Palsy in Switzerland. *The New England Journal of Medicine*, 350(9), 896–903. http://content.nejm.org/cgi/content/short/350/9/896
56. Stiver, H. G., Aoki, F. Y., Allen, U. D., Evans, G. A., Laverdière, M., & Skowronski, D. M. (2015, December 01). *Update on influenza antiviral drug treatment and prophylaxis for the 2015–2016 influenza season.* Association of Medical Microbiology and Infectious Disease Canada. http://www.pulsus.com/scholarly-articles/update-on-influenza-antiviral-drug-treatment-and-prophylaxis-for-the-20152016-influenza-season.pdf
57. Infection and Prevention Control Canada. (IPAC Canada). (2014, October 06). *Pandemic (H1N1) 2009 virus.* Links and Resources. www.ipac-canada.org/links_swineflu.php
58. Public Health Agency of Canada. (2015, April 21). *Avian influenza (H5N1): Global update.* Travel Health Notices. www.phac-aspc.gc.ca/tmp-pmv/notices-avis/notices-avis-eng.php?id=45
59. Infection and Prevention Control Canada. (IPAC Canada). (2014, October 06). *Pandemic (H1N1) 2009 virus.* Links and Resources. www.ipac-canada.org/links_swineflu.php

60. Public Health Agency of Canada. (2016, March 08). *Statement on seasonal influenza vaccine for 2015–2016*. An Advisory Committee Statement (ACS)—National Advisory Committee on Immunization (NACI). www.phac-aspc.gc.ca/naci-ccni/flu-2015-grippe-eng.php#v2

61. Public Health Agency of Canada. (2016, February 12). *Pandemic plans. Canada*. Pandemic Preparedness. Infectious Diseases. www.phac-aspc.gc.ca/influenza/plans-eng.php

62. Borgundvaag, B., Ovens, H., Goldman, B., Schull, M., et al. (2004, November 23). SARS outbreak in the Greater Toronto Area: The emergency department experience. *Canadian Medical Association Journal*, 171(11), 1342–1344.

63. Public Health Agency of Canada. (2015, August 13). *Public health notice: Middle East Respiratory Syndrome Coronavirus (MERS-CoV)*. Public Health Notices. www.phac-aspc.gc.ca/phn-asp/2015/ncoronavirus-eng.php#aug13

64. Ibid.

65. Public Health Agency of Canada. (2014, February 25). *Invasive meningococcal disease*. Vaccine-preventable Diseases. www.phac-aspc.gc.ca/im/vpd-mev/meningococcal-eng.php

66. Pace, D., & Pollard, A. J. (2012). Meningococcal disease: Clinical presentation and sequelae. *Vaccine*, 30 (Suppl 2), B3–B9.

67. Hellenbrand, W., Hanquet, G., Heuberger, S., Nielsen, S., & Stefanoff, P. (2011). What evidence for giving chemopropylaxis to children or students attending the same preschool, school or college as a case of meningococcal disease? *Epidemiology and Infection*, 139(11), 1645–1655.

68. Allen, U. D. (2010). Antifungal agents for the treatment of systemic fungal infections in children. *Paediatric Child Health*, 15(9), 603–608.

69. Public Health Agency of Canada. (2016, March 24). *Meninococcal vaccine*. Active Vaccines. Part 4. Canadian Immunization Guide. www.phac-aspc.gc.ca/publicat/cig-gci/p04-meni-eng.php

70. Ibid.

71. Meningitis Research Foundation of Canada. (n.d.). *Meningococcal disease in college and university residences*. Physicians Corner. www.meningitis.ca/en/MenDiseaseinCollegeandUniRes

72. De Wals, P., Allard, M. A., Guindon, K., Mayrand, L., Simard, S., & Black, R. (2002, April 15). Is vaccination against meningitis useful? The findings of an investigation in the Sherbrooke region, Quebec? *Canada Communicable Disease Report*, 28(8), 61–63. www.ncbi.nlm.nih.gov/pubmed/11974427

73. Government of Canada. (2016, March 16). *Hepatitis*. Diseases. Diseases and Conditions. healthycanadians.gc.ca/diseases-conditions-maladies-affections/disease-maladie/hepatitis-c-hepatite/index-eng.php

74. Public Health Agency of Canada. (2014, September 22). *Hepatitis B—Get the facts*. Blood Borne Pathogens Section. www.phac-aspc.gc.ca/hcai-iamss/bbp-pts/hepatitis/hep_b-eng.php

75. Liver.ca. Canadian Liver Foundation. (2015). *Hepatitis A*. Liver Disease. www.liver.ca/liver-disease/types/viral_hepatitis/Hepatitis_A.aspx

76. Levy, I., Chen, D., Sherman, M., Smith, D., & Krajden, M. (2001). Hepatitis A virus seroprevalence in 1000 university students in Toronto. *Canada Communicable Disease Report*, 27(11), 93–96. www.ncbi.nlm.nih.gov/pubmed/11416942

77. Public Health Agency of Canada. (2015, February 25). *Hepatitis A vaccine. Part 4*. Active Vaccines. Canadian Immunization Guide. www.phac-aspc.gc.ca/publicat/cig-gci/p04-hepa-eng.php

78. Public Health Agency of Canada. (2016, March 07). *Hepatitis B vaccine. Part 4*. Active Vaccines. Canadian Immunization Guide. www.phac-aspc.gc.ca/publicat/cig-gci/p04-hepb-eng.php

79. Government of Canada. (2016, March 16). *Hepatitis C*. Diseases. Diseases and Conditions. healthycanadians.gc.ca/diseases-conditions-maladies-affections/disease-maladie/hepatitis-c-hepatite/index-eng.php

80. Juhas, E., & English III, J. C. (2013). Tattoo-associated complications. *Journal of Pediatric and Adolescent Gynecology*, 26(2), 125–129.

81. Macsween, K. F., Higgins, C. D., McAulay, K. A., Williams, H., Harrisona, N., Swerdlow, A. J., & Crawford, D. H. (2010). Infectious mononucleosis in university students in the United Kingdom: Evaluation of the clinical features and consequences of the disease. *Clinical Infectious Diseases*, 50(5), 699–706.

82. Government of Canada. (2014, February 07). *Methicillin-resistant staphylococcus aureus*. OHS Answers Fact Sheets. Biological Hazards. www.ccohs.ca/oshanswers/biol_hazards/methicillin.html

83. Klevens, R. M., Morrison, M. A., Nadle, J., Petit, S., et al. (2007). Invasive methicillin-resistant Staphylococcus aureus infections in the United States. *Journal of the American Medical Association*, 298(15), 1763–1771.

84. Harbarth, S., Fankhauser, C., Schrenzel, J., Christenson, J., et al. (2008). Universal screening for Methicillin-resistant Staphylococcus aureus at Hospital Admission and nosocomial infection in surgical patients. *Journal of the American Medical Association*, 29(12), 1149–1157.

85. Merkel, T. J., Perera, P. Y., Kelly, V. K., Verman, A., Llewellyn, Z. N., Waldmann, T. A., et al. (2010). Development of a highly efficacious vaccinia-based dual vaccine against smallpox and anthrax, two important bioterror entities. *Proceedings of the National Academy of Sciences*, 107(42), 18091–18096.

86. Saskatchewan Ministry of Health. (2011, March). *Vaginal infections*. Fact Sheet. Communicable Disease. www.publications.gov.sk.ca/details.cfm?p=66742

87. O'Shea, L. (2010). Diagnosing urinary tract infections. *Practice Nurse*, 40(9), 20–25.

88. Public Health Agency of Canada. (2015, February 05). *Sexual health and sexually transmitted Infections*. Infectious Diseases. www.phac-aspc.gc.ca/std-mts/

89. Public Health Agency of Canada. (2013, October 23). The chief public health officer's report on the state of public health in Canada, 2013 infectious disease—the never-ending threat. Reports and Publications. www.phac-aspc.gc.ca/cphorsphc-respcacsp/2013/sti-its-eng.php

90. Starnbach, M. N., & Roan, N. R. (2008). Conquering sexually transmitted diseases. Nature Reviews. *Immunology*, 8(4), 313–317.

91. Marchand, E., Glenn, B. A., & Bastani, R. (2012). Low HPV vaccine coverage among female community college students. *Journal of Community Health*, 37(6), 1136–1144.

92. Caldeira, K. M., Singer, B. J., O'Grady, K. E., Vincent, K. B., & Arria, A. M. (2012). HIV testing in recent college students: Prevalence and correlates. *AIDS Education and Prevention*, 24(4), 363–376.

93. Fehr, S., Vidourek, R. A., & King, K. A. (2015). Intra- and inter-personal barriers to condom use among college students: a review of the literature. *Sexuality and Culture*, 19(1), 103–121.

94. Adefuye, A. S., Abiona, T. C., Balogun, J. A., & Lukobo-Durrell, M. (2009). HIV sexual risk behaviors and perception of risk among college students: Implications for planning interventions. *BMC Public Health, 9*(1), 281–293. www.biomedcentral.com/content/pdf/1471-2458-9-281.pdf

95. Scott-Sheldon, L. A. J., Carey, M. P., & Carey, K. B. (2010). Alcohol and risky sexual behavior among heavy drinking college students. *AIDS Behavior*, 14(4), 845–853.

96. Government of Canada. (2013, April 02). *Chlamydia.* Diseases. Diseases and Conditions. healthycanadians.gc.ca/diseases-conditions-maladies-affections/disease-maladie/chlamyd-eng.php

97. HealthLinkBC. (2015, July 06). *Pelvic inflammatory disease.* Health Topics A-Z. www.healthlinkbc.ca/healthtopics/content.asp?hwid=hw43366

98. Government of Canada. (2013, April 02). *Gonorrhea.* Diseases. Diseases and Conditions. healthycanadians.gc.ca/diseases-conditions-maladies-affections/disease-maladie/gonorrh-eng.php

99. American Sexual Health Association. (2016). NGU (nongonococcal urethritis). *STDs/STIs.* www.ashasexualhealth.org/stdsstis/ngu/

100. Government of Canada. (2015, July 29). Syphilis. *Diseases. Diseases and Conditions.* healthycanadians.gc.ca/diseases-conditions-maladies-affections/disease-maladie/syphilis-eng.php

101. Ibid.

102. Ibid.

103. Government of Canada. (2013, April 02). *Genital herpes.* Diseases. Diseases and Conditions. healthycanadians.gc.ca/diseases-conditions-maladies-affections/disease-maladie/herpes-eng.php

104. Community AIDS Treatment Information Exchange. (CATIE). (n.d.). *Genital herpes.* Fact Sheets. www.catie.ca/en/fact-sheets/sti/genital-herpes

105. Ibid.

106. Morello, C. S., Levinson, M. S., Kraynyak, K. A., & Spector, D. H. (2011). Immunization with herpes simplex virus 2 (HSV-2) genes plus inactivated HSV-2 is highly protective against acute and recurrent HSV-2 disease. *Journal of Virology* 85(7), 3461–3472.

107. Canadian Cancer Society. (2016). *HPV vaccines.* Cancer Information. www.cancer.ca/en/cancer-information/cancer-101/what-is-a-risk-factor/viruses-bacteria-and-other-infectious-agents/hpv-vaccines/?region=bc#ixzz45ep3xrGM

108. Ibid.

109. The Society of Obstetricians and Gynaecologists of Canada (SOGC). (n.d.). *Gardasil 9 HPV vaccine now available in Canada.* News Items. sogc.org/news_items/gardasil-9-hpv-vaccine-now-available-in-canada-2/

110. Lippman, A., Melnychuk, R., Shimmin, C., & Boscoe, M. (2007). Human Papillomavirus, vaccines and women's health: Questions and cautions. *Canadian Medical Association Journal*, 177(5), 484–487.

111. Planned Parenthood Federation of America. (2014). *Chancroid.* STDs. www.plannedparenthood.org/learn/stds-hiv-safer-sex/chancroid

112. Public Health Agency of Canada. (2013, February 01). *Ectoparasitic infestations (pubic lice, scabies).* Canadian Guidelines on Sexually Transmitted Infections. Section 5—Management and Treatment of Specific Infections. www.phac-aspc.gc.ca/std-mts/sti-its/cgsti-ldcits/section-5-3-eng.php

113. UNAIDS (2015). *Fact sheet 2015.* Resources. www.unaids.org/en/resources/campaigns/HowAIDSchangedeverything/factsheet

114. Ibid.

115. World Health Organization. (2016). *Mother-to-child transmission of HIV.* HIV/AIDS. Programs. www.who.int/hiv/topics/mtct/about/en/

116. UNAIDS (2015). *Fact sheet 2015.* Resources. www.unaids.org/en/resources/campaigns/HowAIDSchangedeverything/factsheet

117. Government of Canada (2015, December 01). *HIV and AIDS in Canada: Surveillance report to December 31, 2014.* healthycanadians.gc.ca/publications/diseases-conditions-maladies-affections/hiv-aids-surveillance-2014-vih-sida/index-eng.php?page=8

118. Ibid.

119. Ibid.

120. Ibid.

121. Abionaa, T., Balogunb, J., Yohannesa, E., Adefuyea, A., Yavuz, Y., Amosund, S., & Frantze, J. (2014). HIV/AIDS knowledge, perception of knowledge and sources of information among university students in USA, Turkey, South Africa and Nigeria. *Health Education Journal,* 73(6), 755–767.

122. Canadian Aids Treatment Information Exchange. (CATIE) (n.d.). *Our resources.* About CATIE. www.catie.ca/en/about/resources

123. Government of Canada. (2015, December 01). *HIV and AIDS.* Diseases. Diseases and Conditions. healthycanadians.gc.ca/diseases-conditions-maladies-affections/disease-maladie/hiv-aids-vih-sida/index-eng.php

124. Graffigna, G., & Olson, K. (2009). The ineffable disease: Exploring young peoples discourses about HIV/AIDS in Alberta, Canada. *Qualitative Health Research,* 19(6), 790–801.

125. Maartens, G., Celum, C., & Lewin, S. R. (2014). HIV infection: Epidemiology, pathogenesis, treatment, and prevention. *The Lancet,* 384(9939), 258–271.

126. Ibid.

127. Public Health Agency of Canada. (2011, February 25). HIV/AIDS Epi Updates— July 2010. *Chapter 3: HIV testing and surveillance systems in Canada.* Reports and Publications. www.phac-aspc.gc.ca/aids-sida/publication/epi/2010/3-eng.php

128. Canadian Public Health Association. (CPHA). (n.d.). *What categories and kinds of HIV tests are there?* Testing and Diagnosis. HIV Prevention. www.cpha.ca/en/programs/portals/hiv/prevention/testing/d02.aspx

129. Canadian Aids Society (CAS) and Centre for Infectious Disease Prevention and Control (CIDPC). (2002). *A guide to HIV//AIDS epidemiological and surveillance terms.* Appendix 6. Terminology. Living with HIV/AIDS. General Info and Statistics. librarypdf.catie.ca/PDF/P6/19782.pdf

130. University of San Francisco Medical Center. (2016). *AIDS diagnosis.* Conditions and Treatments. *A–Z.* www.ucsfhealth.org/conditions/aids/diagnosis.html

131. Government of Canada (2015, December 01). *HIV and AIDS in Canada: Surveillance report to December 31, 2014.* healthycanadians.gc.ca/publications/diseases-conditions-maladies-affections/hiv-aids-surveillance-2014-vih-sida/index-eng.php?page=8

132. Government of Canada. (2015, May 26). *The Canadian HIV initiative. (CHVI).* Frequently Asked Questions. www.chvi-icvv.gc.ca/faq-eng.html#Q7

Chapter 10

1. Statistics Canada. (2015, December 10). *The 10 leading deaths in Canada. 2012.* Health Fact Sheets. Publications. Catalogue no. 82-625-X. www.statcan.gc.ca/pub/82-625-x/2015001/article/14296-eng.htm
2. Heart and Stroke Foundation. (2011, October). *What is heart disease?* Health Information. www.heartandstroke.com/site/c.ikIQLcMWJtE/b.3682421/k.48B2/Heart_disease__What_is_heart_disease.htm
3. World Health Organization.(WHO). (2015, January). *Cardiovascular diseases. (CVDs).* Fact Sheet No. 317. Media Centre. www.who.int/mediacentre/factsheets/fs317/en/
4. Heart and Stroke Foundation. (2014). *Creating survivors. 2014 Report on the Health of Canadians.* www.heartandstroke.com/atf/cf/%7B99452D8B-E7F1-4BD6-A57D-B136CE6C95BF%7D/HSF_HMReport2014E_web.pdf
5. Widmaier, E. P., Raff, H., & Strang, K. T. (2006). *Vander's human physiology. The mechanisms of body function.* Boston, MA: McGraw Hill Higher Education.
6. Ibid.
7. Ibid.
8. Ibid.
9. Ibid.
10. Heart and Stroke Foundation. (2009, August). *Anatomy of the heart. What is Heart Disease.* Health Information. www.heartandstroke.com/site/c.ikIQLcMWJtE/b.3532069/k.4265/Heart_disease__Anatomy_of_the_Heart.htm
11. Ibid.
12. Ibid.
13. Ibid.
14. Ibid.
15. Ibid.
16. Ibid.
17. Ibid.
18. Widmaier, E. P., Raff, H., & Strang, K. T. (2006). *Vander's human physiology: The mechanisms of body function.* Boston: McGraw Hill Higher Education.
19. Ibid.
20. Ibid.
21. Ibid.
22. Mayo Clinic. (2016). *Arteriosclerosis/atherosclerosis.* Overview. Diseases and Conditions. www.mayoclinic.org/diseases-conditions/arteriosclerosis-atherosclerosis/home/ovc-20167019
23. Ibid.
24. Heart and Stroke Foundation. (2013, August). *Atherosclerosis.* Heart Disease Conditions. Health Information. www.heartandstroke.com/site/c.ikIQLcMWJtE/b.3484059/k.2FED/Heart_disease__Atherosclerosis.htm
25. Wojciech, S., Wirtwein, M., Trybala, E., & Gruchala, M. (2013). Severity of coronary atherosclerosis and stroke incidence in 7-year follow up. *Journal of Neurology,* 260(7), 1855–1858.
26. Heart and Stroke Foundation. (2009, August). *What is coronary heart disease?* Heart Disease Conditions. Heart Disease. www.heartandstroke.com/site/c.ikIQLcMWJtE/b.3484067/k.6657/Heart_disease__What_is_coronary_artery_disease.htm
27. Musunuru, K., & Kathiresan, S. (2011). Genetics of coronary artery disease. *Annual Review of Genomics and Human Genetics,* 11, 91–108.
28. Patel, A. R., Antkowiak, P. F., Nandalur, K. R., West, A. M., Salerno, M., Arora, V., Christopher, J., Epstein, F. H., & Kramer, C. M. (2011). Assessment of advanced coronary artery disease. Advantages of quantitative cardiac magnetic resonance perfusion analysis. *Journal of the American College of Cardiology, 56*(7), 561–569.
29. Heart and Stroke Foundation. (2014, April). *Signs of heart attack, cardiac arrest and sudden arrhythmia death syndrome (SADS).* Heart Disease. Health Information. www.heartandstroke.com/site/c.ikIQLcMWJtE/b.3483917/k.AA64/Heart_disease__Signs_of_heart_attack_cardiac_arrest_SADS.htm
30. Emslie, C. (2005). Women, men and coronary heart disease: A review of the qualitative literature. *Journal of Advanced Nursing,* 51(4), 382–395.
31. Heart and Stroke Foundation (2014, December). *Getting your blood pressure in check.* High Blood Pressure. Heart Disease Prevention and Risk Factors. www.heartandstroke.com/site/c.ikIQLcMWJtE/b.3484023/k.2174/Heart_disease__High_blood_pressure.htm
32. Chen, S. (2012). Essential hypertension: Perspectives and future directions. *Journal of Hypertension,* 30(1), 42–45.
33. Statistics Canada. (2015, November 27). *High blood pressure, 2013.* Publications. 82-625-X. www.statcan.gc.ca/pub/82-625-x/2014001/article/14101-eng.htm
34. Heart and Stroke Foundation. (2014, December). *Getting your blood pressure in check.* High Blood Pressure. Heart Disease Prevention and Risk Factors. www.heartandstroke.com/site/c.ikIQLcMWJtE/b.3484023/k.2174/Heart_disease__High_blood_pressure.htm
35. Heart and Stroke Foundation. (2016). *Stroke.* Health Information. www.heartandstroke.com/site/c.ikIQLcMWJtE/b.3483933/k.CD67/Stroke.htm
36. Statistics Canada. (2015, December 10). *The 10 leading deaths in Canada. 2012.* Health Fact Sheets. Publications. Catalogue no. 82-625-X. www.statcan.gc.ca/pub/82-625-x/2015001/article/14296-eng.htm
37. Heart and Stroke Foundation. (2013, June). *Stroke report 2013: There is life after stroke.* Reports on Canadians' Stroke Health. www.heartandstroke.com/site/apps/nlnet/content2.aspx?c=ikIQLcMWJtE&b=7498307&ct=13158031
38. Heart and Stroke Foundation. (2014, June). *Transient ischemic attack (TIA or mini-stroke).* Understanding Stroke. www.heartandstroke.com/site/c.ikIQLcMWJtE/b.4847223/k.F294/Stroke__Transient_Ischemic_Attack_TIA_or_ministroke.htm
39. Heart and Stroke Foundation. (2014, July). *Hemorrhagic stroke.* What Is a Stroke? Stroke. www.heartandstroke.on.ca/site/c.pvI3IeNWJwE/b.3581865/k.776F/Stroke__Hemorrhagic_stroke.htm
40. Heart and Stroke Foundation. (2016) *Stroke signs.* Strokes. Health information. www.heartandstroke.com/site/c.ikIQLcMWJtE/b.3483937/k.ED98/Stroke__Stroke_Warning_Signs.htm
41. Heart and Stroke Foundation. (2014). *Creating survivors.* 2014 Report on the Health of Canadians. www.heartandstroke.com/atf/cf/%7B99452D8B-E7F1-4BD6-A57D-B136CE6C95BF%7D/HSF_HMReport2014E_web.pdf
42. Ibid.
43. Mukamal, K. J., & Rimm, E. B. (2008). Alcohol consumption: Risks and benefits. *Current Atherosclerosis Reports: Medicine,* 10(6), 536–543.
44. Zhou, X., Li, C., Xu, W., Hong, X., & Chen, J. (2010). Relation of alcohol consumption to angiographically proved

coronary artery disease in Chinese men. *The American Journal of Cardiology*, 106(8), 1101–1103.

45. Huntgeburth, M., Freyhaus, H., & Rosenkranz, S. (2005). Alcohol consumption and hypertension. *Current Hypertension Reports: Medicine*, 7(3), 180–185.

46. Smyth, A., Teo, K. K., Rangarajan, S., O'Donnell, M., et al. (2015, November 14). Alcohol consumption and cardiovascular disease, cancer injury, admissions to hospital, and mortality: A prospective cohort study. *Lancet*, 386(1007), 1945–1954 (p. 1953).

47. Mukamal, K. J., & Rimm, E. B. (2008). Alcohol consumption: Risks and benefits. *Current Atherosclerosis Reports: Medicine*, 10(6), 536–543.

48. Ford, E., Giles, W., & Dietz, W. (2002). Prevalence of the metabolic syndrome among U. S. adults. Findings from the Third National Health and Nutrition Examination Survey. *Journal of American Medical Association*, 287(3), 356–359.

49. Statistics Canada. (2013, February 13). *Cholesterol levels of Canadians 2009 to 2011*. Catalogue no. 82-625-X. Publications. www.statcan.gc.ca/pub/82-625-x/2012001/article/11732-eng.htm

50. Wierzbicki, A. S., Clarke, R. E., Viljoen, A., & Mikhailidis, D. P. (2012). Triglycerides: A case for treatment. *Current Opinion in Cardiology*, 27(4), 398–404.

51. Ibid.

52. Heartbeats: Graze your way to lower cholesterol. (2002). *Harvard Heart Letter*, 12(9).

53. Heart and Stroke Foundation. (2013, August). *Living with cholesterol: Cholesterol and healthy living*. Living with Cholesterol. Other Resources for Heart Disease. www.heartandstroke.com/site/c.ikIQLcMWJtE/b.3751077/k.FCF7/Heart_disease__Living_with_Cholesterol.htm

54. Heart and Stroke. (2014, September). *Dietary sodium, heart disease and stroke*. Heart and Stroke Position Statements. Healthy Living. www.heartandstroke.com/site/c.ikIQLcMWJtE/b.5263133/k.696/Dietary_sodium_heart_disease_and_stroke.htm

55. Rosenblum, C. (2009, May). *DASHing high blood pressure*. Nutrition Columns. Health Information. Heart and Stroke Foundation. www.heartandstroke.com/site/apps/nlnet/content2.aspx?c=ikIQLcMWJtE&b=4869055&ct=6923125

56. Cohen, D. L., & Townsend, R. R. (2008). What effects does potassium have on blood pressure? *The Journal of Clinical Hypertension*, 10(2), 158–159.

57. Fabry, I., De Paepe, P., Kips, J., Vermeersch, S., & Van Bortel, L. (2011). Different effects of tocolytic medication on blood pressure and blood pressure amplification. *European Journal of Clinical Pharmacology*, 67(1), 11–17.

58. Canadian Diabetes Association. (2016). *Complications research*. Research Funding. www.diabetes.ca/research/research-funding/complications-research

59. McFarlane, S. I., Sica, D. A., & Sowers, J. R. (2005). Stroke in patients with diabetes and hypertension. *Journal of Clinical Hypertension*, 7(5), 286–294.

60. Mason, C., & Katzmarzyk, P. T. (2009). Effect of the site of measurement of waist circumference on the prevalence of the metabolic syndrome. *The American Journal of Cardiology*, 103(12), 1716–1720.

61. Keown, T. L., Smith, C. B., & Harris, M. S. (2009). Metabolic syndrome among college students. *The Journal for Nurse Practitioners*, 5(10), 754–759.

62. Honarbakhsh, S., & Schachter, M. (2009). Vitamins and cardiovascular disease. *British Journal of Nutrition*, 101(8), 1113–1131.

63. Heart and Stroke Foundation. (2013, August). *Living with cholesterol: Cholesterol and healthy living*. Living with Cholesterol. Other Resources for Heart Disease. www.heartandstroke.com/site/c.ikIQLcMWJtE/b.3751077/k.FCF7/Heart_disease__Living_with_Cholesterol.htm

64. Heart and Stroke Foundation of Canada. (2015, November). *Dietary fats, oils and cholesterol*. Healthy Eating. Health Information. www.heartandstroke.com/site/c.ikIQLcMWJtE/b.3484237/k.D734/Healthy_living__Dietary_fats_oils_and__cholesterol.htm

65. Dhaka, V., Gulia, N., Ahlawat, K. S., & Khatkar, B. S. (2011). Trans fats—sources, health risks and alternative approach—a review. *Journal of Food Science and Technology*, 48(5), 534–541.

66. Adolphe, J. L., Whiting, S. J., Juurlink, B. H., Thorpe, L. U., & Alcorn, J. (2010). Health effects with consumption of the flax lignin secoisolariciresinol diglucoside. *British Journal of Nutrition*, 103(7), 929–938.

67. De Leiris, J. D., de Lorgeril, M., & Boucher, F. (2009). Fish oil and heart health. *Journal of Cardiovascular Pharmacology*, 54(5), 378–384.

68. Steffen, L. M. (2006). Eat your fruits and vegetables. *Lancet*, 367(9507), 278–279.

69. Heart and Stroke Foundation. (2014, July). *The DASH diet to lower high blood pressure*. Healthy Eating. Healthy Living. www.heartandstroke.com/site/c.ikIQLcMWJtE/b.3862329/k.4F4/Healthy_living__The_DASH_Diet_to_lower_blood_pressure.htm

70. Jenkins, D. J. A., Jones, P. J. H., Lamarche, B., Kendall, C. W. C., Faulkner, D., Cermakova, L., et al. (2011). Effect of a dietary portfolio of cholesterol-lowering foods given at 2 level of intensity of dietary advice on serum lipids in hyperlipidemia. A randomized controlled trial. *Journal of the American Medical Association*, 306(8), 831–839.

71. Roetert, E. P. (2006). Lifelong physical fitness to prevent heart disease. *National Strength and Conditioning Association*, 28(3), 75–76.

72. Heath, G. W. (2009). Physical activity transitions and chronic disease. *American Journal of Lifestyle Medicine*, 3(1 suppl), 27S–31S.

73. Dalleck, L. C., Allen, B. A., Hanson, B. A., Borresen, E. C., Erickson, M. E., & De Lap, S. L. (2009). Dose-response relationship between moderate-intensity exercise duration and coronary heart disease risk factors in postmenopausal women. *Journal of Women's Health*, 18(1), 105–113.

74. Canadian Society of Exercise Physiology. (CSEP). (2012). *Canadian physical activity guidelines and Canadian sedentary behaviour guidelines*. Publications. www.csep.ca/en/guidelines/get-the-guidelines

75. Lee, I. M., Rexrode, K. M., Cook, N. R., Manson, J. E., & Buring, J. E. (2001). Physical activity and coronary heart disease in women: Is "No pain, no gain" passé? *Obstetrical & Gynecological Survey*, 56(8), 477–479.

76. Tanasescu, M., Leitzmann, M. F., Rimm, E. B., Willett, W. C., Stampfer, M. J., & Hu, F. B. (2001). Exercise type and intensity in relation to coronary heart disease in men. *The Journal of the American Medical Association*, 288(16), 1994–2000.

77. Pfeifer, G. (2011). Collaborative care for diabetes, heart disease and depression. *American Journal of Nursing*, 111(4), 16.

78. Wassertheil-Smoller, S., Shumaker, S., Ockene, J., Talavera, G. A., Greenland, P., Cochrane, B., Robbins, J., Aragaki, A., & Dunbar-Jacob, J. (2004). Depression and cardiovascular sequelae in postmenopausal women. *The Women's Health Initiative (WHI)*, 164(3), 289–298.

79. Zeidenberg, M. (2008). Community colleges under stress: Publicly funded two-year colleges are facing daunting challenges in dealing with surging enrolments of disadvantaged and unprepared students. *Issues in Science and Technology*, 24(4), 53–58.

80. Smith, L. E., (2008). Heart Ed 101. *Journal of American College Health*, 56(6), 698–700.

81. Spencer, L. (2002). Results of a heart disease risk-factor screening among traditional college students. *Journal of American College Health*, 50(6), 291–296.

82. Reid, J. L., Hammond, D., Rynard, V. L., & Burkhalter, R. (2015). *Tobacco use in Canada: Patterns and trends (2015 edition)*. Propel Centre for Population Health Impact, University of Waterloo. www.tobaccoreport.ca/2015/TobaccoUseinCanada_2015.pdf

83. Canadian Cancer Society. (2016). *Tobacco. What is a risk factor?* Cancer 101. www.cancer.ca/en/cancer-information/cancer-101/what-is-a-risk-factor/tobacco/?region=on

84. Canadian Cancer Society. (2016). *Second hand smoke. Tobacco. What is a risk factor?* www.cancer.ca/en/cancer-information/cancer-101/what-is-a-risk-factor/tobacco/second-hand-smoke/?region=on

85. Shields, M., Tremblay, M. S., Connor Gorber, S., & Janssen, I. (2012, June). Abdominal obesity and cardiovascular disease risk factors within body mass index categories. *Health Reports*, 23(2), 7–15.

86. Woo, K. S., Chook, P., Yu, C. W., Sung, R. Y. T., Qiao, M., Leung, S. S. F., Lam, C. W., Metreweli, C., & Celermajer, D. (2004). Effects of diet and exercise on obesity-related vascular dysfunction in children. *Circulation*, 109(16), 1981–1986.

87. Heart and Stroke Foundation. (2014, July). *Risk factors you cannot control.* Heart Disease and Risk Factors. Heart Disease. www.heartandstroke.com/site/c.ikIQLcMWJtE/b.3484043/k.C55/Heart_disease__Risk_factors_you_cant_control.htm

88. Ibid.

89. Heart and Stroke Foundation. (2014, July). *Women and heart disease and stroke.* Heart Disease. Health Information. www.heartandstroke.com/site/c.ikIQLcMWJtE/b.3484041/k.D80A/Heart_disease__Women_and_heart_disease_and_stroke.htm

90. Heart and Stroke Foundation. (2013, August). Heart Smart™ for women: A guide to living with and preventing heart disease and stroke. *Other Resources for Heart Disease.* www.heartandstroke.on.ca/site/c.pvI3IeNWJwE/b.4648513/k.89BC/Heart_Disease__HeartSmart8482_Women_A_guide_to_living_with_and_preventing_heart_disease_and_stroke.htm

91. Christoffersen, M., Frikke-Schmidt, R., Schnohr, P., Jensen, G. B., Nordestgaard, B. G., & Tybjærg-Hansen, A. (2014). Visible age-related signs and risk of ischemic heart disease in the general population. A prospective cohort study. *Circulation*, 129(9), 990–998.

92. Reading, J. (2015). Confronting the growing crisis of cardiovascular disease and heart health among Aboriginal Peoples in Canada. *Canadian Journal of Cardiology*, 9(31), 1077–1080.

93. Chiu, M., Austin, P. C., Manuel, D. G., & Tu, J. V. (2012). Cardiovascular risk factor profiles of recent immigrants vs long-term residents of Ontario: A multi-ethnic study. *Canadian Journal of Cardiology*, 28(1), 20–26.

94. Canadian Cancer Society. (2016). *Staging and grading.* Diagnosis and Treatment. Cancer Information. www.cancer.ca/en/cancer-information/diagnosis-and-treatment/staging-and-grading/?region=on

95. National Cancer Institute. (2015, March 09). *Staging.* Diagnosis and Staging. About Cancer. www.cancer.gov/about-cancer/diagnosis-staging/staging

96. Canadian Cancer Society's Advisory Committee. (2015, June). Canadian Cancer Statistics 2015. Special topic: Predictions of the future burden of cancer in Canada. Toronto, ON. www.cancer.ca/~/media/cancer.ca/CW/cancer%20information/cancer%20101/Canadian%20cancer%20statistics/Canadian-Cancer-Statistics-2015-EN.pdf

97. Ibid.

98. Ibid.

99. Canadian Cancer Society. (2016). *Screening for breast cancer.* Prevention and Screening. www.cancer.ca/en/prevention-and-screening/early-detection-and-screening/screening/screening-for-breast-cancer/?region=bc

100. Ibid.

101. Goss, P. E., Ingle, J. N., Alés-Martínez, J. E., Cheung, A. M., et al. (2011). Exemestane for breast-cancer prevention in postmenopausal women. *The New England Journal of Medicine*, 364(25), 2381–2391.

102. Canadian Cancer Society. (2016). *What is cervical cancer?* Cervical Cancer. Cervical. Cancer Types. www.cancer.ca/en/cancer-information/cancer-type/cervical/cervical-cancer/?region=on

103. Canadian Cancer Society. (2016). *HPV vaccines.* Cancer Information. www.cancer.ca/en/cancer-information/cancer-101/what-is-a-risk-factor/viruses-bacteria-and-other-infectious-agents/hpv-vaccines/?region=bc#ixzz45ep3xrGM

104. Canadian Cancer Society. (2016). *Colorectal cancer statistics.* Statistics. Colorectal. www.cancer.ca/en/cancer-information/cancer-type/colorectal/statistics/?region=on

105. Public Health Agency of Canada. (2015, July 03). *What is lung cancer?* Lung Cancer. Cancer. Chronic Diseases. www.phac-aspc.gc.ca/cd-mc/cancer/lung_cancer-cancer_poumon-eng.php

106. Ibid.

107. Canadian Cancer Society's Advisory Committee. (2015, June). Canadian Cancer Statistics 2015. Special topic: Predictions of the future burden of cancer in Canada. Toronto, ON. www.cancer.ca/~/media/cancer.ca/CW/cancer%20information/cancer%20101/Canadian%20cancer%20statistics/Canadian-Cancer-Statistics-2015-EN.pdf

108. Canadian Cancer Society. (2016). *What's in tobacco smoke?* Tobacco. What Is a Risk Factor? www.cancer.ca/en/cancer-information/cancer-101/what-is-a-risk-factor/tobacco/what-s-in-tobacco-smoke/?region=on

109. McGuiness, T. M. (2009). Update on marijuana. *Journal of Psychosocial Nursing & Mental Health Services*, 47(10), 19–22.

110. Callaghan, R. C., Allebeck, P., & Sidorchuk, A. (2013). Marijuana use and risk of lung cancer: A 40-year cohort study. *Cancer Causes & Control*, 24(10), 1811–1820.

111. Canadian Cancer Society. (2016). *Signs and symptoms of lung cancer.* Signs and Symptoms. Lungs. www.cancer.ca/en/cancer-information/cancer-type/lung/signs-and-symptoms/?region=sk

112. Canadian Lung Association. (2015, April 17). *Treatment. Lung cancer.* Lung Diseases A–Z. www.lung.ca/lung-health/lung-disease/lung-cancer/treatment

113. Ovarian Cancer Canada.(2014). *Ovarian cancer.* Disease Basics. www.ovariancanada.org/about-ovarian-cancer/disease-basics/what-is-ovarian-cancer

114. Philippe, A., Doré, J. F., Eggermont, A. M. M., & Coebergth, J. W. (2011). Epidemiological evidence that UVA radiation is involved in the genesis of cutaneous melanoma. *Current Opinion in Oncology*, 23(2), 189–196.

115. Canadian Cancer Society. (2016). Vitamin D. *Live Well. Prevention and Screening.* www.cancer.ca/en/prevention-and-screening/live-well/vitamin-d/?region=on

116. Public Health Agency of Canada. (2014, May 28). *Non-melanoma skin cancer.* Cancer. Chronic Diseases. www.phac-aspc.gc.ca/cd-mc/cancer/non_melanoma_skin_cancer-cancer_peau_non_melanique-eng.php

117. Public Health Agency of Canada. (2014, May 28). *Melanoma skin cancer.* Cancer. Chronic Diseases. www.phac-aspc.gc.ca/cd-mc/cancer/melanoma_skin _cancer-cancer_peau_melanome-eng.php

118. Melanoma Research Foundation. (2016). *Am I at risk for melanoma?* Melanoma Risk Factors. Preventing Melanoma. www.melanoma.org/understand-melanoma/preventing-melanoma/melanoma-risk-factors

119. Canadian Cancer Society's Advisory Committee. (2015, June). *Special topic: Predictions of the future burden of cancer in Canada.* Canadian Cancer Statistics 2015. Toronto, ON. www.cancer.ca/~/media/cancer.ca/CW/cancer%20information/cancer%20101/Canadian%20cancer%20statistics/Canadian-Cancer-Statistics-2015-EN.pdf

120. Canadian Cancer Society. (2016). *Prostate-specific antigen (PSA) test.* Tests and Procedures. Diagnosis and Treatment. www.cancer.ca/en/cancer-information/diagnosis-and-treatment/tests-and-procedures/prostate-specific-antigen-psa/?region=on

121. Daley, C. M. (2007). College men's knowledge, attitudes, and beliefs about testicular cancer. *American Journal of Men's Health*, 1(3), 173–182.

122. Soerjomataram, I., Oomen, D., Lemmens, V., Oenema, A., Benetou, V., & Trichopoulou, A. (2010). Increased consumption of fruits and vegetables and future cancer incidence in selected European countries. *European Journal of Cancer*, 46(14), 2563–2580.

123. Canadian Cancer Society. (2016). *Diet. What is a risk factor?* Cancer 101. Cancer Information. www.cancer.ca/en/cancer-information/cancer-101/what-is-a-risk-factor/diet/?region=on#

124. Bernstein, L. (2009). Exercise and breast cancer prevention. *Current Oncology Reports*, 11(6), 480–496.

125. Zoeller, R. F. (2009). Lifestyle in the prevention and management of cancer: Physical activity. *American Journal of Lifestyle Medicine*, 3(5), 353–361.

126. Farmer, R. (2008). Prostate cancer: Epidemiology and risk factors. *Urology, Gynaeocology & Sexual Health*, 13(3), 32–34.

127. Canadian Diabetes Association. (2016). *What is diabetes?* Types of Diabetes. About Diabetes. www.diabetes.ca/about-diabetes/types-of-diabetes

128. Canadian Diabetes Association. (2016). *What is diabetes?* Types of Diabetes. About Diabetes. www.diabetes.ca/diabetes-and-you/what/facts/; www.diabetes.ca/about-diabetes/types-of-diabetes

129. Ibid.

130. Ibid.

131. Canadian Diabetes Association. (2016). *Clinical practice guidelines.* Clinical Practice and Education. www.diabetes.ca/clinical-practice-education/clinical-practice-guidelines

132. Canadian Diabetes Association. (2016). *Are you at risk?* Risk Factors. About Diabetes. www.diabetes.ca/about-diabetes/risk-factors/are-you-at-risk

133. Canadian Diabetes Association. (2016). *Children & type 2 diabetes.* Kids, Teens and Diabetes. Diabetes and You. www.diabetes.ca/diabetes-and-you/kids-teens-diabetes/children-type-2-diabetes

134. Panagiotopoulos, C., Riddell, M. C., & Sellers, E. A. (2013, April). Type 2 diabetes in children and adolescents. *Canadian Journal of Diabetes*, 37(Supplement 1), S163–S167.

135. Government of Canada. (2015, December 17). *Type 2 diabetes.* Diseases. Diseases and Conditions. healthycanadians.gc.ca/diseases-conditions-maladies-affections/disease-maladie/diabete-eng.php

136. Urrutia-Rojas, X., & Menchaca, J. (2006). Prevalence of risk for Type 2 diabetes in school children. *Journal of School Health*, 76(5), 189–194.

137. Wood, F. G., Payne-Foster, P., Kelly, R., & Lewis, D. M. (2011). Learning and living diabetes: Development of a college diabetes seminar course. *Diabetes Spectrum*, 24(1), 42–46.

138. Lau, D. C. W., & McFarlane, J. (2010). Diabetes and weight management. *Primary Care Diabetes*, 4 (Supplement 1), S24–S30.

139. Public Health Agency of Canada. (2011, December 15). Chapter 6—Diabetes among First Nations, Inuit, and Métis populations. Diabetes in Canada: Facts and Figures from a Public Health Perspective. *Publications and Statistics.* Ottawa, 2011. www.phac-aspc.gc.ca/cd-mc/publications/diabetes-diabete/facts-figures-faits-chiffres-2011/chap6-eng.php#DIR

Chapter 11

1. Government of Canada. (2015, February 03). *Summary of results for 2013. Canadian Tobacco, Alcohol and Drugs Survey (CTADS).* Data. Science, Research and Data. healthycanadians.gc.ca/science-research-sciences-recherches/data-donnees/ctads-ectad/summary-sommaire-2013-eng.php

2. Ibid.

3. World Health Organization. (WHO). (2013/2016). *Lexicon of alcohol and drug terms published by the World Health Organization.* Management of Substance Abuse. www.who.int/substance_abuse/terminology/who_lexicon/en/

4. Ibid.

5. Kerr, T., Kimber, J., & Rhodes, T. (2007). Drug use settings: An emerging focus for research and intervention. *International Journal of Drug Policy*, 18(1), 1–4.

6. Fortmann, S. P., Burda, B., Senger, C. A., Lin, J. S., & Whitlock, E. (2013). Vitamin and mineral supplements in the primary prevention of cardiovascular disease and cancer: An updated systematic evidence review for the U. S. Preventive Services Task Force. *Annals of Internal Medicine*, 159(12), 824–838.

7. Canadian Generic Pharmaceutical Association. (CGPA). (2014). *2014. The Canadian generic market.* Market Trends. Resources. www.canadiangenerics.ca/en/resources/market_trends.asp

8. Canadian Centre on Substance Abuse. (2016). *Canadian drug trends.* Topics. www.ccsa.ca/Eng/topics/Monitoring-Trends/Canadian-Drug-Trends/Pages/default.aspx

9. Law, M. R., Cheng, L., Dhalla, I., Heard, D., & Morgan, S. G. (2012). The effect of cost on adherence to prescription medications in Canada. *Canadian Medical Association Journal*, 184(3), 297–302.

10. Zullig, K. J., & Divin, A. L. (2012). The association between non-medical prescription drug use, depressive symptoms and suicidality among college students. *Addictive Behaviors*, 37(8), 890–899.

11. Euromonitor International. (2016, January 23). Key global trends in hot drinks from 2015. News and Resources. blog .euromonitor.com/2016/01/key-global-trends-in-hot-drinks -from-2015.html

12. The NPD Group Inc. (2016, February 10). *Canadians love their coffee.* Press Releases. www.npdgroup.ca/wps/portal/npd/ca/ news/press-releases/canadians-love-their-coffee/

13. Ibid.

14. Euromonitor International. (2016, January 23). Key global trends in hot drinks from 2015. News and Resources. blog .euromonitor.com/2016/01/key-global-trends-in-hot-drinks -from-2015.html

15. Food Service and Hospitality. (2014, September 10). *The 2014 coffee and tea report.* http://www.foodserviceandhospitality .com/caffeine-feinds/

16. Coffee Association of Canada. (n.d.). *About coffee.* Home. www.coffeeassoc.com/about-coffee/

17. Government of Canada. (2013, June 11). *Health Canada reminds Canadians to manage their caffeine consumption.* Recalls and Alerts. Healthy Canadians. healthycanadians .gc.ca/recall-alert-rappel-avis/hc-sc/2013/34021a-eng.php

18. Attila, S., & Cakir, B. (2011). Energy-drink consumption in college students and associated factors. *Nutrition*, 27(3), 316–322.

19. Scott, W. H., Coyne, K. M., Johnson, M. M., Lausted, C. G., Sahota, M., & Johnson, A. T. (2002). Effects of caffeine on performance of low intensity tasks. *Perceptual and Motor Skills*, 94(2), 521–532.

20. Pelluchi, C., Tavani, A., & LaVecchia, C. (2008). Coffee and alcohol consumption and bladder cancer. *Scandinavian Journal of Urology and Nephrology*, 42(s218), 37–44.

21. Mayo Clinic. (2016). *Drug addiction. Definition. Basics.* Diseases and Conditions. www.mayoclinic.org/diseases -conditions/drug-addiction/basics/definition/con-20020970

22. Government of Canada. (2015, February 03). *Summary of results for 2013. Canadian Tobacco, Alcohol and Drugs Survey (CTADS).* Data. Science, Research and Data. healthycanadians.gc.ca/science-research-sciences-recherches/ data-donnees/ctads-ectad/summary-sommaire-2013-eng.php

23. Ibid.

24. Canadian Mental Health Association. Ontario. (2016). *Concurrent disorders.* Mental Health Conditions. Mental Health. ontario.cmha.ca/mental-health/mental-health -conditions/concurrent-disorders/

25. Canadian Centre on Substance Abuse. (CCSA). (2009). *Concurrent disorders. Substance abuse in Canada.* www.ccsa.ca/Resource%20 Library/ccsa-011811-2010.pdf

26. Ibid.

27. Dunbar, D., Kushner, H., & Vrecko, S. (2010). Drugs, addiction and society. *BioSocieties*, 5(1), 2–7.

28. Brook, J. S., Whiteman, M., Finch, S., & Cohen, P. (2000). Longitudinally foretelling drug use in the late twenties: Adolescent personality and social-environmental antecedents. *The Journal of Genetic Psychology*, 161(1), 37–51.

29. Bahr, S. J., Hoffmann, J. P., & Yang, X. (2005). Parental and peer influences on the risk of adolescent drug use. *Journal of Primary Prevention*, 26(6), 529–551.

30. Marmorstein, N. R., Iacono, W. G., & McGue, M. (2009). Alcohol and illicit drug dependence among parents: Associations with offspring externalizing disorders. *Psychological Medicine*, 39(1), 149–155.

31. Saywer, T. M., & Stevenson, J. F. (2008). Perceived parental and peer disapproval toward substances: Influences on adolescent decision-making. *Journal of Primary Prevention*, 29(6), 465–477.

32. Government of Canada. (2015, February 03). *Summary of results for 2013. Canadian Tobacco, Alcohol and Drugs Survey (CTADS).* Data. Science, Research and Data. healthycanadians.gc.ca/science-research-sciences-recherches/ data-donnees/ctads-ectad/summary-sommaire-2013-eng.php

33. Weiss, K. G., & Dilks, L. M. (2015). Marijuana, gender, and health-related harms: Disentangling marijuana's contribution to risk in a college "party" context. *Sociological Spectrum*, 35(3), 254–270, DOI: 10.1080/02732173.2015.1021064

34. Government of Canada. (2015, February 03). *Summary of results for 2013. Canadian Tobacco, Alcohol and Drugs Survey (CTADS).* Data. Science, Research and Data. healthycanadians.gc.ca/science-research-sciences-recherches/ data-donnees/ctads-ectad/summary-sommaire-2013-eng.php

35. Martens, M. P., Page, J. C., Mowry, E. S., Damann, K. M., Taylor, K. K., & Cimini, M. D. (2006). Differences between actual and perceived student norms: An examination of alcohol use, drug use, and sexual behaviour. *Journal of American College Health*, 54(5), 295–300.

36. American College Health Association. (2013). American College Health Association—National College Health Assessment II: Canadian Consortium Reference Group Executive Summary Spring 2013. Hanover, MD. www.cacuss .ca/_Library/documents/NCHA-II_WEB_SPRING_2013 _CANADIAN_REFERENCE_GROUP_EXECUTIVE _SUMMARY.pdf

37. American College Health Association. (2015). American College Health Association—National College Health Assessment II: Reference Group Executive Summary Spring 2015. Hanover, M. D. www.acha-ncha.org/docs/NCHA-II _WEB_SPRING_2015_REFERENCE_GROUP_EXECUTIVE _SUMMARY.pdf

38. Jones, S. E., Oeltmann, J., Wilson, T. W., Brener, N. D., & Hill, C. V. (2001). Binge drinking among undergraduate college students in the United States: Implications for other substance use. *Journal of American College Health*, 50(1), 33–38.

39. McMaster University. (2016). *Residence and housing.* Student Life. future.mcmaster.ca/student/residence/

40. Sharp, J. T., & Rosén, L. A. (2007). Recreational stimulant use among college students. *Journal of Substance Use*, 12(2), 71–82.

41. Ibid.

42. Lange, J. E., Reed, M. B., Ketchie Croff, J. M., & Clapp, J. D. (2008). College student use of Salvia divinorum. *Drug and Alcohol Dependence*, 94(1–3), 263–266.

43. Health Canada. (2016, February 11). *Notice—change in legal/ regulatory status of salvia divinorum.* Health Concerns. Controlled Substances. www.hc-sc.gc.ca/hc-ps/substancontrol/ substan/legal-salvia-statut-eng.php

44. Nabors, E. L. (2010). Drug use and intimate partner violence among college students: An in-depth exploration. *Journal of Interpersonal Violence*, 25(6), 1043–1063.

45. Beasley, E. E., & Beirness, D. J. (2012, October). Alcohol and drug use among drivers following the introduction of immediate roadside prohibitions in British Columbia: Findings from the 2012 roadside survey. Ottawa, ON. www2.gov .bc.ca/assets/gov/driving-and-transportation/driving/ publications/bc-roadside-report2012.pdf

46. Volkow, N. D., Chang, L., Wang, G. J., Fowler, J. S., Franceschi, D., Sedler, M. J., Gatley, S. J., et. al. (2001). Higher cortical and lower subcortical metabolism in detoxified

methamphetamine abusers. *American Journal of Psychiatry*, 158(3), 383–389.

47. Government of Canada. (2015, May 04). *Methamphetamine controlled and illegal drugs.* Substance Abuse. healthycanadians.gc.ca/healthy-living-vie-saine/substance-abuse-toxicomanie/controlled-drugs-substances-controlees/methamphetamine-eng.php
48. Royal Canadian Mounted Police. (2011, December 30). *Crystal meth, what you need to know.* Publications. www.rcmp-grc.gc.ca/qc/pub/sens-awar/meth/meth-eng.htm
49. Crystal Meth Addiction.org. (2003–2013). *Crystal meth ingredients.* www.crystalmethaddiction.org/Crystal_Meth_Ingredients.htm
50. Volkow, N. D., Chang, L., Wang, G. J., Fowler, J. S., Franceschi, D., Sedler, M. J., Gatley, S. J., et al. (2001). Higher cortical and lower subcortical metabolism in detoxified methamphetamine abusers. *American Journal of Psychiatry*, 158(3), 383–389.
51. Canadian Centre on Substance Abuse. (2016, April). *Cannabis.* Canadian Drug Summary. www.ccsa.ca/Resource%20Library/CCSA-Canadian-Drug-Summary-Cannabis-2016-en.pdf
52. Arbour-Nicitopoulos, K. P., Kwan, M. Y. W., Lowe, D., Taman, S., & Faulkner, G. E. J. (2011). Social norms of alcohol, smoking and marijuana use within a Canadian university setting. *Journal of American College Health*, 59(3), 191–196.
53. Canadian Centre on Substance Abuse. (2016, April). *Cannabis.* Canadian Drug Summary. http://www.ccsa.ca/Resource%20Library/CCSA-Canadian-Drug-Summary-Cannabis-2016-en.pdf
54. Ibid.
55. Beirness, D. J., & Porath-Waller, A. J. (2015). *Clearing the smoke on Cannabis. Cannabis use and driving—an update.* Canadian Centre on Substance Abuse. www.ccsa.ca/Resource%20Library/CCSA-Cannabis-Use-and-Driving-Report-2015-en.pdf
56. Trezza, V., Cuomo, V., & Vanderschuren, L. J. M. J. (2008). Cannabis and the developing brain: Insights from behaviour. *European Journal of Pharmacology*, 585(2–3), 441–452.
57. Reid, P. T., McLeod, J., & Robertson, J. R. (2010). Cannabis and the lung. *Journal of the Royal College of Edinburgh*, 40(4), 328–333.
58. Mittleman, M. (2001). Triggering myocardial infarction by marijuana. Journal of the *American Medical Association*, 286(6), 655.
59. Aryana, A., & Williams, M. A. (2007). Marijuana as a trigger of cardiovascular events; speculation or scientific certainty? *International Journal of Cardiology*, 118(2), 141–144.
60. Porath-Waller, A. J. (2015). *Clearing the smoke on cannabis. Maternal Cannabis use during pregnancy—an update.* Canadian Centre on Substance Abuse. www.ccsa.ca/Resource%20Library/CCSA-Cannabis-Maternal-Use-Pregnancy-Report-2015-en.pdf
61. Canadian Centre on Substance Abuse. (2016, April). *Cocaine.* Canadian Drug Summary. www.ccsa.ca/Resource%20Library/CCSA-Cocaine-Drug-Summary-2015-en.pdf
62. Phillips, K., Luk, A., Soor, G. S., Abraham, J. R., Leong, S., & Butany, J. (2009). Cocaine cardiotoxicity: A review of the pathophysiology, pathology, and treatment options. *American Journal of Cardiovascular Drugs*, 9(3), 177–196.
63. Shereif, H., Rezkalla, M. D., & Kloner, R. A. (2007). Cocaine-induced acute myocardial infarction. *Clinical Medicine and Research*, 5(3), 172–176.
64. Shine, B. (2000, March). Some cocaine abusers fare better with cognitive-behavioral therapy, others with 12-step programs. *National Institute on Drug Abuse*, NIDA Notes, 15(1).
65. Girard, A. L., & Senn, C. Y. (2008). The role of the new "date rape drugs" in attributions about date rape. *Journal of Interpersonal Violence*, 23(1), 3–20.
66. Németh, Z., Kun, B., & Demetrovics, Z. (2010). Review: The involvement of gamma-hydroxybutyrate in reported sexual assaults: A systematic review. *Journal of Psychopharmacology*, 24(9), 1281–1287.
67. Lwendo, S., Moozwe, M. A., Schensul, J. J., & Kostick, K. M. (2011). The role of MDMA (Ecstasy) in coping with negative life situations among urban young adults. *Journal of Psychoactive Drugs*, 43(3), 199–210.
68. Klein, H., Elifson, K. W., & Sterk, C. (2009). Young adult ecstasy users' enhancement of the effects of their ecstasy use. *Journal of Psychoactive Drugs*, 41(2), 113–120.
69. Government of Canada. (2014, May 04). *Ecstasy.* Controlled and Illegal Drugs. Substance Abuse. healthycanadians.gc.ca/healthy-living-vie-saine/substance-abuse-toxicomanie/controlled-drugs-substances-controlees/ecstasy-eng.php
70. McCardle, K., Luebbers, S., Carter, J. D., Croft, R. J., & Stough, C. (2004). Chronic MDMA (ecstasy) use, cognition and mood. *Psychopharmacology*, 173(3–4), 434–439.
71. Sullam, J. (2011). Your brain on MDMA. *Reason*, 43(2), 8–9.
72. Vorhees, C., Skelton, M., Graham, D., Schaefer, T., Grace, C., Braun, A., & Williams, M. (2010). Effects of age of exposure to 3,4-methylenedioxymethamphetamine (MDMA) in rats on later learning and behaviour. *Neurotoxicology and Teratology*, 32(4), 509.
73. Government of Canada. (2015, May 04). *LSD controlled and illegal drugs.* Substance Abuse. healthycanadians.gc.ca/healthy-living-vie-saine/substance-abuse-toxicomanie/controlled-drugs-substances-controlees/lsd-eng.php
74. Halpern, J. H., & Sewell, R. A. (2005). Hallucinogenic botanicals of America: A growing need for focused drug education and research. *Life Sciences*, 78(5), 519–526.
75. Rickert, V. I., Siqueira, L. M., Dale, T., & Wiemann, C. M. (2003). Prevalence and risk factors for LSD use among young women. *Journal of Pediatric and Adolescent Gynecology*, 16(2), 67–75.
76. Shaw, S. Y., Deering, K. N., Jolly, A. M., & Wylie, J. L. (2010). Increased risk for hepatitis C associated with solvent use among Canadian Aboriginal injection drug users. *Harm Reduction Journal*, 7(1), 16–24.
77. Ibid.
78. Fischer, B., Jones, W., Krahn, M., & Rehm, J. (2011). Differences and over-time changes in levels of prescription opioid analgesic dispensing from retail pharmacies in Canada, 2005–2010. *Pharmacoepidemilogy and Drug Safety*, 20(2011), 1269–1277.
79. Brands, B., Paglia-Boak, A., Sproule, B. A., Leslie, K., & Adlaf, E. M. (2010). Nonmedical use of opioid analgesics among Ontario students. *Canadian Family Physician*, 56(2010), 256–262.
80. Fischer, B., & Keatesa, A. (2012). "Opioid drought," Canadian style? Potential implications of the "natural experiment" of delisting Oxycontin in Canada. *The International Journal of Drug Policy*, 23(6), 495–497.
81. Weeks, C., & Howlett, K. (2016, April 05). Prescriptions of opioid drugs skyrocketing in Canada. *Globe and Mail.* www.theglobeandmail.com/news/national/sales-of-opiod-drug-prescriptionsskyrocketing/article26008639/

82. Friesen, K. J., Woelk, C., & Bugden, S. (2016, April 04). Safety of fentanyl initiation according to past opioid exposure among patients newly prescribed fentanyl patches. *Canadian Medical Association Journal.* DOI: 10.1503/cmaj.150961
83. Talmazan, Y. (2015, August 11). Fentanyl 101: The facts and dangers. *Global News.* www.theglobeandmail.com/news/british-columbia/fentanyl-related-deaths-soar-across-canada-report-says/article25920303/
84. Government of Canada. (2015, May 04). *Heroin.* Controlled and Illegal Drugs. Substance Abuse. healthycanadians.gc.ca/healthy-living-vie-saine/substance-abuse-toxicomanie/controlled-drugs-substances-controlees/heroin-heroine-eng.php
85. Canadian Centre for Substance Abuse. (2015, July). *Prescription opioids.* Canadian Drug Summary. www.ccsa.ca/Resource%20 Library/CCSA-Canadian-Drug-Summary-Prescription-Opioids-2015-en.pdf
86. Government of Canada. (2015, May 04). *PCP.* Controlled and Illegal Drugs. Substance Abuse. healthycanadians.gc.ca/healthy-living-vie-saine/substance-abuse-toxicomanie/controlled-drugs-substances-controlees/pcp-eng.php
87. McCabe, S. E. (2005). Correlates of nonmedical use of prescription benzodiazepine anxioloytics: Results from a national survey of U. C. college students. *Drug and Alcohol Dependence*, 79(1), 53–62.
88. National Institute on Drug Abuse (2016, March). *Drug facts: Anabolic steroids.* Anabolic Steroids. Drug Facts. www.drugabuse.gov/publications/drugfacts/anabolic-steroids
89. Berning, J. M., Adams, K. J., DeBeliso, M., Stamford, B. A., & Newman, I. M. (2008). Anabolic androgenic steroids: Use and perceived use in nonathlete college students. *Journal of American College Health*, 56(5), 499–503.
90. Canadian Centre for Ethics in Sport. (n.d.). *Canadian anti-doping program.* Anti-doping. Home. cces.ca/canadian-anti-doping-program
91. Canadadrugrehab.ca (2014). *Drug addiction treatment options.* www.canadadrugrehab.ca/
92. Wu, L. T., Parrott, A. C., Ringwalt, C. L., Patkar, A. A., Mannelli, P., & Blazer, D. G. (2009). The high prevalence of substance use disorders among recent MDMA users compared with other drug users: Implications for intervention. *Addictive Behaviors*, 34(8), 654–661.
93. Alcoholic Anonymous Worldwide. (2016). Home. www.aa.org/
94. City of Vancouver. (2016). *Four pillars drug strategy.* People and Programs. vancouver.ca/people-programs/four-pillars-drug-strategy.aspx
95. Vancouver Coastal Health. (n.d.). *InSite—Supervised injection site.* Supervisedinjection.vch.ca. Content Management. supervisedinjection.vch.ca/
96. Andresen, M. A., & Jozaghi, E. (2012). The point of diminishing returns: An examination of expanding Vancouver's InSite. *Urban Studies*, 49(16), 3531–3544.
97. Regina Qu'appelle Health Region. (2015). *All Nations' healing hospital. (ANHH).* www.fortquappelle.com/health-emergency/all-nations-healing-hospital
98. Street Works. (n.d.). *About street works.* Professional Site. www.streetworks.ca/pro/index.html
99. Health Canada. (2015, August 07). *Anti-drug strategy initiatives program.* Funding Programs. National Anti-Drug Strategy. healthycanadians.gc.ca/anti-drug-antidrogue/funding-financement/strategy-strategie-initiative-eng.php

Chapter 12

1. Farquharson, V. (2005, August 25). Drinking outside the box. A U. S. journalist finds McGill students have a mature attitude toward booze. *McGill Reporter*, 38. www.mcgill.ca/reporter/38/01/drinking
2. Carlson, S. R., Johnson, S. C., & Jacobs, P. C. (2010). Disinhibited characteristics and binge drinking among university student drinkers. *Addictive Behaviors*, 35(3), 242–251.
3. Balodis, I. M., Potenza, M. N., & Olmstead, M. C. (2009). Binge drinking in undergraduates: Relationships with sex, drinking behaviors, impulsivity, and the perceived effects of alcohol. *Behavioral Pharmacology*, 20(5–6), 518–526.
4. Reid, J. L., Hammond, D., Rynard, V. L., & Burkhalter, R. (2015). *Tobacco use in Canada: Patterns and trends* (2015 edition). Propel Centre for Population Health Impact, University of Waterloo. www.tobaccoreport.ca/2015/TobaccoUseinCanada_2015.pdf
5. International Alliance for Responsible Drinking. (IARD). (2016). *BAC and BrAC Limits.* Policy Tables. www.iard.org/policy-tables/bac-brac-limits/
6. Ministry of Justice. Office of the Superintendent of Motor Vehicles British Columbia (2013, April 11). *Immediate roadside prohibition fact sheet.* www2.gov.bc.ca/assets/gov/driving-and-transportation/driving/publications/factsheet-immediate-roadside-prohibition.pdf
7. MADD Canada. (n.d.). www.madd.ca/
8. Canada Safety Council. (2015, November 30). *National safe driving week.* National Safety Campaigns. canadasafetycouncil.org/news/national-safe-driving-week-2015
9. Government of Canada. (2016, January). *The chief public health officer's report on the state of public health in Canada, 2015: Alcohol consumption in Canada.* Public Health Agency of Canada. healthycanadians.gc.ca/publications/department-ministere/state-public-health-alcohol-2015-etat-sante-publique-alcool/index-eng.php
10. Statistics Canada. (2015, November 27). *Heavy drinking, 2013.* Health Fact Sheets. Publications. Catalogue no. 82-625-X. www.statcan.gc.ca/pub/82-625-x/2014001/article/14019-eng.htm
11. Ibid.
12. Ibid.
13. Intoxication. (2015). In *Merriam-Webster Online Dictionary.* www.merriam-webster.com/dictionary/intoxication
14. Boffetta, P., & Hashibe, M. (2006). Alcohol and cancer. *The Lancet Oncology*, 7(2), 149–156.
15. Boyle, P., & Boffetta, P. (2009). Alcohol consumption and breast cancer risk. *Breast Cancer Research*, 11(3), S3–S3.
16. Mukamal, K. J., & Rimm, E. B. (2008). Alcohol consumption: Risks and benefits. *Current Atherosclerosis Reports*, 10(6), 536–543.
17. Mukamal, K. J., Maclure, M., Muller, J. E., Sherwood, J. B., & Mittlemann, M. A. (2001). Prior alcohol consumption and mortality following acute myocardial infarction. *Journal of the American Medical Association*, 285(15), 1965–1970.
18. Lindberg, M. L., & Amsterdam, E. A. (2008). Alcohol, wine, and cardiovascular health. *Clinical Cardiology*, 31(8), 347–351.
19. Ward, R. J., Lallemand, F., & de Witte, P. (2009). Biochemical and neurotransmitter changes implicated in alcohol-induced brain damage in chronic or "binge drinking" alcohol use. *Alcohol and Alcoholism*, 44(2), 128–135.

20. Bava, S., & Tapert, S. F. (2010). Adolescent brain development and the risk for alcohol and other drug problems. *Neuropsychology Review*, 20(4), 398–413.

21. John, P. D., Snow, W. M., & Tyas, S. L. (2010). Alcohol use among older adults. *Reviews in Clinical Gerontology*, 20(1), 56–68.

22. Government of Canada. (2016, January). *The chief public health officer's report on the state of public health in Canada, 2015: Alcohol consumption in Canada*. Public Health Agency of Canada. healthycanadians.gc.ca/publications/department-ministere/state-public-health-alcohol-2015-etat-sante-publique-alcool/index-eng.php

23. American College Health Association (2015). American College Health Association National College Health Assessment II. Reference Group Executive Summary Fall 2015. Hanover, MD. http://www.acha-ncha.org/docs/NCHA-II_WEB_SPRING_2015_REFERENCE_GROUP_EXECUTIVE_SUMMARY.pdf

24. MADD Canada (n.d.). *The magnitude of the alcohol/drug-related crash problem in Canada: Overview*. Statistics. Overview. Impaired Driving. madd.ca/pages/impaired-driving/overview/statistics/

25. Government of Canada. (2016, January). *The chief public health officer's report on the state of public health in canada, 2015: Alcohol consumption in Canada*. Public Health Agency of Canada. healthycanadians.gc.ca/publications/department-ministere/state-public-health-alcohol-2015-etat-sante-publique-alcool/index-eng.php

26. Ibid.

27. Ibid.

28. Kairouz, S., Gliksman, L., Demers, A., & Adlaf, E. M. (2002). For all these reasons, I do ... drink: A multilevel analysis of contextual reasons for drinking among Canadian undergraduates. *Journal of Studies on Alcohol*, 63(5), 600–608.

29. American College Health Association (2015). American College Health Association National College Health Assessment II. *Group Executive Summary Fall 2015*. Hanover, MD. http://www.acha-ncha.org/docs/NCHA-II_WEB_SPRING_2015_REFERENCE_GROUP_EXECUTIVE_SUMMARY.pdf

30. Ibid.

31. Perkins, H. W., Hains, M. P., & Rice, R. (2005). Misperceiving the college drinking norm and related problems: A nationwide study of exposure to prevention information, perceived norms and student alcohol misuse. *Journal of Studies on Alcohol*, 66(4), 470–478.

32. Lane, D. J. (2012). A comparison of computer-assisted and self-management programs for reducing alcohol use among students in first year experience courses. *Journal of Drug Education*, 42(2), 119–135.

33. Roosen, K. M., & Mills, J. S. (2015). Exploring the motives and mental health correlates of intentional food restriction prior to alcohol use in university students. *Journal of Health Psychology*, 20(6), 875–886.

34. Adlaf, E. M., Demers, A., & Gliksman, L. (Eds.). (2005). *Canadian campus survey 2004*. Toronto, ON: Centre for Addiction and Mental Health. https://www.utsc.utoronto.ca/~facilities/documents/CanadianCampusSurvey2004Report.pdf

35. Balodis, I. M., Potenza, M. N., & Olmstead, M. C. (2009). Binge drinking in undergraduates: Relationships with sex, drinking behaviors, impulsivity, and the perceived effects of alcohol. *Behaviourial Pharmacology*, 20(5–6), 518–526.

36. Kubacki, K., Siemieniako, D., & Rundle-Thiele, S. (2011). College binge drinking: A new approach. *Journal of Consumer Marketing*, 23(3), 225–233.

37. Ibid.

38. Wells, S., Mihic, L., Tremblay, P. F., Graham, K., & Demers, A. (2008). Where, with whom, and how much alcohol is consumed on drinking events involving aggression? Event-level associations in a Canadian national survey of university students. Author Address. *Alcoholism, Clinical and Experimental Research*, 32(3), 522–533.

39. Jones, S., Oeltmann, J., Wilson, T. W., Brener, N. D., & Hill, C. V. (2001). Binge drinking among undergraduate college students in the United States: Implications for other substance use. *Journal of American College Health*, 50(1), 33–38.

40. Adlaf, E. M., Demers, A., & Gliksman, L. (Eds.). (2005). *Canadian campus survey 2004*. Toronto, ON: Centre for Addiction and Mental Health. https://www.utsc.utoronto.ca/~facilities/documents/CanadianCampusSurvey2004Report.pdf

41. Jones, S., Oeltmann, J., Wilson, T. W., Brener, N. D., & Hill, C. V. (2001). Binge drinking among undergraduate college students in the United States: Implications for other substance use. *Journal of American College Health*, 50(1), 33–38.

42. Smith, S. W., LaPlant, C., Novales, W.l., Mayer, W. A., Atkin, C. K., Klein, K., Glazer, E., & Martell, D. (2011). Student-generated protective behaviours to avert severe harm due to high-risk alcohol consumption. *Journal of College Student Development*, 52(1), 101–114. muse.jhu.edu/journals/journal_of_college_student_development/v052/52.1.smith.pdf

43. Ibid.

44. Government of Canada. (2015, June 25). National Native health and drug abuse program (NNADAP). *Funding programs. National anti-drug strategy.* healthycanadians.gc.ca/anti-drug-antidrogue/funding-financement/hc-sc-nnadap-pnlaada-eng.php

45. First Nations Health Authority. (2016). *Together in wellness: 2014–2015*. Home. www.fnha.ca/

46. Cook, J. L., Green, C. R., Lilley, C. M., Anderson, S. M., et al. (2016, February 16). Fetal alcohol spectrum disorder: A guideline for diagnosis across the lifespan. *Canadian Medical Association Journal (CMAJ)*, 188(3), 191–197.

47. Public Health Agency of Canada. (2010, June 02). *Frequently asked questions. Fetal alcohol spectrum disorder*. Programs and Initiatives. www.phac-aspc.gc.ca/hp-ps/dca-dea/prog-ini/fasd-etcaf/faq/index-eng.php

48. Sellman, D., & Connor, J. (2009). In utero brain damage from alcohol: A preventable tragedy. *New Zealand Medical Journal*, 122(1306), 6–8.

49. Foroud, T., Edenberg, H., & Crabbe, J. C. (2010). Genetic research: Who is at risk for alcoholism? *Alcohol Research & Health*, 33(1–2), 64–75.

50. Dom, G., De Wilde, B., Hulgtihn, W., & Sabbe, B. (2007). Traumatic experiences and posttraumatic stress disorders: Differences between treatment-seeking early- and late-onset alcoholic patients. *Comprehensive Psychiatry*, 48(2), 178–185.

51. Johnson, P., & Stone, R. (2009). Parental alcoholism and family functioning: Effects on differentiation levels of young adults. *Alcoholism Treatment Quarterly*, 27(1), 3–18.

52. Currell, C. K., & Jeglic, E. L. (2010). An examination of alcohol and drug use among urban college students. *Journal of Substance Use*, 15(4), 272–282.

53. Fletcher, A. (2001). *Sober for good*. New York: Houghton Mifflin.

54. Dejong, W., & Langford, L. M. (2002). A typology for campus-based alcohol prevention: Moving toward environmental management strategies. (Panel 2: Prevention and treatment of college alcohol problems.) *Journal of Studies on Alcohol*, 63(2), 140–148.

55. Schimpff, S. C., & Gerrans, L. (2013, May 30). *Smokers die ten years sooner than non-smokers.* Medical News Today. www.medicalnewstoday.com/articles/261091.php

56. Wexler, R. K., Elton, T., Pleister, A., & Feldman, D. (2009). Cardio-myopathy: An overview. *American Family Physician*, 79(9), 778–784.

57. Kakafika, A. I., & Mikhailidis, D. P. (2007). Smoking and aortic diseases. *Circulation Journal*, 71(8), 1173–1180.

58. Weinberger, A. H., Mazure, C. M., & McKee, S. A. (2010). Perceived risks and benefits of quitting smoking in non-treatment seekers. *Addiction Research & Theory*, 18(4), 456–463.

59. Lee, Y. H., Shin, M. H., Kweon, S. S., Choi, J. S., Rhee, J. A., Ahn, H. R., Yun, W. J., Ryu, S. Y., Kim, B. H., Nam, H. S., Jeong, S. K., & Park, K. S. (2011). Cumulative smoking exposure, duration of smoking cessation, and peripheral arterial disease in middle-aged and older Korean men. *BMC Public Health*, 11, 94–101.

60. Cornfield, J., Haenszel, W., Hammon, E. C., Lilienfeld, A. M., Shimkin, M. B., & Wynder, E. L. (2009). Smoking and lung cancer: Recent evidence and a discussion of some questions. *International Journal of Epidemiology*, 38(5), 1175–1191.

61. Public Health Agency of Canada. (2015, July 03). *What is lung cancer?* Lung Cancer. Cancer. Chronic Diseases. www.phac-aspc.gc.ca/cd-mc/cancer/lung_cancer-cancer_poumon-eng.php

62. Chappel, H., & Mery, L. (Co-Chairs). Canadian Cancer Society's Steering Committee on Cancer Statistics. (2012). *Canadian cancer statistics 2012*. Toronto, ON. www.cancer.ca/~/media/cancer.ca/CW/cancer%20information/cancer%20101/Canadian%20cancer%20statistics/Canadian-Cancer-Statistics-2012-EN.pdf?la=en

63. Johnson, J. G., Cohen, P., Pine, D. S., Klein, D. F., Kasen, S., & Brook, J. S. (2000). Association between cigarette smoking and anxiety disorders during adolescence and early adulthood. *Journal of American Medical Association*, 284(18), 2348–2351.

64. Reid, J. L., Hammond, D., Burkhalter, R., & Ahmed, R. (2012). *Tobacco use in Canada: Patterns and trends.* Propel Centre for Population Health Impact, University of Waterloo. Waterloo, ON. www.tobaccoreport.ca/2012/TobaccoUseinCanada_2012.pdf

65. Government of Canada. (2014, January 23). *Strong foundation, renewed focus—An overview of Canada's federal tobacco control strategy 2012–17.* Healthy Living. Publications. healthycanadians.gc.ca/publications/healthy-living-vie-saine/tobacco-strategy-2012-2017-strategie-tabagisme/index-eng.php

66. Tindle, H. (2008). Genetics of smoking behaviour. *Current Cardiovascular Risk Reports*, 2(6), 434–438.

67. Wilson, D. B., McClish, D. K., Heckman, C. J., Obando, C. P., & Dahman, B. A. (2007). Parental smoking, closeness to parents, and youth smoking. *American Journal of Health Behavior*, 31(3), 261–271.

68. Wolburg, J. (2009). Misguided optimism among college student smokers: Leveraging their quit-smoking strategies for smoking cessation campaigns. *Journal of Consumer Affairs*, 43(2), 305–331.

69. Bean, M. K., Mitchell, K. S., Speizer, I. S., Wilson, D. B., Smith, B. N., & Fries, E. A. (2008). Rural adolescent attitudes toward smoking and weight loss: Relationship to smoking status. *Nicotine & Tobacco Research: Official Journal of the Society for Research on Nicotine and Tobacco*, 10(2), 279–286.

70. Ling, P. M., & Glantz, A. (2002). Using tobacco-industry marketing research to design more effective tobacco control campaigns. *JAMA*, 287(22), 2983–2989.

71. Non-smoker's Rights Association. Smoking and Health Action Foundation. (2007, February 01). *Why tobacco powerwalls and other forms of retail promotion must be banned.* https://www.nsra-adnf.ca/cms/file/files/pdf/power_walls_should_be_banned_1.pdf

72. Health Canada. (2008, January 10). *The industry: Tobacco marketing makes us sick.* Health Concerns. www.hc-sc.gc.ca/hc-ps/tobac-tabac/youth-jeunes/scoop-primeur/indust-eng.php

73. Ling, P. A., & Glantz, A. (2002). Why and how the tobacco industry sells cigarettes to young adults: Evidence from industry documents. *American Journal of Public Health*, 202(926), 908–916.

74. DiFranza, J. R., Rigotti, N., McNeil, A. D., Ockene, J. K., Savageau, J. A., St. Cyr, D., & Coleman, M. (2000). Initial symptoms of nicotine dependence in adolescents. *Tobacco Control*, 9(3), 313–319.

75. Canadian Cancer Society's Advisory Committee on Cancer Statistics. (2015, June). *Canadian cancer statistics 2015.* Toronto: ON. https://www.cancer.ca/~/media/cancer.ca/CW/cancer%20information/cancer%20101/Canadian%20cancer%20statistics/Canadian-Cancer-Statistics-2015-EN.pdf

76. Reid, J. L., Hammon, D., Rynard, V. L., & Burkhalter, R. (2015). *Tobacco use in Canada: Patterns and trends.* Waterloo, On: Propel Centre for Population Health Impact. University of Waterloo. tobaccoreport.ca/2015/TobaccoUseinCanada_2015.pdf

77. Ibid.

78. Ibid.

79. Berg, C. J., Pratibha, P., Lessard, L., Escoffery, C., Kegler, M., Sterling, K., & Ahluwalia, J. S. (2010). Defining "smoker": College students' attitudes and related smoking characteristics. *Nicotine & Tobacco Research*, 12(9), 963–969.

80. Dierker, L., Lloyd-Richardson, E., Stolar, M., Flay, B., Tiffany, S., Collins, L., Baily, S., Nichter, M., Nichter, M., Clayton, R., & The Tobacco Etiology Research Network (TERN). (2005). The proximal association between smoking and alcohol use among first year college students. *Drug and Alcohol Dependence*, 81(1), 1–9.

81. Beets, M. W., Flay, B. R., Vuchinich, S., Li, K. K., Acock, A., Snyder, F. J., & the Tobacco Etiology Research Network (TERN). (2009). Longitudinal patterns of binge drinking among first year college students with a history of tobacco use. *Drug and Alcohol Dependence*, 103(1–2), 1–8.

82. Wechsler, H., Kelly, K., Seibring, M., Kuo, M., & Rigotti, N. A. (2001). College smoking policies and smoking cessation programs: Results of a survey of college health center directors. *Journal of American College Health*, 49(5), 205–212.

83. Borders, T. F., Xu, K. T., Bacchi, D., Cohen, L., & SoRelle-Miner, D. (2005). College campus smoking policies and programs and students' smoking behaviors. *BMC Public Health*, 5(1), 74–79.

84. Fletcher, P., & Camblin, A. (2009). Preliminary examination of first year female university students: Smoking practices and beliefs in a city with no-smoking legislation. *College Student Journal*, 43(1), 234–240.

85. Hammond, D., Tremblay, I., Chaiton, M., Lessard, E., Collard, C., & The Tobacco on Campus Workgroup. (2005). Tobacco on campus: Industry marketing and tobacco control policy among post-secondary institutions in Canada. *Tobacco Control*, 14(2), 136–140.

86. Ramsay, J., & Hoffman, A. (2004). Smoking cessation and relapse prevention among undergraduate students: A pilot demonstration project. *Journal of American College Health*, 53(1), 11–16.

87. Wong, S. (2016, February 01). Use and misuse of tobacco among Aboriginal peoples. Position statement. *Canadian Paediatric Society*, 11(10), 681–685. www.cps.ca/documents/position/tobacco-aboriginal-people

88. Government of Canada. (2015, February 03). *Summary of results for 2013. Canadian Tobacco, Alcohol and Drugs Survey (CTADS).* Data. Science, Research and Data. healthycanadians.gc.ca/science-research-sciences-recherches/data-donnees/ctads-ectad/summary-sommaire-2013-eng.php

89. Official Position Statement of the Association of Women's Health, Obstetric & Neonatal Nursing. (2010). Smoking and women's health. *Journal of Obstetric, Gynecologic, and Neonatal Nursing*, 39(5), 611–613.

90. Callison, C., Karrh, J. A., & Zillmann, D. (2002). The aura of tobacco smoke: Cigars and cigarettes as image makers. *Journal of Applied Social Psychology*, 32(7), 1329–1343.

91. Government of Canada. (2015, February 03). *Summary of results for 2013. Canadian Tobacco, Alcohol and Drugs Survey (CTADS).* Data. Science, Research and Data. healthycanadians.gc.ca/science-research-sciences-recherches/data-donnees/ctads-ectad/summary-sommaire-2013-eng.php

92. Roskin, J., & Aveyard, P. (2009). Canadian and English students' beliefs about waterpipe smoking: A qualitative study. *BMC Public Health*, 9(1), 10–17.

93. Smith-Simone, S. Y., Curbow, B. A., & Stillman, F. A. (2008). Differing psychosocial risk profiles of college freshmen waterpipe, cigar, and cigarette smokers. *Addictive Behaviors*, 33(12), 1619–1624.

94. Government of Canada. (2015, February 03). *Summary of results for 2013. Canadian Tobacco, Alcohol and Drugs Survey (CTADS).* Data. Science, Research and Data. healthycanadians.gc.ca/science-research-sciences-recherches/data-donnees/ctads-ectad/summary-sommaire-2013-eng.php

95. Schivo, M., Avdalovic, M. VV., & Murin, S. (2014). Non-cigarette tobacco and the lung. *Clinical Reviews in Allergy & Immunology*, 46(1), 34–53.

96. Czoli, C. D., Reid, J. L., Rynard, V. L., & Hammond, D. (2015). *E-cigarettes in Canada: Special supplement.* Tobacco Use in Canada: Patterns and Trends 2015 Edition. Waterloo, ON: Propel Centre for Population Health Impact. University of Waterloo. www.tobaccoreport.ca/2015/TobaccoUseinCanada_2015_EcigaretteSupplement.pdf

97. Ibid.

98. Russell, A. (2016, January 27). Exploding e-cigarettes? Here's what Canadians need to know. *Global News. Canada.* globalnews.ca/news/2481734/exploding-e-cigarettes-heres-what-canadians-need-to-know/

99. Ibid.

100. The Lung Association. (2012, December). The Canadian Lung Association's position statement on electronic cigarettes (E-Cigarettes). www.on.lung.ca/document.doc?id=1519

101. Government of Canada. (2016, January 14). *Second hand smoke.* Avoid Second Hand Smoke. Smoking and Tobacco. healthycanadians.gc.ca/healthy-living-vie-saine/tobacco-tabac/avoid-second-hand-smoke-eviter-fumee-secondaire/second-hand-smoke-fumee-secondaire/index-eng.php

102. Canadian Cancer Society. (2016). *Second hand smoke.* Tobacco. What is a Risk Factor? www.cancer.ca/en/cancer-information/cancer-101/what-is-a-risk-factor/tobacco/second-hand-smoke/?region=on

103. Kelleher, C. C., & Frazer, K. (2014). An international smoking ban—how many lives will be saved? *Current Atherosclerosis Reports*, 16(6), 1–7.

104. Reuters. (2012, December 18). *Tobacco companies, over 17 states settle over payments.* News. www.reuters.com/article/us-tobacco-states-settlement-idUSBRE8BH1BI20121219

105. CBC News. (2005, September 29). *Supreme court rules B. C. clear to sue tobacco companies.* Canada. www.cbc.ca/news/canada/supreme-court-rules-b-c-clear-to-sue-tobacco-companies-1.566154

106. Babbage, M. (2013, May 31). Appeal court gives go-ahead to Ontario's $50-billion lawsuit against big tobacco companies. News. *The National Post.* news.nationalpost.com/news/canada/appeal-court-gives-go-ahead-to-ontarios-50-billion-lawsuit-against-big-tobacco-companies

107. World Health Organization (WHO). (2016). *About the WHO framework convention on tobacco control.* WHO Framework Convention on Tobacco Control. www.who.int/fctc/about/en/

108. Treasury Board of Canada, Secretariat. (2015, November 30). *Federal tobacco control strategy: Plans, spending and results.* Horizontal Results. Organization. 1. www.tbs-sct.gc.ca/hidb-bdih/initiative-eng.aspx?Hi=34

109. Health Canada. (2011, November 21). *Tobacco product labelling.* Legislation. Tobacco. www.hc-sc.gc.ca/hc-ps/tobac-tabac/legislation/label-etiquette/index-eng.php

110. Government of Canada. (2016, January 13). *Quit smoking now.* Smoking and Tobacco. Healthy Living. healthycanadians.gc.ca/healthy-living-vie-saine/tobacco-tabac/quit-cesser/quit-now-cesser-maintenant/index-eng.php

111. Government of Canada. (2012, January 12). *Cost calculator: How much do you spend on cigarettes?* Smoking and Tobacco. Healthy Living. healthycanadians.gc.ca/healthy-living-vie-saine/tobacco-tabac/calculator-calculatrice-eng.php

112. Health Canada. (2014, November 14). *On the road to quitting—guide to becoming a non-smoker.* Healthy Living. Publications. healthycanadians.gc.ca/publications/healthy-living-vie-saine/non-smoker-adult-non-fumeur-adulte/index-eng.php

113. Obermayer, J. L., Riley, W. T., Asif, O., & Jean-Mary, J. (2004). College smoking-cessation using cell phone text messaging. *Journal of American College Health*, 53(2), 71–78.

114. Durkin, A. (2007). Promoting smoking cessation among nursing students: How Faculty can help. *Nursing Education Perspectives*, 28(3), 150–154.

115. Health Canada. (2011, October 20). *Quit smoking aids.* Health Concerns. Smoking and Your Body. www.hc-sc.gc.ca/hc-ps/tobac-tabac/body-corps/aid-eng.php

116. QuitNowca. The Lung Association. (2016). Quitting medications. Preparing to Quit. Quitting Smoking. www.quitnow.ca/quitting/medications

117. QuitNowca. The Lung Association. (2016). *Nicotine patch.* Quitting medications. Preparing to Quit. Quitting Smoking. www.quitnow.ca/quitting/medications/nicotine-patch

Chapter 13

1. Canadian Institute for Health Information. (2015, October 29). *National health expenditure trends.* Spending and Health Workforce. www.cihi.ca/en/spending-and-health-workforce/spending/national-health-expenditure-trends

2. Ibid.

3. Ibid.

4. Ibid.

5. Metcalfe, A., Williams, J., McChesney, J., Patten, S. B., & Jetté, N. (2010). Use of complementary and alternative medicine by those with a chronic disease and the general population—results of a national population based survey. *BMC Complementary and Alternative Medicine*, 10(1), 58–63. bmccomplementalternmed.biomedcentral.com/articles/10.1186/1472-6882-10-58

6. Ardell, D. (1977). *High level wellness: An alternative to doctors, drugs and disease* (10th ed.). Berkeley, CA: Ten Speed Press, p. 94.

7. Romanow, R. J. (2002). *Building on values: The future of health care in Canada—Final report.* Commission on the Future of Health Care in Canada. Government of Canada Publications. publications.gc.ca/site/eng/237274/publication.html

8. Canadian Museum of Civilization. (2010, April 21). Tommy Douglas. Geography. *1939–1948. Making medicare. The history of health care in Canada. Online exhibition.* www.historymuseum.ca/cmc/exhibitions/hist/medicare/medic-3g03e.shtml

9. Health Canada. (2016, February 19). *Canada Health Act annual report 2014–2015.* Canada Health Act Overview. Chapter 1. www.hc-sc.gc.ca/hcs-sss/pubs/cha-lcs/2015-cha-lcs-ar-ra/index-eng.php#c1

10. Ibid.

11. Romanow, R. J. (2002). *Building on values: The future of health care in Canada—Final report.* Commission on the Future of Health Care in Canada. Government of Canada Publications. publications.gc.ca/site/eng/237274/publication.html

12. Health Canada. (2016, February 16). *Canada Health Act annual report 2014–2015.* Canada Health Act Overview. Chapter 1. www.hc-sc.gc.ca/hcs-sss/pubs/cha-lcs/2015-cha-lcs-ar-ra/index-eng.php#c1

13. University of British Columbia. (n.d.). *Current funding.* Evidence and Perspectives on Health Care in Canada. Key Issues. healthcarefunding.ca/key-issues/current-funding/

14. Sutherland, L., & Repin, N. (2014, March). Activity-based funding (ABF) hospital funding models for Canadian provinces. Current Hospital Funding in Canada Policy Brief. Vancouver: UBC Centre for Health Services and Policy Research. healthcarefunding2.sites.olt.ubc.ca/files/2014/03/White-Paper-ABF.pdf

15. University of British Columbia. (n.d.). *Bundled payments.* Evidence and Perspectives on Health Care in Canada. Key Issues. healthcarefunding.ca/key-issues/bundle-test-2/

16. Canadian Institute for Health Information. (2015, September). *Physicians in Canada, 2014: Summary report.* https://secure.cihi.ca/free_products/Summary-PhysiciansInCanadaReport2014_EN-web.pdf

17. Ibid.

18. Ibid.

19. Canadian Institute for Health Information. (2015, June). *Regulated nurses: 2014.* Report. https://secure.cihi.ca/free_products/RegulatedNurses2014_Report_EN.pdf

20. Ibid.

21. Pratt, W. R. (2010). Physician career satisfaction: Examining perspectives of the work environment. *Hospital Topics*, 88(2), 43–52.

22. Angood, P. B. (2013). All physicians are leaders. *American College of Physician Executives*, U.S.A., 39(2), 6–7.

23. The Association of Faculties of Medicine of Canada. (2016). *Admission requirements of Canadian faculties of medicine, 2016.* https://www.afmc.ca/sites/default/files/documents/en/Publications/AdmissionsBook2016-Final-EN.pdf

24. College of Family Physicians of Canada (CFPC), Canadian Medical Association (CMA), Royal College of Physicians and Surgeons of Canada (RCPSC). (2014, December 02). *National physician survey, 2014.* http://nationalphysiciansurvey.ca/surveys/2014-survey/

25. Scott, I., Gowans, M., Wright, B., Brenneis, F. Banner, S., & Boone, J. (2011). De-terminants of choosing a career in family medicine. *Canadian Medical Association Journal*, 183(1), E1–E8.

26. Canadian Nurses Association. (2016). *Becoming an RN.* Home. https://www.cna-aiic.ca/en/becoming-an-rn

27. Lewkonia, R. (2011). Patients' rights and medical education: Clinical principles. *Medical Teacher*, 33(5), 392–396.

28. Canadian Internet Registration Authority (CIRA). (2015). *The Canadian Internet.* CIRA Factbook 2015. cira.ca/factbook/2015/the-canadian-internet.html

29. Tonsaker, T. Bartlett, G., & Trpkov, C. (2014). Health information on the Internet. Gold mine or minefield? *Canadian Family Physician*, 60(5), 407–408.

30. Ibid.

31. National Physician Survey, 2014. (2014, December 02). College of Family Physicians of Canada (CFPC), Canadian Medical Association (CMA), Royal College of Physicians and Surgeons of Canada (RCPSC). nationalphysiciansurvey.ca/surveys/2014-survey/

32. Statista. (2016). Percentage of Canadians who believe their health records are vulnerable to a security breach as of April 2016. Cyber Crime. Internet. www.statista.com/statistics/548412/health-records-security-vulnerability-perception-canada/

33. Underhill, C., & McKeown, L. (2008, November 17). Getting a second opinion: Health information and the Internet. Statistics Canada. Health Reports. *The Daily.* Catalogue no. 82-003-X. Archived. http://www.statcan.gc.ca/daily-quotidien/080221/dq080221c-eng.htm

34. Childs, S. (2005). Judging the quality of internet-based health information. *Performance Measurement and Metrics*, 6(2), 80–96.

35. Ghodse, H., (2010). Watching internet pharmacies. *The British Journal of Psychiatry*, 196(3), 169–170.

36. Government of Canada. (2012, October 19). *Buying drugs over the Internet.* Buying and Using Drug Products Safely. healthycanadians.gc.ca/drugs-products-medicaments-produits/buying-using-achat-utilisation/drugs-internet-medicaments/index-eng.php

37. Montoya, I. D., & Jano, E. (2007). Online pharmacies: Safety and regulatory considerations. *International Journal of Health Services: Planning, Administration, Evaluation*, 37(2), 279–289.

38. National Association of Pharmacy Regulatory Authorities (NAPRA). (2009). Information for consumers about online pharmacies. Pharmacy practice and regulatory resources. napra.ca/pages/Practice_Resources/Practice_ResourcesOnlinePharmacies.aspx

39. British Columbia Medical Association. (n.d.). *Finding health information on the web* (brochure). sci-bc-database.ca/wp-content/uploads/Finding-Health-Information-on-the-Internet.pdf

40. Wilson, P. (2002). How to find the good and avoid the bad or ugly: A short guide to tolls for rating quality of health information on the Internet. Education and debate. *British Medical Journal*, 324, 598–602.

41. Gagliardi, A., & Jadad, A. R. (2002). Examination of instruments used to rate quality of health information on the Internet: Chronicle of a voyage with an unclear destination. *British Medical Journal*, 324, 569–573.

42. Pilapitiya, S. (2013). Issues in clinical trials in complementary and alternative medicine (CAM). *Current Opinion in Pharmacology*, 13(2), 311–312.

43. Esmail, N. (2007, May). Complementary and alternative medicine in Canada: Trends in use and public attitudes 1997–2006. *Fraser Institute, Public Policy Sources*, 87, 3–53. www.fraserinstitute.org/studies/complementary-and-alternative-medicine-in-canada-trends-use-and-public-attitudes-1997-2006

44. Ibid.

45. Metcalfe, A., Williams, J., McChesney, J., Patten, S. B., & Jetté, N. (2010). Use of complementary and alternative medicine by those with a chronic disease and the general population—results of a national population based survey. *BMC Complementary and Alternative Medicine*, 10(1), 58–63. bmccomplementalternmed.biomedcentral.com/articles/10.1186/1472-6882-10-58

46. Falci, L., Shi, Z., & Greenlee, H. (2016, May 05). Multiple chronic conditions and use of complementary and alternative medicine among US adults: Results from the 2012 National Health Interview Survey. *Preventing Chronic Disease*, 2016, (13):150501. DOI: dx.doi.org.ezproxy.library.uvic.ca/10.5888/pcd13.150501

47. Littlewood, R. A., & Vanable, P. A. (2008). Complementary and alternative medicine use among HIV-positive people: Research synthesis and implications for HIV care. *Aids Care*, 20(8), 1002–1018.

48. Busse, J. W., Heaton, G., Wu, P., Wilson, K. R., & Mills, E. J. (2005). Disclosure of natural product use to primary care physicians: A cross-sectional survey of naturopathic clinic attendees. *Mayo Clinic Proceedings*, 80(5), 616–623.

49. Mak, J. C. S., Mak, L. Y., Shen, Q., & Faux, S. (2009). Perceptions and attitudes of rehabilitation medicine physicians on complementary and alternative medicine in Australia (PARP-CAMA). *Internal Medicine Journal*, 39(3), 164–169.

50. Quartey, N. K., Ma, P. H., Chung, V. C. H., & Griffiths, S. M. (2012). Complementary and alternative medicine education for medical profession: Systematic review. *Evidenced Based Complementary and Alternative Medicine, 2012*. Article ID 656812.13

51. The College of Physicians and Surgeons of Ontario. (2011, November). *Complementary/alternative medicine*. Policies and Publications. www.cpso.on.ca/policies-publications/policy/complementary-alternative-medicine

52. Frass, M. Strassl, R. P., Friehs, H., Müller, M., Kundi, M., & Kaye, A. D. (2012). Use and acceptance of complementary and alternative medicine among the general population and medical personnel: A systematic review. *The Oshsner Journal*, 12(1), 45–56.

53. Winslow, L. C., & Shapiro, H. (2002). Physicians want education about complementary and alternative medicine to enhance communication with their patients. *Archives of Internal Medicine*, 162(10), 1176–1181.

54. WHO. (2013). *WHO Traditional medicine strategy, 2014 to 2023*. Essential Medicines and Health Products. Programmes. www.who.int/medicines/publications/traditional/trm_strategy14_23/en/

55. Ramsay, C. (2009, September 10). *Unnatural regulation: Complementary and alternative medicine policy in Canada*. Studies in Health Care Policy. Fraser Institute. www.fraserinstitute.org/sites/default/files/UnnaturalRegulation.pdf

56. Esmail, N. (2007, May). Complementary and alternative medicine in Canada: Trends in use and public attitudes 1997–2006. *Fraser Institute, Public Policy Sources*, 87, 3–53. www.fraserinstitute.org/sites/default/files/ComplementaryAlternativeMedicine.pdf

57. Ramsay, C. (2009, September 10). *Unnatural regulation: Complementary and alternative medicine policy in Canada*. Studies in Health Care Policy. Fraser Institute. www.fraserinstitute.org/sites/default/files/UnnaturalRegulation.pdf

58. Turner, L., Singh, K., Garritty, C., Tsertsvadze, A., Manheimer, E., Wieland, S., Galipeau, J., & Moher, D. (2011). An evaluation of the completeness of safety reporting in reports of the complementary and alternative medicine trials. *BMC Complementary and Alternative Medicine*, 11(1), 67–77.

59. IN-CAM Canada. (2014). *About IN-CAM*. www.incamresearch.ca/content/about-cam

60. Nahin, R., & Straus, S. (2001). Research into complementary and alternative medicine: Problems and potential. *British Medical Journal*, 33(7279), 161.

61. Canadian College of Homeopathic Medicine. (2015). *Regulation of homeopathic medicine*. The College. www.homeopathycanada.com/regulation-homeopathy

62. Registered Massage Therapists' Association of Ontario. (2016). *Massage therapy in Canada*. Massage Therapy—Regulation of MT. secure.rmtao.com/massage_therapy/regulation_of_mt/massage_therapy_in_canada.htm

63. De Guzman, M. L. (2015, November 24). *Manitoba approves regulation of massage therapy profession*. Massage Therapy Canada. Regulation, Education. www.massagetherapycanada.com/regulations/manitoba-approves-regulation-of-massage-therapy-profession-3107

64. Association des Acupunctures des Québec. (2016). *The acupuncture profession*. Discover Acupuncture. www.acupuncture-quebec.com/en/discover-acupuncture/acupuncture-profession.html

65. Vogel, L. (2010). Hodge-podge regulation of alternative medicine in Canada. *Canadian Medical Association Journal*, 182(12), E569–E570.

66. Health Canada. (2016, March 14). *About natural health product regulation in Canada*. Drug and Health Products. www.hc-sc.gc.ca/dhp-mps/prodnatur/about-apropos/index-eng.php

67. Health Canada. (2016, March 24). *About natural health products*. Drug and Health Products. www.hc-sc.gc.ca/dhp-mps/prodnatur/about-apropos/cons-eng.php

68. Mehl-Madrona, L. (2008). Narratives of exceptional survivors who work with Aboriginal Healers. *Journal of Alternative and Complementary Medicine*, 14(5), 497–504.

69. The Chinese Medicine and Acupuncture Association of Canada (CMAAC). (2014). Home. www.cmaac.ca/

70. Cummings. M. (2001). Commentary: Controls for acupuncture—Can we finally see the light? *British Medical Journal*, 322(7302), 1578.

71. Reflexology Association of Canada. (2015). Home. www.reflexologycanada.org/en/

72. International Institute of Ayurveda and Complimentary Medicines Inc. (IIACM). (2016). *Ayurveda courses*. www.iiacm.com/index.html

73. The College of Holistic International Studies. (2010). *Biofeedback*. Home. cihs.albodigital.net/about-cihs.php

74. Canadian Chiropractic Association. (2016). *Canadian chiropractors*. About Chiropractic. www.chiropractic.ca/about-chiropractic/canadian-chiropractors/

75. Haller, C., & Benowitz, N. (2000). Adverse cardiovascular and central nervous system events associated with dietary

supplements containing ephedra alkaloids. *New England Journal of Medicine*, 343(25), 1833–1838.

76. Canadian College of Homeopathic Medicine. (2015). *Why study with CCHM?* The College. www.homeopathycanada.com/why-study-cchm
77. Canadian Kinesiology Alliance. (n.d.). *Who are kinesiologists?* What Is the Scope of Practice for Kinesiologists in Canada? www.cka.ca/faq-questions-inline
78. Canadian Massage Therapist Alliance. (CMTA). (2016). National standards of practice. www.crmta.ca/?page=22
79. Chaitow, L. (2006). What is naturopathic physical medicine? *Journal of Bodywork and Movement Therapies*, 11(1), 1–2.
80. Walji, R., Weeks, L., Cooley, K., & Seely, D. (2010). Naturopathic medicine and Aboriginal health: An exploratory study at Anishnawbe health Toronto. *Canadian Journal of Public Health*, 101(6), 475–480.
81. Canadian Association of Naturopathic Doctors. (n.d). *Regulation in provinces and territories.* Common Questions: Education and Regulation. www.cand.ca/common-questions-education-and-regulation/#regulation-in-provinces-and-territories
82. Canadian Association of Naturopathic Doctors. (n.d.). *Education and training.* Common Questions: Education and Regulation. www.cand.ca/common-questions-education-and-regulation/#education-and-training
83. Canadian Physiotherapy Association. (2012). *Description of physiotherapy in Canada 2012.* About Physiotherapy. www.physiotherapy.ca/About-Physiotherapy/Description-of-Physiotherapy
84. Canadian Physiotherapy Association. (2012). *Physiotherapy education.* About Physiotherapy. www.physiotherapy.ca/About-Physiotherapy/Careers-in-Physiotherapy

Chapter 14

1. Keeling, R. (2002, September). Risks to students' lives: Setting priorities. *Journal of American College Health*, 51(2), 53–56.
2. Thompson Rivers University. (2010). *Working and learning safely at TRU.* Health and Safety. www.tru.ca/hsafety/workinglearningsafely.html
3. University of Waterloo. (n.d.). *Personal safety guide.* Police. Home. Offices and Services. uwaterloo.ca/police/personal-safety-guide/all-times
4. Statistics Canada. (2015, June 24). Canadian community health survey: Combined data, 2013/2014. *The Daily.* www.statcan.gc.ca/daily-quotidien/150624/dq150624b-eng.htm
5. Billette, J. M., & Janz, T. (2011, June 28). *Injuries in Canada: Insights from the Canadian community health survey.* Health at a Glance. Catalogue No. 82-624-X. Publications. Statistics Canada. www.statcan.gc.ca/pub/82-624-x/2011001/article/11506-eng.htm
6. Accreditation Canada, Canadian Institute for Health Information and Canadian Patient Safety Institute. (2014). *Preventing falls: From evidence to improvement in Canadian health care.* Ottawa, ON: CIHI. accreditation.ca/sites/default/files/falls-joint-report-2014-en.pdf
7. Canada Safety Council. (2012, November 06). *National senior safety week. Drug safety for seniors.* National Safety Campaigns. canadasafetycouncil.org/campaigns/national-senior-safety-week-drug-safety-seniors
8. Parachute. (n.d.). *Poison prevention.* Injury Topics. www.parachutecanada.org/policy/item/261
9. Knowledge is the best medicine (KiBM). (2016). App. MyMedRec. Create Your Own Record. Institute for Safe Medication Practices Canada (ISMP Canada). www.knowledgeisthebestmedicine.org/index.php/en/app
10. Canadian Red Cross. (1999–2016). *First aid kit.* Kit Contents. First Aid Tips. www.redcross.ca/training-and-certification/first-aid-tips-and-resources-/first-aid-tips/kit-contents
11. Ibid.
12. Naim, K., & Sana, K. (2013). Disaster resiliency and culture of preparedness for university and college campuses. *Administration and Society*, 45(1), 3–37.
13. Longo, P. J. (2010). Stalking on campus: Ensuring security with rights and liberties. *College Student Journal*, 44(2), 309–325.
14. Sookman, J. (2012, January 19). Guardly launches free mobile emergency phone service to students at 67 universities and colleges across Canada: Connects students, faculty and staff to campus security instantly with mobile app for smartphones, available anywhere on campus. Marketwire L. P. Toronto, Canada. guardly.com/blog/2012/01/19/guardly-launches-free-mobile-emergency-phone-service-to-students-at-67-universities-and-colleges-across-canada/index.html
15. Infrastructure Health and Safety Association (IHSA). (2016). *Safe job procedures.* Safe Work Practices. Tools and Resources. www.ihsa.ca/resources/safe_practices_procedures.aspx
16. Health Canada. (2012, November 02). *Environmental and workplace health.* Home. www.hc-sc.gc.ca/ewh-semt/index-eng.php
17. Canadian Centre for Occupational Health and Safety (CCOHS). (2016, May 13). Home. Government of Canada. www.ccohs.ca/
18. Transport Canada. (2016, May 10). *Canadian motor vehicle traffic collision statistics 2014.* Statistics and Data. Motor Vehicle Safety. Road Transportation. www.tc.gc.ca/eng/motorvehiclesafety/resources-researchstats-menu-847.htm
19. Ibid.
20. Transport Canada. (2014, July 11). *Road safety in Canada.* Road and Motor Vehicle Safety Publications. Road Transportation. www.tc.gc.ca/eng/motorvehiclesafety/tp-tp15145-1201.htm
21. Ibid.
22. Canadian Council of Motor Transport Administrators. (CCMTA). (2016). *Road safety measures.* Canada's Road Safety Strategy 2015. crss2015.ccmta.ca/search-initiatives.php?action=s&cf1=1&keyword=
23. Ibid.
24. Canadian Association of Road Safety Professionals. (2016). *Front air bags.* High-Tech Vehicle Safety Systems. www.carsp.ca/research/resources/high-tech-vehicle-safety-systems/front-air-bags/
25. Canadian Association of Road Safety Professionals. (2016). *Side air bags.* High-Tech Vehicle Safety Systems. www.carsp.ca/research/resources/high-tech-vehicle-safety-systems/side-air-bags/
26. Transport Canada. (2012, January 27). Airbag deactivation: What you need to know to make an informed decision. *Road & Motor Vehicle Safety Publications. Road Transportation.* www.tc.gc.ca/eng/roadsafety/tp-tp13178-menu-124.htm
27. Ibid.
28. Brown, S. W., Valar, W. G. M., & Robertson, R. D. (2015, December). Alcohol and drug-crash problem in Canada. 2012 report. *CCMTA Road Safety Research Report Series. Canadian Council of Motor Transport Administrators (CCMTA).* http://ccmta.ca/images/publications/pdf//2012_Alcohol__Drug_Crash_Problem_Report_ENG.pdf
29. Ibid.
30. Ibid.

31. Traffic Injury Research Foundation. (2015, December). *The road safety monitor 2015. Drinking and driving in Canada.* Ottawa, ON. tirf.ca/publications/PDF_publications/RSM_2015_Drinking_Driving_Eng_7.pdf

32. Statistics Canada. (2013, January 10). *Impaired driving in Canada in 2011.* Juristat. Publications. Catalogue no. 85-002-X. Canadian Centre for Justice Statistics. www.statcan.gc.ca/pub/85-002-x/2013001/article/11739-eng.pdf

33. Weschler, H., Lee, J. E., Nelson, T. F., & Lee, H. (2005). Drinking and driving among college students: The influence of alcohol-control policies. *American Journal of Preventive Medicine*, 25(3), 212–218.

34. Ibid.

35. MADD Parkland. (2016). *MADD youth in Canada. Let's keep each other alive.* Youth. Services and Programs. maddchapters.ca/parkland/services-programs/youth/

36. Students Against Drinking and Driving Alberta. (n d.). SADD Alberta. www.saddalberta.com/

37. ICBC. (2016). *ICBC driving tips.* Safe Drivers and Passengers. Road Safety. www.icbc.com/road-safety/safer-drivers/Pages/Default.aspx

38. Brown, S. W., Valar, W. G. M., & Robertson, R. D. (2015, December). *Alcohol and drug-crash problem in Canada. 2012 report.* CCMTA Road Safety Research Report Series. Canadian Council of Motor Transport Administrators (CCMTA). http://ccmta.ca/images/publications/pdf//2012_Alcohol__Drug_Crash_Problem_Report_ENG.pdf

39. Ibid.

40. Dawe, M., Fischer, B., McGuire, F., Rehm, J., & Shield, K. D. (2011). Driving under the influence of cannabis or alcohol in a cohort of high-frequency cannabis users: Prevalence and reflections on current interventions. *Canadian Journal of Criminology and Criminal Justice,* 53(2), 247–259.

41. Ministry of Transportation Ontario. (2015, November 04). *Impaired driving.* Driving Safety. www.mto.gov.on.ca/english/safety/impaired-driving.shtml

42. Pashley, C. R., Robertson, R. D., & Vanlaar, W. G. M. (2013, September). *The road safety monitor 2013. Drugs and driving.* Traffic Injury Research Foundation. Ottawa, ON. www.tirf.ca/publications/PDF_publications/2013_RSM_Drugs&Driving_6.pdf

43. Brown, S. W., Valar, W. G. M., & Robertson, R. D. (2015, December). *Alcohol and drug-crash problem in Canada. 2012 report.* CCMTA Road Safety Research Report Series. Canadian Council of Motor Transport Administrators (CCMTA). http://ccmta.ca/images/publications/pdf//2012_Alcohol__Drug_Crash_Problem_Report_ENG.pdf

44. Ibid.

45. Canadian Wireless Telecommunications Association (CWTA). (2016). *Wireless phone subscribers in Canada.* CWTA Facts and Figures. cwta.ca/facts-figures/

46. Canadian Automobile Association. (CAA). (n.d.). *Crash odds.* Education Topics. distracteddriving.caa.ca/education/crash-odds.php

47. Johnson, T. D., (2012). Distracted driving: Stay focused when on the road. *The Nation's Health*, 42(1), 28.

48. Caird, J. K., Willness, C. R., Steel, P., & Scialfa, C. (2008). A meta-analysis of the effects of cellphones on driver performance. *Accident Analysis & Prevention*, 40(4), 1282–1293.

49. Seo, D. C., & Torabi, M. R. (2004). The impact of in-vehicle cellphone use on accidents or near-accidents among college students. *Journal of American College Health*, 53(3), 101–108.

50. Canadian Automobile Association. (CAA). (n.d.). *Distracted driving laws in Canada.* Education Topics. distracteddriving.caa.ca/education/distracted-driving-laws-in-canada.php

51. Insurance Corporation of British Columbia. (ICBC). (2016). *Distracted driving.* Road Safety. www.icbc.com/road-safety/crashes-happen/Distracted-driving/Pages/default.aspx

52. Traffic Injury Research Association (TIRA). (2014). *The issues. Belt use.* Young and New Driver Resource Centre. yndrc.tirf.ca/issues/beltuse.php

53. Transport Canada. (2015). *Canadian motor vehicle traffic collision statistics 2014.* Road & Motor Vehicle Safety Publications. Road Transportation. www.tc.gc.ca/media/documents/roadsafety/cmvtcs2014_eng.pdf

54. Government of Canada. (2014, July 11). *Road safety in Canada.* Motor Vehicle Safety Publications. Motor Vehicle Safety. Transport Canada. www.tc.gc.ca/eng/motorvehiclesafety/tp-tp15145-1201.htm#s31

55. Stephenson, J. (2002). Backseat seat belts. *Journal of the American Medical Association*, 287(6), 706.

56. Canadian Automobile Association. (CAA). (2011). *Bicycle statistics.* Cyclists. bikesafety.caa.ca/cyclists/bicycle-statistics.php

57. Canada Safety Council. (2002, July). *Helmets: Attitudes and actions. Survey finds most kids wear helmets, most adults don't.* Sports and Active Living. https://canadasafetycouncil.org/sports-active-living/helmets-attitudes-and-actions

58. Letovsky, E., Rowe, B. H., Friedman, S. M., Snider, C., & Sullivan, E. (2014). Improving bicycle safety in Canada. *Canadian Journal of Emergency Medicine,* 17(3), 323–327. caep.ca/sites/caep.ca/files/caep/PositionStatments/caep_position_statement_-_improving_bike_safety_-_english.pdf

59. Ibid.

60. Brown, S. W., Valar, W. G. M., & Robertson, R. D. (2015, December). *Alcohol and drug-crash problem in Canada. 2012 report.* CCMTA Road Safety Research Report Series. Canadian Council of Motor Transport Administrators (CCMTA). http://ccmta.ca/images/publications/pdf//2012_Alcohol__Drug_Crash_Problem_Report_ENG.pdf

61. Canada Safety Council. (n.d.). *Expect the unexpected. Safety in the great outdoors.* Safety Info. canadasafetycouncil.org/sports-active-living/safety-great-outdoors

62. Ibid.

63. Canadian Institute for Health Information. (2012, January 17). *More than 5,600 Canadians seriously injured from winter activities. Skiing and snowboarding lead to twice as many hospitalizations as hockey.* Winter Injuries. Trauma Injuries. Types of Care. www.cihi.ca/en/types-of-care/specialized-services/trauma-and-injuries/more-than-5600-canadians-seriously-injured

64. Canadian Standards Association (CSA). (2014). Z263.1-14 - *Recreational alpine skiing and snowboarding helmets.* Detailed Information. Injury Prevention. shop.csa.ca/en/canada/injury-prevention/z2631-14/invt/27028372014

65. Canada West Ski Areas Association (CWSAS) (2016). *Position statement. Snow sports helmet usage.* Policy. https://cwsaa.org/policy/ski-helmet-usage/

66. Brown, S. W., Valar, W. G. M., & Robertson, R. D. (2015, December). *Alcohol and drug-crash problem in Canada. 2012 report.* CCMTA Road Safety Research Report Series. Canadian Council of Motor Transport Administrators (CCMTA). http://ccmta.ca/images/publications/pdf//2012_Alcohol__Drug_Crash_Problem_Report_ENG.pdf

67. Canadian Council of Snowmobile Organizations. (2015). *Zero-alcohol—Your smart choice.* Safety. www.ccso-ccom.ca/zero-alcohol/

68. Canada Safety Council. (n.d.). *Boating safety.* Safety Info. canadasafetycouncil.org/sports-active-living/boating-safety

69. Ibid.

70. Transport Canada. (2016, May 12). Office of Boating Safety. *The safe boating guide.* www.tc.gc.ca/eng/marinesafety/debs-obs-menu-1362.htm

71. Boatsmart! (2015, May 05). *Know the facts about drinking and boating in Canada!* Favourites. www.boatsmartexam.com/know-the-facts-about-drinking-and-boating-in-canada/

72. Government of Canada. (2014, May 29). *Skin cancer.* Sun Safety. Environmental Health. www.healthycanadians.gc.ca/healthy-living-vie-saine/environment-environnement/sun-soleil/skin-cancer-peau-eng.php

73. Neenan, A., Lea, C. S., & Lesesky, E. B. (2012). Reasons for tanning bed use: A survey of community college students in North Carolina. *North Carolina Medical Journal,* 73(2), 89–92.

74. Government of Ontario. (2014, May 01). *The skin cancer prevention act (tanning beds), 2013.* Ministry of Health and Long-Term Care. www.health.gov.on.ca/en/public/programs/tanning/

75. Health Canada. (2013, January 23). *Extreme cold.* Healthy Living. Environment. www.hc-sc.gc.ca/hl-vs/iyh-vsv/environ/cold-extreme-froid-eng.php

76. Ibid.

77. Parachute. (2015, August 25). *Why pay attention to injuries?* About Injuries. Injury Topics. www.parachutecanada.org/injury-topics

78. Ibid.

79. Ibid.

80. Parachute. (2015, June). *The cost of injury in Canada.* Knowledge Translation. www.parachutecanada.org/downloads/research/Cost_of_Injury-2015.pdf

81. Peltzer, K., & Pengpid, S. (2015). Factors associated with unintentional injury among university students in 26 countries. *Public Health Nursing,* 32(5), 440–452.

82. Keeling, R. P. (2002). Risks to students' lives: Setting priorities. *Journal of American College Health,* 51(2), 53–56.

83. Canadian Safety Council. (2003, May). *Traffic congestion steams Canadian drivers.* Safety Information. canadasafetycouncil.org/traffic-safety/traffic-congestion-steams-canadian-drivers

84. Park, A. (2005). Can you push yourself too hard? You bet! Just ask the athletes who run the world's most brutal races. (Getting fit/Extreme sports). *Time,* 165(23), 69.

85. World Health Organization. (2016). *Injuries.* Children's Environmental Health. www.who.int/ceh/risks/cehinjuries2/en/

86. Parachute. (2015, August 25). *Why pay attention to injuries?* About Injuries. Injury Topics. www.parachutecanada.org/injury-topics

87. Parachute. (2015, June). *The cost of injury in Canada.* Knowledge Translation. www.parachutecanada.org/downloads/research/Cost_of_Injury-2015.pdf

88. Boyce, J. (2015, November 30). *Police-reported crime statistics in Canada, 2014.* Juristat. Publications. Catalogue no. 85-002-x. http://www5.statcan.gc.ca/olc-cel/olc.action?ObjId=85-002-X201500114211&ObjType=47&lang=en&limit=0

89. Ibid.

90. Ibrahim, D., & Burczycka, M. (2016, January 21). *Family violence in Canada: A statistical profile, 2014.* Canadian Centre for Justice Statistics. Juristat. Catalogue no. 85-002-X. www.statcan.gc.ca/pub/85-002-x/2016001/article/14303-eng.pdf

91. Ibid.

92. Ibid.

93. Devarics, C. (2006). Crime creeping higher on campuses. *Diverse: Issues in Higher Education,* 23(20), 12–13.

94. Floreno, J. (2011). Computer crimes. *American School & University,* 83(6), 34–36.

95. Ibrahim, D., & Burczycka, M. (2016, January 21). *Family violence in Canada: A statistical profile, 2014.* Canadian Centre for Justice Statistics. Juristat. Catalogue no. 85-002-X. www.statcan.gc.ca/pub/85-002-x/2016001/article/14303-eng.pdf

96. Fitzgerald, N. (2002). Safety on campus: Most schools are safe havens for learning. But dangers—crime, alcohol use, hazards—do exist. Knowing the realities can help you protect yourself. *Careers & Colleges,* 22(4), 18–21.

97. Allen, M. (2015, June 09). *Police-reported hate crimes in Canada, 2013.* Canadian Centre for Justice Statistics. Juristat. Catalogue no. 85-002-X. www.statcan.gc.ca/access_acces/alternative_alternatif.action?l=eng&loc=/pub/85-002-x/2015001/article/14191-eng.pdf

98. Ibid.

99. Paling, E. (2016, April 14). Hate crimes against Muslims double in Canada (and it's not a coincidence). Anti-Muslim Hate Crimes. *The Huffington Post Canada.* www.huffingtonpost.ca/

100. Ibid.

101. Perry, B. (2011). Identity and hate crime on Canadian campuses. *Race and Justice,* 1(4), 321–340.

102. Gonzales, A. R., Schofield, R. B., & Schmitt, G. R. (2005, December). *Sexual assault on campus: What colleges and universities are doing about it.* National Institute of Justice. https://www.ncjrs.gov/pdffiles1/nij/205521.pdf

103. Mastropasqua, K. (2015, September 22). *Sexual assault and rape on U. S. college campuses: Research roundup.* Journalists Resource. journalistsresource.org/studies/society/public-health/sexual-assault-rape-us-college-campuses-research-roundup

104. Ibid.

105. Kane, L. (2016, April 27). Sexual misconduct on B. C. campuses subject of proposed law. *The Canadian Press.* www.cbc.ca/news/canada/british-columbia/sexual-assault-bc-universities-law-1.3556142

106. Victims of Violence. (2016). *Acquaintance rape.* Research Library. www.victimsofviolence.on.ca/research-library/acquaintance-rape/

107. Lawyer, S., Resnick, H., Bakanic, V., Burkett, T., & Kilpatrick. D. (2010). Forcible, drug-facilitated, and incapacitated rape and sexual assault among undergraduate women. *Journal of American College Health,* 58(5), 453–460.

108. Tamburri, R., & Samson, M. (2014, October 20). *Ending sexual violence on campus.* University Affairs. www.universityaffairs.ca/features/feature-article/ending-sexual-violence-campus/

109. Barnett, L., MacKay, L., & Valiquet, D. (2007, October 29). *Bill C-2: An act to amend the criminal code and to make consequential amendments to other acts.* Parliament of Canada. www.lop.parl.gc.ca/About/Parliament/Legislative Summaries/Bills_ls.asp?lang=F&ls=c2&Parl=39&Ses=2&source=library_prb#part2

110. Rape Victims Support Network. (2016). *Sexual assault statistics.* Sexual Assault. assaultcare.ca/sexual-assault/sexual-assault-statistics/

111. Women Against Violence Against Women (WAVAW). (2014). *Rape myths*. Mythbusting. www.wavaw.ca/mythbusting/rape-myths/

112. Canadian Federation of Students. (n.d.). *No means no*. The Issues. cfs-fcee.ca/issues/no-means-no/

113. Sleath, E., & Bull, R. (2010). Male rape victim and perpetrator blaming. *Journal of Interpersonal Violence*, 25(6), 969–988.

114. Elklit, A., & Christiansen, D. M. (2010). ASD and PTSD in rape victims. *Journal of Interpersonal Violence, 25*(8), 1470–1488.

115. Government of Canada. (2016, March 24). *Family violence and prevention program*. Social Programs. Indigenous and Northern Affairs Canada. www.aadnc-aandc.gc.ca/eng/1100100035253/1100100035254

Chapter 15

1. Gerontologist. In *Medical Dictionary. The Free Dictionary*. (2011). www.thefreedictionary.com/gerontologist

2. Aging. In *Medical Dictionary. The Free Dictionary*. (2011). www.thefreedictionary.com/aging

3. Onedera, J. D., & Stickle, R. (2008). Healthy aging in later life. *The Family Journal: Counseling and Therapy for Couples and Families*, 16(1), 73–77.

4. Statistics Canada. (2015, September 29). Canada's population estimates: Age and sex, July 1, 2015. *The Daily*. www.statcan.gc.ca/daily-quotidien/150929/dq150929b-eng.htm

5. Ibid.

6. Ibid.

7. Ibid.

8. Ibid.

9. Statistics Canada. (2015, September 29). *Population by sex and age group*. Population Estimates and Projections. Summary Tables. www.statcan.gc.ca/tables-tableaux/sum-som/l01/cst01/demo10a-eng.htm

10. World Health Organization. (WHO). (2016). *Statistics*. Countries. Canada. www.who.int/countries/can/en/

11. Beatty, B. B., & Berdahl, L. (2011). Health care and Aboriginal seniors in urban Canada: Helping a neglected class. *The International Indigenous Policy Journal*, 2(1), 1–16.

12. Canadian Institute for Health Information (2011). *A focus on seniors and aging*. Health Care in Canada, 2011. https://secure.cihi.ca/free_products/HCIC_2011_seniors_report_en.pdf

13. Roizen, Michael. Personal interview.

14. *The Free Dictionary*. (2016). Chronological aging. *Medical Dictionary*. medical-dictionary.thefreedictionary.com/chronological+age

15. *The Free Dictionary*. (2016). Functional aging. *Medical Dictionary*. medical-dictionary.thefreedictionary.com/functional+age

16. *The Free Dictionary*. (2011). Psychological aging. Medical Dictionary. medical-dictionary.thefreedictionary.com/psychological+age

17. Charles, S. T., & Carstensen, L. L. (2010). Social and emotional aging. *Annual Review of Psychology*, 61(1), 383–409.

18. Active Living Coalition for Older Adults. (2016, March 23). Home page. www.alcoa.ca/e/index.htm

19. Buford, T. W., Anton, S. D., Clark, D. J., Higgins, T. J., & Cooke, M. B. (2014). Optimizing the benefits of exercise on physical function in older adults. *Physical Medicine & Rehabilitation*, 6(6), 528–543.

20. Gremeauxa, V., Gaydaa, M., Leperse, R., Sosnera, P., Juneaua, M., & Nigama, A. (2012). Exercise and longevity. *Maturitas*, 73(4), 312–317.

21. Lin, J. S. (2010). Encouraging physical activity among frail older adults. *American Family Physician*, 82(3), 230.

22. Cheitlin, M. D. (2003). Cardiovascular physiology—Changes with aging. American *Journal of Geriatric Cardiology*, 12(1), 9–13.

23. Heart and Stroke Foundation. (2011, March). *Physical activity needs of seniors*. Health Information. www.heartandstroke.com/site/c.ikIQLcMWJtE/b.3484257/k.EB1C/Healthy_living__Physical_activity_needs_of_seniors.htm

24. Active Living Coalition for Older Adults. (2013, August 03). Homepage. www.alcoa.ca/e/index.htm

25. Sharatt, M. T. (2004, October). *Physical activity and coronary heart disease. It's never too late to benefit*. Research Update. Active Living Coalition for Older Adults (ALCOA). www.alcoa.ca/research_u_docs/2004_10oct_en_update.pdf

26. Canadian Society of Exercise Physiology (CSEP). (2011). *Canadian physical activity guidelines for older adults 65 years & older*. Physical Activity. www.csep.ca/CMFiles/Guidelines/CSEP_PAGuidelines_older-adults_en.pdf

27. Close, G. L., Kayani, A., Vasilaki, A., & McArdle, A. (2005). Skeletal muscle damage with exercising and aging. *Sports Medicine*, 35(5), 413–427.

28. *The Free Dictionary*. (2016). Sarcopenia. *The Medical Dictionary*. medical-dictionary.thefreedictionary.com/sarcopenia

29. Lexell, J., Downham, D., & Sjöström, M. (1986). Distribution of different fibre types in human skeletal muscles. Fibre type arrangement in m. vastus lateralis from three groups of healthy men between 15 and 83 years. *Journal of Neurological Sciences*, 72(2–3), 211–222.

30. Goodpaster, B. H., Park, S. W., Harris, T. B., Kritchevsky, S. B., Nevitt, M., Schwartz, A. V., Simonsick, E. M., Tylaysky, F. A., Visser, M., & Newman, A. B. (2006). The loss of skeletal muscle strength, mass, and quality in older adults: The health, aging and body composition study. *Journal of Gerontology Series A Biological Sciences and Medical Sciences*, 61(10), 1059–1064.

31. Ploutz-Snyder, L., Druger, M., & Manini, T. M. (2005). Misconceptions about strength exercise among older adults. *Journal of Aging and Physical Activity*, 13(4), 422–433.

32. Osteoporosis Canada. (2016). *Osteoporosis facts and statistics*. Osteoporosis and You. www.osteoporosis.ca/osteoporosis-and-you/osteoporosis-facts-and-statistics/

33. Osteoporosis Canada. (2016). *Drug treatments*. Osteoporosis and You. www.osteoporosis.ca/osteoporosis-and-you/drug-treatments/

34. BC Women's OSTEOFIT Program. (2016). *OSTEOFIT*. Population Health Promotion. www.bcwomens.ca/our-services/population-health-promotion/osteofit/

35. Ambrosea, A. F., Paula, G., & Hausdorffb, J. M. (2013). Risk factors for falls among older adults: A review of the literature. *Maturitas*, 75(1), 51–61.

36. Chang, H. J., Lynm, C., & Glass, R. M. (2010). Falls and older adults. JAMA Patient Page. *Journal of the American Medical Association*, 303(3), 288.

37. da Costa, T. C., Locks, R. R., Koppe, S., Yamaguti, A. M., & Formiga, A. C. (2013). Strength and stretching training and detraining on flexibility of older adults. *Topics in Geriatric Rehabilitation*, 29(2), 142–148.

38. Wilkins, C. H., Sheline, Y. I., Roe, C. M., Birge, S. J., Morris, J. C. (2006). Vitamin D deficiency is associated with low mood and worse cognitive performance in older adults. *American Journal of Geriatric Psychiatry*, 14(12), 1032–1040.

39. Ramage-Morin, P. L., & Garriguet, D. (2013, March). Nutritional risk among older Canadians. *Health Reports*, 24(3), 3–13.

40. Smee, D. J., Pumpa, K., Falchi, M., & Lithander, F. E. (2015, December). The relationship between diet quality and falls risk, physical function and body composition in older adults. *The Journal of Nutrition, Health and Aging*, 19(10), 1037–1042.

41. Riddle, D. R., & Schindler, M. K. (2007). Brain aging research. Reviews in Clinical *Gernontology*, 17(4), 225–239.

42. Rowe, John. Personal interview.

43. Cameron, B., & Landreth, G. E. (2010). Inflammation, microglia, and Alzheimer's disease. *Neurobiology of Disease*, 37(3), 503–509.

44. Ballard, C., Gauthier, S., Corbett, A., Brayne, C., Aarsland, D., & Jones, E. (2011). Alzheimer's disease. *The Lancet*, 377(9770), 1019–1031.

45. Government of Canada. (2016, April 12). *Dementia*. Diseases. Diseases and Conditions. healthycanadians.gc.ca/diseases-conditions-maladies-affections/disease-maladie/dementia-demence/index-eng.php

46. Alzheimer's of Canada. (2014, December 16). *Day to day living. Living with dementia*. www.alzheimer.ca/en/Living-with-dementia/Day-to-day-living

47. Menopauseandu.ca. (n.d.). *Am I in menopause?* Society of Obstetricians and Gynaecologists of Canada. (SOGC). http://menopauseandu.ca/am-i-in-menopause_e.aspx

48. Schenck-Gustafsson, K., Brincat, M., Erel, C. T., Gambaccani, M., Lambrinoudaki, I., Moen, M. H., et al. (2011). EMAS position statement: Managing the menopause in the context of coronary heart disease. *Maturitas*, 68(1), 94–97.

49. Britt, K. (2012). Menarche, menopause, and breast cancer risk. *The Lancet Oncology*, 13(11), 1071–1072.

50. Hlatky, M., Boothroyd, D., Vittinghoff, E., Sharp, P., & Whooley, M. A. (2002). Quality of life and depressive symptoms in postmenopausal women after receiving hormone therapy: Results from the heart and estrogen/progestin replacement study (HERS) trial. *Journal of the American Medical Association*, 287(5), 591–597.

51. Potera, C. (2011). The safety of HRT remains unsettled. *The American Journal of Nursing*, 11(1), 15.

52. National Institutes of Health (NIH). (2004, June 22). *WHI study finds no heart disease benefit, increased stroke risk with estrogen alone*. Press Releases. News and Resources. www.nhlbi.nih.gov/news/press-releases/2004/whi-study-finds-no-heart-disease-benefit-increased-stroke-risk-with-estrogen-alone

53. Stevenson, J. C., Hodisb, H. N., Pickarc, J. H., & Loboc, R. A. (2009). Coronary heart disease and menopause management: The swinging pendulum of HRT. Review. *Atherosclerosis*, 207(2), 336–340.

54. Eggertson, L. (2009). New clinical guidelines say misconceptions have surrounded hormone therapy. *Canadian Medical Association Journal*, 180(5), 504–505.

55. Canadian Psychological Association. (CPA). (2014). *"Psychology works" fact sheet: Depression among seniors*. www.cpa.ca/docs/File/Publications/FactSheets/PsychologyWorksFactSheet_DepressionAmongSeniors.pdf

56. Ibid.

57. McCormack, B., Boldy, D., Lewin, G., & McCormack, G. R. (2011). Screening for depression among older adults referred to home care services: A single-item depression screener versus the geriatric depression scale. *Home Health Care Management & Practice*, 23(1), 13–19.

58. Government of Canada. (2015, February 06). *Facts on psychological and emotional abuse of seniors*. Elder Abuse Awareness. Programs and Initiatives. www.seniors.gc.ca/eng/pie/eaa/psychologicalandemotional.shtml

59. Wade, T. J., & Pevalin, D. J. (2004, June). Marital transitions and mental health. *Journal of Health and Social Behaviour*, 45, 155–170.

60. Buchanan, D., Tourigny-Rivard, M. F., Cappeliez, P., Frank, C., et al. (2006). National guidelines for seniors' mental health: The assessment and treatment of depression. *The Canadian Journal of Geriatrics*, 9(S2), S52–S58. www.ccsmh.ca/pdf/final%20supplement.pdf

61. Motle, R. W., Konopack, J. F., McAuley, E., Elavsky, S., Jerome, G. J., & Marquez, D. X. (2005). Depressive symptoms among older adults: Long-term reduction after a physical activity intervention. *Journal of Behavioral Medicine*, 28(4), 385–394.

62. Transport Canada. (2014). Canadian Motor Vehicle Traffic Collision Statistics. Catalogue no: T45-3E-PDF. www.tc.gc.ca/media/documents/roadsafety/cmvtcs2014_eng.pdf

63. Turcotte, M. (2012, January 23). *Profile of seniors' transportation habits*. Statistics Canada. Publications. Catalogue no. 11-008-X. www.statcan.gc.ca/pub/11-008-x/2012001/article/11619-eng.htm

64. Reid, J. L., Hammon, D., Rynard, V. L., & Burkhalter, R. (2015). *Tobacco use in Canada: Patterns and trends, 2015 edition*. Waterloo, ON: Propel Centre for Population Health Impact, University of Waterloo. tobaccoreport.ca/2015/TobaccoUseinCanada_2015.pdf

65. The Lung Association. (2008). *COPD BreathWorks plan*. Chronic Obstructive Pulmonary Disease (COPD). Resources. www.lung.ca/lung-health/lung-disease/chronic-obstructive-pulmonary-disease-copd/resources

66. Ibid.

67. Gellert, C., Schöttker, B., Müller, H., Holleczek, B., & Brenner, H.(2013). Impact of smoking and quitting on cardiovascular outcomes and risk advancement periods among older adults. *Cardiovascular Disease*, 28(8), 649–658.

68. The Lung Association (Canada). (2014, October 17). *Treatment*. COPD Lung Diseases A–Z. www.lung.ca/lung-health/lung-disease/copd/treatment

69. Ontario Ministry of Health and Long Term Care. (2015, December 10). *MedsCheck. Resources for pharmacists*. Health Care Professionals. Public Information. www.health.gov.on.ca/en/pro/programs/drugs/medscheck/resources.aspx

70. Public Health Agency of Canada. (2014, October 09). Chapter 3: The health and well-being of Canadian seniors. *The chief public health officer's report on the state of public health in Canada 2010*. Reports and Publications. Home. www.phac-aspc.gc.ca/cphorsphc-respcacsp/2010/fr-rc/index-eng.php

71. Sartre, D. (2015). Alcohol and drug use problems among older adults. *The Journal of Applied Gerontology*, 28(2), 235–255.

72. Lindau, S. T., Schumm, L. P., Laumann, E. O., Levinson, W., O'Muircheartaigh, C. A., & Waite, L. J. (2007). A student of sexuality and health among older adults in the United States. *New England Journal of Medicine*, 357(8), 762–774.

73. Ibid.

74. Ginsberg, T. B., Pomerantz, S. C., & Kramer-Feeley, V. K. (2005). Sexuality in older adults: Behaviours and preferences. *Age and Ageing*, 34(5), 475–480.

75. Revera Living.com. (2012, June 20). *Tech-savvy seniors bridging the digital divide: Revera report.* News release. www.reveraliving.com/revera/files/e1/e1b42975-8ec3-4728-8a82-08328cedb021.pdf

76. Sum, S., Matthews, R. M., Hughes, I., & Campbell, A. (2008). Internet use and loneliness in older adults. *CyberPsychology & Behavior*, 11(2), 208–211.

77. Heo, J., Kim, J., & Won, Y. S. (2011). Exploring the relationship between internet use and leisure satisfaction among older adults. *Activities, Adaptation & Aging*, 35(1), 43–54.

78. Hill, R. S. (2015, February 12). *Insight into Canada's Internet.* News. About Us. CA Community Investment Program. https://cira.ca/80-canadians-see-importance-keeping-seniors-connected-through-internet-technology

79. Public Health Agency of Canada. (2010, October 28). Chapter 3: The health and wellbeing of Canadian seniors. *The chief public health officer's report on the state of public health in Canada 2010.* Reports and Publications. Home. www.phac-aspc.gc.ca/cphorsphc-respcacsp/2010/fr-rc/cphorsphc-respcacsp-06-eng.php

80. Kübler-Ross, E. (1975). *Death: The final stage of growth.* Englewood Cliffs, NJ: Prentice Hall.

81. Bischoff, K. E., Sudore, R., Miao, Y., Boscardin, W. J., & Smith, A. K. (2013). Advance care planning and the quality of end-of-life care in older adults. *Journal of the American Geriatrics Society*, 61(2), 209–214.

82. Spoelhof, G. D., & Elliot, B. (2012, March 01). Implementing advance directives in office practice. *American Family Physician*, 85(5), 461–468.

83. Caregiving Matters. (2013, June 17). Canadians 65+ have highest suicide rate of any group in the country. *Caregiver News.* www.caregivingmatters.ca/canadians-65-and-older-have-highest-suicide-rate-of-any-group-in-the-country/

84. Bhara, S. S., & Brown, G. K. (2012). Treatment of depression and suicide in older adults. *Cognitive and Behavioral Practice*, 19(1), 116–125.

85. Cukrowicz, K. C., Duberstein, P. R., Vannoy, S. D., Lynch, T. R., McQuoid, D. R., & Steffens, D. C. (2009). Course of suicide ideation and predictors of change in depressed older adults. *Journal of Affective Disorders*, 113(1–2), 30–36.

86. Parliament of Canada. (2016, April 14). *Bill C-14.* House of Commons. Parliamentary Business. www.parl.gc.ca/HousePublications/Publication.aspx?DocId=8183660&Language=E&Mode=1

87. Parliament of Canada. (2016, June 17). *Bill C-14. Royal assent.* House of Commons. Parliamentary Business. http://www.parl.gc.ca/housepublications/publication.aspx?Language=E&Mode=1&DocId=8384014

88. Berzoff, J. (2011). The transformative nature of grief and bereavement. *Clinical Social Work Journal*, 39(3), 262–269.

89. Vickio, C. J. (2008). Designing and conducting grief workshops for college students. *New Directions for Student Services*, 121, 41–50.

Chapter 16

1. IPCC. (2014). *Climate change 2014: Synthesis report.* Contribution of working groups I, II and III to the fifth assessment report of the intergovernmental panel on climate change [Core Writing Team, R. K. Pachauri and L. A. Meyer (eds.)]. IPCC, Geneva, Switzerland, 151 pp. www.ipcc.ch/report/ar5/syr/

2. Luck, G. W., Chan, K. M. A., Eser, U., Goméz-Baggethun, E., Batzdof, B., Norton, B., & Potshcin, M. B. (2012). Ethical considerations in on-ground applications of the ecosystem services concept. *BioScience*, 62(12), 1020–1029.

3. Hsu, A., et al. (2016). *Environmental performance index.* New Haven, CT. Yale University. issuu.com/2016yaleepi/docs/epi2016_final

4. Ibid.

5. EPR Canada. (2015, October 01). *BC's overall grade climbs to A in EPR Canada's 2015 scored report card on implementation of producer responsibility programs.* News Release. eprcanada.ca/reports/2014/2015-EPR-News-Release-EN.pdf

6. Ibid.

7. David Suzuki Foundation. (n.d.). *What is climate change?* Issues. Science & Policy. www.davidsuzuki.org/issues/climate-change/science/climate-change-basics/climate-change-101-1/

8. Hodgson, P. (2008). On climate change. *Modern Age*, 50(4), (p. 345).

9. Centre for Climate and Energy Solutions (C2ES).(2011). *Climate change 101.* Overview. The Basics. Science and Impacts. www.c2es.org/publications/climate-change-101/overview

10. Hodgson, P. (2008). On climate change. *Modern Age*, 50(4), 345–352.

11. Centre for Climate and Energy Solutions (C2ES). (n.d.). *The basics.* Science and Impacts. www.c2es.org/science-impacts/basics

12 David Suzuki Foundation. (2014). *What is climate change?* Issues. Science & Policy. www.davidsuzuki.org/issues/climate-change/science/climate-change-basics/climate-change-101-1/

13. David Suzuki Foundation. (2014). *Greenhouse gases.* Issues. Climate Change Basics. www.davidsuzuki.org/issues/climate-change/science/climate-change-basics/greenhouse-gases/

14. Centre for Climate and Energy Solutions (C2ES). (2011, January). *Climate change 101.* Science and Impacts. www.c2es.org/docUploads/climate101-science.pdf

15. Government of Canada. (2016, April 04). *Greenhouse gas emissions by province and territory.* Greenhouse Gas Emissions. Environmental Indicators. Environment and Climate Change Canada. www.ec.gc.ca/indicateurs-indicators/default.asp?lang=en&n=18F3BB9C-1

16. National Aeronautics and Space Administration. (NASA). (2016, January 20). *NASA, NOAA analyses reveal record-shattering global warm temperatures in 2015.* NASA News & Feature Releases. http://www.giss.nasa.gov/research/news/20160120/

17. Centre for Climate and Energy Solutions (C2ES). (2011). *Climate change 101.* Science and Impacts. www.c2es.org/docUploads/climate101-science.pdf

18. Weaver, A. (2008). *Keeping our cool: Canada in a warming world.* Toronto, ON: Penguin Group.

19. Knutson, T. R., Mcbride, J. I., Chan, J., Emanuel, K., Holland, G., Landsea, C., Held, I., Kossin, J. P., Srivastava, A. K., & Sugi, M. (2010). Tropical cyclones and climate change. *Nature Geoscience*, 3, 157–163.

20. Rosenthal, J. (2010). EU connections in climate research. *Policy Review*, 162, 37–51.

21. National Geographic. (2016). *Effects of global warming. Signs are everywhere.* Environment. environment.nationalgeographic.com/environment/global-warming/gw-effects/

22. Sharma, R., Ve'lez-espino, L. A, Wertheimer, A. C., Mantua, N., & Francis, R. C. (2013). Relating spatial and temporal scales of climate and ocean variability to survival of Pacific

Northwest Chinook salmon (Oncorhynchus tshawytscha). *Fisheries Oceanography*, 22(1), 14–31.

23. Canadian Press. (2016, January 26). *High River says Alberta 2013 flood response inadequate, damage remains.* Environment. globalnews.ca/news/2478010/high-river-says-alberta-2013-flood-response-inadequate-damage-remains/
24. Bartko, K, & Mertz, E. (2016, May 04). *Fort McMurray wildfire: Alberta government declares provincial state of emergency*. Global News. Environment. globalnews.ca/news/2679178/fort-mcmurray-wildfire-how-many-homes-have-been-lost-in-the-fire/
25. Guo, L., & Ma, H. (2009). Greenhouse effect international cooperation: Rethink Kyoto protocol. *Journal of Sustainable Development*, 2(2), 54–57.
26. Edward, P. (2007). Equity and the Kyoto protocol. *Politics*, 27(1), 8–15.
27. Clémençon, R. (2008). The Bali road map. A first step on the difficult journey to a post-Kyoto protocol agreement. *The Journal of Environment & Development*, 17(1), 70–94.
28. Rajamani, L. (2010). The making and unmaking of the Copenhagen accord. *International and Comparative Law Quarterly*, 59(3), 824–843.
29. Sandler, L. M., & Schiffman Kymer, R. I. (2010). Copenhagen Accord: Next steps, and business implications. *Environmental Claims Journal*, 22(2), 144–149.
30. Rogelj, J., Nabel, J., Chen, C., Hare, W., Markmann, K., Meinshausen, M., Schaeffer, M., Macey, K., & Hohne, N. (2010). Copenhagen accord pledges are paltry. *Opinion. Nature*, 464(7292), 1126–1128.
31. Thompson, A. (2010). Development ethics and the Copenhagen Accord: How important are the global poor? *Ethics, Place and Environment*, 13(2), 191–196.
32. United Nations Sustainable Development Knowledge Platform (n.d.). *United Nations conference on sustainable development, Rio120.* Intergovernmental Process. sustainabledevelopment.un.org/rio20.html
33. Center for Climate Energy and Solutions (C2ES). (2015, December). *Outcomes of the U. N. climate change conference in Paris.* Publications Library. www.c2es.org/international/negotiations/cop21-paris/summary
34. Kindornay, S., & Venkatesh, J. (2015, December 21). *The Paris agreement: Implications for Canada.* Canadian International Development Platform. cidpnsi.ca/the-paris-agreement-implications-for-canada/
35. Suzuki Foundation. (n.d.). *Carbon offsets.* Climate Change. Issues. www.davidsuzuki.org/issues/climate-change/science/climate-change-basics/carbon-offsets/
36. Bramley, M. (2009). *Key questions for a Canadian cap and trade system.* The Pembina Institute. Sustainable Energy Solutions. www.pembina.org/pub/2015
37. Indigenous Environmental Network. (2015). Home. indigenousrising.org/lakota-youth-running-500-miles-in-opposition-of-dakota-access-pipeline/
38. Sierra Club BC. (n.d.). Home. sierraclub.bc.ca/
39. Ibid.
40. Carson, R. (1962). *Silent spring.* Boston: Houghton Mifflin.
41. National Women's History Museum. (n.d.). *Rachel Carson (1907–1964).* Biography Index. Biography. www.nwhm.org/education-resources/biography/biographies/rachel-carson/
42. Lear, L. (2008, September 15). *Rachel Louise Carson.* Biography. www.rachelcarson.org/Bio.aspx
43. Gore, A. (1992). *Earth in the balance: Ecology and the human spirit.* Boston: Houghton Mifflin.
44. Gore, A. (2006). *An inconvenient truth: The planetary emergency of global warming and what we can do about it.* Emmaus, PA: Rodale.
45. Gore, A. (2013). *The future: Six drivers of global change.* New York: Random House.
46. Penn, B. (2015). *The real thing: The natural history of Ian McTaggart Cowan.* Canada: Rocky Mountain Books Ltd.
47. Ibid.
48. David Suzuki Foundation. (n.d.). *About us.* www.davidsuzuki.org/about/
49. David Suzuki Foundation. (n.d.). *What you can do.* www.davidsuzuki.org/what-you-can-do/
50. Andrew Weaver (n.d.). *Meet Andrew Weaver.* Andrew Weaver Oak Bay-Gordon Head MLA. www.andrewweavermla.ca/meet-andrew-weaver/
51. Canada Green Building Council. (n.d.). *Going green with LEED.* LEED. www.cagbc.org/CAGBC/LEED/CAGBC/Programs/LEED/Going_green_with_LEE.aspx?hkey=54c44792-442b-450a-a286-4aa710bf5c64
52. Greene, H., & Greene, M. (2008). Sustainable admissions: How prospective students are tracking down institutions' environmental records and using them in the college decision-making process. *University Business*, 11(7), 57–58.
53. Common Energy UBC. (n.d.). Home. commonenergyubc.com/
54. Recycling Council of British Columbia. (2016). *Retailer take back programs.* Recycling Programs and Resources. www.rcbc.ca/recycling-programs/retailer-take-back
55. Commoner, B. (1971). *The closing circle: Nature, man and technology.* New York: Knopf.
56. Global Footprint Network. (2016, May 01). *Footprint calculator.* Resources. www.footprintnetwork.org/en/index.php/GFN/page/calculators/
57. Environmental Paper Network. (2012). *Paper calculator.* c.environmentalpaper.org/home
58. Canadian Automobile Association. (n.d.). *Driving cost calculator.* caa.ca/car_costs/
59. Live Smart BC. (n.d.). *Lifestyle carbon calculator.* Live Smart at Home. BC Home. www.livesmartbc.ca/homes/h_calc.html
60. Hancock, T. et al. (2015, May). *Global change and public health: Addressing the ecological determinants of health.* Canadian Public Health Association (CPHA). www.cpha.ca/uploads/policy/edh-discussion_e.pdf
61. Office of Disease Prevention and Health Promotion (ODPHP). (2016, May 05). *Environmental Health.* 2020 Topics and Objectives. www.healthypeople.gov/2020/topics-objectives/topic/environmental-health
62. Prüss-Ustün, A., Bonjour, S., & Corvalán, C. (2008). The impact of the environment on health by country: A meta-synthesis. *Environmental Health*, 7(1), 7–16.
63. Fung, I. Y., Doney, S. C., Swann, A. L., Levis, S., & Bonan, G. B. (2010). Changes in Artic vegetation amplify high-latitude warming through the greenhouse effect. *Proceedings of the National Academy of Sciences*, 107(4), 1295–1300.
64. Hess, J. J., Malilay, J. N., & Parkinson, A. J. (2008). Climate change. The importance of place. *American Journal of Preventive Medicine*, 25(5), 468–478.
65. Environment and Climate Change Canada. (2016, February 05). *Air quality health index.* Air Quality. Air. www.ec.gc.ca/cas-aqhi/default.asp?lang=En&n=CB0ADB16-1

66. Government of Canada. (2014, July 21). *Smog and your health.* Air Quality. Environmental Health. healthycanadians.gc.ca/healthy-living-vie-saine/environment-environnement/air/smog-eng.php

67. Natural Resources Canada. (2015, December 04). *Emission impacts resulting from vehicle idling transportation initiatives. Communities and Infrastructure.* www.nrcan.gc.ca/energy/efficiency/communities-infrastructure/transportation/idling/4397

68. Health Canada. (2015, January 27). *Drinking water.* Environmental and Workplace Health. www.hc-sc.gc.ca/ewh-semt/water-eau/drink-potab/index-eng.php

69. Health Canada. (2013, December 05). *Frequently asked questions about bottled water.* Food and Nutrition. www.hc-sc.gc.ca/fn-an/securit/facts-faits/faqs_bottle_water-eau_embouteillee-eng.php

70. Ohnishi, T., Goto, K., Kanda, T., Kanazawa, Y., Ozawa, K., et al. (2013). Microbial contamination associated with consumption and the growth in plastic bottled beverage. *Journal of Environmental Science and Health, Part A: Toxic/Hazardous Substances and Environmental Engineering,* 48(7), 781–790.

71. Government of Canada. (2015, June 09). *Health risks of asbestos.* Indoor Air Contaminants. Air Quality. healthycanadians.gc.ca/healthy-living-vie-saine/environment-environnement/air/contaminants/asbestos-amiante-eng.php

72. Health Canada. (2013, February 04). *What is lead?* Lead. Environmental and Work Place Health. www.hc-sc.gc.ca/ewh-semt/contaminants/lead-plomb/index-eng.php

73. Health Canada. (2009, March 02). *Mercury and human health.* Environment. It's Your Health. Healthy Living. www.hc-sc.gc.ca/hl-vs/iyh-vsv/environ/merc-eng.php

74. Government of Canada. (2016, January 12). *Residential indoor air quality guideline: Carbon monoxide.* Healthy Living. Publications. healthycanadians.gc.ca/publications/healthy-living-vie-saine/carbon-monoxide-carbone/index-eng.php

75. Agriculture and Agri-Food Canada. (2016, March 07). *Canada's soft drink, bottled water and ice industry.* Processed Food and Beverages. By Product and Sector. www.agr.gc.ca/eng/industry-markets-and-trade/statistics-and-market-information/by-product-sector/processed-food-and-beverages/canadas-soft-drink-bottled-water-and-ice-industry/?id=1172167862291

76. Wolf-Wylie, W. (2014, August 08). *How private companies are using Ontario's public water. Canada.com.* o.canada.com/news/how-private-companies-are-using-ontarios-public-water

77. The Water Project. (2016). *Bottled water is wasteful.* Learn. thewaterproject.org/bottled_water_wasteful

78. Ibid.

79. Queen's University. (2012, September 04). *Queen's bans water bottle sales.* Queen's Gazette. www.queensu.ca/gazette/content/queens-bans-bottled-water-sales

80. Health Canada. (2016, April 15). *Fluoride and human health.* Healthy Living. Environment. www.hc-sc.gc.ca/hl-vs/iyh-vsv/environ/fluor-eng.php

81. Ibid.

82. Ibid.

83. Nova Scotia Canada. (2014, March 31). *Reducing or eliminating trihalomethanes (THMs) in drinking water.* Drinking Water. www.novascotia.ca/nse/water/thm.asp

84. Government of Canada. (2015, January 30). *Use pesticides safely.* About Pesticides. Using Pesticides. www.healthycanadians.gc.ca/product-safety-securite-produits/pest-control-products-produits-antiparasitaires/pesticides/about-au-sujet/use-utilisation-eng.php

85. Aboriginal Affairs and Northern Development. (2010, March). *Persistent Organic Pollutants (POPs) fact sheet series: Dichlorodiphenyltrichloroethane (DDT).* Persistent Organic Pollutants (POPs). Publications. www.aadnc-aandc.gc.ca/eng/1316102914633/1316103004743

86. U. S. Environmental Protection Agency. (2015, November 05). *DDT—A brief history and status.* Learn the Issues. www.epa.gov/ingredients-used-pesticide-products/ddt-brief-history-and-status

87. Fox, M., Curriero, F., Kulbicki, K., Resnick, B., & Burke, T. (2010). Evaluting the community health legacy of WWI chemical weapons testing. *Journal of Community Health,* 35(1), 93–103.

88. David Suzuki Foundation. (2010, October). *What's inside? That counts: A survey of toxic ingredients in our cosmetics.* Reports. Publications. www.davidsuzuki.org/publications/downloads/2010/DSF-report-Whats-inside-that-counts.pdf

89. Health Canada. (2015, May 28). *Safety of cosmetic ingredients.* Consumer Product Safety. www.hc-sc.gc.ca/cps-spc/cosmet-person/labelling-etiquetage/ingredients-eng.php

90. David Suzuki Foundation. (2014). *"Dirty dozen" cosmetic chemicals to avoid.* Issues. www.davidsuzuki.org/issues/health/science/toxics/dirty-dozen-cosmetic-chemicals/?gclid=CPvOnqzyxcwCFVFgfgodUFkN3Q

91. UL. (2016). *EcoLogo TM certification.* Environment. industries.ul.com/environment/certificationvalidation-marks/ecologo-product-certification

92. Leslie, H. A. (2014). Review of microplastics in cosmetics. Scientific background on a potential source of plastic particulate marine litter to support decision making. ICM Institute for Environmental Studies. Report R14/29. ivm.vu.nl/en/Images/Plastic_ingredients_in_Cosmetics_07-2014_FINAL_tcm234-409704.pdf

93. U. N. Centre News. (2015, June 16). *UN environment agency urges ban of microplastics in cosmetics and personal care products.* News. www.un.org/apps/news/story.asp?NewsID=51169#.VyzYMU32bIV

94. David Suzuki Foundation. (2014). *Electromagnetic radiation and fields.* Issues. www.davidsuzuki.org/issues/health/science/enviro-health-policy/electromagnetic-radiation-and-fields/

95. Health Canada. (2012, November 07). *Electric and magnetic fields from power lines and electrical appliances.* Home and Garden Safety. Environmental Health. healthycanadians.gc.ca/healthy-living-vie-saine/environment-environnement/home-maison/emf-cem-eng.php

96. National Cancer Institute. (2016, March 28). *Cell phones and cancer risk.* Radiation. Risk Factors. www.cancer.gov/about-cancer/causes-prevention/risk/radiation/cell-phones-fact-sheet

97. World Health Organization (WHO). (2011, May 31). *IARC classifies radiofrequency electromagnetic fields as possibly carcinogenic to humans.* Press Release No. 208. International Agency for Research on Cancer. www.iarc.fr/en/media-centre/pr/2011/pdfs/pr208_E.pdf

98. Health Canada. (2006, December 19). *Safety of exposure to electric and magnetic fields from computer monitors and other video display terminals.* Products. It's Your Health. Healthy Living. www.hc-sc.gc.ca/hl-vs/iyh-vsv/prod/monit-eng.php

99. Health Canada. (2015, June 22). Limits of human exposure to radiofrequency electromagnetic energy in the frequency range from 3 kHz to 300 GHz. Consultations. Environmental and Workplace Health. www.hc-sc.gc.ca/ewh-semt/consult/_2014/safety_code_6-code_securite_6/final_finale-eng.php

100. World Health Organization. (2014, October). *Electromagnetic fields and public health: mobile phones.* Fact Sheet No. 193. Media Centre. www.who.int/mediacentre/factsheets/fs193/en/

101. Ibid.

102. Ibid.

103. Boice, J. D., & Tarone, R. E. (2011). Cellphones, cancer and children. *Journal of the National Cancer Institute*, 103(16), 1211–1213.

104. Canadian Food and Inspection Agency. (2014, March 22). *Food Irradiation.* Fact Sheets. Information for Consumers. www.inspection.gc.ca/food/information-for-consumers/fact-sheets/irradiation/eng/1332358607968/1332358680017

105. Orriolsa, R., Costa, R., Cuberase, G., Jacasf, C., Castelle, J., & Sunyerg, J. (2009). Brain dysfunction in multiple chemical sensitivity. *Journal of the Neurological Sciences*, 287(1–2), 72–78.

106. Feder, K., Michaud, D., Ramage-Morin, P., & McNamee, J., & Beauregard, Y. (2015, July 15). Prevalence of hearing loss among Canadians aged 20 to 79: Audiometric results from the 2012/2013 Canadian Health Measures Survey. *Health Reports*, 26(7), 18–25. Statistics Canada, Catalogue no. 82-003-X. www.statcan.gc.ca/pub/82-003-x/2015007/article/14206-eng.pdf

107. Hoover, A., & Krishnamurti, S. (2010). Survey of college students' MP3 listening: Habits, safety issues, attitudes, and education. *American Journal of Audiology*, 19(1), 73–83.

108. Statistics Canada.(2015, November 27). *Hearing loss of Canadians, 2012 and 2013.* Health Fact Sheets. Publications. Catalogue no. 82-625-X. www.statcan.gc.ca/pub/82-625-x/2015001/article/14156-eng.htm

Chapter 17

1. Shahjahan, R. A. (2004). Centering spirituality in the academy: Toward a transformative way of teaching and learning. *Journal of Transformative Education*, 2(4), 294–312.

2. Cragun, R. T., Henry, P., Mann, M., & Russell Krebs, S. (2014). Chapel use on college and university campuses. *Journal of College & Character*,. 15(2), 103–118. DOI: 10.1515/jcc-2014-0014

3. Reyman, L. S., Fialkowski, G. M., & Stewart-Sicking, J. A. (2015). Exploratory study of spirituality and psychosocial growth in college students. *Journal of College Counseling*, 18(2), 103–115.

4. Stoyles, G., Chadwick, A., & Caputi, P. (2015). Purpose in life and well-being: The relationship between purpose in life, hope, coping and inward sensitivity among first-year university students. *Journal of Spirituality in Mental Health*, 17(2), 119–134. DOI: 10.1080/19349637.2015.985558

5. Travis, J. W., & Ryan, R. S. (2004). *Wellness workbook* (3rd ed.). Berkley, CA: Celestial Arts Ten Speed Press.

6. Erriker, C., & Erriker, J. (Eds.). (2001). *Contemporary spiritualities: Social and religious contexts.* London and New York: Continuum, p. xv.

7. Scherurs, A. (2002). *Psychotherapy and spirituality: Integrating the spiritual dimension into therapeutic practice.* London: Jessica Kingsley Publishers.

8. Tisdell, E. J. (2003). *Exploring spirituality and culture in adult and higher education.* San Francisco: Jossey Bass.

9. National Institute for Healthcare Research. (1997). *Final report. Scientific progress in spiritual research.* Rockville, MD: Author. As quoted in Mytko, J. J., & Knight, S. J. (2004). Body, mind and spirit: Towards the integration of religiosity and spirituality in cancer quality of life research. *Psycho-Oncology*, 8, 439–450.

10. Hunglemann, J., Kenkel-Rossi, E., Klassen, L., & Stollenwork, R. (1996). Focusing on spiritual well-being: Harmonious interconnectedness of mind–body–spirit use of the JAREL spiritual well-being scale. *Geriatric Nursing*, 17(6), 262–266.

11. Kulchyski, P., McCaskill, D., & Newhouse, D. (Eds.). (1999). *In the words of elders: Aboriginal cultures in transition.* Toronto, ON: University of Toronto Press.

12. National Wellness Institute, Inc. (n.d.). *Six dimensional model.* c.ymcdn.com/sites/www.nationalwellness.org/resource/resmgr/docs/sixdimensionsfactsheet.pdf

13. Berry, D. (2005). Methodological pitfalls in the study of religiosity and spirituality. *Western Journal of Nursing Research*, 27(5), 626–647.

14. Estanek, S. M. (2006). Redefining spirituality: A new discourse. *College Student Journal*, 40(2), 270–282.

15. Ingersoll, R. E., & Bauer, A. L. (2004). An integral approach to spiritual wellness in school/counseling settings. *Professional School Counseling*, 7(5), 301–308.

16. Maheshwari. N. (2015). Spiritual intelligence: Occupational commitment. *Journal of Indian Management*, 12(2), 29–38.

17. Berry, D. (2005). Methodological pitfalls in the study of religiosity and spirituality. *Western Journal of Nursing Research*, 27(5), 626–647.

18. Starbuck, E. D. (1899). *The psychology of religion: An empirical study of the growth of religious consciousness.* New York: Scribner.

19. James, W. (1902). *The varieties of religious experience: A study of human nature.* New York: Random House.

20. Jung, C. G. (1923). *Psychological types: Or the psychology of the individuation.* Translated by H. Godwin Baynes. London: Kegan Paul, Trench, Trubner.

21. Frankl, V. E. (1959). *Man's search for meaning.* New York: Pocket Books.

22. Seeman, T. E., Dubin, L. F., & Seeman, M. (2003). Religiosity/spirituality and health: A critical review of the evidence for biological pathways. *American Psychologist*, 58(1), 53–63.

23. Cousins, N. (1979). *Anatomy of an illness.* New York: Norton.

24. Cousins, N. (1989). *Head first: The biology of hope and the healing power of the human spirit.* New York: Dutton.

25. Fosarelli, P. (2002). Fearfully wonderfully made: The interconnectedness of body– mind–spirit. *Journal of Religion and Health*, 41(3), 207–229.

26. Freeman, R. (2004). Richard Freeman on yoga as a path to physical and spiritual health. Interview by Bonnie Harrigan. *Alternative Therapies in Health and Medicine*, 10(2), 64–72.

27. Robbins, J. A., & Dewar, J. (2011). Traditional Indigenous approaches to healing and the modern welfare of traditional knowledge, spirituality and lands: A critical reflection on practices and policies taken from the Canadian Indigenous example. *The International Indigenous Policy Journal*, 2(4), 1–17.

28. Subia Bigfoot, D., & Fundeburk, B. W. (2011). Honoring children, making relatives: The cultural translation of parent–child therapy for American Indian and Alaska native families. *Journal of Psychoactive Drugs*, 43(4), 309–318.

29. Wagemakers Schiff, J., & Moore, K. (2006). The impact of the sweat lodge ceremony on dimensions of well-being. *American Indian and Alaska Native Health Research*, 13(3), 48–69.

30. Bopp, J., Bopp, M., Brown, L., & Lane, P. Jr. (1985). *The sacred tree.* Lethbridge, AB: Four Worlds International Institute for Human and Community Development. www.4worlds.org

31. Ibid., p. 7.

32. Ibid., p. 7.
33. Ibid., p. 22.
34. Ibid., p. 22.
35. Ibid., p. 23.
36. Ibid., p. 24.
37. Ibid., pp. 81–82.
38. Kumar, M. B., & Janz, T. (2014, April 23). *An exploration of cultural activities of Métis in Canada.* Canadian Social Trends. Publications. Statistics Canada. No. 89. Archived. Catalogue no. 11-008-X.
39. Inuit Art Alive. (2016). *Spirituality.* The North. www.inuitartalive.ca/index_e.php?p=119
40. Love, K. L. (2008). Interconnectedness in nursing: A concept analysis. *Journal of Holistic Nursing*, 26(4), 255–265.
41. Meditation and Buddhism Kadampa Centre of Canada. (2015). *Meditations for world peace.* Classes. kadampa.ca/mondays/
42. Tuttle, W. (2015, August 28). *Our ability to sense profound interconnectedness is vital to peace.* The World Peace Diet. www.worldpeacediet.com/2015/08/our-ability-to-sense-profound-interconnectedness-is-vital-to-peace/
43. McGee, M., Nagael, L., & Moore, M. K. (2003). A study of university classroom strategies aimed at increasing spiritual health. *College Student Journal*, 37(4), 583–595.
44. Faver, C. A. (2004). Relational spirituality and social caregiving. *Social Work*, 49(2), 241–249.
45. Kabatt-Zinn, J. (1990). *Full catastrophe living: Using the wisdom of your mind to face stress, pain and illness.* New York: Dell.
46. Kabatt-Zinn, J. (1982). An outpatient program in behavorial medicine for chronic pain patients based on the practice of mindfulness meditation: Theoretical considerations and preliminary results. *General Hospital Psychiatry*, 4, 33–47.
47. Thera, N. (1962). *The heart of Buddhist meditation: A handbook of mental training based on the Buddha's way of mindfulness.* London: Rider and Company.
48. Niemiec, R. M., Rashid, T., & Spinella, M. (2012). Strong mindfulness: Integrating mindfulness and character strength. *Journal of Mental Health Counseling*, 34(3), 240–254.
49. Scott, R., Lau, M., Shapiro, S., Carlson, L., Anderson, N. C., Carmody, J., Segal, Z., Abbey, S., Speca, M., Velting, D., & Devins, G. (2004). Mindfulness: A proposed operational definition. *Clinical Psychology: Science and Practice*, 11(3), 230–241.
50. Palmer, A., & Rodger, S. (2009). Mindfulness, stress, and coping among university students. *Canadian Journal of Counselling*, 43(3), 198–212.
51. Evans, M., & Atkins, M. J. (2007). Making meaning using creativity and spirituality. *Journal of Creativity in Mental Health*, 2(1), 35–46.
52. Kiesling, C., Sorell, G. T., Montgomery, M. J., & Colwell, R. K. (2008). Identity and spirituality: A psychosocial exploration of the sense of spiritual self. *Developmental Psychology*, 42(6), 1269–1277.
53. Pecchenino, R. A. (2008). Becoming: Identity and spirituality. *Journal of Socio-Economics*, 38(1), 31–36.
54. Lydon-Lam, J. (2012). Models of spirituality and consideration of spiritual assessment. *International Journal of Childbirth Education* 27(1), 18–22.
55. Bondar, R. (1994). *Touching the earth.* Toronto: Key Porter Books, pp. 76–77.
56. Faver, C. A. (2004). Relational spirituality and social caregiving. *Social Work*, 49(2), 241–249.
57. Rosmarin, D. H., Wachholz, A., & Ai, A. (2011). Beyond descriptive research: Advancing the study of spirituality and health. *Journal of Behavioral Medicine*, 34(6), 409–413.
58. Seeman, T. E., Dubin, L. F., & Seeman, M. (2003). Religiosity, spirituality and health: A critical review of the evidence for biological pathways. *American Psychologist*, 58(1), 53–63.
59. Koenig, H. G. (2012). Religion, spirituality, and health: The research and clinical implications. Review article. *ISRN Psychiatry*, 2012 (4), 1–33.
60. Jim, H. S., Pustejovsky, J. E., Park, C., Danhauer, S. C., et al. (2015). Religion, spirituality, and physical health in cancer patients: A meta-analysis. *Cancer*, 121(21), 3760–3768. DOI: 10.1002/cncr.29353
61. Bhui, K., (2010). Culture, religion and health care. *International Journal of Integrated Care, Conceptual Explorations on Person-centered Medicine*, 2010 (10 Suppl), 57–59.
62. Sullivan, W. P. (2009). Spirituality: A road to mental health or mental illness. *Journal of Religion & Spirituality*, 29(1–2), 84–98.
63. Hutchins, D., Hutchins, E., Pursley, R. J., & Nelms, L. W. (2007). Spirituality and the health of college students. *Journal of Religion and Health*, 46(2), 249–265.
64. Balbeuna, L., Baetz, M., & Bowen, R. (2013). Religious attendance, spirituality, and major depression in Canada: A 14 year follow-up study. *Journal of Psychiatry*, 58(4), 225–232.
65. Baker, S., & Morrison, R. (2008). Environmental spirituality: Grounding our response to climate change. *European Journal of Science and Theology*, 4(2), 35–50.
66. Montes, S. (1996). Uses of natural settings to promote, maintain and restore human health. In B. L. Driver, D. Dustin, T. Baltic, G. Elsner, and G. Peterson (Eds.), *Nature and the human spirit: Toward an expanded land management ethic.* (pp. 105–115). State College, PA: Venture Publishing, Inc.
67. Elsner, G., Snell, F., Lewis, D., & Spitzer, W. (1996). The role of public lands in maintaining and rejuvenating the human spirit. In B. L. Driver, D. Dustin, T. Baltic, G. Elsner, and G. Peterson (Eds.), *Nature and the human spirit: Toward an expanded land management ethic.* (pp. 10–13). State College, PA: Venture Publishing, Inc.
68. Suzuki, D. (2003). *The David Suzuki reader: A lifetime of ideas from a leading activist and thinker.* Vancouver: Greystone Books, p. 11.
69. Hammond, H., & Judy, S. (1996). Belief, wholeness, and experience: Sensitizing professional land managers to spiritual values. In B. L. Driver, D. Dustin, T. Baltic, G. Elsner, and G. Peterson (Eds.), *Nature and the human spirit: Toward an expanded land management ethic.* (pp. 367–381). State College, PA: Venture Publishing, Inc.
70. Paredes-Collins, K. (2013). Cultivating diversity and spirituality: A compelling interest for institutional priority. *Christian Higher Education*, 12(1–2), 122–137.
71. Subbiondo, J. L. (2011). Bottom line: Spirituality on campus. The emergence of a postsecular age in American higher education. *About Campus*, 16(5), 30–32.
72. Sorrentino, P. V. (2010). What do college students want? A student-centered approach to multifaith involvement. *Journal of Ecumenical Studies*, 45(1), 79–98.
73. Livingston, K. A., & Cummings, A. L. (2009). Spirituality and young women in transition: A preliminary investigation. *Counseling and Values*, 53(3), 224–236.

74. Shores, C. I. (2010). Spiritual perspectives of nursing students. *Nursing Education*, 3(1), 8–12.

75. Levy, Abe. (2004, August 28). Campus religious groups offer prayer meetings, discussions for students. *The Wichita Eagle. Knight-Ridder/Tribune Business News.*

76. Adams, T. B., Bezner, J. R., Drabbs, M. E., Zambarano, R. J., & Steinhardt, M. A. (2000). Conceptualization and measurement of the spiritual and psychological dimensions of wellness in a college population. *Journal of American College Health*, 48(4), 165–173.

77. Kuh, G. D., & Gonyea, R. M. (2006, Winter). Spirituality, liberal learning and college student engagement. *Liberal Education*, 92(1), 40–47.

78. Shahjahan, R. A. (2004). Centering spirituality in the academy: Toward a transformative way of teaching and learning. *Journal of Transformative Education*, 2(4), 294–312.

79. Nagel, E., & Sgoutas-Emch, S. (2007). The relationship between spirituality, health beliefs, and health behaviours in college students. *Journal of Religion and Health*, 46(1), 141–154.

80. Sargeant, D. M. (2009). Teaching spirituality in the physical therapy classroom and clinic. *Journal of Physical Therapy Education*, 23(1), 29–35.

81. McGee, M., Nagel, L., & Moore, M. K. (2003). A study of university classroom strategies aimed at increasing spiritual health. *College Student Journal*, 37(4), 583–595.

82. Dalton, A. M. (2007, December). Religion and ecology. Academic Matters. *The Journal of Higher Education.* Ontario: Confederation of University Faculty Association.

83. Religion in Canada Institute. (2015). Trinity Western University. www.twu.ca/research/institutes-and-centres/university-institutes/religion-in-canada-institute/

84. Bowker, J. (Ed.). (2003). *The concise Oxford dictionary of world religions.* New York: Oxford University Press. www.oxfordreference.com/view/10.1093/acref/9780192800947.001.0001/acref-9780192800947

85. Ibid.

86. Angus Reid Institute. (2015, March 26). *Religion and faith in Canada today: Strong belief, ambivalence and rejection define our views.* Canadian Public Opinion Poll. angusreid.org/faith-in-canada/

87. *Religions in Canada* (2nd ed.). (2008). Publications. National Defence and the Canadian Forces (March 2011). Archived. publications.gc.ca/collections/collection_2011/dn-nd/D2-147-2008-eng.pdf

88. *The Canadian Encyclopedia, Historica Dominion Institute.* (2013, December 16). Buddhism. www.thecanadianencyclopedia.ca/en/article/buddhism/

89. His Holiness, The 14th Dalai Lama of Tibet. (n.d.). *The Dalai Lama.* www.dalailama.com/biography

90. *Religions in Canada* (2nd ed.). (2008). Publications. National Defence and the Canadian Forces (March 2011). Archived. publications.gc.ca/collections/collection_2011/dn-nd/D2-147-2008-eng.pdf

91. Statistics Canada. (2015, Decemeber 22). 2011 National Household Survey: Immigration, place of birth, citizenship, ethnic origin, visible minorities, language and religion. Catalogue no. 99-010-X. www12.statcan.gc.ca/nhs-enm/2011/as-sa/99-010-x/99-010-x2011001-eng.cfm#a6

92. God's Ten Laws.com. (2016). *The ten commandments listed.* Ten Commandments. Home. www.godstenlaws.com/ten-commandments/#.Vyf2lk32bIU

93. Bowker, J. (Ed.). (2003). *The concise Oxford dictionary of world religions.* New York: Oxford University Press. www.oxfordreference.com/view/10.1093/acref/9780192800947.001.0001/acref-9780192800947

94. Cheng, C. Y. (2010). Developing Confucian onto-ethics in a postmodern world/age. *Journal of Chinese Philosophy*, 37(1), 3–17.

95. *Religions in Canada* (2nd ed.). (2008). Publications. National Defence and the Canadian Forces (March 2011). Archived. http://publications.gc.ca/collections/collection_2011/dn-nd/D2-147-2008-eng.pdf

96. Ibid.

97. Ibid.

98. *The Canadian Encyclopedia, Historica Dominion Institute.* (2015, July 10). Islam. www.thecanadianencyclopedia.ca/en/article/islam/

99. Ibid.

100. *Religions in Canada* (2nd ed.). (2008). Publications. National Defence and the Canadian Forces (March 2011). Archived. publications.gc.ca/collections/collection_2011/dn-nd/D2-147-2008-eng.pdf

101. Ibid.

102. Brym, R. J. (2008). Religion, politics, and suicide bombing: An interpretive essay. *Canadian Journal of Sociology*, 33(1), 89–108.

103. Bowker, J. (Ed.). (2003). *The concise Oxford dictionary of world religions.* New York: Oxford University Press. www.oxfordreference.com/view/10.1093/acref/9780192800947.001.0001/acref-9780192800947

104. Ibid.

105. *The Canadian Encyclopedia. Historica Dominion Institute.* (2015, March 04). Judaism. www.thecanadianencyclopedia.ca/en/article/judaism/

106. Ibid.

107. Bowker, J. (Ed.). (2003). *The concise Oxford dictionary of world religions.* New York: Oxford University Press. www.oxfordreference.com/view/10.1093/acref/9780192800947.001.0001/acref-9780192800947

108. Ibid.

109. *The Canadian Encyclopedia, Historica Dominion Institute.* (2014, October 28). Sikhism. www.thecanadianencyclopedia.ca/en/article/sikhism/

110. Raz, G. (2012). *The emergence of Daoism: Creation of tradition.* New York: Abingdon, OX.

111. Ibid.

112. The Unitarians. (2014). *Unitarianism explained.* Home. www.unitarian.org.uk/pages/unitarianism-explained

113. McKanan, D. (2013). Unitarianism, universalism, and Unitarian universalism. *Religion Compass*, 7(1), 15–24.

Index